# Imaging of Orthopaedic Fixation Devices and Prostheses

# Imaging of Orthopaedic Fixation Devices and Prostheses

**Thomas H. Berquist, MD, FACR**

Professor of Diagnostic Radiology
Mayo Clinic College of Medicine
Rochester, Minnesota;
Consultant in Diagnostic Radiology
Mayo Clinic Jacksonville
Jacksonville, Florida

Wolters Kluwer | Lippincott Williams & Wilkins
Health

Philadelphia • Baltimore • New York • London
Buenos Aires • Hong Kong • Sydney • Tokyo

*Acquisitions Editor:* Lisa McAllister
*Managing Editor:* Ryan Shaw
*Project Manager:* Alicia Jackson
*Manufacturing Coordinator:* Kathleen Brown
*Senior Marketing Manager:* Angela Panetta
*Designer:* Stephen Druding
*Cover Designer:* Larry Didona
*Production Services:* Laserwords Private Limited, Chennai, India



**530 Walnut Street**
**Philadelphia, PA 19106 USA**
**LWW.com**



Printed in China

---

**Library of Congress Cataloging-in-Publication Data**
Imaging of orthopaedic fixation devices and prostheses / editor, Thomas H. Berquist.
p. ; cm.
Includes bibliographical references and index.
ISBN-13: 978-0-7817-9252-3 (alk. paper)
ISBN-10: (invalid) 0-7817-9252-3 (alk. paper)
1. Orthopedic apparatus—Imaging. 2. Musculoskeletal system—Diseases—Imaging. 3. Musculoskeletal system—Diseases—Surgery. I. Berquist, Thomas H. (Thomas Henry), 1945-
[DNLM: 1. Musculoskeletal Diseases—diagnosis. 2. Diagnostic Imaging. 3. Musculoskeletal Diseases—surgery. 4. Orthopedic Fixation Devices. WE 141 I301 2009]
RD755.5.I38 2009
617′.9—dc22

2008024236

---



10 9 8 7 6 5 4 3 2 1

I dedicate this text to my loving wife, Mary,
for her continued support and understanding.

# Preface

In 1995 we published an Atlas of Orthopaedic Appliances and Prostheses. This was a work dedicated to bridging the gap between orthopaedic surgeons and imagers. I have continued to dedicate efforts to improve the understanding of orthopaedic procedures and "what the surgeon needs to know" when ordering preoperative and postoperative imaging studies.

Orthopaedic instrumentation and prostheses continue to evolve, making it difficult for imagers to keep up with all possible implants that may appear on radiographs or other imaging modalities. With this in mind, it is essential for surgeons and radiologists to work closely and we, as imagers, need to become familiar with the instrumentation systems our surgeons prefer.

This edition is designed to be more concise than the prior atlas with no attempt to demonstrate every possible fixation device or prostheses. We review the important clinical and image features of orthopaedic devices including clinical concepts and patient selection, the normal appearance of orthopaedic devices and the image features, and most appropriate modalities for evaluating complications.

Chapter 1 is a concise review of image modalities that may play a role in evaluation of orthopaedic fixation devices and prostheses. Chapter 2 provides a list and definitions of commonly used orthopaedic terms and an overview of general fixation devices including screws, plates, intramedullary nails, wires and cables, and soft tissue anchors. These chapters serve to reduce redundancy in later chapters where these devices may be used. Chapters 3 through 13 are anatomically oriented and focus on fixation devices, prostheses, and procedures for a given anatomic region. Emphasis is placed on indications, clinical data and decision making, as well as preoperative and postoperative imaging and complications. Each chapter includes trauma, orthopaedic classifications where appropriate, and joint replacement and other common orthopaedic procedures related to the anatomic region covered in the chapter. Chapter 14 reviews clinical data, staging, and preoperative and postoperative imaging in patients with musculoskeletal neoplasms.

This text will be most useful to practicing radiologists and radiologists in training. Other physicians who deal with orthopaedic problems will also find the information provided in this text extremely useful.

# Acknowledgments

Preparation of this text required the support of numerous individuals and colleagues. I first wish to thank my colleagues in musculoskeletal imaging at Mayo Jacksonville, Laura Bancroft, Mark Kransdorf, and Jeffrey Peterson for their support and assistance in providing the necessary images needed to fulfill the mission of this text. I also want to thank my colleagues in orthopaedic surgery, Mark Broderson, Stephen Trigg, Cedric Ortiguera, Peter Murry, Mary O'Connor, Kurtis Blasser, and Joseph Whalen for their consultative support.

Daniel Huber and John Hagen were instrumental in providing images and art required to demonstrate anatomy, normal and abnormal image features for devices described in this text. The vendors of orthopaedic devices were also very helpful in providing photographs and artwork to assist with demonstration of devices and their indications to use along with the images in this text.

Finally, I wish to thank Ryan Shaw, Lisa McAlliser, and Kerry Barrett from Lippincott Williams & Wilkins for their assistance and support with this project.

# Contents

# 1
# Imaging Techniques

Appropriate use of imaging techniques is essential for diagnosis, treatment planning, and follow-up of orthopaedic procedures. Basic techniques will be discussed in this chapter to avoid redundancy in anatomic chapters.

## Routine Radiographs

Routine radiographs remain the primary screening examination for musculoskeletal disorders. Appropriate evaluation of radiographs may provide the diagnosis or allow selection of the next imaging procedure to completely evaluate the clinical problem. Specifically, radiographs are essential for proper interpretation of magnetic resonance (MR) images.

Currently, screen-film radiography is being replaced with computed radiography (CR) at many institutions. Regardless of the system used, it is essential to ensure proper patient positioning and accurate chronologic labeling of images. Multiple views (two to four) are required to evaluate osseous and articular anatomy. Specific views will be discussed in subsequent anatomic chapters. In certain cases, fluoroscopically positioned images are useful to optimize positioning and reduce bony overlap. This approach is useful in the foot and wrist. The technique is also appropriate to evaluate interfaces of arthroplasty components, fixation devices, and evaluate pin tracts when infection is suspected clinically. Fluoroscopic positioning is also useful when performing stress tests to assure that the joint is properly positioned. Stress studies are most often performed on the ankle, elbow, knee, and wrist (see Fig. 1-1).

### Suggested Reading


Bender CE, Berquist TH, Stears JG, et al. Diagnostic techniques. In: Berquist TH, ed. *Imaging of orthopaedic trauma*, 2nd ed. New York: Raven Press; 1992:1–37.

Bontrager KL. *Textbook of radiographic positioning and related anatomy*, 5th ed. Mosby: St. Louis; 2001.


## Computed Tomography

Computed tomography (CT) is a fast and efficacious technique for evaluating musculoskeletal disorders. New systems are even faster which allows more flexibility for reconstruction in multiple image planes. There are also improved techniques for evaluating patients with orthopaedic fixation devices or joint replacements. The basic components of a CT scanner include a gantry that houses the detectors and a movable patient table. Common CT terminology is summarized as follows:

**Multislice:** Number of images generated

**Multidetector:** Number of detector rows to register data

**Multichannel:** Ability to register data during gantry rotation using a data acquisition system, typically 16 channels

**Detector array:** Multichannel CT systems have a slip-ring design system that allows electronic manipulation of the x-ray beam into multiple channels of data

**Beam collimation:** Metal collimators near the x-ray source are adjusted to control the width of the beam directed to the patient

**Section collimation:** Smallest section thickness that can be reconstructed from the acquired data and is based on how detectors are configured to channel the data

**Effective section thickness:** Related to beam collimation for single channel CT or width of the detector row for multichannel CT

**Pitch:** Table translation in millimeters per gantry rotation divided by beam collimation

CT is particularly suited for evaluating complex skeletal anatomy in the spine, shoulder, pelvis, foot, ankle, hand, and wrist. Thin-section images allow reformatting in multiple image planes and three-dimensional reconstruction. Pre- and postcontrast images (intravenous iodinated contrast) are useful for evaluation of soft tissue lesions. Imaging of patients with orthopaedic implants requires special attention to detail to minimize metal artifacts.

Metal-related artifacts can cause significant image degradation in patients with orthopaedic implants. Certain metals

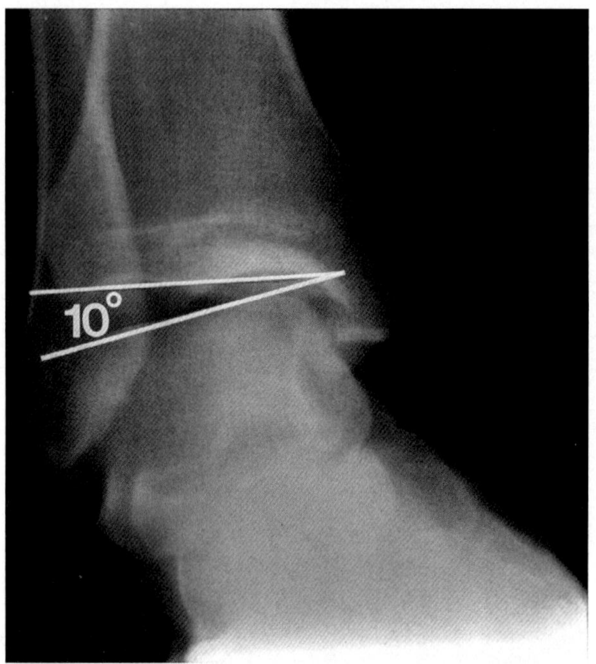


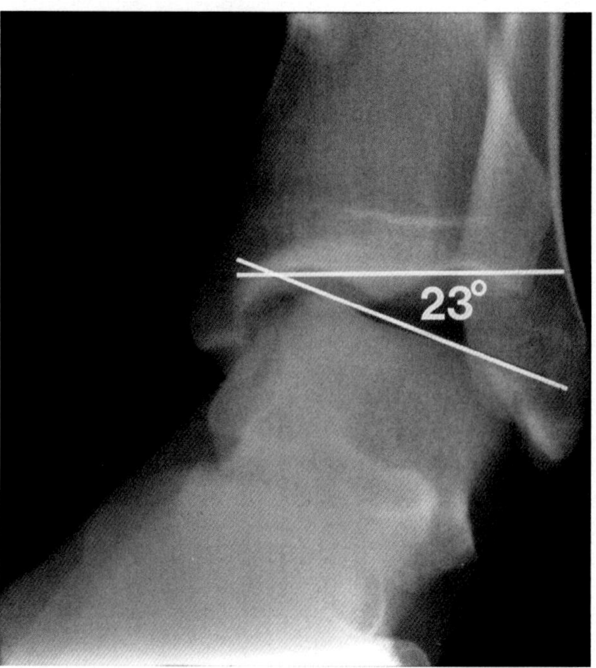


Fig. 1-1 Stress views of the ankle done with valgus positioning of the normal (A) and involved ankle (B) for comparison. The tibiotalar angle on the abnormal side (B) opens 13 degrees more than the normal side indicating tears of the anterior talofibular and calcaneofibular ligaments (>5 degrees indicates one ligament is disrupted and >10 degrees indicates both ligaments are disrupted).

are more problematic. Implants with lower beam attenuation coefficients such as titanium produce fewer artifacts than stainless steel and cobalt-chromium implants. Artifact reduction can be accomplished by modifying parameters such as milliampere-seconds, kilovolt peak (kVp), and reconstruction algorithms. Higher kilovolt peak increases metal penetration. Several authors recommend using 140 kVp. Increasing the tube current may also reduce metal artifacts. Multichannel scanners can collect redundant data by using a lower pitch setting. This also reduces metal artifact (see Fig. 1-2).

## Suggested Reading

Berland LL, Smith KL. Multidetector array CT. Once again technology creates new opportunities. *Radiology*. 1998;209:327–329.

Douglas-Akinwande AC, Buckwalter KA, Rydberg J, et al. Multichannel CT: Evaluating the spine in postoperative patients with orthopaedic hardware. *Radiographics*. 2006;26:S97–S110.

Memarsadeghi M, Breitenseher MJ, Schaefer-Prokop C, et al. Occult scaphoid fractures: Comparison of multidetector CT and MR imaging-initial experience. *Radiology*. 2006;240:169–176.

Ohashi K, El-Khoury GY, Bennett DL, et al. Orthopaedic hardware complications diagnosed with multidetector row CT. *Radiology*. 2005;237:570–577.

## Magnetic Resonance Imaging

Magnetic resonance imaging (MRI) is a proven technique with expanding musculoskeletal applications. Most imaging is performed at 1.5 Tesla (T). However, 3 T units are being used with increasing frequency. There are also multiple open bore and extremity configurations at lower field strengths for musculoskeletal imaging.

Before considering MRI as an imaging option one must consider certain patient screening and safety issues. A written questionnaire is preferred with specific, easy to answer questions to improve detection of patients who may be at risk during MRI examinations. Information regarding obvious risk factors such as cardiac pacemakers, certain cerebral aneurysm clips, metallic foreign bodies, and electrical devices can be obtained from the questionnaire and/or by verbal clarification with the patient. When metallic foreign bodies are suspected, radiographs or CT should be obtained for confirmation.

Metallic implants may create artifacts that significantly degrade image quality, especially if they contain ferromagnetic impurities. Fortunately, most orthopaedic implants are made of alloys that do not contain ferromagnetic material. The size of the implant and its configuration may still cause problems. Image quality can be improved in several ways. Increasing the bandwidth and number of acquisitions decreases metal artifact. One can also set the frequency encoding direction along the axis of the metal. Unfortunately, this is not always possible. T1-weighted, fast spin-echo (SE) and fast short T1 inversion

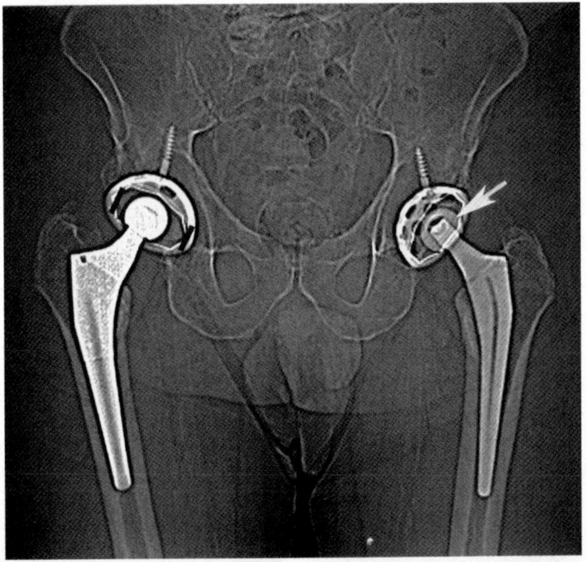

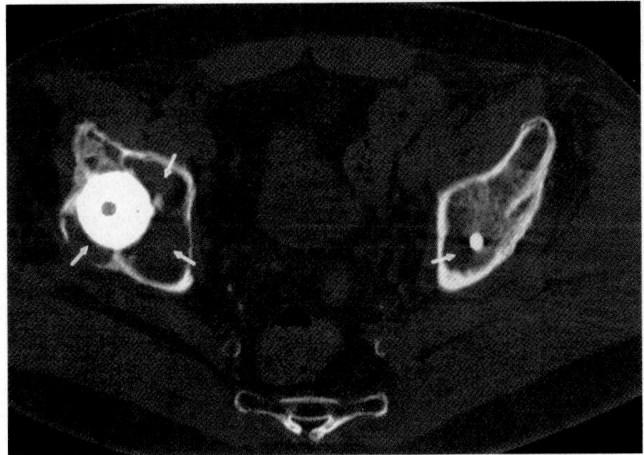

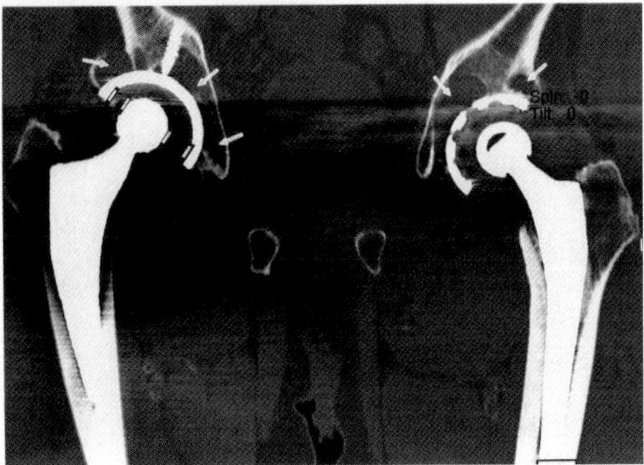

Fig. 1-2 A: Computed tomographic (CT) scout image demonstrating bilateral hip arthroplasties with metal and polyethylene components on the right and a modular ceramic head (*arrow*) on the left. There is slight asymmetry of the femoral heads noted by *black lines* on the right. Axial (B) and coronal (C) CT images with artifact reduction techniques clearly demonstrate the bilateral osteolysis (*arrows*) and femoral head asymmetry (*lines*).

recovery (STIR) sequences may be useful to improve image quality (see Fig. 1-3). Gradient echo sequences should be avoided. Metal artifact is also less of an issue at lower field strengths. Cast material and methyl methacrylate do not cause artifacts.

## Patient Monitoring and Sedation

Patient age, clinical status, and length of MRI examination must be considered before determining whether sedation or pain medication is required. Patient monitoring including blood pressure, heart rate, respiratory rate, skin temperature, and oxygen saturation can be accomplished in the MR gantry. Claustrophobia, a problem with high-field units, is a less significant problem with lower field strength open units.

When sedation is required, oral medications are used whenever possible. Patient monitoring is usually not required in this setting. Chloral hydrate is an effective oral medication, especially in children younger than 2 years of age. Alprazolam (Xanax), diazepam (Valium), and ketorolac tromethamine (Toradol) can be used in adults with anxiety or claustrophobia. The main disadvantages of oral medication are the time of onset and unpredictable effect.

Intravenous sedation requires patient monitoring, but the effects are more predictable. The authors use midazolam (Versed), fentanyl, and, for the elderly patient, diphenhydramine (Benadryl) for intravenous sedation. Patients given sedation should not drive for 24 hours and must be accompanied if travel is required following the examination.

## Patient Positioning and Coil Selection

Patient positioning considerations include patient size, body part and structures to be examined, and examination time. The patient should be studied with the most closely coupled coil (smallest coil that covers the anatomy of interest) to achieve the optimal signal-to-noise ratio and spatial resolution. The torso coil is used for the trunk, pelvis, and thigh regions. Patients

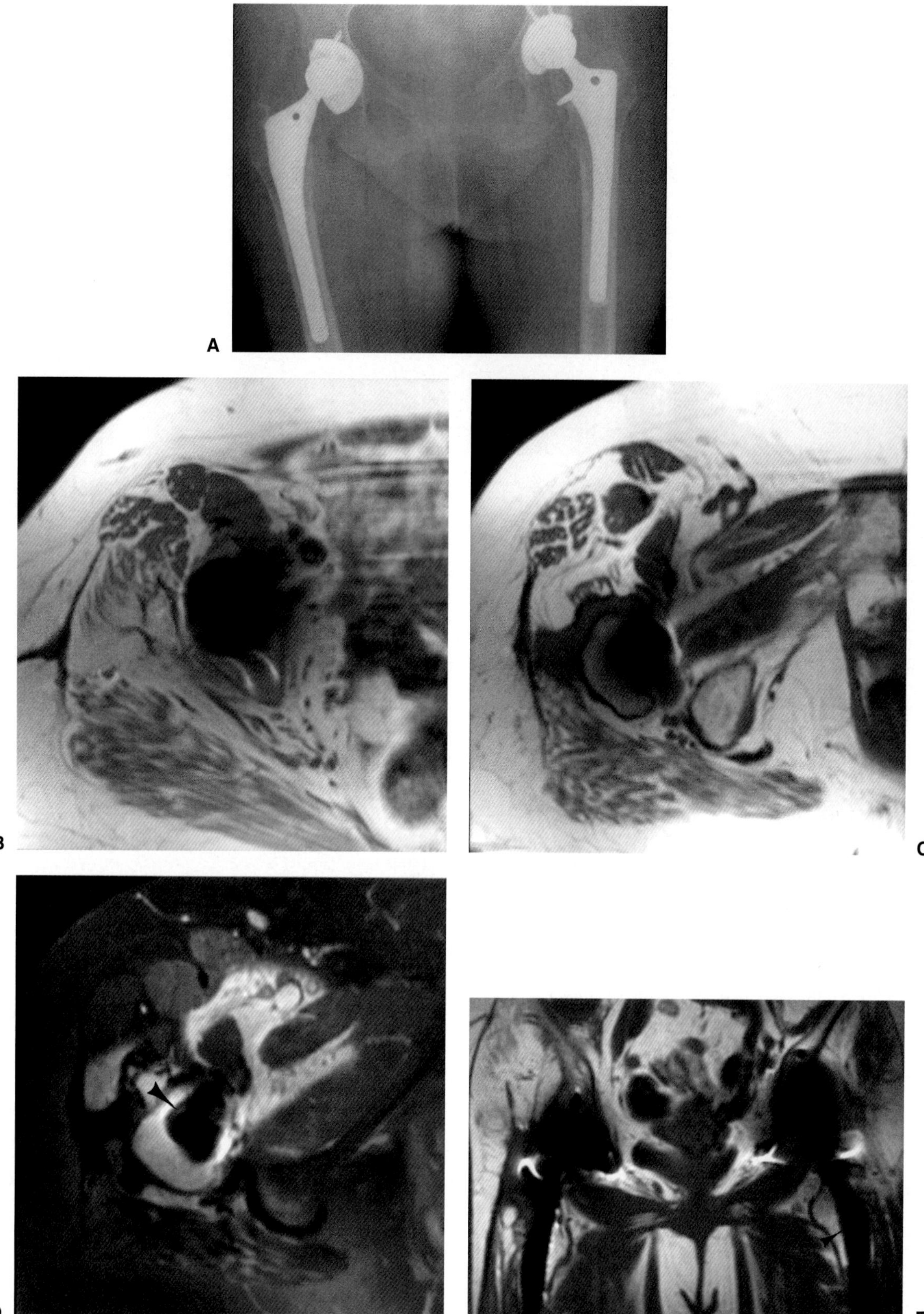


Fig. 1-3 A: Radiograph of the pelvis and hips demonstrating bilateral uncemented hip replacements in a patient with hip pain. Axial T1-weighted (B and C), proton density weighted (D), and coronal T1-weighted (E) images show some degree of artifact. However, the metal bone interfaces are well seen with fibrous tissue demonstrated along the implant (*arrowheads*).

can be placed in the gantry in the prone or supine position. The prone position is preferred for posterior pathology, as soft tissue compression is avoided. Claustrophobic patients also may tolerate the prone position more easily.

Most extremity examinations are performed with circumferential, partial volume, or flat coils. Open or flat coils allow more flexibility for positioning and motion studies. However, signal drop-off can occur with small flat coils (depth of view limited to approximately one half the coil radius). Newer coils, including dual switchable coils, allow simultaneous examination of both extremities.

### Pulse Sequences and Slice Selection

Pulse sequences should be selected to optimize anatomic display, enhance lesion conspicuity, and characterize lesions. In many cases, conventional T1-weighted (SE 500/10) SE and dual echo T2-weighted (SE 2000/80, 20) sequences are adequate for lesion detection and characterization. Fast SE sequences can be performed more quickly and substituted for conventional T2-weighted SE sequences. Subtle lesions may be more easily appreciated with STIR sequences, fat suppression, or intravenous or intra-articular gadolinium. At least two image planes are obtained to define the extent of lesions. Slice thickness can range from 1 to 5 mm depending on the size of the lesion and detail required.

## Suggested Reading

Berquist TH. General technical considerations. In: Berquist TH, ed. *MRI of the musculoskeletal system*, 5th ed. Philadelphia: Lippincott Williams & Wilkins; 2006:61–97.

Glueker TM, Bongartz G, Ledermann HP, et al. MR angiography of the hand with subsystolic cuff-compression optimization of injection parameters. *AJR Am J Roentgenol.* 2006;187:905–910.

Magee TH, Williams D. Sensitivity and specificity in detection of labral tears with 3.0 T MRI of the shoulder. *AJR Am J Roentgenol.* 2006;187:1448–1452.

Tehranzadeh J, Ashikyan O, Anavim A, et al. Enhanced MR imaging of tenosynovitis of the hand and wrist in inflammatory arthritis. *Skeletal Radiol.* 2006;35:814–822.

## Radionuclide Scans/Positron Emission Tomography

Multiple agents are available for bone imaging. Radiopharmaceuticals may be used alone or in combination.

The agents selected and imaging techniques vary with the clinical indication for the examination.

### Bone Scans

Patients are injected intravenously with 10 to 20 mCi (370 to 740 MBq) of technetium-labeled diphosphonate (see Table 1-1). Images are obtained 3 to 4 hours after injection.

**Indications:** Primary or metastatic bone lesions
Subtle fractures, that is, stress fractures
Battered child
Bone pain

Three-phase bone scans are performed using the same radiopharmaceutical, but with a different imaging sequence. Blood flow images are obtained in the initial 60 seconds after injection, followed by blood pool images 2 to 5 minutes after injection, and delayed images at 3 to 5 hours.

Table 1-1

RADIOPHARMACEUTICALS FOR MUSCULOSKELETAL IMAGING

| RADIOPHARMACEUTICAL | DOSE | PHYSICAL HALF-LIFE (HOURS) | REMARKS |
|---|---|---|---|
| Technetium 99m diphosphonate | 10–20 mCi (370–740 MBq) | 6 | 50%–60% in bone at 3–4 h |
| Technetium 99m sulfur colloid | 4–6 mCi (48–222 MBq) | 6 | Localization—liver 80%–90%, spleen 5%–10%, marrow 1%–5% |
| Indium 111–labeled leukocytes | 0.5–1.0 mCi (18.5–37 MBq) | 67 | Localization—spleen 30%, liver 30%. Elimination mainly through decay with 1% excreted by Gastrointestinal (GI) tract and kidney in 24 h. |
| Gallium 67 citrate | 2–6 mCi (74–222 MBq) | 78 | Accumulates in breast milk; renal excretion in the first 24 h, then gastrointestinal excretion |
| Fluorine-18-deoxyglucose | 15 mCi (555 MBq) | 1.83 (110 min) | Excreted by kidneys; high uptake in cerebral cortex; variable uptake in myocardium, bowel, tonsils, parotid glands, and muscles of mastication |

**Indications:** Stress fractures
Differentiation of osteomyelitis from cellulitis
Detection of infarction or avascular necrosis
Evaluation of reflex sympathetic dystrophy
Evaluation of peripheral vascular disease

Single-photon emission CT can be used in addition to conventional delayed bone imaging to define subtle lesions, such as pars defects in patients with low back pain. Computers reconstruct images in multiple planes.

### Bone Marrow Imaging

Patients are injected intravenously with 10 to 15 mCi (370 to 555 MBq) of technetium-labeled sulfur colloid. Images are obtained approximately 15 minutes after injection. Lead shields are placed over the abdomen to delete counts from the liver and spleen.

**Indications:** Identify marrow replacement by neoplasms
Define marrow replacement around joint prostheses

### Infection

Special approaches may be required for specific indications, such as infection. Several radiopharmaceuticals have been used in this setting. Three-phase bone scans are sensitive, but not specific. White blood cells labeled with Gallium citrate Ga 67 and Indium In 111 or Technetium Tc 99m provide more specificity.

In 111–labeled leukocyte scans are performed 18 to 24 hours after intravenous injection of 500 mCi (18.5 MBq). Tc-labeled white cell or antigranulocyte antibody imaging can be performed in 2 to 4 hours. This isotope is more available, and image resolution is superior to that obtained by In 111 studies. A disadvantage of technetium is biliary excretion into bowel, which may obscure portions of the spine and pelvis.

Ga 67 citrate scans are performed after 5 to 10 mCi (185 to 370 MBq) of Ga 67 citrate is injected intravenously. Scanning is performed 24 to 72 hours after injection.

### Combined Studies

Use of multiple radiopharmaceuticals may be required for special clinical situations, such as failed joint prosthesis or osteomyelitis. Remember, conventional techniteum scans can be positive for up to a year after joint arthroplasty. Combined technetium sulfur colloid and In 111–labeled leukocytes is useful for evaluating loosening or infection of joint prostheses. Combined Tc 99m diphosphonate and In 111–labeled leukocytes or techniteum antigranulocyte antibody scans are useful for osteomyelitis (see Fig. 1-4).

### Positron Emission Tomography

Positron emission tomography (PET) has provided a new physiologic approach to imaging musculoskeletal disorders, specifically infection and neoplasms. Positron emitting agents include Fluorine-18-deoxyglucose, L-methyl-carbon 11-methronin, and oxygen 15. Fluorine-18 has a half-life of 110 minutes compared to the shorter half-life of 20 and 21 minutes, respectively, for the other agents. Therefore Fluorine-18 is used clinically. Fluorine-18 fluorodeoxyglucose imaging demonstrates increased glucose utilization seen with these active processes. Patients must be fasting for 4 hours before the examination. No sugared beverages should be taken. Normal blood sugar levels are optimal. Scanning is performed 1 hour after injection. Images are evaluated and uptake ratios of abnormal to normal tissues can be calculated. Early studies demonstrate that PET imaging is more accurate than combined studies described earlier for evaluating infection, chronic infection, and infection associated with joint replacement arthroplasties. PET, especially combined with CT (PET/CT), is also more useful than conventional radionuclide studies for detection of tumor activity and metastasis.

## Suggested Reading

De Winter F, Van de Wiele C, Vogelaers D, et al. Fluorine-18 fluorodeoxyglucose-positron emission tomography: A highly accurate imaging modality for the diagnosis of chronic musculoskeletal infections. *J Bone Joint Surg*. 2001;83A:651–660.

McAfer JG. Update on radiopharmaceuticals for medical imaging. *Radiology*. 1989;171:593–601.

Mettler FA, Guiberteau MJ. *Essentials of nuclear medicine*, 5th ed. Philadelphia: WB Saunders; 2005.

## Ultrasound

The term ultrasound refers to mechanical vibrations for which frequencies are above human detection. Ultrasound imaging utilizes frequencies from 2 to 12 MHz. Most musculoskeletal structures examined are superficial, requiring a 7- to 12-MHz transducer. Doppler ultrasound used for peripheral vascular disease is performed at approximately 8 MHz.

Musculoskeletal applications for ultrasound have expanded considerably in recent years. The joints, soft tissues, and vascular structures are particularly suited to ultrasound examination. Evaluation of cortical and trabecular bone is now feasible and permits examination of the calcaneus for osteoporosis. Because of its low cost and availability, ultrasound is now being used more frequently to evaluate various conditions, as listed in Table 1-2.

## Suggested Reading

Jacobson JA, Van Holsbeek MT. Musculoskeletal ultrasonography. *Orthop Clin North Am*. 1998;29:135–167.

Lin J, Fassell DP, Jacobson JA, et al. An illustrated tutorial of musculoskeletal ultrasound. Part I, introduction and general principles. *AJR Am J Roentgenol*. 2000;175:637–645.

## Interventional Procedures

Interventional procedures are used preoperatively to localize symptoms and confirm the source of pain. Postoperatively, these techniques are useful to evaluate potential complications of orthopaedic procedures.

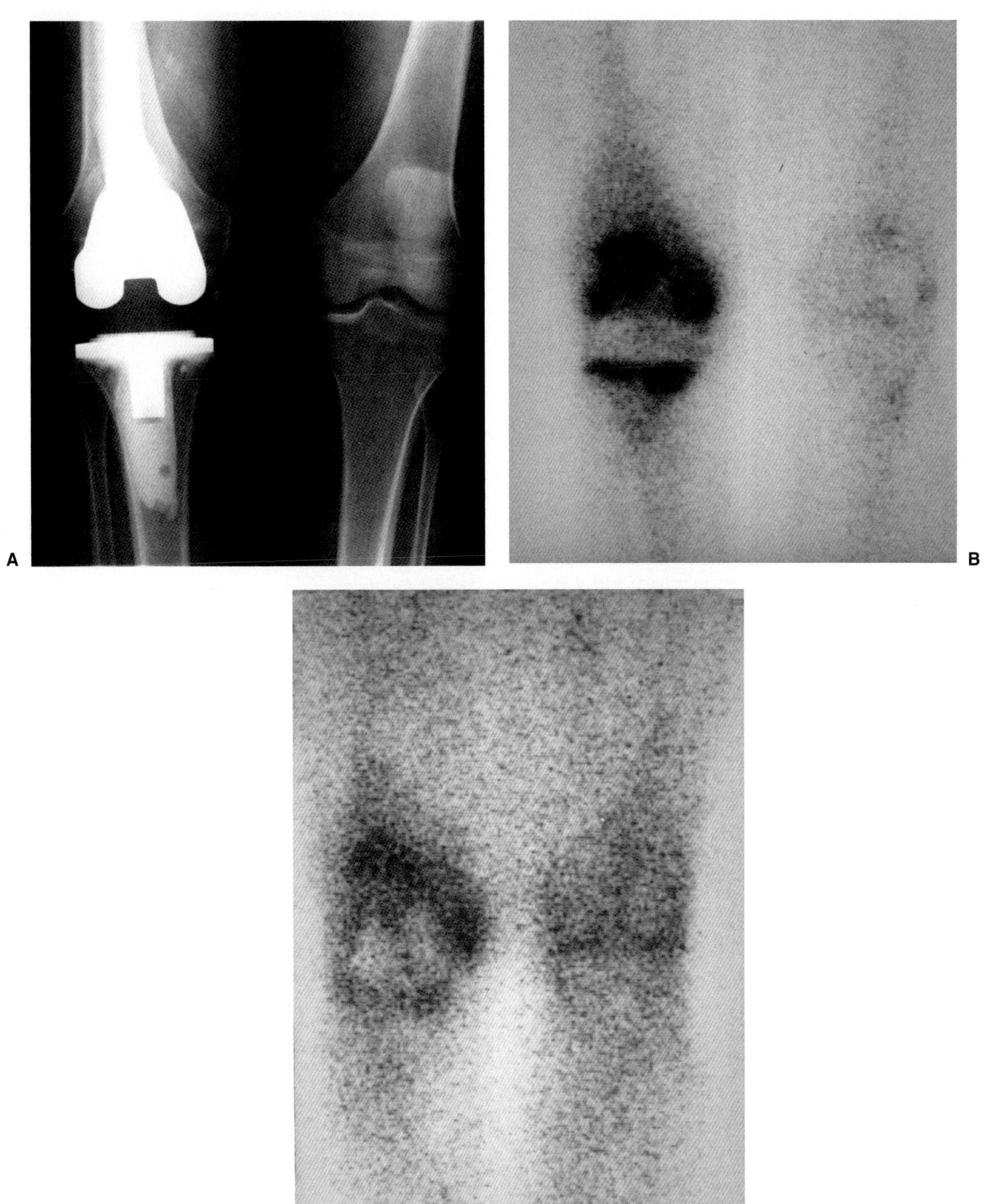


Fig. 1-4 Patient with painful right knee arthroplasty. Anteroposterior (AP) radiograph (A) is normal. Technetium 99m methylene-diphosphonate (MDP) (B) and indium-labeled white blood cell scans (C) demonstrate increased tracer about the components on the right due to infection.

**Table 1-2**

INDICATIONS FOR MUSCULOSKELETAL ULTRASOUND

- Soft tissue masses
- Vascular disease
- Ligament/tendon tears
- Bone
  - Osteoporosis
  - Fractures
- Articular disorders
  - Cartilage
  - Effusions
- Foreign bodies
- Joint aspirations

## Arthrography/Diagnostic-Therapeutic Injections

Conventional arthrography has largely been replaced with MRI or MR arthrography. However, arthrograms are still useful to evaluate capsular and articular anatomy, aspirate fluid for culture and laboratory analysis, distend joints in patients with adhesive capsulitis, and localize symptoms with anesthetic injection. In certain preoperative cases, anesthetic is combined with steroids to provide more therapeutic results.

Most commonly these procedures are preformed to confirm the source of pain and exclude infection. Most procedures are performed with fluoroscopic guidance although ultrasound can also be used to guide needle placement. Subtraction arthrography is a useful technique in patients with joint replacements. Digital techniques can exclude metal components allowing the injected contrast material to be more effectively evaluated along the components or the cement bone interfaces. Table 1-3 summarizes locations and common indications for interventional musculoskeletal procedures.

## Facet Injections

Facet injections are performed most commonly in the lumbar spine. This technique is useful for treatment, preoperative planning, localization of the source of pain, and postoperative evaluation. Patients with facet syndrome present with low back pain that may radiate to the gluteal region or lower extremity.

Routine radiographs and CT should be reviewed, if available, to assess the extent of facet joint abnormalities. The facet joints to be injected are selected, and the patient is placed on the fluoroscopic table in the prone position. The patient is rotated with the involved side up to align the facet joint. Each joint to be injected should be positioned carefully. Sterile preparation is used, and local anesthetic is injected over the involved joint(s). A 22-gauge spinal needle generally is adequate to enter the joint. Contrast medium can be used to confirm needle position. One milliliter of bupivacaine can be injected if the technique is purely diagnostic. For therapeutic injections, a 2:1 mixture of bupivacaine and betamethasone is used.

**Table 1-3**

MUSCULOSKELETAL INTERVENTIONAL PROCEDURES

| ANATOMIC REGION | INDICATIONS |
|---|---|
| Spine | Facet syndrome<br>Discography<br>Painful instrumentation (i.e., hooks, wires)<br>Localize source of pain<br>Aspirate fluid for infection |
| Shoulder | Rotator cuff tears<br>Adhesive capsulitis<br>Subacromial bursitis<br>Aspiration of calcium deposits<br>Localize joint symptoms/aspiration<br>Aspirate fluid for infection |
| Elbow | Capsule/ligament tears<br>Loose bodies<br>Bursitis<br>Localize joint symptoms/aspiration |
| Hand and wrist | Ligament tears<br>Triangular fibrocartilage tears<br>Tendonitis<br>Localize joint symptoms/aspiration |
| Pelvis and hips | Synovial chondromatosis<br>Labral tears<br>Snapping iliopsoas tendon<br>Sacroiliac pain or instability<br>Pubic symphysis pain<br>Localize joint symptoms/aspiration |
| Knee | Proximal tibiofibular joint pain<br>Aspirate joint effusions<br>Localize joint symptoms/aspiration |
| Foot and ankle | Ligament tears<br>Tendon tears<br>Tendonitis<br>Localize joint symptoms/aspiration |

## Discography

Discography has been a controversial technique over the years, but it does play a useful role in assessing disc morphology and localizing patient symptoms. This is especially important following spinal instrumentation when patients develop new symptoms adjacent to the operative site. Confirming the site(s) of pain is critical if additional surgery may be required (see Fig. 1-5). Combined CT and discography can be particularly useful for evaluating lumbar disorders.

Patients are positioned in a manner similar to that used for facet injections. A posterolateral approach is used most often, after sterile preparation and local anesthetic is injected along the needle entry path. The L5-S1 disc is more difficult to enter and may require a coaxial needle approach. The first needle is advanced to the margin of the disc and a second Chiba needle

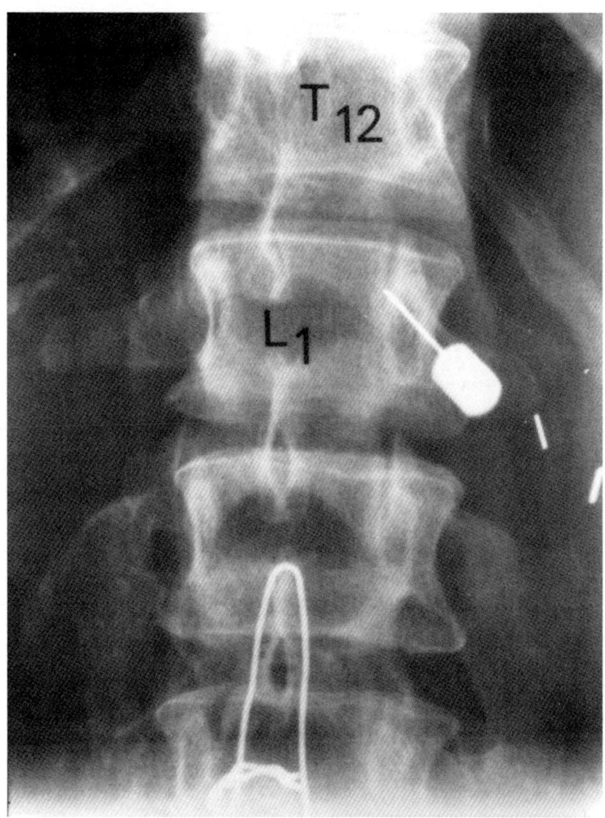


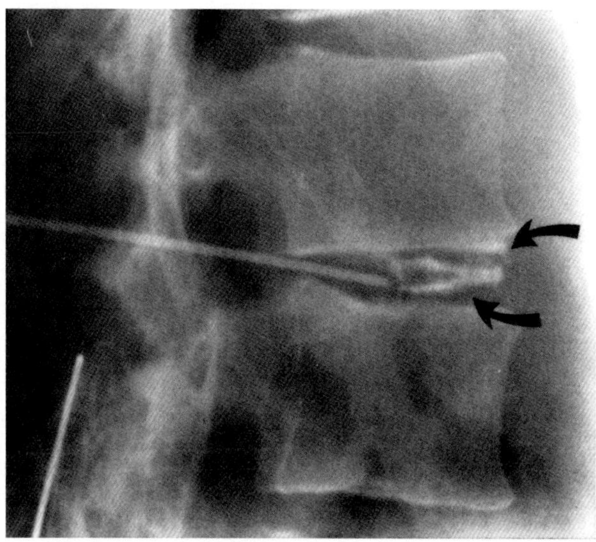

A B

Fig. 1-5 Patient with prior fusion T12 to L1 with new pain above the fusion site. A: Frontal fluoroscopic image demonstrates needle in place for facet injection to confirm the source of pain. B: Discogram demonstrates normal filling (*curved arrows*).

with a slight distal bend is placed through the first needle and into the disc.

The normal disc will accept 2 to 2.5 mL of contrast medium. Antibiotic is often added to the contrast medium. A degenerative disc may accept a larger volume. In this setting, contrast may extend into the annulus and beyond. Distension of the disc space may recreate or exaggerate the patient's symptoms.

### Complications of Interventional Procedures

Arthrography and diagnostic injections are relatively benign procedures. The main concerns are the contrast media and drug allergies. Infection is rare due to use of sterile technique. Painful effusions can occur due to acute eosinophilic synovitis. The effusions usually occur shortly (<12 hours) after injection and may require joint aspiration to relieve symptoms.

Injections in certain regions, specifically in the spine or near nerve roots, may cause inadvertent nerve block with numbness and reduced function. These problems are generally transient and resolve after the anesthetic effect has worn off.

## Suggested Reading

Berquist TH. Diagnostic and therapeutic injections. *Semin Intervent Radiol.* 1993;10:326–343.

Berquist TH. *Imaging atlas of orthopaedic appliances and prostheses.* New York: Raven Press; 1995:1–43.

Berquist TH. Imaging of the postoperative spine. *Radiol Clin North Am.* 2006;44(3):407–418.

Peterson JJ, Fenton DS, Czervionke LF. *Image-guided musculoskeletal intervention.* Philadelphia: Elsevier Science; 2007.

# 2 Common Orthopaedic Terminology and General Fixation Devices

Appropriate use of terminology is critical when communicating with orthopaedic surgeons. Common definitions, descriptive terms, eponyms, and proper description of common orthopaedic fixation devices will be discussed in this chapter to avoid redundancy in later anatomic chapters. For ease of discussion, we will review terminology in sections with terms in alphabetic order.

## Fracture/Dislocations

**Bone bruise:** Marrow edema pattern without a fracture line or cortical disruption best seen on magnetic resonance (MR) images (see Fig. 2-1)

**Closed fracture:** Osseous disruption with intact overlying soft tissues and no penetrating wound

**Complete fracture:** Structural break involving both cortices (see Fig. 2-2)

**Diastasis:** Complete separation of adjacent bones, such as the tibia and fibula, at the syndesmosis or rupture of a nonmobile or minimally mobile articulation such as the sacroiliac joint or pubic symphysis (see Fig. 2-3)

**Dislocation:** Complete displacement of the articular surfaces of a given joint (see Fig. 2-4)

**Fatigue fracture:** Fracture resulting from abnormal muscle tension on normal bone (see also "Stress fracture")

**Incomplete fracture:** Structural break involving only one cortex (see Fig. 2-5)

**Incongruency:** Asymmetry of the articular surfaces of a joint with minimal or no subluxation (see Fig. 2-6)

**Insufficiency fracture:** Osseous injury due to normal stress or muscle tension acting on a bone with abnormal elastic resistance; may only be visible on radionuclide scan, computed tomography (CT), or magnetic resonance imaging (MRI); common locations include the sacrum, acetabulum, pubic rami, and femoral neck (see Fig. 2-7)

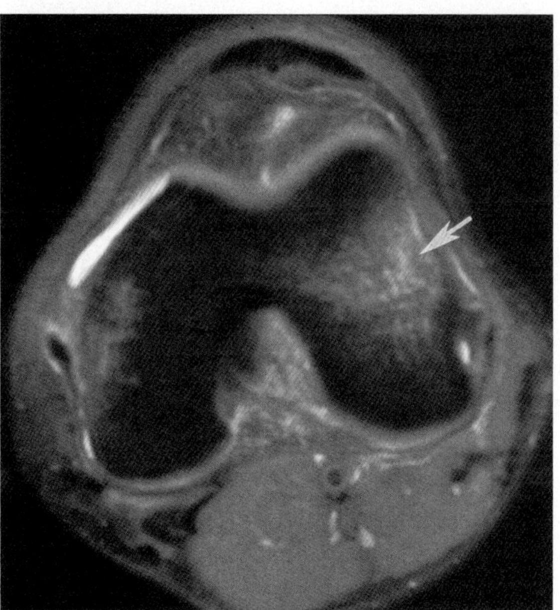

**Fig. 2-1** Bone bruise. Axial fat-suppressed T2-weighted magnetic resonance (MR) image demonstrating marrow edema in the femoral condyle (*arrow*) in a patient with an anterior cruciate ligament tear.

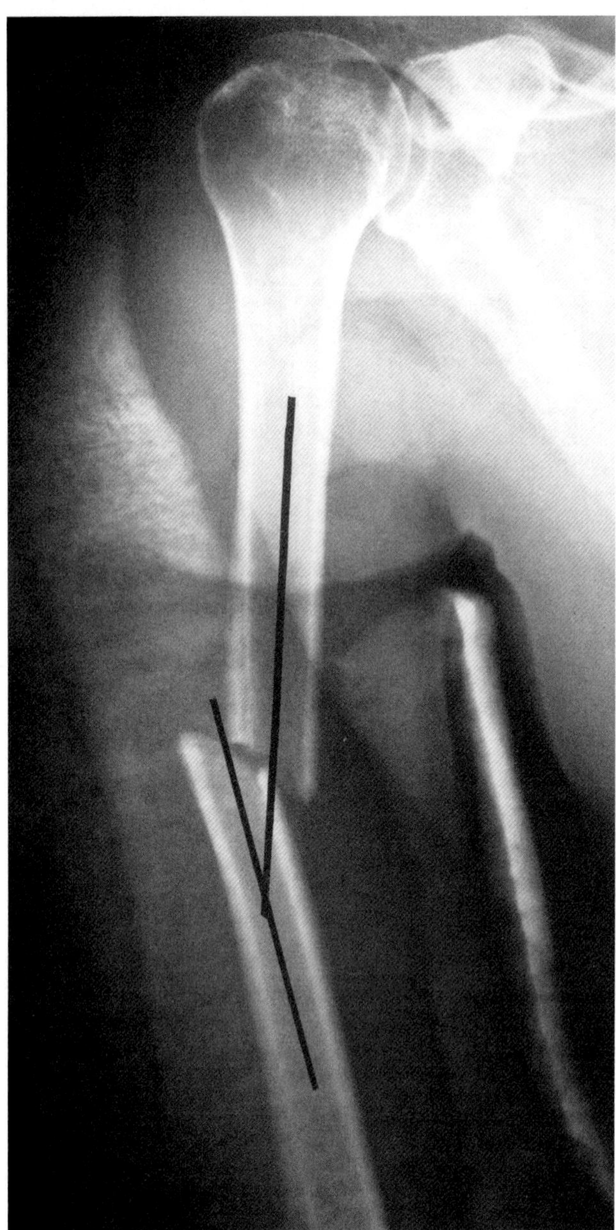

**Fig. 2-2** Complete fracture. Oblique fracture of the mid-humerus involving both cortices with lateral angulation (*lines*). Image taken in a hanging cast.

**Open fracture:** Lack of continuity of skin due to fracture fragment penetration or penetrating wound (see Fig. 2-8)

**Stress fracture:** Variety of fractures that result from repetitive stress of lesser magnitude than required for an acute fracture; may only be visible on radionuclide scan or MRI (see Fig. 2-9)

**Subluxation:** Partial displacement of articular surfaces of a joint (see Fig. 2-10)

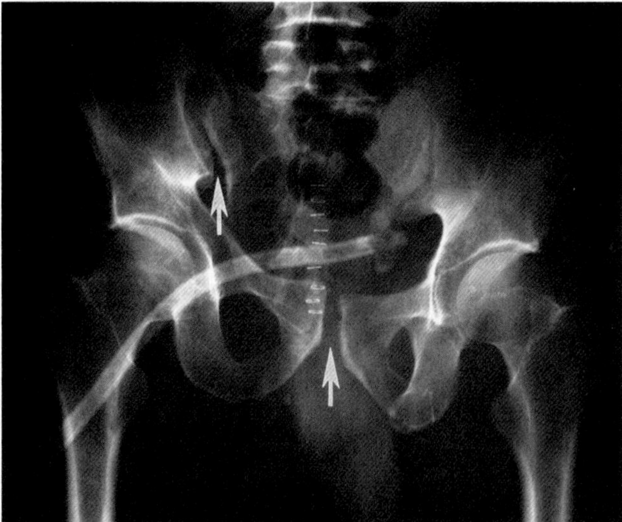

**Fig. 2-3** Diastasis. Vertical shearing injury to the pelvis with diastasis and step off of the pubic symphysis and right sacroiliac joint (*arrows*). There are also pubic rami fractures on the left and a suprapubic tube in the bladder.

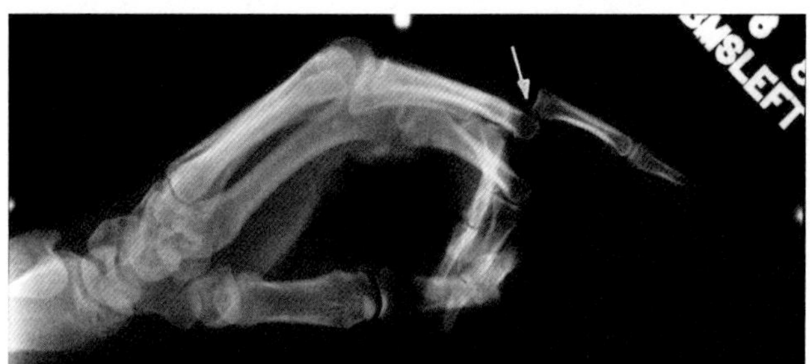

**Fig. 2-4** Dislocation. Lateral radiograph of the hand demonstrating a dorsal dislocation of the interphalangeal joint (*arrow*) with complete loss of articular contact.

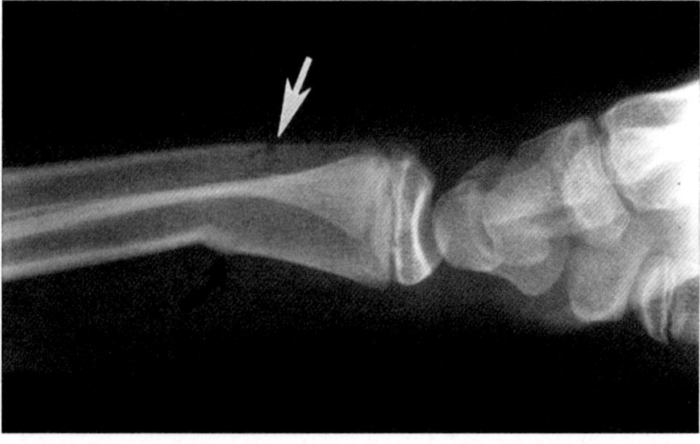

**Fig. 2-5** Incomplete fracture. Incomplete fractures of the ulna (*white arrow*) and radius (*curved black arrow*). The radial fracture is a torus or buckle fracture.

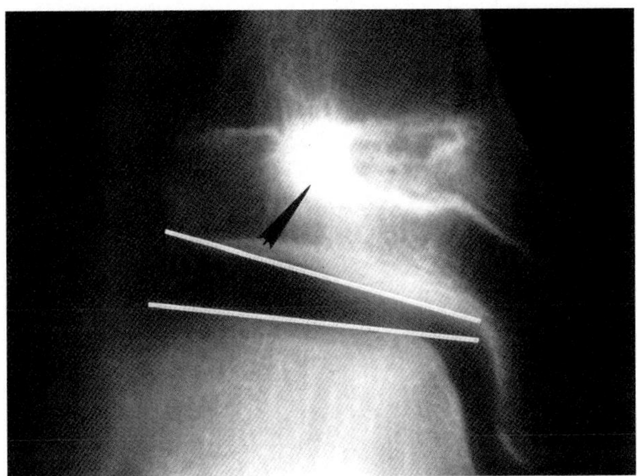

Fig. 2-6 Incongruency. Anteroposterior (AP) radiograph of the ankle with physeal bar after prior growth plate fracture (*arrowhead*) with resulting joint space asymmetry (*lines*).

## Descriptive Fracture Terminology

**Alignment:** Fracture fragment position related to the normal long axis of the involved bone (see Fig. 2-11A–C and E)

**Angulated:** Loss of normal alignment described by apex direction or displacement of the distal fragment (Fig. 2-11D and F and see Fig. 2-12)

**Apophyseal fracture:** Avulsion fracture through an apophysis or bony prominence (see Fig. 2-13)

**Apposition:** Degree of bone contact at the fracture site (see Fig. 2-14)

**Avulsion fracture:** Fracture caused by abrupt muscle contraction or at a ligament attachment associated with joint separation (Fig. 2-13)

**Bayonet position:** Fragments touch and overlap, but are in good alignment (Fig. 2-11E)

**Burst:** Fracture of the vertebral body with multiple fragments and expansion of the vertebral body, usually into the spinal canal (see Fig. 2-15)

**Butterfly fracture:** Triangular fragment displaced from a long bone fracture (see Fig. 2-16)

**Comminution:** Fracture with more than two fragments (see Fig. 2-17)

**Compression:** Trabecular fracture with loss of height usually reserved for spinal injuries (see Fig. 2-18)

**Condylar:** Fracture involving the condyle of the distal humerus or femur (see Fig. 2-19)

**Depression:** Calvarial or articular fracture with the fragment displaced below the calvarial table or in the case of a joint, below the articular surface (see Fig. 2-20)

**Diaphyseal:** Fracture of the shaft or diaphysis of a long bone (Figs. 2-8, 2-12, and 2-14)

**Displaced:** Fracture fragments angulated, rotated, or separated by >2 mm (Fig. 2-11)

**Distraction:** Separation of the fragments; may be associated with soft tissue interposition or excessive traction (Fig. 2-11C)

**Extracapsular:** Fracture near, but outside of the joint capsule

**Flake fracture:** Linear fracture fragment due to ligament or tendon injury (peroneal tendon dislocation may cause a fibular flake fracture) (see Fig. 2-21)

**Impaction:** Fracture compressed so the fragment is driven into the adjacent fragment (Fig. 2-11B)

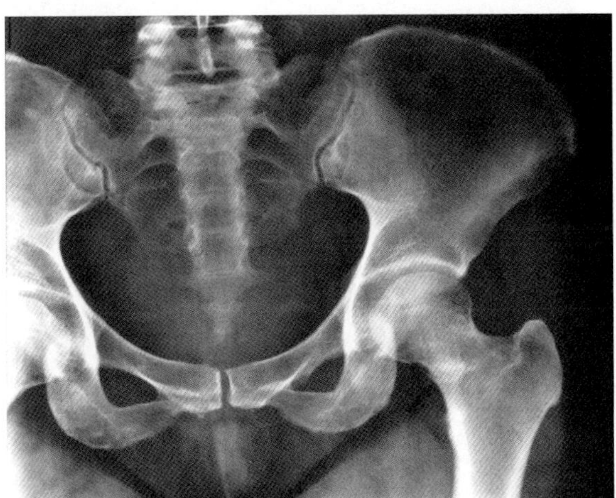


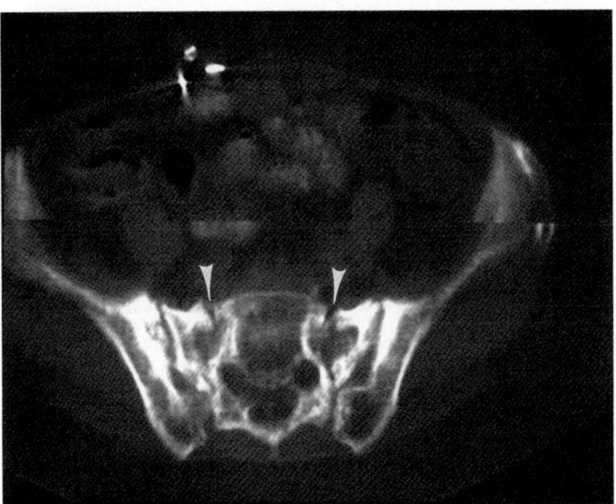


Fig. 2-7 Insufficiency fracture. A: Anteroposterior (AP) radiograph of the hip demonstrating a femoral neck insufficiency fracture (*arrow*). B: Axial computed tomography (CT) image of the pelvis demonstrating bilateral sacral insufficiency fractures (*arrowheads*).

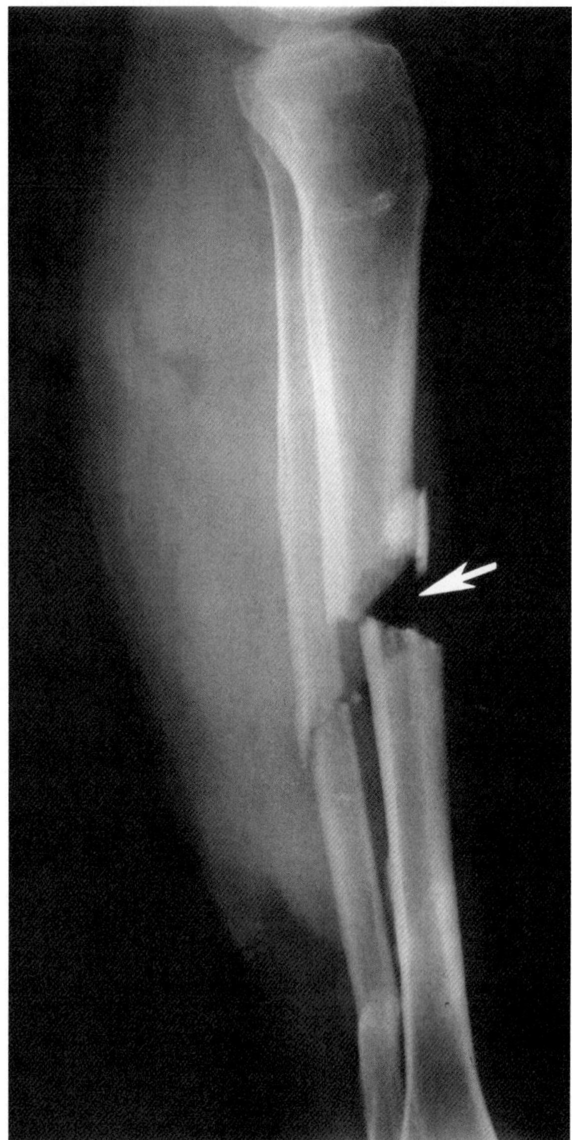

Fig. 2-8 Open fracture. Comminuted fractures of the mid-tibia and fibula with an open wound and air in the wound (*arrow*) at the fracture site.

**Infraction (pseudofracture):** Lucent line in abnormal bone, usually metabolic, such as osteomalacia (see Fig. 2-22)

**Intra-articular:** Fracture line enters the joint surface (Fig. 2-20)

**Intracapsular:** Fracture of the osseous portion of bone within the capsule, but not involving the articular surface (see Fig. 2-23)

**Linear:** Straight transverse or longitudinal fracture line (see Fig. 2-24A)

**Metaphyseal:** Fracture involving the metaphysis

**Oblique:** Fracture line oriented at an angle to the axis of a long bone (Fig. 2-24B)

**Occult:** Fracture not visible on radiographs, but may be seen on MRI or radionuclide scans (see Fig. 2-25)

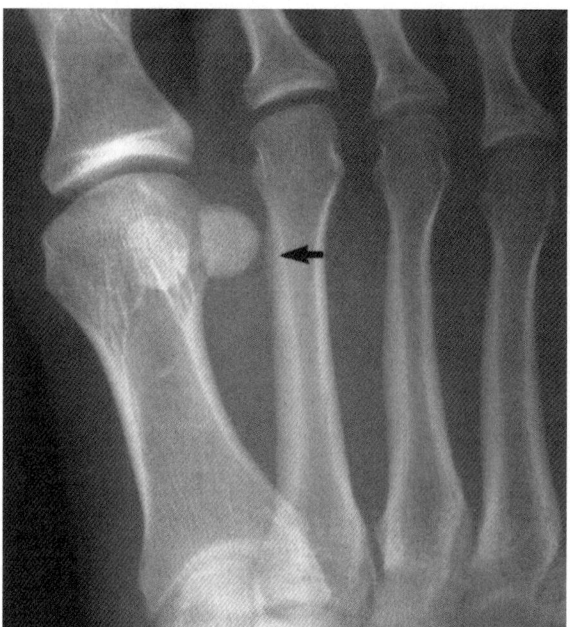

Fig. 2-9 Stress fracture. Radiograph of the foot demonstrating subtle periosteal reaction (*arrow*) due to a stress fracture of the distal second metatarsal. See also march fracture (Fig. 2-77).

**Osteochondral:** Fracture involving the cartilage and bone of a joint surface (see Fig. 2-26)

**Pathologic:** Fracture through abnormal bone (see Fig. 2-27)

**Physeal:** Fracture through the physis or growth plate; classified by Salter and Harris (see Fig. 2-28)

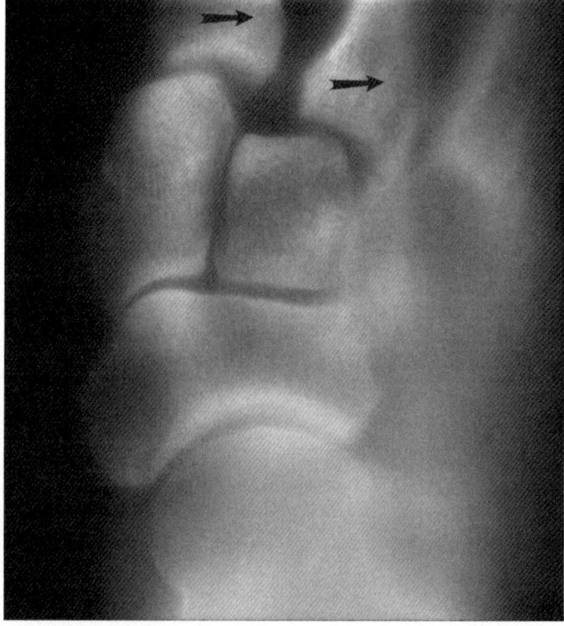

Fig. 2-10 Subluxation. Lisfranc injury with partial lateral displacement of the first and second metatarsals (*arrows*).

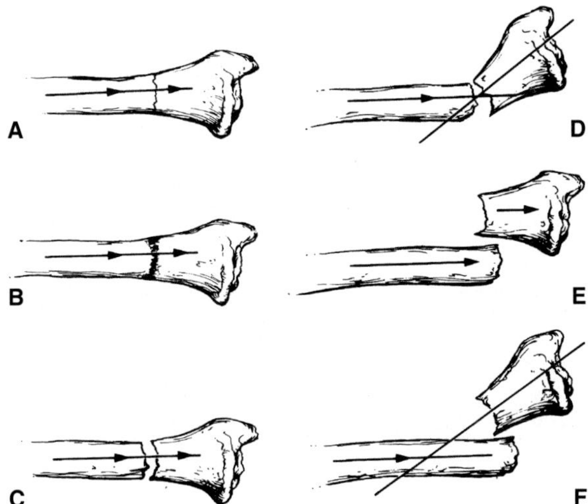


Fig. 2-11 Illustration of fracture descriptive terms. A: An undisplaced, complete fracture with normal alignment and no angulation, shortening, or rotation. B: An impacted complete fracture with minimal shortening, but normal alignment and no angulation or rotation. C: A complete fracture with distraction, normal alignment, and no angulation or rotation. D: A complete fracture with dorsal displacement of the distal fragment or volar angulation. E: Displaced overriding fracture with shortening, but alignment is maintained (*arrows* mark longitudinal axis). F: A complete fracture with displacement, angulation, and shortening.

**Type I**—fracture through the physis without metaphyseal or epiphyseal involvement
**Type II**—fracture of the physis that exits through the metaphysis
**Type III**—fracture of the physis that exits through the epiphysis
**Type IV**—fracture line extends through the metaphysis, physis, and epiphysis
**Type V**—growth plate or physeal impaction or compression

**Rotation:** Fragment turned on the opposing fragment, usually internal or external rotation (see Fig. 2-29)

**Secondary:** Fracture in pathologic or weakened bone (Fig. 2-27)

**Segmental:** Several large fracture fragments in the same long bone (see Fig. 2-30)

**Shortening:** Loss of length of the involved bone (Fig. 2-11E and F and 2-12)

**Spiral:** Fracture line rotates obliquely about the bone, usually due to twisting or rotation injury (Fig. 2-24C)

**Stellate:** Numerous fracture lines radiating from the central point of injury (see Fig. 2-31)

**Subchondral:** Fracture beneath the articular surface of the joint, commonly seen with abnormal bone and stress or insufficiency injuries (see Fig. 2-32)

**Torus:** Incomplete fracture of childhood with cortical buckling (see Fig. 2-33)

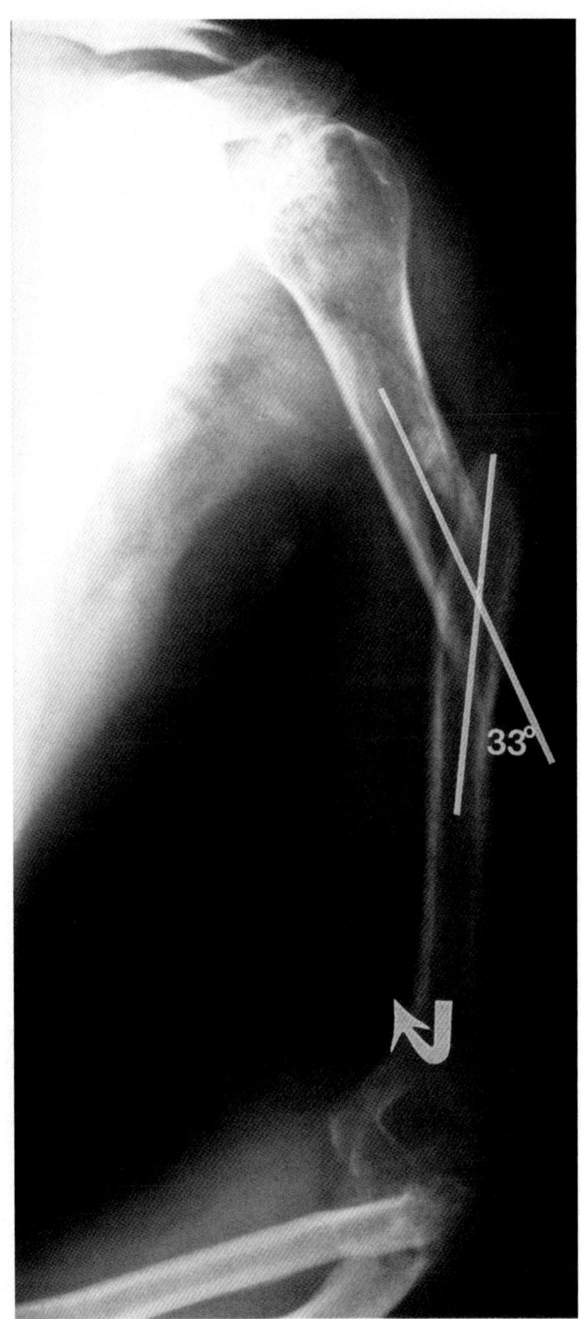


Fig. 2-12 Angulation. Spiral fracture of the mid-humerus with 33 degrees of lateral angulation. There is also overriding of the fragments with shortening and internal rotation of the distal fragment (*curved arrow*).

**Transcondylar:** Fracture that crosses the condyles of the distal humerus or femur

**Transverse:** Fracture line perpendicular to the axis of a long bone (Fig. 2-24A)

**Tuft:** Fracture of the distal aspect of the distal phalanx in the hand or foot (see Fig. 2-34)

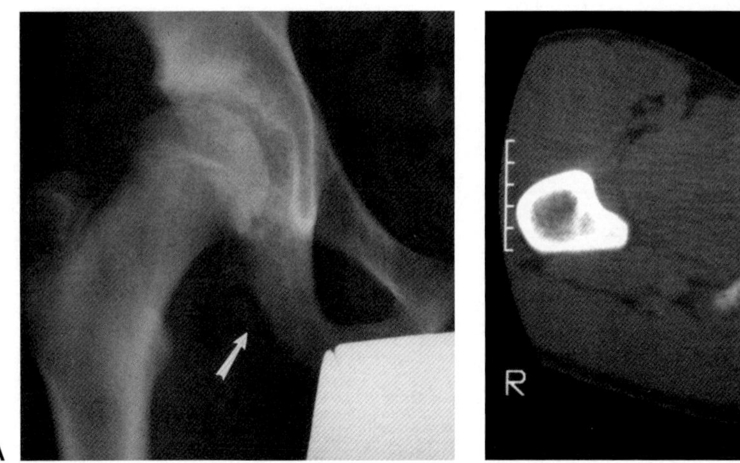

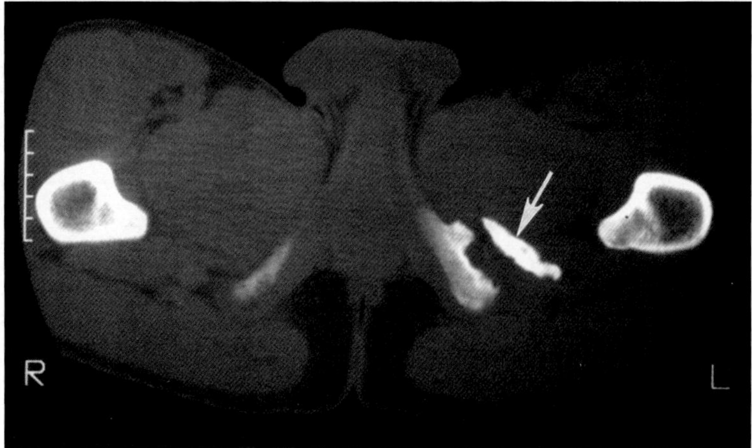


Fig. 2-13 Avulsion fracture. Anteroposterior (AP) radiograph (**A**) and axial computed tomographic (CT) image (**B**) of ischial apophysis avulsion fractures (*arrows*) in an adolescent due to hamstring muscle pull.

Fig. 2-14 Apposition. **A**: Anteroposterior (AP) radiograph of the leg demonstrating displaced fractures of the tibia and fibula (*arrows*) with no cortical apposition of the fracture margins (*lines*). Splint in place. **B**: Fractures of the tibia and fibula with minimal apposition (*lines*). See Figure 2-11A which demonstrates 100% apposition.

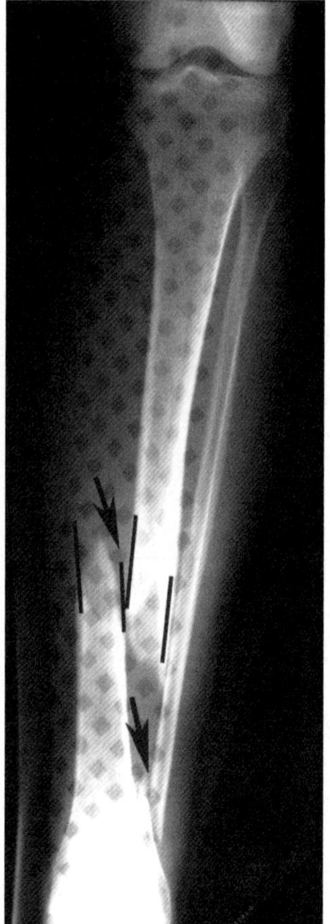

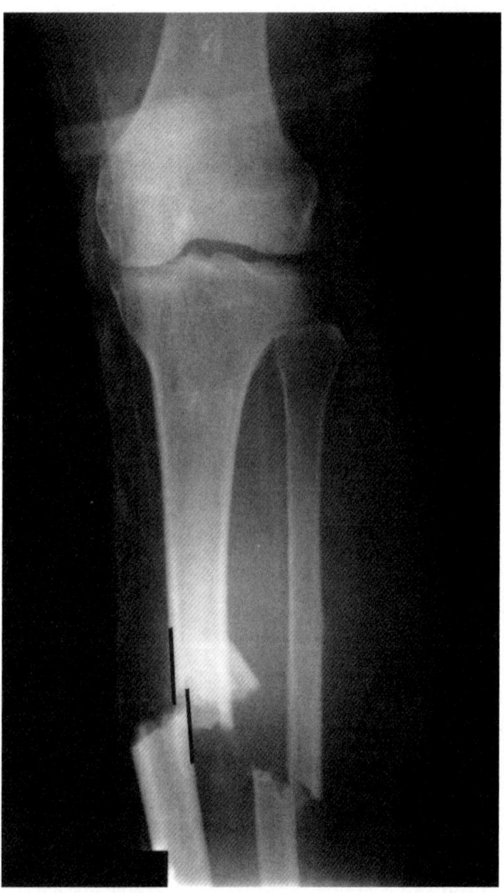

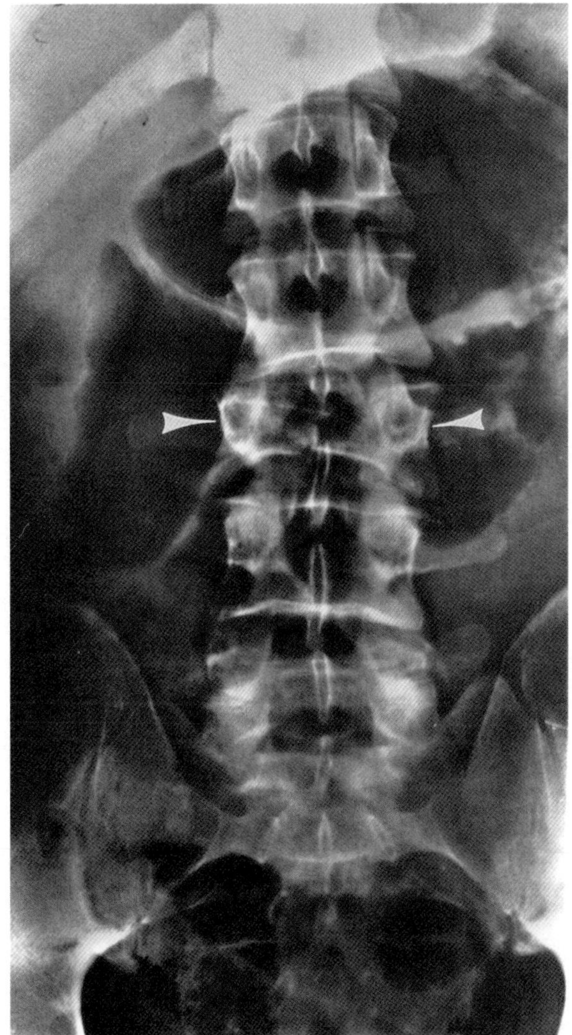
A

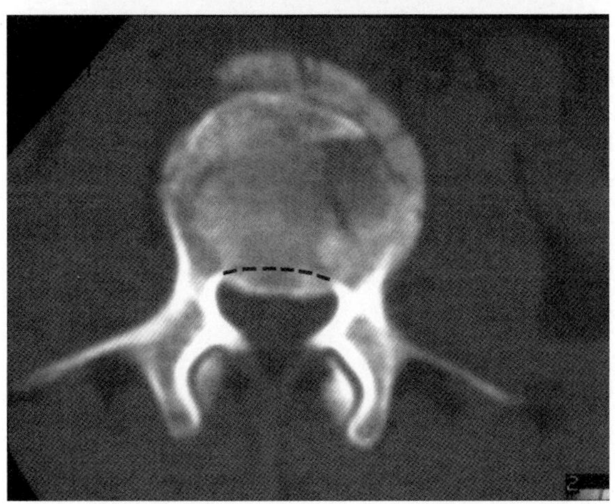
B

Fig. 2-15 Burst fracture. A: Anteroposterior (AP) radiograph of the lumbar spine demonstrating an L3 burst fracture with loss of height and lateral displacement of the pedicles and vertebral margins (*arrowheads*). B: Axial computed tomographic (CT) image shows comminution of the vertebral body with posterior extension into the spinal canal (*broken line* marks normal body configuration).

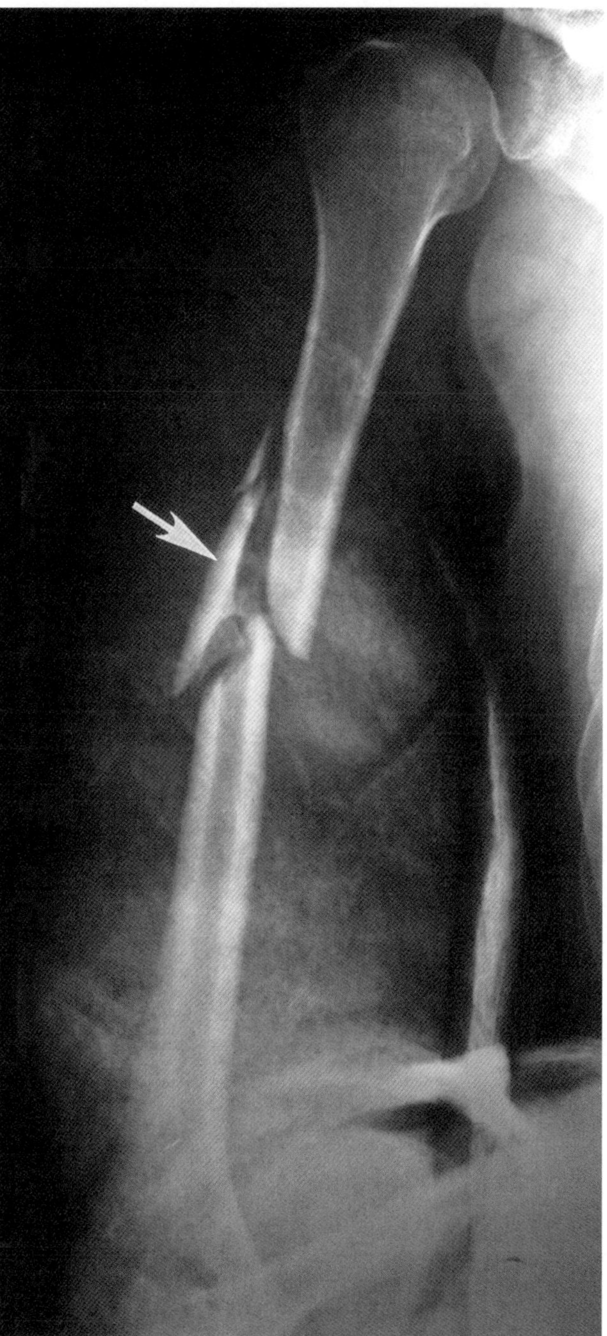

Fig. 2-16 Butterfly fracture. Comminuted midshaft fracture of humerus with a triangular displaced fragment (*arrow*). Hanging cast in place.

## Fracture Healing Terminology

**Bone union:** *Clinical*—no pain or motion at fracture site; *radiographic*—fracture site bridged by trabecular bone and/or callus

**Callus formation:** Radiographically identifiable periosteal bone formation at the fracture site (see Fig. 2-35)

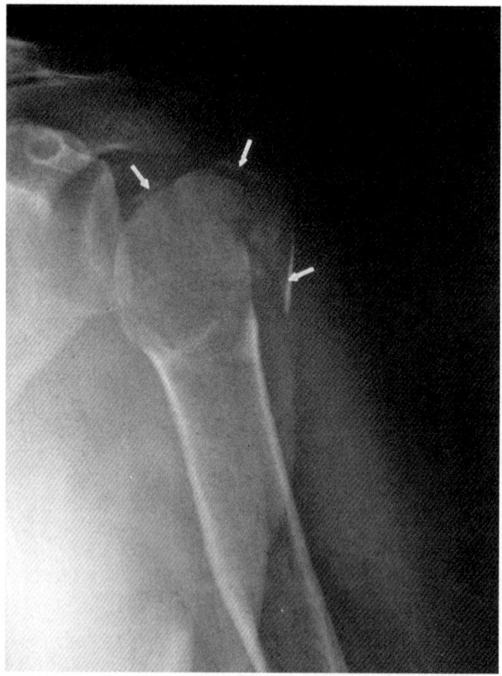

Fig. 2-17 Comminuted fracture. Anteroposterior (AP) radiograph of the humerus demonstrating a displaced, comminuted fracture (*arrows*).

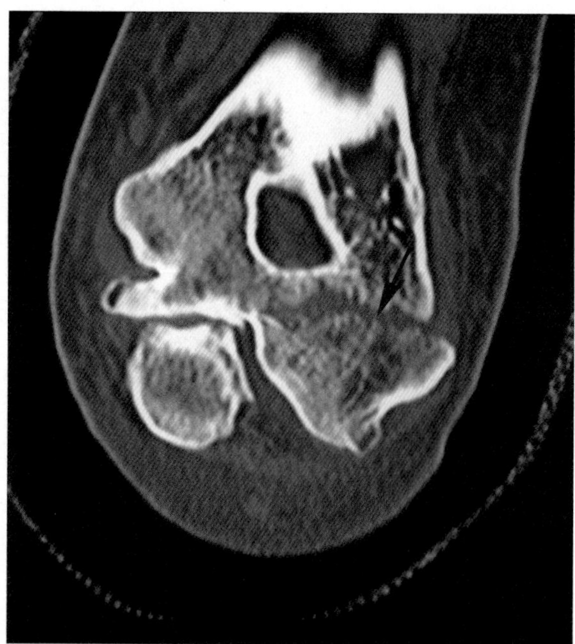

Fig. 2-19 Condylar fracture. Coronal computed tomographic (CT) image demonstrating a condylar fracture of the distal humerus (*arrow*).

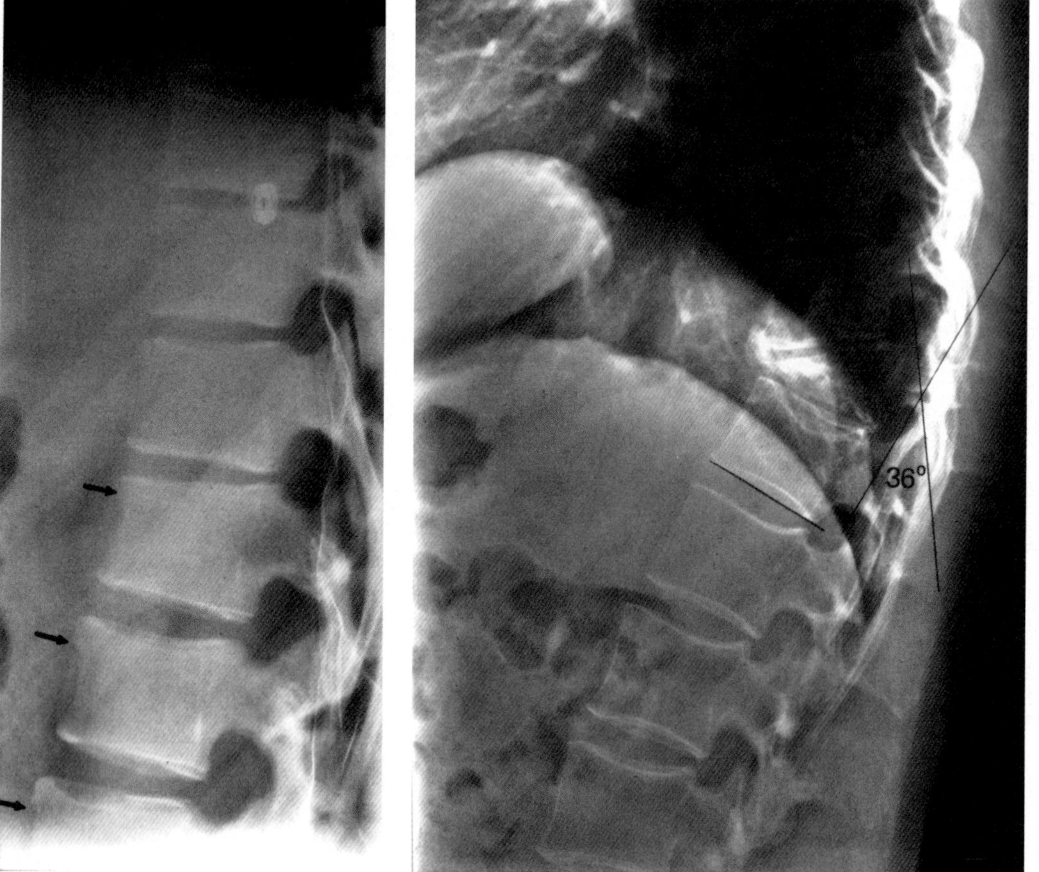


Fig. 2-18 Compression fracture. A: Lateral view of the thoracolumbar junction demonstrating subtle compression fractures (*arrows*) with buckling of the anterior cortex. B: Marked compression of T11 with 36 degrees of kyphotic angulation.

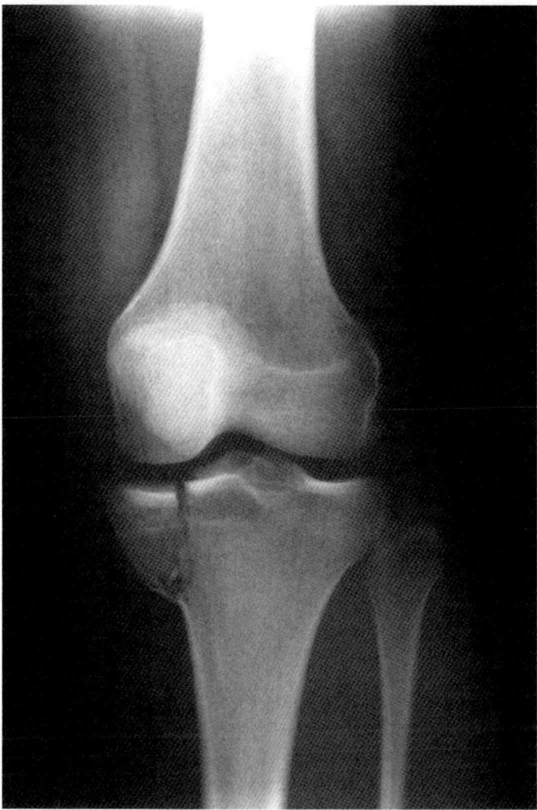

Fig. 2-20 Depression fracture. Anteroposterior (AP) radiograph of the knee demonstrating a depressed intra-articular fracture of the medial tibial plateau.

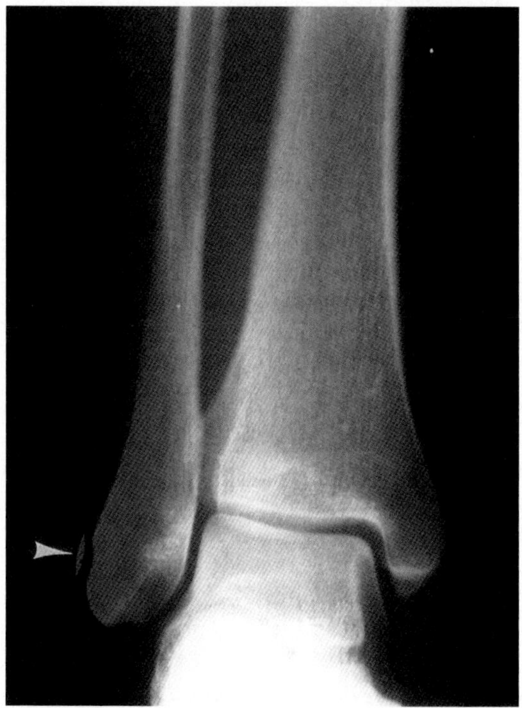

Fig. 2-21 Flake fracture. Mortise view of the ankle demonstrating a flake fracture of the fibula (*arrowhead*) due to peroneal tendon dislocation.

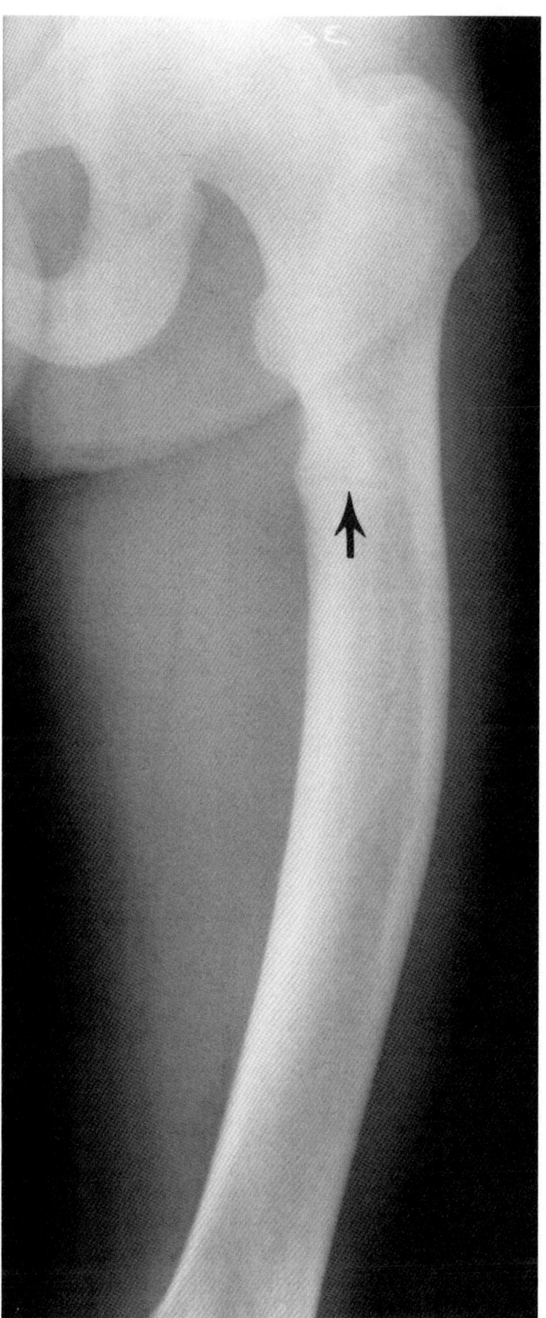

Fig. 2-22 Radiograph of the femur demonstrating a lucent infraction or pseudofracture in a patient with osteomalacia.

**Delayed union:** Union (healing) which takes more than the average time for a given anatomic site; fracture ends may be sclerotic on radiographs or CT (see Fig. 2-36)

**Early union:** Appearance of trabeculae across the fracture site earlier than expected for a given anatomic site

**Established union:** Cortical callus organization and remodeling begin (Fig. 2-35C–I)

**Fibrous union:** No pain at the fracture line with clinical stability; lucent line persists radiographically with low signal intensity on T1- and T2-weighted MR images

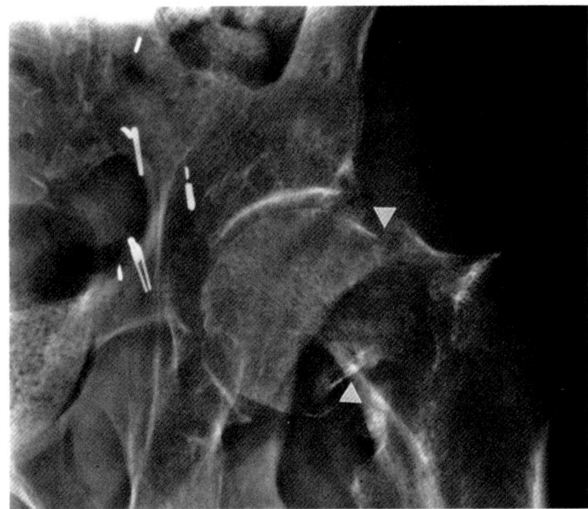

Fig. 2-23 Intracapsular fracture. Anteroposterior (AP) radiograph demonstrating a displaced intracapsular fracture of the femoral neck (*arrowheads*) without articular involvement.

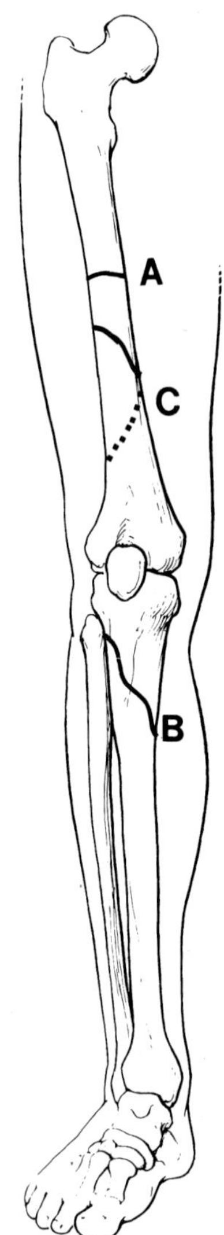


Fig. 2-24 Illustration of transverse (A), oblique (B), and spiral (C) fractures.

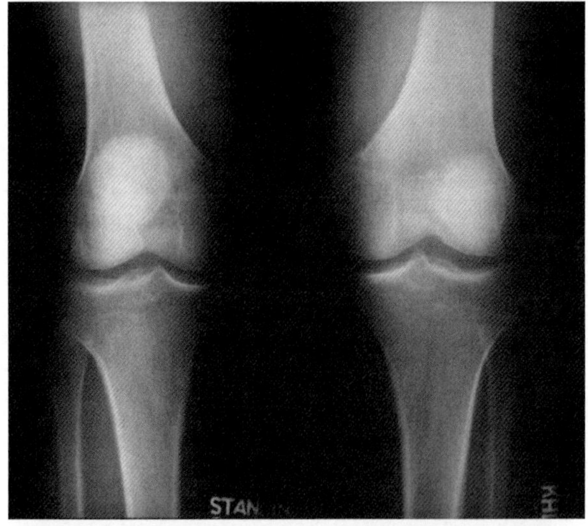


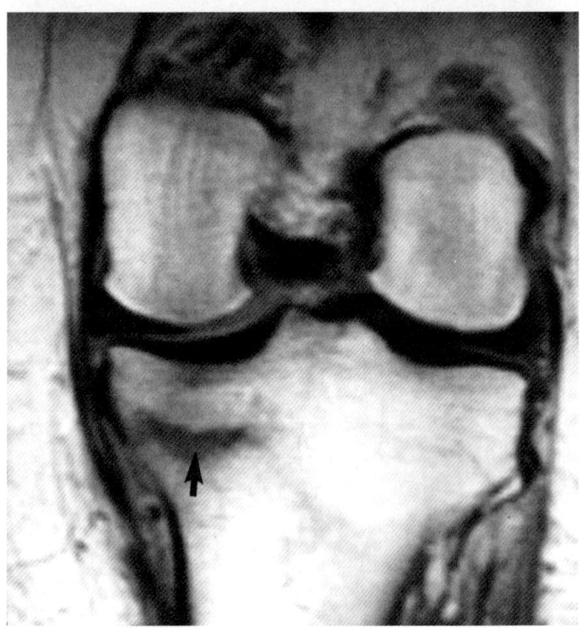


Fig. 2-25 Occult fracture. A: Standing radiographs of the knee in a patient with left knee pain are normal. B: T1-weighted magnetic resonance (MR) image demonstrates a linear stress fracture (*arrow*).

**Malunion:** Fracture heals in poor or nonanatomic position (see Fig. 2-37)

**Nonunion:** Diagnosed by clinical evaluation due to failure to heal properly; radiographic features:

- **Atrophic**—atrophy of fracture ends (see Fig. 2-38)
- **Hypertrophic**—prominent hypertrophic nonbridging callus at the fracture site (see Fig. 2-39)

**Phases of healing:** There are three phases of fracture healing (Fig. 2-35)

- **Reactive phase**—fracture and inflammatory phase; granulation tissue formation; first 10% of healing process
- **Reparative phase**—callus formation and lamellar bone deposition; second 40% of healing process

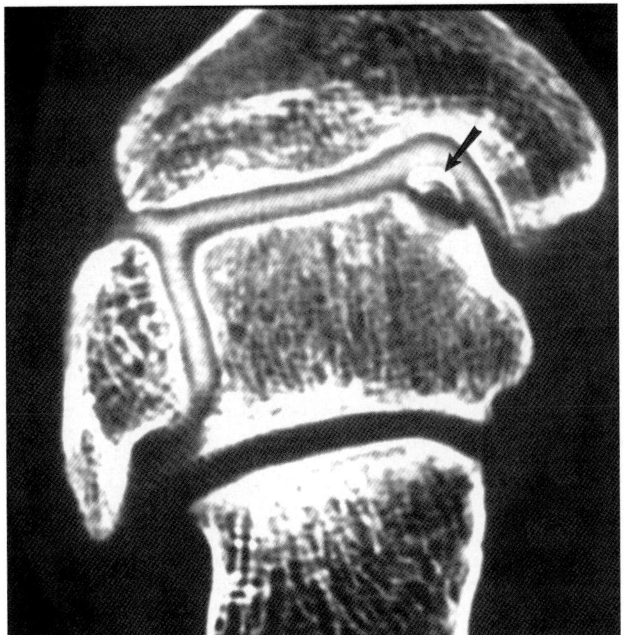

Fig. 2-26 Osteochondral fracture. Coronal computed tomographic (CT) arthrogram demonstrating a displaced osteochondral fracture (*arrow*) of the talar dome.

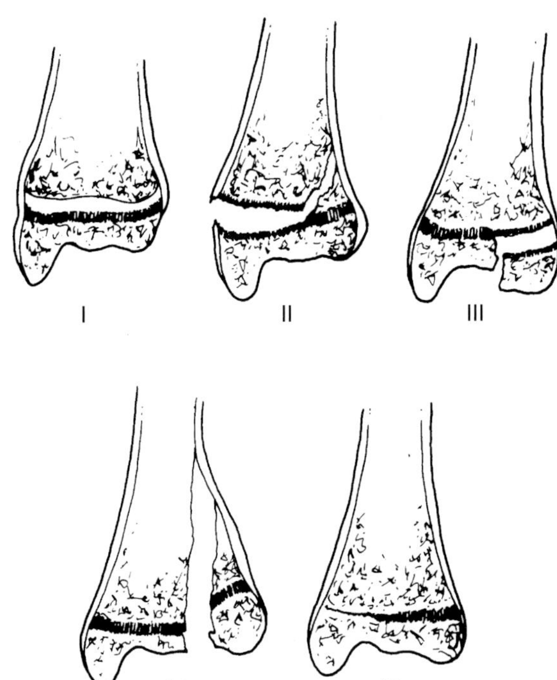


Fig. 2-28 Physeal fractures. Illustration of the Salter-Harris classification for physeal fractures. Type I fracture through the physis, type II physeal fracture exiting through the metaphysis, type III physeal fracture exiting through the epiphysis, type IV fracture extending through the metaphysis, epiphysis, and growth plate, type V physeal compression.

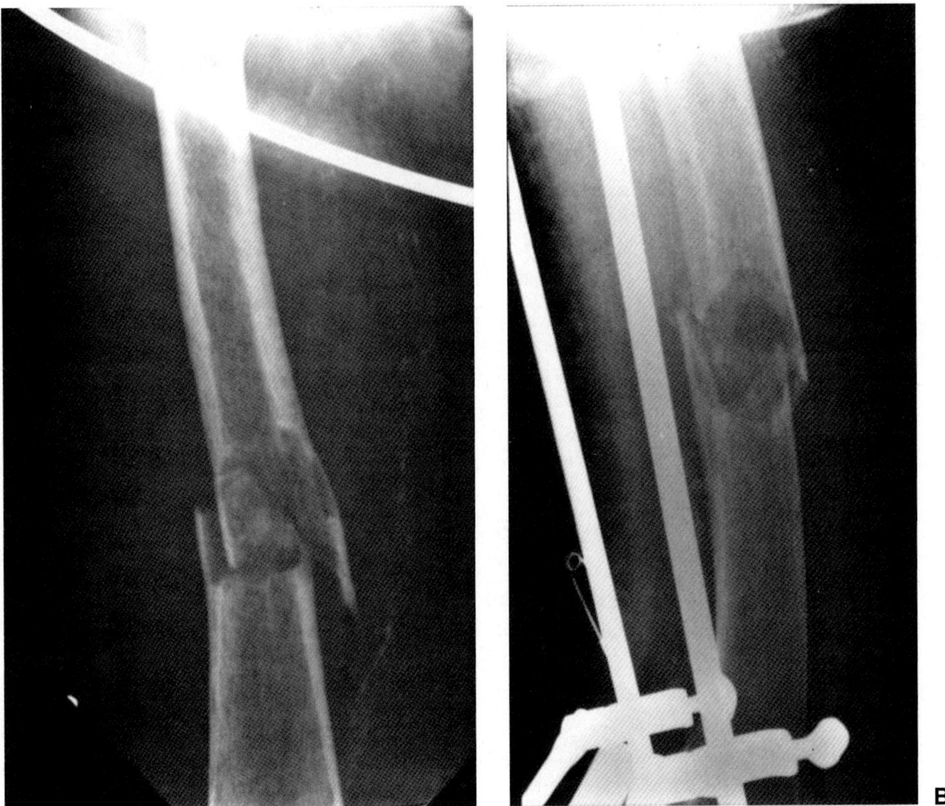


Fig. 2-27 Pathologic fracture. Anteroposterior (AP) (A) and lateral (B) radiographs demonstrating a fracture through a femoral metastasis. Traction in place.

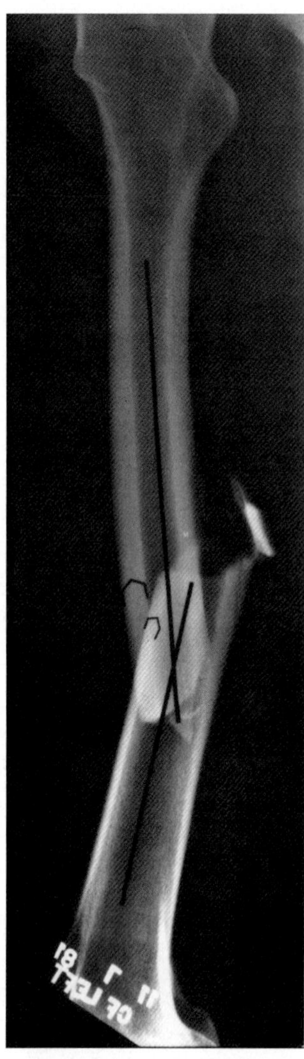

Fig. 2-29 Rotation. Comminuted fracture of the femur with external rotation of the distal fragment (the knee is directed to the right) and angulation (*lines*). Note the difference in cortical thickness (*brackets*) at the fracture site.

**Remodeling phase**—remodeling of original bone contour; 70% of healing process

**Pseudarthrosis:** Nonunion with formation of a synovial lined capsule in the fracture line

## Fracture/Dislocation Eponyms

**Ankle mortise diastasis:** Separation of the distal tibia and fibula due to syndesmotic and interosseous ligament tears; may be associated with dislocations (see Fig. 2-40)

**Archer's shoulder:** Recurrent posterior subluxation or dislocation of the shoulder

**Aviator's astragalus:** A variety of fractures of the talus caused by impaction of the foot into the ankle; may be associated with subtalar or tibiotalar dislocations (see Fig. 2-41)

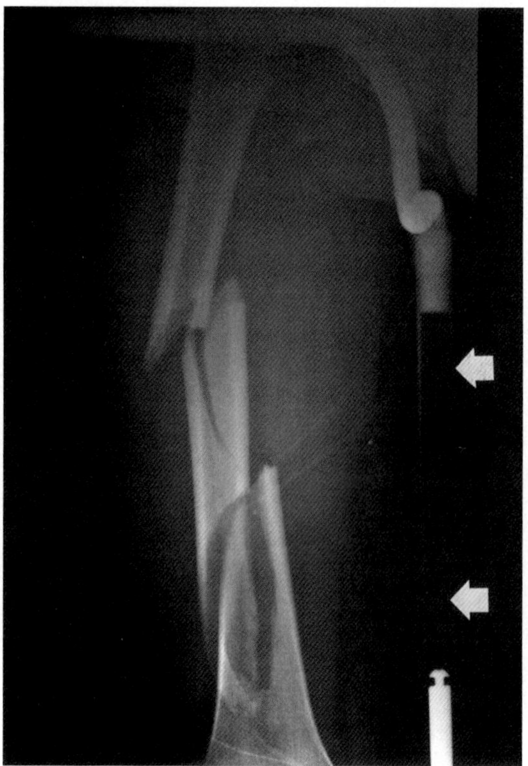

Fig. 2-30 Segmental fracture. Anteroposterior (AP) radiograph of the femur demonstrating three large shaft fragments.

**Bankart:** Anterior-inferior glenoid rim or labral detachment seen with anterior dislocations (see Fig. 2-42)

**Barton:** Intra-articular fracture of the dorsal or volar lip of the distal radius (see Fig. 2-43)

**Baseball finger:** Hyperflexion injury of the distal interphalangeal joint due to extensor tendon avulsion, which may have

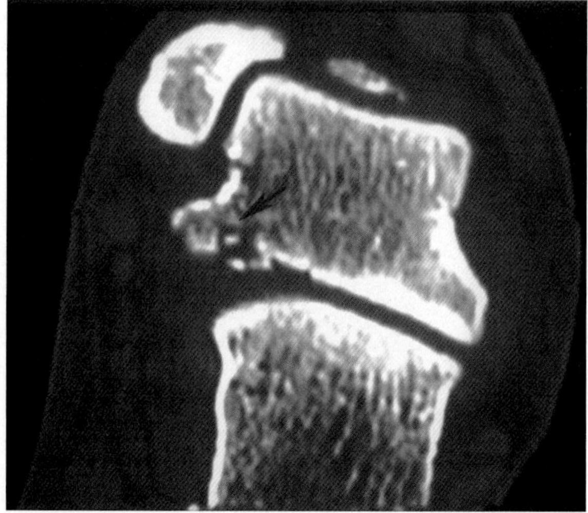

Fig. 2-31 Stellate fracture. Coronal computed tomographic (CT) image demonstrating a stellate fracture (*arrow*) with multiple small fragments in the medial talus.

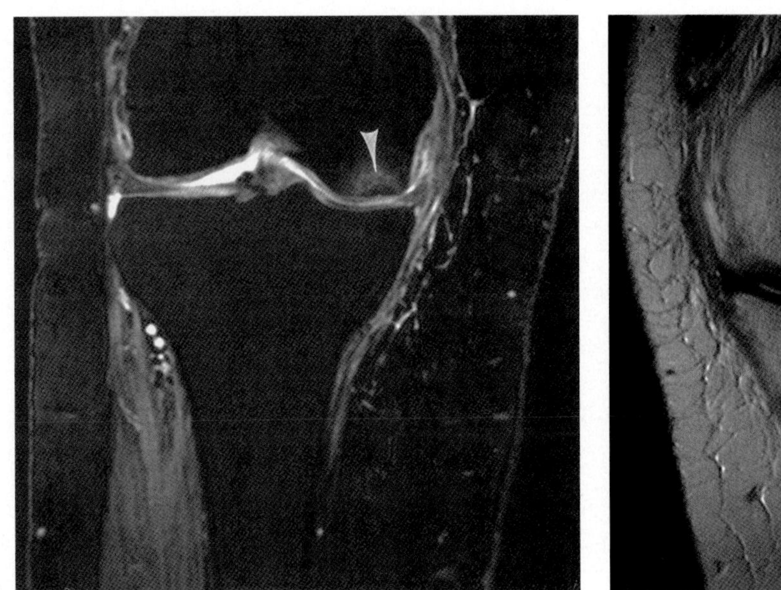


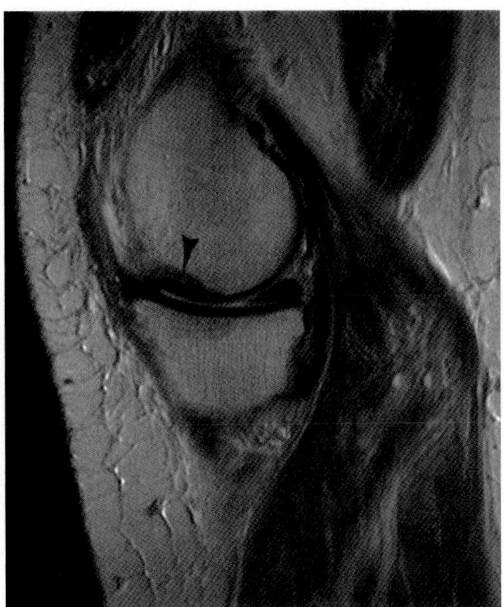


**Fig. 2-32** Subchondral fracture. Coronal double echo steady state (DESS) (A) and sagittal T1-weighted (B) magnetic resonance (MR) images demonstrating a subchondral fracture (*arrowheads*).

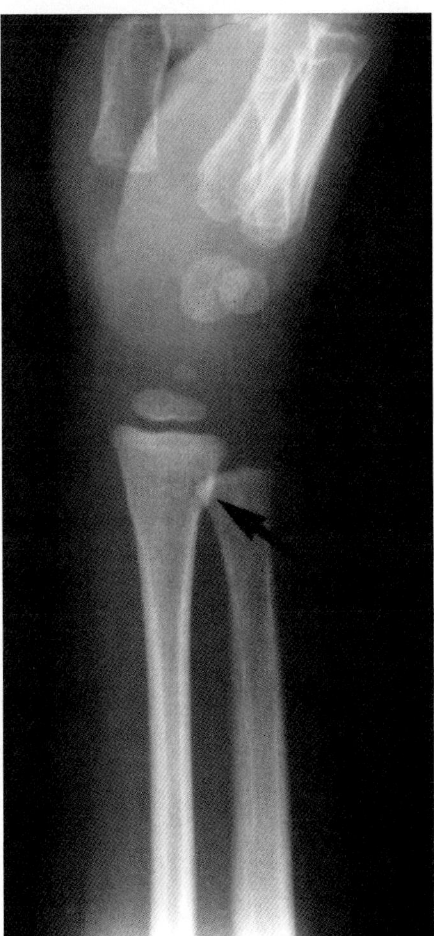

**Fig. 2-33** Torus fractures. Oblique radiograph demonstrating subtle buckling of the radial cortex (*arrow*). Also see Figure 2-6.

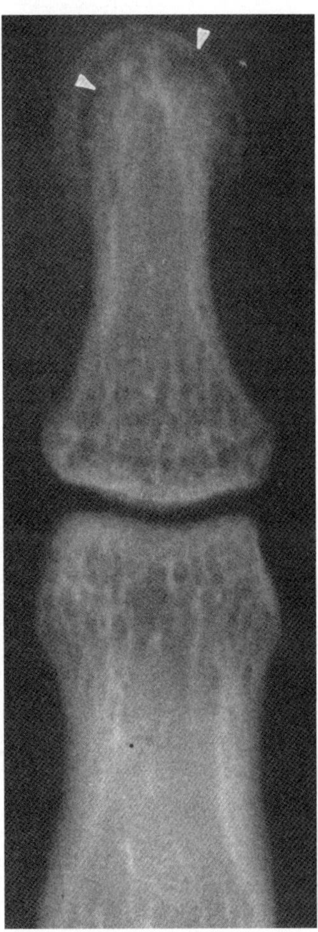

**Fig. 2-34** Tuft fracture. Posteroanterior (PA) radiograph of the finger demonstrating a comminuted fracture of the phalangeal tuft (*arrowheads*).

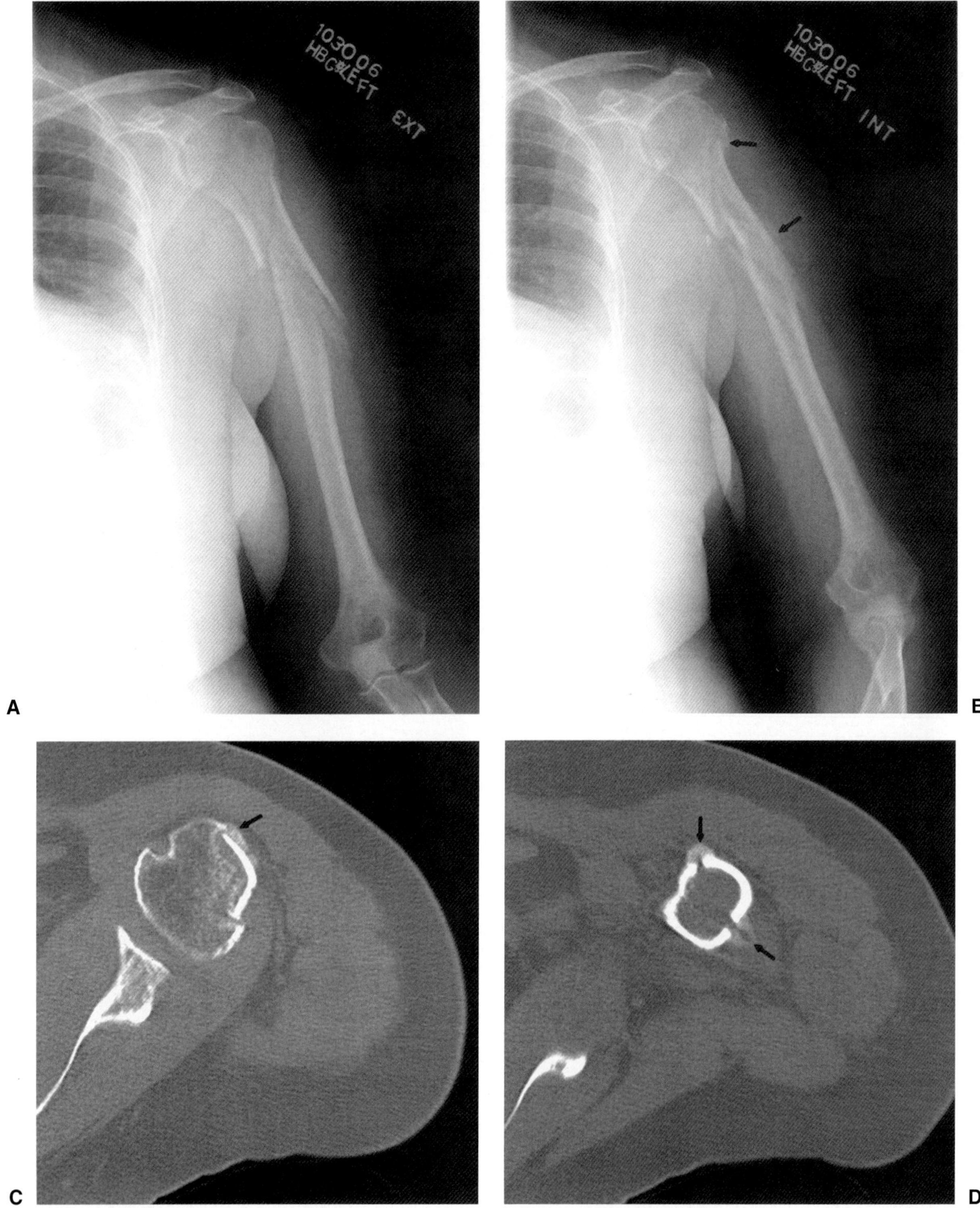


**Fig. 2-35** Callus formation. Radiographs of the humerus (**A** and **B**) demonstrate a comminuted fracture with slight callus formation (*arrows*) along a portion of the fracture. The extent of callus formation is difficult to evaluate. Axial computed tomographic (CT) images (**C–E**) show developing callus (*arrows*), which is most obvious along the regions where fracture separation is the least. Reformatted and three-dimensional CT images (**F–I**) demonstrate the degree of callus formation (*arrows*) more clearly.

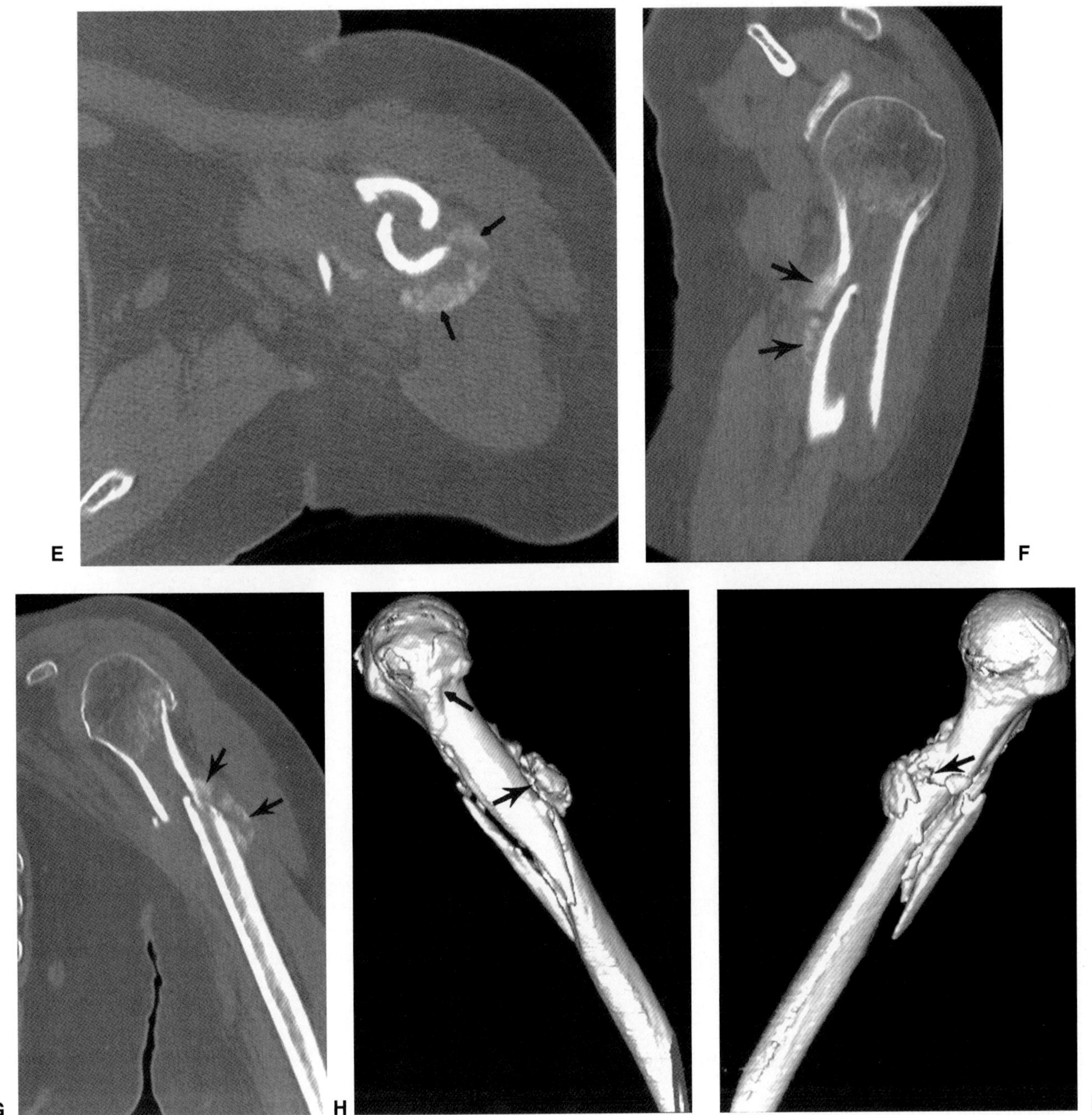


Fig. 2-35 (*Continued*)

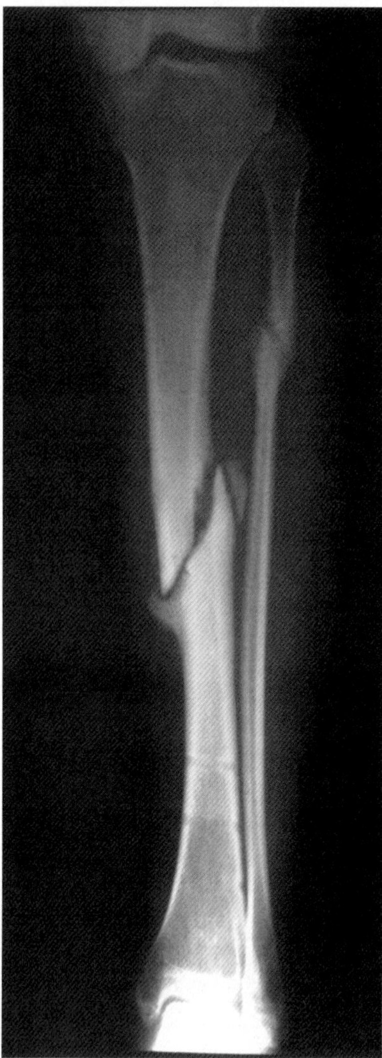

Fig. 2-36 Delayed union. Anteroposterior (AP) radiograph demonstrates a mid-tibial fracture with sclerotic margins and hypertrophic nonbridging callus 5 months after injury.

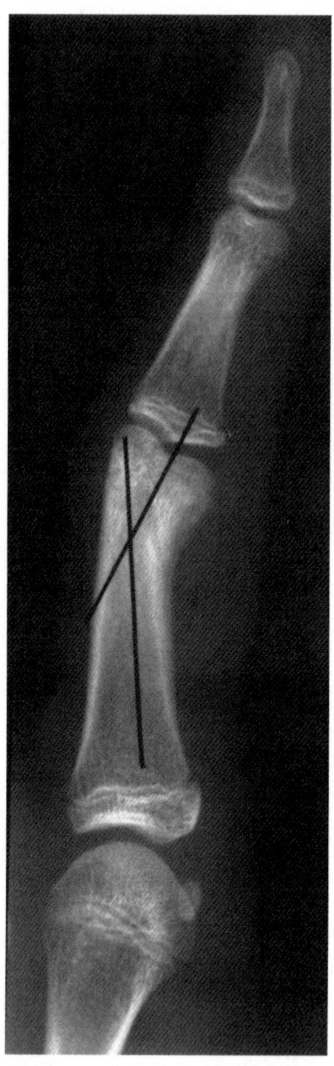

Fig. 2-37 Malunion. Healed fracture of the proximal phalanx with angulation (*lines*) rotation and articular incongruency.

an associated osseous fragment (dropped or mallet finger) (see Fig. 2-44)

**Basketball foot:** Subtalar dislocation (see Fig. 2-45)

**Bennett:** Intra-articular fracture of the base of the first metacarpal with volar ulnar fragment due to the attachment of the strong ulnar oblique ligament (see Fig. 2-46)

**Boot top:** Fractures of the distal third of the tibia and fibula at the level of the top of a ski boot (see Fig. 2-47)

**Bosworth:** Fracture dislocation of the ankle with an oblique distal fibular fracture with locking of the distal fragment behind the tibia

**Boutonniere deformity:** Hyperflexion of the proximal interphalangeal joint of the finger with hyperextension of the distal interphalangeal joint due to disruption of the central extensor tendon (see Fig. 2-48)

**Boxer:** Fracture of the fifth metacarpal neck with palmar displacement of the metacarpal head and dorsal angulation at the fracture site (see Fig. 2-49)

**Boxer's elbow:** Chip fracture of the olecranon due to rapid extension of the elbow

**Bucket handle:** Vertical shear injury to the pelvis with fracture of the anterior pubic rami and opposite ilium or sacroiliac (SI) joint diastasis (see Fig. 2-50)

**Bumper:** Fracture of the tibia or femur due to a direct blow to the tibial tuberosity region caused by car bumper; may be bilateral

**Bunkbed:** Childhood fracture involving the intra-articular base of the first metatarsal

**Buttonhole:** Perforation fracture of bone associated with penetrating injury such as a gunshot wound (see Fig. 2-51)

**Cedell:** Fracture of the posterior talar process (see Fig. 2-52)

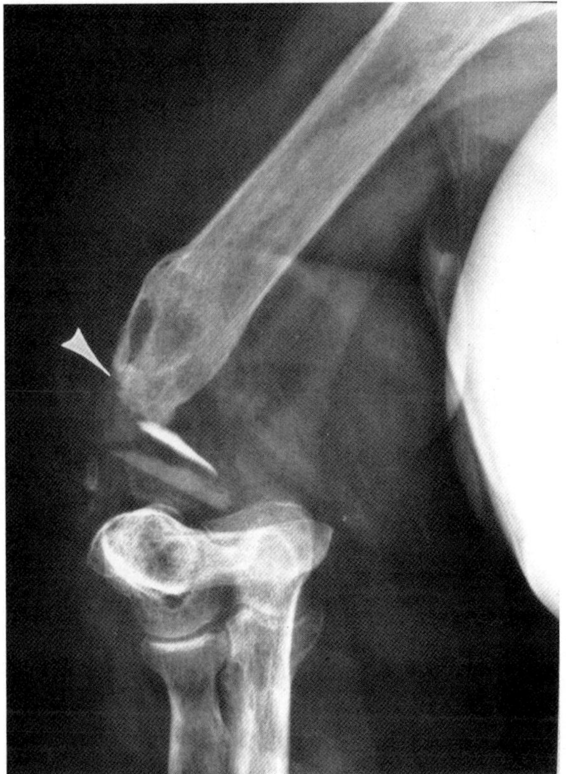


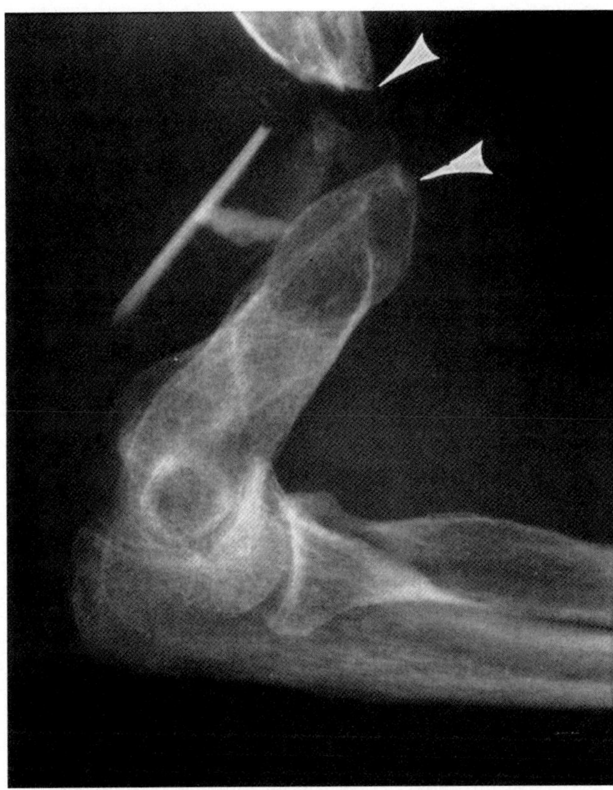


Fig. 2-38 Nonunion. Atrophic nonunion of the distal humerus demonstrated on frontal (**A**) and lateral (**B**) radiographs. Note the atrophy of the fracture ends (*arrowheads*). Compare to Figure 2-39 which is hypertrophic nonunion.

**Chance:** Flexion distraction injury of the spine with posterior ligament injury and fracture and associated, although often mild, anterior vertebral compression; usually at L1 or the thoracolumbar junction; associated with lap seat belts (see Fig. 2-53)

**Chaput:** Fracture of the anterior tubercle of the distal tibia due to avulsion of the distal anterior tibiofibular ligament

**Chauffeur:** Intra-articular fracture of the radial styloid; also called *backfire fracture* (see Fig. 2-54)

**Chisel:** Intra-articular fracture of the radial head with extension distally approximately 1 cm from the central articular surface (see Fig. 2-55)

**Chopart:** Fracture dislocation of the talonavicular and calcaneocuboid articulations; derived from surgical amputation at these joints described by Chopart (see Fig. 2-56)

**Clay shoveler:** Isolated or multiple fractures of the spinous processes; most often affecting the lower cervical and upper thoracic spine (see Fig. 2-57)

**Coach's finger:** Dorsal dislocation of the proximal interphalangeal joint (Fig. 2-4)

**Colles:** Fracture of the distal radial metaphysis with dorsal displacement of the distal fragment; may or may not have associated ulnar styloid fracture (see Fig. 2-58)

**Cotton:** Trimalleolar ankle fracture with the posterior and superior displacement of the posterior tibial fragment

**Dashboard:** Fracture of the posterior acetabular rim caused by force transmitted from the knee to the femur and hip during a motor vehicle accident (see Fig. 2-59)

**De Quervain:** Fracture of the scaphoid with volar displacement of the proximal fragment and lunate

**Desault:** Dislocation of the distal radioulnar joint; best demonstrated on axial CT or MR images in neutral, pronation, and supination (see Fig. 2-60)

**Descot:** Fracture of the distal posterior margin of the tibia (third malleolus) (see Fig. 2-61)

**Die punch:** Depression fracture of the lunate fossa of the distal radius with proximal migration of the lunate

**Dupuytren:** Fracture of the distal fibula above the joint due to pronation-external rotation; associated tears of the tibiofibular and deltoid ligaments; similar to Maisonneuve but fibular fracture more distal with Dupuytren

**Duverney:** Isolated iliac wing fracture (see Fig. 2-62)

**Essex-Lopresti:** Comminuted fracture of the radial head with dislocation of the distal radioulnar joint

**Galeazzi:** Fracture of the distal radial shaft with associated dislocation of the distal radioulnar joint (see Fig. 2-63)

**Gamekeeper:** Disruption of the ulnar collateral ligament of the thumb at the metacarpal phalangeal joint; there may be an associated avulsion fracture (see Fig. 2-64)

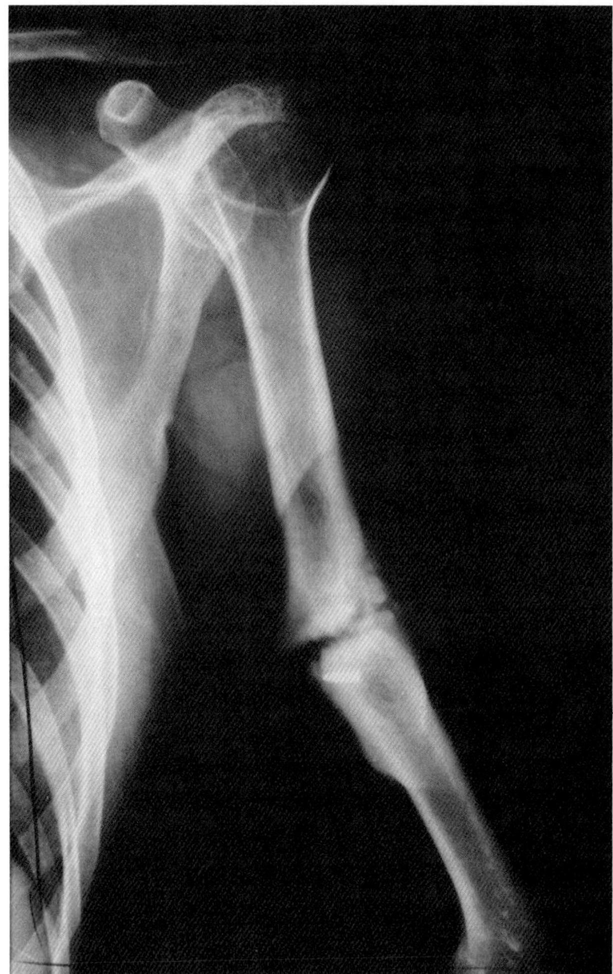

Fig. 2-39 Nonunion. Hypertrophic nonunion of a humeral fracture with hypertrophy and dense nonbridging callus.

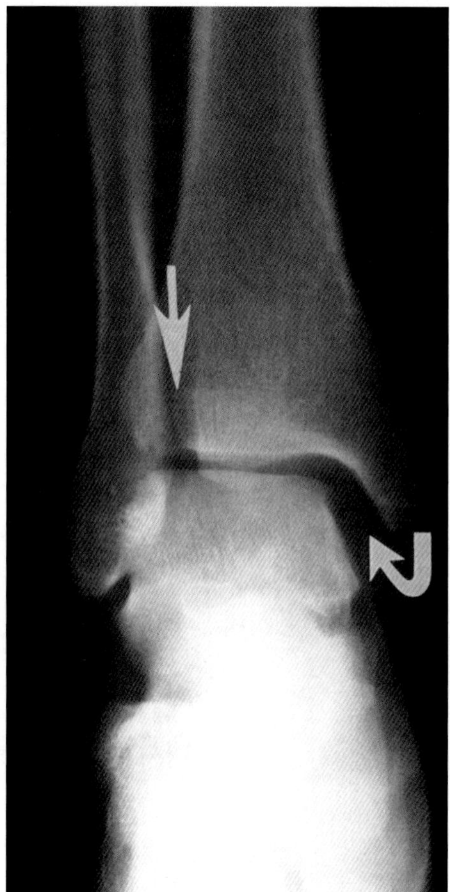

Fig. 2-40 Ankle diastasis. Anteroposterior (AP) radiograph demonstrates widening of the syndesmosis (*arrow*) with associated disruption of the deltoid ligament (*curved arrow*).

**Gosselin:** Intra-articular "V" shaped fracture of the distal tibia

**Greenstick:** Incomplete long bone fracture with cortical disruption on the tension side and bowing on the compression side (see Fig. 2-65)

**Hangman's (hanged man's):** Fracture of the neural arch of C2 due to a distraction-hyperextension injury (see Fig. 2-66)

**Hill-Sachs:** Impaction fracture of the posterolateral humeral head associated with anterior shoulder dislocation (Fig. 2-42)

**Hill-Sachs reverse:** Impaction fracture in the anterior medial humeral head associated with posterior dislocations (see Fig. 2-67)

**Hoffa:** Coronal fracture of the medial femoral condyle

**Holstein-Lewis:** Fracture of the humeral shaft at the junction of the mid and distal thirds associated with radial nerve injury due to proximity of nerve to fracture (see Fig. 2-68)

**Horseback rider's knee:** Posterior dislocation of the fibular head due to striking the knee against the gate post

**Jefferson:** Burst fracture of the ring of C1 due to axial compression injury (see Fig. 2-69)

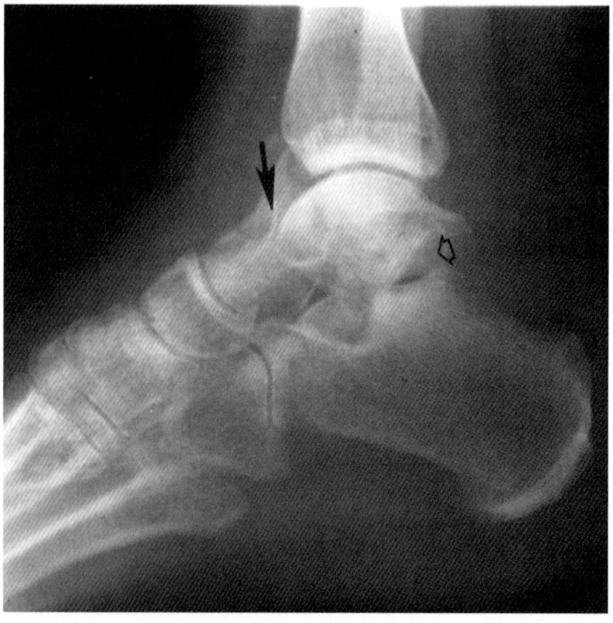

Fig. 2-41 Aviator's astragalus. Radiograph of the ankle in a patient with a displaced talar neck fracture (*arrow*) and subtalar dislocation (*open arrow*).

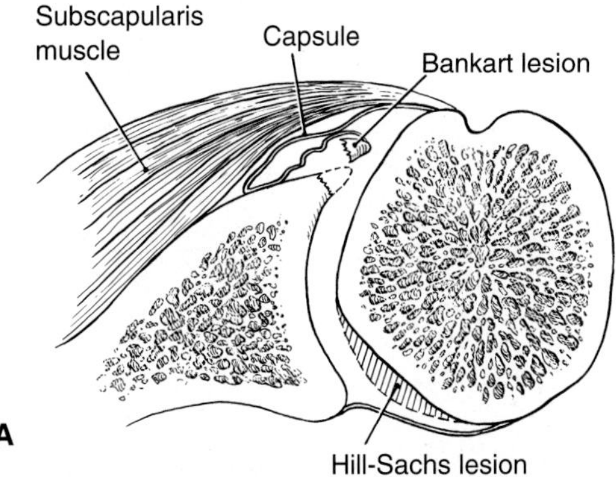


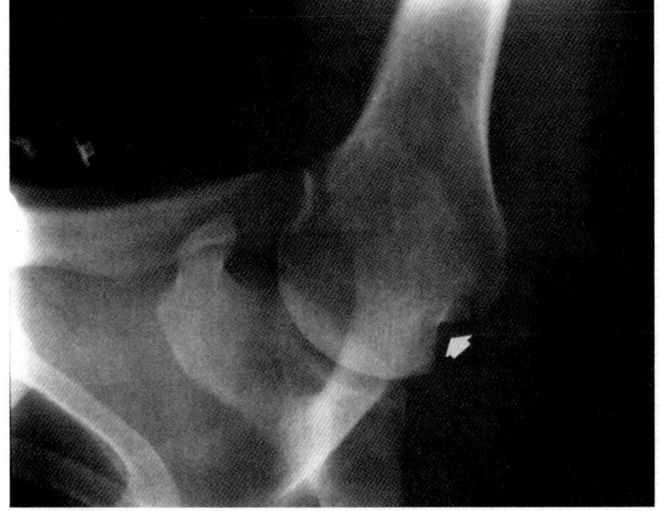


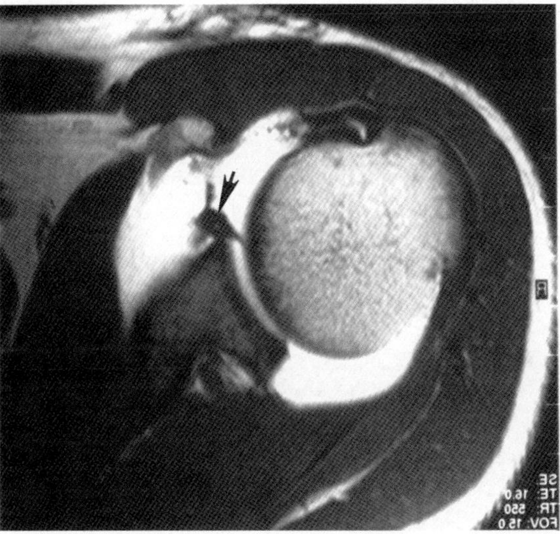


Fig. 2-42 Bankart and Hill-Sachs lesions. A: Illustration of the Bankart lesion, which may involve the labrum or the labrum plus a glenoid margin fracture and the Hill-Sachs lesion which is impaction of the posterolateral humeral head. B: Stryker notch view demonstrating a Hill-Sachs lesion (*arrow*). Axial magnetic resonance (MR) arthrogram demonstrating an enlarged capsule from prior dislocation and an anterior labral tear (*arrow*)—Bankart lesion.

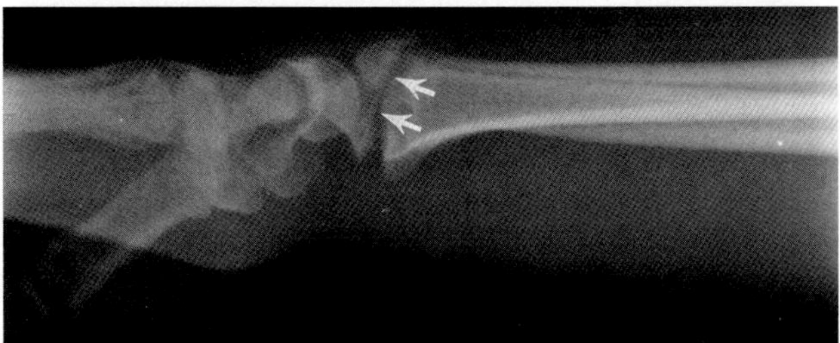

Fig. 2-43 Barton fracture. Lateral radiograph demonstrating a dorsal lip fracture of the distal radius (*arrows*).

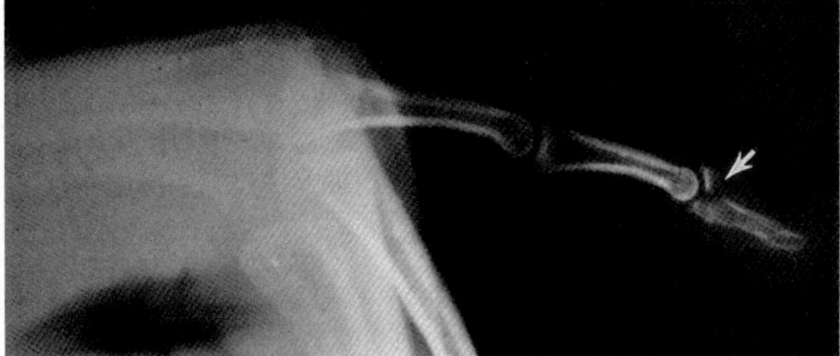

Fig. 2-44 Baseball finger (Mallet). Lateral radiograph of the finger with a dorsal avulsion of the distal phalanx (*arrow*) and flexion deformity of the distal interphalangeal joint.

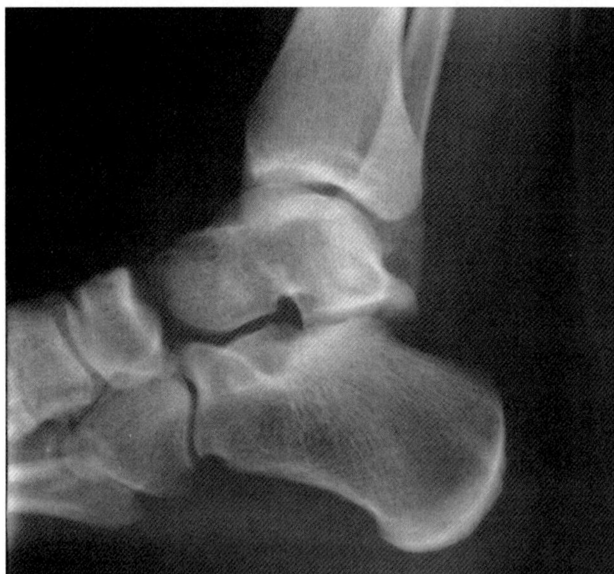

Fig. 2-45 Basketball foot. Lateral radiograph demonstrates subluxation or the subtalar and talonavicular joints. The dislocations have partially reduced.

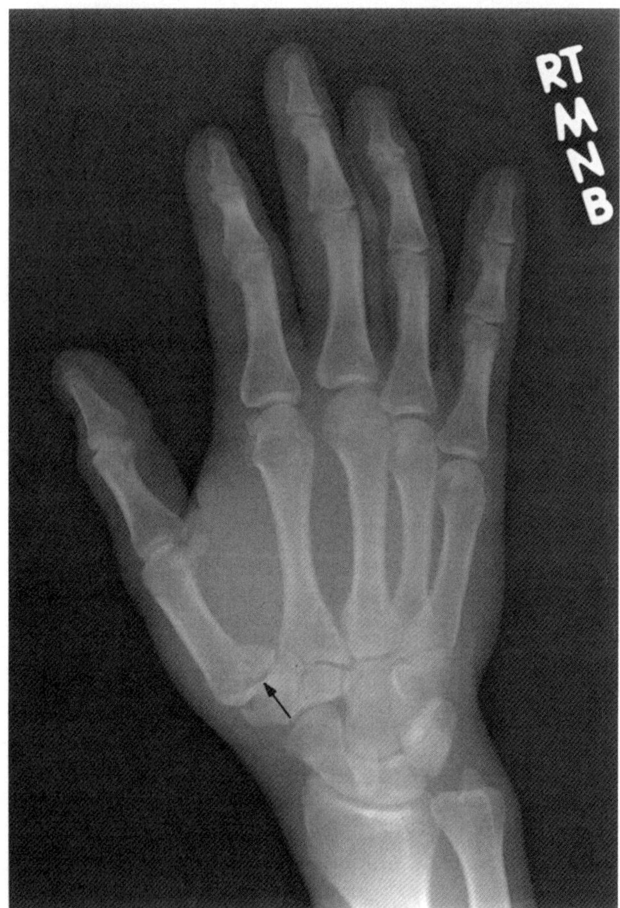


Fig. 2-46 Bennett fracture. Radiograph of the hand demonstrating an oblique intra-articular fracture at the base of the first metacarpal (*arrow*).

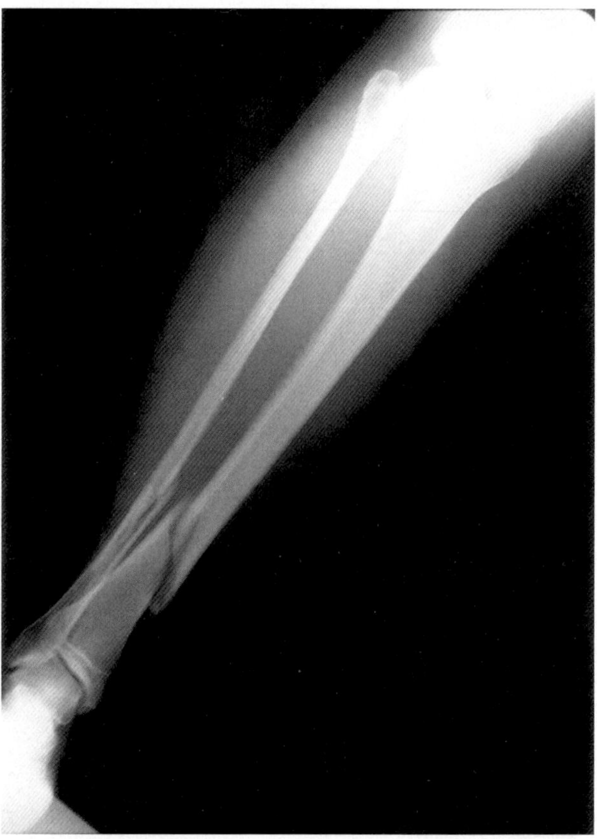

Fig. 2-47 Boot-top fracture. Anteroposterior (AP) radiograph of the leg demonstrating fractures at the junction of the mid and distal thirds of the tibia and fibula.

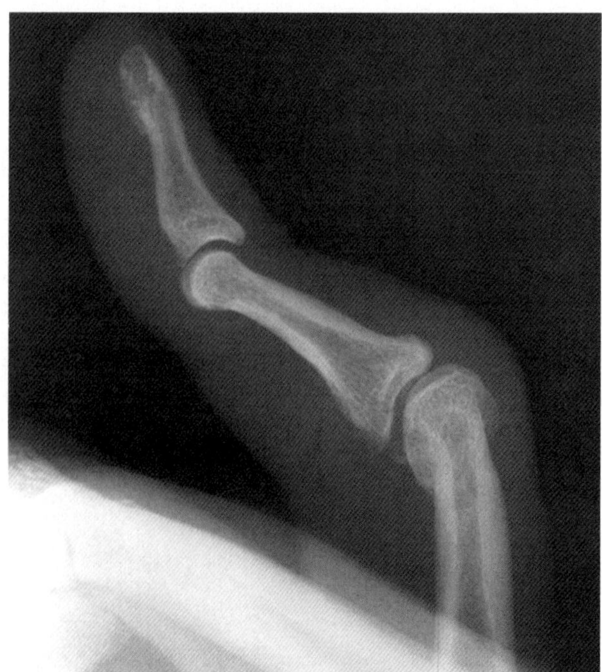

Fig. 2-48 Boutonniere deformity. Lateral radiograph of the finger demonstrating hyperflexion of the proximal interphalangeal joint and hyperextension of the distal interphalangeal joints.

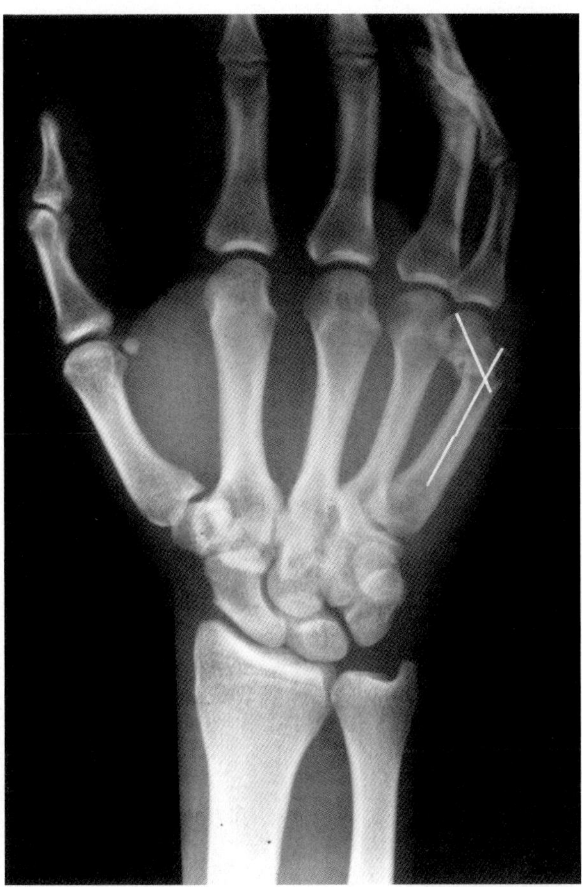

Fig. 2-49 Boxer's fracture. Radiograph demonstrating a dorsally angulated fracture (*lines*) of the distal fifth metacarpal neck.

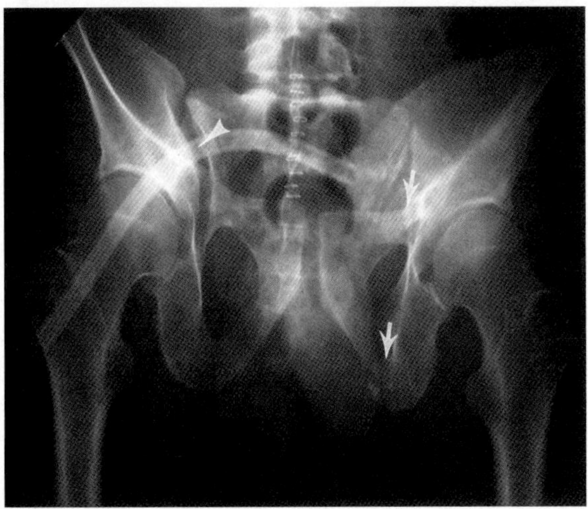

Fig. 2-50 Bucket handle fracture of the pelvis. Radiograph of the pelvis demonstrating pubic rami fractures on the left (*arrows*) and diastasis of the right sacroiliac joint (*arrowhead*).

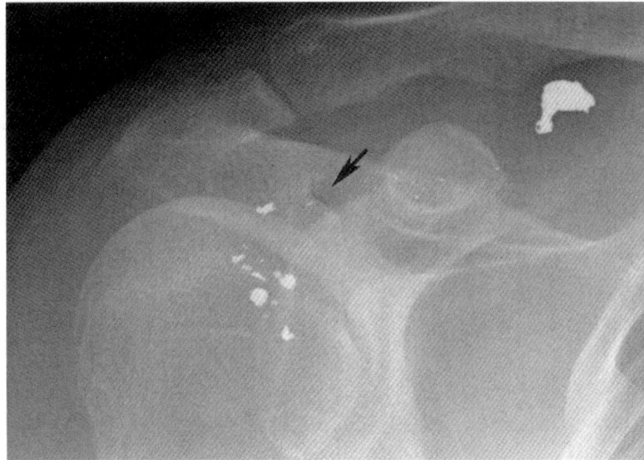

Fig. 2-51 Buttonhole fracture. Shoulder radiograph after a gunshot wound demonstrating the bullet hole in the scapular spine (*arrow*) and residual bullet fragments.

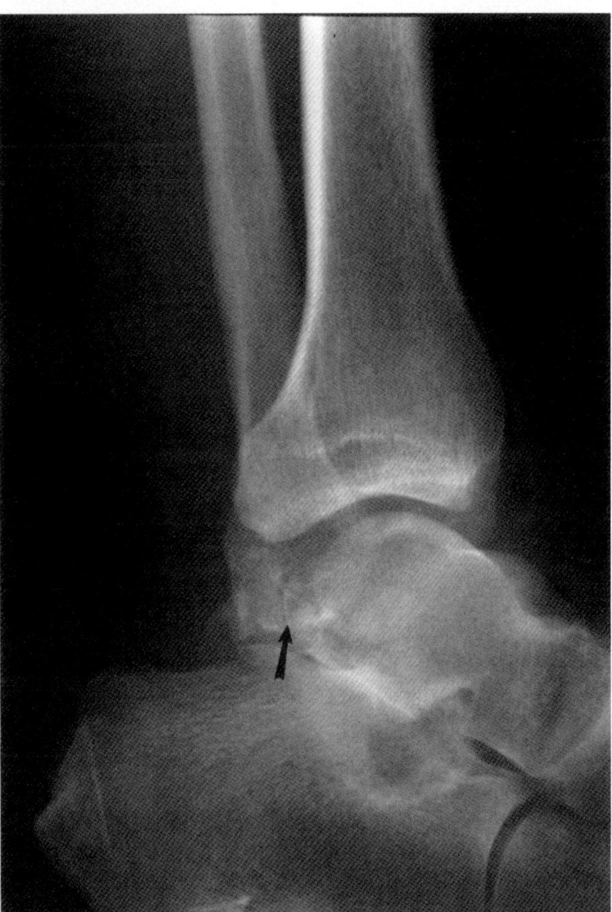

Fig. 2-52 Cedell fracture. Lateral radiograph of the ankle demonstrating a posterior talar process fracture (*arrow*). Note the associated subtalar subluxation.

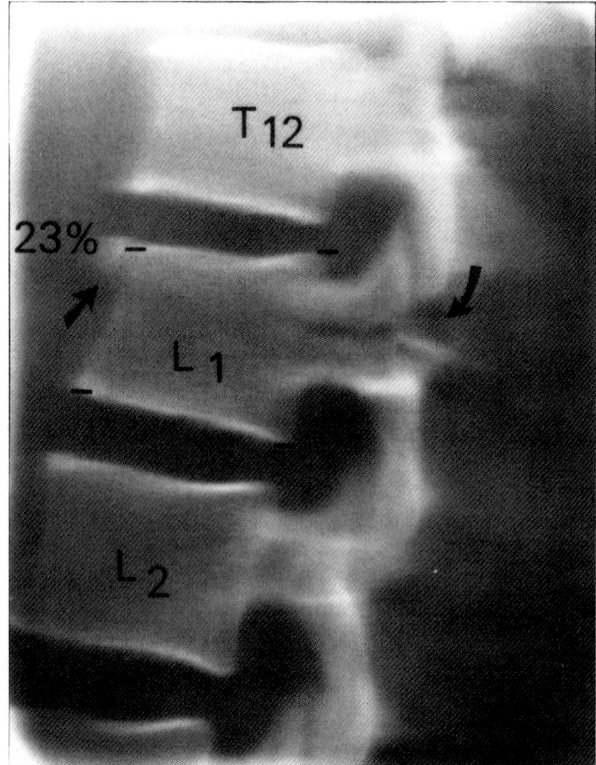


Fig. 2-53 Chance fracture. Lateral radiograph of the spine demonstrating mild compression of L1 (*arrow*) with a fracture line extending through the posterior elements (*curved arrow*).

**Jones:** Fracture of the proximal fifth metatarsal just distal to the tuberosity; now considered zone 2 (see Fig. 2-70)

**Juvenile Tillaux:** Salter-Harris III fracture of the lateral aspect of the distal tibia seen in children aged 12 to 14 years (see Fig. 2-71)

**Kocher:** Intra-articular fracture of the capitellum of the distal humerus (see Fig. 2-72)

**Kohler:** Childhood fracture with avascular necrosis of the tarsal navicular (see Fig. 2-73)

**Laugier:** Fracture of the trochlea of the distal humerus

**Lead pipe:** Long bone fracture with buckling of one cortex (torus fracture) and an incomplete fracture of the opposite cortex

**Le Fort:** Avulsion fracture of the fibular attachment of the anterior distal tibiofibular ligament

**Lisfranc:** Fracture dislocations of the tarsometatarsal joints; derived from surgeon Lisfranc's amputation through this region (see Fig. 2-74)

**Maisonneuve:** Spiral fracture in the proximal fibula associated with disruption of the interosseous membrane and syndesmosis (see Fig. 2-75)

**Malgaigne (humerus):** Hyperextension supracondylar fracture of the distal humerus

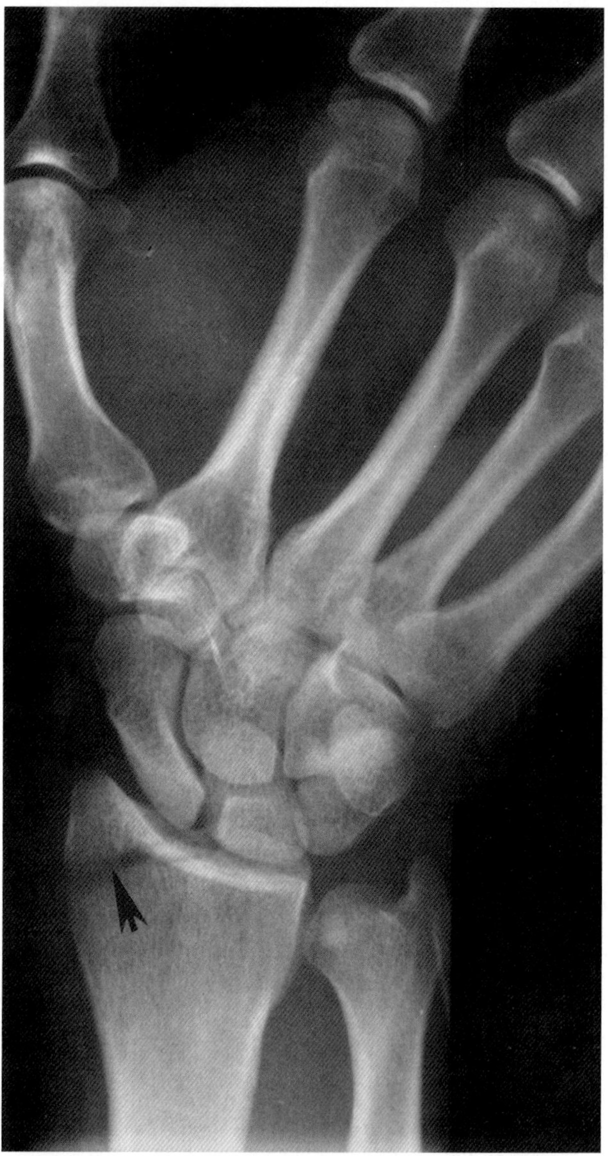

Fig. 2-54 Chauffeur fracture. Radiograph demonstrating a minimally displaced intra-articular fracture of the radial styloid (*arrow*).

**Malgaigne (pelvis):** Unilateral pubic rami fractures with associated iliac or sacral fracture or diastasis of the sacroiliac joint due to vertical shearing injury (see Fig. 2-76)

**Mallet:** Fracture of the dorsal aspect of the distal phalanx or extensor avulsion; same as baseball finger (Fig. 2-44)

**March:** Metatarsal stress fracture seen in military recruits (see Fig. 2-77 and also Fig. 2-9)

**Microfracture:** Bowing, usually the radius and ulna; fracture line may not be evident on radiographs (see Fig. 2-78)

**Midnight:** Oblique fracture of the proximal phalanx of the fifth toe, may be open

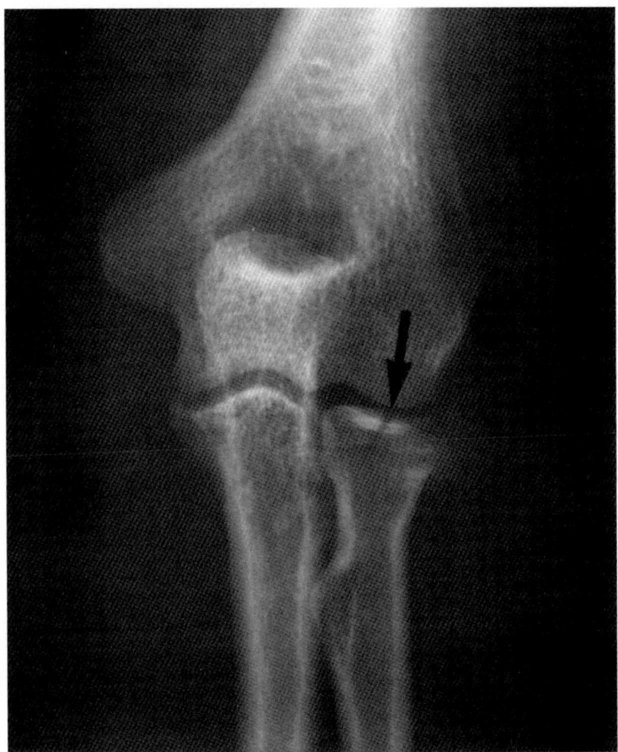

Fig. 2-55 Chisel fracture. Radiograph demonstrates an intra-articular fracture of the radial head with extension distally approximating 1 cm.

**Monteggia:** Fracture of the proximal third of the ulna with radial head dislocation (see Fig. 2-79)

**Montercaux:** Fracture of the fibular neck with associated diastasis of the distal tibia and fibula

**Nightstick:** Isolated ulnar fracture due to direct blow (see Fig. 2-80)

**Nursemaid elbow:** Dislocation of the radial head in a toddler caused by lifting the child by the hands or wrists; typically reduced during radiographic positioning so radiographs are frequently unremarkable

**Parachute knee:** Anterior dislocation of the fibular head due to landing (see Fig. 2-81)

**Piedmont:** Oblique fracture of the distal radius with distal fragments pulled into the ulna; requires surgical reduction; described at Piedmont Orthopaedic Society

**Pilon:** Comminuted intra-articular fracture of the distal tibia (see Fig. 2-82)

**Pitcher's elbow:** Avulsion of the medial epicondyle in skeletally immature pitchers (see Fig. 2-83)

**Plafond:** Articular surface fracture of the distal tibia (see Fig. 2-84)

**Posada:** Transcondylar fracture of the distal humerus with anterior displacement of the distal fragment and posterior dislocation of the radius and ulna

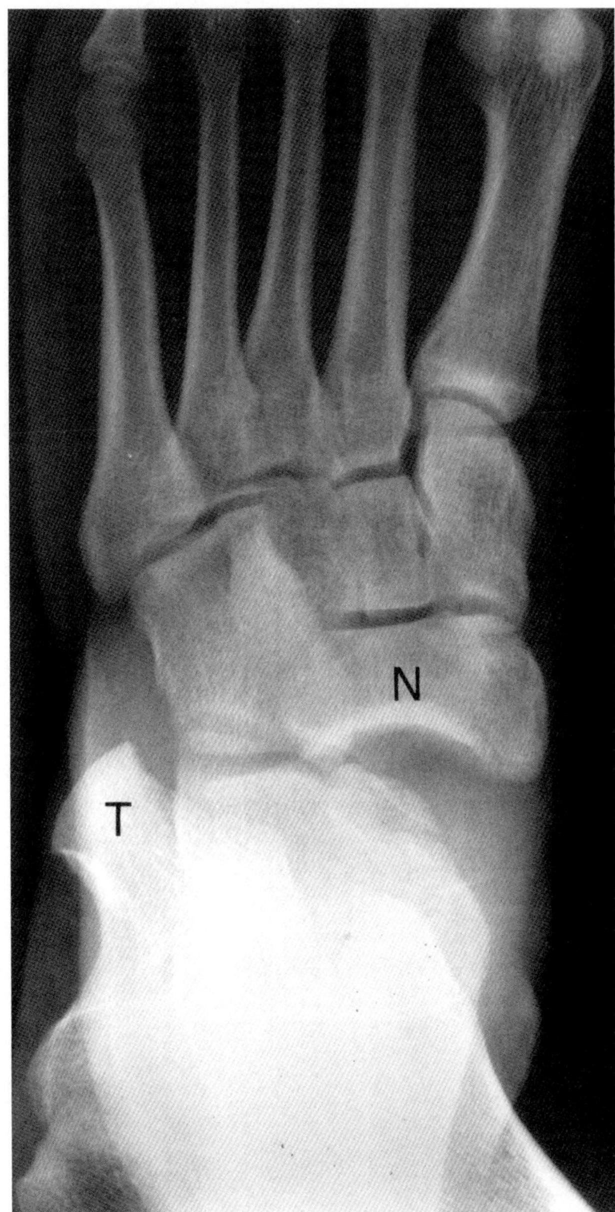


Fig. 2-56 Chopart fracture/dislocation. Radiograph demonstrating a fracture dislocation of the talonavicular joint (*T*-talus, *N*-navicular). The calcaneocuboid joint is not clearly demonstrated.

**Rolando:** Comminutes "Y" or "T" shaped fracture of the base of the first metacarpal (see Fig. 2-85)

**Segond:** Avulsion fracture of the lateral tibial condyle at the lateral capsular ligament attachment; usually associated with anterior cruciate ligament tears (see Fig. 2-86)

**Shepherd:** Fracture of the lateral tubercle of the posterior talar process; may simulate an os trigonum (see Fig. 2-87)

**Sideswipe:** Comminuted fracture of the distal humerus due to direct blow; may involve the radius and ulna

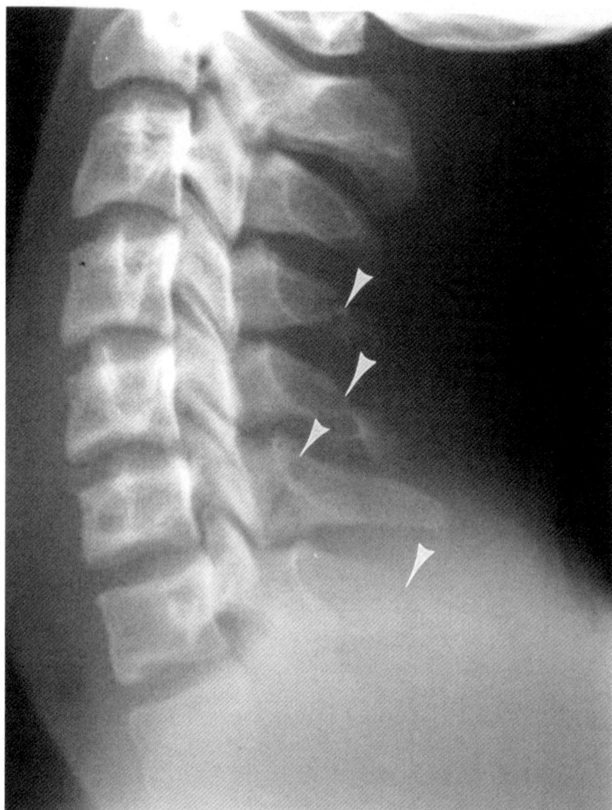

Fig. 2-57 Clay shoveler's fracture. Lateral radiograph demonstrating spinous process fractures from C4-7 (*arrowheads*).

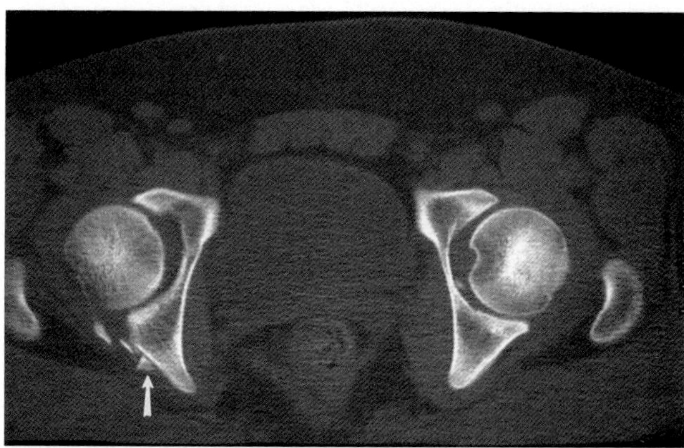

Fig. 2-59 Dashboard fracture. Axial computed tomographic (CT) image demonstrating a posterior acetabular rim fracture (*arrow*).

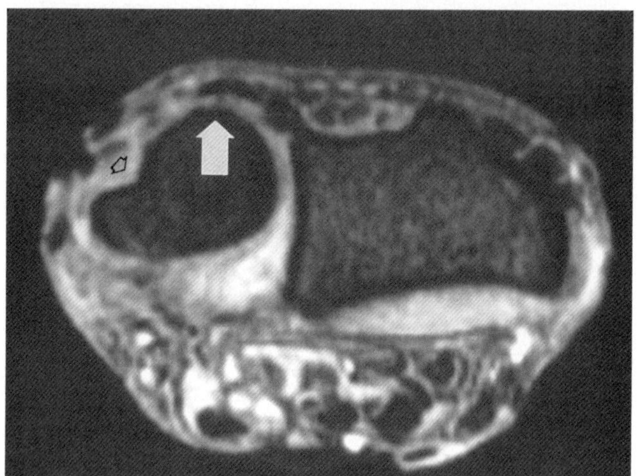

Fig. 2-60 Desault. Axial fast spin-echo T2-weighted magnetic resonance (MR) image demonstrating dorsal subluxation of the ulna (*large white arrow*) and dislocation of the extensor carpi ulnaris tendon (*open arrow*).

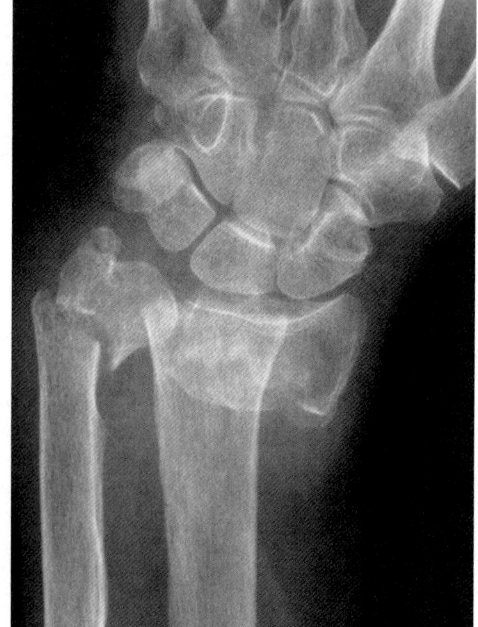

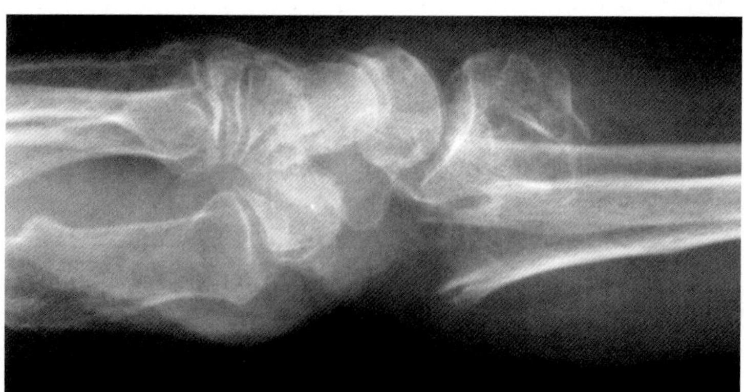



Fig. 2-58 Colles fracture. Posteroanterior (PA) (A) and lateral (B) radiographs demonstrate fractures of the distal radius and ulna with dorsal displacement of the distal fragments.

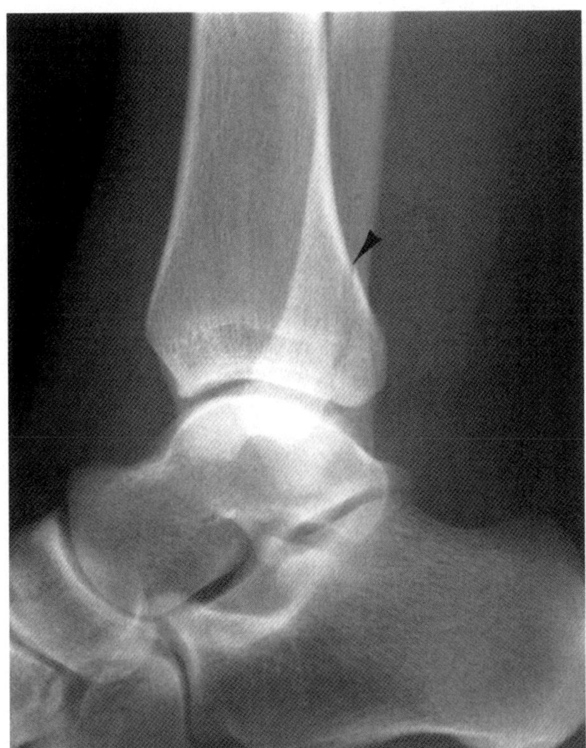

Fig. 2-61 Descot fracture. Lateral radiograph demonstrates a posterior tibial fracture (*arrowhead*).

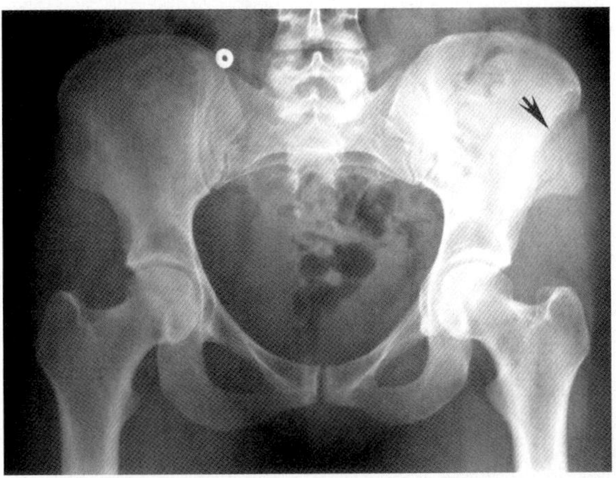

Fig. 2-62 Duverney fracture. Anteroposterior (AP) radiograph of the pelvis demonstrating an isolated iliac wing fracture (*arrow*).

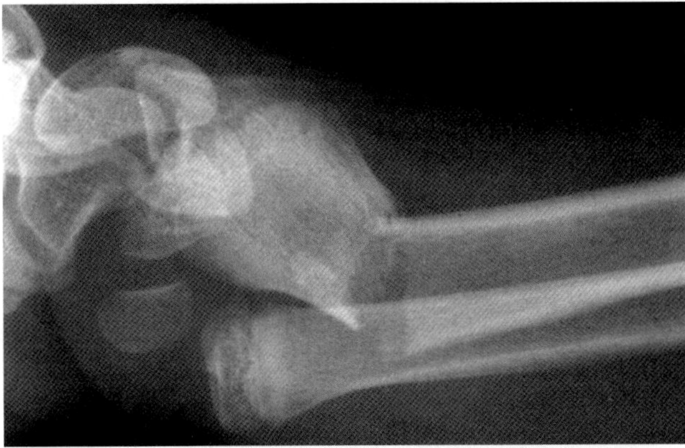

Fig. 2-63 Galeazzi fracture. Lateral radiograph demonstrates a distal radial fracture with dislocation of the distal radioulnar joint.

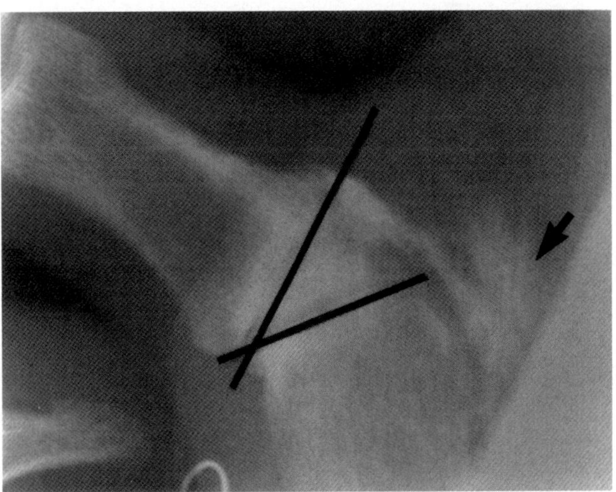

Fig. 2-64 Gamekeeper thumb (ski pole thumb). Stress arthrogram shows opening of the ulnar side of the joint (*lines*) with contrast extravasation outside the joint (*arrow*) due to an ulnar collateral ligament tear.

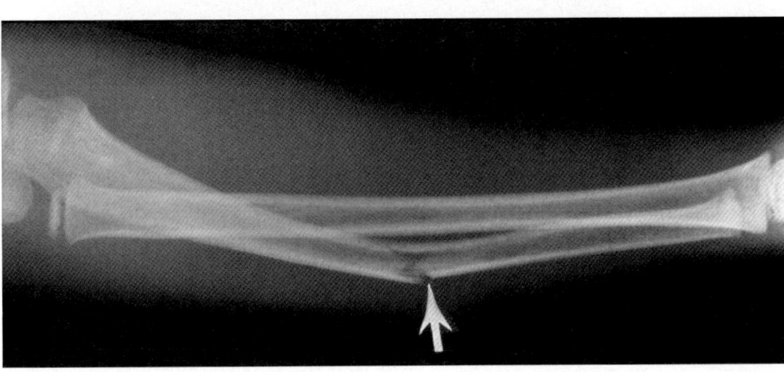

Fig. 2-65 Greenstick fracture. Radiograph of the forearm demonstrating an incomplete fracture of the mid-ulna (*arrow*).

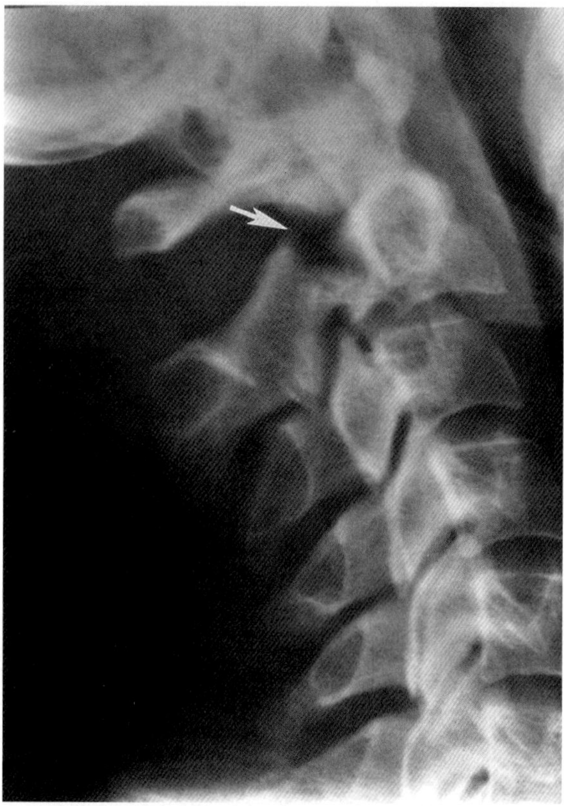

Fig. 2-66 Hangman's (hanged man's) fracture. Lateral radiograph of the cervical spine demonstrating a displaced C2 neural arch fracture (*arrow*) with subluxation of C2 on C3.

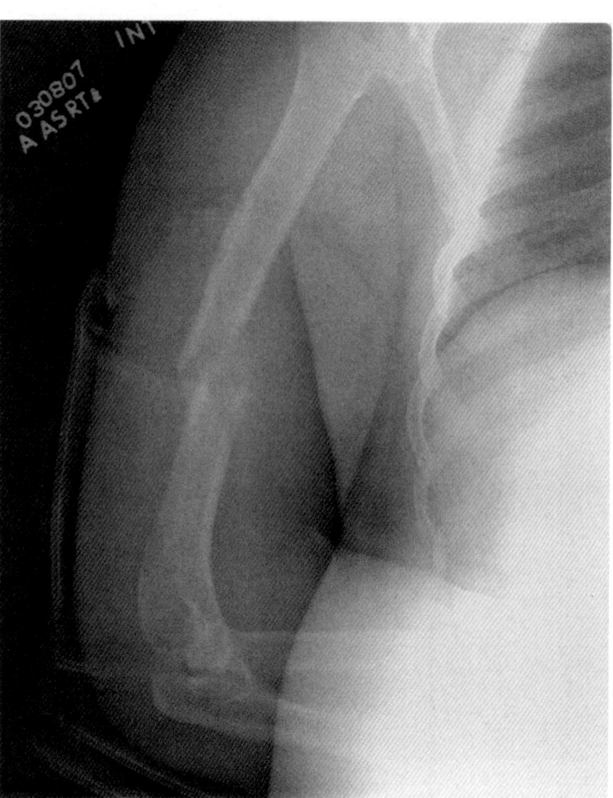


Fig. 2-68 Holstein-Lewis fracture. Radiograph demonstrating a fracture of the humerus at the junction of the mid and distal thirds with radial nerve injury.

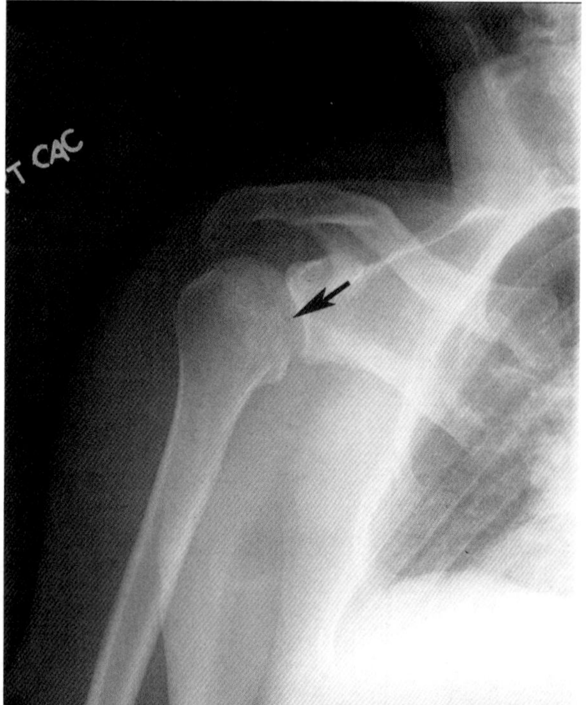


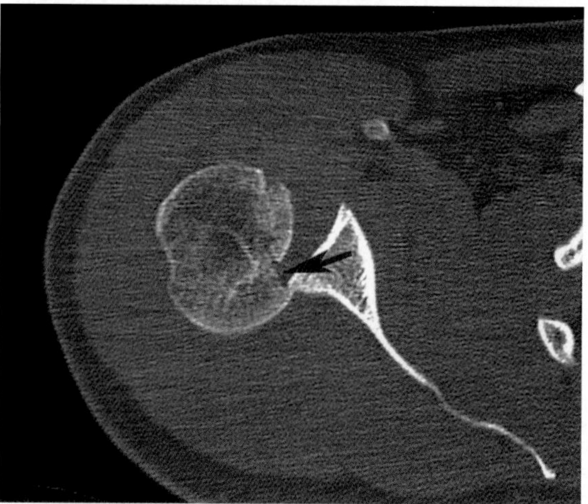


Fig. 2-67 Hill-Sachs reverse. Radiograph (A) and computed tomographic (CT) (B) images of a posterior dislocation with an impaction fracture of the anteromedial humeral head (*arrows*).

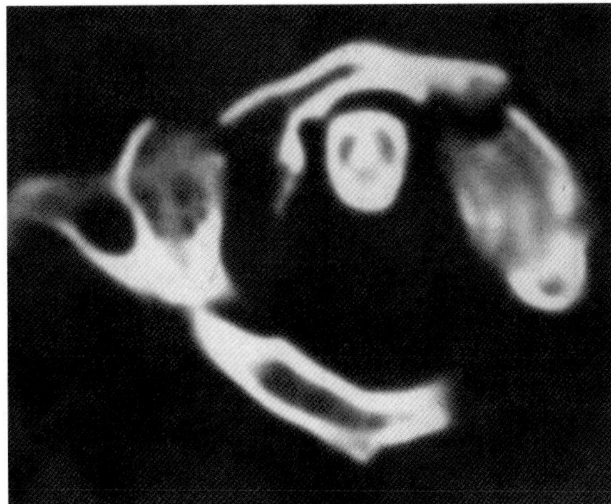

Fig. 2-69 Jefferson fracture. Axial computed tomographic (CT) image demonstrating multiple breaks in the ring of C1.

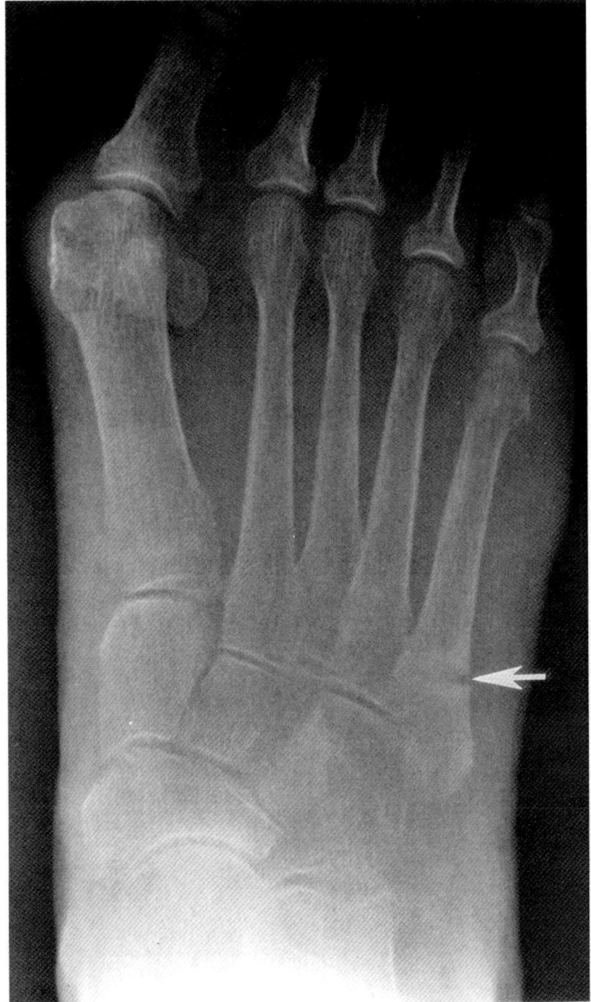

Fig. 2-70 Jones fracture. Frontal radiograph demonstrates a fracture of the proximal fifth metatarsal (*arrow*) with sclerosis developing along the fracture due to delayed union.

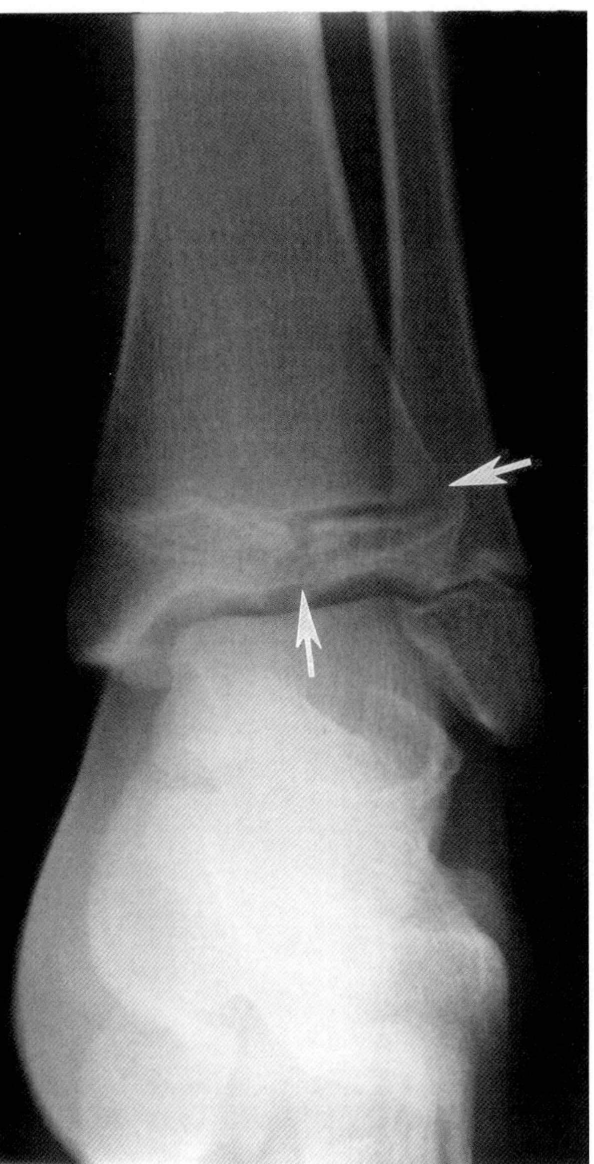

Fig. 2-71 Juvenile Tillaux fracture. Anteroposterior (AP) radiograph of the ankle demonstrating a Salter-Harris III fracture involving the lateral tibia (*arrows*).

**Smith:** Fracture of the distal radius which may be intra-articular and displaces volarly; opposite the displacement of a Colles fracture (see Fig. 2-88)

**Sprinter:** Avulsion fracture of the anterior superior or anterior inferior iliac spine due to sprinting (see Fig. 2-89)

**Stieda:** Avulsion of the medial femoral condyle at the site of medial collateral ligament attachment; may ossify later leading to Pellegrini-Stieda disease (see Fig. 2-90)

**Straddle:** Bilateral superior and inferior pubic rami fractures (see Fig. 2-91)

**Teardrop:** Comminuted vertebral fracture with anteriorly displaced fragment (see Fig. 2-92)

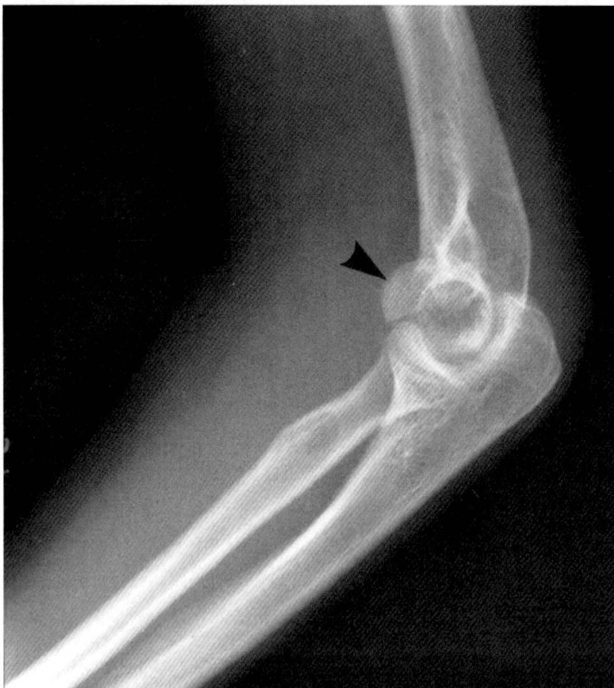

Fig. 2-72 Kocher fracture. Lateral radiograph demonstrating an intra-articular fracture of the capitellum (*arrowhead*) with anterior displacement.

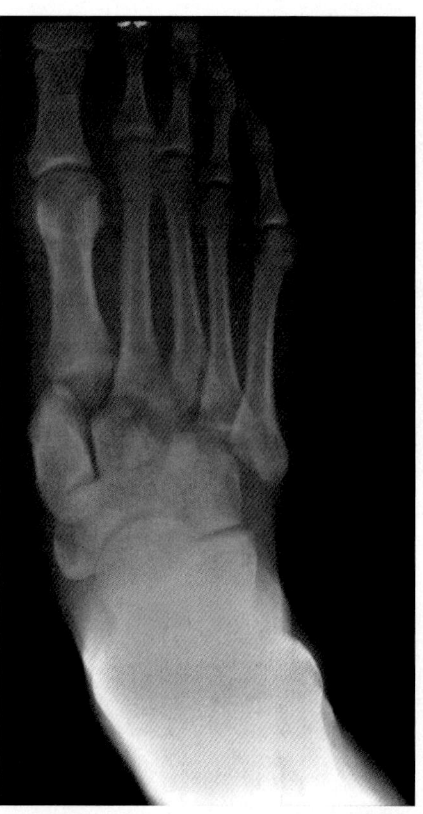

Fig. 2-74 Lisfranc fracture dislocation. Frontal radiograph of the foot demonstrating lateral displacement of all metatarsals in relation to the tarsal bones.

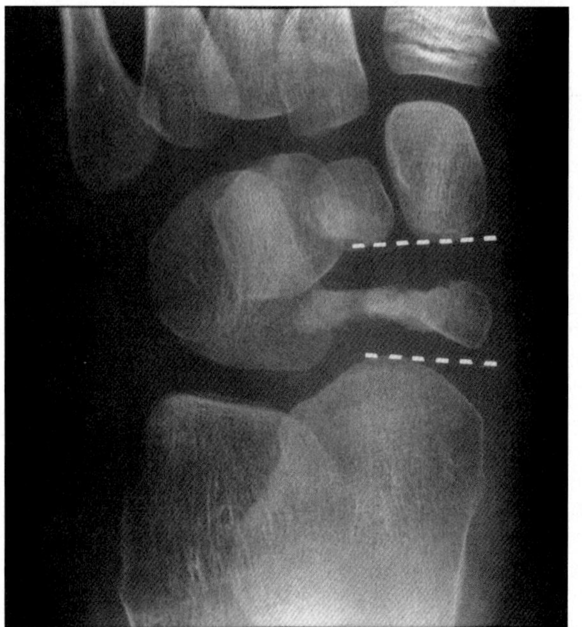


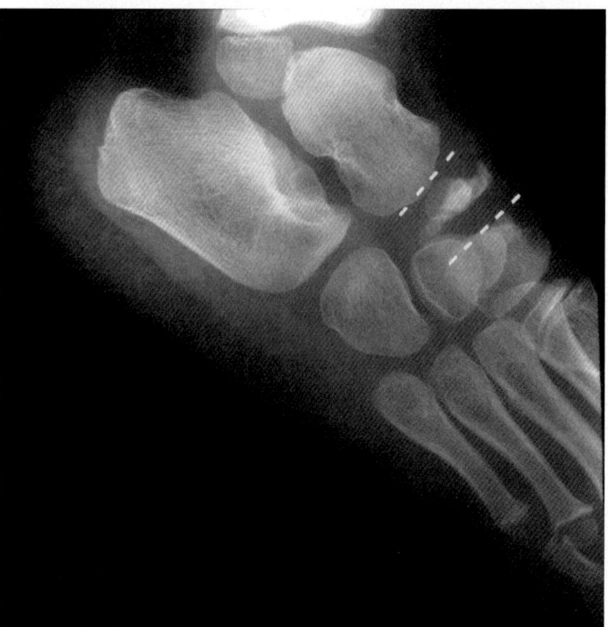


Fig. 2-73 Kohler. Frontal (A) and lateral (B) radiographs in a child with avascular necrosis and marked flattening of the navicular. Normal space marked with broken lines.

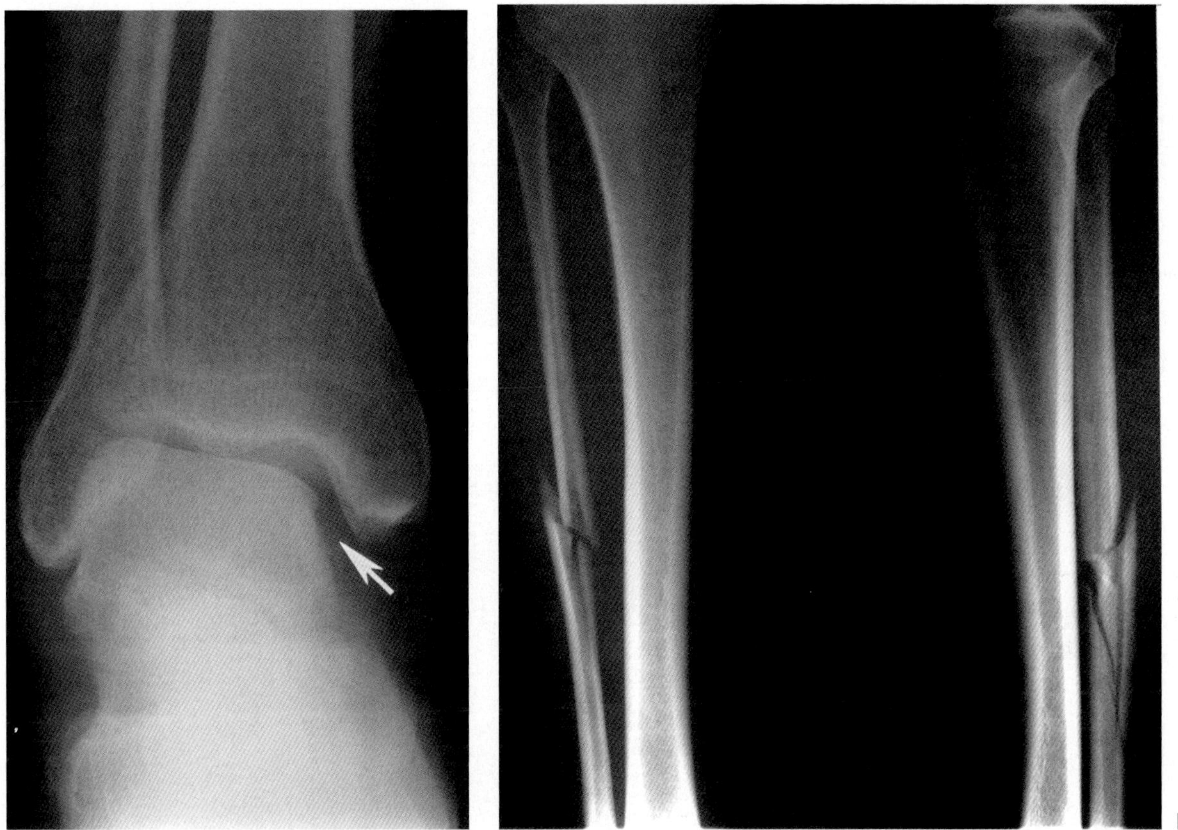


Fig. 2-75 Maisonneuve fracture. Anteroposterior (AP) radiograph of the ankle (**A**) demonstrates widening of the medial mortise (*arrow*) due to ligament tear. The high fibular fracture is demonstrated on radiographs (**B**) of the leg.

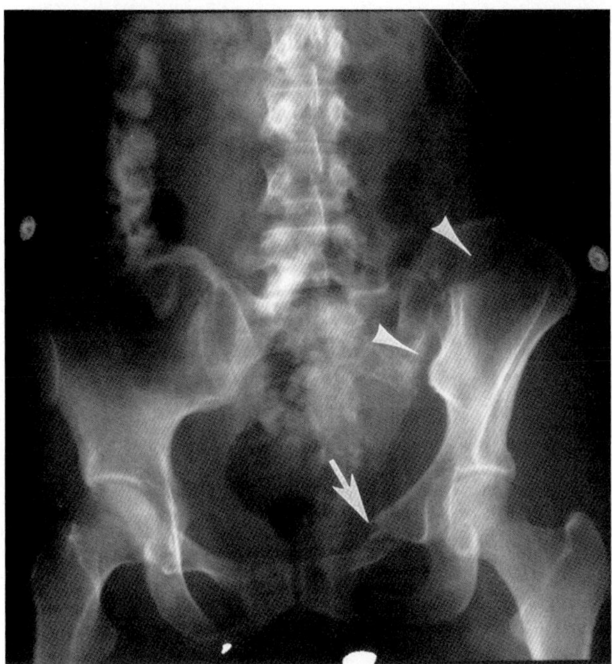

Fig. 2-76 Malgaigne (pelvis) fracture. Anteroposterior (AP) radiograph of the pelvis with pubic rami fractures on the left (*arrow*), diastasis of the sacroiliac joint, and an iliac fracture on the left (*arrowheads*).

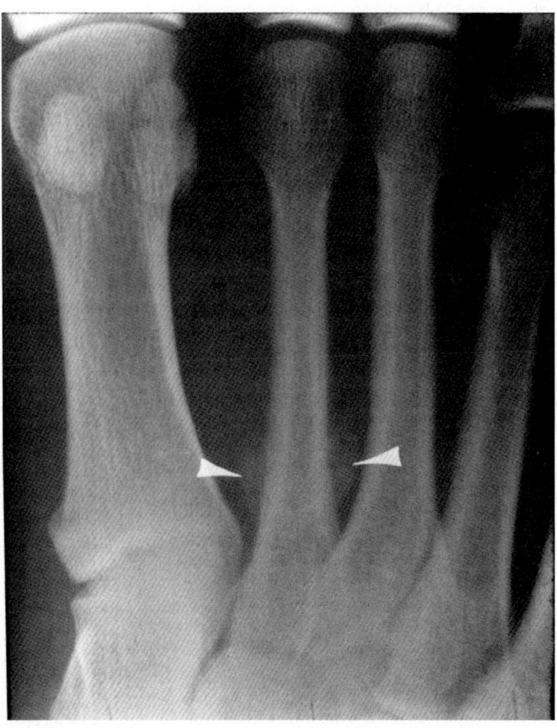

Fig. 2-77 March fracture. Radiograph of the foot demonstrating a healing stress fracture (*arrowheads*) of the second metatarsal.

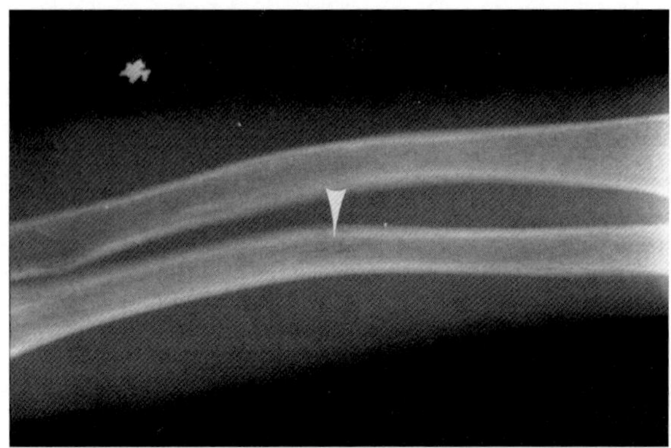

Fig. 2-78 Microfracture. Radiograph of the forearm demonstrating bowing deformities with a subtle fracture (*arrowhead*).

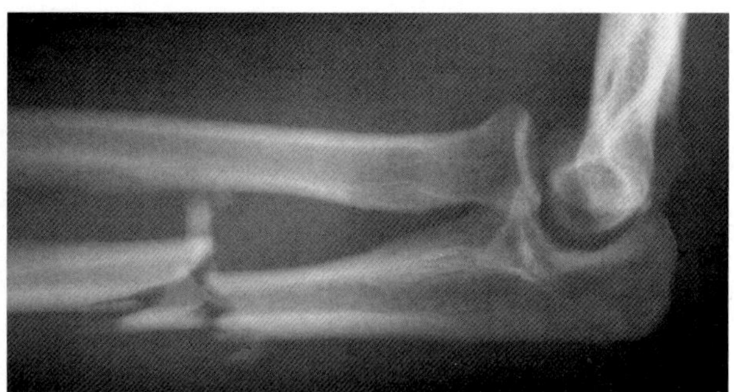

Fig. 2-79 Monteggia fracture. Lateral radiograph demonstrating a proximal ulnar fracture with dislocation of the radial head.

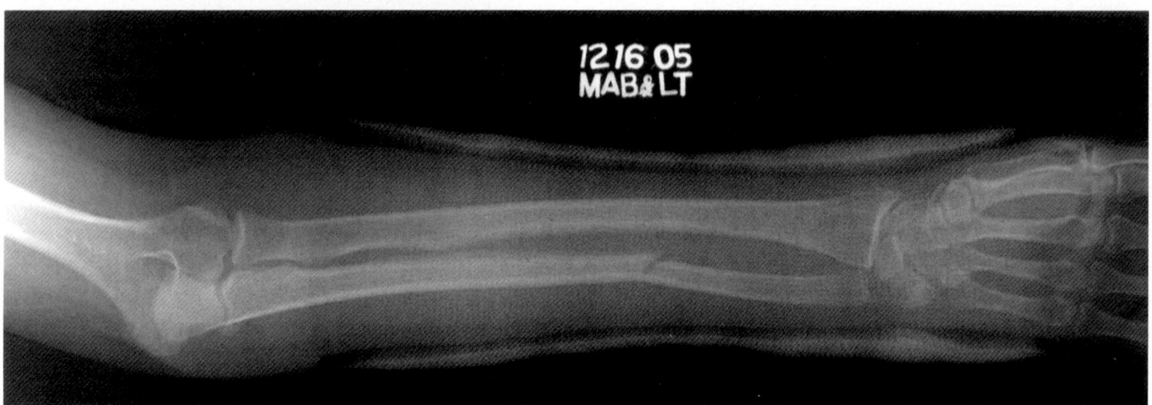


Fig. 2-80 Nightstick fracture. Radiograph of the forearm demonstrating an isolated ulnar fracture. Immobilization with a short arm cast.

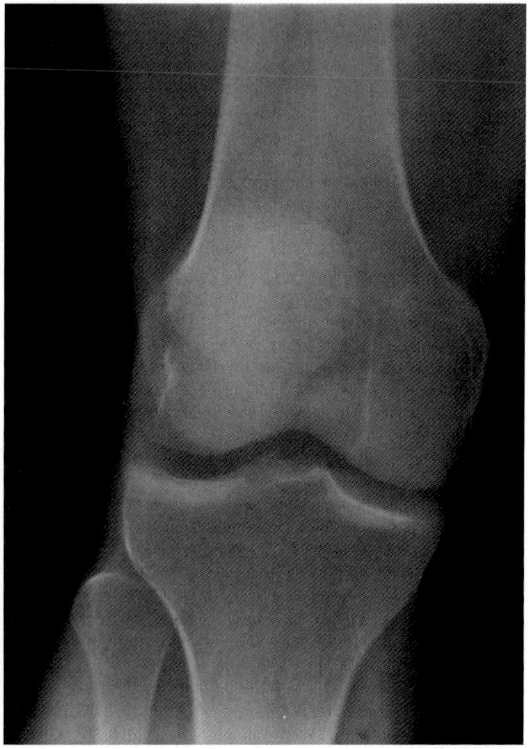


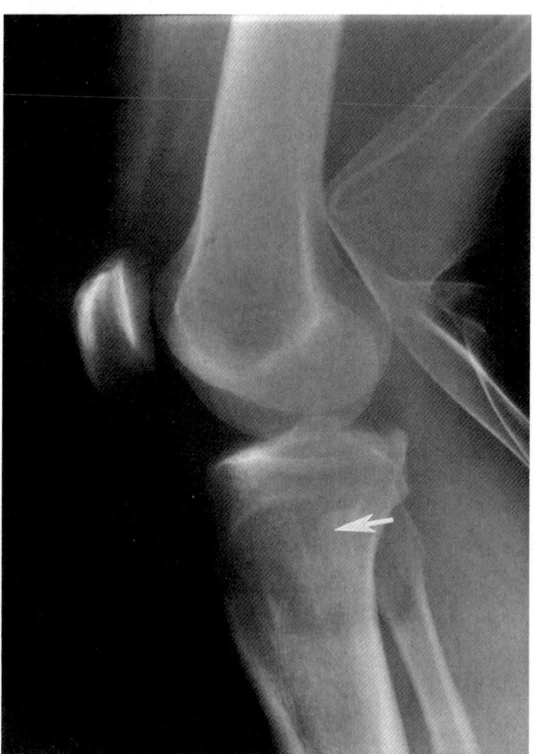


Fig. 2-81 Parachute knee. Anteroposterior (AP) (A) and lateral (B) radiographs of the knee. The fibular head is dislocated anteriorly (*arrow*) on the lateral view.

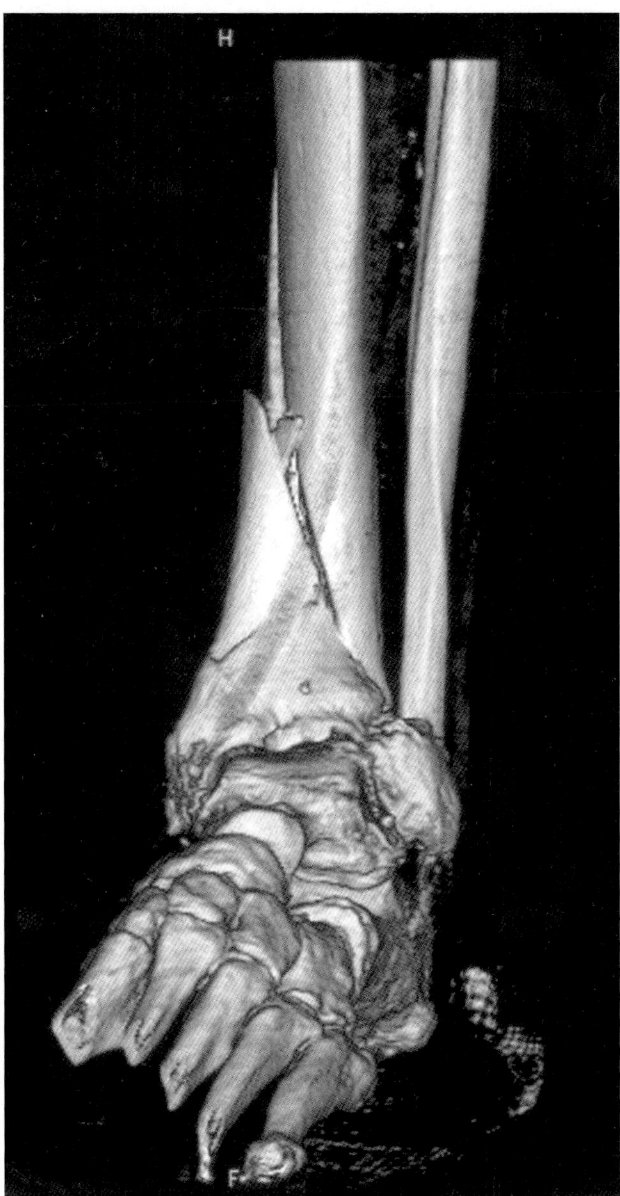


**Fig. 2-82** Pilon fracture. Three-dimensional computed tomographic (CT) image of a complex distal tibial fracture extending with complex articular involvement.

**Toddler:** Undisplaced tibial fracture in a toddler; usually spiral (see Fig. 2-93)

**Tongue:** Horizontal fracture of the posterior superior calcaneus (see Fig. 2-94)

**Triplane:** Adolescent ankle fracture involving the physes with three fragments—tibial shaft, anterolateral epiphysis, and remaining epiphysis with the posterior metaphyseal fragment (see Fig. 2-95)

**Unciform:** Hook of the hamate fracture; due to direct blow

**Wagon wheel:** Traumatic separation of the distal femoral epiphysis (see Fig. 2-96)

**Wagstaff-Le Fort:** Avulsion fracture of the distal fibula at the site of anterior tibiofibular ligament attachment

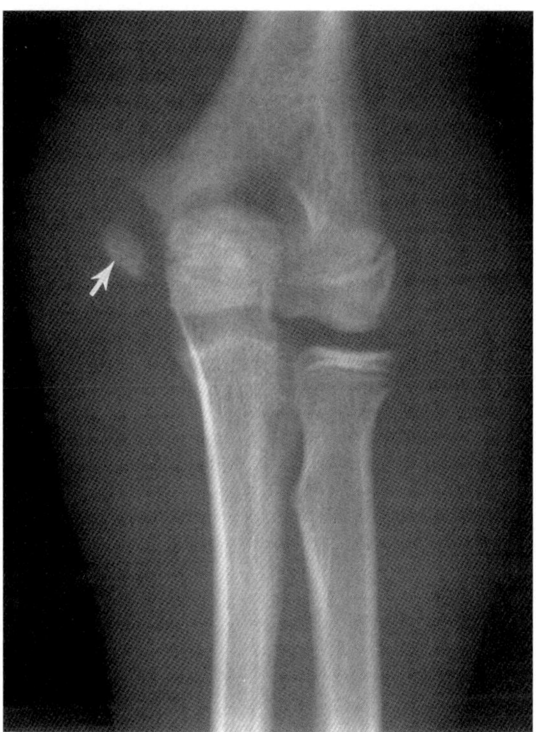

**Fig. 2-83** Pitcher's elbow. Anteroposterior (AP) radiograph of the elbow with avulsion of the medial epicondyle (*arrow*).

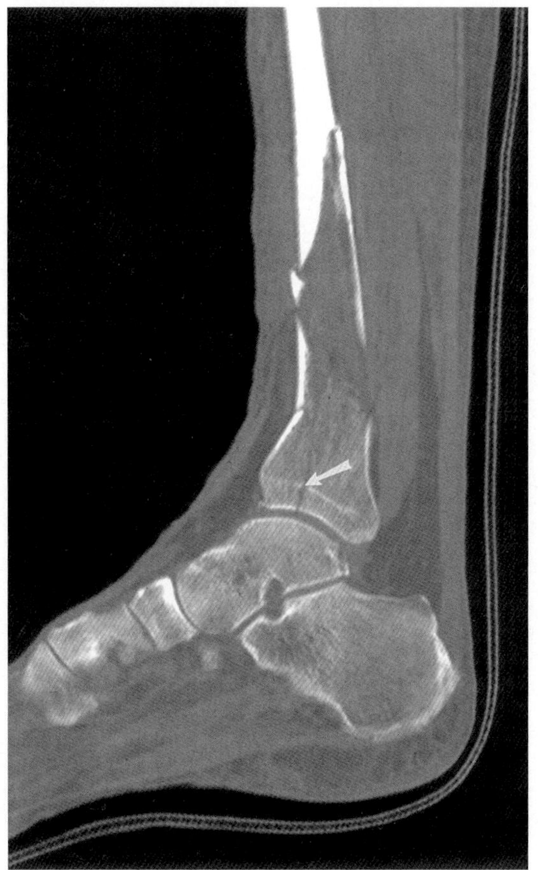

**Fig. 2-84** Plafond fracture. Sagittal computed tomographic (CT) image demonstrating a distal tibial fracture that enters the tibial plafond (*arrow*).

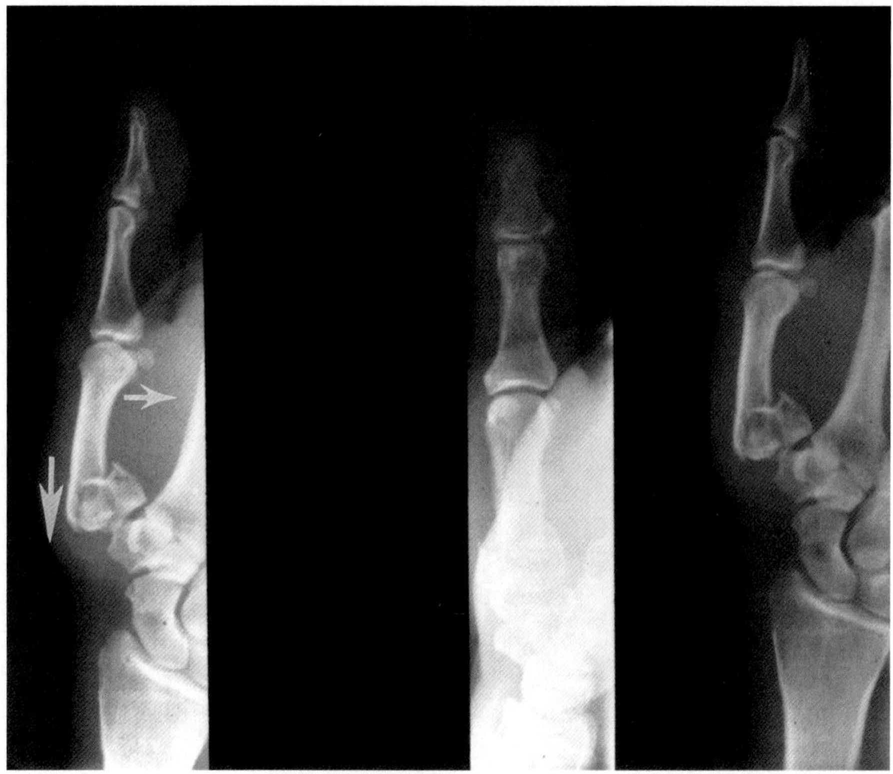

Fig. 2-85 Rolondo fracture. Radiographs of the thumb demonstrate a "Y" shaped intra-articular fracture with displacement (*arrows*) due to ligaments holding the medial fragment and muscle forces.

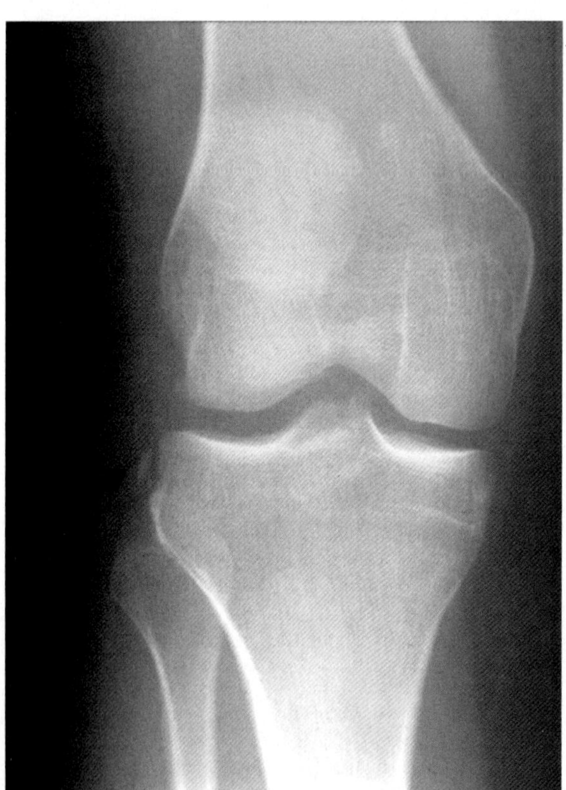

Fig. 2-86 Segond fracture. Anteroposterior (AP) radiograph demonstrates a small flake fracture (*arrow*) from the proximal lateral tibia.

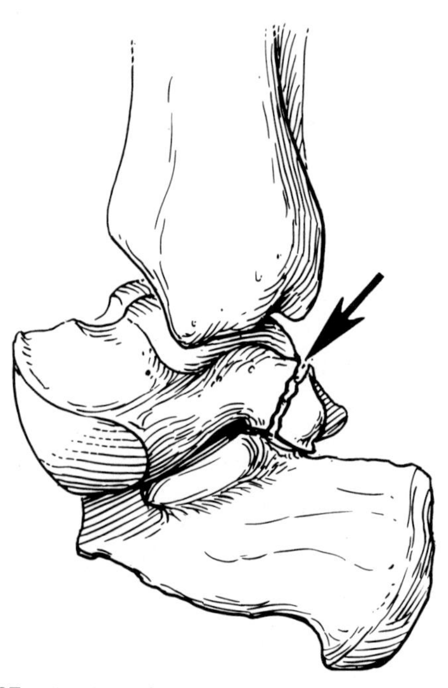

Fig. 2-87 Shepherd fracture. Illustration demonstrating a fracture (*arrow*) of the posterior lateral talar process.

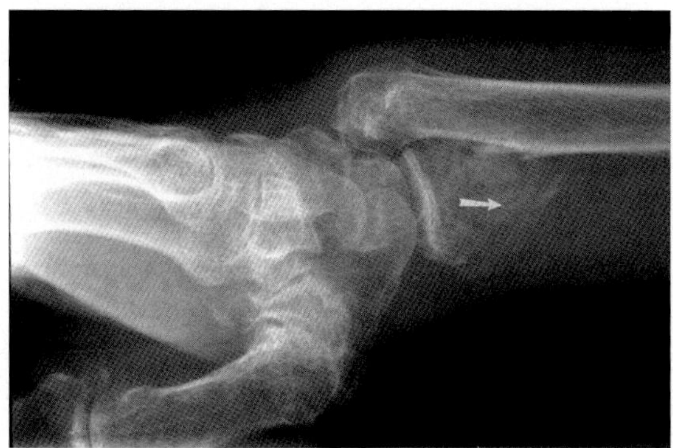

Fig. 2-88 Smith fracture. Lateral radiograph demonstrating a distal radial fracture with volar and proximal (*arrow*) displacement.

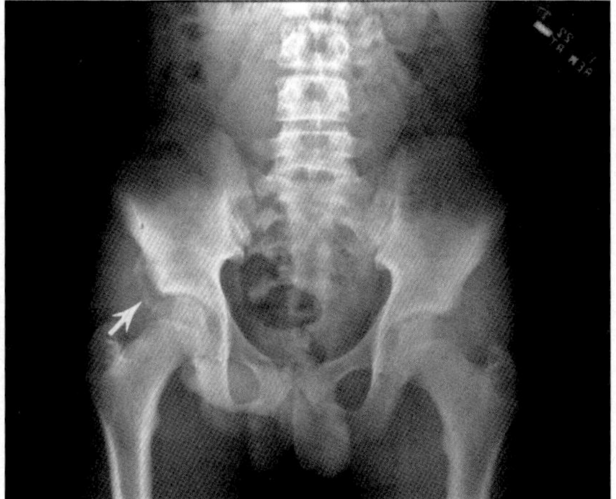

Fig. 2-89 Sprinter's fracture. Radiograph of the pelvis showing an avulsion of the anterior inferior iliac spine (*arrow*).

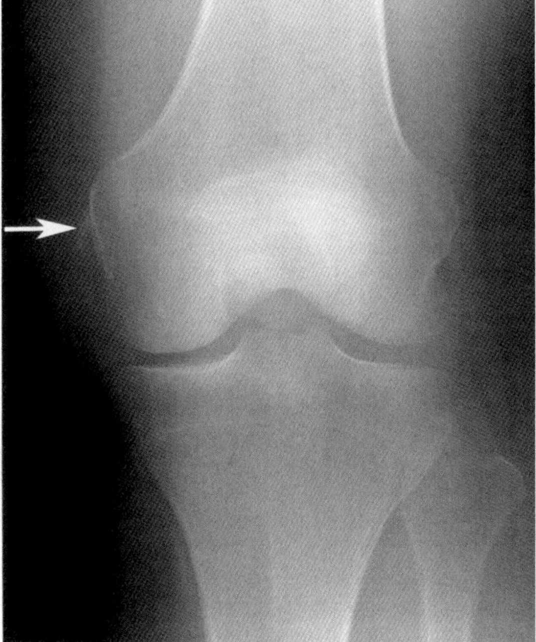

Fig. 2-90 Steida (Pelligrini-Steida). Anteroposterior (AP) radiograph of the knee demonstrating heterotopic ossification at the origin of the medial collateral ligament.

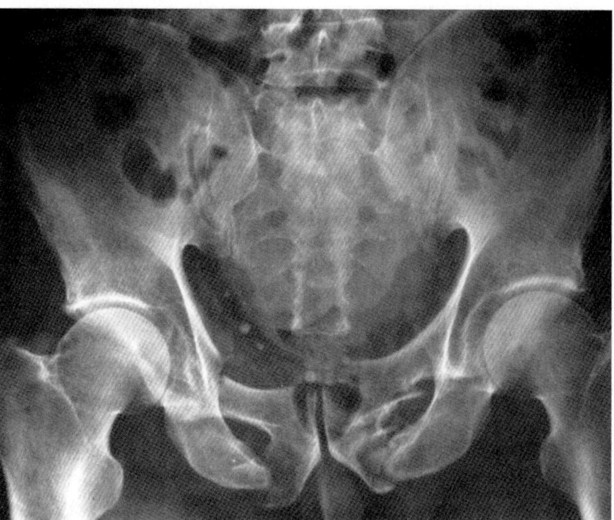

Fig. 2-91 Straddle fracture. Radiograph demonstrating displaced pubic rami fractures bilaterally.

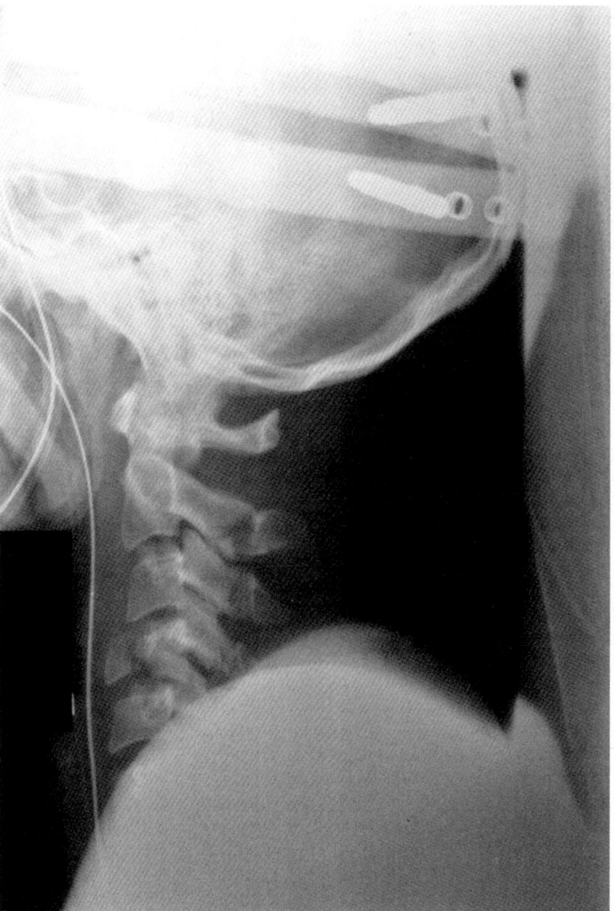

Fig. 2-92 Teardrop fracture. Lateral radiograph of the cervical spine taken in halo support shows an anteriorly displaced fragment in C4.

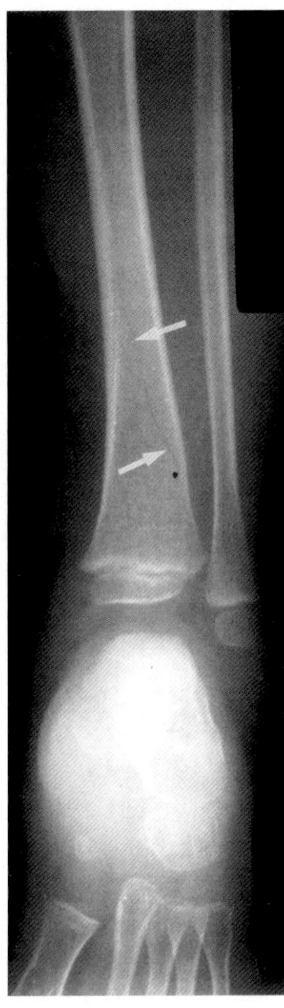

Fig. 2-93 Toddler fracture. Subtle spiral fracture (*arrows*) of the tibia.

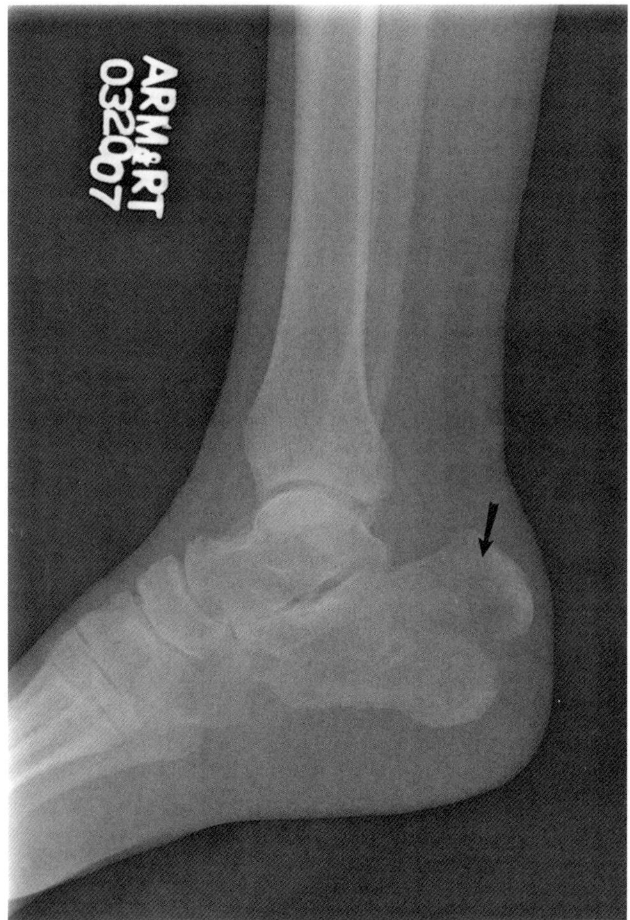


Fig. 2-94 Tongue fracture. Lateral radiograph shows a displaced fracture of the posterior superior calcaneus (*arrow*).

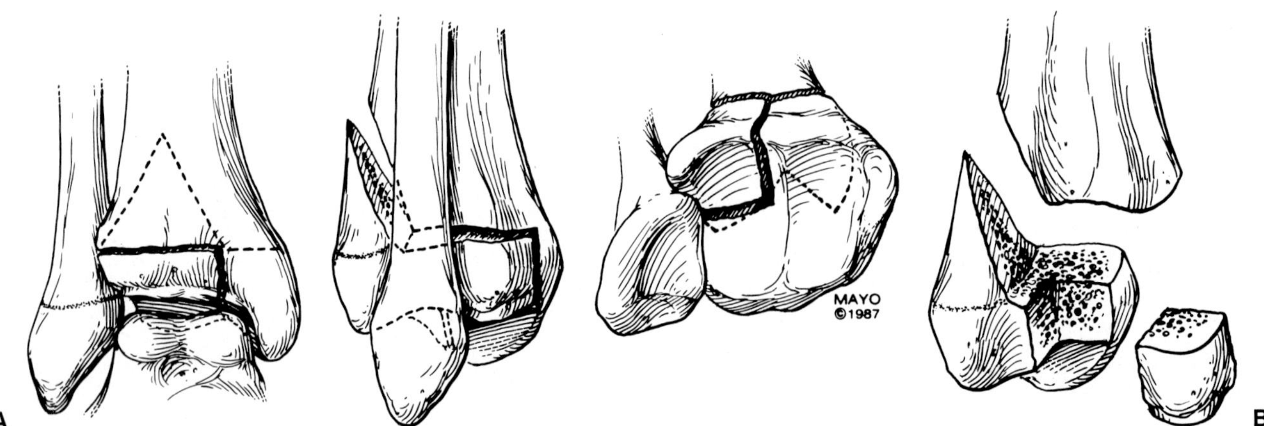


Fig. 2-95 Triplane fracture. Illustrations in the frontal and lateral planes (A) and from below with fragments separated (B) demonstrating physeal fractures resulting in three fragments.

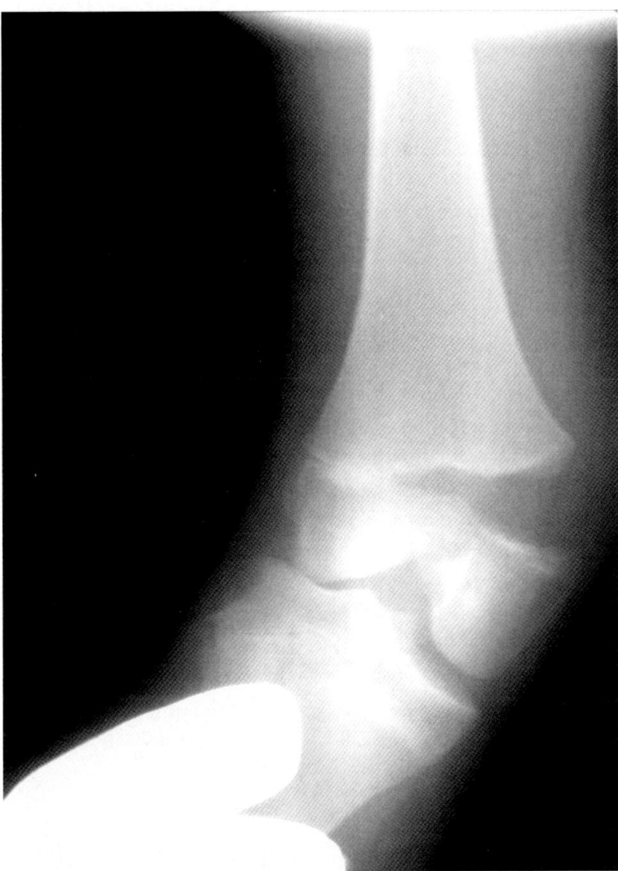

Fig. 2-96 Wagon wheel fracture. Stress image of the knee showing separation of the distal femoral epiphysis.

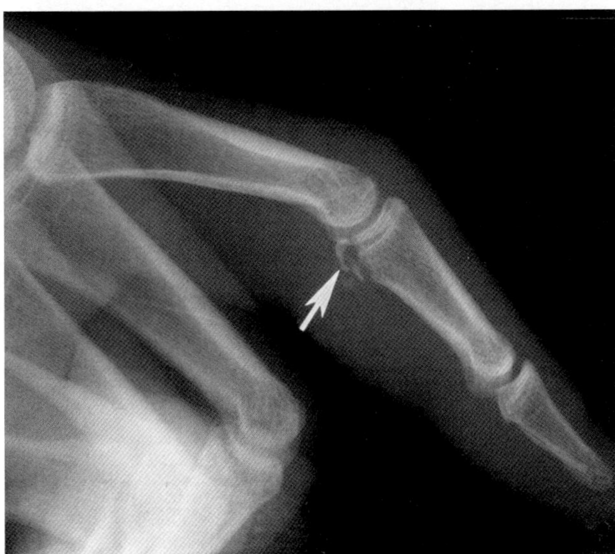

Fig. 2-97 Wilson fracture. Lateral radiograph shows avulsion of the volar plate of the middle phalanx (*arrow*) due to hyperextension injury.

**Walther:** Transverse fracture of the ilioacetabular region involving the acetabulum and ischial spine

**Wilson:** Fracture of the volar plate of the middle phalanx of the finger; hyperextension injury (see Fig. 2-97)

## Suggested Reading


Berquist TH. *Imaging of orthopaedic trauma*, 2nd ed. New York: Raven Press; 1992:39–81, 881–894.

Blauvelt CT, Nelson FRT. *A manual of orthopaedic terminology*, 6th ed. St. Louis: Mosby; 1998.

Daffner RH. Stress fractures. *Skeletal Radiol.* 1978;2:221–229.

Hoppenfeld S. *Physical examination of the spine and extremities*. Norwalk: Connecticut, Appleton-Century-Crofts; 1976.

Kilcoyne RF, Farrar E. *Handbook of orthopaedic terminology*. Boca Raton: CRC Press; 1991.

Salter RB, Harris R. Injuries to the physeal plate. *J Bone Joint Surg*. 1963;45A:587–622.

Schultz RJ. *The language of fractures*. Baltimore: Williams & Wilkins; 1972.

Starkey C, Ryan J. *Evaluation of orthopaedic and athletic injuries*, 2nd ed. Philadelphia: FA Davis Co; 2002.


# General Orthopaedic Fixation Devices

Fixation devices are often poorly understood by radiologists. Fixators may be used for trauma or reconstructive procedures. Selection of the proper device to fit the injury, osteotomy, or reconstructive procedure is critical to achieve proper healing and maintain function. This section will review immobilization procedures, general fixation devices, terminology, and complications related to their use. Devices designed for specific anatomic regions will be more fully discussed in later anatomic chapters.

## Cast/Splint Immobilization

When possible, fractures are reduced and position maintained with closed reduction techniques (cast, brace, or splint immobilization). This approach can be used with undisplaced or reducible fractures that are not at risk for progressive displacement due to muscle, tendon, or ligament stresses.

Casts, splints, and slings are configured with plaster or synthetic materials such as fiberglass and metal. Casts and splints are used to restore and maintain anatomic position with limited mobility of the supported structures. Braces are used to provide limited motion for joints after trauma or surgery. Common terminology is described in the subsequent text:

**Airplane splint:** Removable cast or metal device used to hold the arm in abduction (see Fig. 2-98)

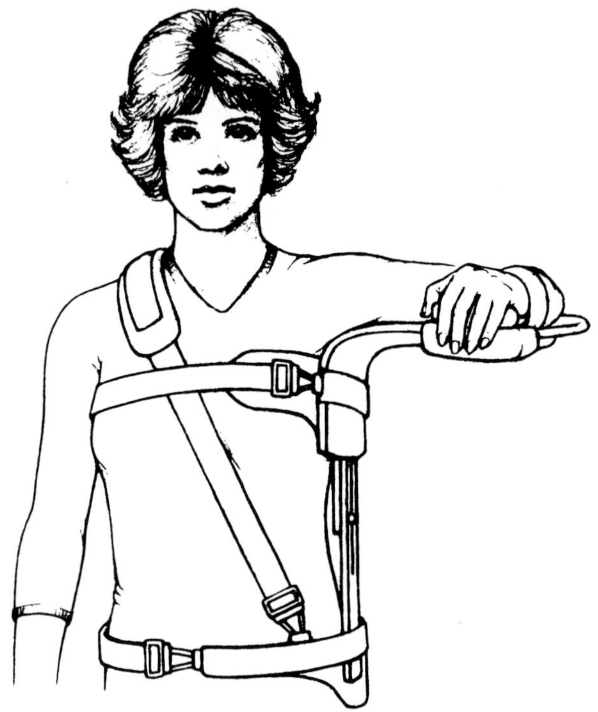

Fig. 2-98 Illustration of a patient with an airplane splint holding the arm in 90 degrees of abduction.

**Aluminum foam splint:** Flexible aluminum splint covered with foam used for hand and finger injuries

**Arm cylinder:** Long arm cast with elbow flexed and wrist not included

**Baseball splint:** Metal splint applied to the distal forearm and hand, which positions the hand as if holding a baseball

**Batchelor:** Hip spica that holds the hip in internal rotation used for developmental dysplasia of the hip

**Bivalve cast:** Cast cut on opposite sides to make two halves; performed to release pressure or permit removal for therapy or imaging; edges may be cut with jagged margins to allow improved locking with frequent removal and repositioning—Boston bivalve cast

**Body cast:** Circumferential cast of the trunk used for spinal immobilization for treatment of conditions such as scoliosis or following surgical procedures

**Cast boot:** Commercially produced devices that strap on and serve as a short leg cast

**Cylinder cast:** Cast from the thigh to just above the ankle used for knee injuries

**Dehne cast:** Thumb cast with separate extenders for the second and third fingers used for treatment of scaphoid fractures

**Delbert cast:** Short leg cast with trimmed anterior ankle and posterior ankle and heel to allow slight dorsal and plantar flexion with medial and lateral stability maintained

Fig. 2-99 Fenestrated cast. Anteroposterior (AP) (A) and lateral (B) radiographs demonstrating mid-tibia and fibular fractures and an open wound. There is cast immobilization with a window or fenestration (*arrowheads*) to allow wound access.

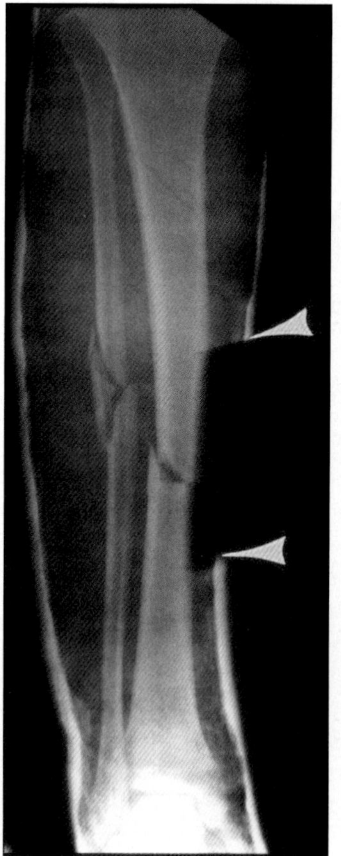



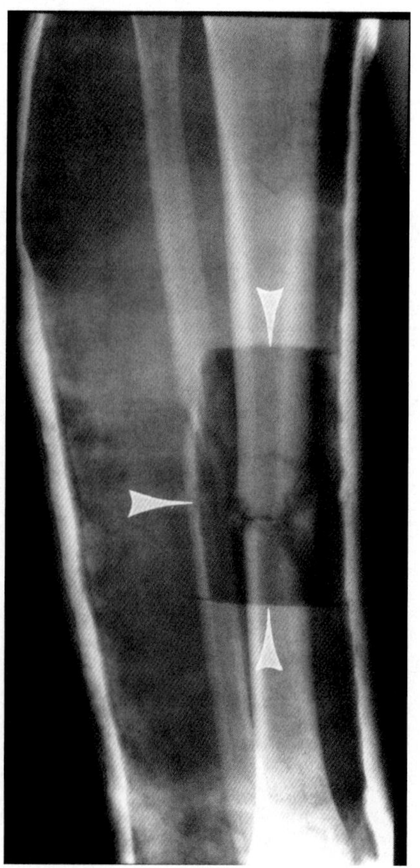

**Fenestrated cast:** Cast with window cut into it to allow wound access (see Fig. 2-99)

**Gauntlet cast:** Short cast from proximal to the wrist to the mid-palm with attachments to control position of metacarpal or phalangeal fractures or dislocations

**Gel cast:** Semisolid cast applied to the foot and ankle for injuries and swelling

**Gutter splint:** Semicircular splint formed around the injured structures (see Fig. 2-100)

**Halo cast:** Cast from the pelvis to over the shoulders with metal extenders to attach to metal halo attached to the head (Fig. 2-92)

**Hanging arm cast:** Long arm cast with associated sling to cause traction on a humeral fracture (Fig. 2-2)

**Hip spica cast:** Cast applied to the lower trunk and pelvis with extension to one or both lower extremities

**Long leg cast:** Cast applied from the upper thigh to the toes for knee injuries and associated fractures of the tibia and fibula; a rubber sole may be attached to the heel to create a walking cast

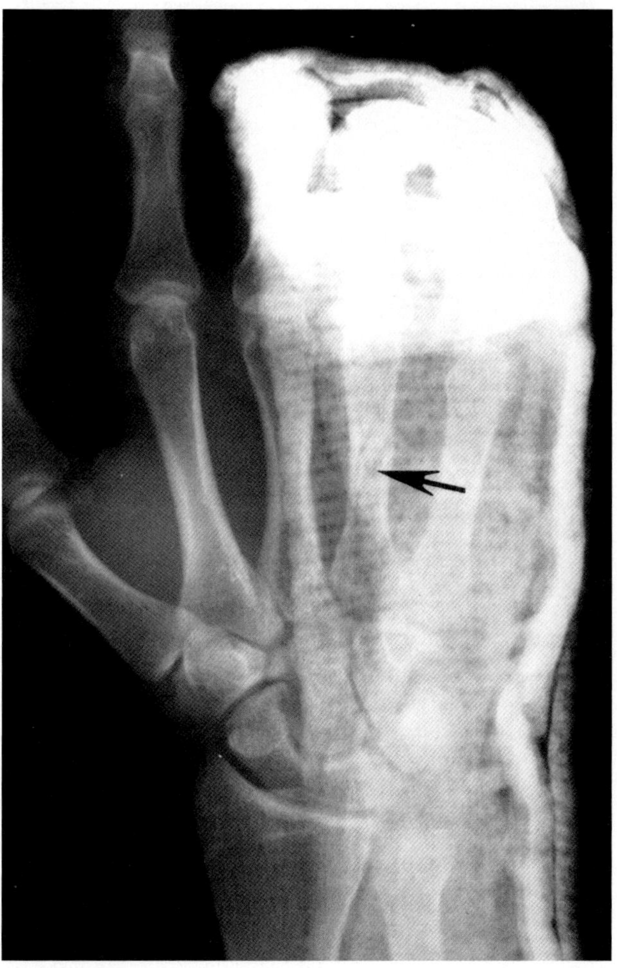

Fig. 2-100 Gutter splint. Radiograph of the hand and wrist with semicircular splint after reduction of a third metacarpal fracture (*arrow*).

**Minerva jacket:** Cast extending from the back of the head and incorporating the head with extension down the back to the hip region; for neck fractures and scoliosis

**Pneumatic compression sleeve or boot:** Allows intermittent compression to prevent deep venous thrombosis

**Quengel cast:** Cast of the thigh and leg to ankle with open hinged portion at the knee to allow motion

**Short arm cast:** Cast extending from the elbow to the palm; used for forearm fractures (Fig. 2-80)

**Short leg cast:** Cast from below the knee to the toes for lower leg and ankle fractures

**Shoulder spica cast (airplane):** Cast applied to the trunk and humerus to keep the humerus abducted (similar to Fig. 2-98)

**Spica cast:** Cast that includes the body and adjacent extremity; most common in the hip, shoulder, and thumb

**Sugar tong splint:** Long piece of plaster applied to the injured area and attached with an outer dressing; used for the shoulder, arm, and forearm

**Thumb spica cast:** Cast incorporating the forearm and thumb

**Univalve cast:** Cast cut on one side to relieve pressure

**Universal gutter splint:** Wire mesh splint for lower extremity fractures

**Volar splint:** Splint applied to anterior or volar forearm

**Wedge casts:** Casts modified by cutting and changing the position before recasting the cut portion to maintain the new bone position; cut area can be widened (opening wedge) or narrowed (closing wedge)

**Window:** Opening produced in the cast; usually square or rectangular to allow wound access (see "Fenestrated cast") (Fig. 2-99)

## Internal Fixation Devices

The goals of fracture management and many reconstructive procedures are to restore normal anatomy and maintain function. Table 2-1 summarizes the indications for internal fixation.

Internal fixation may be accomplished with single or multiple systems including screws, plates, pins and wires, intramedullary nails, staples, and cables. Specific instrumentation, such as for the spine, will be discussed in later chapters.

Table 2-1

| INDICATIONS FOR INTERNAL FIXATION |
|---|
| Failed closed reduction |
| Soft–tissue forces will prevent maintenance of reduction |
| Displaced intra-articular fractures |
| Pathologic fractures |
| Early mobility |
| Cost reduction |

## Screws

Orthopaedic screws may be used alone or in combination with other fixation devices. Screws may be fully or partially threaded with different pitch and configuration. Pitch is the distance between the threads. The distance is greater with cancellous screws. Screws may also be cannulated, have different head configurations, and designed to be inserted with or without tapping and predrilling. Screws are typically made of stainless steel or titanium, but new bioabsorbable screws are also available. Screws may be used with washers in areas of thin cortical bone such as the tibial metaphysic and epiphysis. Nuts may also be used to increase stability in osteoporotic bone or provide additional compression. Methacrylate may also be used to improve hold in osteoporotic bone.

**Cortical screws:** Designed for placement in cortical bone; fully threaded, smaller thread diameter, and pitch; should penetrate both cortices and project approximately 2 mm beyond the distal cortex (see Fig. 2-101)

**Cancellous screws:** Designed for cancellous bone; deeper threads, greater pitch, and more often partially threaded (Fig. 2-101)

**Malleolar screws:** Partially threaded screw with threads similar to cortical screws; trocar tip (cortical screws are blunt) and finer thread pattern (see Figs. 2-102 and 2-103)

**Non–self-tapping screw:** Screw that requires a tapping procedure in a predrilled guide hole before insertion; tapping cuts the threads before insertion (Fig. 2-103)

**Self-tapping screw:** A guide hole is drilled the same diameter as the screw and the screw cuts its own threads with insertion; tapped screws are thought to provide better hold (Fig. 2-103)

**Cannulated screws:** Cannulated screws have a hollow shaft that allows insertion over a guide wire; these screws do not penetrate the opposite cortex; if cortical penetration is a concern, contrast can be injected to detect cortical or articular penetration (see Fig. 2-104)

**Interfragmentary screws:** Screw that crosses a fracture line; should be placed perpendicular to the fracture line (see Fig. 2-105)

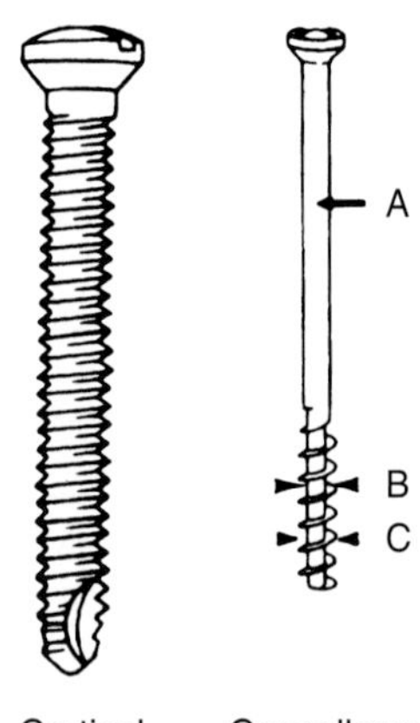


Fig. 2-101 Illustration of the two basic screws; cortical fully threaded and partially threaded cancellous screws. A: Shank. B: Core diameter. C: Thread diameter. (Courtesy of Zimmer, Warsaw, Indiana.)

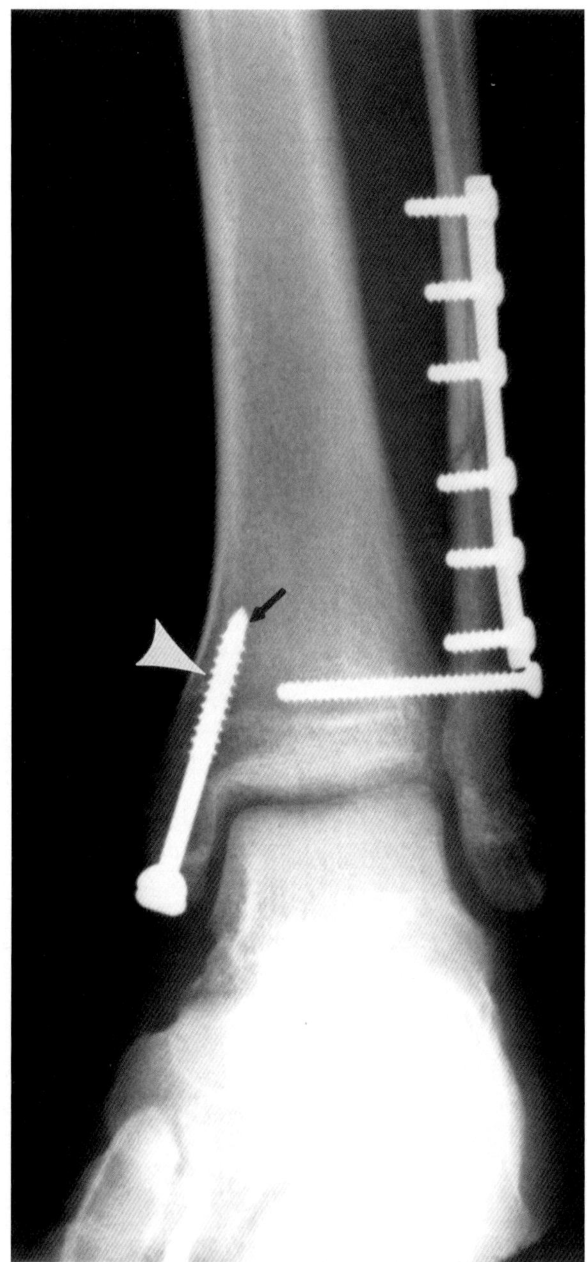

Fig. 2-102 Malleolar screw. Anteroposterior (AP) radiograph after reduction of a pronation-lateral rotation injury. There are two malleolar screws for fixation of the medial malleolar fracture. Note the threads (*white arrowhead*) are similar to a cortical screw, but there is a trocar tip (*black arrow*). There is also a screw across the syndesmosis (syndesmotic screw) and one third tubular plate and cortical screws for fixation of the fibular fracture.

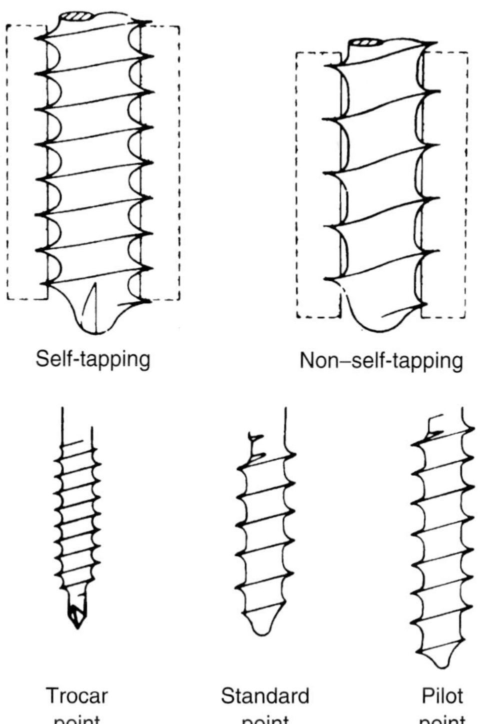


Fig. 2-103 Illustration of screw points and self-tapping and non–self-tapping screws. Self-tapping can be inserted after a pilot hole has been drilled. The screw must cut its own threads. Non–self-tapping screws require a pilot hole and tapping to precut the threads.

**Schanz screws:** Larger diameter and less deep self-cutting threads

**Herbert screws:** Lacks a head, cannulated and threaded at both ends; wider pitch proximally than distally; threads run in the same direction to permit compression of the fracture fragments; commonly used in the scaphoid (see Fig. 2-106)

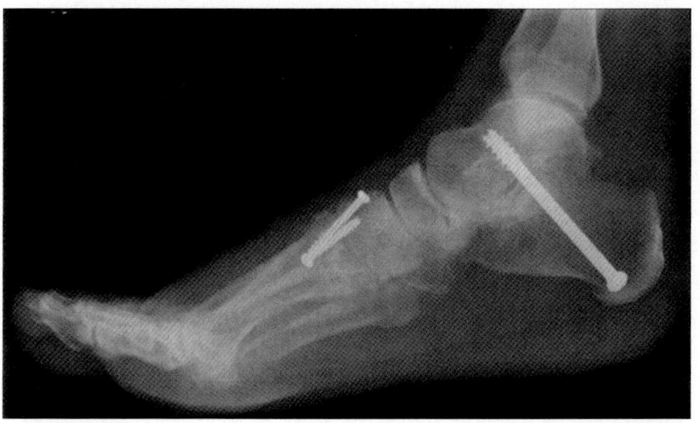

Fig. 2-104 Cannulated screws. Tarsometatarsal and subtalar fusions with cannulated screws for fixation. The ends are open and the screws hollow to allow passing them over a guide wire.

**Acutrak screws:** Used similar to the Herbert screw; cannulated, but fully threaded, no head (see Fig. 2-107)

**Interference screws:** Headless, short fully threaded screws commonly used for cruciate ligament repair; screws are placed in predrilled tunnels to hold bone blocks at the ends of the graft in place (see Fig. 2-108)

**Syndesmotic screws:** Screws used to maintain position of the distal tibia and fibula after ligament disruption; usually removed after ligament healing (see Fig. 2-109)

**Dynamic compression screws:** Partially threaded distally; placed in the barrel of a side plate to allow compression of the fragments; commonly used for intertrochanteric fractures (see Fig. 2-110)

## Fixation Plates

Orthopaedic plates come in various sizes and shapes with different lengths, numbers, and types of screw holes. Most

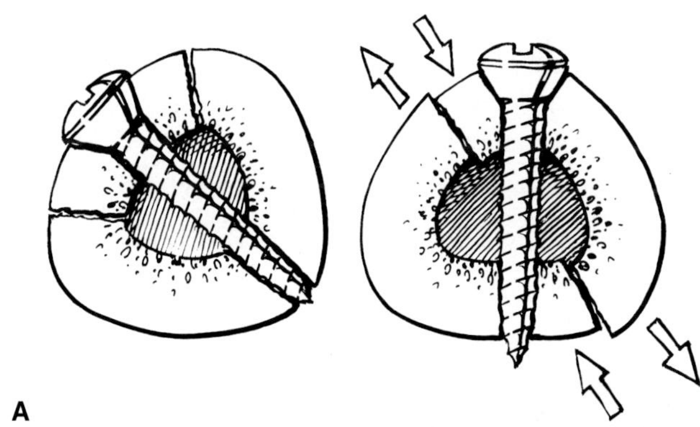


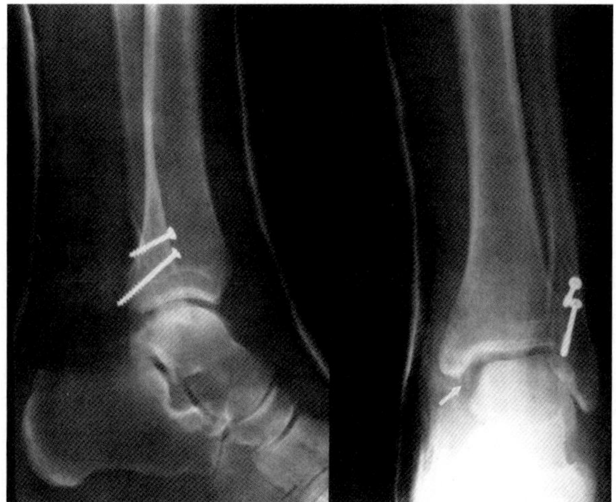


Fig. 2-105 Interfragmentary screws. **A:** Illustration of properly (*left*) and improperly (*right*) placed interfragmentary screws. The screw should be perpendicular to the fracture line. **B:** Lateral and anteroposterior (AP) radiographs after placement of two partially threaded interfragmentary screws in the oblique distal fibular fracture. There is cast immobilization and a small avulsion fracture (*arrow*) of the medial malleolar tip.

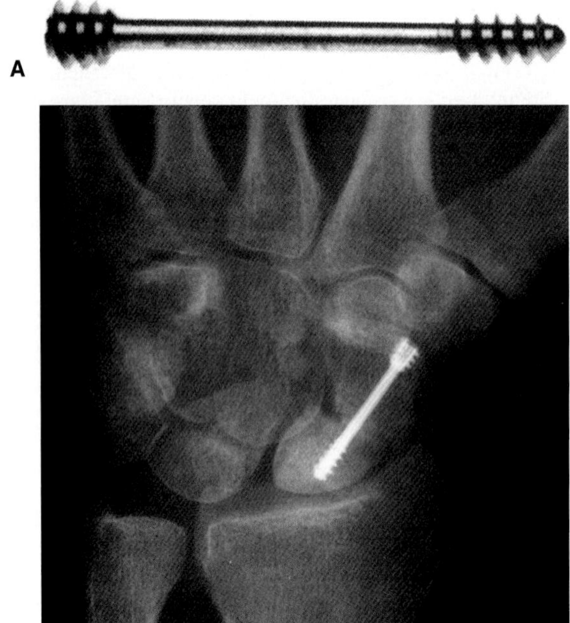

Fig. 2-106 Herbert screw. A: The screw is threaded at both ends with wider pitch proximally and threads run in the same direction to allow compression of fragments. B: Radiograph of a Herbert screw for fixation of a scaphoid fracture. The proximal pole is sclerotic, indicating avascular necrosis.

plates are configured of stainless steel or titanium, although new bioabsorbable plates are also available. There are several basic types of plates. Compression plates are designed to stabilize fractures or osteotomies with compression forces. Dynamic compression plates have oval holes (see Fig. 2-111) that are beveled to draw the fragments together when screws are placed. These plates are tightly applied to bone, which can reduce periosteal blood flow. New low-contact compression plates improve vascularity in the region of the plate. The less invasive stabilization system (LISS) allows the plate to be placed through a small incision and the screw (placed percutaneously) lock to the plate improving vascularity to the bone and reducing soft tissue and periosteal trauma.

Neutralization plates are designed to protect osseous structures from bending, rotational, and axial forces. These plates are often used with interfragmentary screws in addition to the screws in the plate. Buttress plates support structures unstable to compression or axial loading such as at the metaphysis of the tibia.

**Compression plates:** Designed for fractures stable in compression; frequently used with lag or interfragmentary screws

**Dynamic compression plates:** Oval beveled holes to draw the fragments together (Fig. 2-111)

**Low-contact dynamic compression plates:** Reduced area of contact with plate and bone; preserves periosteal blood flow (see Fig. 2-112)

**Semitubular plates:** Designed for areas such as the distal fibula where there are lower tension forces; edges dig into the adjacent bone (see Fig. 2-113)

**Reconstruction plates:** Plates with scored edges allowing plates to be reshaped to fit the anatomic region; acetabulum, calcaneus, mandible, and distal humeral fixation (see Fig. 2-114)

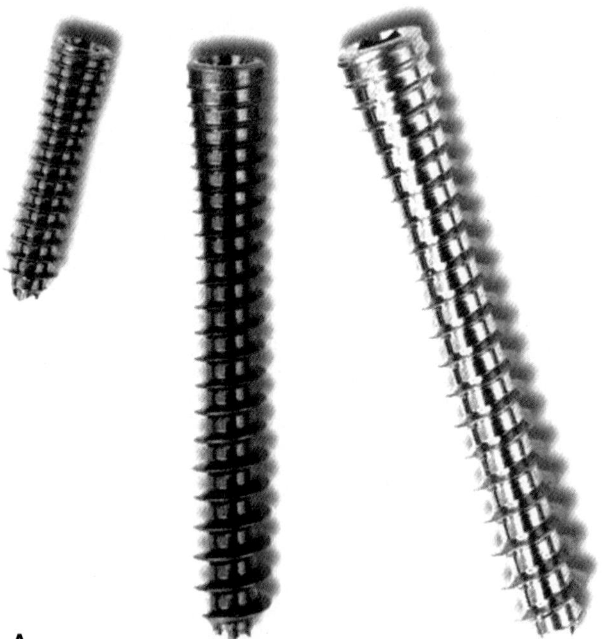

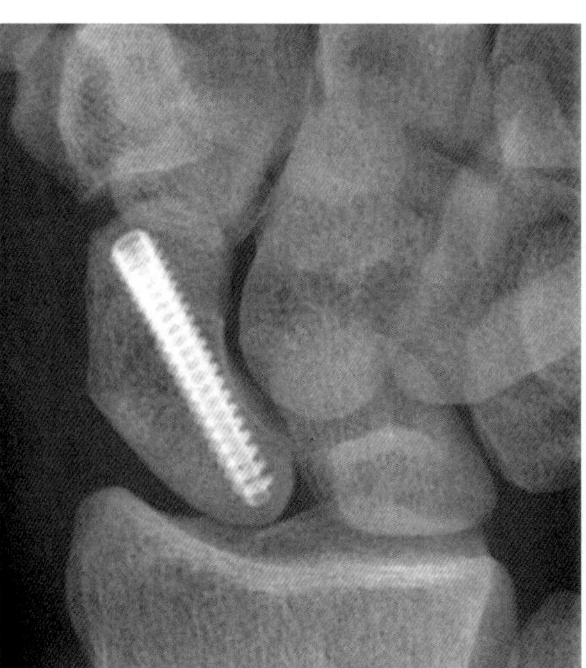

Fig. 2-107 Acutrak screw. A: Acutrak headless screws of different sizes for different anatomic locations. (Courtesy Acumed, Hillsboro, Oregon.) B: Radiograph of the wrist with Acutrak screw fixation of the scaphoid. The screw is fully threaded with no head.

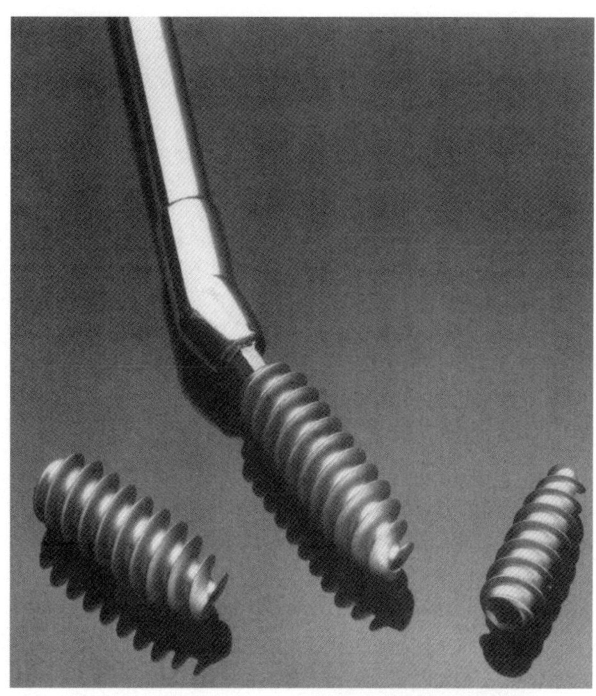


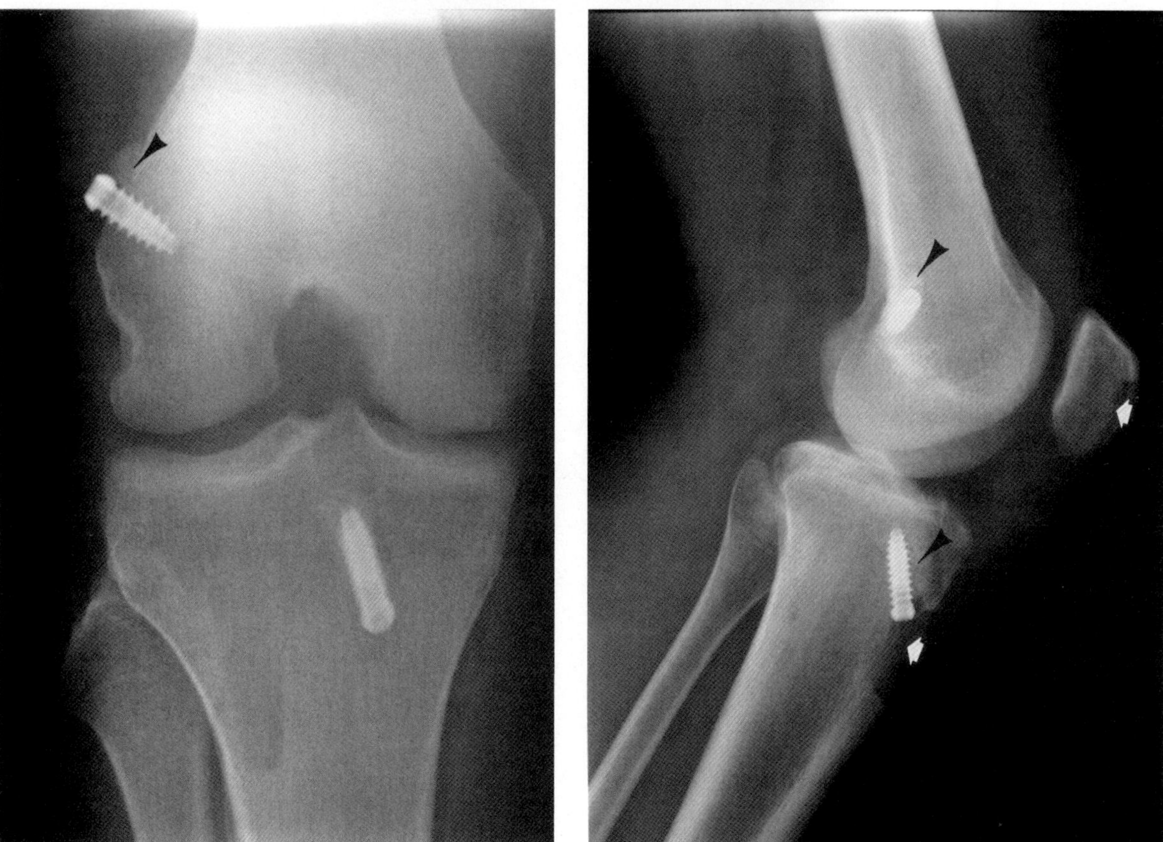


Fig. 2-108 Interference screws. A: Headless interference screws with insertion device. Notch (B) and lateral (C) views following anterior cruciate ligament repair with patellar tendon graft. Note the donor sites (*white arrows*). The interference screws secure the bond plugs from the patella and tuberosity in the femoral and tibial tunnels (*arrowheads*).

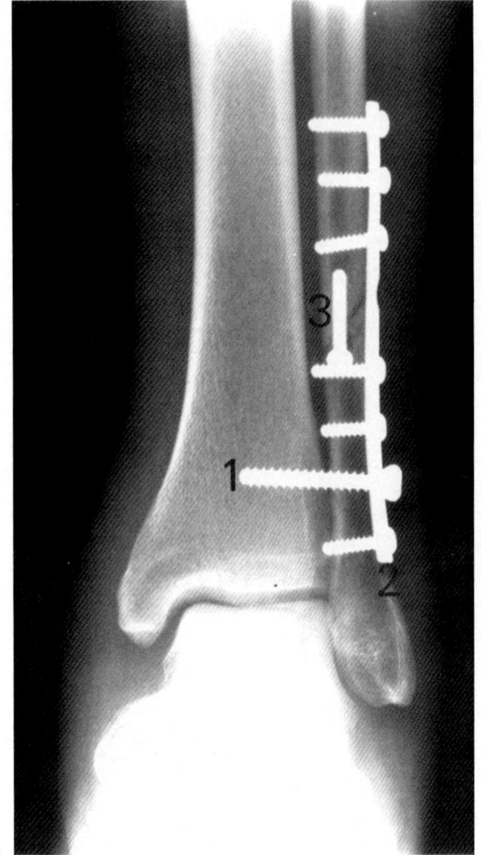


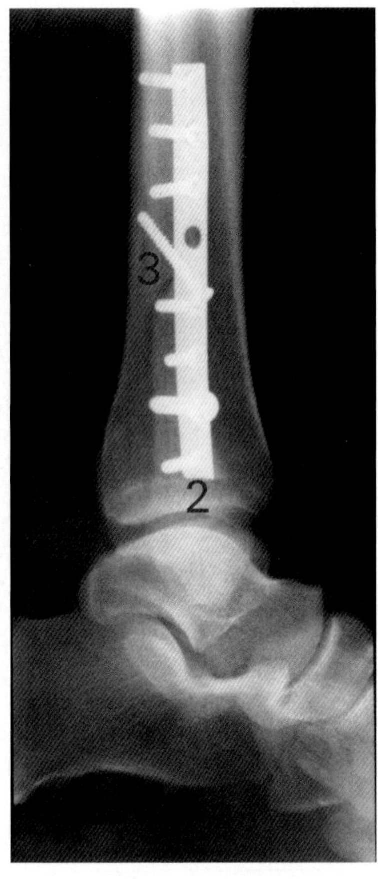


**Fig. 2-109** Syndesmotic screw. Anteroposterior (AP) (**A**) and lateral (**B**) radiographs after pronation-lateral rotation injury. There is a syndesmotic screw (*1*) crossing the distal tibia and fibula. In addition, there is fixation of the fibular fracture with a one third tubular plate (*2*) and cortical screws and an interframentary (lag) screw (*3*) placed perpendicular to the fracture line.

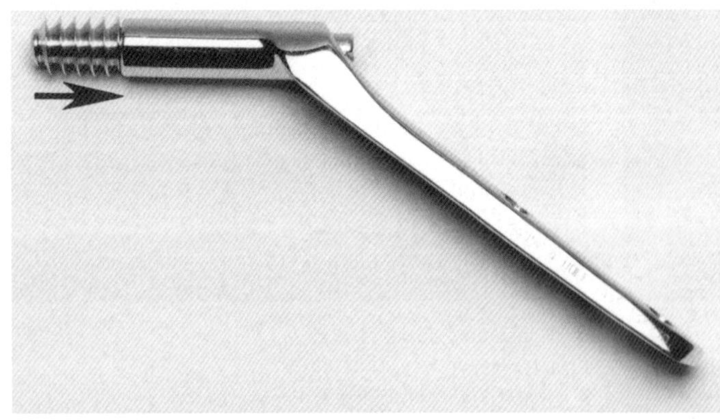


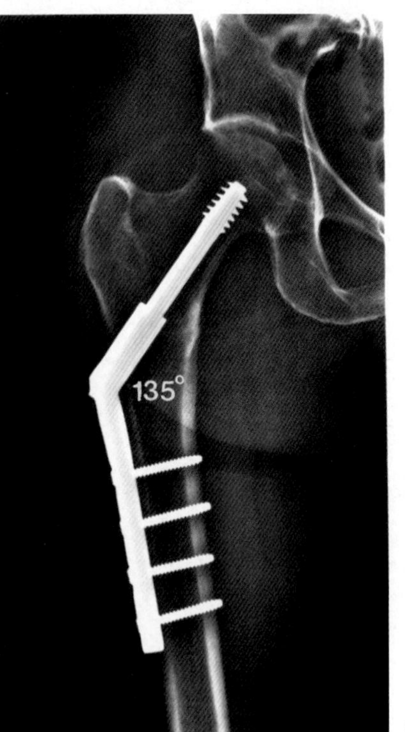


**Fig. 2-110** Dynamic hip screw. Dynamic compression screw in the barrel of the side plate (**A**) and with compression into the barrel (*arrow* in **B**). **C:** Anteroposterior (AP) radiograph of a dynamic hip screw with four-hole 135-degree side plate.

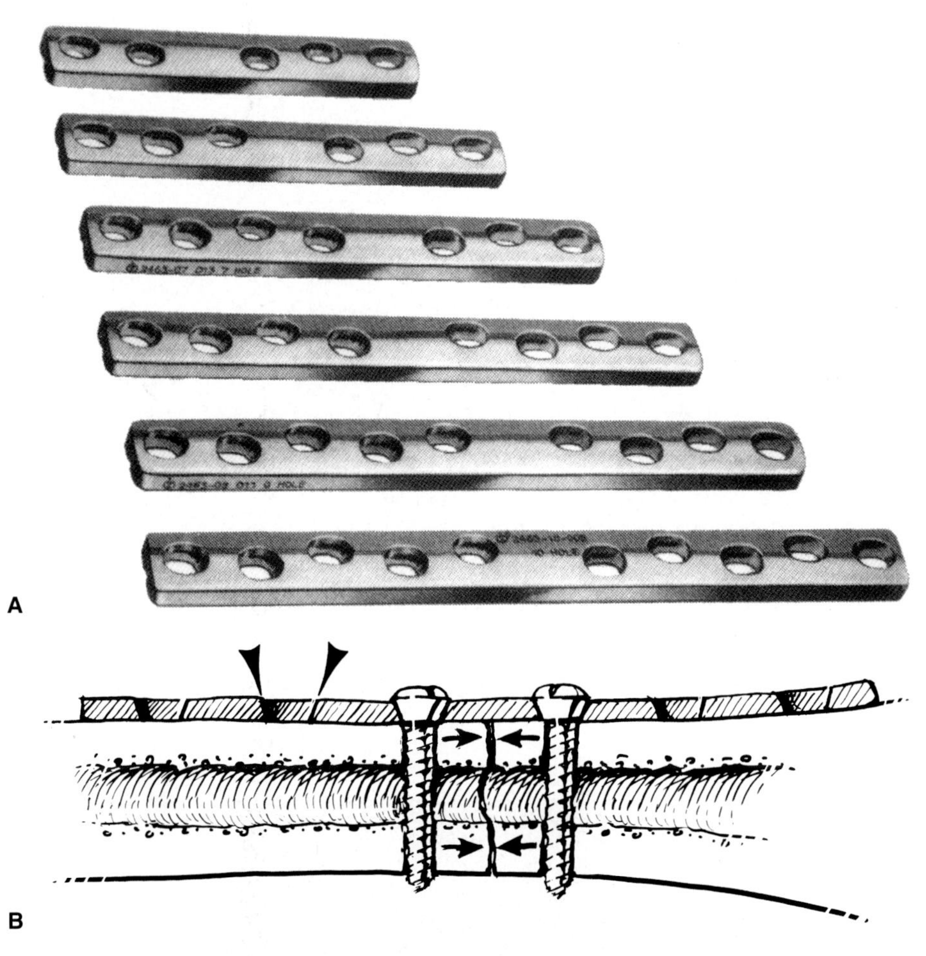


**Fig. 2-111** A: Dynamic compression plates with oval holes in different sizes (5 to 10 offset holes). (Courtesy of Zimmer, Warsaw, Indiana.) B: Illustration of dynamic compression plate with beveled holes (*arrowheads*) that draw the fragments together with screw insertion (*arrows*).

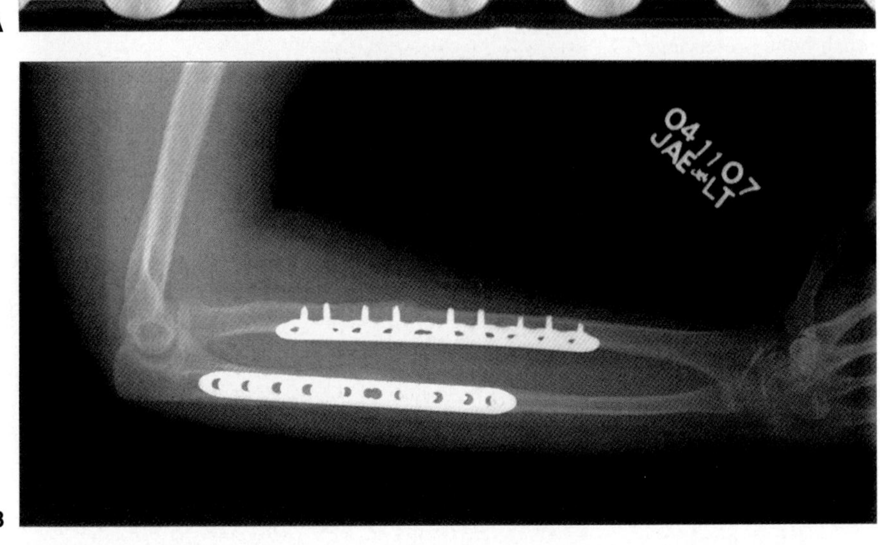


**Fig. 2-112** Photograph of a low-contact dynamic compression plate. B: Radiograph of the forearm with radial and ulnar shaft fractures treated with 3.5-mm low-contact dynamic compression plates and screws.

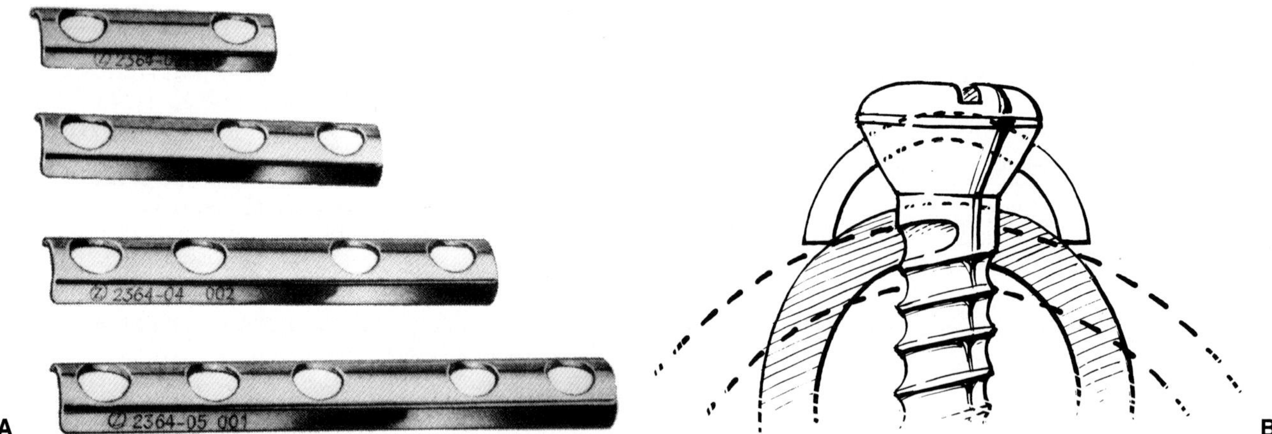


**Fig. 2-113** One third tubular plates. **A:** One third tubular plates with two to five holes and curved edges. (Courtesy of Zimmer, Warsaw, Indiana.) **B:** Cross-sectional illustration of a tubular plate and cortical engagement when screws are placed. See radiographs in Figure 2-108.

**Blade plates:** Blade plates have angled ends for specific uses; 130-degree angled plates for the proximal femur; condylar blade plates for the distal and proximal femoral osteotomies; pediatric blade plates for femoral osteotomies (see Fig. 2-115)

**T and L plates:** Buttress plates commonly used in the proximal tibia (see Fig. 2-116)

**Spoon plates:** Designed for use in the distal anterior tibia; shaped for large posterior fragment fixation

**Cloverleaf plates:** Designed for small fragment fractures of the tibial metaphysic (see Fig. 2-117)

**Cobra head plates:** Designed for hip fusion procedures (see Fig. 2-118)

**Bridge plates:** Designed for complex diaphyseal fractures; minimal soft tissue damage and exposure; screws placed near the ends of the plate only

**LISS plate:** Designed for the distal femur and proximal tibia; configured to the bone shape; need not touch bone preserving vascular supply and less invasive surgical approach; unicortical screws lock to plate and are inserted with less invasive approach (see Fig. 2-119)

**Miniplates:** Designed for the small bones of the hand and foot (see Fig. 2-120)

## Intramedullary Fixation

Intramedullary fixation devices may be hollow or solid (see Fig. 2-121). They are available in different lengths and configurations for different diaphyseal regions. Solid devices are typically termed *nails* and may not require prereaming of the medullary space. Hollow devices are usually termed *rods* and may have round, triangular, or cloverleaf cross-sectional configuration. These rods require prereaming of the medullary canal. Intramedullary fixation does not require surgical exposure of the fracture site so it is less invasive. Also, rods or nails can be inserted antegrade or retrograde depending upon the fracture site. These fixation systems are most frequently used in the femur, tibia, and humerus. Screw fixation may be added to reduce rotation and shortening. Dynamic technique (screws at one end) allows the fragments to impact; static technique places screws at both ends of the rod (see Fig.2-122).

**Rush rod:** The tip is beveled so no reaming is required; shepherd's crook at the end; typically used in small bones such as the fibula (see Fig. 2-123)

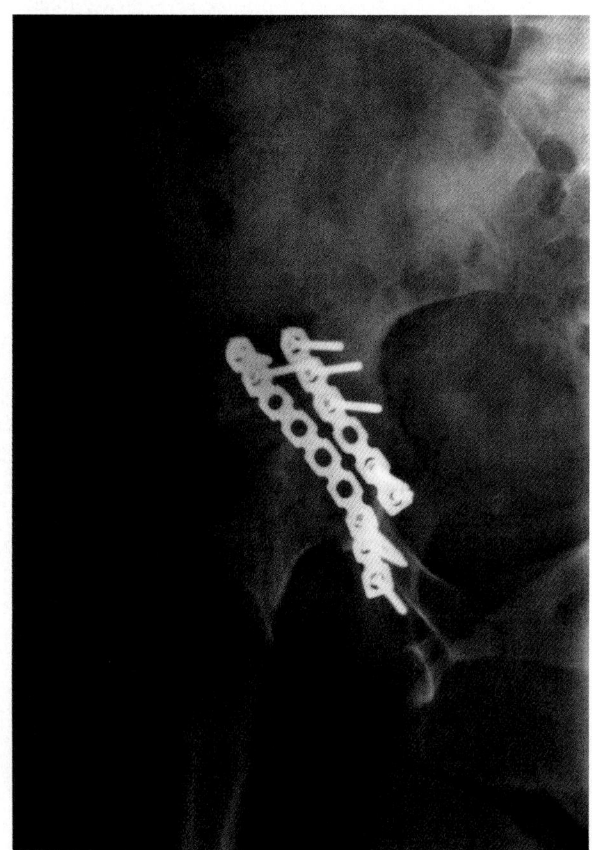

**Fig. 2-114** Reconstruction plates. Radiograph demonstrating acetabular fracture fixation using two reconstruction plates and screws. Plates are notched to allow shaping to fit the anatomic region.

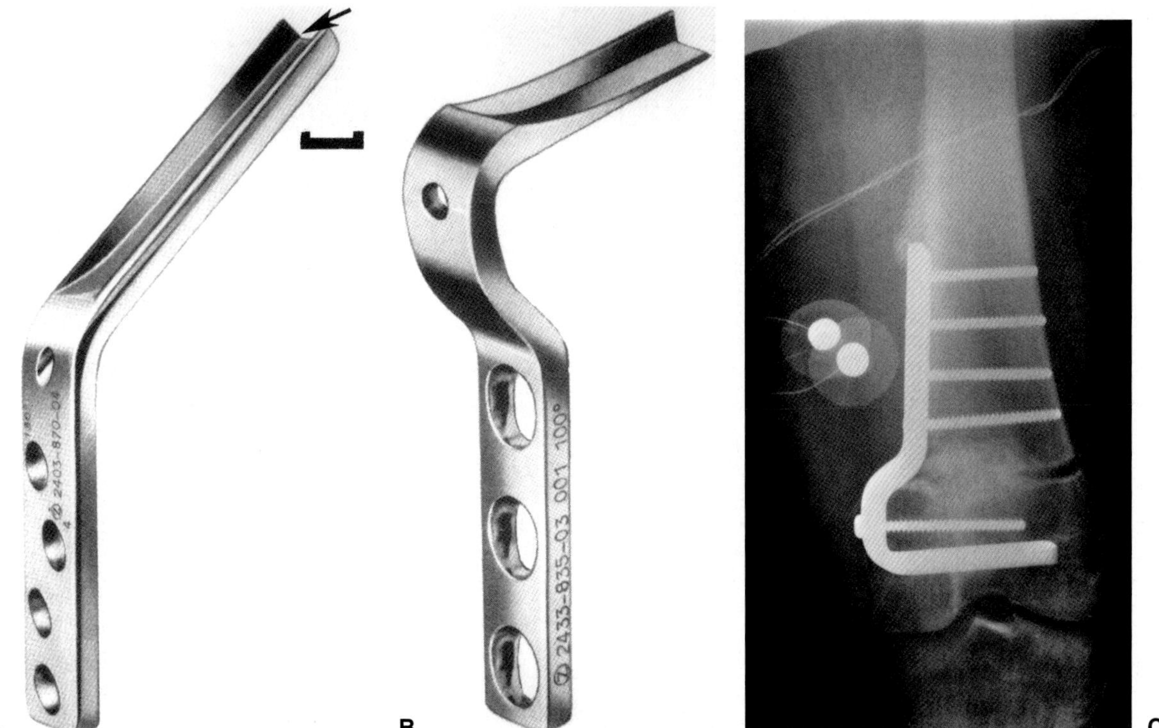


Fig. 2-115 Blade plates. A: 130-degree blade plate for proximal femoral fixation. Note the shape of the blade (*arrow*) to prevent rotation. B: A 100-degree pediatric blade plate for trochanteric osteotomies. (Courtesy of Zimmer, Warsaw, Indiana.) C: Radiograph of a distal femoral osteotomy with blade plate and screw fixation.

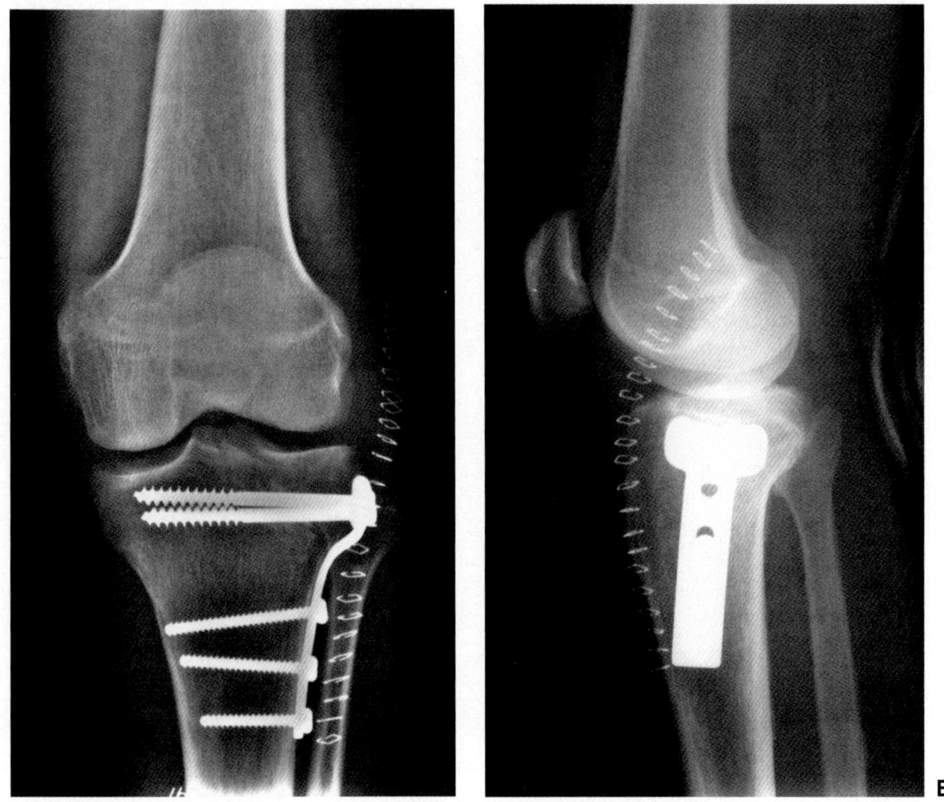


Fig. 2-116 T and L buttress plates. Anteroposterior (AP) (A) and lateral (B) radiographs of a T buttress plate and screws for fixation of a tibial plateau fracture. AP (C) and lateral (D) radiographs of an L buttress plate for fixation of a tibial osteotomy.

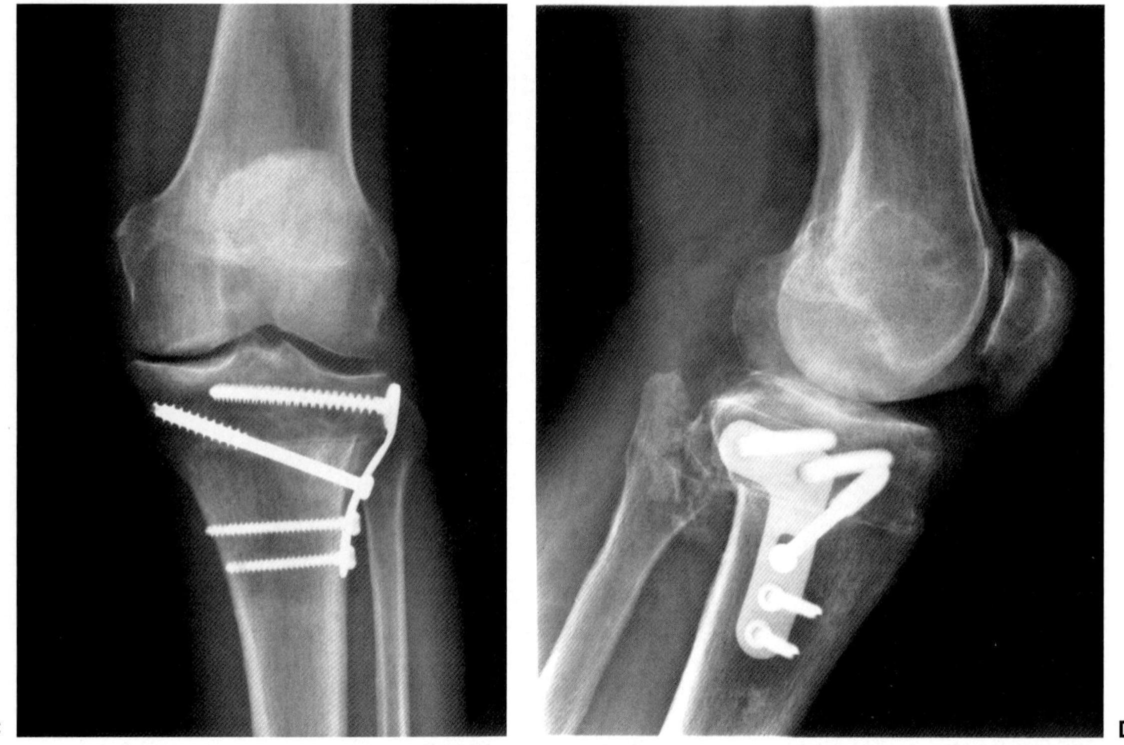

Fig. 2-116 (*Continued*)

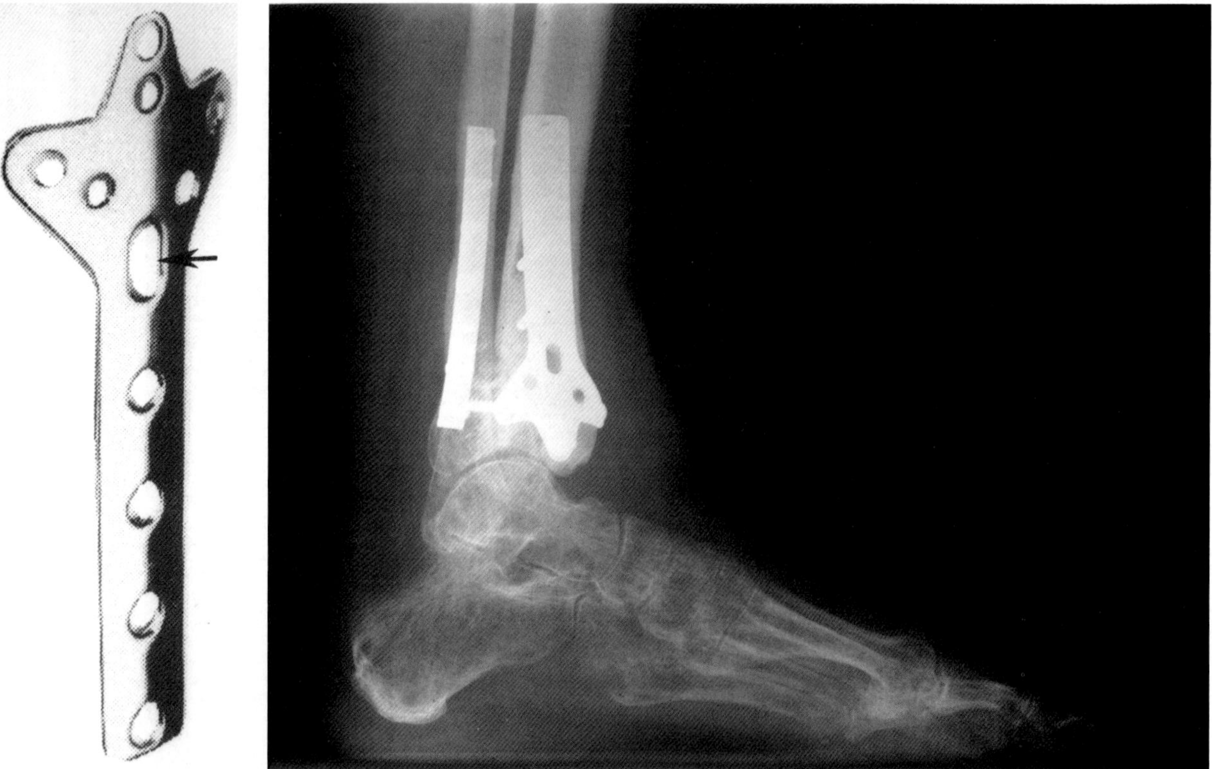

Fig. 2-117 Cloverleaf plates. **A:** Cloverleaf plate with elongated hole (*arrow*) near the base of the cloverleaf. **B:** Radiograph of the ankle demonstrating a cloverleaf plate for fixation of the distal tibial fracture. The fibular fracture is secured with a one third tubular plate.

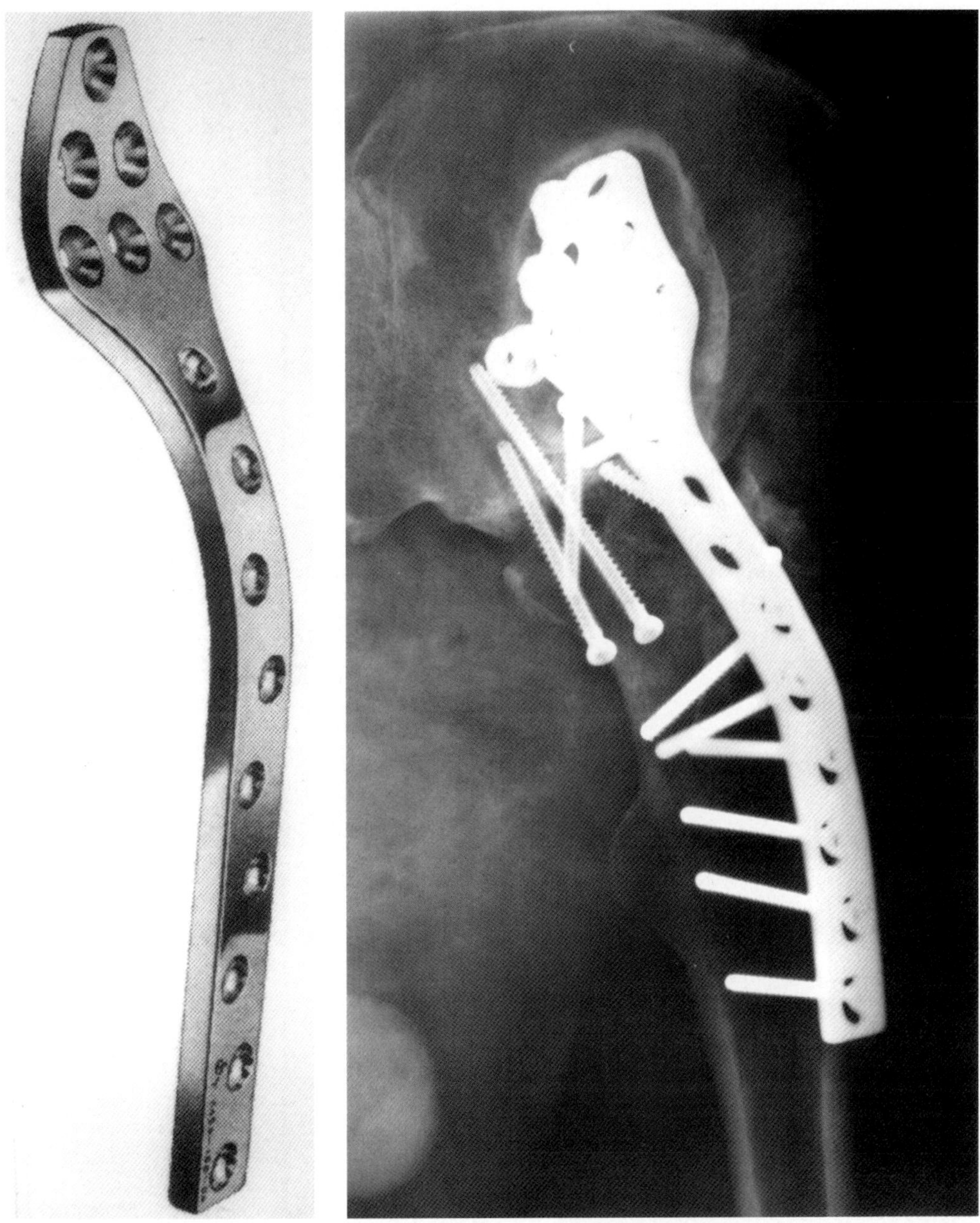


Fig. 2-118 Cobra head plates. A: Cobra head plate for hip arthrodesis. (Courtesy of Zimmer, Warsaw, Indiana.) B: Radiograph of hip arthrodesis with cobra head plate and screw fixation. There is lucency and sclerosis about the iliac portion of the plate due to loosening.

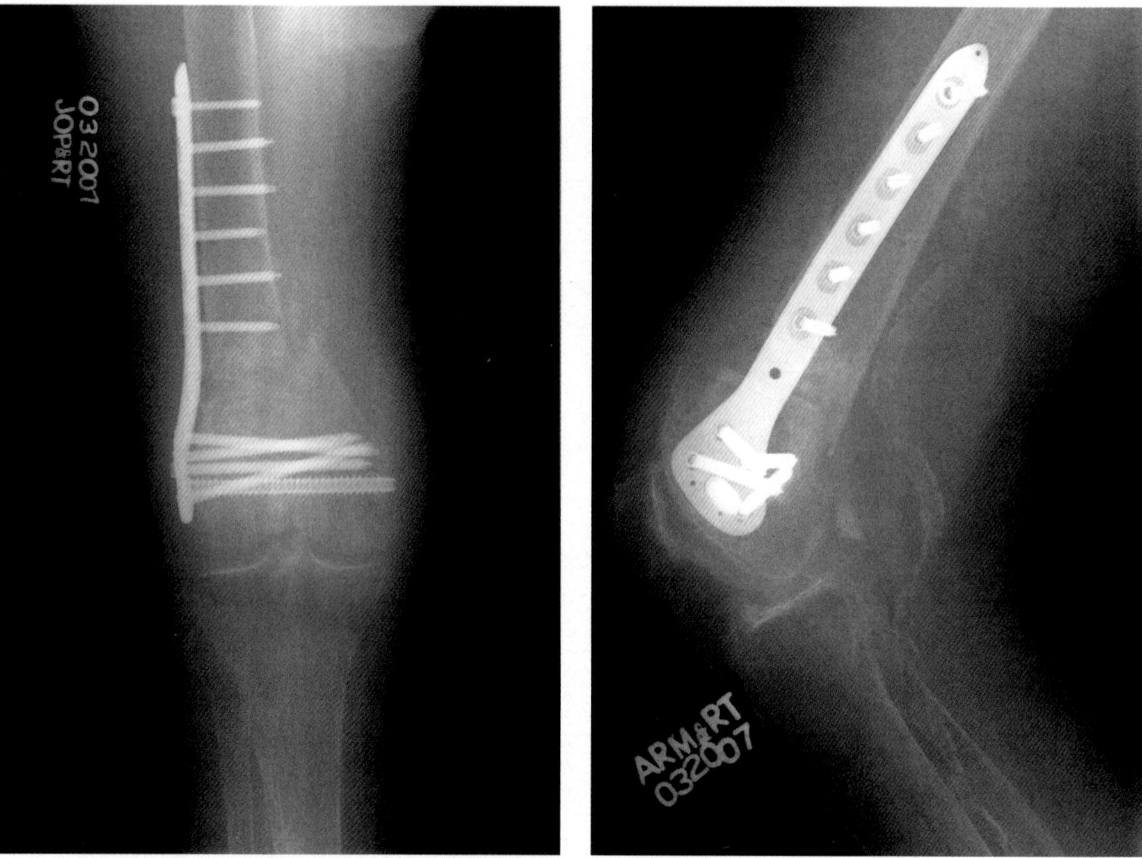


Fig. 2-119 Less invasive stabilization system (LISS). Anteroposterior (AP) (A) and lateral (B) radiographs of the distal femur after LISS fixation of an osteopenic fracture. Note that the plate does not contact the bone distally. There is also bone graft material in and about the fracture site.

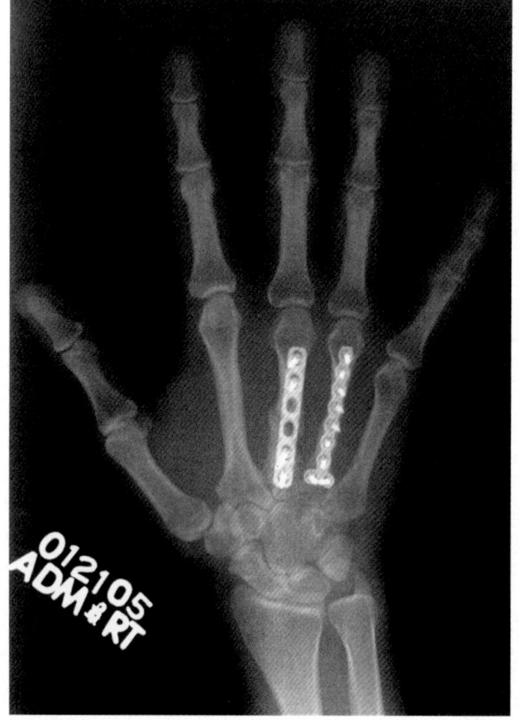


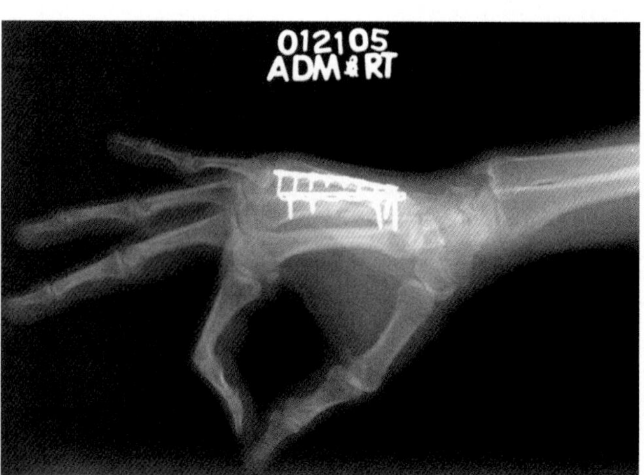


Fig. 2-120 Miniplates. Anteroposterior (AP) (A) and lateral (B) radiographs of the hand with miniplate and screw fixation of third and fourth metacarpal fractures.

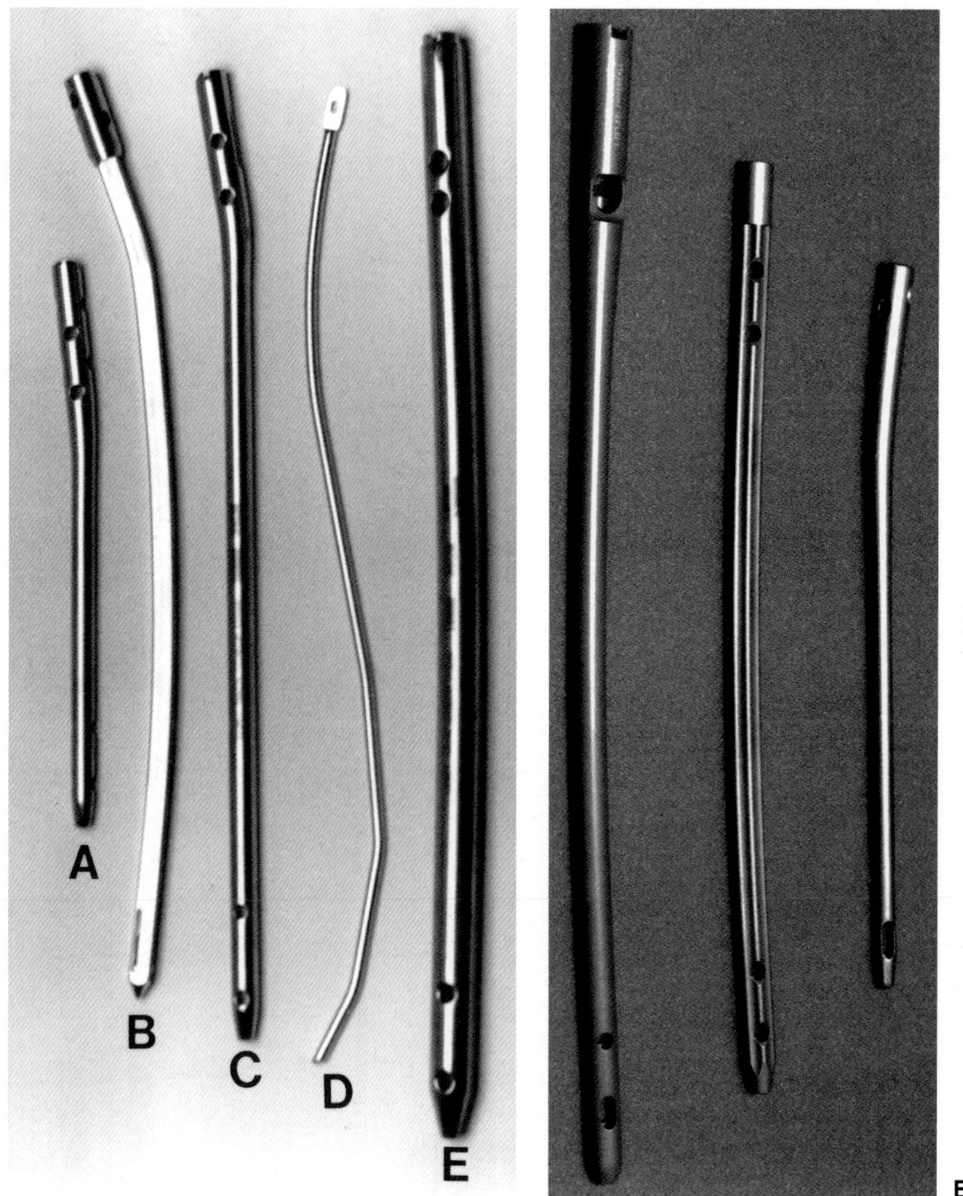


Fig. 2-121 Intramedullary fixation devices. A: *A*—hollow round interlocking humeral rod, *B*—solid square Hansen-Street nail, *C*—hollow interlocking tibial rod, *D*—Ender rod, *E*—hollow interlocking femoral rod. B: Newer generation T2 intramedullary nails. (B Courtesy of Stryker Orthopaedics, Mahwah, New Jersey.)

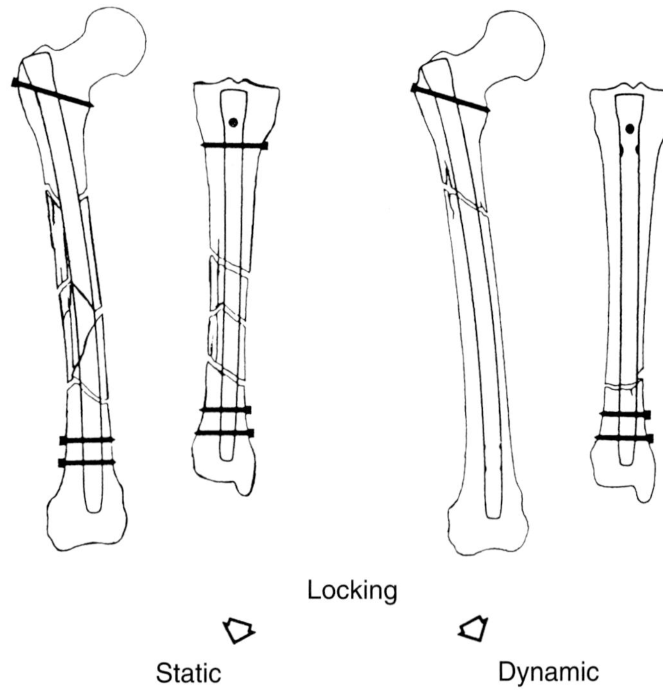


**Fig. 2-122** Illustration of static (screws at both ends) and dynamic (screws at one end) approaches with intramedullary nails.

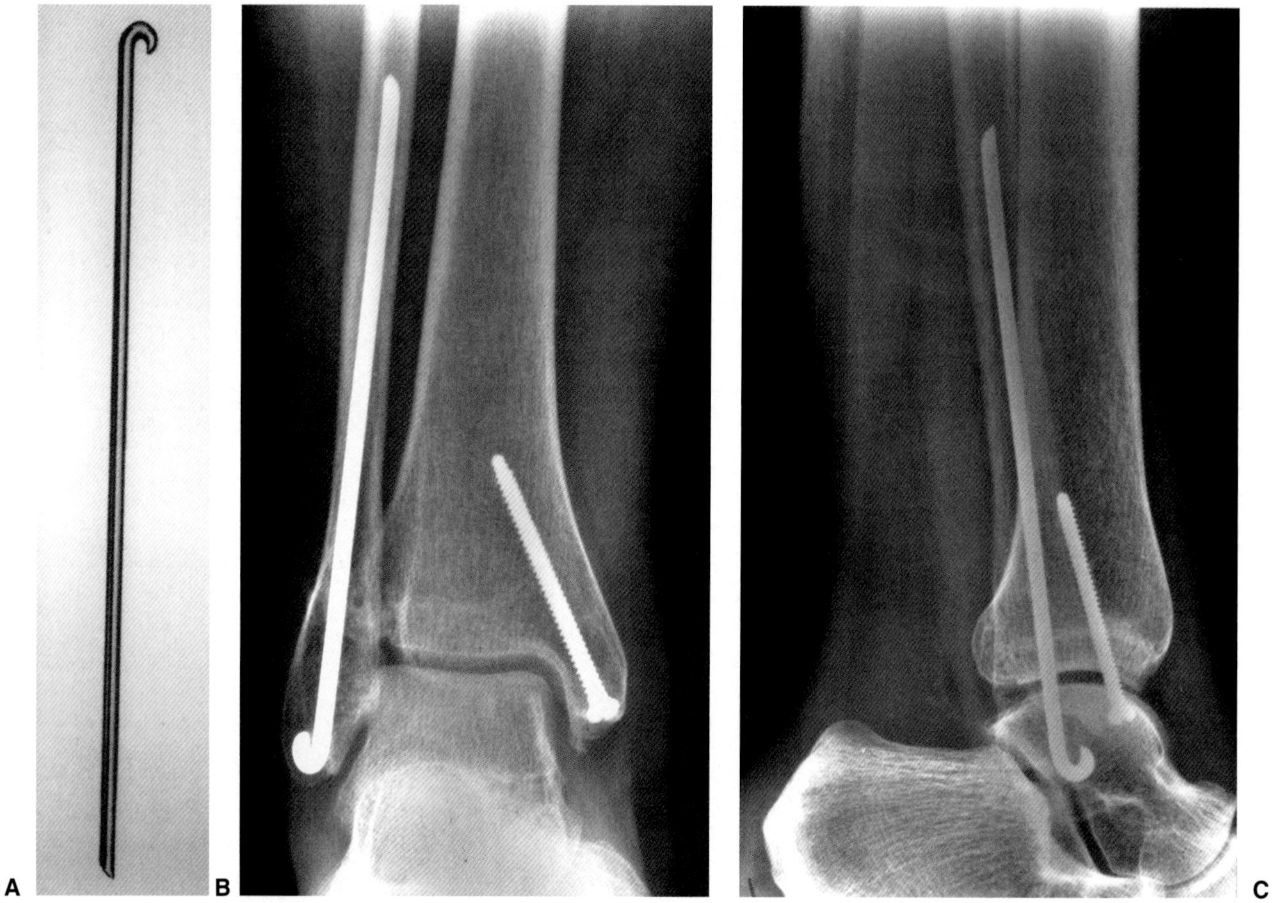

**Fig. 2-123** Rush rod. A: Rush rod. Anteroposterior (AP) (B) and lateral (C) radiographs of the ankle demonstrating healed fracture with a Rush rod in the fibula and a medial malleolar screw.

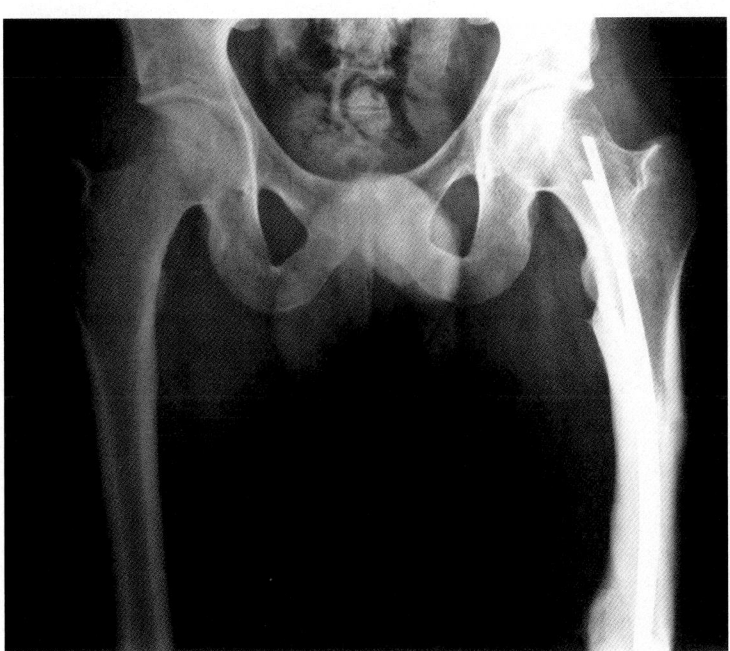
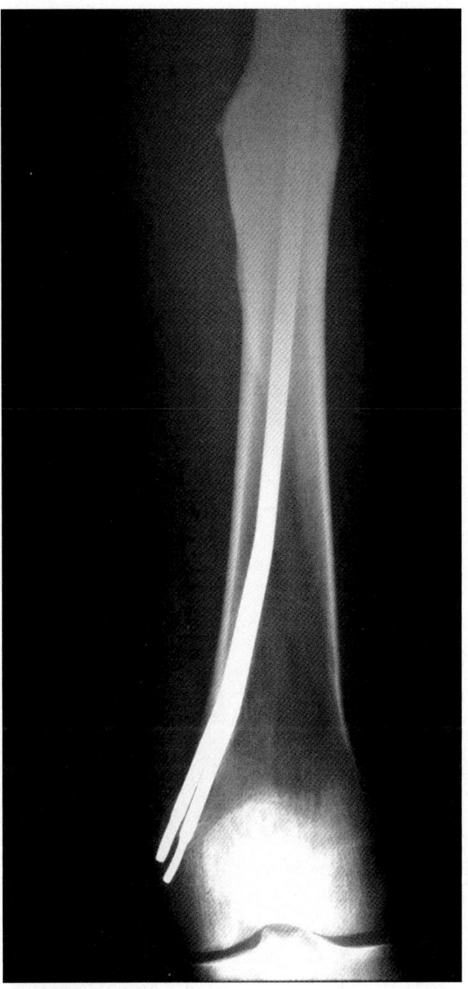

Fig. 2-124 Ender nails. Anteroposterior (AP) radiographs (A and B) of the femur with two Ender rods and a healed femoral midshaft fracture (also see label D in Fig. 2-121A).

**Ender nail:** Solid with oval cross section; multiple rods used to fill the medullary canal; does not prevent rotation of fragments (see Fig. 2-124 and also Fig. 2-121A)

**Sampson rod:** Rigid thick-walled fluted rod that prevents rotation; used for knee arthrodesis

**Kuntscher nail:** Hollow rod with cloverleaf cross-sectional configuration; providing a press fit in the medullary canal

**Zickel nail:** Solid nail with triphalanged Smith-Peterson pin for subtrochanteric fractures (see Fig. 2-125)

**Interlocking nails:** Designed to be used with pins, screws, or expanding blades; static fixation at both ends; dynamic fixation at one end (Fig. 2-122); shorter interlocking systems are available for intertrochanteric and subtrochanteric femoral fractures (see Fig. 2-126)

## Wires and Cables

Wires may be used in different configurations described in the subsequent text. Cables, such as Dall-Miles, come in different sizes with compressible fixation clamps. Parham bands are flat metal strips used for fixation of cortical fragments. Wires and cables may be used alone, but more commonly they are used to provide additional fixation in conjunction with other systems.

**Cerclage wires:** Used for diaphyseal fragment fixation; often in combination with other systems (see Fig. 2-127)

**Tension-band wires:** Used with straight K-wires for patellar or olecranon fractures (see Fig. 2-128)

**K-wires (Kirschner):** Used for small fragment fixation or with tension-banding (see Fig. 2-129 and also Fig. 2-128)

**Dall-Miles cables:** Used for diaphyseal fractures or to secure on-lay bone grafts (Fig. 2-127B)

**Cable-claw systems:** Used to reattach the greater trochanter after hip arthroplasty or fracture fixation (see Fig. 2-130)

**Parham bands:** Flat metal strips used to secure diaphyseal fragments (Fig. 2-125B)

## Pins

There are multiple configurations for pins including solid, cannulated, and variations in the extent and type of threads

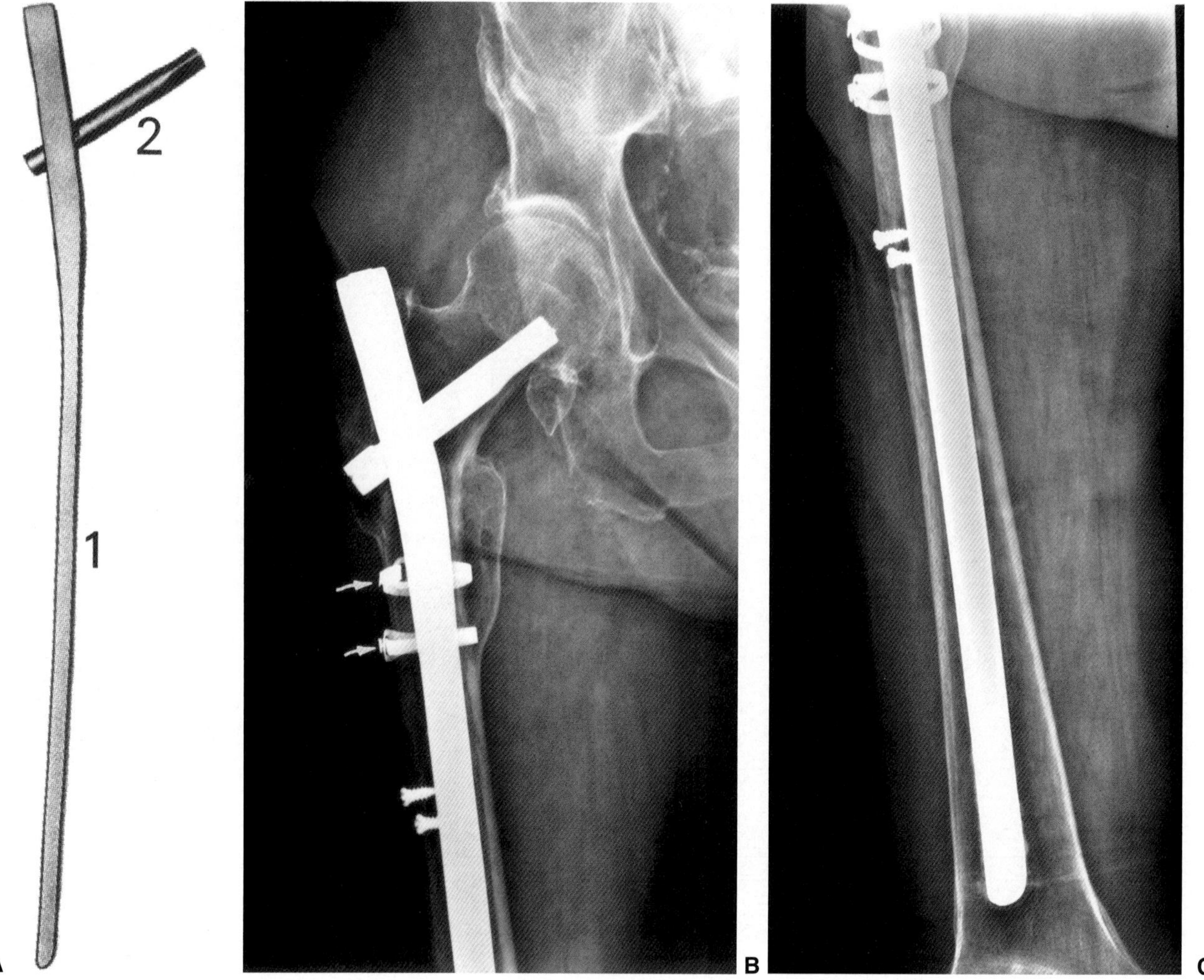


**Fig. 2-125** Zickel nails. **A:** Zickel nail (*1*) with Smith-Peterson triphalaned pin (*2*). Anteroposterior (AP) radiographs (**B** and **C**) demonstrating a Zickel nail and Parham bands (*arrows*) for subtrochanteric fracture fixation.

(Knowles, Hagie, and Steinman). Pins may also be smooth without threads. Most pins are used for femoral neck fractures (see Fig.2-131). Steinman pins are large bore wires with or without threads and used for traction or fracture fixation (see Fig. 2-132).

## Staples

Staples are available with smooth and barbed ends. The latter reduces the pulling out after insertion. Special configurations include the stepped osteotomy staple and the table staple that has four prongs. The table stable is used for ligament repairs and patellar tendon surgery (see Fig. 2-133).

## Soft Tissue Anchors

Soft tissue anchors are used to provide a mechanism for anchoring sutures to bone for soft tissue repairs such as rotator cuff, labral, and capsular repairs. Anchors have barbs or threads to prevent pullout (see Fig. 2-134). Mitek anchors are constructed of nickel-titanium alloy and inserted in a predrilled hole. They come with multiple barb configurations, most commonly two or four.

Threaded systems are also available. Anchors may have fine or cancellous type threads and are inserted into predrilled pilot holes (see Fig. 2-135). New biodegradable anchors are also available. Biodegradable anchors cause less image distortion on MRI examinations.

## Bone Grafts

Bone graft materials are used in many situations to improve healing, replace bone loss, and provide direct antibiotic implantation. Grafts may be autografts, allografts, or synthetic in nature.

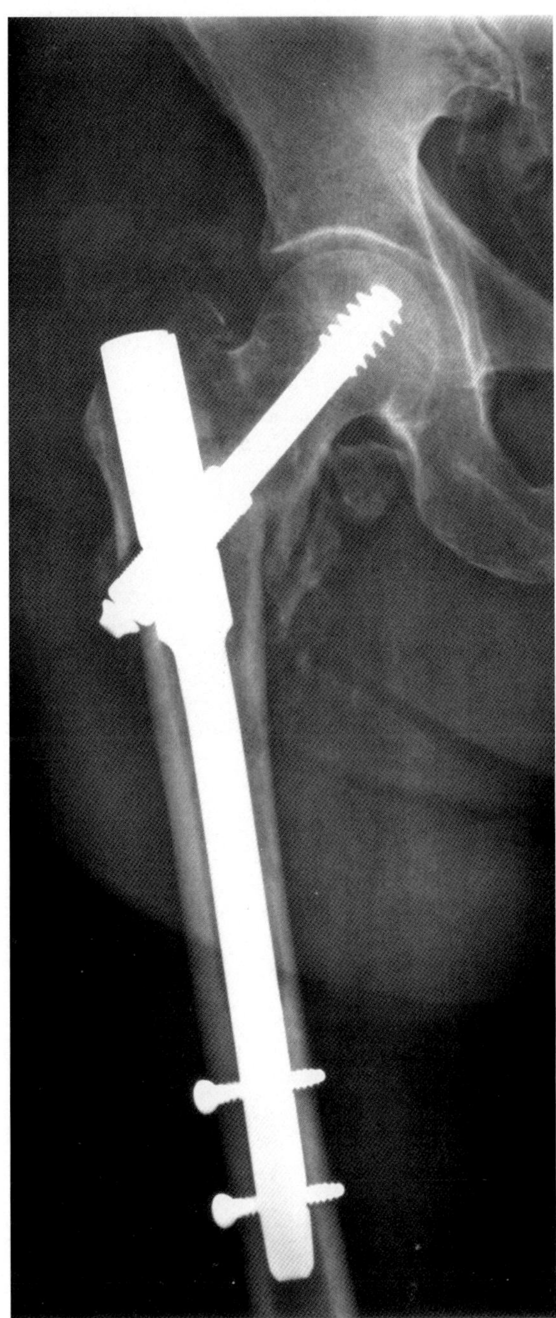

Fig. 2-126 Short interlocking nail. Anteroposterior (AP) radiograph showing a short interlocking nail for fixation of a comminuted intertrochanteric fracture.

**Autograft:** Bone obtained from the patient; grafts may be cancellous, cancellous and cortical, cortical and vascularized, or nonvascularized

**Allograft:** Bone graft from a cadaver bank (see Fig. 2-136)

**Synthetic substitutes:** Demineralized bone matrix, ceramics, or composite materials

Autografts are most frequently obtained from the iliac crest and fibula. However, other sites including the long bones, femoral head, and ribs may also be used. The graft may be applied intact (Fig. 2-127A) or in the form of paste, chips, and blocks. Although autogenous graft is superior in many ways there are limitations including the amount of graft material required and morbidity at the donor site.

Allografts provide flexibility in the amount of graft material needed (Fig. 2-136). However, disadvantages include disease transmission, immunogenicity, and reduced mechanical properties due to processing.

Disadvantages of autografts and allografts have increased the interest in synthetic substitutes. Substitutes have been used for fracture augmentation, vertebroplasty, fracture nonunion, and filling in defects after infection and/or debridement. Antibiotic impregnated methacrylate in the form of beads or spacers are also used in patients with infected joint replacements or to fill bone defects in osteomyelitis.

## External Fixation

External fixation systems should achieve three goals. First, allow access to injured areas. Second, they should be used in situations where there is no danger of injury to vital tissues. Third, the system should meet the mechanical demands of the injury.

External fixation systems come in different configurations depending upon the anatomic site and indication. Some fixation systems are designed to allow motion at the joint, others for more rigid fracture fixation or lengthening procedures. External fixation is the technique of choice for open fractures, complex fractures with soft tissue injury, patients with multiple traumas, and for arthrodesis.

External fixation systems may be unilateral, bilateral, ring (see Fig. 2-137A), or hybrid in configuration (see Figs. 2-137 and 2-138). In recent years, the trend has been toward simpler unilateral designs. Fixation systems are attached to pins (threaded or unthreaded) or wires that are placed percutaneously. The pins or wires must penetrate both cortices, avoid the joint, and not cause soft tissue or neurovascular injury.

### Advantages

Three-dimensional stability
Limited soft tissue injury with insertion
Pins can be used as handles to position bone fragments
Early motion of involved joints
Wound access for open injuries

### Disadvantages

Pin tract infection
Damage to soft tissue or neurovascular structures
Fixation failure leading to open procedure

## Traction

Traction systems are usually designed for temporary treatment. Both skin (see Fig. 2-139) and skeletal (see Fig. 2-140) traction

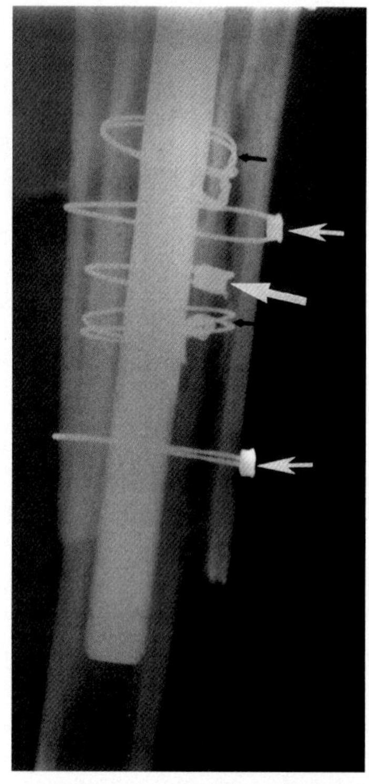

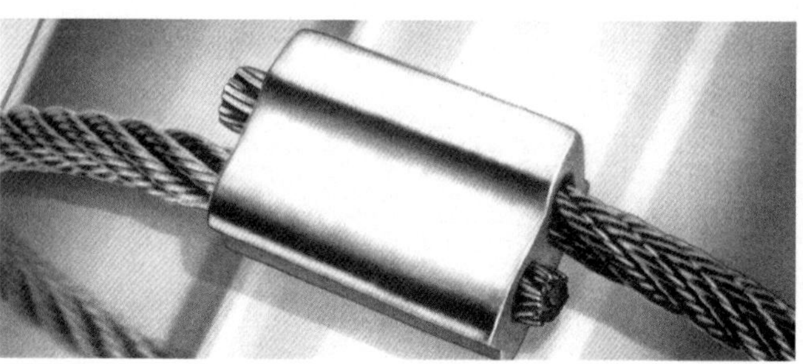

Fig. 2-127 Cerclage wires and Dall-Miles cables. A: Radiograph of the femur in a patient with a hip arthroplasty supported by cerclage wires (*black arrows*). Later cortical bone grafts were applied supported by Dall-Miles cables (*white arrows*). B: Dall-Miles cable. (Courtesy of Howmedica, Rutherford, New Jersey.)

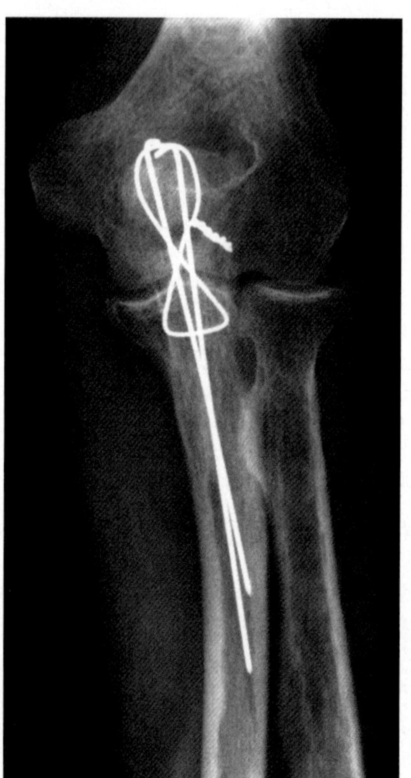

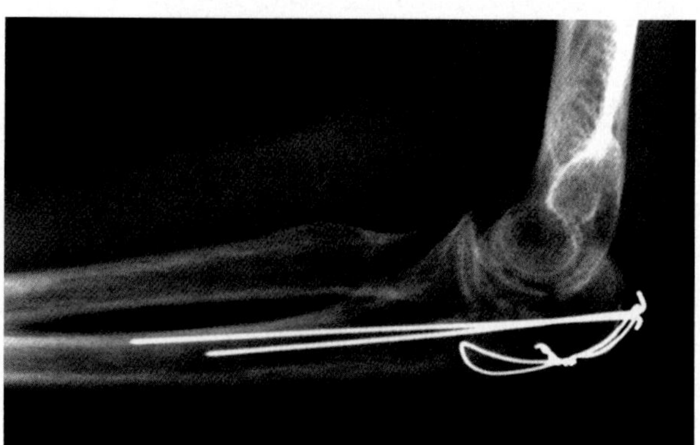

Fig. 2-128 K-wires and tension band fixation of an olecranon fracture demonstrated on anteroposterior (AP) (A) and lateral (B) radiographs.

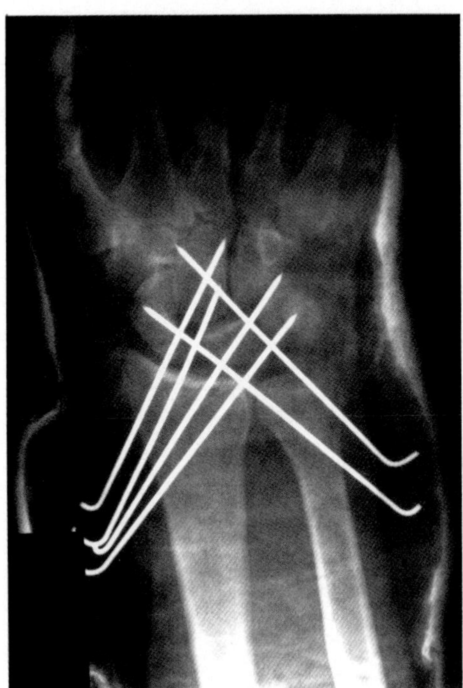

Fig. 2-129 K-wires. Radiograph of the wrist after carpal dislocation reduced with K-wires and cast immobilization.

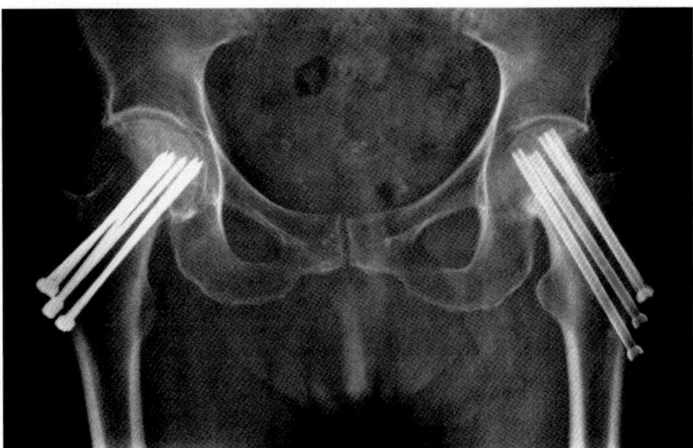

Fig. 2-131 Hip pins. Radiograph of the pelvis and hips in a patient with bilateral femoral neck fractures internally fixed with four Knowles pins on the right and four cannulated Ace pins on the left.

techniques are available. Traction is designed for fracture reduction or for longer periods to improve fragment position before more definitive therapy.

Skeletal traction can be accomplished using threaded Steinman pins, smooth pins, or K-wires. The latter cause less soft tissue damage but tend to cut through bone. Occasionally, two

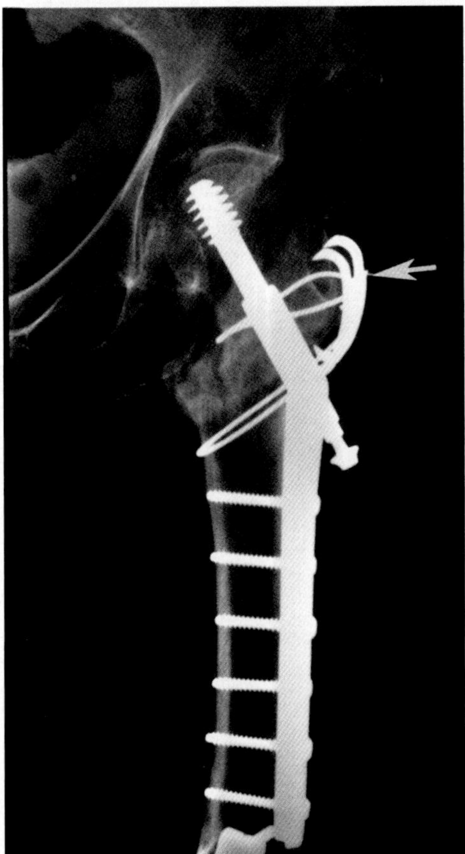



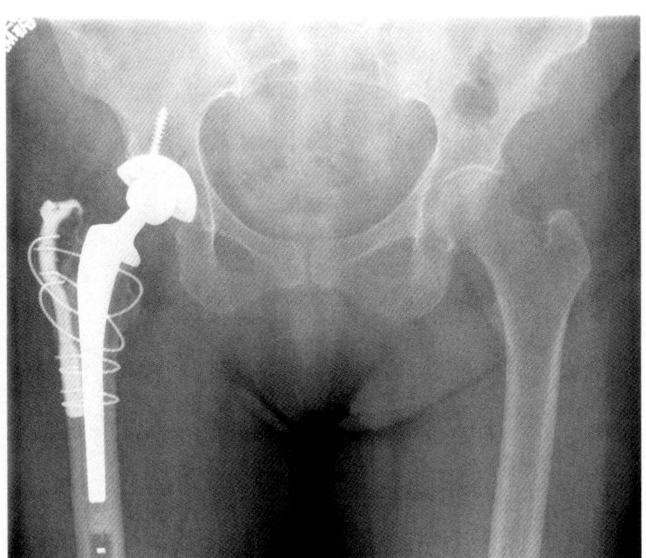



Fig. 2-130 Cable-claw systems. A: Radiograph following reduction of an intertrochanteric fracture using a dynamic hip screw with a Dall-Miles cable-claw system (*arrow*) for greater trochanteric fixation. B: Radiograph following hip arthroplasty with a Zimmer claw system for trochanteric fixation.

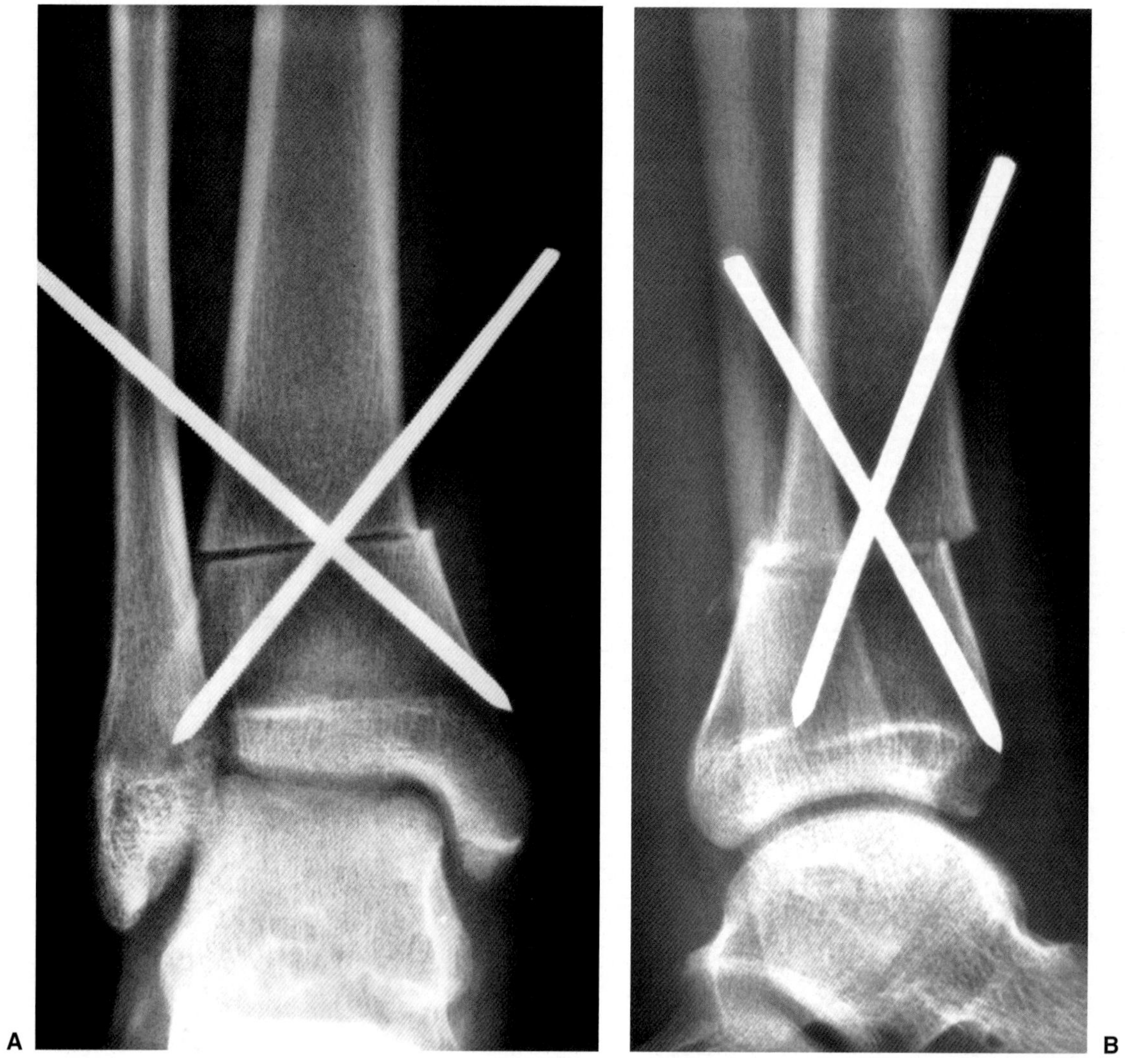

Fig. 2-132 Steinman pins. Anteroposterior (AP) (A) and lateral (B) radiographs following a distal tibial osteotomy with crossed threaded Steinman pins for fixation.

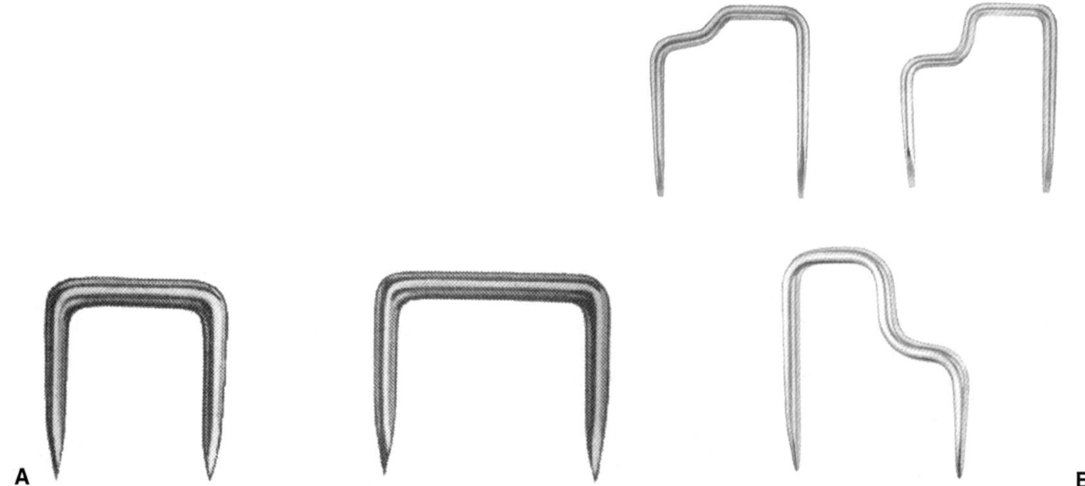


Fig. 2-133 Staples. Orthopaedic staple configurations include fracture staples (A), osteotomy staples (B), barbed staples (C), and table staples (D). Radiographs of the knee demonstrating an osteotomy staple (E) and table staple (F).

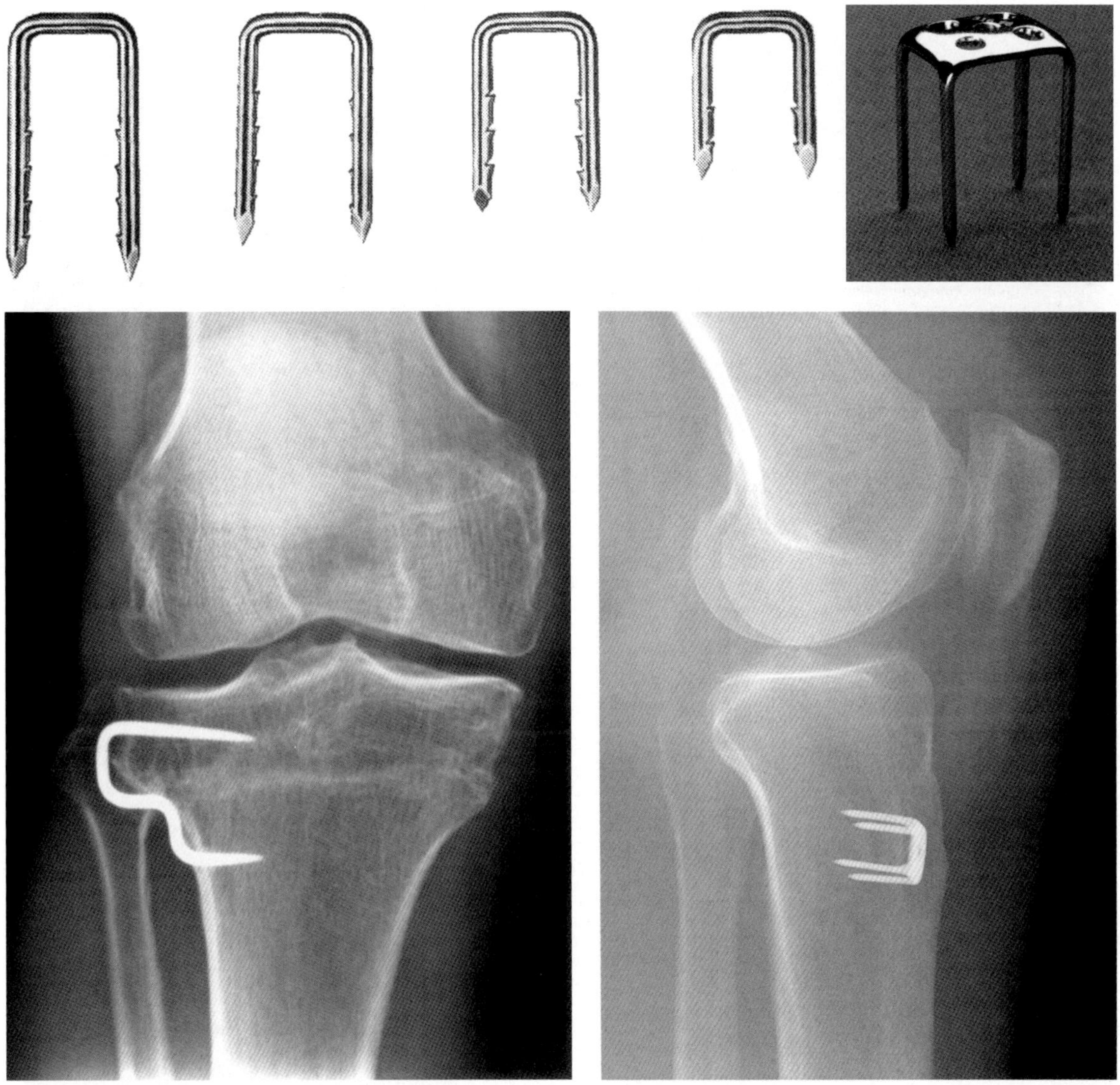

C D E F

Fig. 2-133 *(Continued)*

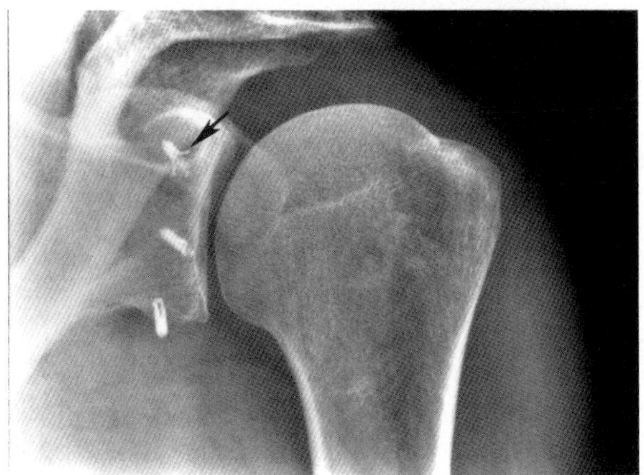

Fig. 2-134 Mitek soft tissue anchors. Radiograph of the shoulder after labral repair with three Mitek soft tissue anchors. The position of the two barbs is seen superiorly (*arrow*).

pins are used depending upon the thickness of cortical bone. The most common indication for traction is complex distal femoral fractures. However, traction is also used for certain humeral fractures. Traction pins in the lower extremity can be placed in one of three sites—supracondylar region of the femur, proximal tibia, and calcaneus. The proximal tibia is most often selected as the site for pin placement (Fig. 2-140). A disadvantage of distal femoral traction pins is quadriceps scarring that may lead to decreased knee function. Calcaneal traction should be avoided due to the increased risk of infection.

## Complications

Complications related to orthopaedic fixation devices vary with anatomic region and the type of procedure. More indepth discussion of complications will be reviewed in subsequent anatomic chapters. However, basic problems are summarized in the subsequent text.

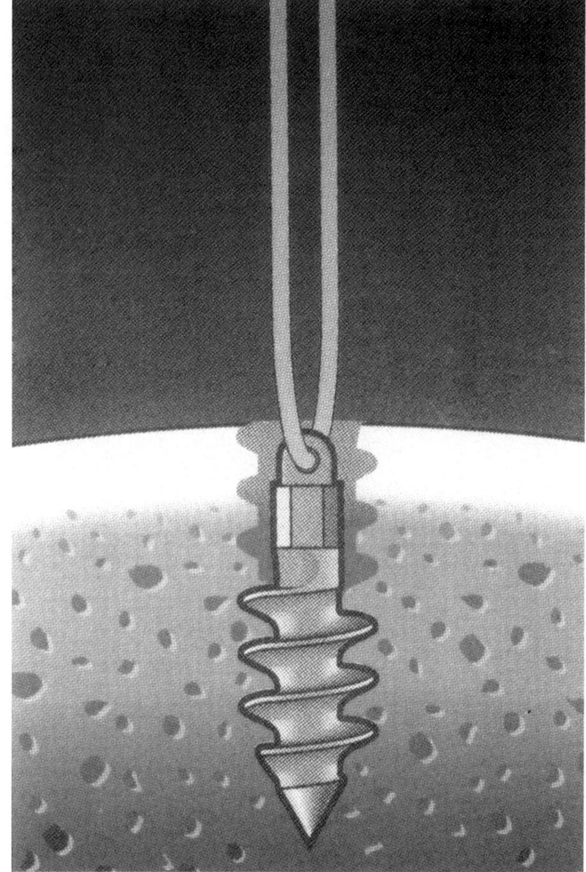


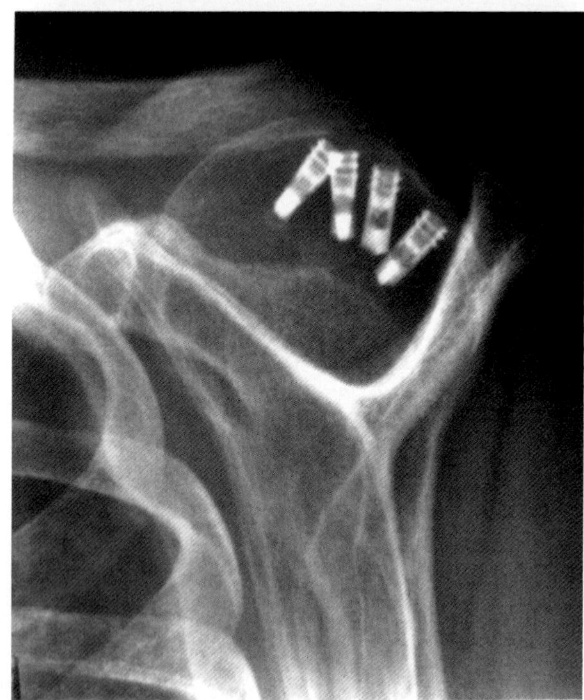


Fig. 2-135 Threaded soft tissue anchors. A: Cancellous Revo soft tissue anchor. (Courtesy CONMED Linvatec, Largo, Florida.) B: Radiograph of the shoulder with four threaded soft tissue anchors for rotator cuff repair.

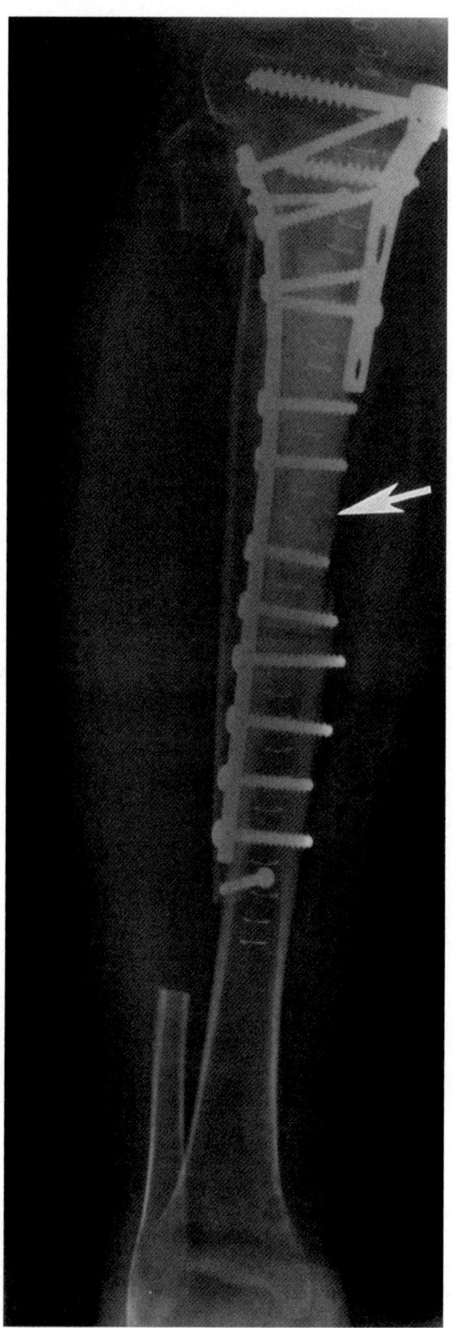

Fig. 2-136 Limb salvage procedure. Anteroposterior (AP) radiograph demonstrates resection of the upper femur and a long section of the fibula with a proximal tibial allograft (*arrow*) and plate and screw fixation.

## Internal Fixation

### Screws and plate-screw fixation

Loosening and screw pullout (see Fig. 2-141)
Soft tissue irritation by protruding screws
Stress risers in screw holes leading to fracture
Infection (see Fig. 2-142)
Delayed union, malunion, nonunion

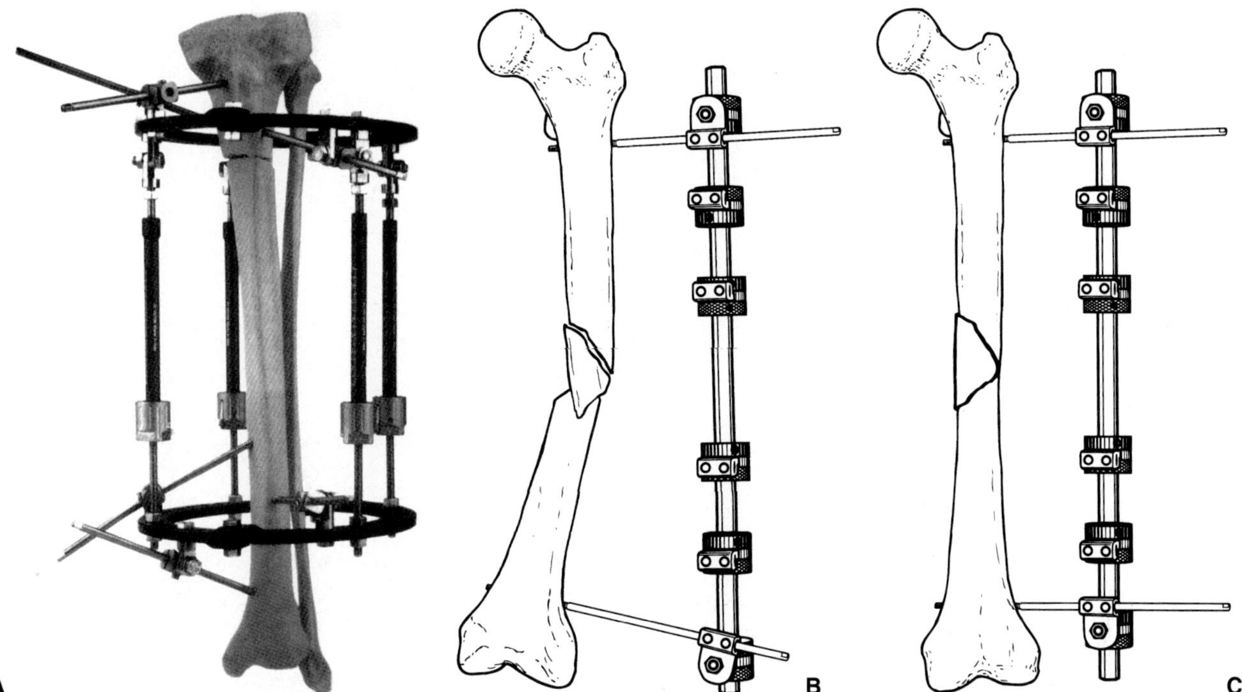


Fig. 2-137 A: Illustration of the Ilizarov ring fixator. B and C: Unilateral Hex-Fix external fixator with pins used to reduce and improve fracture alignment. (Courtesy of Smith and Nephew Richards, Memphis, Tennessee.)

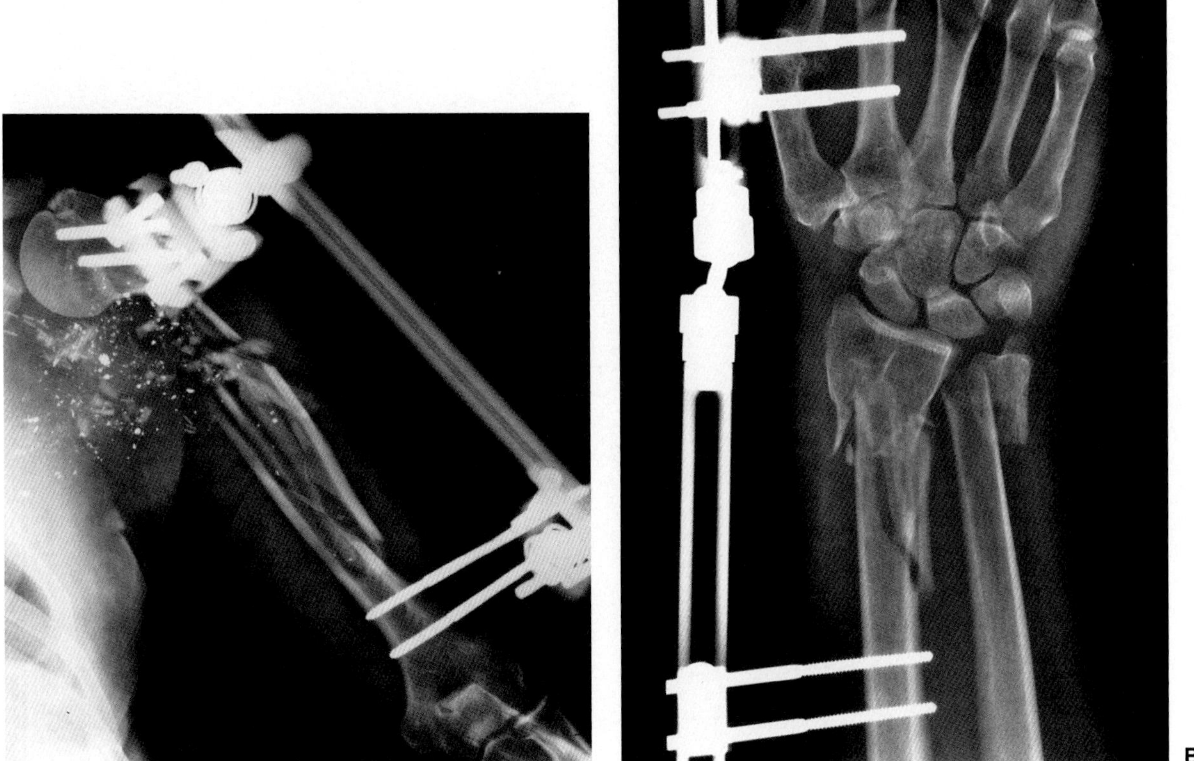


Fig. 2-138 External fixation of the humerus (A) with a unilateral fixator for a complex gunshot wound with severe comminution and (B) a unilateral hinged wrist fixator for complex distal radius and ulnar fractures.

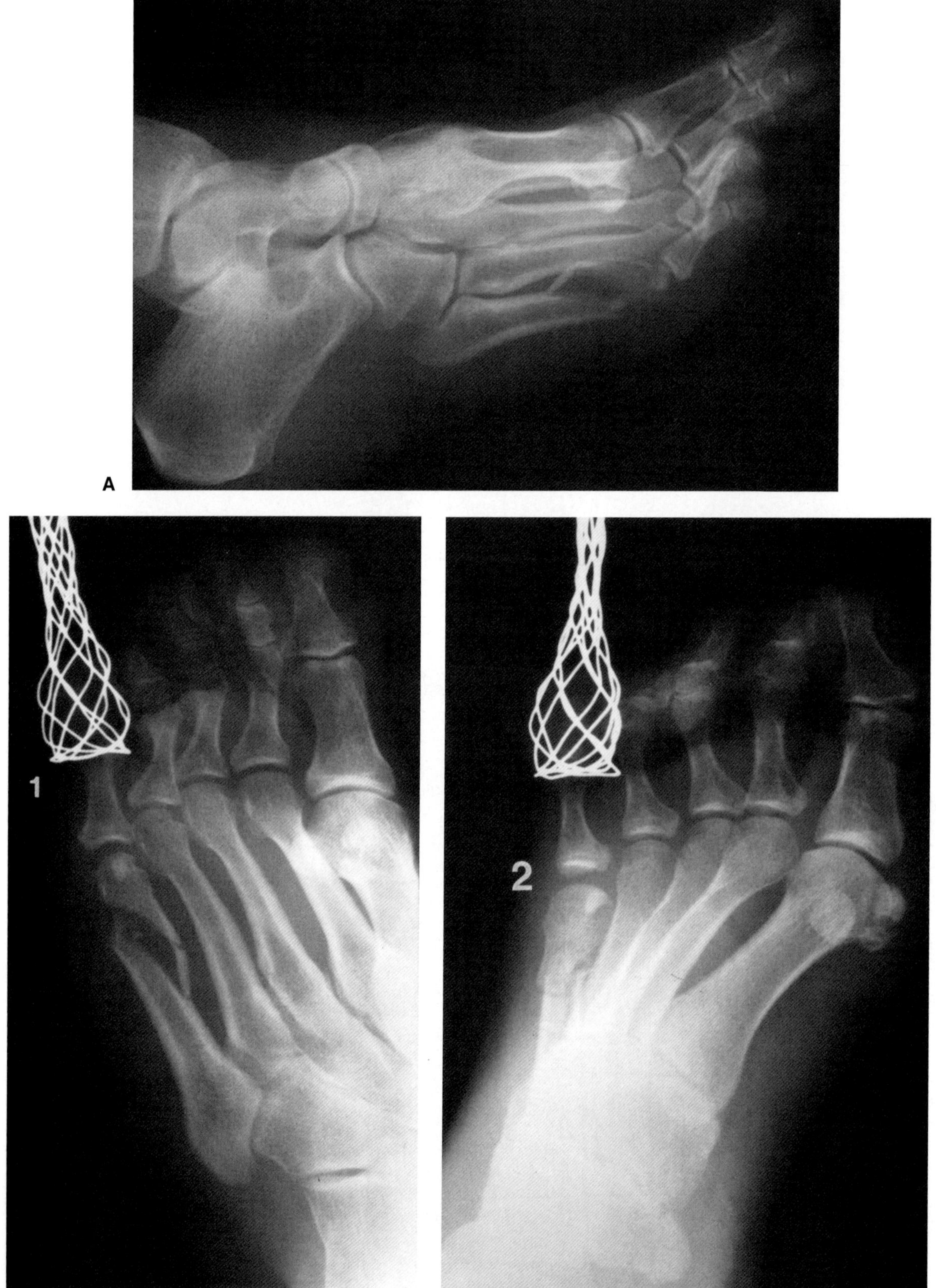


Fig. 2-139 Skin traction. Radiograph of the foot (A) demonstrating a complex distal fifth metatarsal fracture. Sequential images (B and C) obtained during traction to improve alignment before casting.

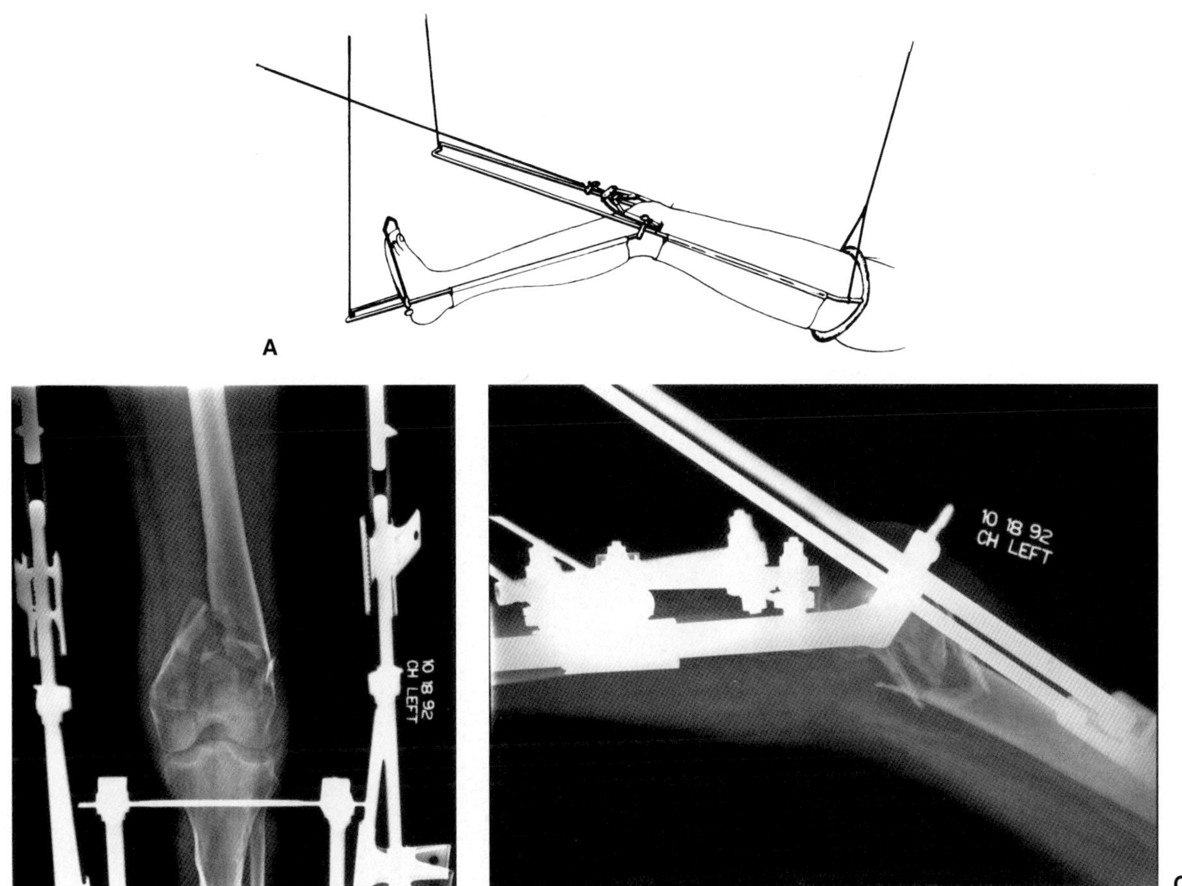


Fig. 2-140 A: Illustration of a skeletal traction system. (Courtesy of Zimmer, Warsaw, Indiana.) Anteroposterior (AP) (B) and lateral (C) radiographs of a complex distal femoral fracture with proximal tibial threaded traction pin.

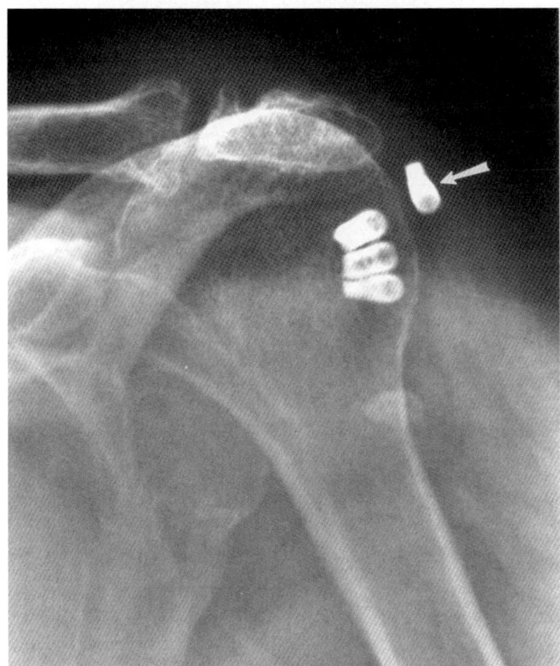

Fig. 2-141 Radiograph of the shoulder in a patient with a failed rotator cuff repair and pulling out one of the soft tissue anchor (*arrow*).

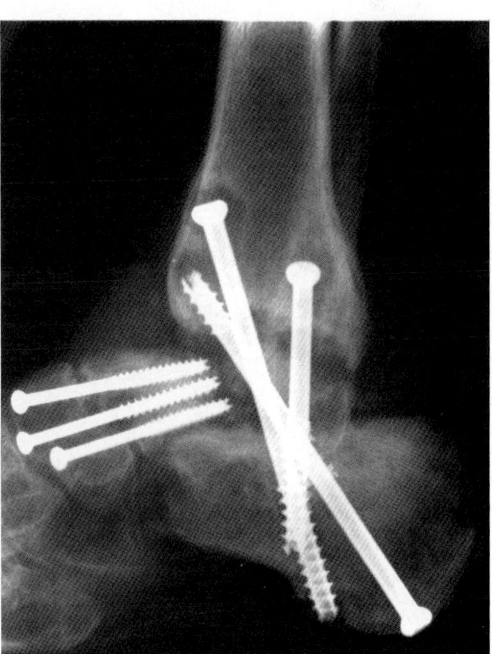

Fig. 2-142 Radiograph of the ankle after tibiocalcaneal and talonavicular arthrodesis. There is considerable lucency about the cannulated tibiocalcaneal screw and irregularity of the distal tibia and remaining talus due to infection and screw loosening.

### Intramedullary rods/nails

- Shortening at the fracture site
- Rotation of fragments
- Instrument failure
- Implant migration (see Fig. 2-143)
- Infection
- Delayed union, nonunion

### Traction/external fixators

- Pin tract infection
- Pin loosening
- Instrument failure
- Delayed union, malunion, nonunion

Implant removal may be required as the result of failure of persistent symptoms related to the implant. Ideally, implants should be left in place until the process requiring the implant has healed. In children, implants are generally removed once they are no longer required to avoid stress shielding and allow more complete bone remodeling. Implants are left in place in elderly and osteopenic patients. In addition, implants in the upper extremity or non–weight bearing bones, the proximal femur and single metaphyseal screws, are also

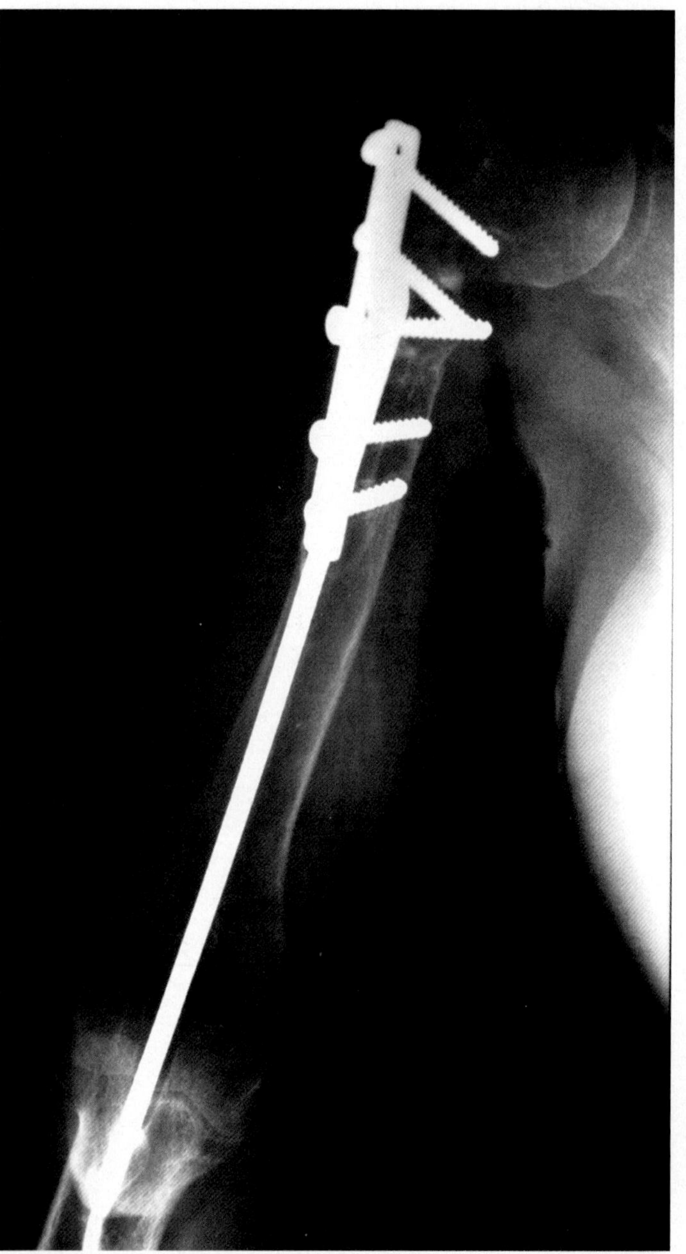


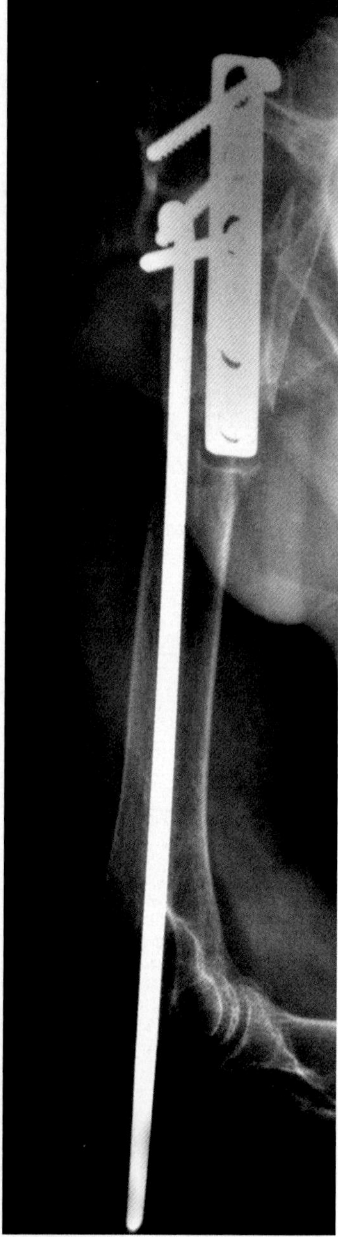


Fig. 2-143 Failed intramedullary fixation of the humerus. A: Anteroposterior (AP) radiograph of the humerus with proximal plate and screw fixation and a long Rush rod. The distal tip of the rod is not clearly seen. B: Lateral radiograph demonstrates that the rod has migrated distally and extended through the elbow and soft tissues.

left in place. More detail is provided in specific anatomic chapters.

## Suggested Reading

Beaman FD, Bancroft LW, Peterson JJ, et al. Imaging characteristics of bone graft materials. *Radiographics*. 2006;26:373–388.

Behrens F. A primer of fixation devices and configurations. *Clin Orthop*. 1989;241:5–14.

Behrens F. General theory and principles of external fixation. *Clin Orthop*. 1989;241:15–23.

Berquist TH, Broderson MP. General orthopaedic fixation devices. In: Berquist TH, ed. *Imaging atlas of orthopaedic appliances and prostheses*. New York: Raven Press; 1995:45–107.

Fragomen AT, Rozbruch R. The mechanics of external fixation. *HSS Journal*. 2007;3:13–29.

Kubiak EN, Fulkerson E, Strauss E, et al. The evolution of locking plates. *J Bone Joint Surg*. 2006;88A:189–200.

Taljanovic MS, Jones MD, Ruth JT, et al. Fracture fixation. *Radiographics*. 2003;23:1569–1590.

Ziran BH, Smith WR. Anglen JO, et al. External fixation: How to make it work. *J Bone Joint Surg*. 2007;89A:1620–1632.

# 3 Spinal Instrumentation

The goals of spinal instrumentation are to provide stability, reduce deformity by restoring and improving anatomic alignment, and reduce pain. Spinal instrumentation techniques have expanded dramatically over the last decade. Fixation devices are designed for the cervical, thoracic, and lumbosacral spine using a variety of surgical techniques involving anterior, posterior, transverse, and combined approaches. In most cases, bone grafting is also performed because instrument failure will eventually result if solid bony fusion is not obtained.

Imaging plays an important role in pre- and postoperative imaging of patients who may be candidates for surgical intervention. Postoperative imaging is particularly important to determine the position of the implants, follow bone graft incorporation or fusion, and to define potential complications. It is critical that radiologists be familiar with surgical techniques, the normal appearance of spinal instrumentation devices, and potential complications associated with the different procedures. Proper use of imaging techniques and knowledge of their advantages and limitations are essential for optimal patient care.

This chapter will focus on spinal instrumentation, including diagnosis, basic clinical data, and imaging of common conditions including scoliosis, trauma, degenerative disease, and spondylolisthesis. Treatment of malignant conditions will be included in Chapter 14.

## Suggested Reading


Berquist TH. Imaging of the postoperative spine. *Radiol Clin North Am.* 2006;44:407–418.


## Scoliosis

Scoliosis is a spinal deformity that can result in complex rotational and lateral curvature of the spine. Deformities may involve isolated or multiple segments. Scoliosis may be congenital (usually vertebral anomalies from birth), idiopathic (infantile, juvenile, or adolescent) or occur in adults following skeletal maturity. Idiopathic adolescent scoliosis is the most common form and is felt to be inherited with incomplete penetrance. Table 3-1 summarizes the etiologies of scoliosis.

### Idiopathic Scoliosis

#### Infantile scoliosis

- Aged 3 years or younger
- More common in males

**Table 3-1**

ETIOLOGY OF SCOLIOSIS

- Idiopathic
  - Infantile
  - Juvenile
  - Adolescent
- Congenital
  - Hemivertebrae
  - Wedge vertebrae
  - Unilateral bars
  - Bilateral bar (block)
  - Neuroskeletal developmental disorders
    - Myelodysplasia
    - Diastematomyelia
    - Meningocele
  - Extraspinal disorders
    - Rib fusions
    - Myositis ossificans progressiva
- Neuromuscular disorders
  - Cerebral palsy
  - Neurofibromatosis
  - Syringomyelia
  - Myopathies
- Skeletal dysplasias
- Trauma
- Metabolic disease
- Neoplasms

- Left curve most common
- Curve <30 degrees usually resolve
- Curves with the progressive form have >70-degree curve by age 10
- Significant curves may cause cardiorespiratory compromise

### Juvenile scoliosis

- More common in females
- Right curve is more common
- Curve progression more common than infantile

### Adolescent scoliosis

- Occurs at or near onset of puberty
- Includes idiopathic scoliosis diagnosed after age 10
- Curve must be >10 degrees
- Occurs in 2% to 3% of children in the age-group of 10 to 16 years
- Family history in 15% to 20% of cases
- Curves <30 degrees at maturity usually do not progress
- Treatment more often required in females

### Adult scoliosis

- Scoliosis occurring after maturity
- Multiple etiologies (Table 3-1)
- Thoracic curves most often treated
- Curve progression and pain are indications for surgery

### Congenital scoliosis

- Commonly caused by vertebral anomalies (Table 3-1)
- Unilateral bars progress most rapidly
- Prognosis also less favorable for multiple hemivertebrae
- Other organ anomalies are not uncommon
- Lumbar curves more commonly associated with genitourinary and lower extremity anomalies
- Thoracic curves more often associated with cardiac anomalies

## Clinical Features

Scoliosis is relatively common and 70% to 80% of cases are idiopathic. Therefore, school screening has been performed across the country for quite some time. On examination, there is back asymmetry and there may be a noticeable deformity of the ribs. There may also be tilt of the shoulders and/or pelvis. Clinical curve measurements of >10 degrees are considered significant.

Measured on radiographs, curves of <10 degrees are not considered scoliosis. Two percent to 3% of children in the age-group of 10 to 16 will have scoliotic curves >10 degrees. The male to female ratio is approximately equal with smaller curves. However, measurements of >30 degrees are much more common in females. Whether curves progress depends on growth potential and specific curve patterns to be discussed later. Curve changes tend to be most significant during growth spurts. Curves ≤30 degrees typically do not progress after skeletal maturity. However, larger curves frequently progress into adulthood. Curves from 10 to 30 degrees should be followed approximately every 6 months as progression tends to occur at approximately 1 degree per month. Radiographic measurements may normally vary by 4 degrees due to human error. Therefore, the 6-month rule was established to more accurately evaluate curve progression.

Progressive curvature may result in significant cosmetic deformity and secondary effects on other organ systems such as the heart and lungs. Current treatment options include observation for small curves, electrical stimulation, braces, and surgical intervention. Curves of 30 to 50 degrees are initially treated conservatively with braces to reduce progression. Curves >50 degrees generally require surgical intervention.

## Suggested Reading


Berquist TH, Currier BL, Broderick DF. The spine. In: Berquist TH, ed. *Imaging atlas of orthopaedic appliances and prostheses*. New York: Raven Press; 1995:109–215.

Connolly PJ, Von Schroeder HP, Johnson GE, et al. Adolescent scoliosis. *J Bone Joint Surg*. 1995;77A:1210–1215.

Jarvis JG, Greene RN. Adolescent idiopathic scoliosis. *J Bone Joint Surg*. 1996;78A:1707–1713.

Lonstein JE. Scoliosis: Surgical versus nonsurgical treatment. *Clin Orthop*. 2006;443:248–259.

Oestreich AE, Young LW, Poussaint TY. Scoliosis circa 2000: Radiologic imaging perspective. I. Diagnosis and pretreatment evaluation. *Skeletal Radiol*. 1998;27:591–605.


## Scoliosis Terminology

**Compensatory curve:** A secondary curve located above or below the structural curve; develops to maintain body alignment

**Decompensation:** Loss of the spinal balance when the thoracic cage is not centered over the pelvis

**Dextroscoliosis:** Curve convexity is to the right

**Double curve:** Two curves in the same spine

**Functional curve:** Nonstructural or correctable by active or passive lateral bending or corrects when in the supine position

**Kyphoscoliosis:** Structural scoliosis associated with round back deformity

**Kyphosis:** Posterior convex angle of the spine seen in the sagittal plane

**Levoscoliosis:** Scoliosis with curve convex to the left

**Lordoscoliosis:** Lateral curvature of the spine associated with swayback

**Lordosis:** Anterior curvature of the spine in the saggital plane

**Lumbar curve:** Spinal curve with the apex between L1 and L4

**Lumbosacral curve:** Lateral curve with the apex at L5 or below

**Major curve:** Structural

**Minor curve:** Nonstructural curve

**Nonstructural curve:** Curve that is not fixed

**Primary curve:** First or earliest curve to appear

**Scoliosis:** Lateral curvature of the spine >10 degrees on radiographs

**Structural curve:** Lateral curve that is fixed

**Thoracic curve:** Lateral curve with apex between T2 and T11

**Thoracolumbar curve:** Lateral curve with the apex at T12 or L1

## Suggested Reading

Dangerfield PH. The classification of spinal deformities. *Pediatr Rehabil.* 2003;6:133–136.

Oestreich AE, Young LW, Poussaint TY. Scoliosis circa 2000: radiologic imaging perspective. I. Diagnosis and pretreatment evaluation. *Skeletal Radiol.* 1998;27:591–605.

Scoliosis Research Society. *Definition of Scoliosis Terms.* 2007.

## Classification/Curve Measurements

Scoliosis may be classified by age of onset, underlying pathology, anatomic involvement, or curve patterns. For the purpose of this discussion, the focus will be on classifications systems and measurements. There are multiple measurement approaches to include curve and rotational deformities. The Cobb method is most commonly used to measure curves and can be applied to single, double, or triple curves.

### Cobb Measurement Method

- Select upper and lower end vertebrae; vertebrae directed maximally to the concavity of the curve
- Vertebrae included have widened disc spaces on the convex side
- Lines are drawn along the most superior and inferior endplates or pedicles of the selected end vertebrae (see Fig. 3-1)
- For large angles the lines may cross; for smaller angles, lines are drawn perpendicular to the end vertebral lines to form the angle

### Rotational Measurements

- Use apex vertebra in the curve and determine the position of the pedicles or spinous process (see Fig. 3-2)
- Pedicle method is preferred

### Kyphosis Measurements

- The end vertebrae that are maximally directed to the convexity are selected
- Lines are drawn along the superior end plate of the upper end vertebrae and inferior endplate of the lower end vertebrae (see Fig. 3-3)
- For large curves the lines will cross

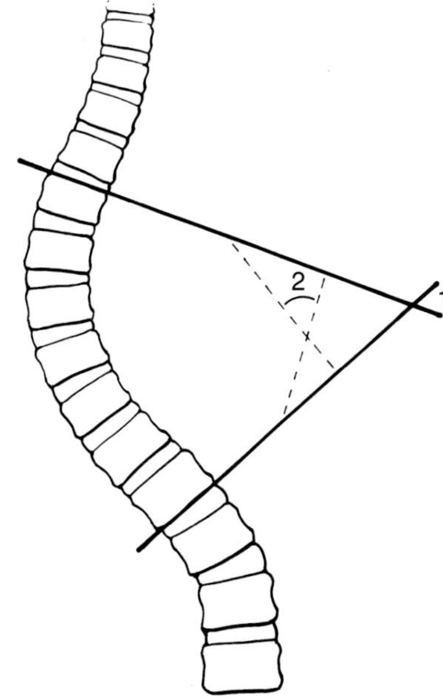


Fig. 3-1 Cobb method for measuring spinal curves. Lines are drawn along the upper vertebral margin or pedicles of the superior end vertebra and lower margin or pedicle of the inferior end vertebra. For larger curves the lines may cross giving the angle (*1*), for smaller curves lines are drawn perpendicular to the end vertebral lines to provide the angle (*2*).

- For smaller kyphotic deformities lines are drawn perpendicular to the end vertebral lines resulting in the measurement

### King Classification

Useful for predicting extent of spinal fusion; it is two dimensional and ignores sagittal profile. There are five curve categories, which are as follows.

**Type I:** "S" shaped with both thoracic and lumbar curves crossing midline; lumbar more severe and thoracic more flexible (see Fig. 3-4A)

**Type II:** Similar to type I except that thoracic curve is larger (Fig. 3-4B)

**Type III:** Lumbar curve does not cross the midline and is centered over the sacrum (Fig. 3-4C)

**Type IV:** Long thoracic curve with L5 centered over the sacrum and L4 tilted to the thoracic curve (Fig. 3-4D)

**Type V:** Double thoracic curve with T1 tilted to the concavity of the upper curve, which is structural (Fig. 3-4E)

### Lenke Classification

Defines six curve types with modifiers for the lumbar spine in the frontal plane and thoracic spine in the sagittal plane

**Lumbar modifier:** Based on relationship of apex of the curve to central vertical sacral line (CVSL) (see Fig. 3-5) A-minimal lumbar curve, B-moderate lumbar curve, C-large lumbar curve

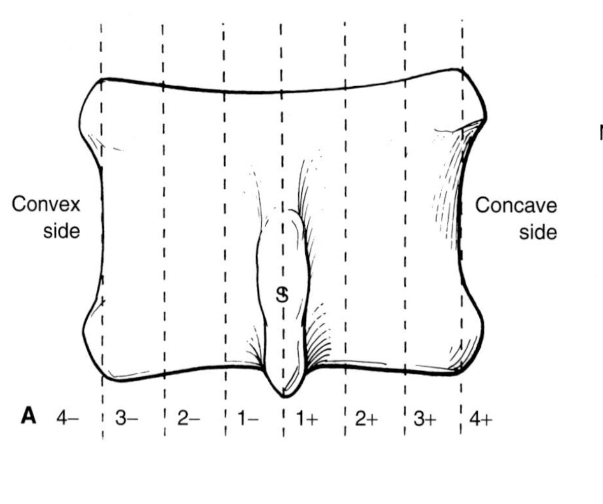


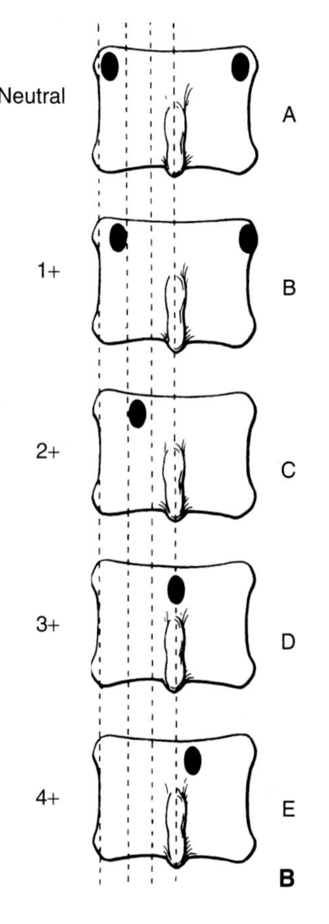


**Fig. 3-2** Rotational measurements. **A:** Spinous process method. The vertebral body is divided into six segments (*vertical broken lines*). Neutral is used when the spinous process is midline. Positive is used for rotation toward the concavity and negative toward the convexity of the curve with grading from 1 to 4. **B:** Pedicle method. *A*—pedicles in normal position, *B*—right pedicle moves toward the midline and left at vertebral margin, *C*—right pedicle moves closer to midline and left not seen, *D*—right pedicle at midline and left not seen, *E*—right pedicle beyond the midline and left not seen.

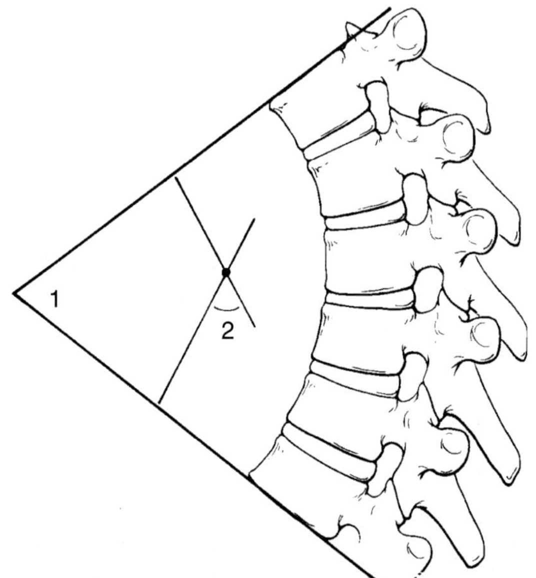


**Fig. 3-3** Kyphosis measurement. The upper and lower end vertebrae are selected in a manner similar to scoliosis measurements. Lines are drawn along the endplates. For larger angles the line may cross (*1*), for smaller angles perpendicular lines are drawn to the end vertebral lines resulting in the measurement (*2*).

**Thoracic modifier:** Based on the sagittal curve measurement from T5-12 minus curve of <+10 degrees, neutral curve of 10 to 40 degrees, positive curve of >+40 degrees (see Fig. 3-6)

- **Type 1:** Main thoracic—main thoracic curve is the major curve and proximal thoracic and thoracolumbar curves are minor or nonstructural
- **Type 2:** Double thoracic—main thoracic curve is major curve, the proximal thoracic curve is minor and structural, and the thoracolumbar curve is minor and nonstructural
- **Type 3:** Double major—main thoracic and thoracolumbar curves are structural, whereas the proximal thoracic curve is nonstructural
- **Type 4:** Triple major—proximal, main thoracic, and thoracolumbar are all structural; either of the latter two may be the major curve
- **Type 5:** Thoracolumbar/lumbar—thoracolumbar/lumbar curve is the major curve and structural; proximal thoracic and main thoracic are nonstructural
- **Type 6:** Thoracolumbar/lumbar-main thoracic; thoracolumbar/lumbar curve is the major curve and measures ≥5 degrees more than the main thoracic curve that is structural; proximal thoracic curve is nonstructural

## Three Dimensional Classification

It includes scoliosis, kyphosis, and sagittal and curve profiles plus rotational component

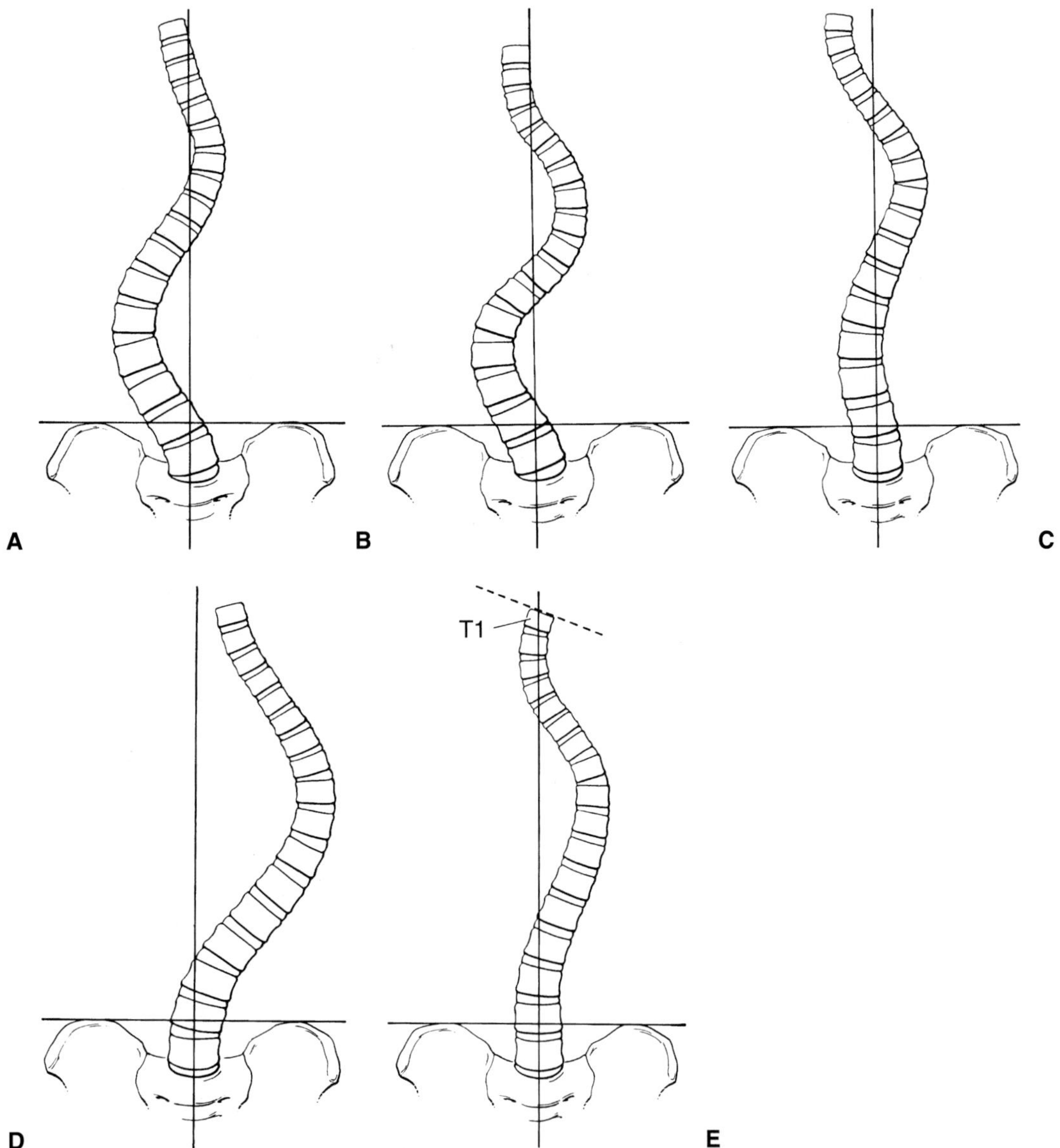


Fig. 3-4 King classification of curve patterns. A: Type I—"S" shaped pattern with both the thoracic and lumbar curves crossing the midline. The lumbar curve is larger and less flexible. B: Type II—"S" shaped curve with more severe and less flexible thoracic component. C: Type III—lumbar curve does not cross the midline and is centered over the sacrum. D: Type IV—long thoracic curve with L4 directed to the thoracic curve. E: Type V—double thoracic curve with T1 directed to the concavity of the upper curve. The upper curve is the structural curve.

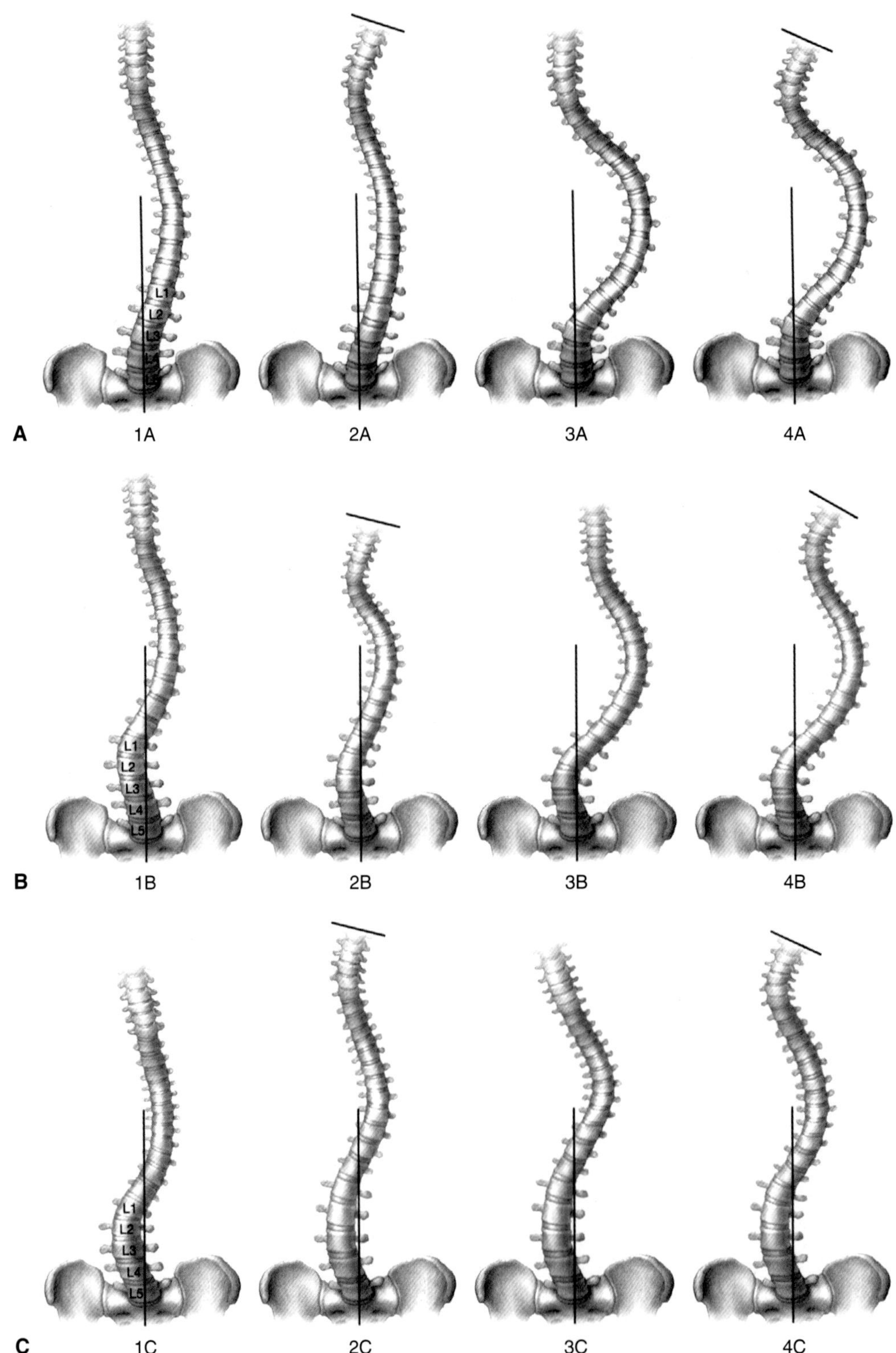


Fig. 3-5 Lumbar modifiers. **A:** Type A—minimal lumbar curve: 1A—major thoracic curve, 2A—double thoracic, 3A—double major curves, 4A—triple major. **B:** Type B—moderate lumbar curve: 1B—major thoracic curve, 2B—double thoracic curve, 3B—double major curves, 4B—triple major. **C:** Type C—large lumbar curve: 1C—major thoracic curve, 2C—double thoracic, 3C—double major curves, 4C—triple major curves.

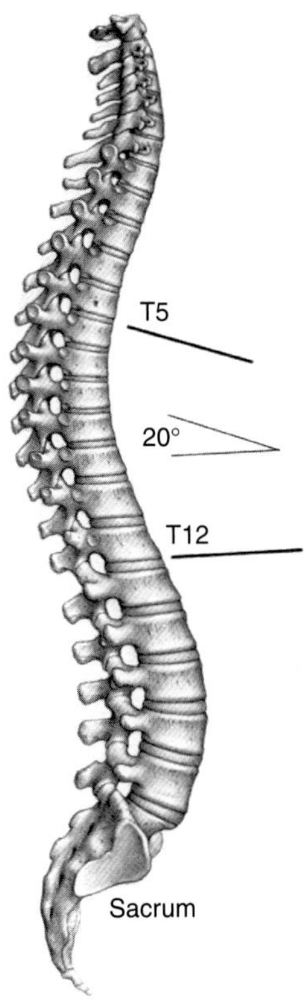


Fig. 3-6 Sagittal thoracic modifiers. Measurements from T5 to T12. Minus curve <10 degrees, neutral curve 10 to 40 degrees, positive curve >40 degrees. In this example the curve is 20 degrees therefore falls in the neutral curve range.

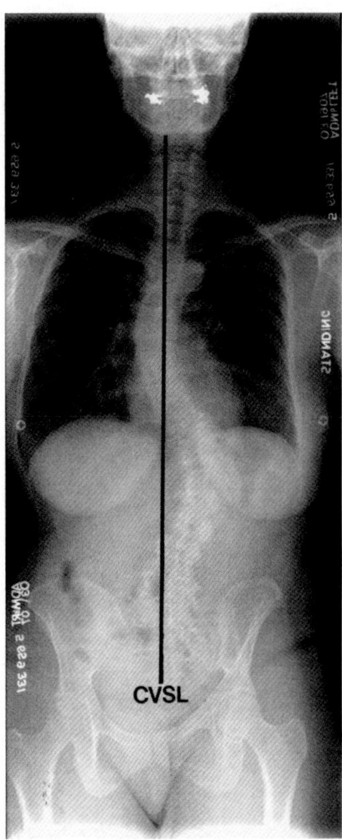


Fig. 3-7 Standing posteroanterior (PA) radiograph with thoracic and lumbar curves. The central vertical sacral line (CVSL) extends vertically through the mid-sacrum. Both curves cross the midline with the lumbar curve being more exaggerated.

## Suggested Reading

Dangerfield PH. The classification of spinal deformities. *Pediatr Rehabil.* 2003;6:133–136.

King HA, Moe JH, Bradford DS, et al. The selection and fusion levels in thoracic idiopathic scoliosis. *J Bone Joint Surg.* 1983;65A:1302–1313.

Lenke LG, Betz RR, Harms J, et al. Adolescent idiopathic scoliosis: A new classification to determine the extent of spinal arthrodesis. *J Bone Joint Surg.* 2001;83A:1169–1181.

Poncet P, Dansereau J, Labelle H. Geometric torsion in idiopathic scoliosis: Three-dimensional analysis and proposal for a new classification. *Spine.* 2001;26:2235–2243.

### Imaging of Scoliosis

Imaging of scoliosis begins with quality full-length standing radiographs of the entire spine. Radiographs are essential for curve measurement, classification, and treatment planning. Detection of congenital anomalies can also be accomplished radiographically. The number and type of views may vary with the patient's age, clinical status, and type of curve detected clinically. Orthopaedic surgeons rely on the standing anteroposterior (PA), lateral, and lateral bending views. The latter allow assessment of curves to determine if they are fixed (structural) in which case they do not change, or nonstructural in which case they correct when bending to the convex side.

**Posteroanterior (PA) radiograph:** Should include the occiput to the sacrum (see Fig. 3-7)
- Use central vertical sacral line to evaluate curves
- Cobb method to measure curves (Fig. 3-1)
- Pedicle or spinous process method to measure rotation (Fig. 3-2)

**Lateral bending radiographs:** Same field of view as PA radiographs
- Measure changes in curves using same end vertebrae
- With multiple curves, the degree of correction is important
- If lumbar correction exceeds thoracic, only the thoracic is fused
- When lumbar correction is less than thoracic both are fused

**Lateral radiograph:** Should include occiput to hips (see Fig. 3-8)
- Evaluate lumbar lordosis using L1-5
- Evaluate thoracic kyphosis T4-12
- T9 offset using vertical line from the hip
- Sacral slope
- Pelvic tilt
- Vertebral height T9-S1
- Disc space height and symmetry

**Special studies:** In certain cases computed tomography (CT) or magnetic resonance imaging (MRI)

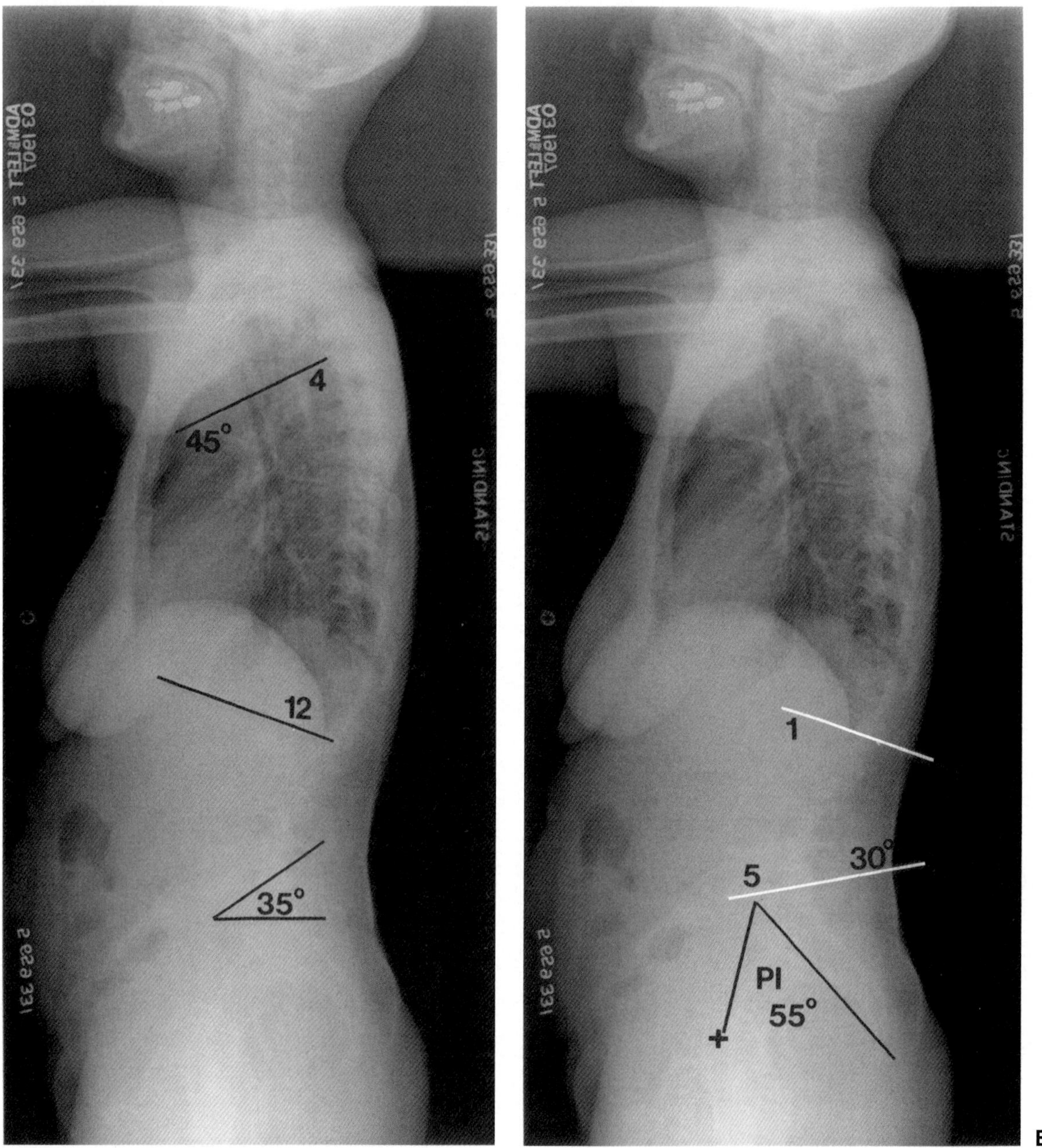


Fig. 3-8 Standing lateral radiograph of the spine. A: Sacral slope is the angle formed by a horizontal line and the end plate of S1 (range 17 to 63 degrees, mean 42 degrees); in this case it is 35 degrees. Thoracic kyphosis measured from the endplates of T12 and T4 (mean 41 degrees, range 0 to 69 degrees); in this case 45 degrees. B: Lumbar lordosis measured from the endplates of L1 and L5 (14 to 69 degrees, mean 43 degrees); in this case 30 degrees. The pelvic incidence (PI) is a key parameter for spinal balance and is measured by a line perpendicular to the center of the sacral end plate and a second line from the central femoral axis (+) to the center of the sacral end plate (range 33 to 82 degrees, mean 55 degrees) in this case 55 degrees.

may be required to fully evaluate the curves, spinal canal, or associated congenital anomalies. Thin-section CT with reformatting in the sagittal, coronal, and oblique planes or three-dimensional reconstructions may be required. On occasion, discograms and facet injections may be required to confirm symptomatic levels.

## Suggested Reading

Berquist TH. Imaging of the postoperative spine. *Radiol Clin North Am.* 2006;44:407–418.

Lenke LG, Betz RR, Harms J, et al. Adolescent idiopathic scoliosis: A new classification to determine the extent of spinal arthrodesis. *J Bone Joint Surg.* 2001;83A:1169–1181.

Oestreich AE, Young LW, Poussaint TY. Scoliosis circa 2000: Radiologic imaging perspective. I. Diagnosis and pretreatment evaluation. *Skeletal Radiol.* 1998;27:591–605.

Vialle R, Levassor N, Rillardon L, et al. Radiographic analysis of the sagittal alignment and balance of the spine in asymptomatic subjects. *J Bone Joint Surg.* 2005;87A:260–267.

## Treatment of Scoliosis

Management of scoliosis may be complex requiring multiple or combined approaches depending on the degree of involvement and the likelihood of curve progression. Treatment options include simple observation and follow-up, bracing, and surgical intervention with spinal arthrodesis. The most important initial decision is whether or not the curve will progress if not treated. The risk of progression is increased with larger curves and in females. In children and adolescents, curves up to 30 degrees tend not to progress. Curves of 30 to 39 degrees in a child are a good indication for bracing as 68% progress. Curves >45 to 50 degrees usually progress and are an indication for surgical arthrodesis. A brace treated curve that progresses 45 to 50 degrees is also an indication for surgical intervention. In adults, there is often associated degenerative disease and concern regarding cosmetic appearance and pain. For purposes of this text the focus will be on options for operative instrumentation. Instrumentation may include short or long segments and anterior, posterior, or combined approaches.

### Anterior Instrumentation

Usually used for short-segment scoliosis or in combination with other systems. Examples include the following:

**Dwyer instrumentation** (see Fig. 3-9)

**Indications**

Lumbar and thoracic idiopathic scoliosis
Neurogenic scoliosis
Lordotic spinal deformities

**Instrumentation:** Flexible titanium cable; cancellous screws cannulated for the cable and staples

**Advantages:** Excellent correction of primary curve

**Disadvantages:** Cable rupture; kyphotic affect; not effective for multiple curves

**Zielke instrumentation**

**Indications:** Idiopathic and degenerative lumbar or thoracic scoliosis

**Instrumentation:** Similar to Dwyer except that cable replaced with stainless steel rod

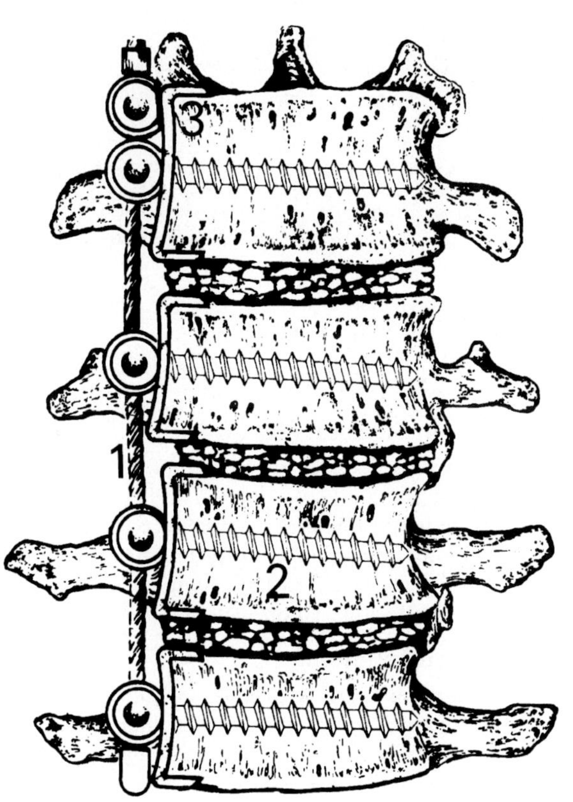


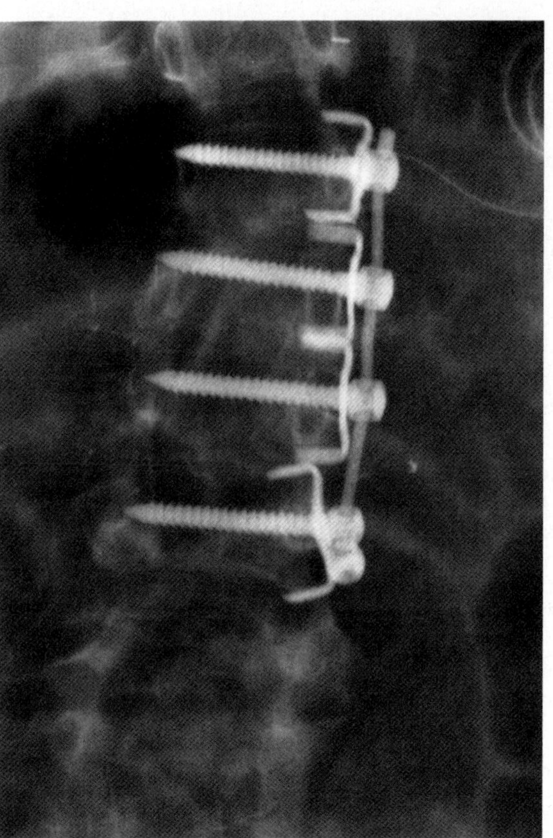


Fig. 3-9 Dwyer instrumentation. A: Illustration of Dwyer fixation with flexible cable (*1*), cancellous screw with central hole in the head for cable (*2*), vertebral staple (*3*). (Courtesy of Zimmer, Warsaw, Indiana.) B: Anteroposterior (AP) radiograph on a patient with Dwyer instrumentation.

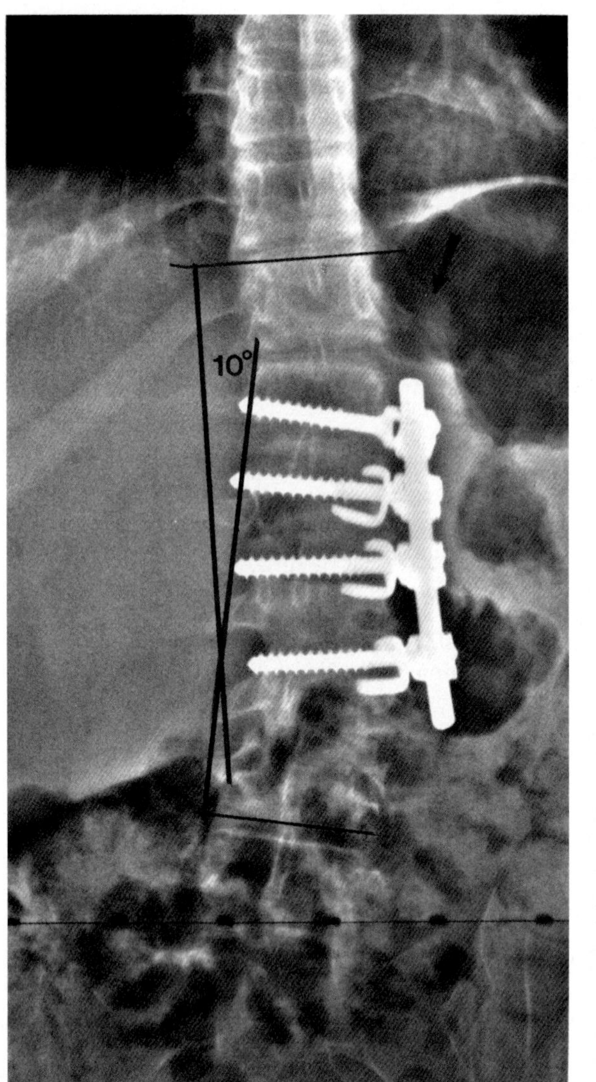


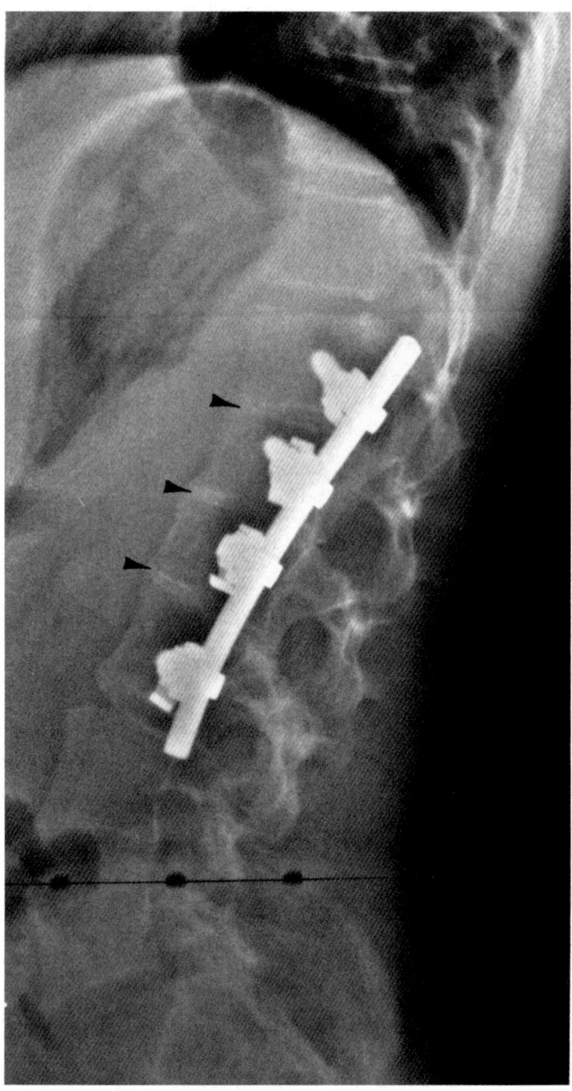


**Fig. 3-10** Texas Scottish Rite Hospital (TSRH) instrumentation. Anteroposterior (AP) (**A**) and lateral (**B**) radiographs after anterior TSRH instrumentation. Note the rod replaces the cable used in the Dwyer system. The twelfth rib (*arrow* in **A**) has been resected and used for interbody fusion (*arrowheads*).

**Advantages:** Improved derotation capability; avoids excess kyphosis

**Disadvantages:** More difficult procedure; solid fusion more difficult to obtain with larger curves

### Texas Scottish Rite Hospital Instrumentation (see Fig. 3-10)

Similar to the description in the preceding text; uses a single rod, screws, staples, and washers

## Posterior Instrumentation

Usually used for longer segment scoliosis procedures; multiple systems available

### Harrington instrumentation (see Fig. 3-11)

**Indications:** Longer segment thoracic and lumbar scoliosis

**Instrumentation:** Two rod systems, one for distraction and one for compression; distraction has collar on one end and ratches on the other; compression rod is threaded; hooks are attached to create compression or distraction

### Moe instrumentation

**Indications:** Long-segment thoracic or lumbar scoliosis

**Instrumentation:** Similar to Harrington except that the rod is square distal to the collar and hooks have square holes to reduce rotation

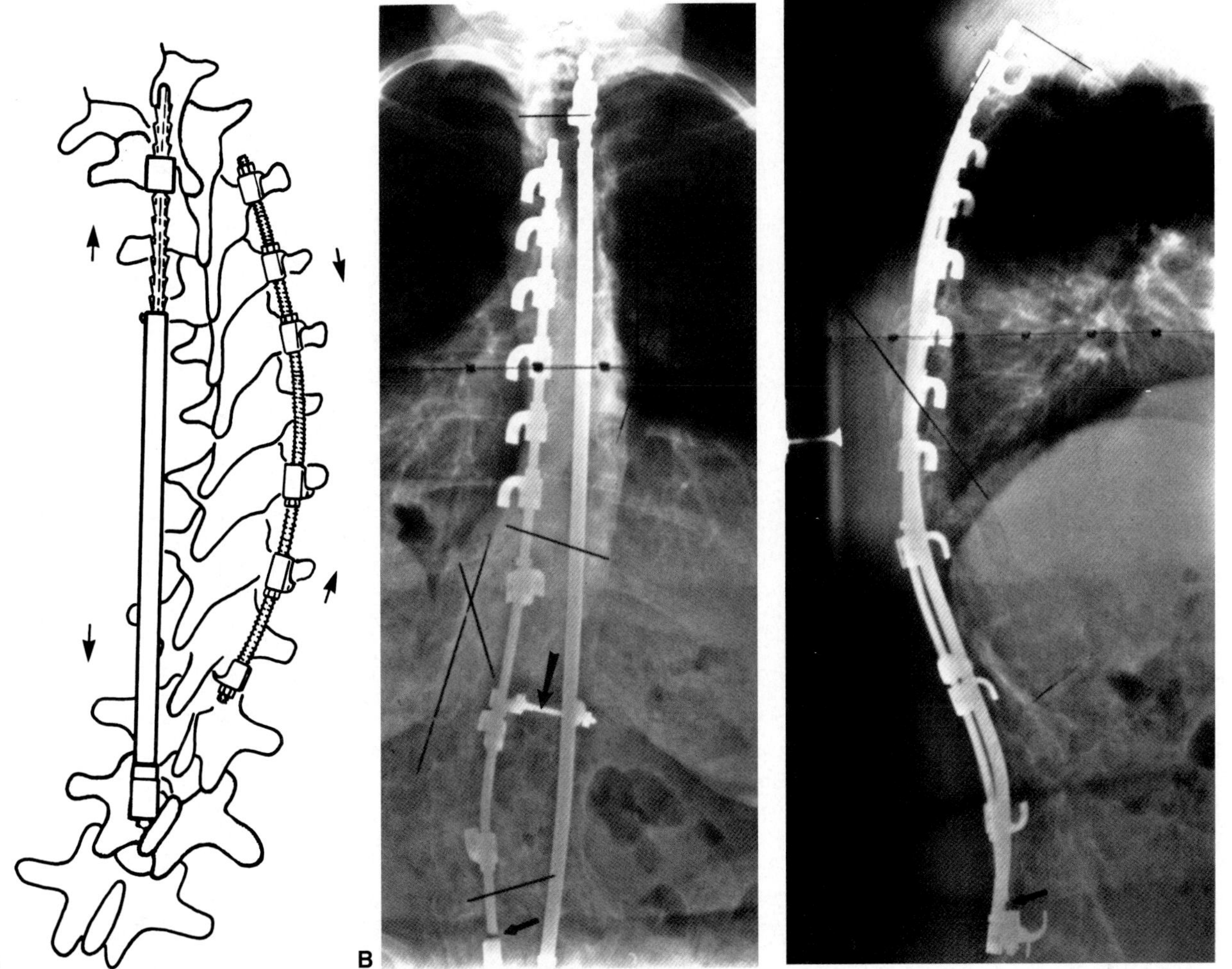


Fig. 3-11 Harrington instrumentation. A: Illustration of Harrington instrumentation with a threaded compression rod on the right (*arrows*) and a distraction rod on the left (*arrows*) with ratchets superiorly. Anteroposterior (AP) (B) and lateral (C) radiographs with compression rod on the right and distraction rod on the left. There is a cross-link for stability (*arrow*) and a fracture in the distal compression rod (*small black arrow*).

## Luque Instrumentation (see Fig. 3-12)

**Indications:** Scoliosis and congenital deformities

**Instrumentation:** Smooth straight or "L" shaped rods with sublaminar wires instead of hooks

**Advantages:** Corrective forces applied at each vertebral level

**Disadvantages:** Sublaminar wires may cause neurologic damage

### Wisconsin Instrumentation

Similar to Luque instrumentation except that wires pass through the base of the spinous process with paired buttons to protect the bone

## Corel-Dubousset Instrumentation (see Fig. 3-13)

**Indications:** Long-segment scoliosis

**Instrumentation:** Diamond knurled coated rods to improve hook fixation; hooks similar to Harrington system but have set screws to improve fixation to rod and designed for lamina, pedicle, or transverse process placement; transverse crosslinks for three-dimensional stability

**Advantages:** Improved frontal plane correction and kyphosis; maintains lumbar lordosis; postoperative bracing not needed

**Disadvantages:** Rigid fixation may stress the spine to be shielded; increased instrumentation decreases space for bone graft

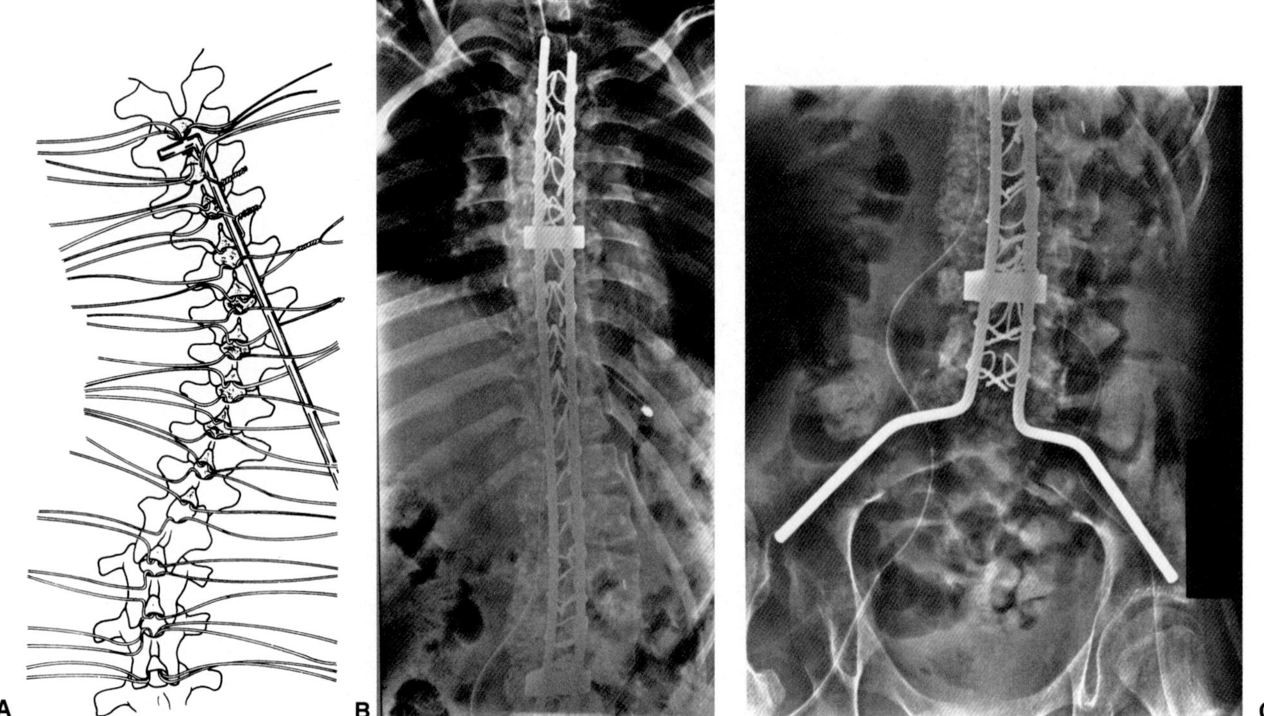

Fig. 3-12 Luque instrumentation. A: Illustration of sublaminar wires and rod placement. The rod is smooth with no ratchets or hooks. Anteroposterior (AP) radiographs (B and C) after Luque rod and sublaminar wire placement for scoliosis. Note the extensive bone grafting on the right.

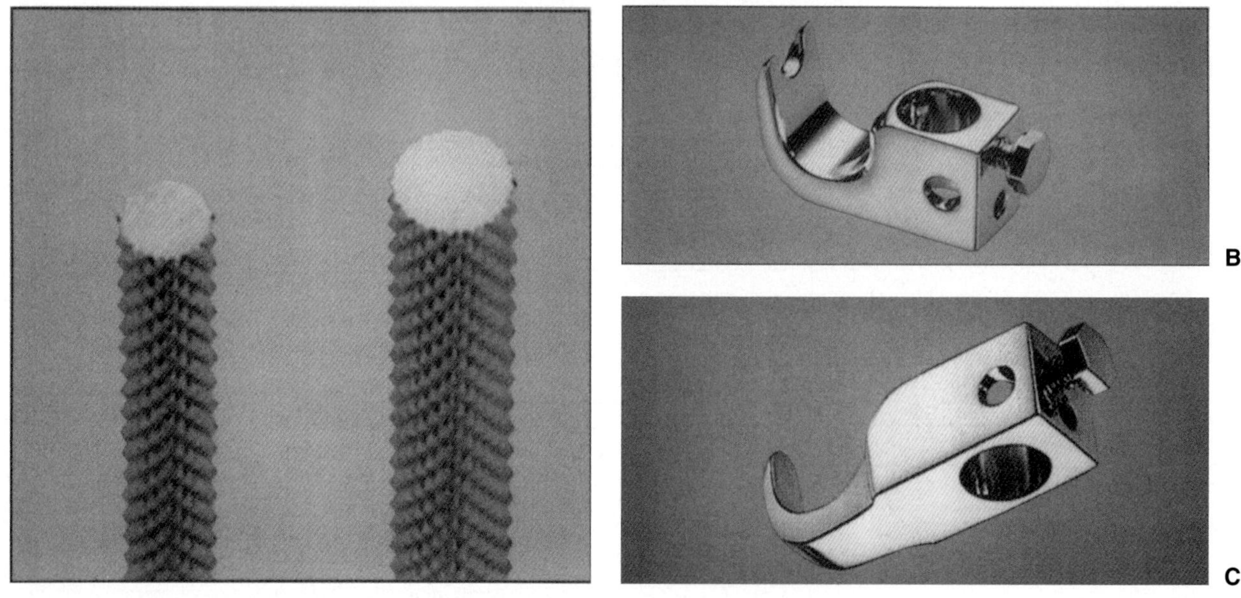

Fig. 3-13 Cotrel-Dubousset instrumentation. Diamond-pointed rod surface (A), various hook configurations with set screws to secure the hook to the rod (B and C), sacral screws (D) and crosslinks (E), and system attached to bone model (F). (Courtesy of Stuart Specialty, Spine Division, Greensburg, Pennsylvania.) Anteroposterior (AP) (G) and lateral (H) radiographs after Cotrel-Duboussett instrumentation with transverse stabilizers proximally and distally.

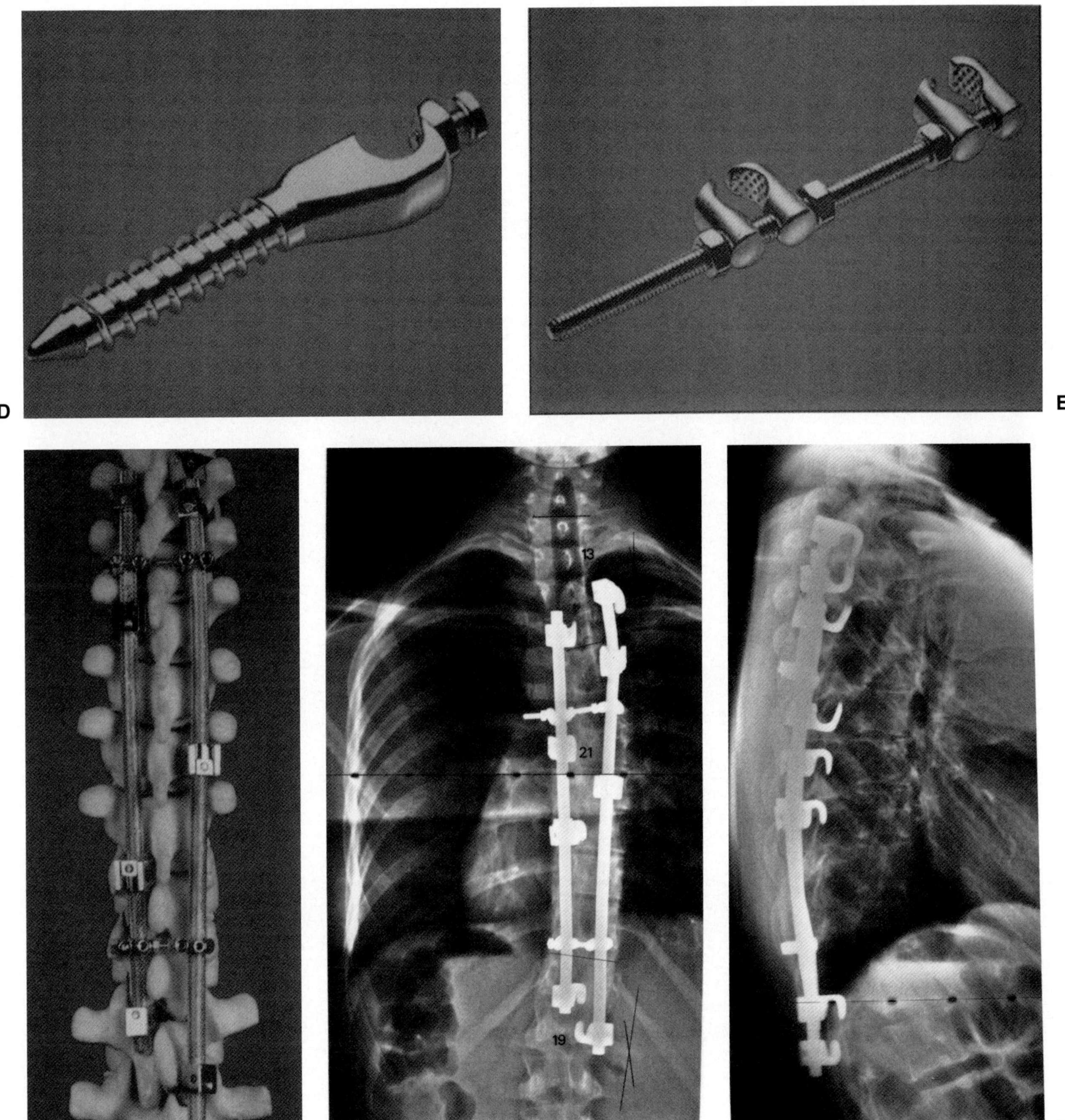


Fig. 3-13 *(Continued)*

### Texas Scottish Rite Hospital Instrumentation

**Indications:** Long- or short-segment scoliosis; may be used anteriorly or posteriorly

**Instrumentation:** Rods smooth with hexagonal ends, hooks, eye bolt connectors for crosslinks, cancellous screws

### ISOLA Instrumentation (see Fig. 3-14)

Designed to simplify the number of implants and improve sacral fixation

**Instrumentation**: Multiple rod configurations, hooks, cancellous screws, rod connectors, crosslinks, spacers, and washers

**Advantages**: Three-dimensional stability and minimal postoperative support required

**Minimally Invasive Spine Instrumentation System:** Similar to the description in the preceding text with ability to use rods, hooks, and pedicle screws. Instruments inserted through small incisions with screws placed percutaneously over guide wires (see Fig. 3-15)

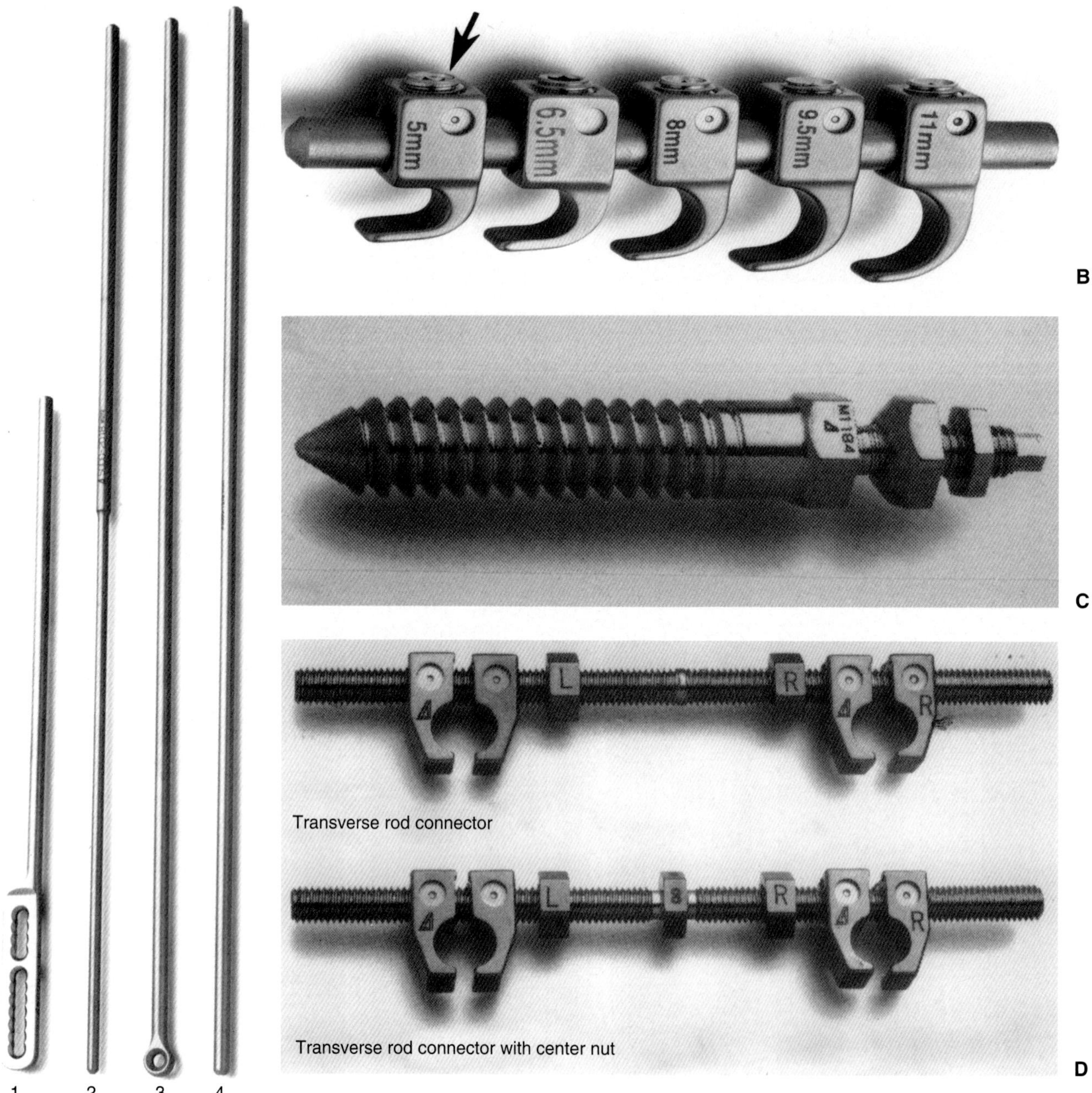


Fig. 3-14 ISOLA instrumentation. A: Rods: (*1*) plate rod, (*2*) dual diameter rod, (*3*) eye rod, (*4*) smooth rod. B: Hooks with end tightening screw (*arrow*). C: Cancellous sacral screw. D: Transverse connector rods. (Courtesy of Acromed, Cleveland, Ohio.) Posteroanterior (PA) (E) and lateral (F) radiographs after ISOLA instrumentation for scoliosis.

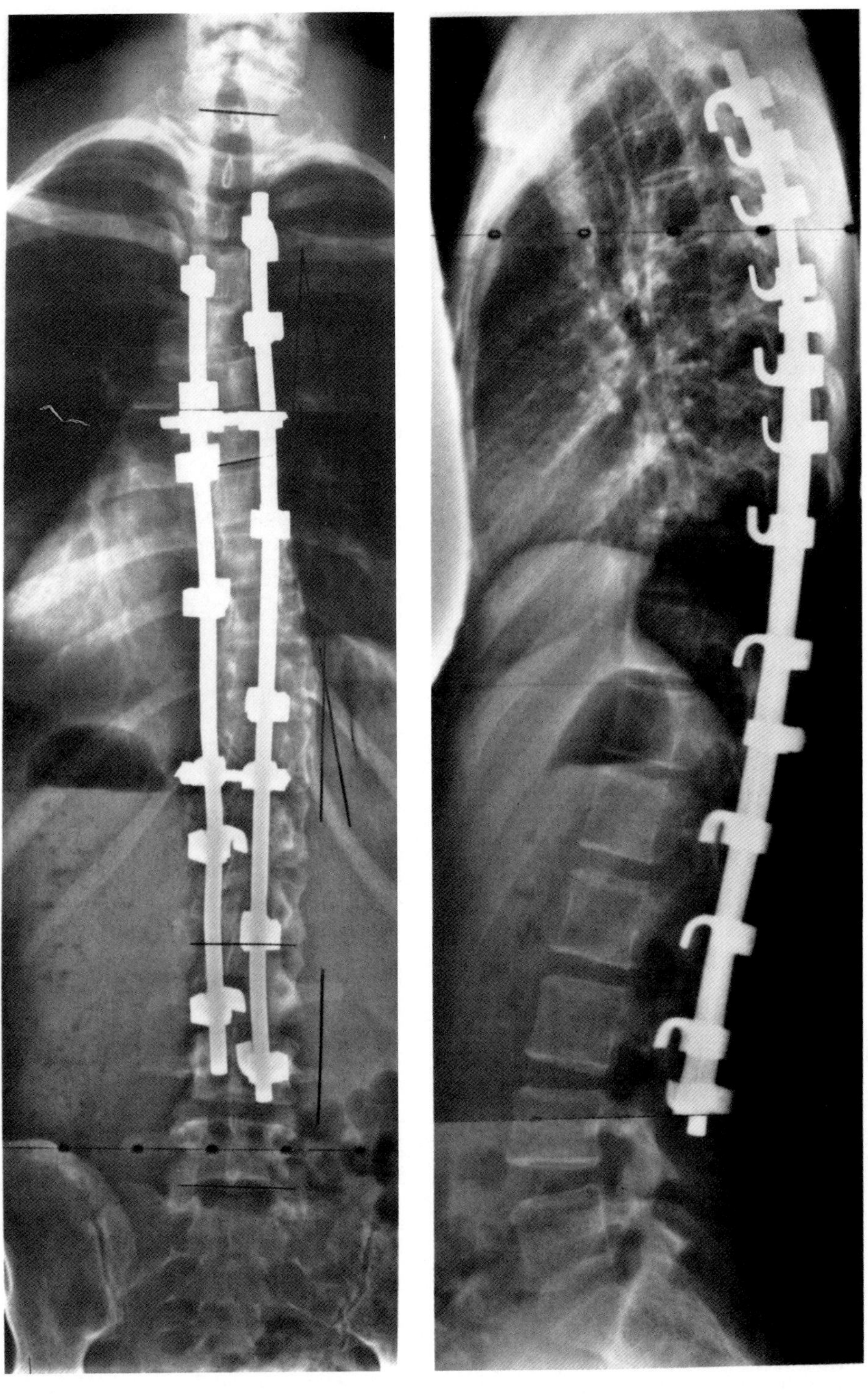

Fig. 3-14 *(Continued)*

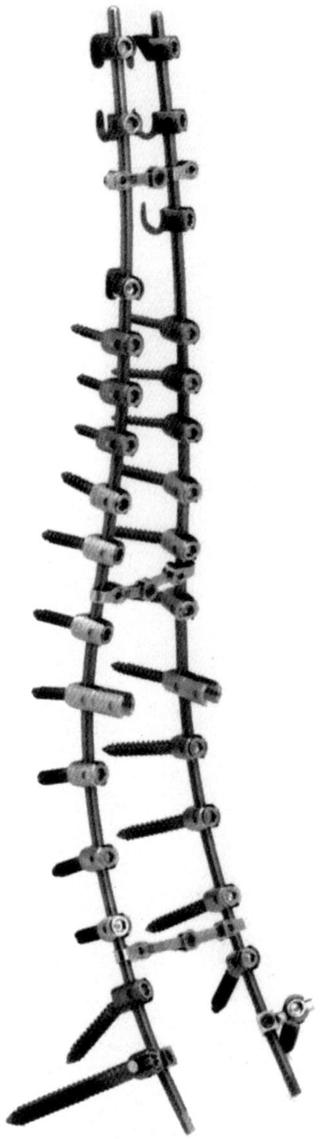

Fig. 3-15 Minimally invasive spinal instrumentation. Photograph of the ZODIAC system. Note the difference in appearance of the pedicle screws compared to the other examples (see Figs. 3-11 to 3-14). (Courtesy of Alphatec Spine, Inc. Carlsbad, California.)

## SUGGESTED READING

Asher M, Lai SM, Burton D, et al. Safety and efficacy of ISOLA instrumentation and arthrodesis for adolescent idiopathic scoliosis: Two-12-year follow-up. *Spine.* 2004;29:2013–2023.

Berquist TH. Imaging of the postoperative spine. *Radiol Clin North Am.* 2006;44:407–418.

Kim YJ, Lenke LG, Cho SK, et al. Comparative analysis of pedicle screw versus hook instrumentation in posterior spinal fusion of adolescent idiopathic scoliosis. *Spine.* 2004;29:2040–2048.

Lonstein JE. Scoliosis: Surgical versus nonsurgical treatment. *Clin Orthop.* 2006;443:248–259.

Remes V, Helenius I, Schlenzka D, et al. Cotrel-Dubousset (CD) or Universal Spine System (USS) instrumentation in adolescent idiopathic scoliosis (AIS): Comparison of midterm clinical, functional and radiologic outcomes. *Spine.* 2004;29:2024–2030.

## Imaging of Postoperative Complications

Complications associated with scoliosis instrumentation vary with the type of procedure and patient status. Complications may be directly related to the procedure and occur intraoperatively, perioperatively, or later in the course of follow-up. Complications may also be related to other organ systems. Certain complications may be increased if postoperative immobilization or casting is required. Fortunately, new techniques have reduced the need for long-term postoperative support.

Intraoperative complications include the following:

- Laminar fracture
- Nerve injury (sublaminar wires, pedicle screws)
- Improper screw placement
- Sensory loss at hook sites
- Dural tears

Immediate postoperative complications include the following:

- Pneumonia and pleural effusion or hemothorax
- Pneumothorax
- Gastrointestinal-adynamic ileus, duodenal ulcer, superior mesenteric artery syndrome (midline compression due to supporting devices such as body casts)
- Deep infection
- Deep venous thrombosis
- Reoperation due to suboptimal instrument placement

Delayed complications include the following:

- Loss of correction
- Instrument failure
  - Rod fracture (see Figs. 3-16, 3-11B and C)
  - Hook displacement (Fig. 3-16)
  - Screw pullout
  - Cable rupture
- Deep infection
- Pseudarthrosis
- Chronic pain
- Neurologic

Imaging of complications requires appropriate selection of techniques. Serial radiographs are most useful to evaluate correction of curves and changes in deformity. Evaluation of bone graft may require CT, radionuclide scans, or MRI.

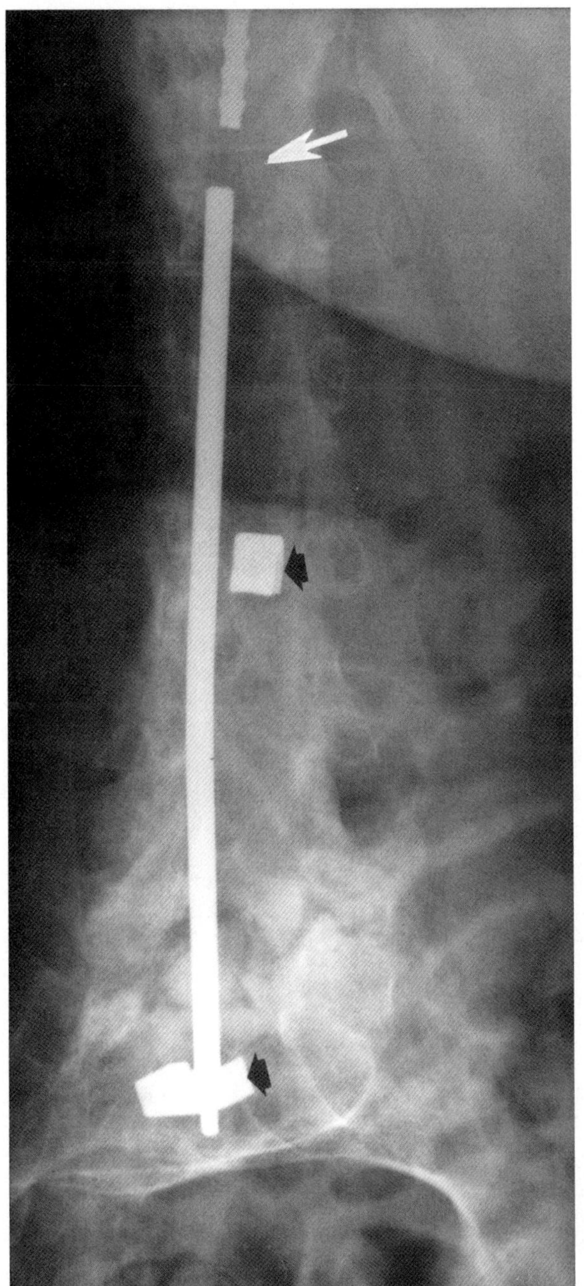

Fig. 3-16 Anteroposterior (AP) radiograph demonstrating fracture of the Harrington rod (*arrow*) and displaced hooks (*black arrows*).

Typically graft fusion requires 6 to 9 months. Pseudarthrosis is the most feared complication and is reported in 5% to 32% of patients depending on the extent of the procedure. Deep infection is reported in 1% to 3% of cases. Table 3-2 summarizes complications and imaging approaches.

Table 3-2

SCOLIOSIS INSTRUMENTATION COMPLICATIONS

| Imaging Approaches | |
|---|---|
| **Primary complications** | **Imaging techniques** |
| Loss of curve correction | Serial radiographs |
| Rod fracture | Serial radiographs (Fig. 3-11) |
| Cable rupture | Serial radiographs |
| Hook placement | Fluoroscopic spot views (Fig. 3-16) |
| Screw pullout/loosening | Serial radiographs |
| Screw position | CT |
| Pseudarthrosis | CT, radionuclide scans |
| Neurological | MRI |
| Infections | Serial radiographs, MRI, CT |
| Local pain | Diagnostic anesthetic injections |
| **Secondary complications** | |
| Pneumonia, pneumothorax, hemothorax | Radiographs |
| Deep venous thrombosis | Ultrasound |

CT, computed tomography; MRI, magnetic resonance imaging.

## Suggested Reading


Ali RM, Boachie-Adjei O, Rawlins BA. Functional and radiographic outcomes after surgery for adult scoliosis using third generation instrumentation techniques. *Spine.* 2003;28:1163–1169.

Asher M, Lai SM, Burton D, et al. Safety and efficacy of Isola instrumentation and arthrodesis for adolescent idiopathic scoliosis: Two to 12 year follow-up. *Spine.* 2004;29: 1013–2023.

Hedequist DJ, Hall JE, Emans JB. The safety and efficacy of spinal instrumentation in children with congenital spine deformities. *Spine.* 2004;29:2081–2086.

Kim YJ, Lenke LG, Samuel K, et al. Comparative analysis of pedicle screw versus hook instrumentation in posterior spinal fusion of adolescent idiopathic scoliosis. *Spine.* 2004;29:2040–2048.

Oestreich AE, Young LW, Poussaint TY. Scoliosis circa 2000: Radiologic imaging perspective. II. Treatment and follow-up. *Skeletal Radiol.* 1998;27:651–656.

Remes V, Helenius I, Schlenzka D, et al. Cotrel-Dubousset (CD) or Universal Spine System (USS) instrumentation in adolescent idiopathic scoliosis (AIS): Comparison of midterm clinical, functional and radiologic outcomes. *Spine.* 2004;29:2024–2030.

# Spondylolisthesis and Degenerative Disease

Surgical techniques for treatment of cervical and lumbar degenerative changes have changed dramatically over the last decades. Clinical features, treatment options, and the role of pre- and postoperative imaging and complications will be reviewed in this section.

## Lumbar Spondylolisthesis and Degenerative Disease

Spondylolisthesis may occur at any level. Subluxation at L5-S1 is commonly associated with an L5 pars defect (spondylolisis). Spondylolisis is bilateral in 74% of patients and occurs in 5% to 7.2% of the general population. Degenerative spondylolisthesis occurs most commonly (80%) at L4-5. Multiple levels are involved in more than 5% of patients. The etiology of spondylolisthesis has been debated for years. Most feel that both acquired and congenital causes are implicated. A recent classification is summarized in Table 3-3.

The high dysphasic type refers to disorders at L5-S1, which usually become symptomatic during adolescence. There is frequently a dome-shaped articular surface or vertical sacral angle. Low dysplastic spondylolisthesis is frequently associated with spinal bifida occulta and becomes symptomatic in the young adult years. Subluxation in the low dysplastic form occurs without kyphotic angulation at L5-S1.

Degenerative disease may be associated with spondylolisthesis. The spine can be anatomically divided into two or three columns. For purposes of degenerative disease two columns may be preferred. The anterior column consists of the vertebral body, intervertebral discs, and longitudinal ligaments. The posterior column consists of the posterior bony structures, including the transverse processes and the attaching ligaments and muscles. Degenerative disease may affect one or both columns and typically involves multiple levels. This section will focus on the lumbar and cervical degenerative disease and surgical treatment approaches.

**Table 3-3**

**MARCHETTI-BARTOLOZZI CLASSIFICATION OF SPONDYLOLISTHESIS**

| ACQUIRED | DEVELOPMENTAL |
|---|---|
| Traumatic | High dysplastic |
| Acute fracture | With lysis |
| Stress fracture | With elongation |
| Post surgical | Low dysplastic |
| Direct | With lysis |
| Indirect | With elongation |
| Pathologic | |
| Local | |
| Systemic | |
| Degenerative | |
| Primary | |
| Secondary | |

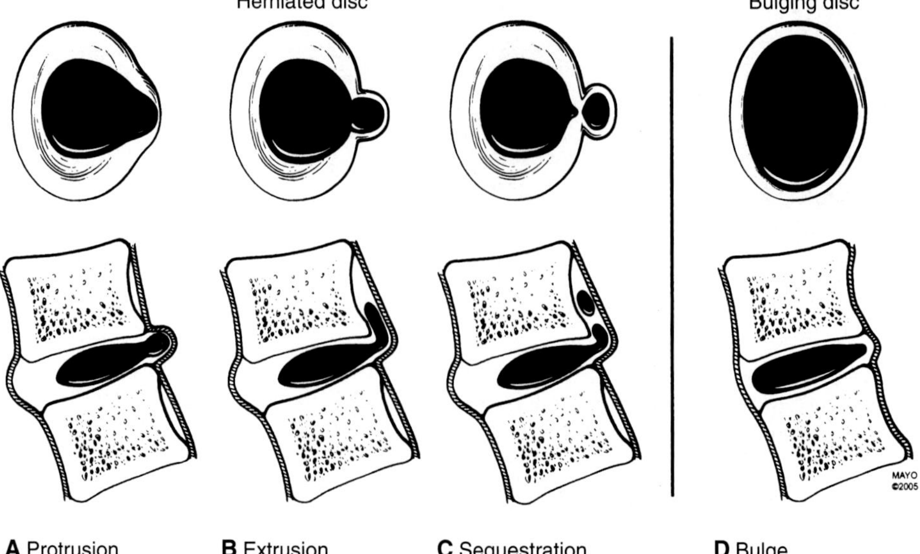


**Fig. 3-17** Disc bulge, protrusion, extrusion, and sequestration based on consensus terminology. (From Witte RJ, Lane JI, Miller GM, et al. Spine. In: Berquist TH, ed. *MRI of the musculoskeletal system,* 5th ed. Philadelphia: Lippincott Williams & Wilkins; 2006:121–202.)

## Common Terminology

**Ankylosis:** Nonsurgical joint fusion seen with several arthropathies including ankylosing spondylitis

**Arthrodesis:** Surgical immobilization of a joint or disc space

**Disc disorders** (see Fig. 3-17)

**Disc bulge**—broad-based expansion of the circumference of the disc due to loss of interspace height with extension beyond the confines of the adjacent vertebral body secondary to laxity of the annular fibers without evidence of concentric tear (see Figs. 3-17D and 3-18).

**Disc protrusion**—focal broad-based expansion of disc material that is confined by the outer annular layers. On axial and sagittal MR images it is seen only at the disc level (see Figs. 3-17A and 3-19).

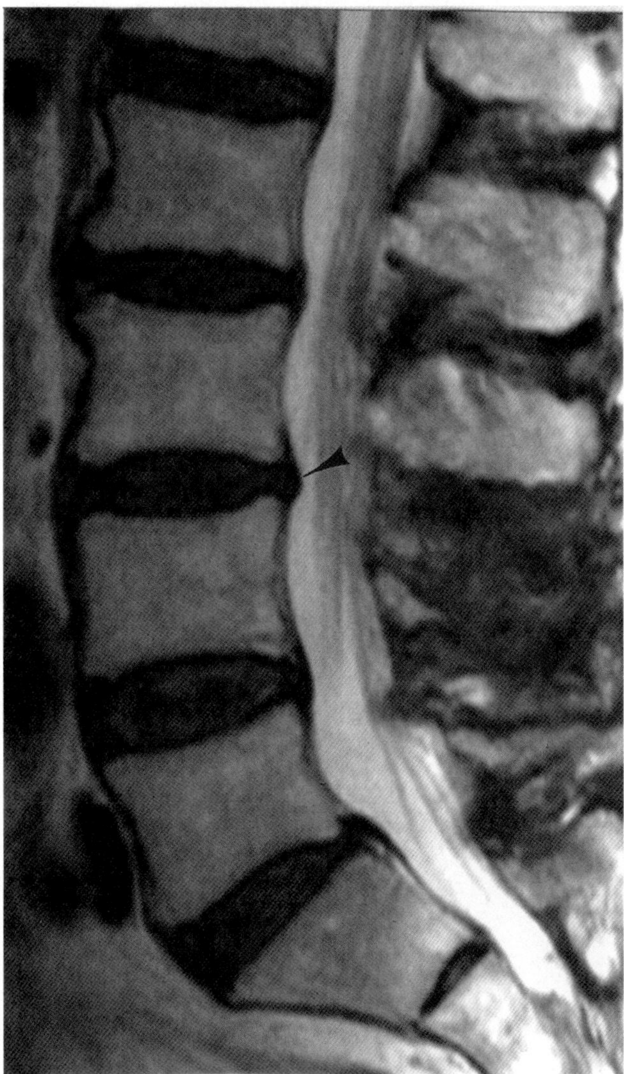

Fig. 3-18 Disc bulges. Sagittal magnetic resonance (MR) image demonstrating a disc bulge at L3-4 (*arrowhead*).

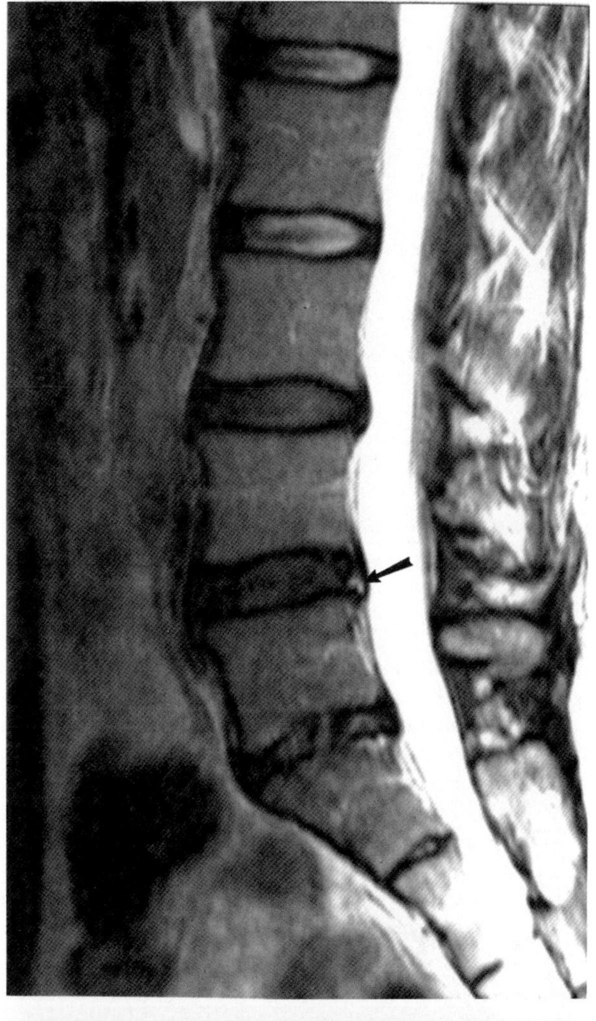

A

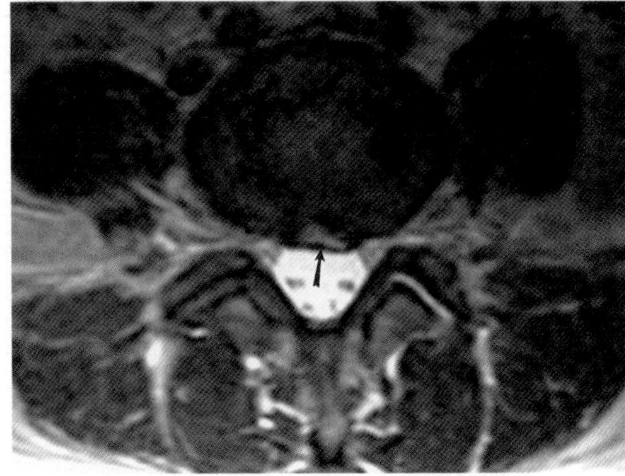

B

Fig. 3-19 Disc protrusion. Sagittal (A) and axial (B) magnetic resonance (MR) images demonstrating a disc protrusion at L4-5. On the sagittal T2-weighted image (A) there is increased signal intensity in the posterior annulus (*arrow*) compatible with an annular tear. The axial image (B) demonstrates a focal defect (*arrow*) with flattening of the ventral thecal sac.

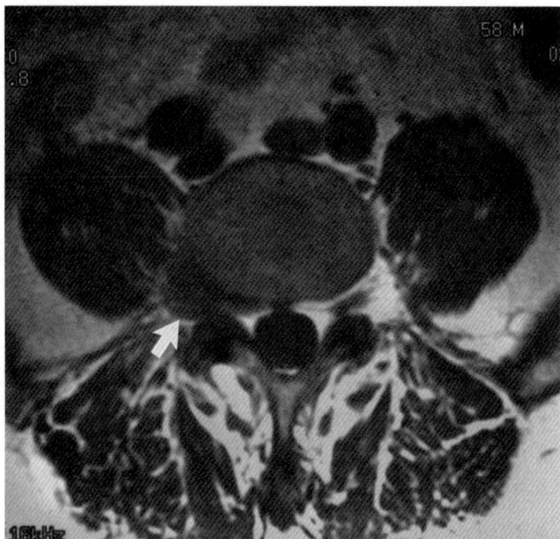

Fig. 3-20 Disc extrusion. Axial magnetic resonance (MR) image demonstrating a lateral fragment (*arrow*) displacing the L4 nerve root.

**Disc extrusion**—herniation of nucleus pulposus through all layers of the annulus. A small extrusion is difficult to differentiate from a disc protrusion. The disc extrusion appears as a focal soft tissue mass that may displace the thecal sac or adjacent nerve roots (see Figs. 3-17B and 3-20).

**Disc sequestration**—disc material that has herniated through all layers of the annulus and is no longer connected to the parent disc. The sequestered fragment may migrate several disc levels superiorly or inferiorly (see Figs. 3-17C and 3-21).

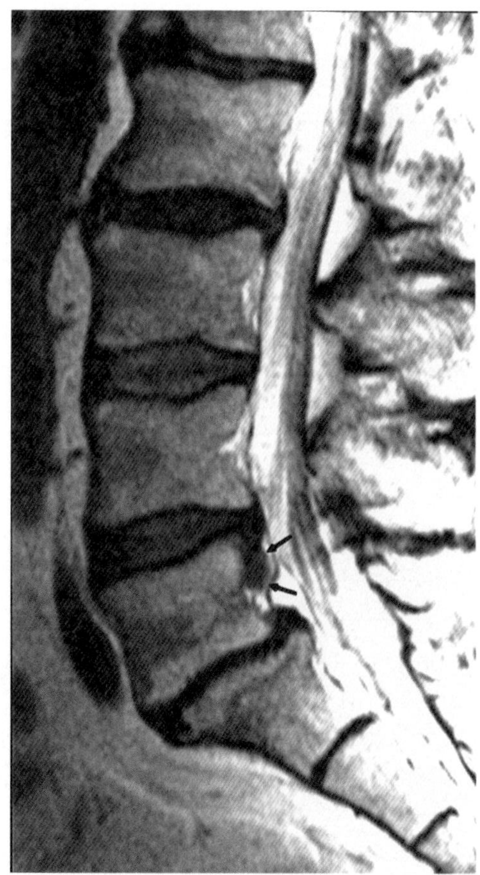

Fig. 3-21 Disc sequestration. Sagittal magnetic resonance (MR) image demonstrating a posterior disc fragment posterior to the L5 vertebral body (*arrows*) and displaced from the parent disc.

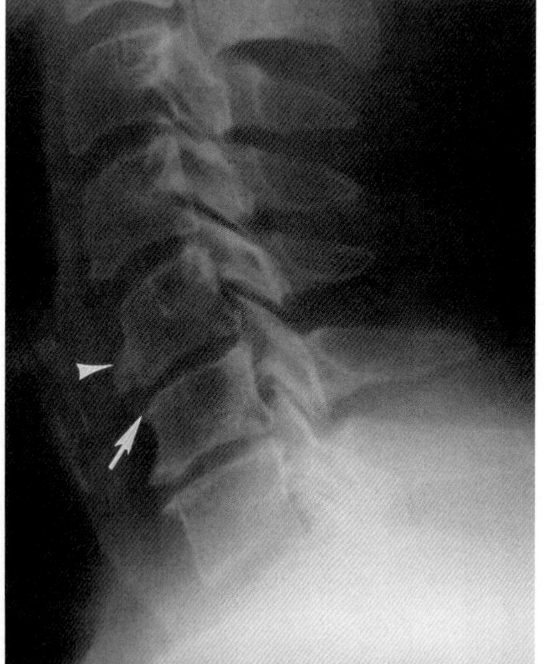

A

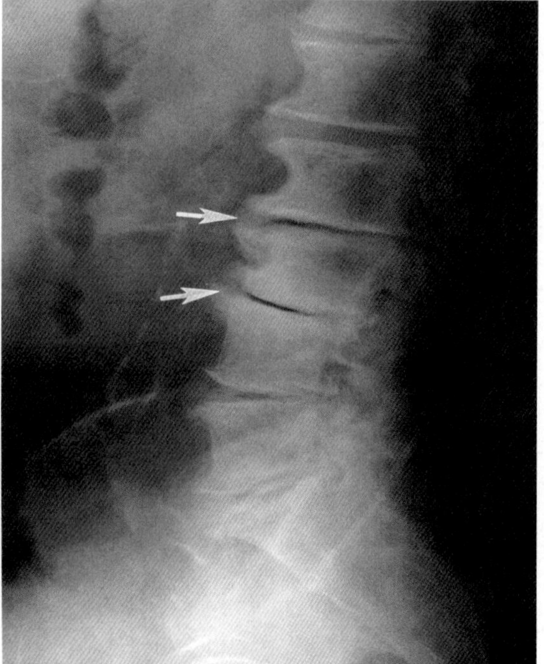

B

Fig. 3-22 Osteophytes. Lateral radiographs of the cervical (A) and lumbar spine (B) demonstrating marginal (*arrows* in A and B) and nonmarginal (*arrowhead* in A) osteophytes. There is also vacuum disc phenomenon and advance degenerative change in the lumbar spine (B).

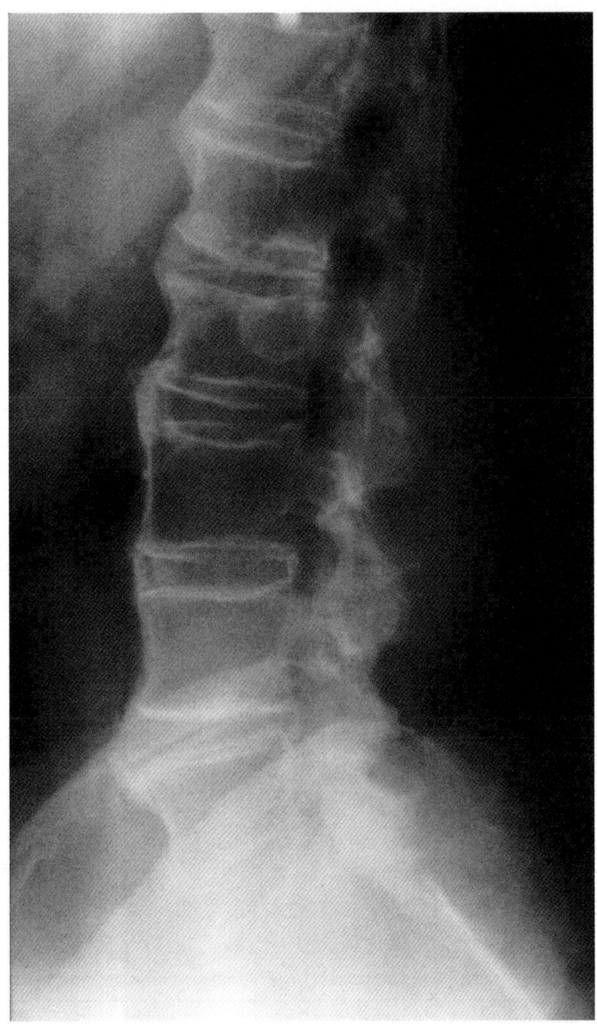

Fig. 3-23 Diffuse idiopathic skeletal hyperostosis (DISH). Lateral radiograph of the lumbar spine demonstrating ossification of the paraspinal soft tissues with normal disc spaces.

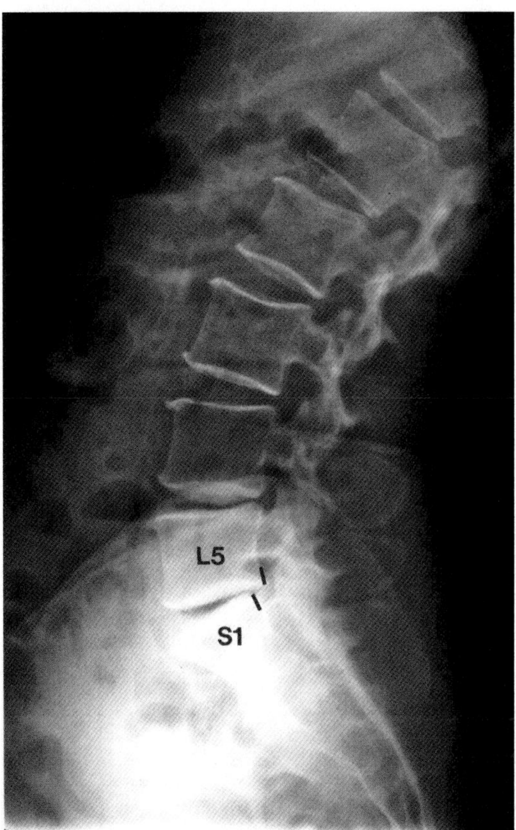


Fig. 3-24 Lateral radiograph of the lumbar spine demonstrating posterior displacement of L5 on S1 (*lines*).

**Osteophytes:** Pathologic bony outgrowth

- **Marginal osteophyte**—horizontal bony projection from the vertebral end plate seen in degenerative spine disease (see Fig. 3-22)
- **Nonmarginal osteophyte**—bone projection several millimeters away from the vertebral end plate (Fig. 3-22A)
- **Paraspinal osteophyte**—paraspinal ossification in the soft tissues surrounding the vertebra seen in diffuse idiopathic skeletal hyperostosis (DISH) (see Fig. 3-23)

**Retrolisthesis:** Posterior displacement or subluxation of a vertebral body on the inferior adjacent vertebra (see Fig. 3-24)

**Spondylolisthesis:** Anterior displacement of a vertebral body on the adjacent body below (see Fig. 3-25)

**Spondylolisis:** Used to describe disruption of the pars (Fig. 3-25)

**Spondylosis:** Used to describe any of a variety of degenerative changes in the spine

**Syndesmophyte:** Vertically oriented ossification bridging the vertebral bodies seen with ankylosing spondylitis and other spondyloarthropathies (see Fig. 3-26)

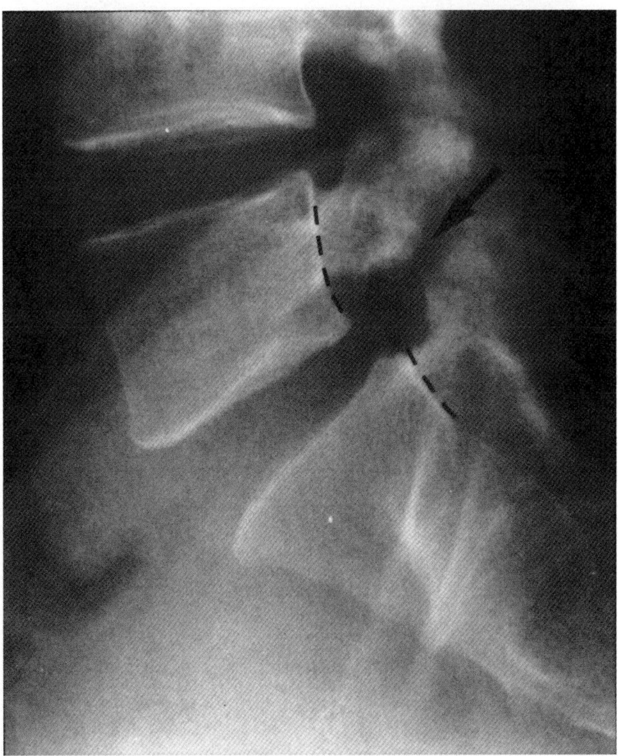

Fig. 3-25 Spondylolisthesis. Lateral radiograph of the spine demonstrating anterior displacement of L5 on S1 (*broken lines*) due to pars defect (*arrow*) at L5.

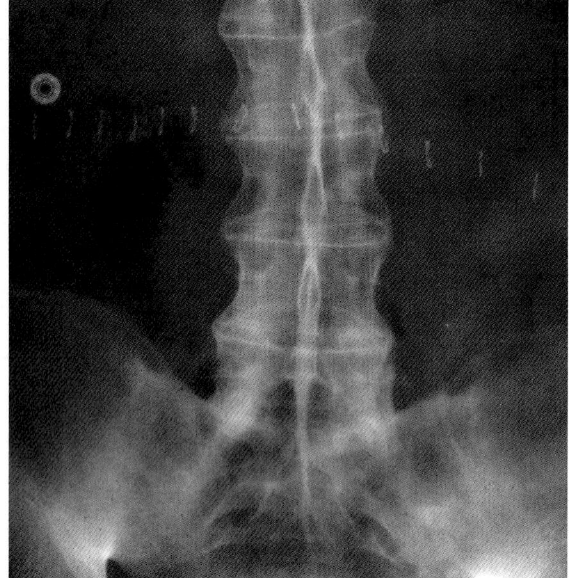

A

B

Fig. 3-26 Syndesmophyte. Anteroposterior (AP) radiograph of the lower lumbar spine and sacroiliac joints (**A**) demonstrating ankylosis of the sacroiliac joints and smooth vertical syndesmophytes along the vertebral margins. Lateral radiograph of the cervical spine (**B**) demonstrating uniform smooth ossification of the anterior longitudinal ligament.

## Suggested Reading

Hammerberg KW. New concepts in pathogenesis and classification of spondylolisthesis. *Spine*. 2005;30(S6):S4–S11.

Milette P. The proper terminology for reporting lumbar intervertebral disk disorders. *AJNR Am J Neuroradiol*. 1997;18: 1859–1866.

Witte RJ, Lane JI, Miller GM, et al. Spine. In: Berquist TH, ed. *MRI of the musculoskeletal system*, 5th ed. Philadelphia: Lippincott Williams & Wilkins; 2006:121–202.

### Preoperative Imaging

Radiographic imaging of the spine provides valuable information on stability and levels of involvement. In addition to radiographs, CT, MRI, or diagnostic injections in the facets or discs may be required for operative planning

**Lumbar radiographs:** AP, lateral, coned down lateral lower lumbar spine, obliques, flexion-extension and lateral bending views.

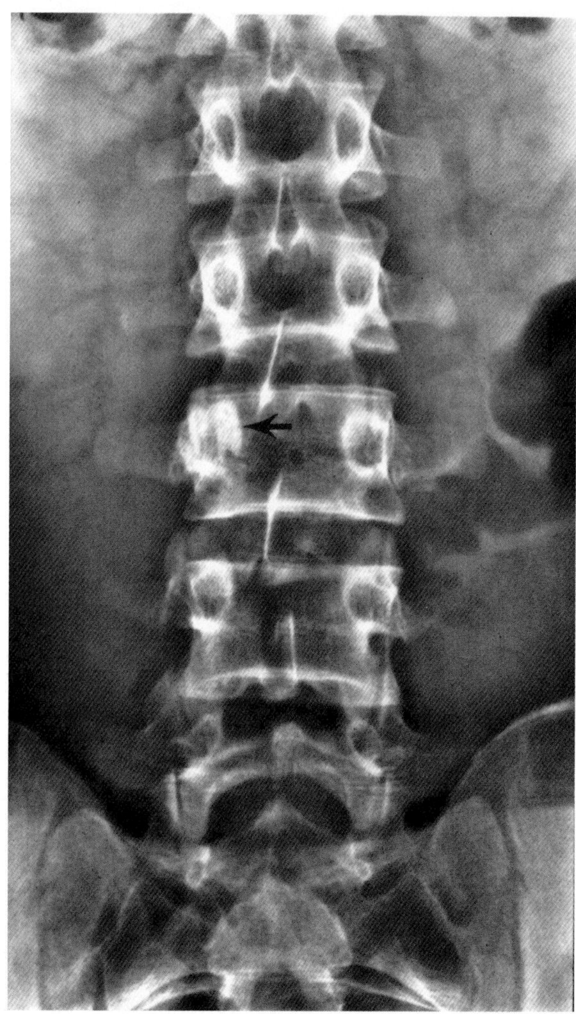

A

Fig. 3-27 Pedicle sclerosis. Anteroposterior (AP) radiograph of the lumbar spine demonstrates a sclerotic pedicle at L3 on the right (*arrow*) due to a pars defect on the left demonstrated on the oblique view (*arrow* in **B**).

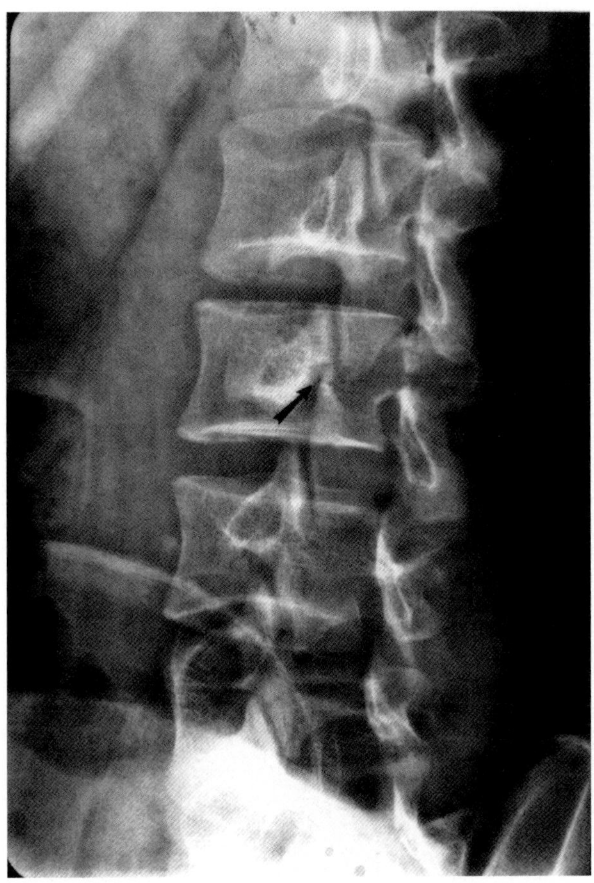


Fig. 3-27 (*Continued*)

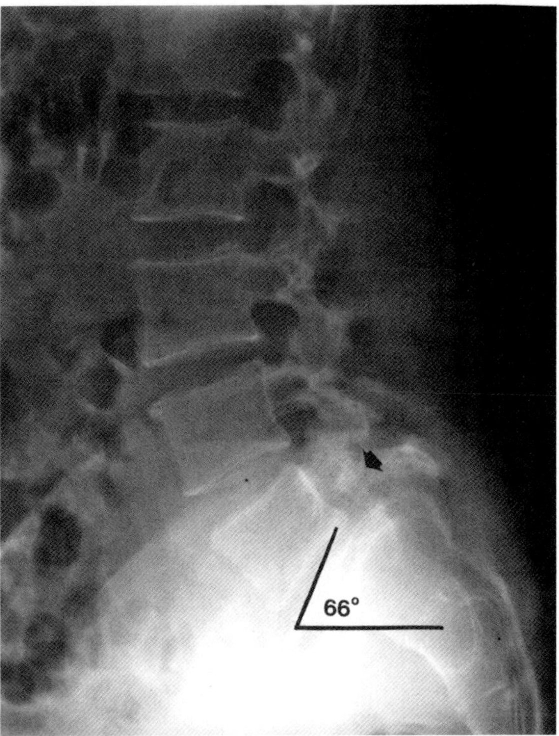


Fig. 3-29 Sacral angle (slope). Lateral radiograph measuring the sacral angle by drawing a line along the upper end plate of S1 and the horizontal (range 17 to 63 degrees, mean 42 degrees). In this case the sacral angle is 66 degrees. Note the pars defect and sclerosis (*arrow*) and grade I anterior subluxation of L5 on S1.

- **AP view**—sclerotic pedicle may be seen with contralateral pars defect (see Fig. 3-27)
- Angled AP view (30 degrees to the head) may assist in defining pars defects
- **Lateral view**—classify spondylolisthesis (Meyerding) (see Fig. 3-28)
- Measure sacral angle (slope) (see Fig. 3-29) and slip angle (see Fig. 3-30)
- **Oblique views**—facet arthrosis and pars defects (see Fig. 3-31)
- **Motion studies**—evaluate stability, disc space, and curve changes (see Fig. 3-32)

**CT:** Clarify pars defects (see Fig. 3-33), spinal stenosis

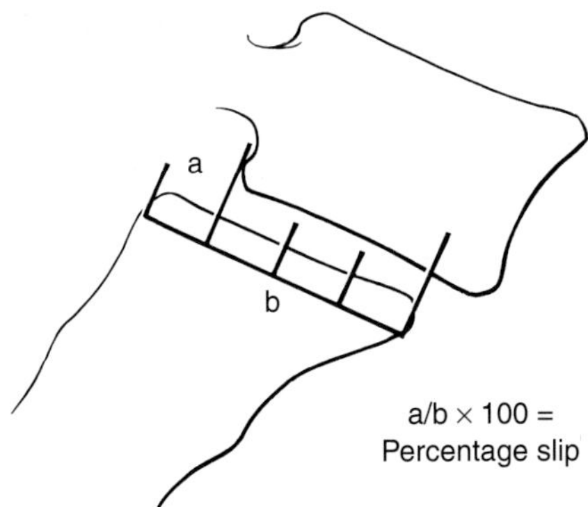


Fig. 3-28 Meyerding classifiction for spondylolisthesis. The vertebral end plate is divided into four equal segments and graded I to IV depending on the degree of slip. Illustration of the Meyerding system at L5-S1. In this case the degree of slip is 25% or grade I.

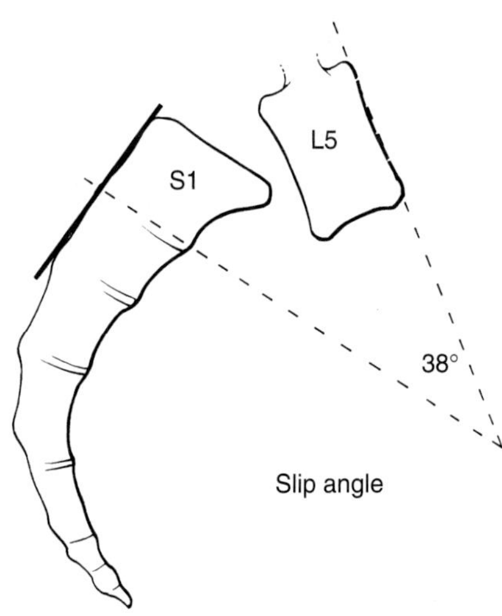


Fig. 3-30 Slip angle. The slip angle is measured by a line along the upper endplate of L5 and the second line perpendicular to the posterior aspect of the sacrum. A high slip angle indicates greater risk for instability, progression of slip, and reduced healing potential.

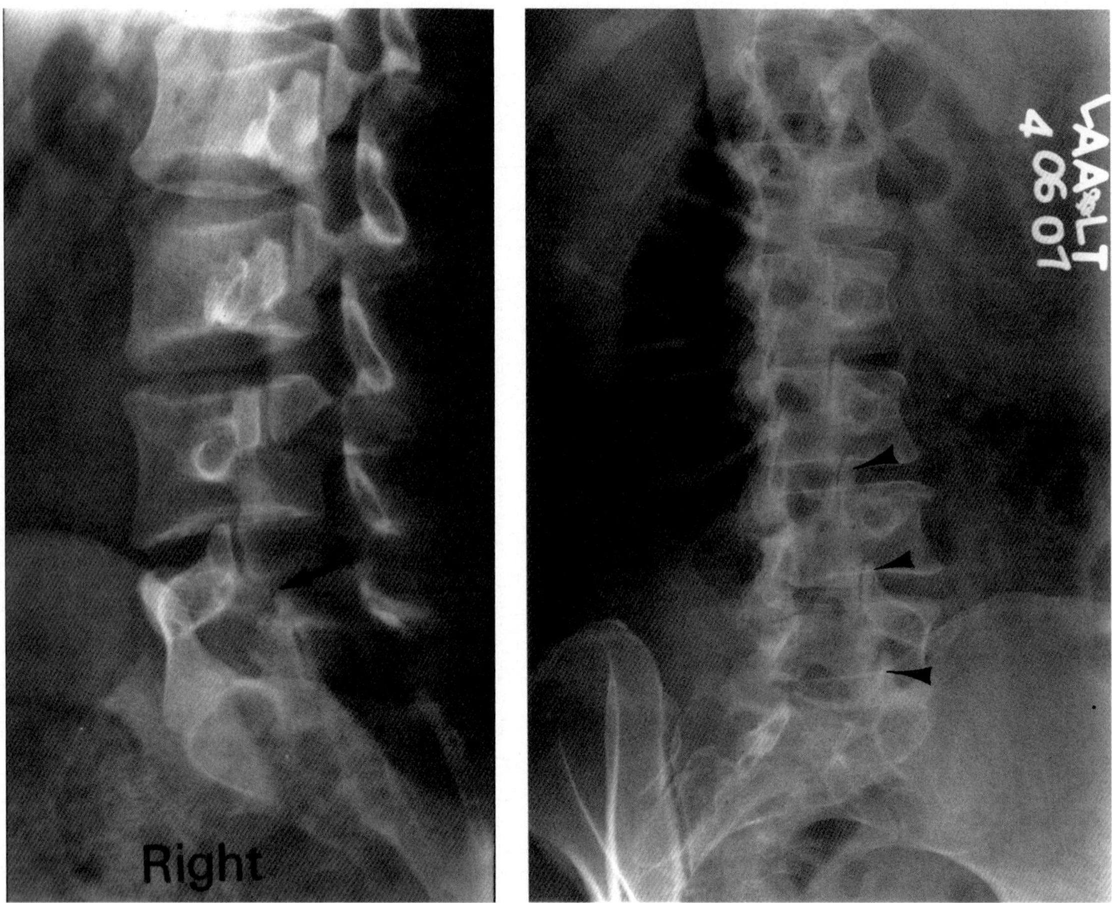


Fig. 3-31 Oblique views. A: Right oblique radiograph demonstrating a pars defect at L5 (*arrow*). B: Oblique radiograph demonstrating advanced facet arthropathy with sclerosis, joint space narrowing, and marginal osteophytes (*arrowheads*) at multiple levels.

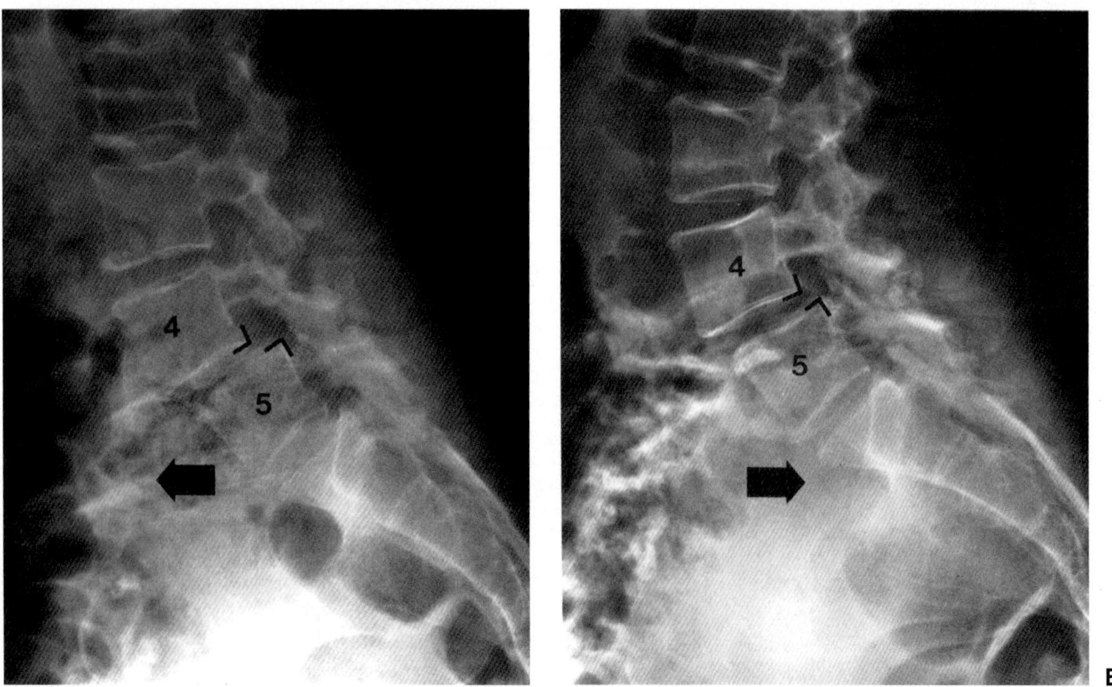


Fig. 3-32 Motion studies. Flexion (A) and extension (B) radiographs in a patient with grade I degenerative subluxation of L4 on L5 that increases with flexion.

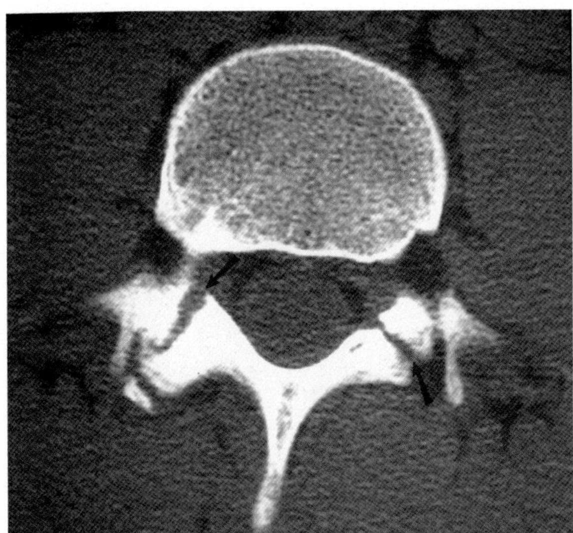

Fig. 3-33 Computed tomographic (CT) image demonstrating bilateral pars defects (*arrows*).

**MRI:** Evaluates disc morphology, neural structures (Figs. 3-18 to 3-21)

**Diagnostic injections of facets or discs:** Confirm source of pain and levels of involvement

## Suggested Reading

Berquist TH. Imaging of the postoperative spine. *Radiol Clin North Am.* 2006;44:407–418.

### Surgical Approaches to Lumbar Degenerative Diseases

Surgical approaches to degenerative disease and spondylolisthesis vary with the extent of involvement including disc disease and the number of segments affected. Posterior, anterior, transverse, and combined approaches may be used.

The clinical setting in lumbar degenerative disease is critical in selection of appropriate treatment options. Pain may be related to disc degeneration, spinal deformity, instability, or abnormal loading with or without abnormal motion. Conservative treatment is attempted initially. Specifically for disc disease, less invasive techniques such as intradiscal electrothermal therapy (IDET), radiofrequency ablation, percutaneous endoscopic laser discectomy (PELD), and cryoablation may also be affective.

Indications for arthrodesis include the following:

Spondylolisthesis grade II or higher
Failed discectomy (two or more)
Instability (subluxation or translation >3 mm)
Established mechanical pain
Failed decompression procedures

Most approaches seek solid fusion to reduce motion. However, more recently dynamic stabilization is now being investigated in patients who have pain with no demonstrable motion on radiographs. This suggests pain is related to abnormal load as opposed to instability. Approaches to surgical intervention are summarized in the subsequent text.

#### Posterolateral arthrodesis

- Autogenous bone graft without instrumentation (see Fig. 3-34)
- Bone graft from spinous processes applied to lamina
- Bone graft with posterior instrumentation

#### Pedicle screw instrumentation

- May be used with rods or plates (see Fig. 3-35)
- Usually combined with bone grafting
- Rods allow more space for bone graft placement

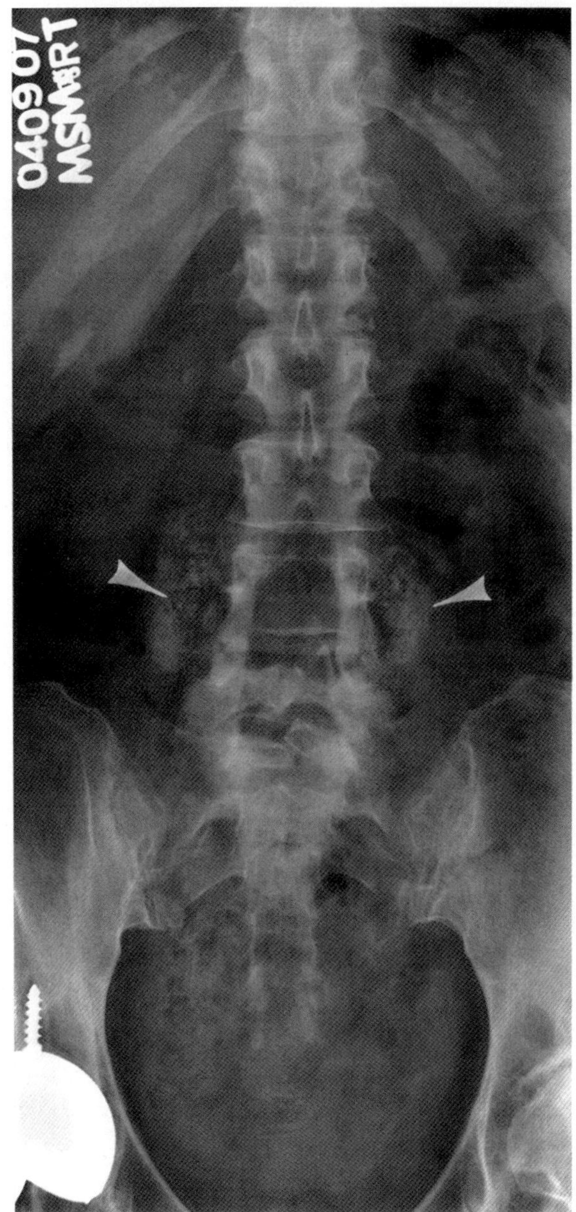


Fig. 3-34 Anteroposterior (AP) radiograph after L4-5 laminectomies with posterolateral bone graft (*arrowheads*), but no instrumentation.

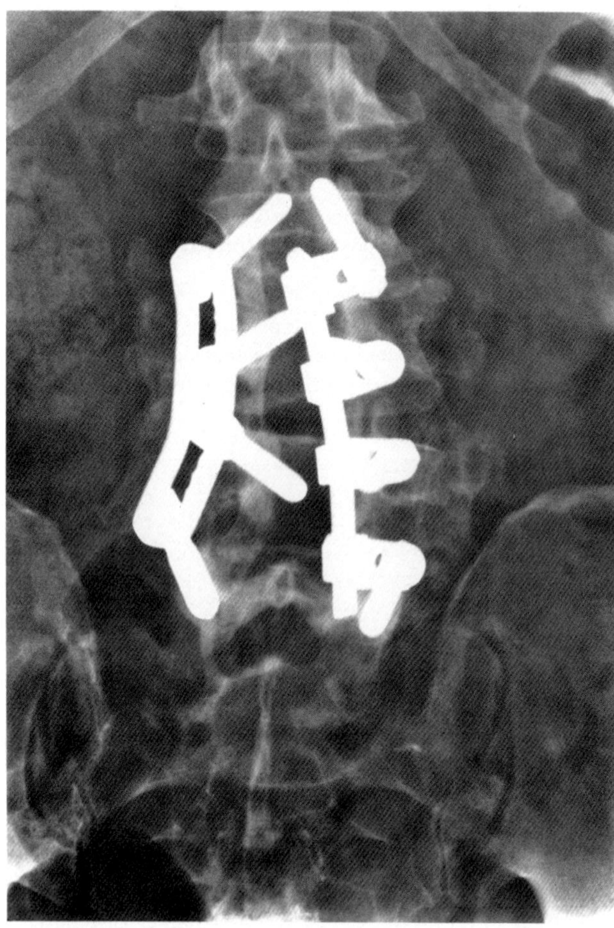

Fig. 3-35 Anteroposterior (AP) radiograph with posterior instrumentation using a Steffee plate on the right and rod on the left, both with pedicle screws.

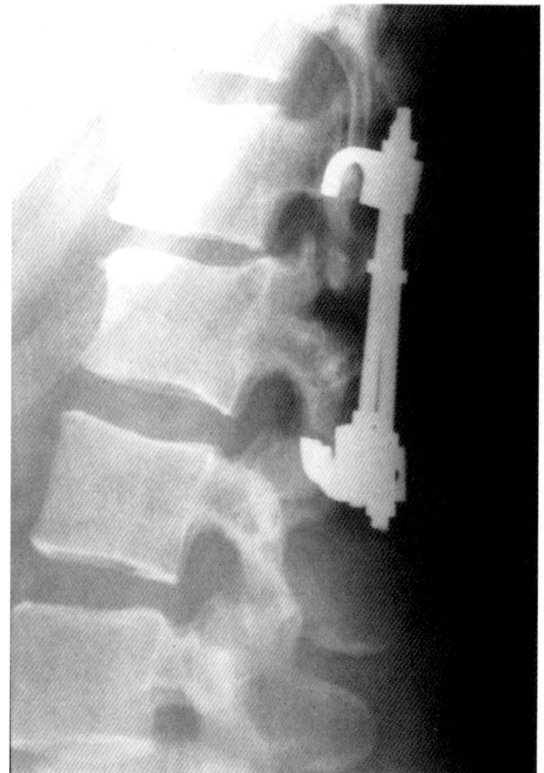

Fig. 3-36 Lateral radiograph with threaded rods and compression hooks for fusion of T12-L1.

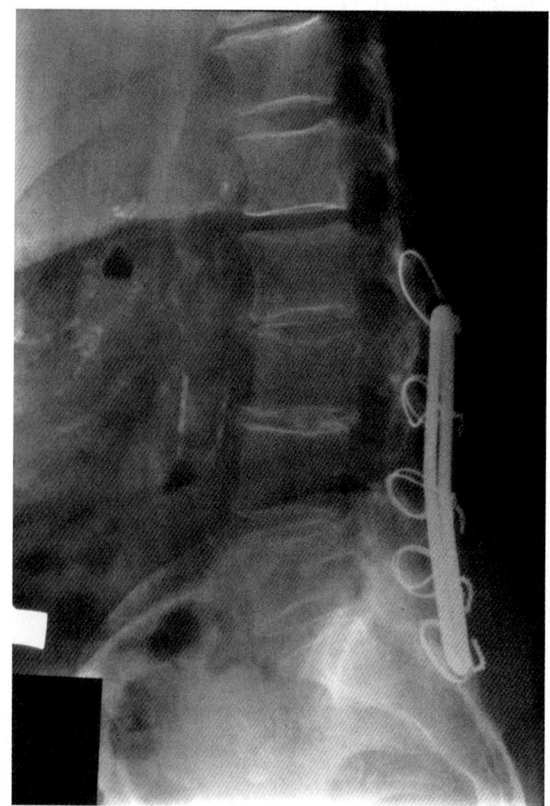

Fig. 3-37 Lateral radiograph after posterior fusion using a Luque rectangle and sublaminar wires L2 to the sacrum.

## Sublaminar wires and/or hooks

- Hooks or sublaminar wires may be used with rods (see Fig. 3-36)
- Sublaminar wires may also be used with Luque rectangles (see Fig. 3-37)
- Usually combined with bone grafting

## Interspinous process instrumentation

- Minimally invasive procedure
- Device placed between the spinous processes to limit extension
- Designed for older patients with neurogenic claudication and spinal stenosis
- Placed at symptomatic disc levels (see Fig. 3-38)

## Lumbar interbody arthrodesis

- Disc considered primary source of pain
- Disc removal
- Fusion accomplished with bone graft
- Graft reestablishes disc height

## Anterior lumbar interbody arthrodesis

- Direct removal of disc without posterior paraspinal muscle dissection

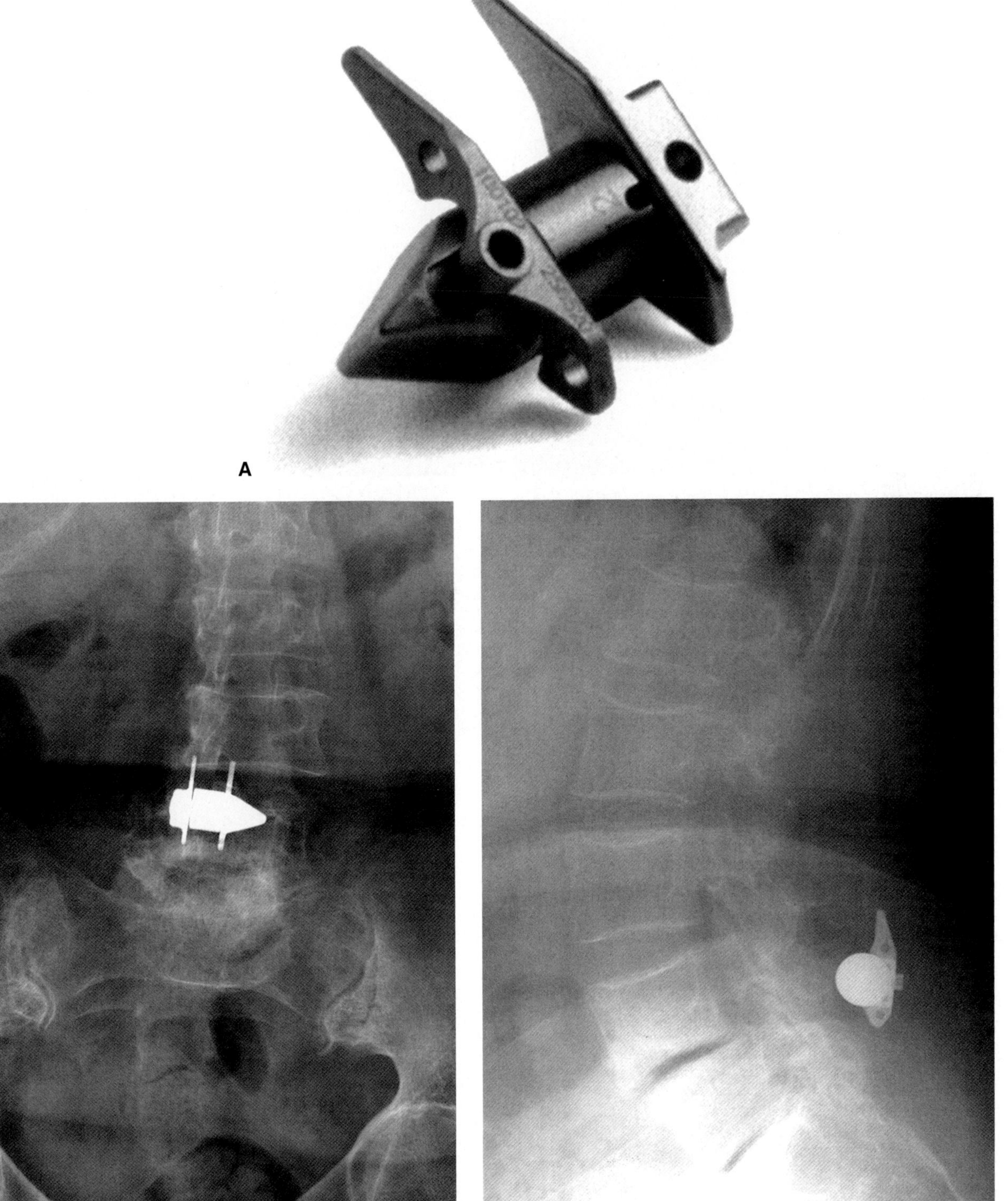

Fig. 3-38 A: Illustration of the X-STOP interspinous process device. (Courtesy of Kyphon, Sunnyvale, California.) Anteroposterior (AP) (B) and lateral (C) radiographs of an X-STOP device placed between the L4-5 spinous processes. Degenerative disc disease at L4-5 and L5-S1.

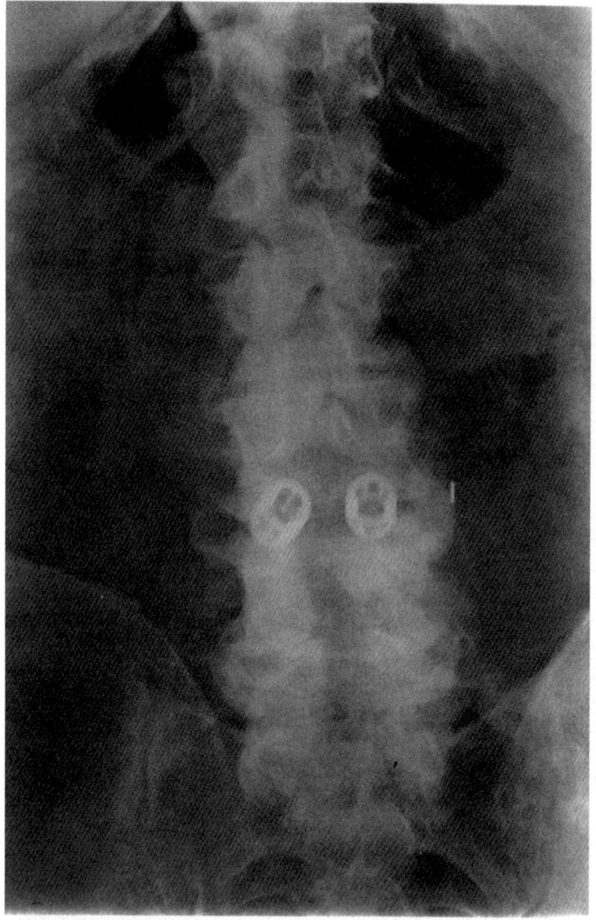

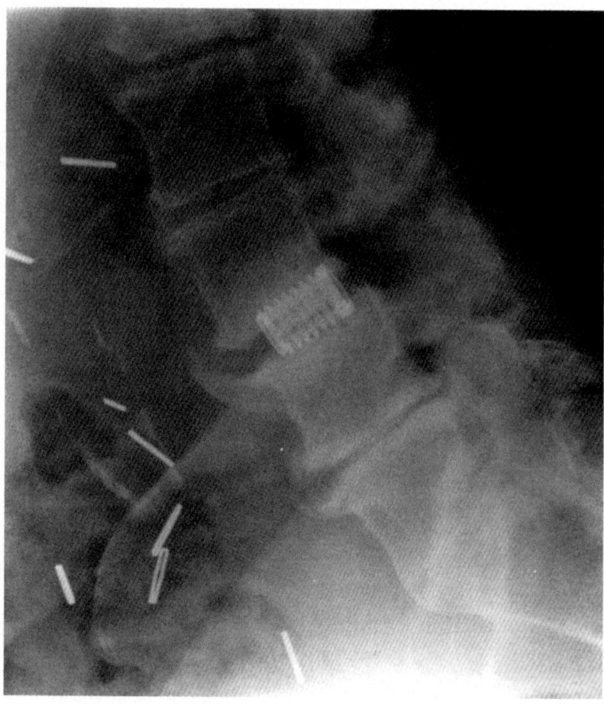

Fig. 3-39 Anteroposterior (AP) (A) and lateral (B) radiographs demonstrate two interbody fusion cages at L3-4 in a patient with advanced arthrosis and laminectomies L3-5.

- More complete excision of disc
- May injure presacral plexus

**Interbody fusion cages**

- Multiple configurations (see Fig. 3-39)
- Titanium commonly employed
- Used with bone graft

**Disc prostheses** (see Fig. 3-40)

- Disc disease alone
- Multiple configurations
- Must not transfer load to facets
- Hydraulic, elastic, and mechanical properties

**Combined procedures**

- Combined anterior disc spacers and posterior instrumentation (see Fig. 3-41)
- Bone graft or cages with posterior rods and pedicle screws commonly used
- Multiple segments commonly fused

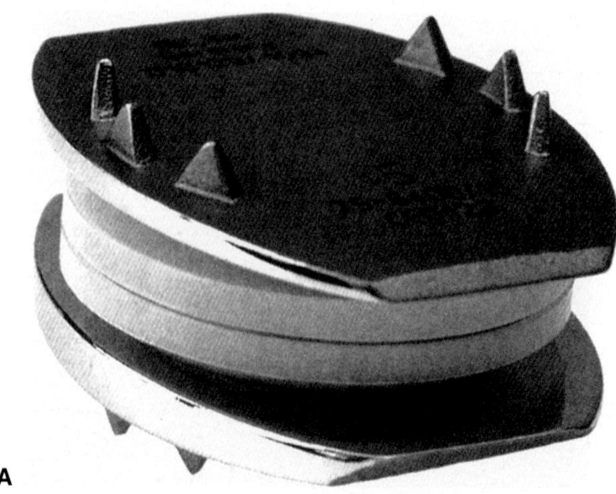

Fig. 3-40 Charite disc prosthesis. Anteroposterior (AP) (A) and lateral (B) radiographs of a Charite disc replacement at L5-S1. (Courtesy of DePuy Spine, Raynham, Massachusetts.)

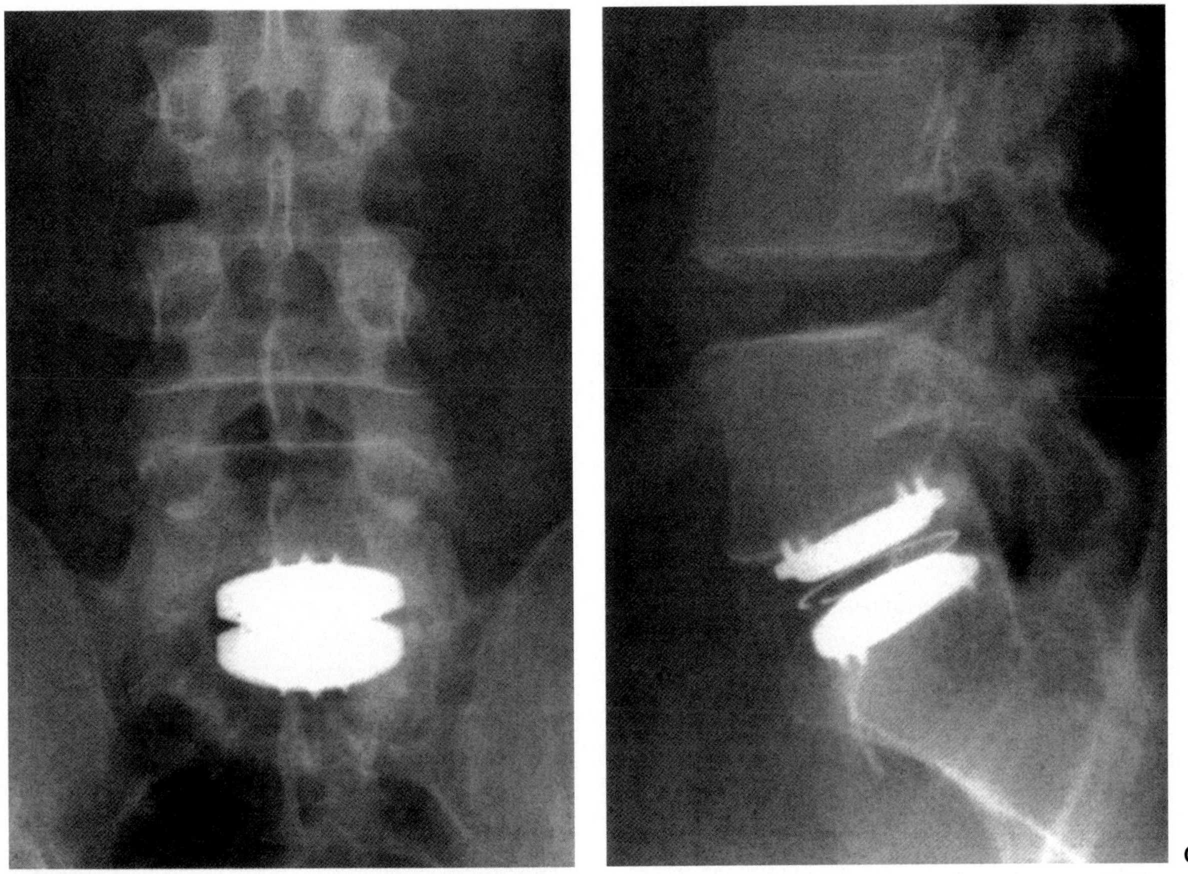


Fig. 3-40 *(Continued)*

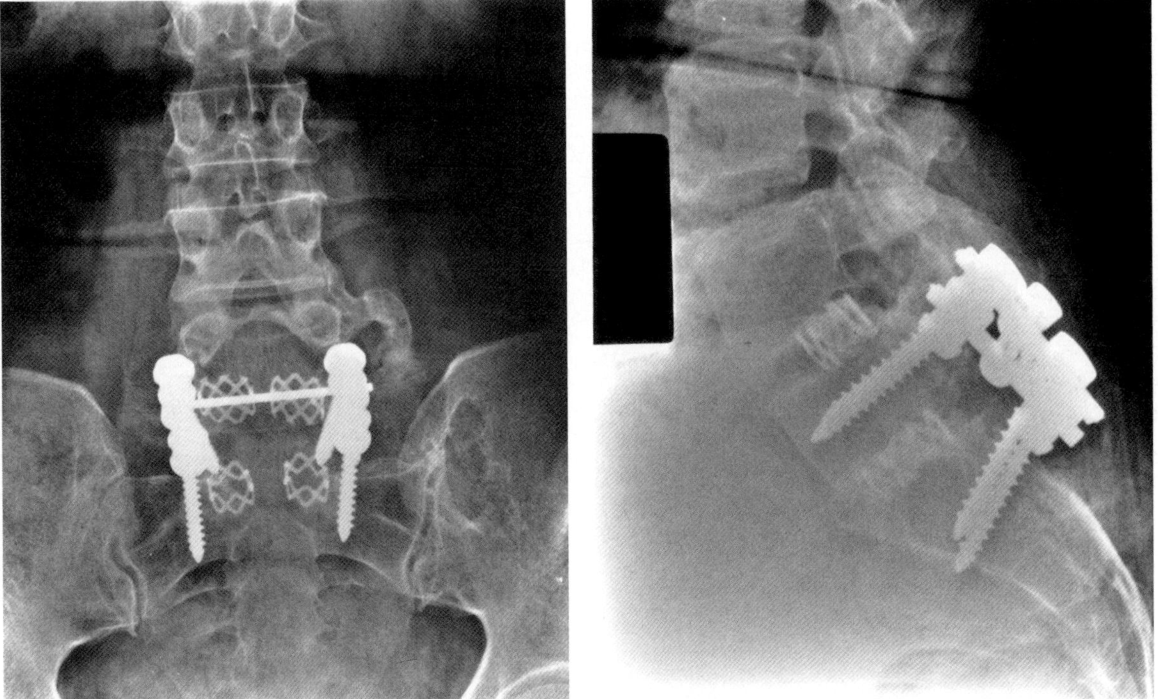


Fig. 3-41 Anteroposterior (AP) (A) and lateral (B) radiographs following rod and pedicle screw instrumentation with anterior spacers at L4-5 and L5-S1. There is solid bone graft posterolaterally.

## Suggested Reading

Bridwell KH, Edwards CC, Lenke LG. The pros and cons to saving the L5-S1 motion segment in a long scoliosis fusion. *Spine*. 2003;28:S234–S242.

Hammerberg KW. New concepts on the pathogenesis and classification of spondylolisthesis. *Spine*. 2005;30:S4–S11.

Hanley EN, David SM. Lumbar arthrodesis for the treatment of back pain. *J Bone Joint Surg*. 1999;81A:716–731.

McAfee PC. Interbody fusion cages in reconstructive operations on the spine. *J Bone Joint Surg*. 1999;81A:859–879.

Nockels RP. Dynamic stabilization in the surgical management of painful spinal disorders. *Spine*. 2005;30:S68–S72.

Petersilge CA. Lumbar disc replacement. *Semin Musculoskelet Radiol*. 2006;10:22–29.

Weidenbaum M. Considerations for focused surgical intervention in the presence of adult spinal deformity. *Spine*. 2006;31:S139–S143.

### Cervical Degenerative Disease

The intervertebral discs provide strength between adjacent segments and limit motion by resisting compressive, shearing, and rotational forces. The cervicooccipital junction is more mobile and comprises synovial joints supported by capsular ligamentous structures. Although instability can result from trauma, rheumatoid arthritis, infection, congenital causes, degenerative disease is also implicated.

Cervical spine degenerative disease is common in adults with spondylotic myelopathy representing the leading cause of cord dysfunction in the adult population. Up to 61% of patients have radicular symptoms, 16% myelopathic symptoms, and 23% a combination of the two. Conservative treatment with collar support and modification of activities can be effective in patients with mild symptoms. However, surgical intervention is beneficial in patients with more severe symptoms or failed conservative management.

The goals of surgical management include decompression of the spinal cord and stabilization of levels with abnormal motion that may contribute to the myelopathy.

## Suggested Reading

Phillips FM, Garfin SR. Cervical disc replacement. *Spine*. 2005;30:S27–S33.

Rao RD, Gourab K, David KS. Operative treatment of cervical spondolytic myelopathy. *J Bone Joint Surg*. 2006;88A: 1619–1639.

Stock GH, Vaccaro AR, Brown AK, et al. Contemporary posterior occipital fixation. *J Bone Joint Surg*. 2006;88A:1642–1649.

#### Preoperative Imaging

As with the lumbar spine, radiographs provide significant information regarding levels of involvement and stability. CT and MRI provide additional data specific to subtle osseous, soft tissue, and disc and spinal canal abnormalities.

**Cervical radiographs:** AP, lateral, oblique, open-mouth odontoid and flexion/extension views

- **AP radiograph**—alignment and interspinous distance; facet and lateral mass abnormalities (see Fig. 3-42)
- **Lateral radiograph**—alignment; disc space narrowing; midsagittal spinal canal measurement (normal 17 to 18 mm C3-7) (see Fig. 3-43)
- **Oblique radiographs**—foraminal encroachment; facet osteophytes
- **Flexion/extension radiographs**—subluxation >3.5 mm; dynamic canal narrowing <12 mm (see Fig. 3-44)

**CT:** Spinal canal measurements and osseous abnormalities (see Fig. 3-45)

**MRI:** Disc, spinal cord, and ligament abnormalities (see Fig. 3-46)

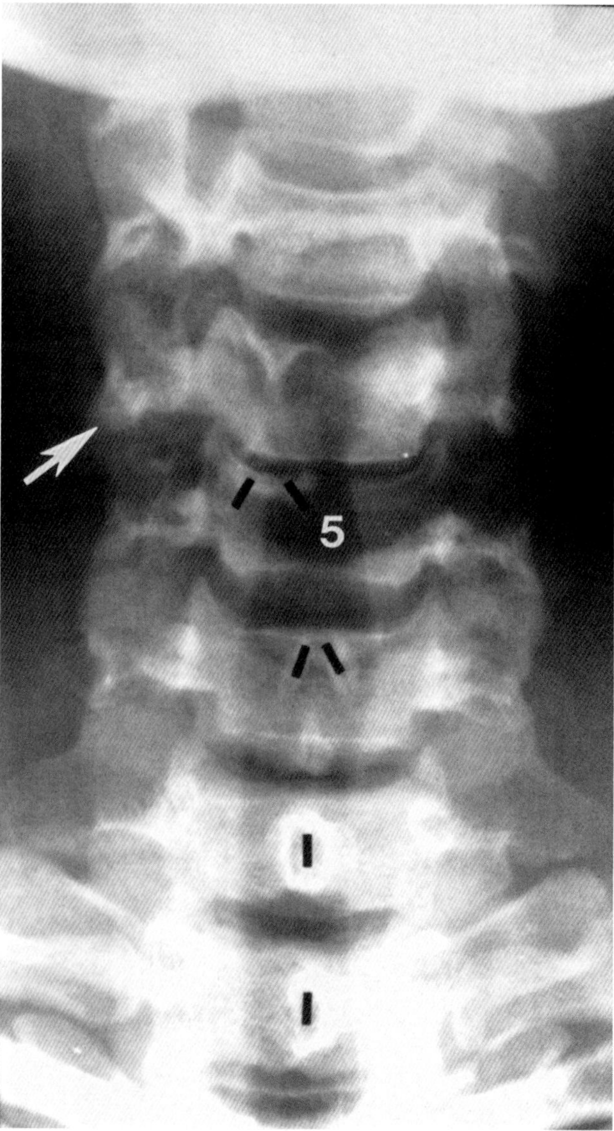


**Fig. 3-42** Anteroposterior (AP) radiograph demonstrating rotation of C5 on C6 with facet asymmetry (*arrow*). Note the bifid spinous processes (*lines*) at C5 and C6.

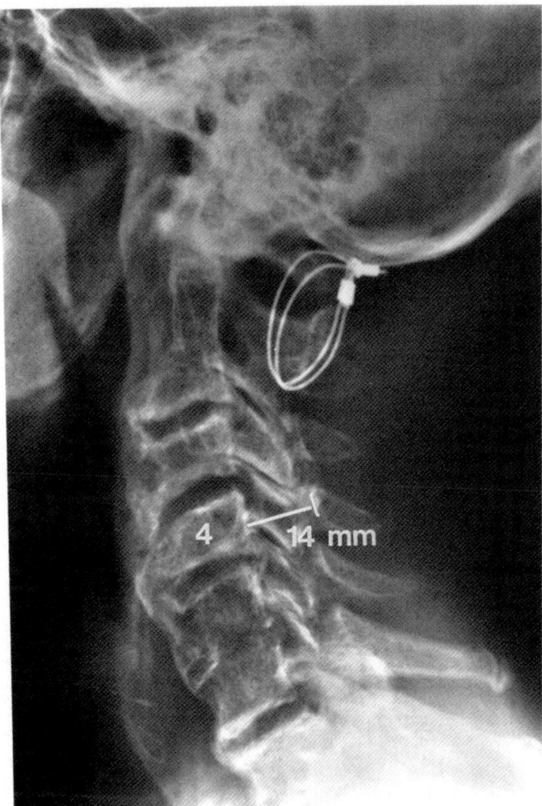


Fig. 3-43 Lateral radiograph of the cervical spine in a patient with advanced degenerative changes and prior C1-2 fusion with Songer cables. The mid-sagittal diameter of the spinal canal is measured from the mid-posterior vertebral body to the spinolaminar line (normal 17 to 18 mm, <13 mm considered stenosis), and in this case measured at C4 it is 14 mm.

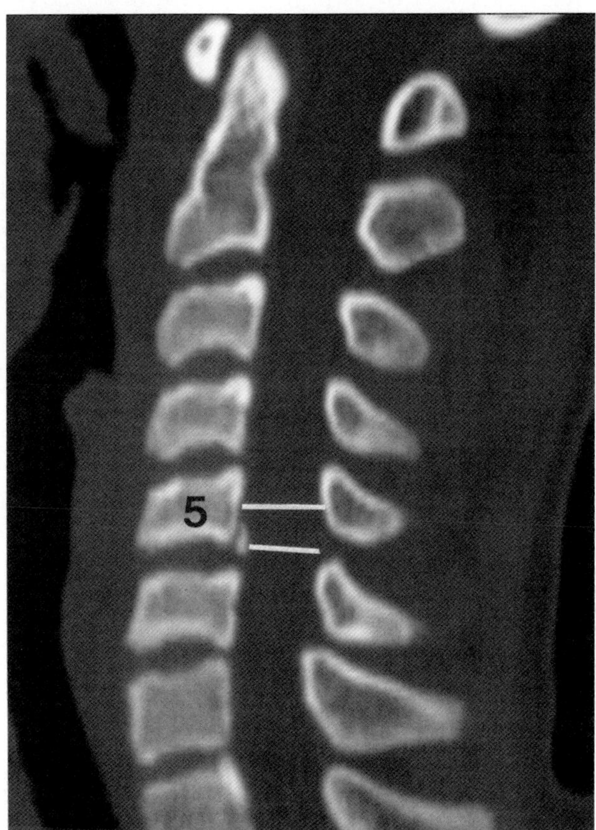


Fig. 3-45 Sagittal computed tomographic (CT) image demonstrating ossification posterior to C5 and anteroposterior (AP) dimension of the spinal canal at the mid vertebral level and narrowing at the level of ossification.

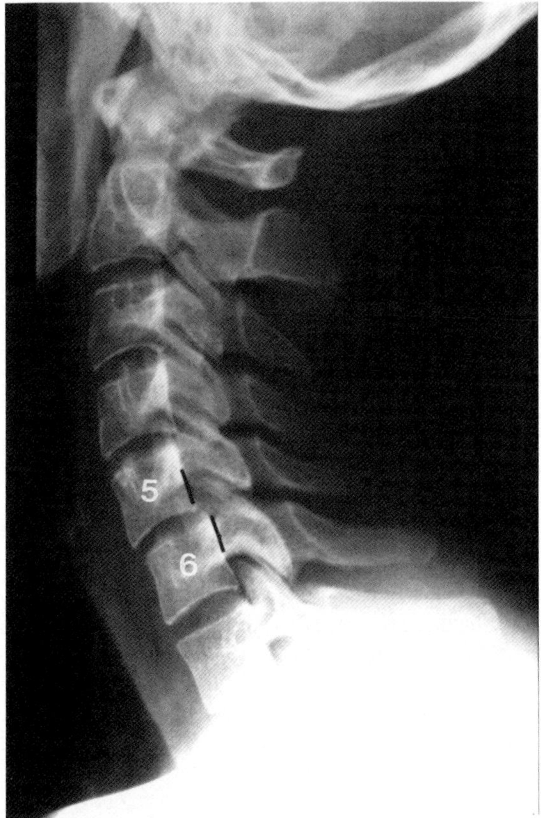


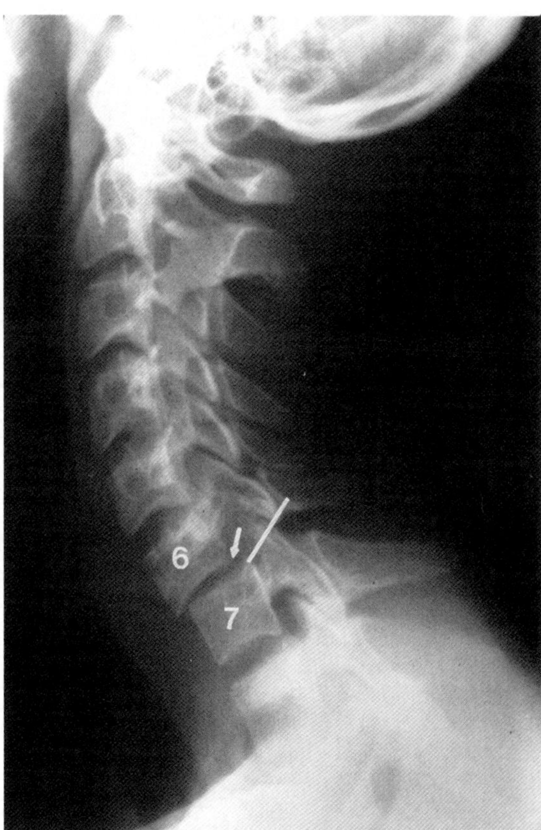


Fig. 3-44 A: Lateral radiograph demonstrates mild displacement of C5 on C6 (*black lines*) and slight disc space narrowing. B: Lateral radiograph in flexion shows subluxation of C6 on C7 measuring 4 mm (normal <3 mm) (*arrow*) with narrowing of the spinal canal (*white line*) measured from the vertebral margin to the adjacent laminar line (<12 mm dynamic stenosis).

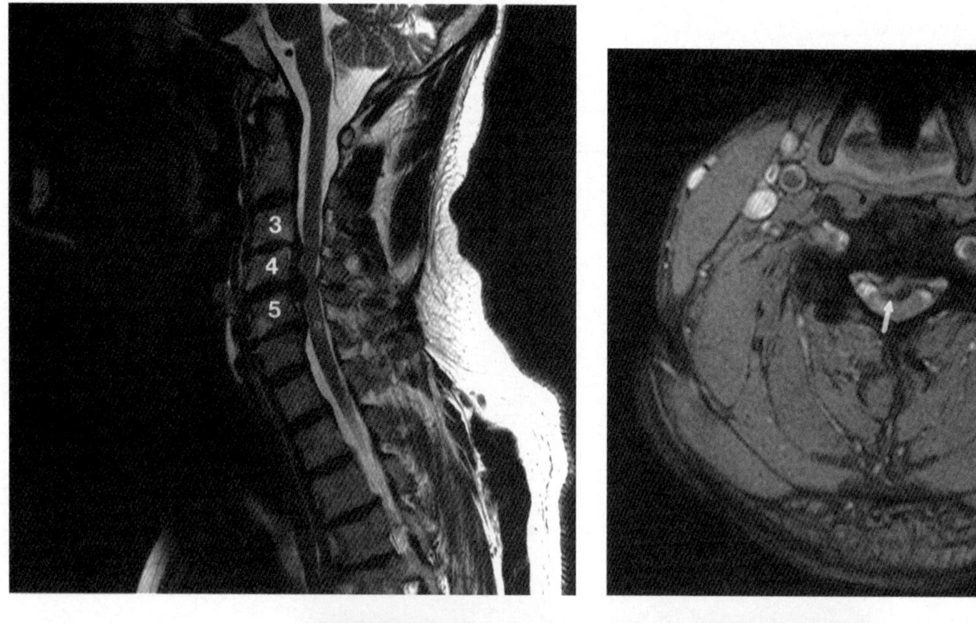


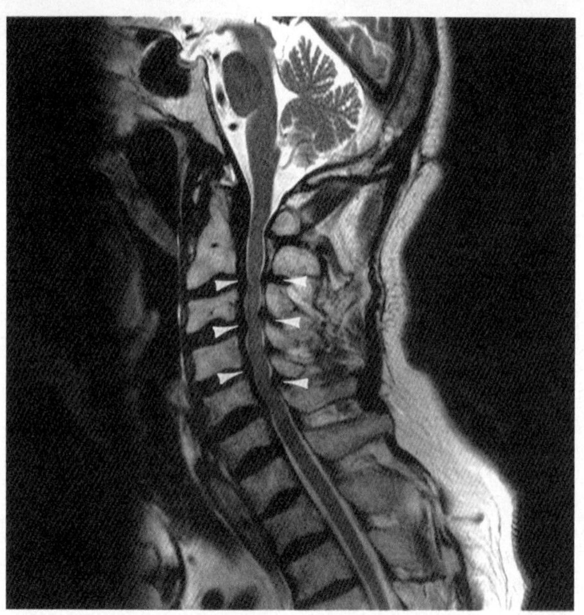


**Fig. 3-46** Magnetic resonance (MR) images demonstrating prominent disc extrusions and multilevel spinal stenosis. Sagittal (**A**) and axial (**B**) images demonstrating a large central disc extrusion at C4-5 (*arrow* in **B**) and smaller extrusions at C3-4 and C5-6. **C**: Sagittal MR image demonstrating multilevel stenosis due to disc changes and hypertrophy of the ligamentum flavum (*arrowheads*).

## Suggested Reading

Berquist TH, Currier BL, Broderick DF. The spine. In: Berquist TH, ed. *Imaging atlas of orthopaedic appliances and prostheses*. New York: Raven Press; 1995:109–215.

Rao RD, Gourab K, David KS. Operative treatment of cervical spondylotic myelopathy. *J Bone Joint Surg*. 2006;88A:1619–1639.

### Surgical Approaches to Cervical Degenerative Disease

The primary goals of surgical intervention for cervical degenerative disease are expansion (decompression) of the spinal canal and stability with fusion. Anterior, posterior, and combined approaches may be employed depending on spinal alignment, levels of involvement, and the presence of prior surgery. Patients with reversal or straightening of the spinal alignment do not allow translation of the cord away from the anterior compression

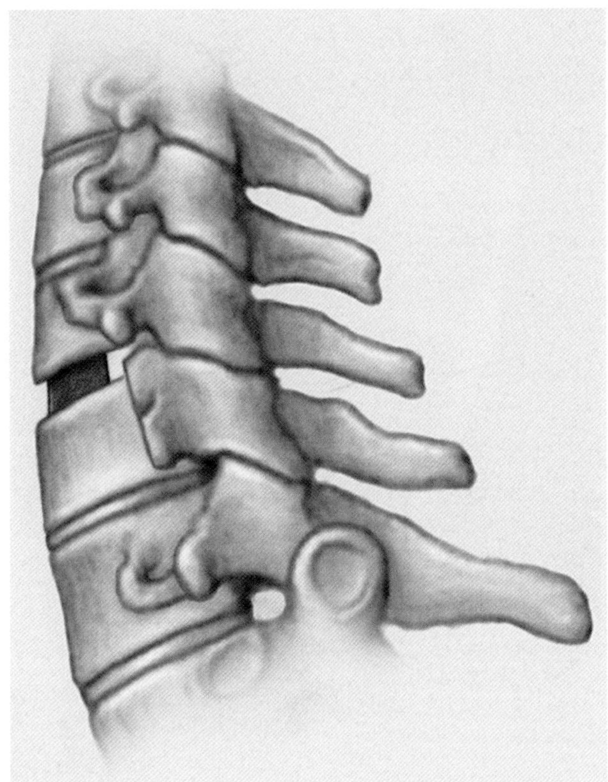


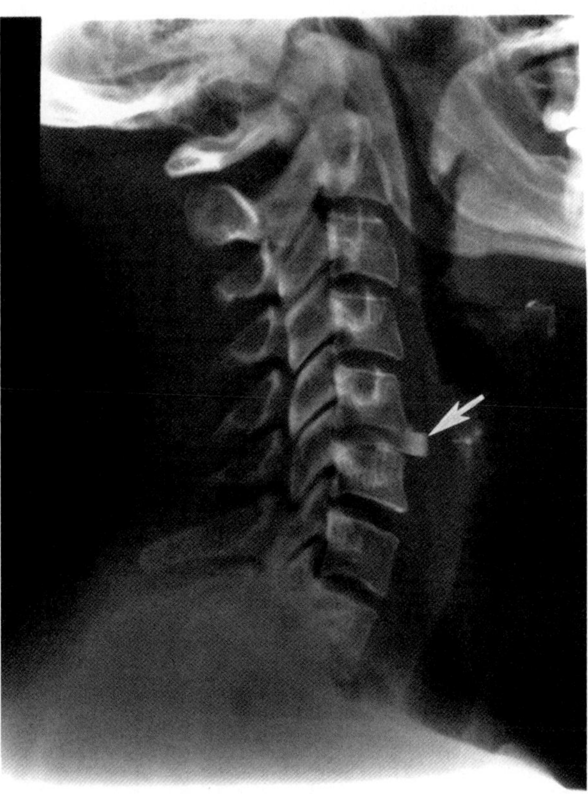


Fig. 3-47 A: Illustration of anterior discectomy and bone graft fusion. B: Lateral radiograph demonstrates anterior displacement of the bone graft (*arrow*).

if a posterior approach is used. When one or two levels are involved most surgeons prefer an anterior approach. Dysphagia and graft complications increase with increasing levels of involvement using the anterior approach. In patients with prior surgery with an anterior or posterior approach, the reoperation may be most easily accomplished by using a different approach to avoid scar tissue from the prior procedure.

ANTERIOR OPTIONS

**Anterior discectomy and fusion** (see Fig. 3-47)
- Removes disc and posterior osteophytes
- Bone graft (>2 mm thick) distracts disc for indirect decompression
- Protects stability, less exposure of spinal cord
- Not recommended with severe spinal stenosis

**Anterior discectomy, fusion, and anterior plating** (see Fig. 3-48)
- Improves the rate of fusion compared to bone graft fusion alone
- Reduces postoperative immobilization
- Decreases graft-related complications (see Fig. 3-47B)
- Reduces progressive kyphosis, especially with multilevel fusions
- Plate selected to keep proximal and distal ends 5 mm away from the vertebral end plate to reduce postoperative heterotopic ossification

**Anterior decompression with corpectomy** (see Fig. 3-49)
- Removal of anterior midline vertebral body to posterior longitudinal ligament and cephalad and caudad discs
- Allows removal of osteophytes
- Wide trough allows for larger bone graft or cage
- Iliac crest commonly used for bone graft
- Fibular strut graft for multisegment corpectomies
- Anterior plate fixation

POSTERIOR OPTIONS

**Laminoplasty** (see Fig. 3-50)
- Single or double lamina lifted dorsally to enlarge the spinal canal
- Leaves bone and ligamentum flavum covering; therefore, less instability
- Spinous process bone graft and/or mini plates to secure position

**Laminectomy and fusion** (see Fig. 3-51)
- Bone removed to junction of lamina and lateral masses
- May also perform foraminotomy in patients with foraminal encroachment
- Posterior fusion with rods and sublaminar facet wires or screws

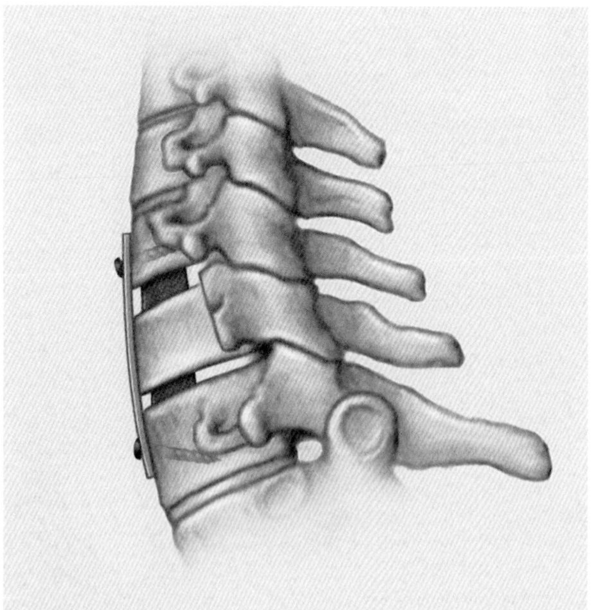

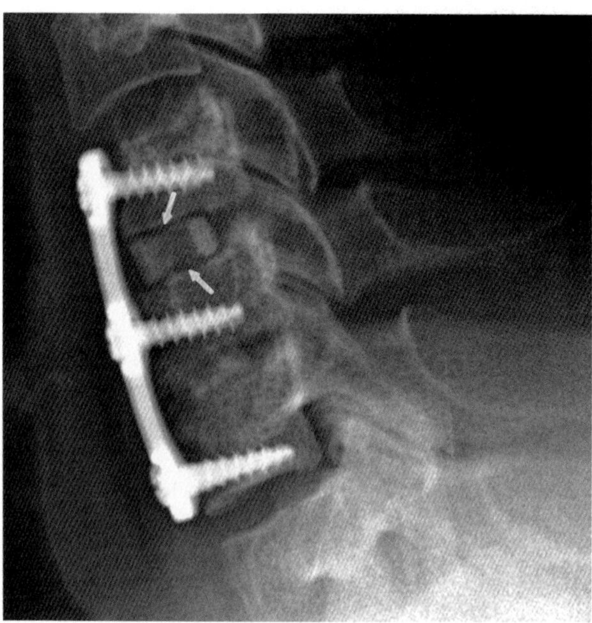

A B

Fig. 3-48 A: Illustration of multilevel discectomy, bone grafts, and anterior plate and screw fixation. B: Lateral radiograph after multilevel fusion with anterior plate and screw fixation from C5-7. The bone graft at C6-7 has incorporated into the adjacent vertebrae. There is lucency about the graft at C5-6 indicating lack of fusion (*arrows*).

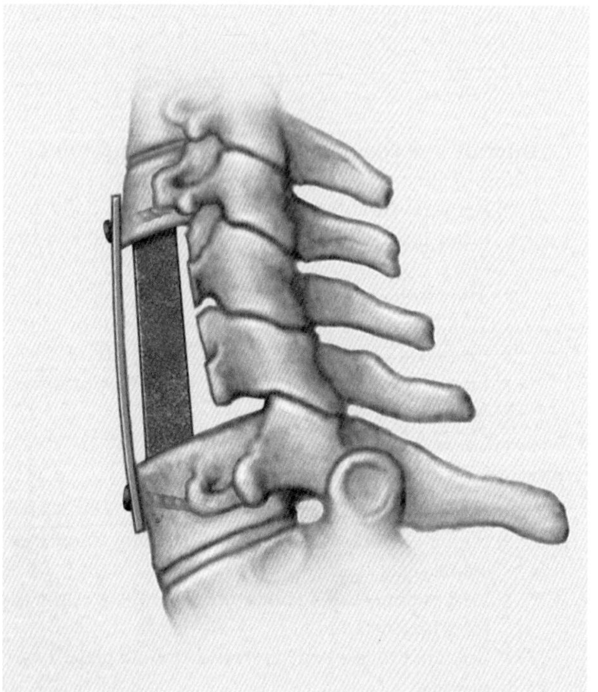

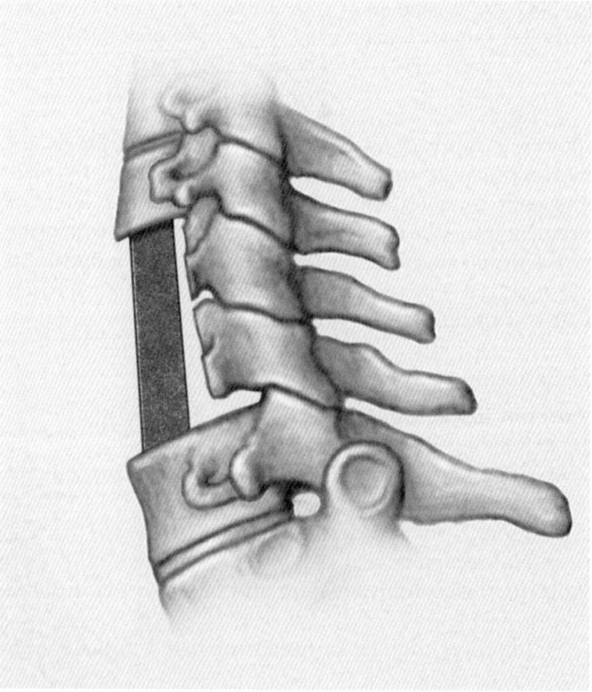

A B

Fig. 3-49 Illustrations of corpectomy with strut graft fusion without (A) and with (B) plating. C: Lateral radiograph demonstrating strut graft from C4-6 with anterior plating. D: Several months later the lateral radiograph demonstrates displacement (*arrow*) of the distal graft anteriorly.

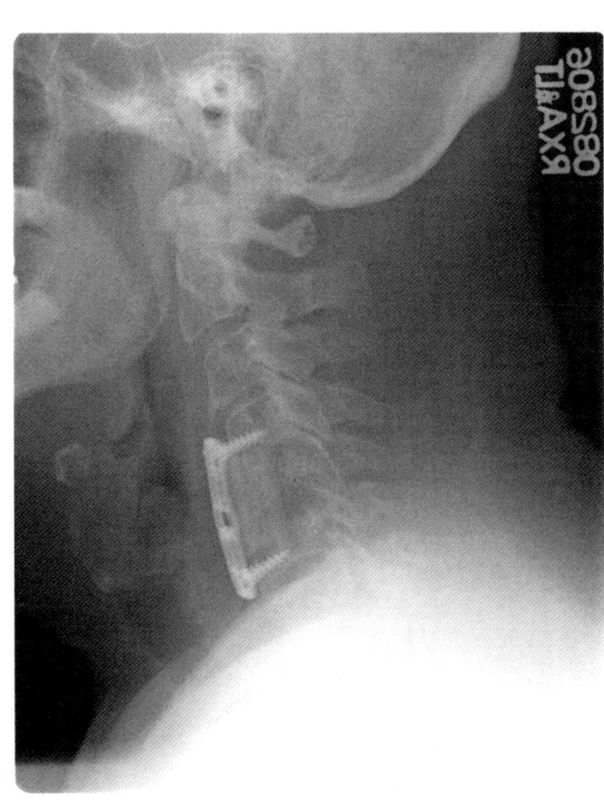
C

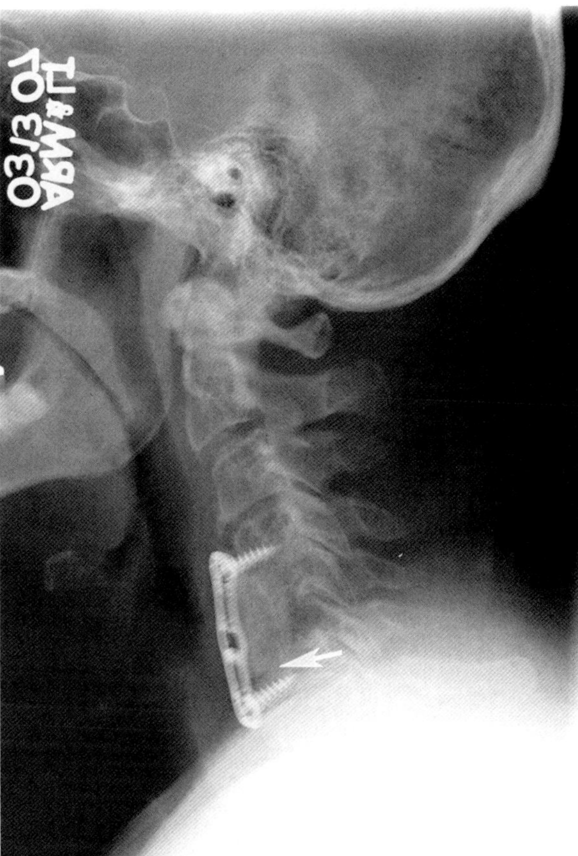
D

Fig. 3-49 *(Continued)*

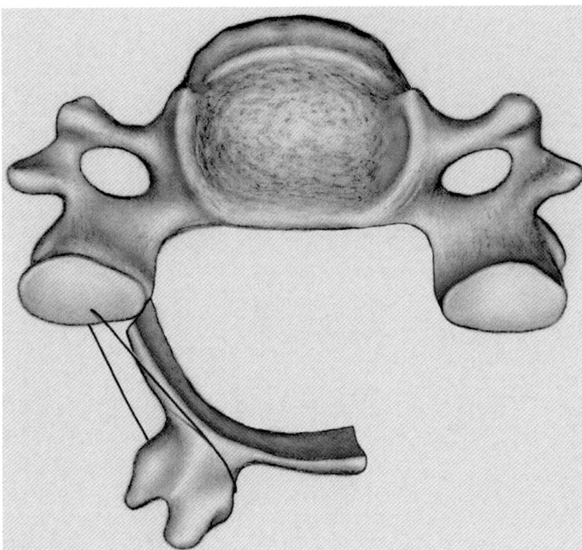
A

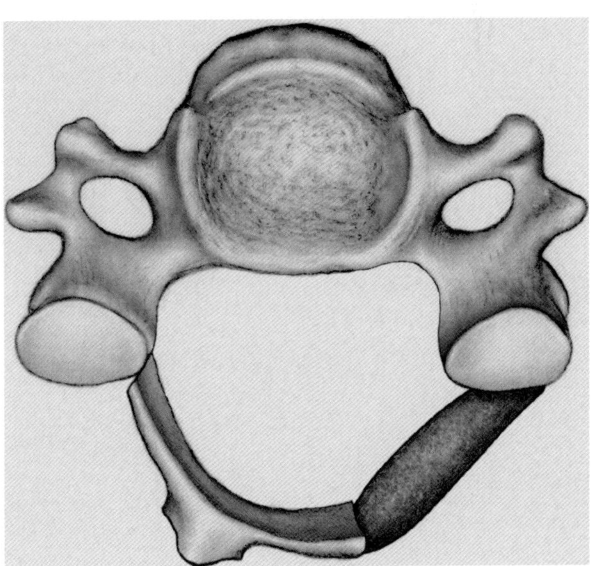
B

Fig. 3-50 Illustration of laminoplasty (A) with bone graft (B) or mini plate (C) to maintain position. D: Bilateral (double door) laminoplasty with bone graft to maintain position. E: Axial computed tomographic (CT) myelogram after laminoplasty with miniplate fixation. There is contrast posteriorly (*arrow*) due to a leak of cerebrospinal fluid (CSF).

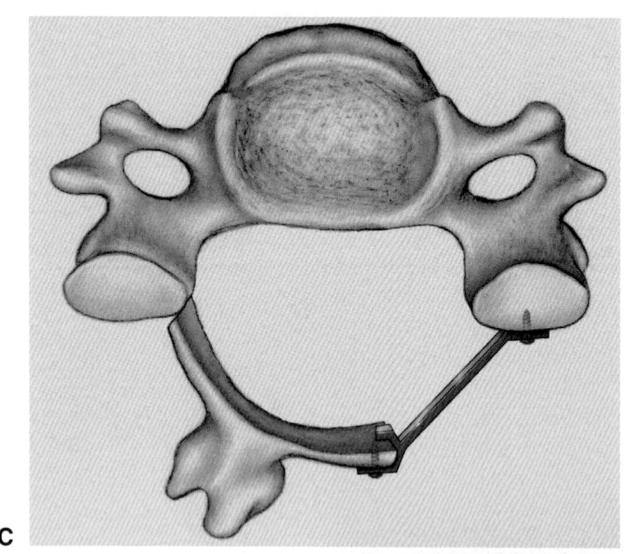
C

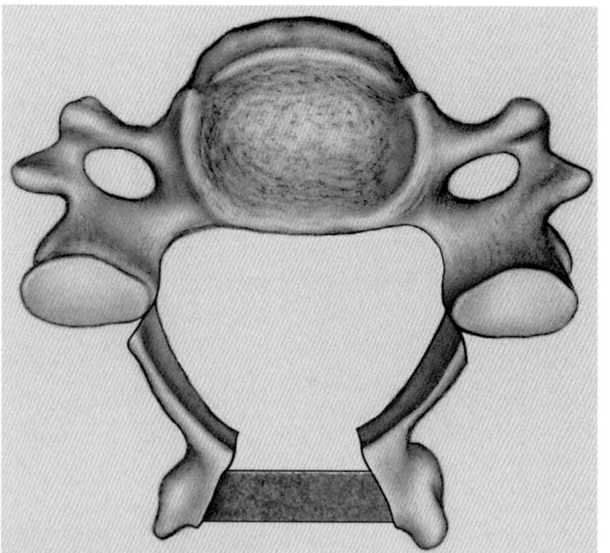
D

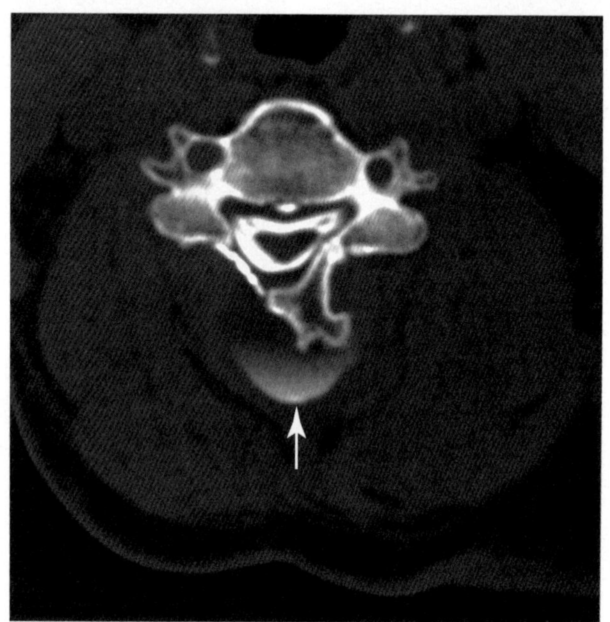
E

Fig. 3-50 *(Continued)*

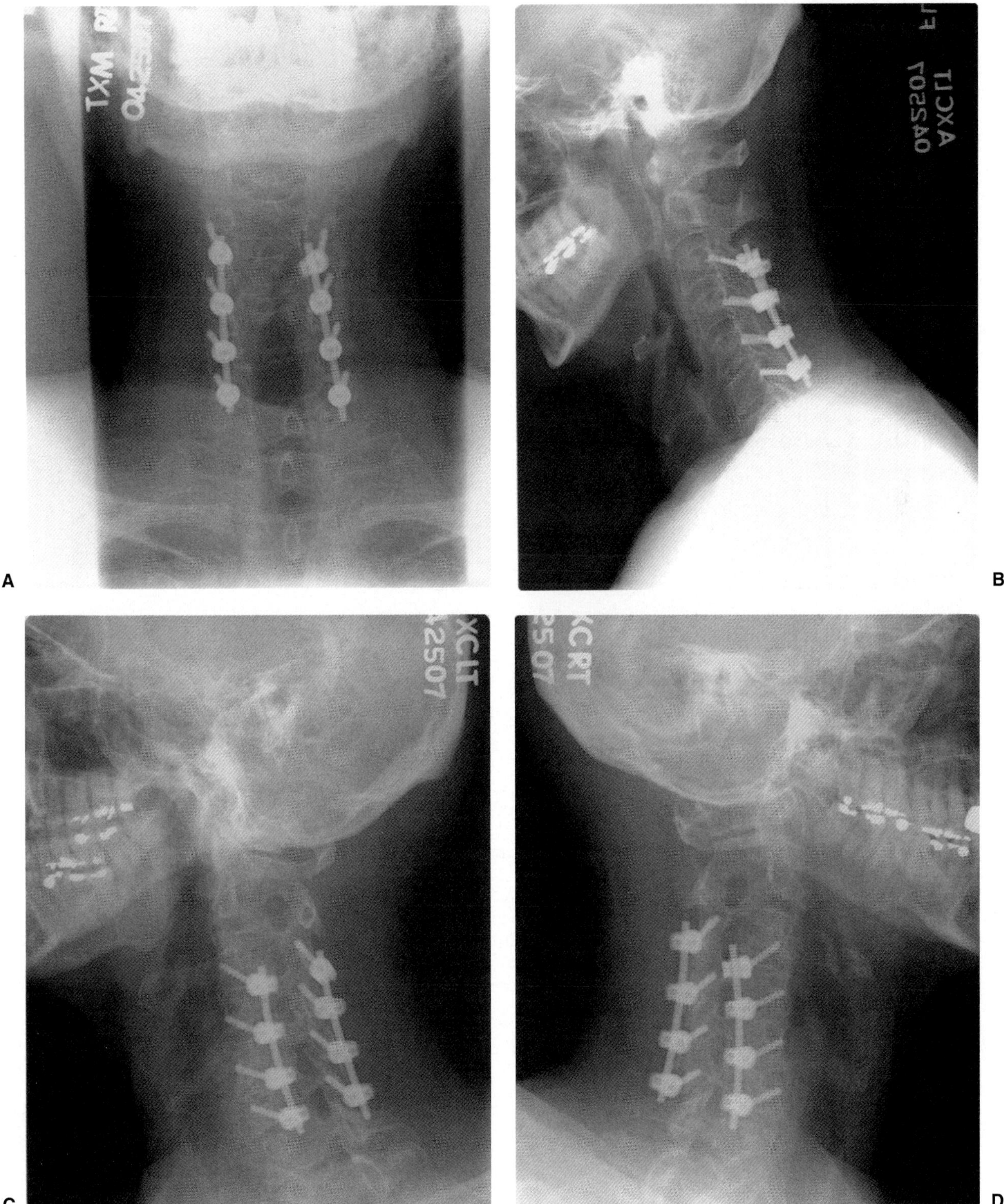

Fig. 3-51 Posterior laminectomy and fusion. Anteroposterior (AP) (A), lateral (B), and oblique radiographs (C and D) after laminectomy and fusion C3-6 with posterior rod and lateral mass screws for fixation.

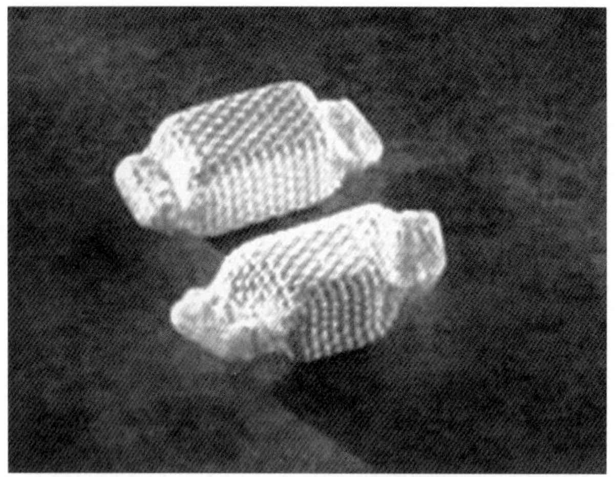

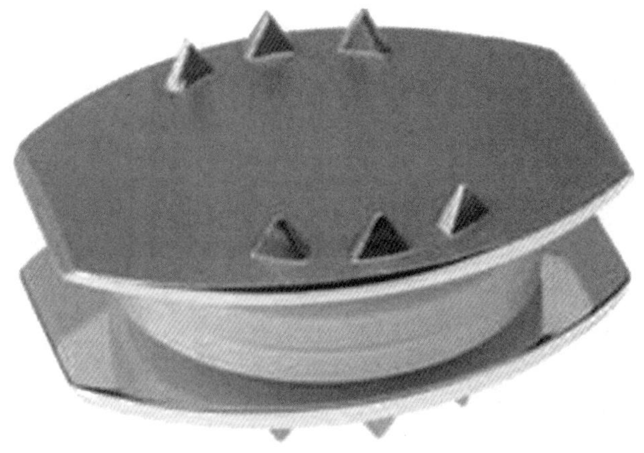

**Fig. 3-52** Disc replacement options. **A:** Prosthetic disc nucleus with hydrogel core and woven polyethylene jacket (Courtesy Raymedica, Bloomington, Mn.) **B:** Acroflex disc with rubber core and titanium endplates (Courtesy DePuy Acromed, Raynham, Ma.) **C:** Link SB Charite disc with biconvex ultra–high molecular weight polyethylene and end plates coated with titanium and hydroxyapatite to promote bone in growth. Use in the lumbar spine (Courtesy DePuy Spine, Raynham, Ma).

**DISC REPLACEMENT**

- Lower incidence of adjacent degeneration when motion maintained at operated disc level
- Multiple implant designs, which must resist fatigue with load (see Fig. 3-52)
- Implants fixed to adjacent vertebrae
- Current data promising but preliminary

## Suggested Reading

Phillips FM, Garfin SR. Cervical disc replacement. *Spine.* 2005;30:S27–S33.

Rao RD, Goubar K, David KS. Operative treatment of cervical spondylotic myelopathy. *J Bone Joint Surg.* 2006;88A: 1619–1639.

### Imaging of Postoperative Complications

Complications may occur during the procedure or later related to multiple factors including inadequate surgical technique, surgical approach (anterior vs. posterior), and anatomic region. Imaging plays a vital role in evaluating potential complications following spinal fusion with or without instrumentation. Postoperative evaluation of lumbar and cervical procedures requires knowledge of the normal appearance of instrumentation and graft material as well as an understanding of the potential complications with each type of device.

Postoperative imaging begins with baseline radiographs when the patient can tolerate the examination. Images should include AP, lateral, and oblique images, and after adequate immobilization flexion and extension images. Serial radiographs remain the primary screening technique for evaluation of instrument failure and graft abnormalities. CT, radionuclide scans, MRI, ultrasound, and diagnostic injections may also be indicated. Complications may be slightly different in the cervical and lumbar spine.

INTRAOPERATIVE COMPLICATIONS

## Cervical spine

- **Nerve root injury**—sublaminar wires, pedicle screws (0.6%)
- **Vertebral artery injury**—more common with anterior approach
- **Cord injury**—due to ischemia, stretching, direct trauma, or hypothermia
- **Dural tears**—more common with posterior approach

## Lumbar spine

- **Posterior approach**—radiculopathy, dural tears, nerve root injury with sublaminar wires or pedicle screws
- **Anterior approach**—vascular injury, genitourinary complications

POSTOPERATIVE COMPLICATIONS Symptoms following cervical and lumbar arthrodesis vary with the location and extent of surgery. Following cervical laminoplasty, up to 60% of patients complain of neck and shoulder pain and 72% complain of neck stiffness. Following laminectomy without fusion, up to 30% of patients develop kyphosis and 21% will develop new neurologic symptoms due to instability. Up to 40% of patients develop radiculopathy following cervical arthrodesis. Dysphagia and recurrent laryngeal nerve palsy may also follow cervical fusion. However, the former usually resolves over the course of a year. Following lumbar procedures recurrent pain is not uncommon. Nerve root irritation and cauda equina syndrome may also develop in these patients.

Pseudarthrosis or nonunion (see Fig. 3-53) is among the most significant complications following spinal arthrodesis. The incidence varies with the anatomic region and number of segments included. The incidence has been reported as high as 56%. Pseudarthrosis associated with scoliosis instrumentation is 30%, lumbar arthrodesis without instrumentation 31.5%, lumbar arthrodesis with instrumentation 13.5%, and cervical arthrodesis up to 26%. If bony fusion fails the instrumentation will also eventually break down. Up to 50% of patients with nonunion may be asymptomatic. In symptomatic patients, treatment options include electrical stimulation, bracing, and reoperation (see Fig. 3-54).

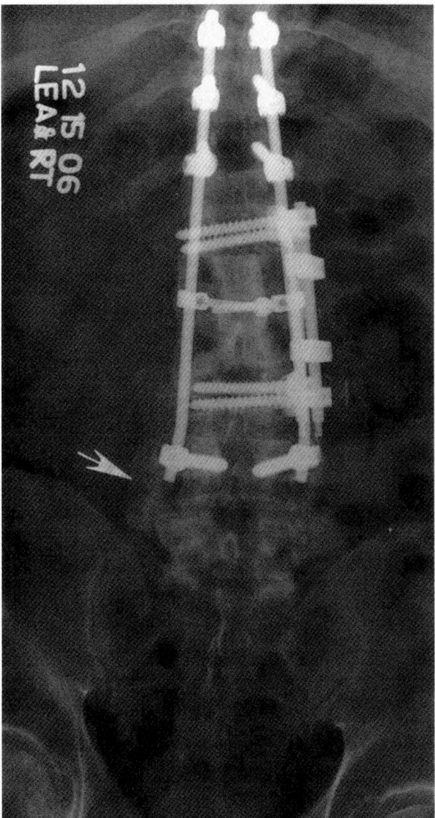

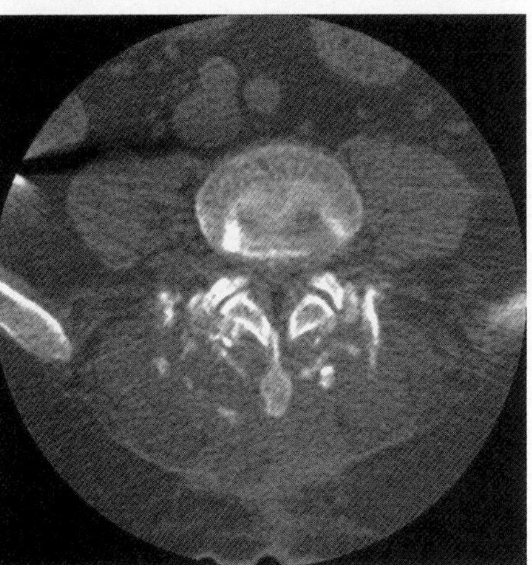


Fig. 3-53 Pseudarthrosis or nonunion. A: Anteroposterior (AP) radiograph demonstrating combined anterior and posterior instrumentation from T10-L4 with corpectomy and strut graft at L2 and posterolateral bone graft (*arrow*). B: SPECT radionuclide images demonstrate intense uptake in the posterolateral bone graft (*arrows*) at L4 bilaterally. Axial (C) image demonstrates resorption and failure of incorporation of the posterolateral bone graft. SPECT, single photon emission computed tomography.

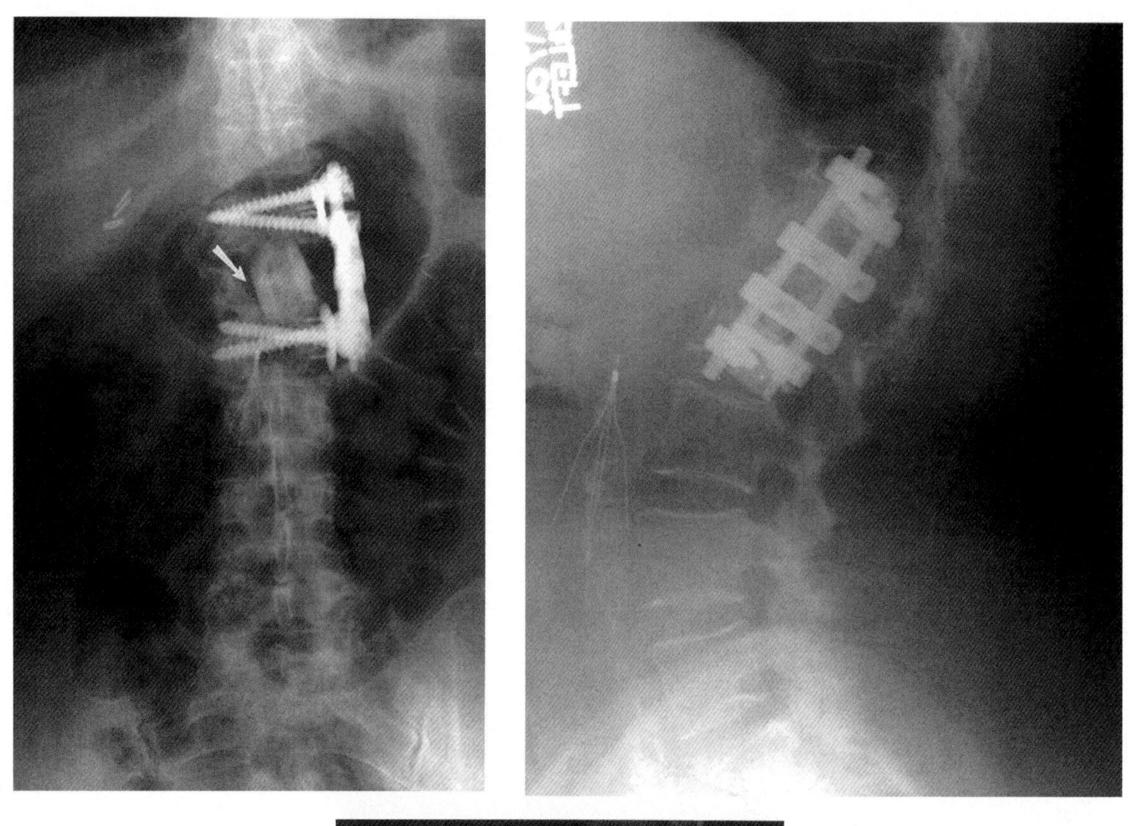

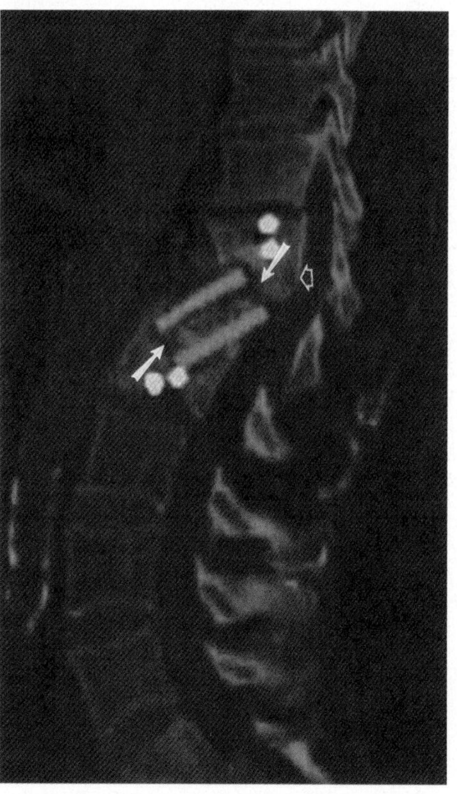

Fig. 3-54 L1 partial corpectomy with strut graft and anterior instrumentation. Anteroposterior (AP) (A) and lateral (B) radiographs demonstrate lucency about the strut graft (*arrow*) and posterior subluxation of T12. C: Sagittal reformatted computed tomographic (CT) image demonstrates the oblique position of the graft with lucency (*arrows*) and lack of incorporation with posterior displacement of T12 (*open arrow*). AP (D) and lateral (E) radiographs after reoperation with rods and pedicle screws from T9 to L4. Note the new compression fracture of L4 (*arrow*).

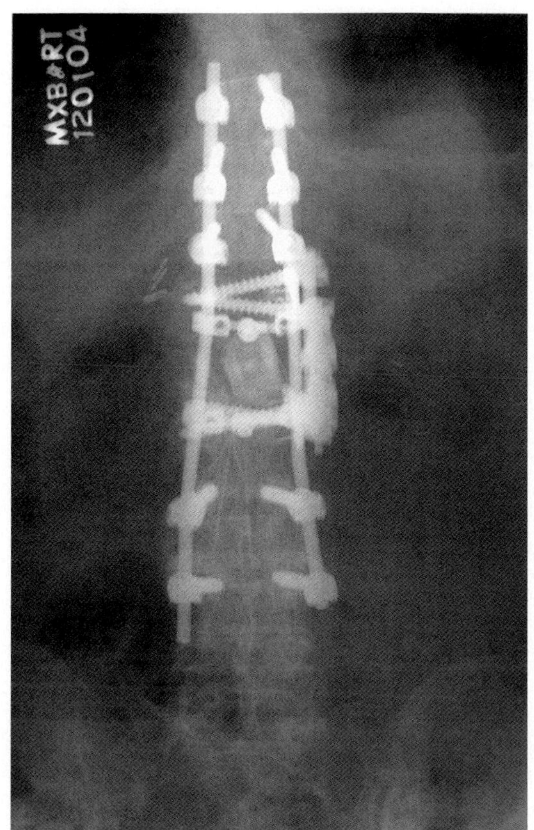


D

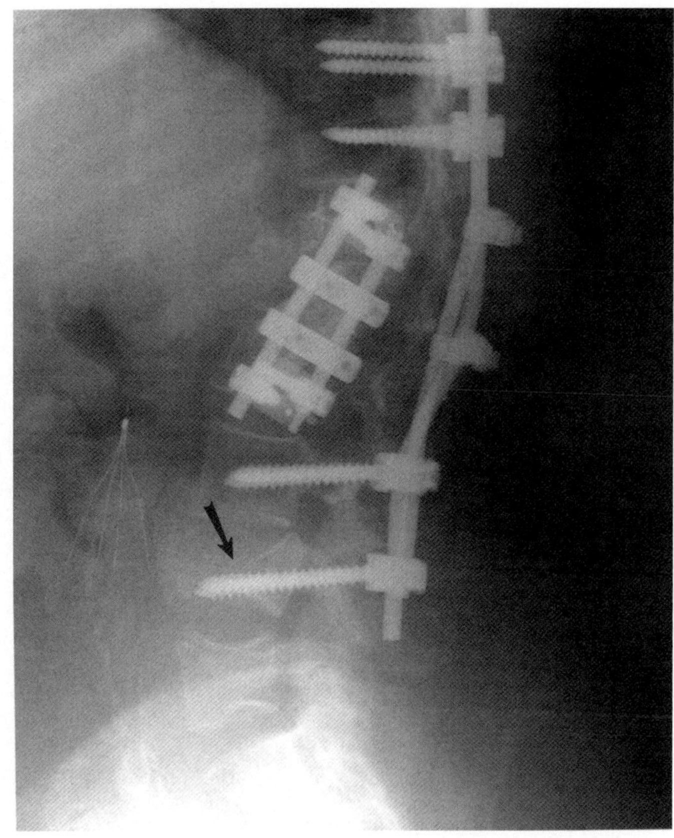

E

Fig. 3-54 *(Continued)*

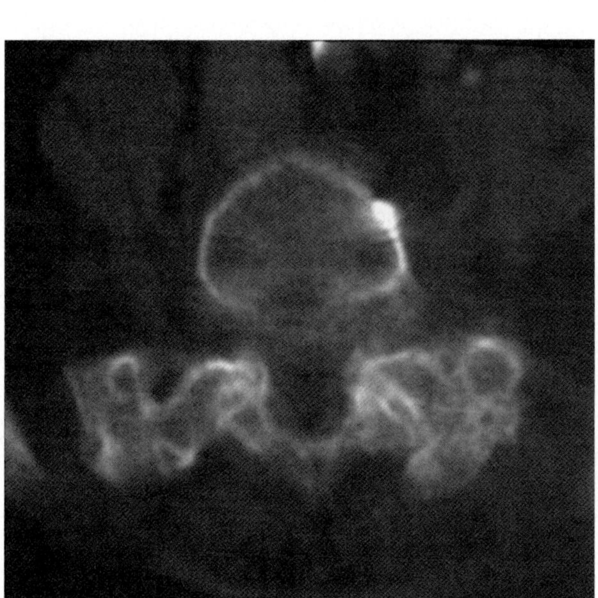

A

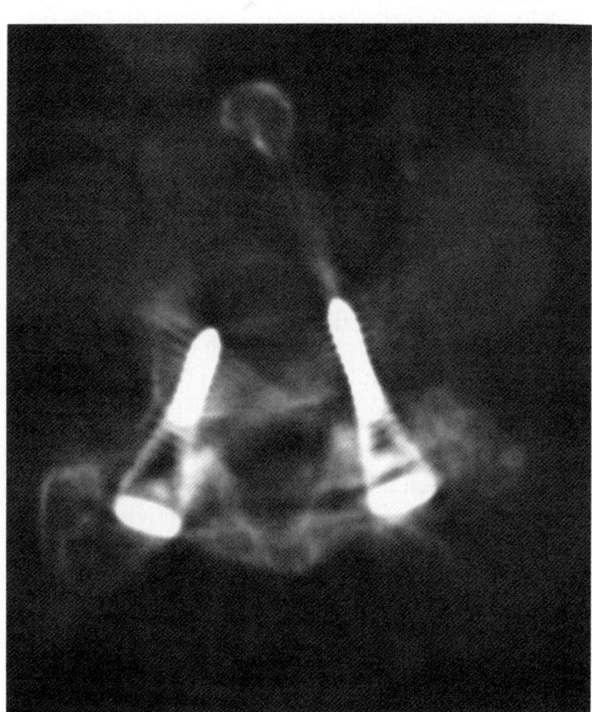

B

Fig. 3-55 Axial computed tomographic (CT) images (A and B) demonstrating solid bone graft fusion posterolaterally with rod and pedicle screw instrumentation.

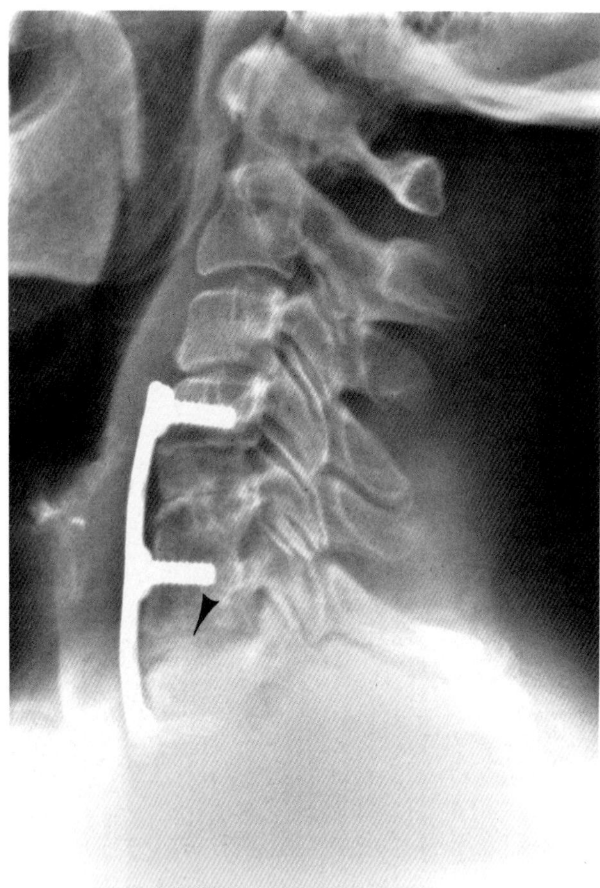

Fig. 3-56 Prior anterior discectomy and fusion C4-7. There is loss of height and sclerosis of the graft at the lower fused disc space (*arrowhead*).

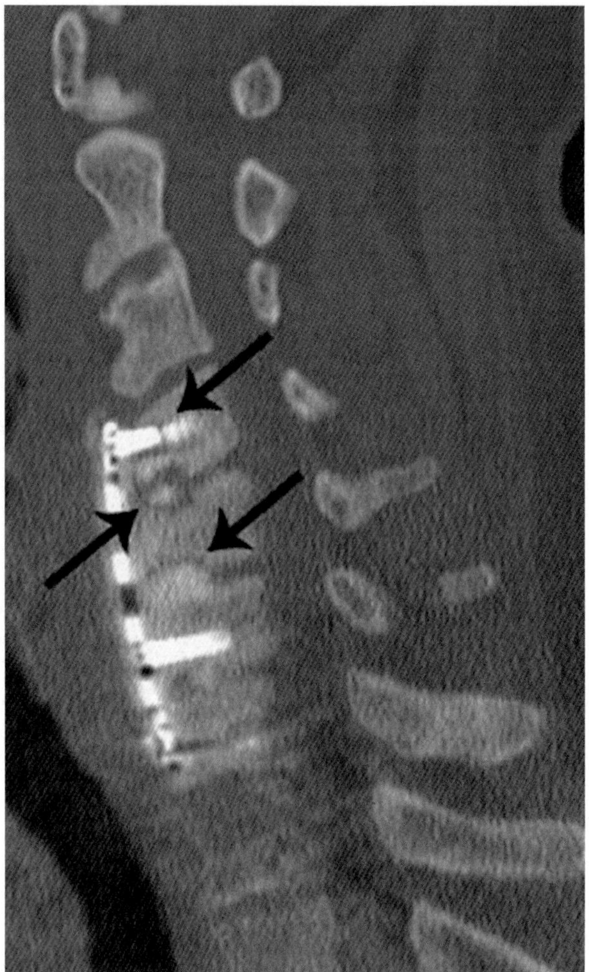

Fig. 3-57 Sagittal computed tomography (CT) of the cervical spine after multilevel discectomy and fusion with anterior plate fixation. The upper screws (*upper arrow*) have fractured due to graft failure. There is resorption of the graft at C3-4 with end plate fracture (*middle anterior arrow*) and endplate fracture by the graft at C4-5 (*lower arrow*).

### Indications of solid fusion

- Bone graft bridges the fused segments or disc space (see Fig. 3-55)
- No motion or <3 degrees angulation on flexion and extension
- No lucency about the disc graft (Fig. 3-48B)
- No disc graft sclerosis (see Fig. 3-56)
- No endplate or graft fracture (see Fig. 3-57)

### Pseudarthrosis or nonunion: Haggness and Esses Classification

- **Atrophic**—graft resorption (Fig. 3-54C to E )
- **Transverse**—horizontal discontinuity of graft material (see Fig. 3-58)
- **Shingle**—oblique discontinuity
- **Complex**—multiple adjacent graft defects

### Image features of pseudarthrosis or nonunion

- **Radiographs**—lucency about screws (see Fig. 3-59), broken or uncoupled implants (see Fig. 3-60), progressive vertebral subluxation, motion on flexion extension images, graft displacement
- **CT**—discontinuity in graft material or failure to incorporate into lamina or disc endplates; use metal artifact reduction filters (Fig. 3-54)
- **MRI**—abnormal high signal intensity about the disc spacer or through the posterior bone graft on T2-weighted images; metal artifact reduction sequences and techniques
- **Radionuclide scans**—abnormal tracer accumulation at the site of graft failure (Fig. 3-53B)
- **Ultrasound**—clefts in graft or fluid collections
- **Diagnostic injection**—anesthetic injection of defect to confirm source of pain

Instrument failure or uncoupling typically occurs with failure of bony fusion. This may include fracture of wires, rods, plates or screws, screw loosening or pull out, and hook dislodgement (Fig. 3-60). Detection of these complications is usually

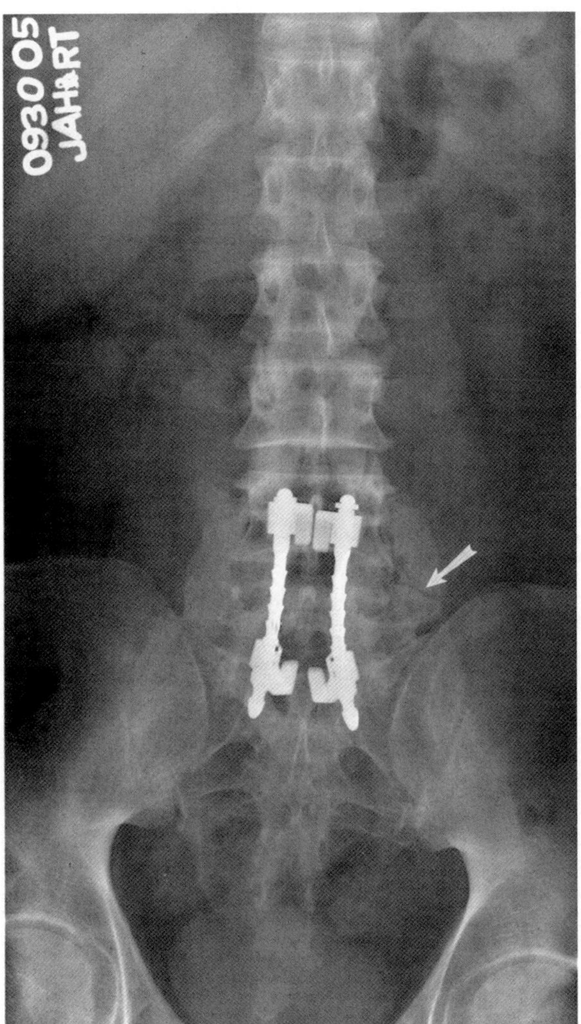

Fig. 3-58 Anteroposterior (AP) radiograph following Harrington rod and hook instrumentation L4-S1 with transverse interruption of bone graft (*arrow*) at L5 on the left.

accomplished with serial radiographs or computed radiographic (CR) images. In certain cases, fluoroscopic positioning may be required to fully evaluate the position of hooks. CT is preferred to evaluate pedicle and lateral mass screw position and complications.

Most statistical data is available for pedicle screws or in the case of the cervical spine and lateral mass screws (see Fig. 3-51). Figure 3-61 demonstrates the normal position for lumbar pedicle screws. Lateral mass screws in the cervical spine cause nerve root irritation in 0.6% of cases. Vertebral artery injuries are uncommon with lateral mass screws. Pedicle screw complications are summarized in the subsequent text (see Figs. 3-62 to 3-64).

**Pedicle screw complications:** 2.4%
- Screw malposition 5% (Figs. 3-59 and 3-64)
- Screw fractures 2.2% (65% have pseudarthrosis) (Fig. 3-62)
- Cut out of cortex during insertion 1.4% (Fig. 3-63)
- Dural tears 1%
- Nerve root irritation 1%

Anterior bone graft, struts, cages, spacers, and disc prostheses present another area for image evaluation. Bone grafts are typically harvested from the iliac crest or fibula for strut grafts (autografts). However, allografts may also be used. The collapse rate is higher for allografts (28%). Failure rates for anterior grafts increase with multilevel fusions. The fusion rate for single-level grafts is 89% compared to 73% for two levels and 50% to 71% for three-level strut grafts. When combined with posterior fusion the failure rates are reduced. Graft position can be easily evaluated on serial radiographs (see Fig. 3-65, also Fig. 3-47B) and when necessary CT or MRI may be required to assess graft changes or neural involvement (see Fig. 3-66).

### Indications of solid fusion

- Bone graft bridges the fused segments or disc space
- No motion or <3 degrees angulation on flexion and extension

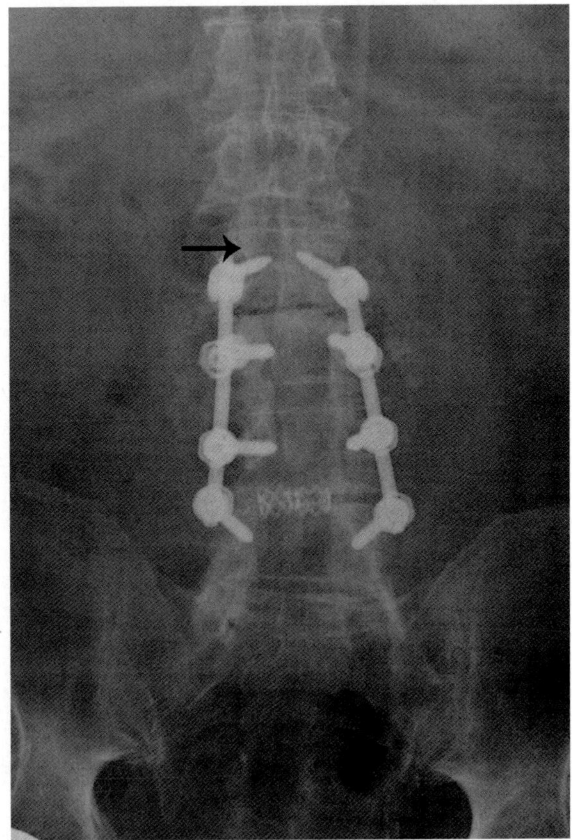


Fig. 3-59 Screw loosening with surrounding lucency. **A:** Anteroposterior (AP) radiograph after laminectomy and rod and pedicle screw instrumentation L2-5 with anterior cage at L4-5. There is lucency about the proximal pedicle screws (*arrow*). Lateral radiographs at 2 (**B**) and 4 months (**C**) following the procedure demonstrate progressive disc space deterioration and retrolisthesis at L2-3.

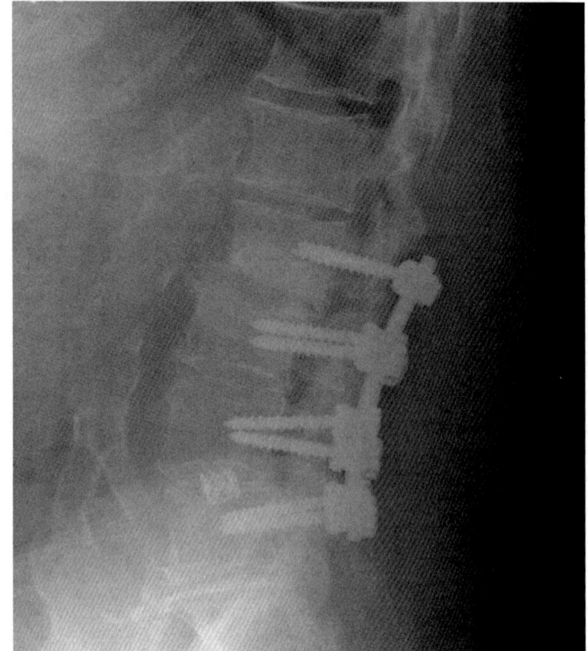

B

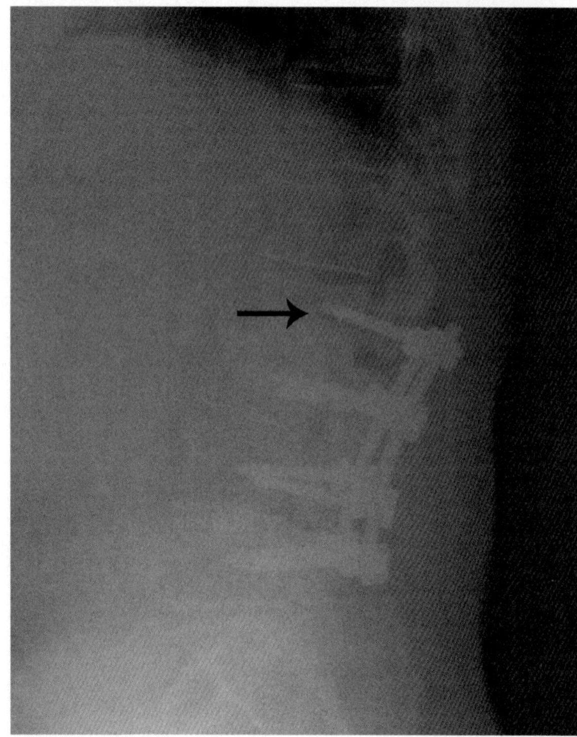

C

Fig. 3-59 *(Continued)*

- No lucency about the disc graft (Fig. 3-48B)
- No disc graft sclerosis (Fig. 3-57)
- No endplate or graft fracture

Interbody fusion cages (Fig. 3-39) can be evaluated in a similar manner. Disc height, displacement, endplate fracture and motion at the fused segment indicate lack of fusion. Two percent to 9% of interbody fusion cages displace. Disc prostheses are now being used in the lumbar and cervical spine primarily in patients with isolated disc disease. Preliminary results are promising. Disc prosthesis can be imaged similar to other anterior graft material or cages. Heterotopic ossification about the disc occurs in 4.3% of cases.

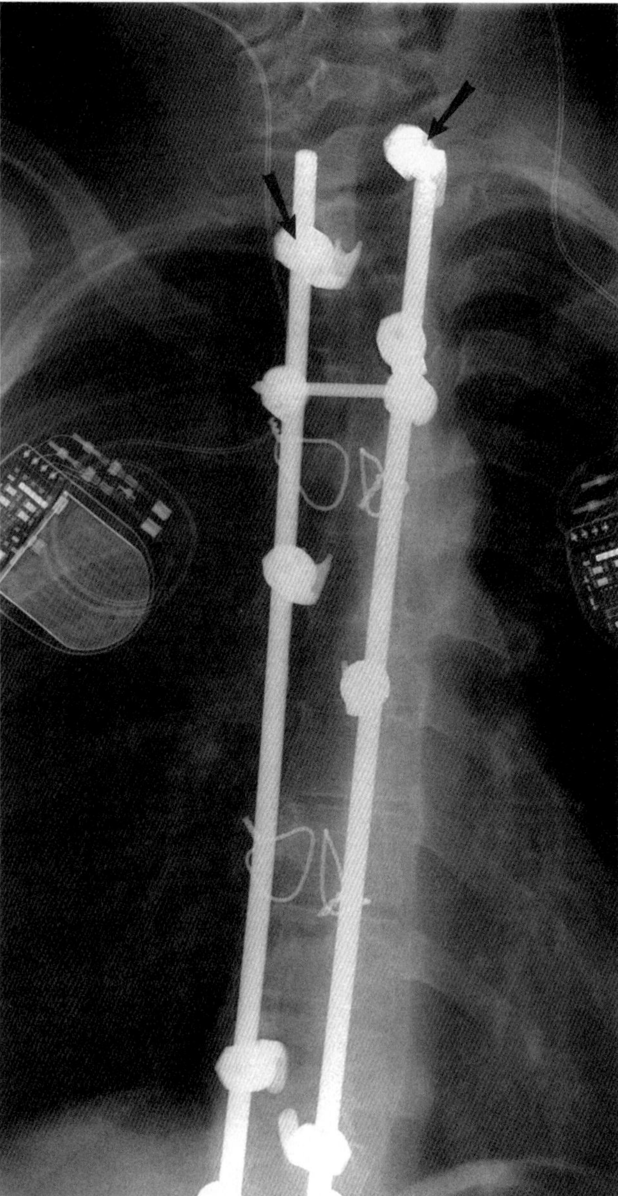

Fig. 3-60 Hook dislodgement. Anteroposterior (AP) radiograph after rod and hook instrumentation with dislodging of the two proximal hooks (*arrows*).

Adjacent segment disease (ASD) is common following spinal arthrodesis. This occurs due to stress transferred adjacent to the fused segments. The incidence 3 years after fusion varies from 5% to 100%. This disorder is also more common with

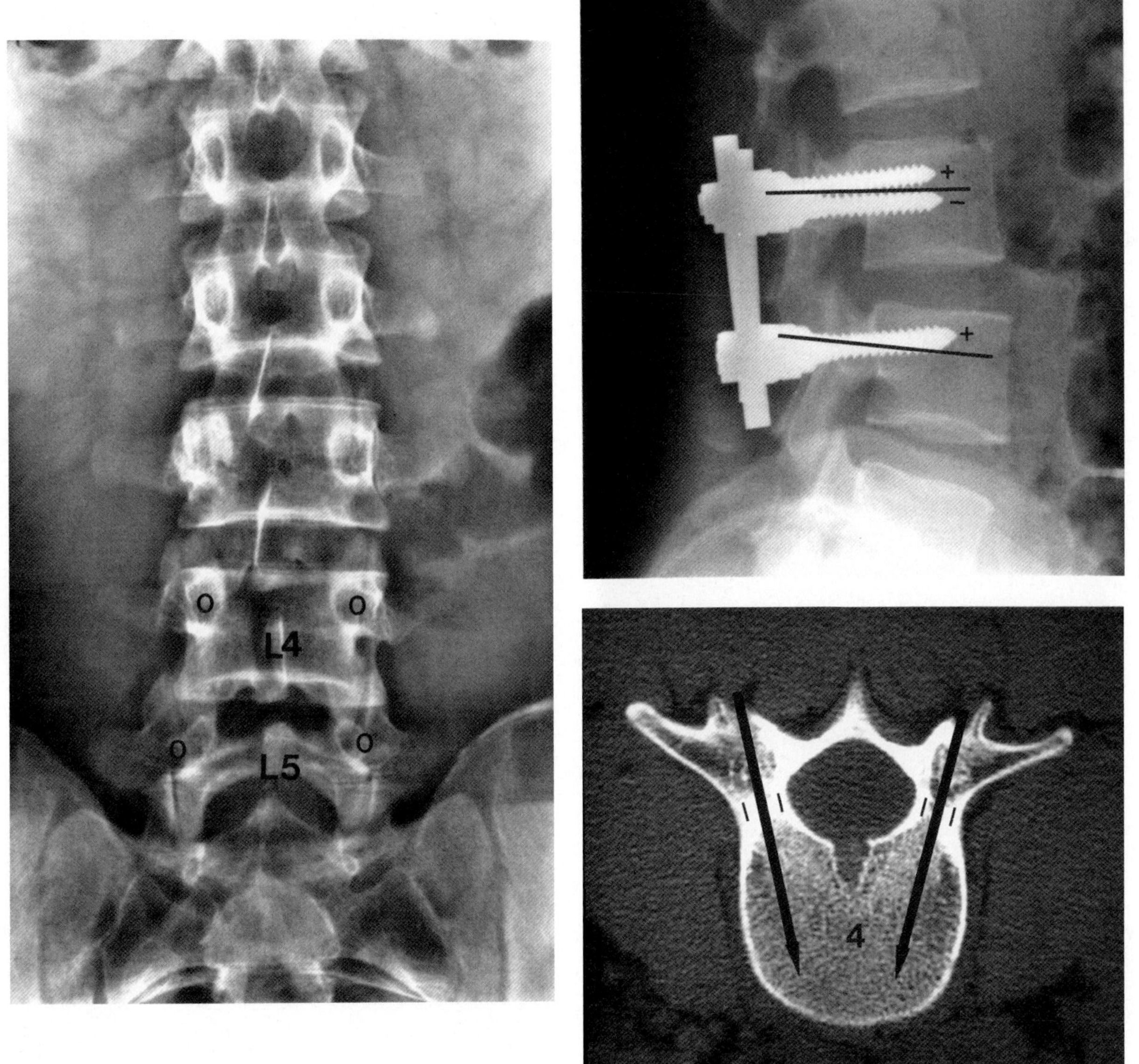


Fig. 3-61 Normal lumbar pedicle screw position. A: Anteroposterior (AP) radiograph demonstrating the normal entry sites for pedicle screws. Normally the screw enters the pedicle near the inferior end of the facet (0, at L4). The screws are usually angled medially 5 to 10 degrees at L1 increasing to 20 degrees to 25 degrees at L5. Therefore, a slightly more lateral entry site may be selected at L5. B: Lateral view of the spine with rod and pedicle screw instrumentation. The *black lines* represent normal (neutral) position. The screws in L4 are angled slightly superiorly (positive position). One of the screws in L3 is positive and one negative in position. Computed tomography (CT) is ideal for evaluation of screw position. C: Axial image at L4 demonstrating the normal position just below the anterior cortex. The screws should not be too large or pedicle fracture may occur.

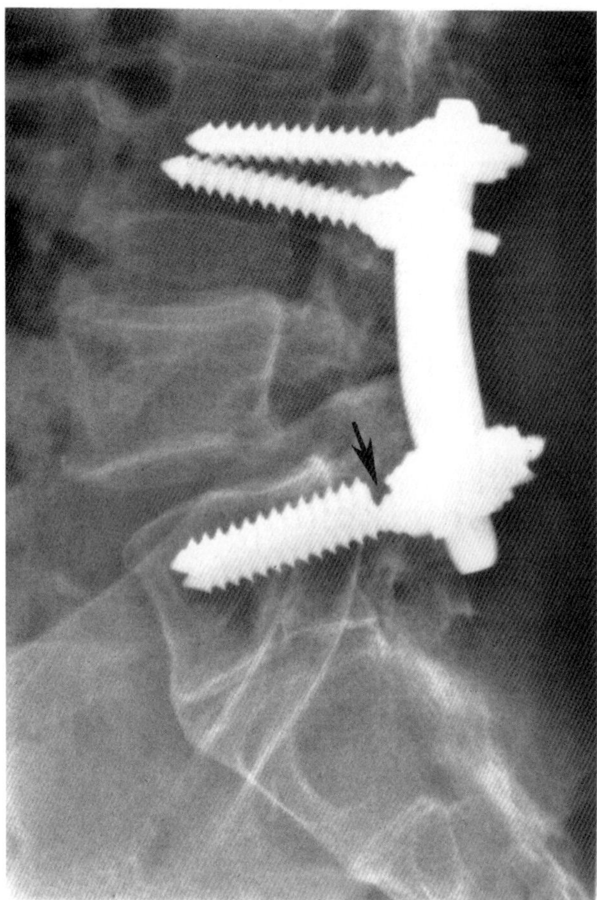

Fig. 3-62 Lateral radiograph following plate and pedicle screw instrumentation from L3 to L5. There is fracture (*arrow*) of one of the lower screws.

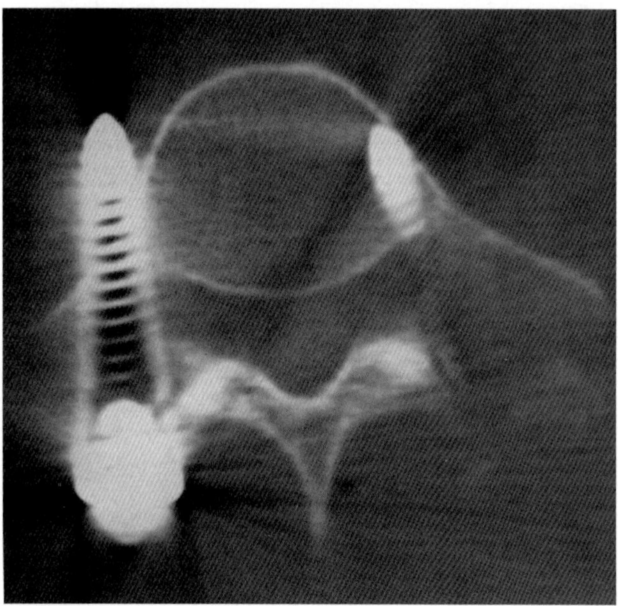

Fig. 3-63 Axial computed tomographic (CT) image of a pedicle screw that was placed too far laterally and has broken through the lateral cortex.

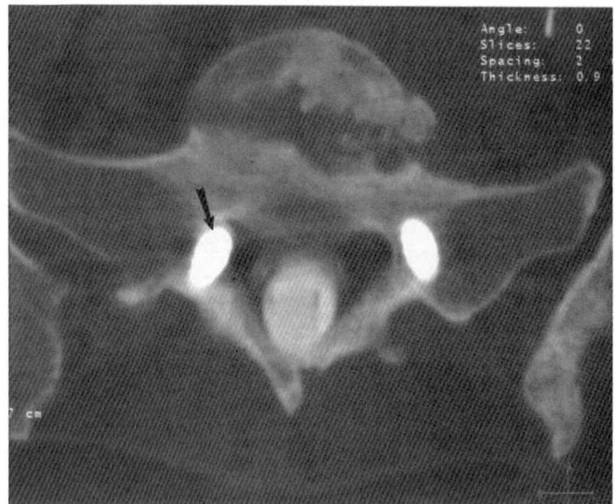


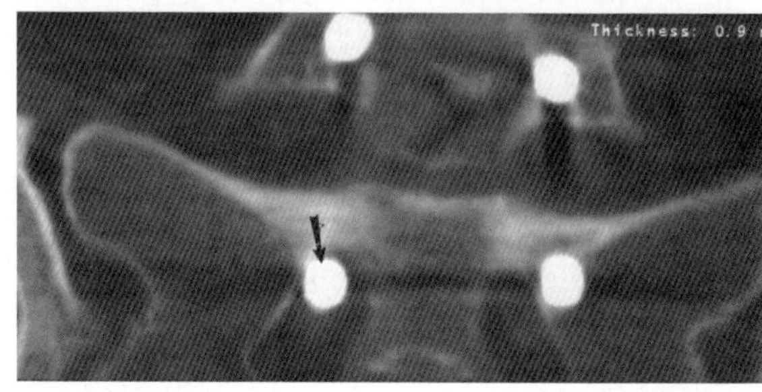


Fig. 3-64 Axial (A) and coronal (B) computed tomographic (CT) images demonstrate the pedicle screw entering the sacral foramen (*arrow*).

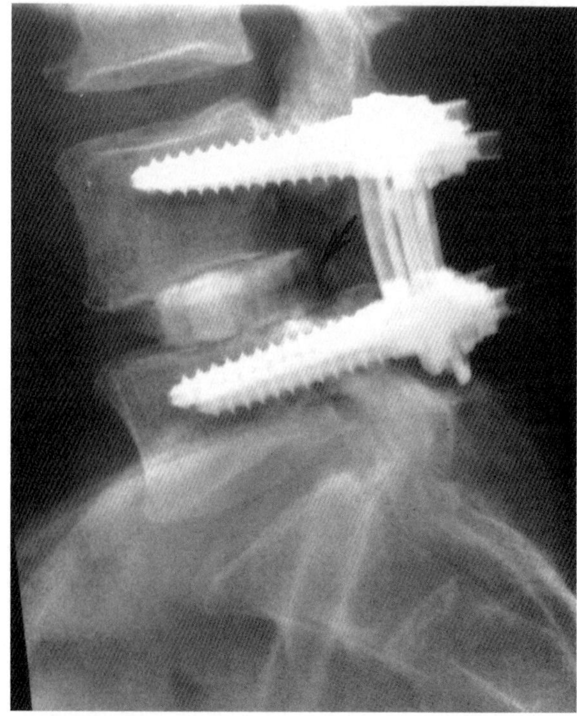

Fig. 3-65 Lateral radiograph after posterior instrumentation at L4-5 with an anterior bone graft. The graft has displaced posteriorly (*arrow*) resulting in nerve root compression and radiculopathy.

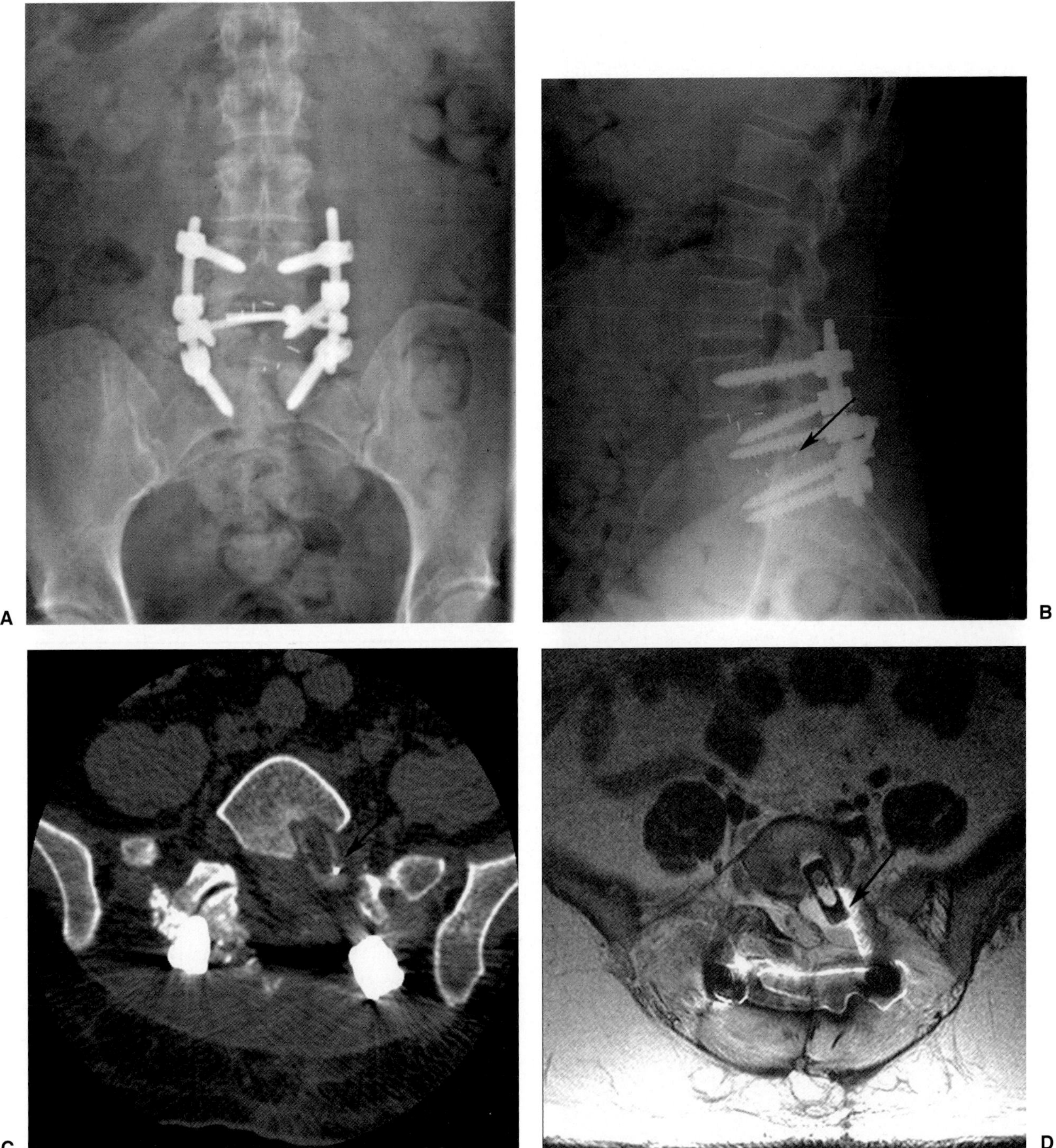


Fig. 3-66 Anteroposterior (AP) (A) and lateral (B) radiographs with posterior rod and pedicle screw instrumentation L4-S1 and anterior spacers at L4-5 and L5-S1. The spacer at L5-S1 has displaced posteriorly (*arrow*). Axial computed tomographic (CT) (C) and magnetic resonance (D) images demonstrate the spacer (*arrow*) which caused nerve root compression.

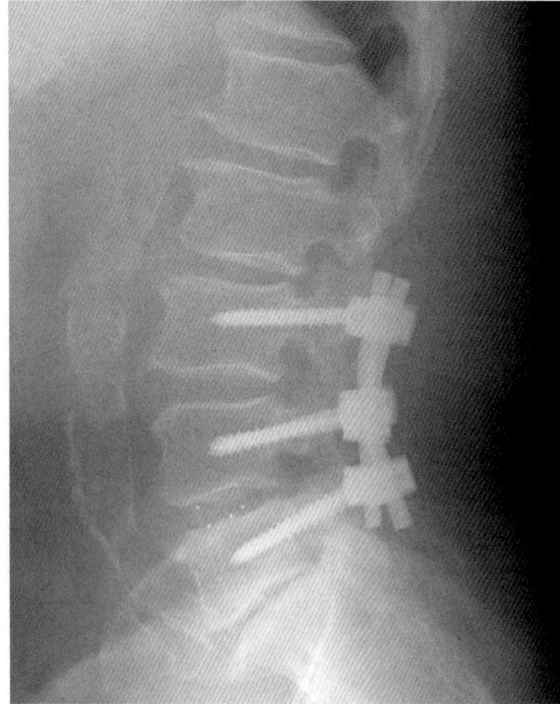

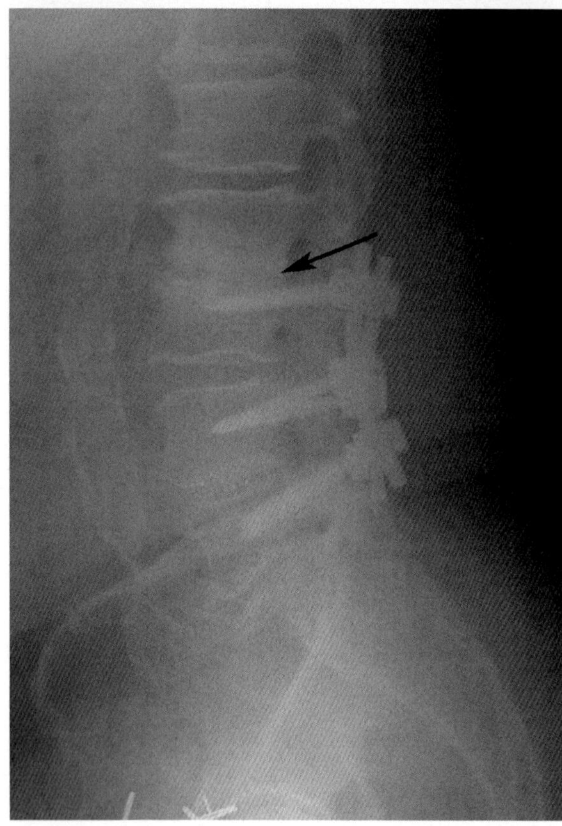

Fig. 3-67 Adjacent segment disease (ASD). Lateral radiographs after L3-5 fusion obtained in the immediate postoperative period (A) and 7 months later (B) demonstrating advanced degenerative disc disease with endplate sclerosis (*arrow*) at the segment above the fusion.

**Table 3-4**

**IMAGING OF COMPLICATIONS FOLLOWING CERVICAL AND LUMBAR PROCEDURES FOR DEGENERATIVE DISEASES**

| IMAGING TECHNIQUE | COMPLICATION |
|---|---|
| Serial radiographs | Instrument failure, ASD*, infection failed fusion |
| Motion studies | ASD*, instability, failed fusion |
| Fluoroscopic spot views | Instrument position |
| Radionuclide scans/PET | Infection, pseudarthrosis/ nonunion |
| Ultrasound | Fluid collections, pseudarthrosis |
| CT | Instrument position (pedicle screws) pseudarthrosis, infection, fragments spinal canal, vertebral alignment, spacer position |
| MRI | Infection, failed back, recurrent disc pseudarthrosis |
| Diagnostic injections, discograms | Confirm source of pain, aspirate for infection |

ASD, adjacent segment disease.

multisegment fusions (78%). Data specific to the cervical spine indicate that ASD occurs most commonly following C6-7 fusions (25.6%). Image features described in the subsequent text do not always correlate with clinical symptoms.

**Image features of ASD** (see Fig. 3-67)

- Disc height decrease of >3 mm
- Posterior opening of the disc space by >5 degrees with flexion
- Subluxation >3.5 mm
- Endplate sclerosis and marginal osteophytes
- Progressive deformity

Table 3-4 summarizes complications and imaging approaches for cervical and lumbar procedures for degenerative disease.

## Suggested Reading

Berquist TH. Imaging of the postoperative spine. *Radiol Clin North Am*. 2006;44:407–418.

Chang SD, Lee MJ, Munk PL, et al. MRI of spinal hardware: Comparison of conventional T1-weighted sequence with new metal artifact reduction sequence. *Skeletal Radiol.* 2001;30:213–218.

Douglas-Akinwande AC, Buckwalter KA, Ryberg J, et al. Multidetector CT: Evaluating the spine in postoperative patients with orthopaedic hardware. *Radiographics*. 2006;26:S97–S110.

Hanley EN, David SM. Lumbar arthrodesis for treatment of back pain. *J Bone Joint Surg*. 1999;81A:716–731.

Lee C, Doreil J, Radomisli TE. Nonunion of the spine: A review. *Clin Orthop*. 2004;419:71–75.

McAfee P. Interbody fusion cages in reconstructive operations of the spine. *J Bone Joint Surg*. 1999;81A:859–879.

Ohashi K, El-Khoury GY, Bennett DL, et al. Orthopaedic hardware complications diagnosed with multidetector CT. *Radiology*. 2005;237:570–577.

Okada S, Iwasaki M, Miyauchi A, et al. Risk factors for adjacent segment disease after PLIF. *Spine*. 2004;29:1535–1540.

Olgilvie JW. Complications in spondylolisthesis surgery. *Spine*. 2005;30:S97–S101.

Park P, Garton H, Gula VC, et al. Adjacent segment disease after lumbar and lumbosacral fusion: Review of the literature. *Spine*. 2004;29:1938–1944.

Rao RD, Goubar K, David KS. Operative treatment of cervical spondylotic myelopathy. *J Bone Joint Surg*. 2006;88A: 1619–1639.

Tortolani PJ, Cunningham BW, McAfee PC, et al. Prevalence of heterotopic ossification following total disc replacement. *J Bone Joint Surg*. 2007;89A:82–88.

Yahiro MA. Comprehensive literature review: Pedicle screw fixation devices. *Spine*. 1994;20:S2274–S2278.

# Trauma

There are approximately 30,000 spinal injuries in the United States each year. Up to 50% of injuries result in neurologic deficit. Injuries may be severe or even fatal. Imaging plays a significant role in detection and classification of spinal injuries. Closed or open techniques are selected for therapy depending on the type, location, and extent of injuries demonstrated on radiographs, CT, and MR images.

Acutely injured patients with suspected spinal injury must be immobilized until the extent of injury and stability are determined. This requires close communication between the radiologist and referring physician to assure that appropriate sequence of imaging techniques is performed to detect fractures and soft tissue injuries and prevent patient deterioration.

**Goals for management of spine trauma**

- Early detection
- Appropriate classification
- Stabilization
- Evaluate distant injuries
- Avoid complications

Radiographs remain the primary screening technique for detection of spinal injuries, although multichannel CT is considered the best technique for evaluation of the cervical spine. The cervical spine trauma series includes AP, lateral, and open-mouth odontoid views, although many institutions still add oblique views. AP and lateral views are typically performed for thoracic and lumbar injuries. CT with coronal and sagittal reformatting is essential to define the extent of injury in an increasing number of cases. MRI should also be performed to evaluate cord injury in patients with neurologic symptoms even in the presence of normal radiographs. Specific techniques will be discussed more completely when specific injuries are reviewed.

The goals of spinal injury treatment include anatomic reduction, rigid fixation, and neurologic decompression.

## Suggested Reading

Bagley LJ. Imaging of spinal trauma. *Radiol Clin North Am*. 2006;44:1–12.

## Cervical Spine Trauma

Trauma to the cervical spine is usually the result of blunt trauma due to motor vehicle accidents, significant falls, or sports injuries. The goals for cervical spine management include early detection, appropriate classification, stabilization, evaluation of distant injuries, and avoidance of complications.

The first decision is when imaging should be required. The Canadian Rules Study employs clinical features to determine whether images are required. This approach is 100% sensitive.

**Canadian rule study for low-risk patients**

- Ambulatory
- No midline tenderness or immediate onset of pain
- Able to attain sitting position
- Able to turn head 45 degrees in both directions
- 100% sensitivity

**Indications for imaging**

- High-risk mechanism of injury
- Neurologic symptoms
- Pain or spasm in cervical region
- Altered mental status
- Image entire spine in multiple trauma (15% to 20% multiple-segment injuries)

Screening of the cervical spine can be accomplished with radiographs using AP, lateral, and open-mouth odontoid views (American College of Radiology [ACR] appropriateness criteria). Oblique views are also obtained at certain institutions. More recently multichannel CT has been recommended as a screening tool to increase accuracy. Radiographs may overlook 20% to 33% of injuries, especially at the craniocervical and cervicothoracic junctions. This can result in delayed diagnosis and patient deterioration in more than 10% of patients. Therefore, multichannel CT with coronal and sagittal reformatting is becoming more popular as a screening tool.

| IMAGING TECHNIQUE | SENSITIVITY (%) | SPECIFICITY (%) |
|---|---|---|
| Radiographs | 39–94 | 72–89 |
| CT | 90–99 | 72–98 |

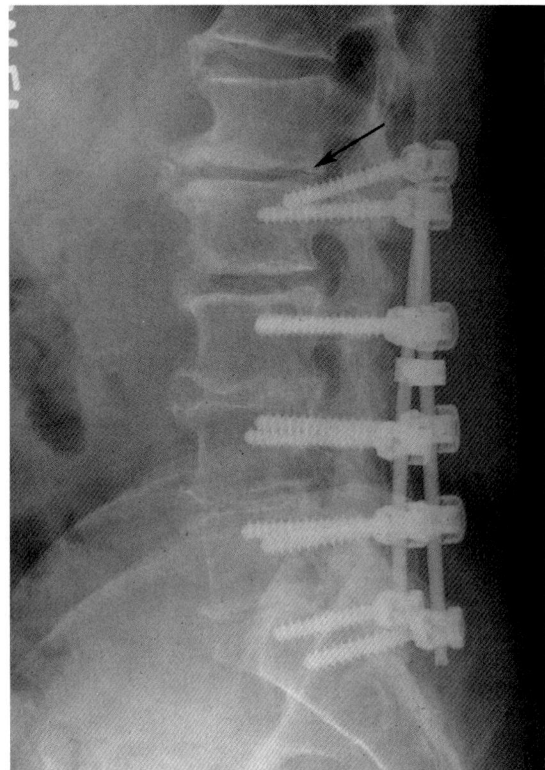


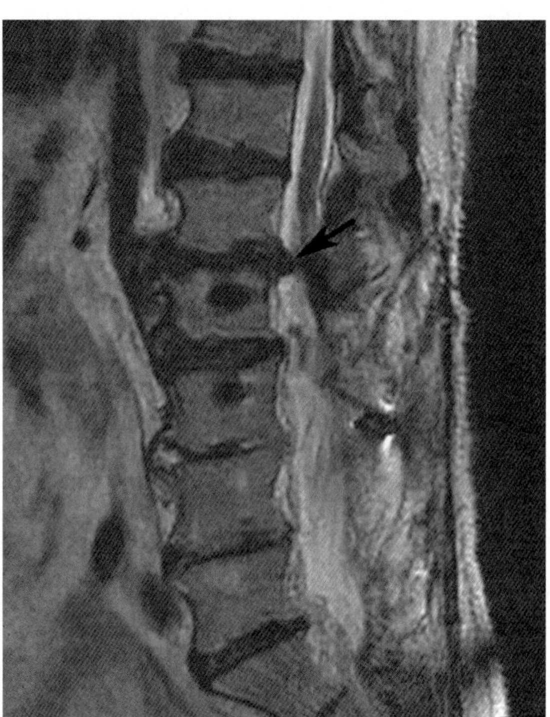


Fig. 3-68 A: Lateral radiograph following posterior rod and pedicle screw instrumentation from L2-S1. There is degenerative disc disease at L1-2 (*arrow*). B: Sagittal T1-weighted magnetic resonance (MR) image shows little artifact from the pedicle screws with a disc extrusion at L1-2 (*arrow*).

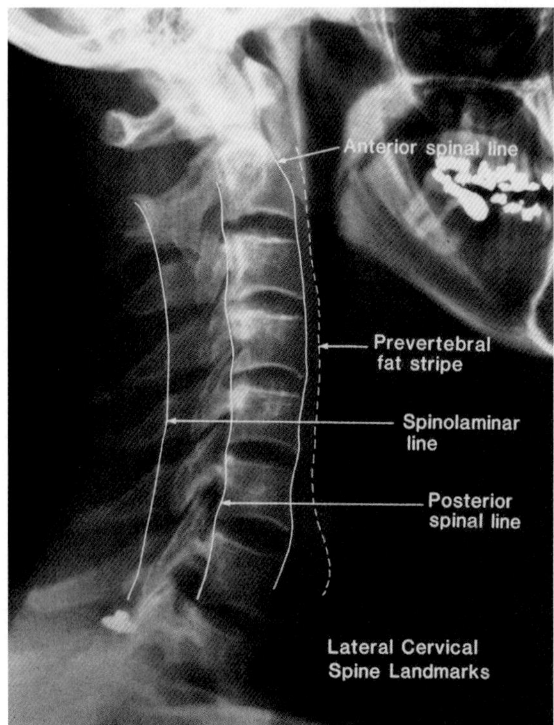


Fig. 3-69 Lateral radiograph demonstrating the prevertebral fat stripe (*broken line*) and anterior, posterior, and spinolaminar lines. The interspinous distance decreases from cephalad to caudad.

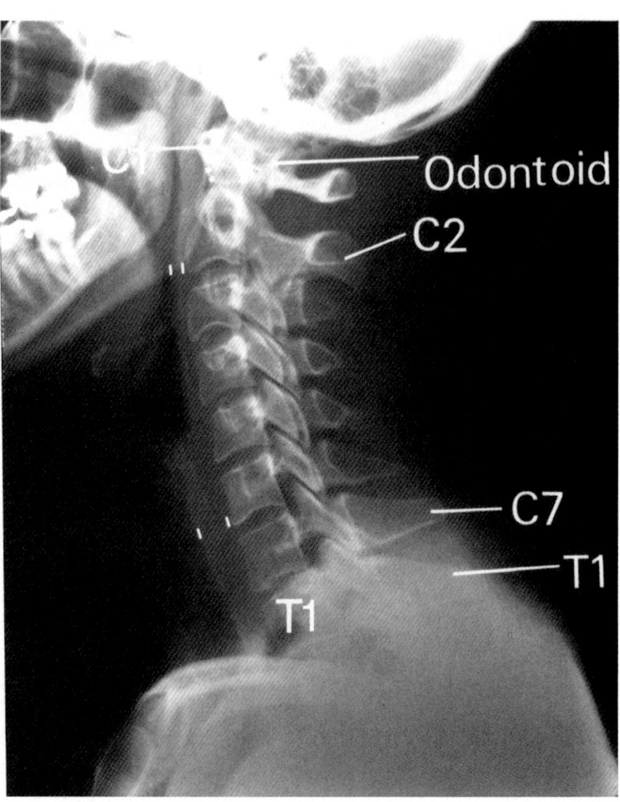


Fig. 3-70 Lateral radiograph demonstrating the points to measure C1-odontoid, C2, and C6 soft tissues.

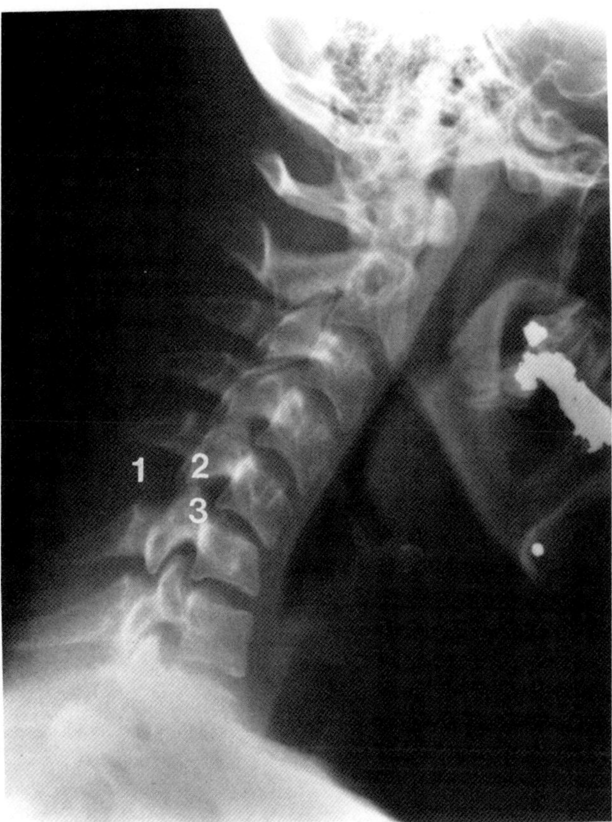


Fig. 3-71 Lateral radiograph of the cervical spine following a distractive hyperflexion injury with no fracture but posterior ligament tears with widening of the interspinous distance at C5-6 (*1*), facet subluxation (*2*), and asymmetric disc space (*3*) with posterior widening.

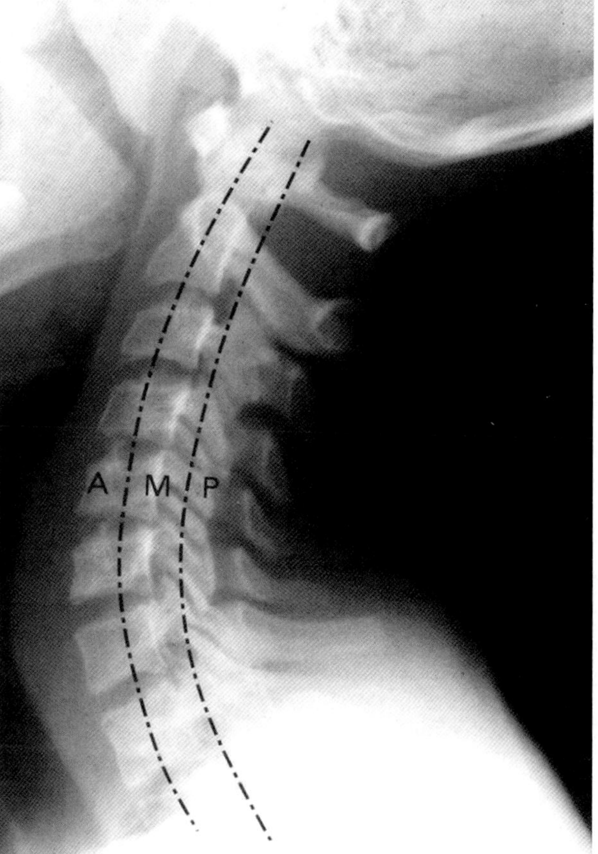


Fig. 3-72 Three-column approach of Denis demonstrated on lateral radiograph. Anterior column—anterior longitudinal ligament, anterior body, and disc; middle column—posterior body and disc and posterior longitudinal ligament; posterior column—posterior ligaments, facet joints, and neural arch.

Image evaluation of radiographs should be systematic to achieve management goals listed in the preceding text. Each view should be evaluated with specific features in mind.

**Lateral view** (see Fig. 3-68)

- Most important view; mechanism of injury classified in 90%; identifies 95% of significant injuries
- Must include C7 and T1; if not seen use swimmers view or CT
- **Alignment**—prevertebral fat stripe, anterior spinal line, posterior spinal line, spinal laminar line, interspinous distance decreases C3-7 (see Fig. 3-69)
- **Measurements**—C1-odontoid—2 mm in adults and 4 mm in children
  Anterior inferior C2 to pharynx—7 mm
  Anterior inferior C6 to trachea—14 mm in children and 22 mm in adults (see Fig. 3-70)
- Disc height should be the same anteriorly and posteriorly; asymmetry may be seen with hyperextension or hyperflexion injuries (see Fig. 3-71)
- **Stability**—multiple approaches to evaluation

## Definitions

**Stability:** Ability of the spine under physiologic loads to maintain its pattern of displacement; therefore, no initial or neurologic deficit, or deformity or incapacitating pain

**Instability:** Pathologic process that can lead to displacement of vertebrae beyond their physiologic limits

**Denis three-column approach:** The spine is divided into anterior, middle, and posterior columns; involvement of two columns indicates instability (see Fig. 3-72)

**Four-column approach:** Spine divided into anterior, posterior, and right and left lateral mass columns. A score (0 to 20, 0 to 5 for each column) is calculated depending on the degree of osseous and soft tissue injury in each column. The former approach is easier to use

**AP view** (see Fig. 3-73)

- Lateral masses should be smooth; spinous processes midline and equal distance apart; midspinous processes may be bifid (see Fig. 6-73)

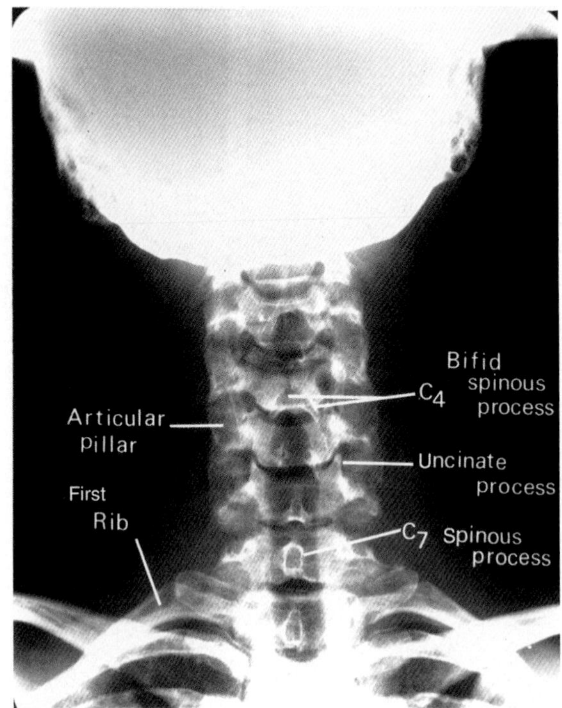


Fig. 3-73 Normal anteroposterior (AP) radiograph of the cervical spine.

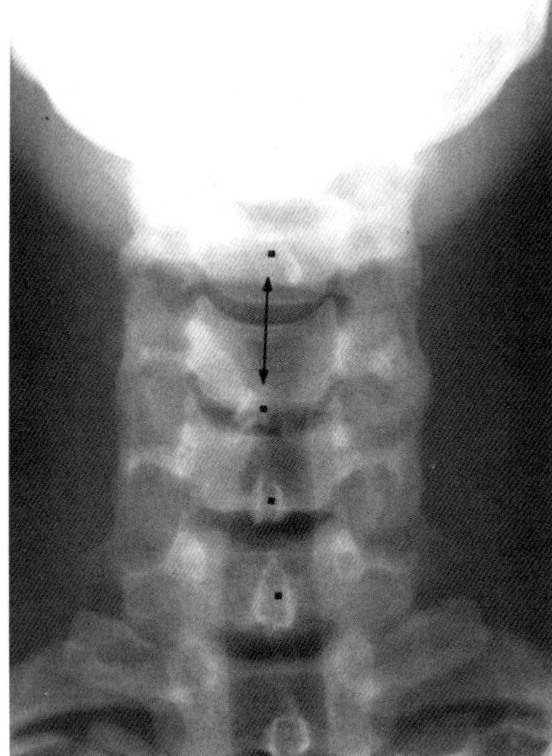

Fig. 3-74 Increased interspinous distance (*double arrow* between dots on spinous processes) indicates a posterior ligament injury, in this case bilateral locked facets.

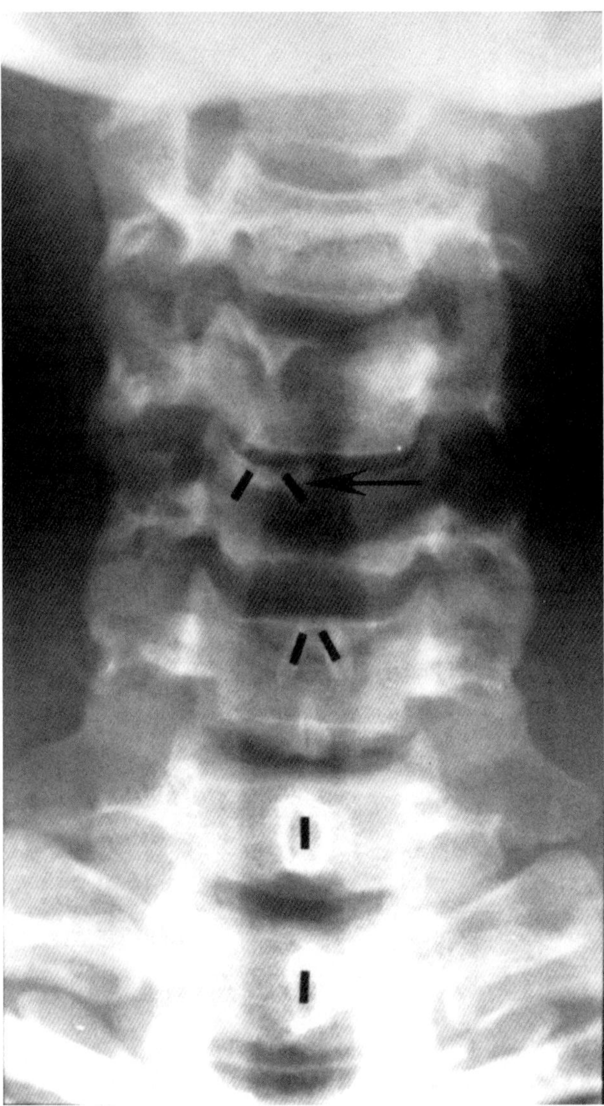

Fig. 3-75 Anteroposterior (AP) radiograph demonstrating rotation of the spinous process of C5 (*arrow, lines* indicate bifid spinous process) due to a unilateral locked facet.

- Widened interspinous distance indicates posterior ligament injury (see Fig. 3-74)
- Rotation of a spinous process indicates a flexion-rotation injury (see Fig. 3-75)
- Double spinous process indicates a spinous process fracture (see Fig. 3-76)

**Open-mouth odontoid view** (see Fig. 3-77)

- Odontoid centered between the lateral masses of C1
- Evaluate symmetry of joint spaces and lateral masses (see Fig. 3-78)
- If question of rotation or fracture, CT with coronal and sagittal reformatting

**Flexion/extension views** (see Fig. 3-79)

- Useful to confirm soft tissue injury in the absence of fracture

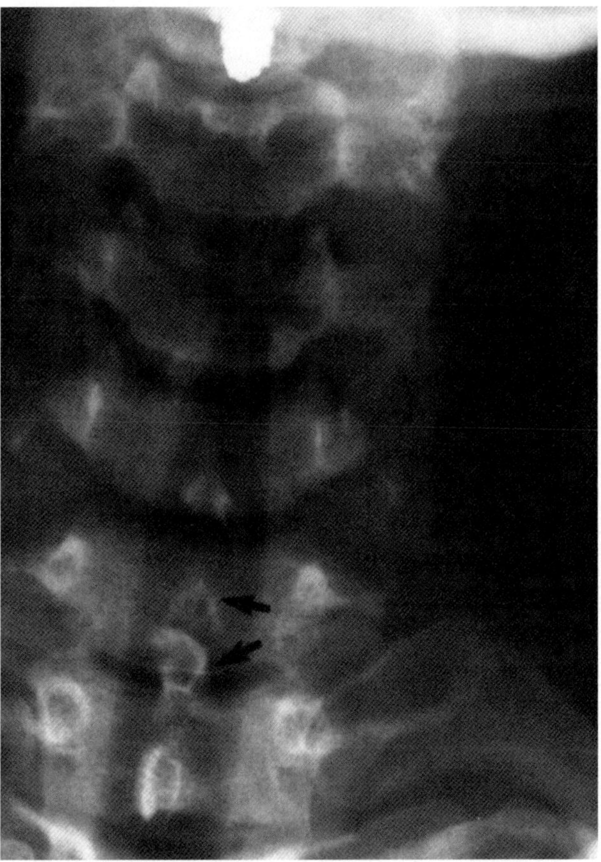

Fig. 3-76 Anteroposterior (AP) radiograph with a double spinous process at C7 (*arrows*) due to a spinous process fracture.

- Perform after thorough orthopaedic or neurologic examination
- May be falsely negative in the acute setting due to spasm; therefore, cervical support and examination after 48 hours may be necessary

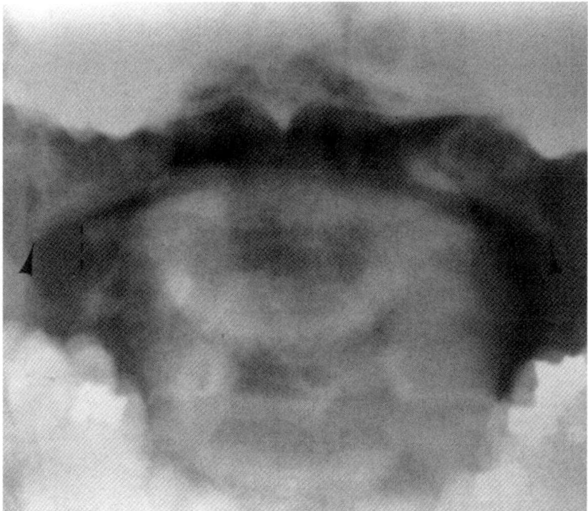

Fig. 3-78 Open-mouth odontoid view demonstrates displacement of the lateral masses bilaterally (*arrowheads* and *broken lines*) due to a Jefferson fracture.

- Perform with fluoroscopic guidance to properly position and stop motion if instability is demonstrated
- Voluntary flexion and extension by the patient

**Multichannel CT** (see Fig. 3-80)

- Thin sections with coronal and sagittal reformatting
- May be used for screening, especially if there are cervical symptoms or impaired mental status
- Average examination time 12 minutes compared to 22 minutes for radiographs
- Improved visualization of the craniocervical and lower cervical regions where radiographs may be more difficult to interpret

**MRI** (see Fig. 3-81)

- Suspected cord injury or neurologic findings
- Suspected ligament injury
- Unconscious for more than 48 hours

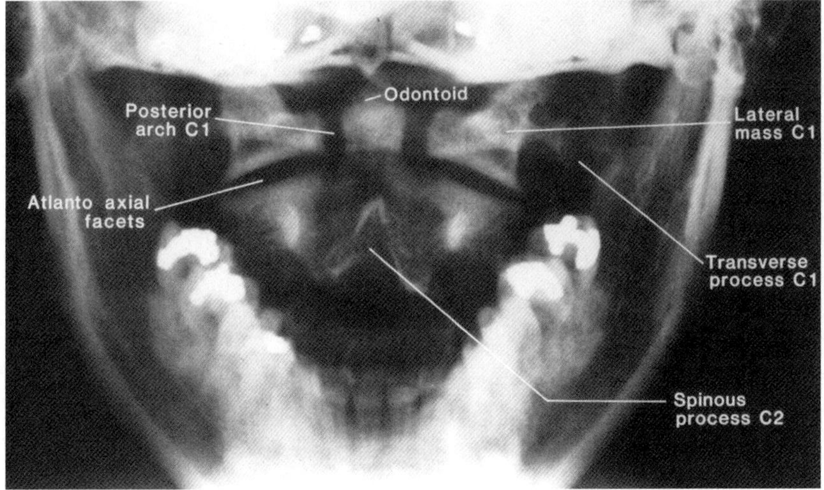


Fig. 3-77 Normal open-mouth odontoid view with anatomy labeled.

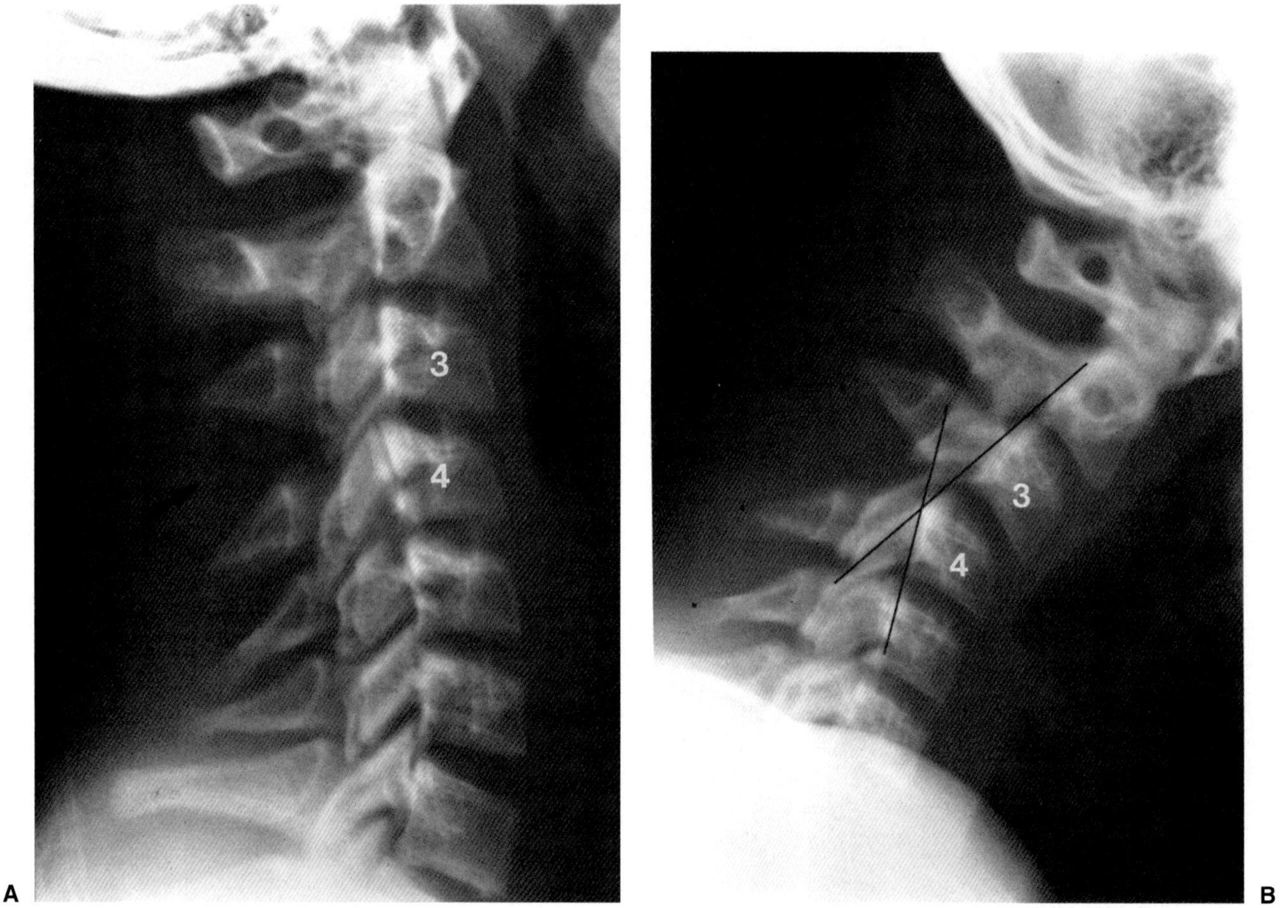

Fig. 3-79 Flexion/extension study. A: Extension image shows limited motion with widening of the C3-4 interspinous distance (*arrow*) and disc asymmetry at C3-4. B: Flexion demonstrates increasing angular deformity (*lines*), further widening of the interspinous distance, facet subluxation, and subluxation of C3 on 4.

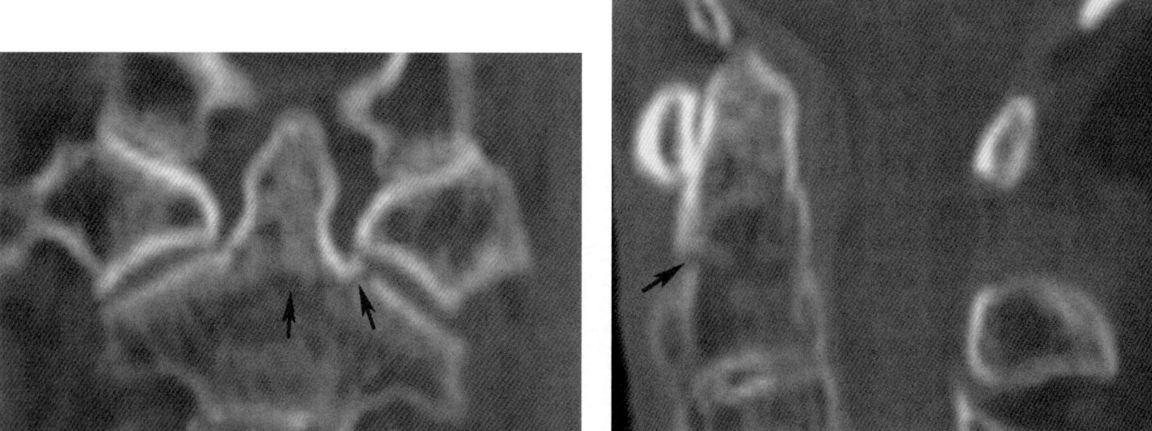

Fig. 3-80 Coronal (A) and sagittal (B) reformatted images demonstrating a type III odontoid fracture (*arrows*).

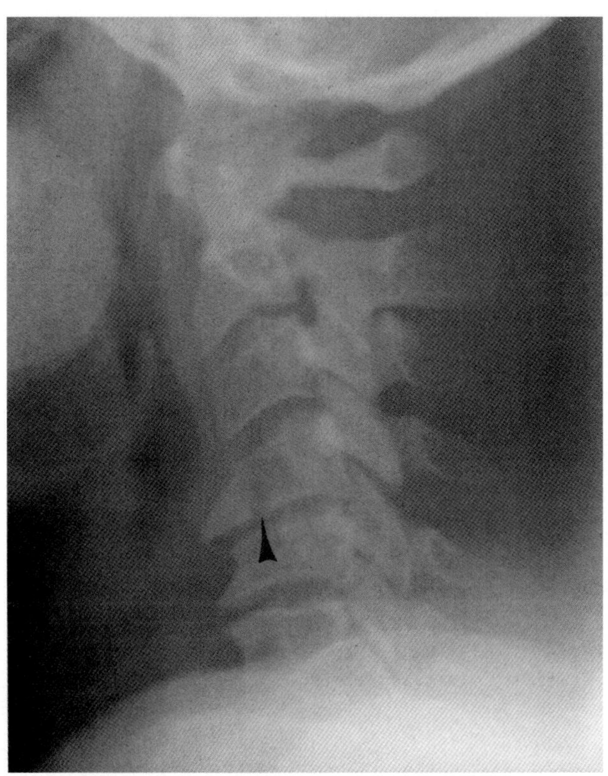


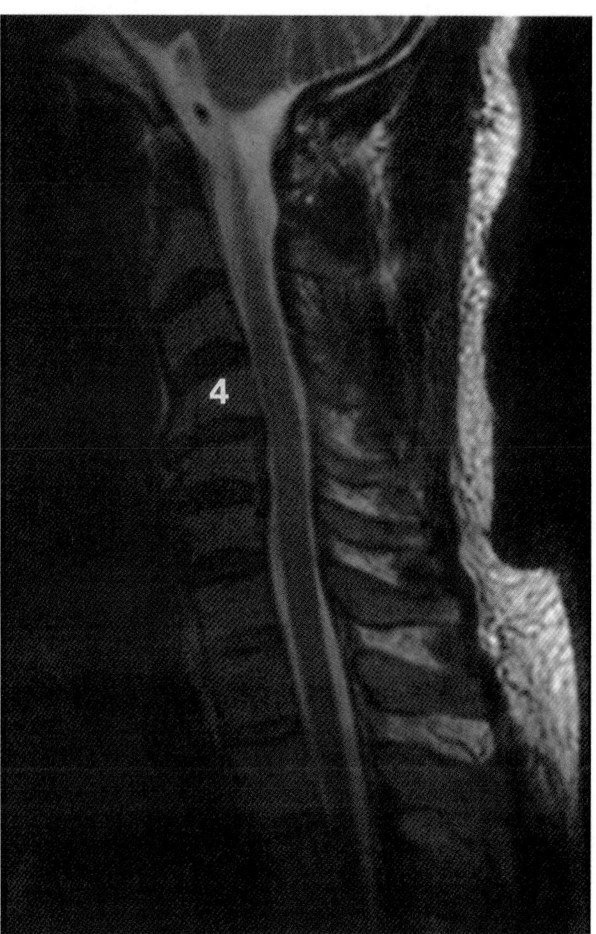


Fig. 3-81 A: Radiograph demonstrating a burst fracture of C4 (*arrowhead*). B: Sagittal T2-weighted magnetic resonance (MR) image shows minimal displacement of the thecal sac and cord.

## SUGGESTED READING


Anderson PA, Moore TA, Davis KW, et al. Cervical spine injury severity score: Assessment of reliability. *J Bone Joint Surg*. 2007;89A:1057–1065.

Blackmore CC, Mann FA, Wilson AJ. Helical CT in the primary trauma evaluation of the cervical spine: An evidence based approach. *Skeletal Radiol*. 2000;29:632–639.

Griffen MM, Frykberg ER, Kerwin AJ, et al. Radiographic clearance of blunt cervical spine injury: Plain radiograph or computed tomography scan? *J Trauma*. 2003;55:222–227.

Hanson JA, Blackmore CC, Mann FA, et al. Cervical spine injury: A clinical decision rule to identify high-risk patients before helical CT. *AJR Am J Roentgenol*. 2000;174:713–717.

McCulloch PT, France J, Jones DL, et al. Helical computed tomography alone compared with plain radiographs with adjunct computed tomography to evaluate the cervical spine after high-energy trauma. *J Bone Joint Surg*. 2005;87A:2388–2395.

Nguyen GK, Clark R. Adequacy of plain radiography in the diagnosis of cervical spine injuries. *Emerg Radiol*. 2005;11:158–161.

Stiell IG, Wells GA, Vandemheen KL, et al. The Canadian C-spine rule for radiography in alert and stable patients. *JAMA*. 2001;286:1841–1848.


## Mechanisms of Injury and Specific Injuries

The mechanism of injury in the cervical spine is rarely pure, but more often due to a combination of forces. In adults, most injuries (75%) involve the lower cervical spine with 20% to 25% involving the occipital condyles to C2. The opposite is true in children. Understanding the mechanism of injury and image features is critical to determining stability and managing patients with cervical spine injuries. Percentages listed in the subsequent text total more than 100% in some cases due to multiple studies and combined injuries.

### Mechanisms of injury

- Hyperflexion
- Hyperextension
- Axial compression
- Rotation
- Shearing
- Combination

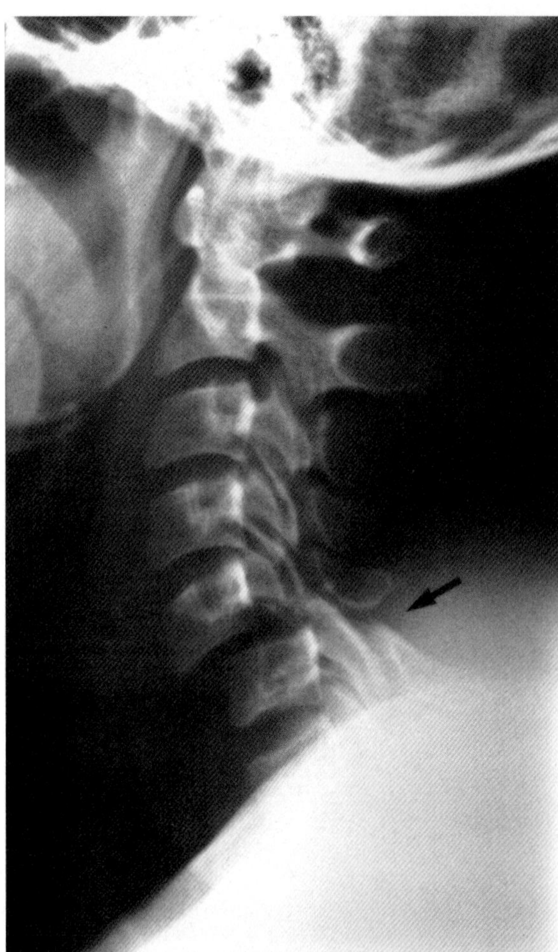

Fig. 3-82 Lateral radiograph demonstrating >50% displacement of C5 on C6 due to bilateral locked facets (*arrow*).

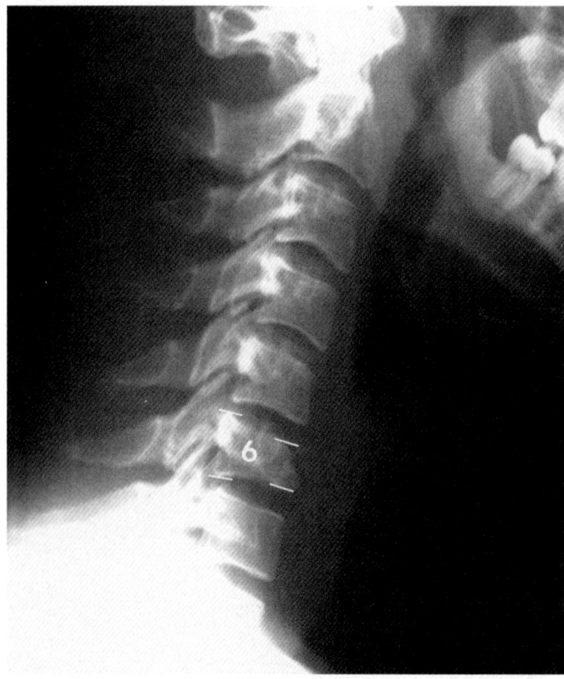


Fig. 3-83 Flexion compression injury with anterior compression of C6.

## Hyperflexion Mechanisms and Image Features (46% of spinal injuries)

**Hyperflexion/distraction (disruptive):** 41% of flexion injuries
- Posterior ligament injury with widened interspinous distance (Fig. 3-71)
- Posterior soft tissue injury with locked facets (see Fig. 3-82) vertebral subluxation
- Spinous process fractures
- Minimal vertebral compression compared to compression injuries

**Hyperflexion/compression:** 40% of flexion injuries
- Anterior vertebral compression (see Fig. 3-83)
- Teardrop fractures (see Fig. 3-84)
- Burst fractures (see Fig. 3-85)
- Fracture dislocations (see Fig. 3-86)

**Hyperflexion/shearing:** 3% of flexion injuries
- Occipitoatlantal subluxation/dislocation (see Fig. 3-87)
- C1-2 subluxation/dislocation
- Odontoid fracture (see Fig. 3-88)

**Hyperflexion/lateral compression:** 16% of flexion injuries
- Transverse process fractures
- Uncinate process fractures
- Lateral mass fractures (see Fig. 3-89)
- Lateral vertebral compression
- Laterally displaced odontoid fractures

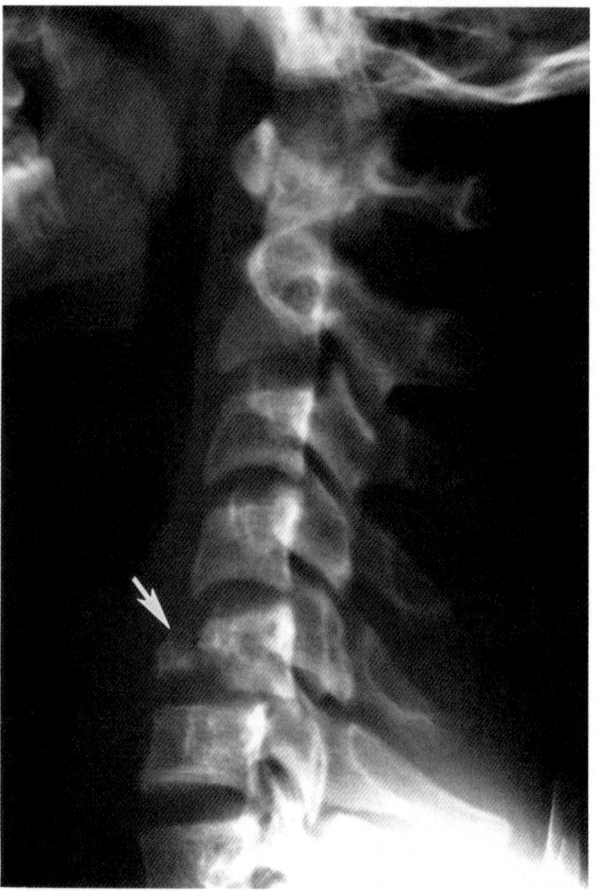

Fig. 3-84 Lateral radiograph demonstrating a flexion teardrop fracture of C5 (*arrow*).

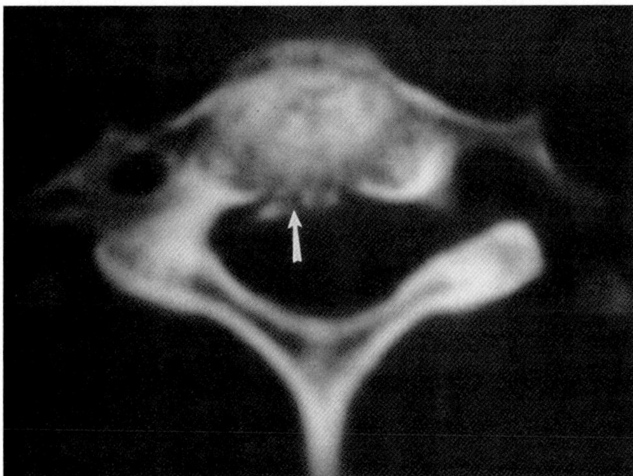

Fig. 3-85 Axial computed tomographic (CT) image demonstrating posterior displacement of bone fragments (*arrow*) following a burst fracture.

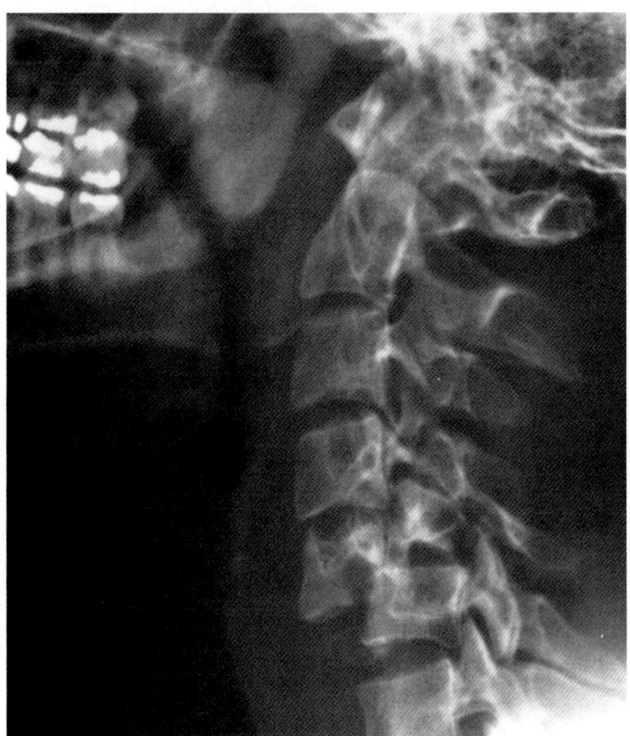

Fig. 3-86 Fracture/dislocation at C5-6.

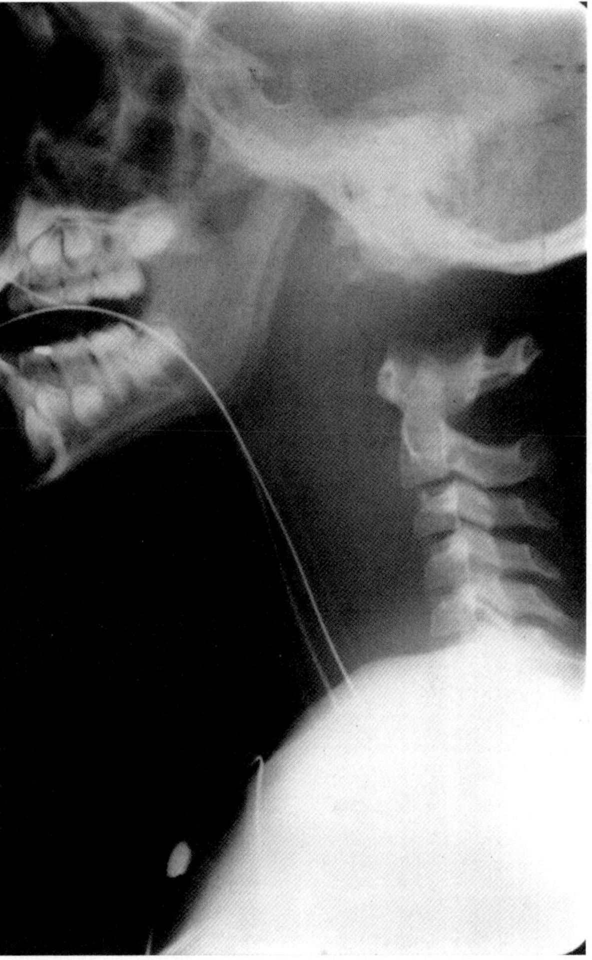

Fig. 3-87 Lateral radiograph demonstrating dislocation of the occipital condyles on C1. There is a large prevertebral hematoma.

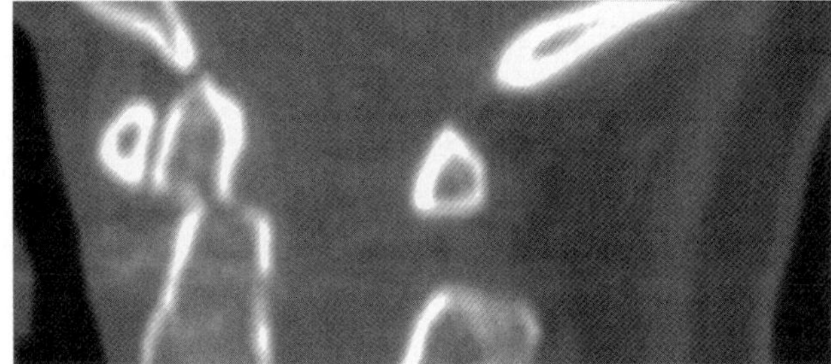

Fig. 3-88 Sagittal computed tomographic (CT) image of an anteriorly displaced type II odontoid fracture due to a flexion/shearing injury.

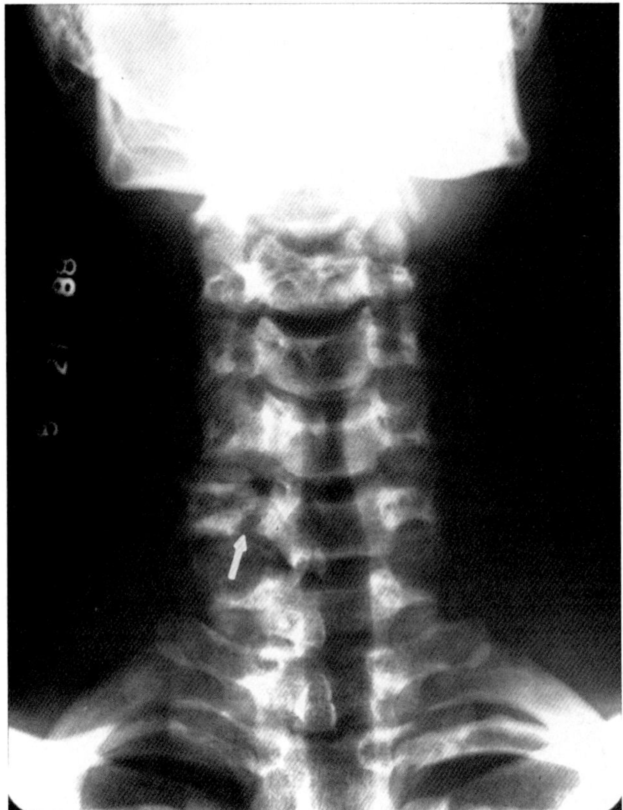

Fig. 3-89 Lateral compression injury with fracture of the right lateral mass of C6 (*arrow*).

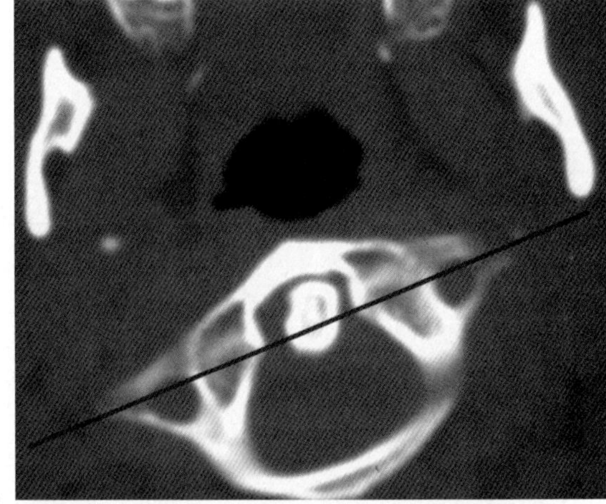

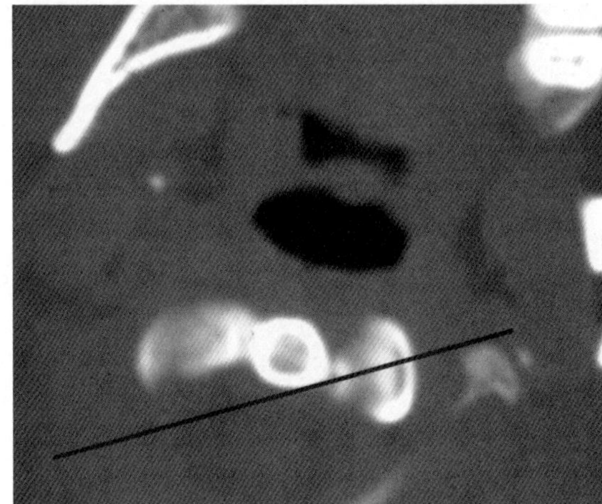

Fig. 3-91 Axial computed tomographic (CT) images (A and B) demonstrating rotational subluxation of C1 on C2 (*lines*) due to rotational injury.

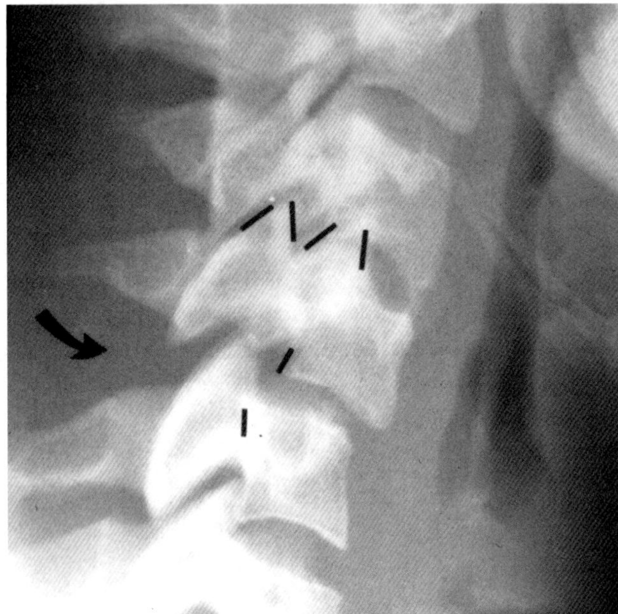

Fig. 3-90 Lateral radiograph after flexion rotation injury with slight subluxation of C4 on 5 and widening of the interspinous distance (*curved arrow*). There is a "bow tie" sign (*oblique lines*) due to rotation of C4 and unilateral locked facets.

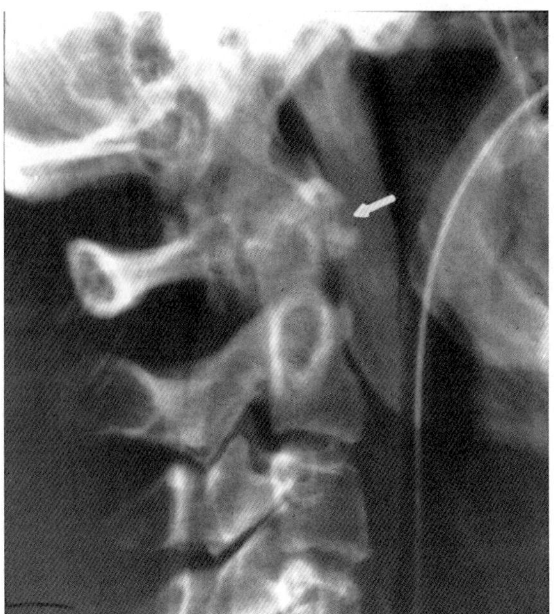

Fig. 3-92 Lateral radiograph demonstrating an avulsion of the anterior ring of C1 (*arrow*) due to distractive hyperextension injury.

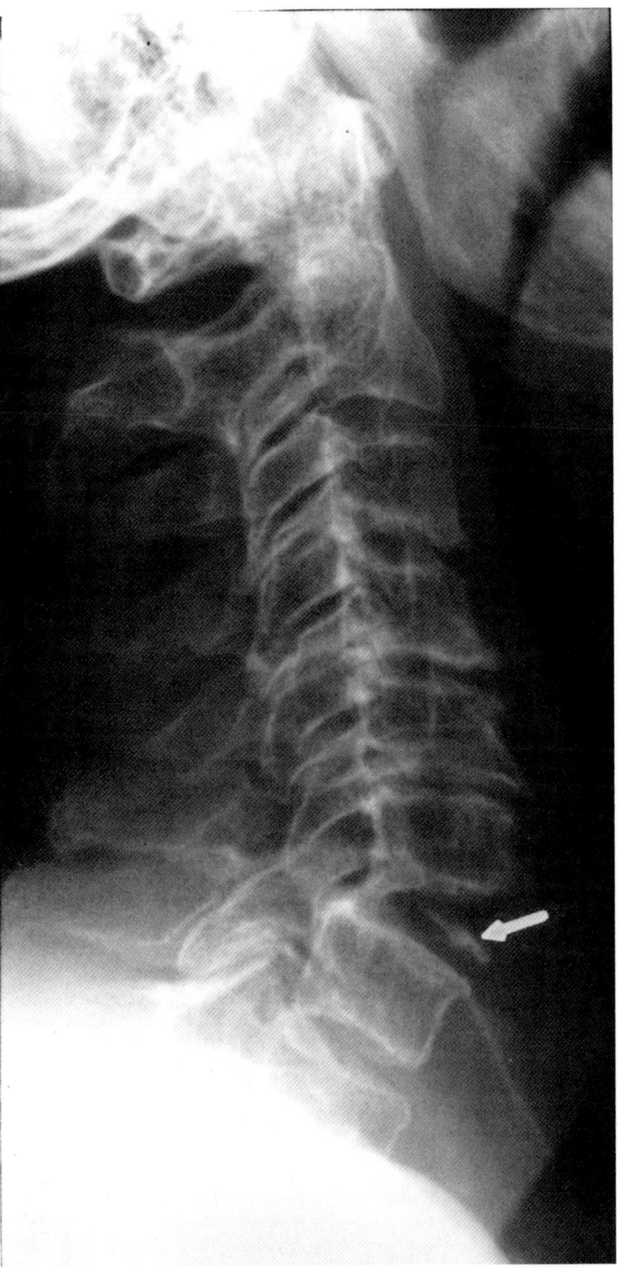

Fig. 3-93 Lateral radiograph following a distractive hyperextension injury with widening of the C6-7 disc anteriorly and an avulsed fragment (*arrow*).

**Hyperflexion/rotation:** 12% of flexion injuries

- Unilateral locked or perched facets (see Fig. 3-90)
- C1-2 rotary fixation or subluxation (see Fig. 3-91)

## Hyperextension Mechanisms and Image Features (38% of spinal injuries)

**Hyperextension/distraction:** 54% of hyperextension injuries

- Anterior ring C1 avulsion (see Fig. 3-92)
- Anterior disc-space widening (see Fig. 3-93)
- Displaced or obliterated anterior fat stripe

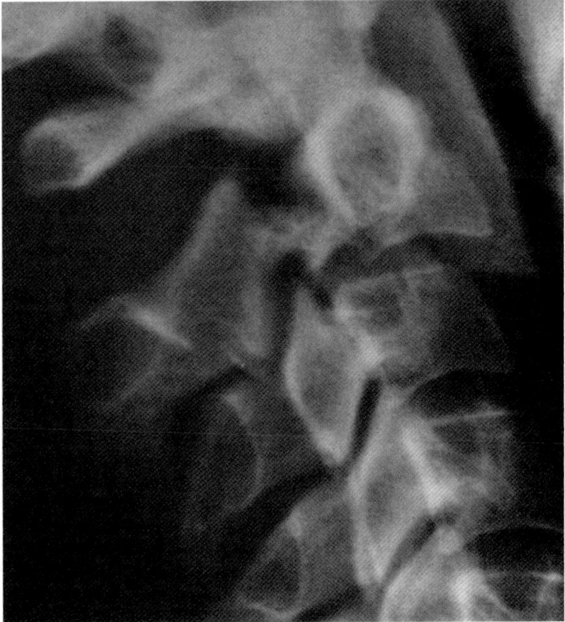

Fig. 3-94 Lateral radiograph demonstrating a displaced posterior arch fracture of C2 (Hanged man).

- Anterior-inferior body margin fracture
- Hanged man's fracture (see Fig. 3-94)

**Hyperextension/compression:** 46% of hyperextension injuries

- Posterior arch fractures (see Fig. 3-95)
- Posteriorly displaced odontoid fractures

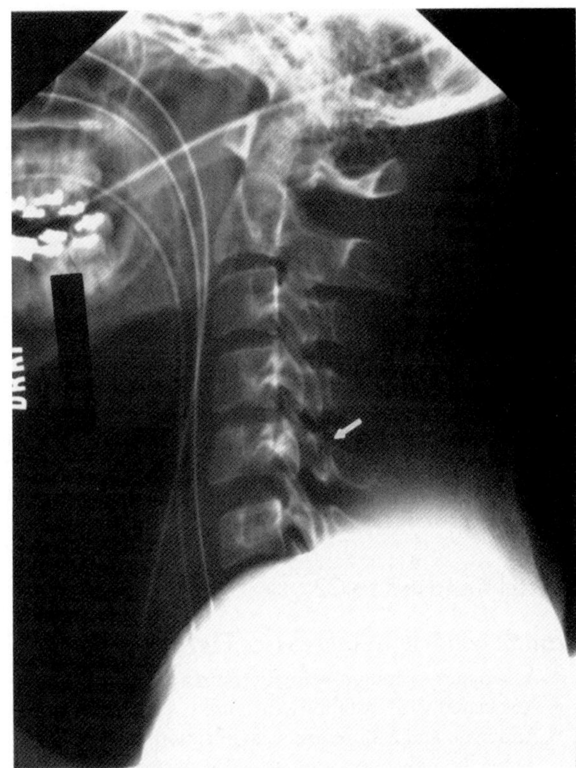

Fig. 3-95 Lateral radiograph shows widening of the disc space at C5-6 with a posterior arch fracture (*arrow*) at C5.

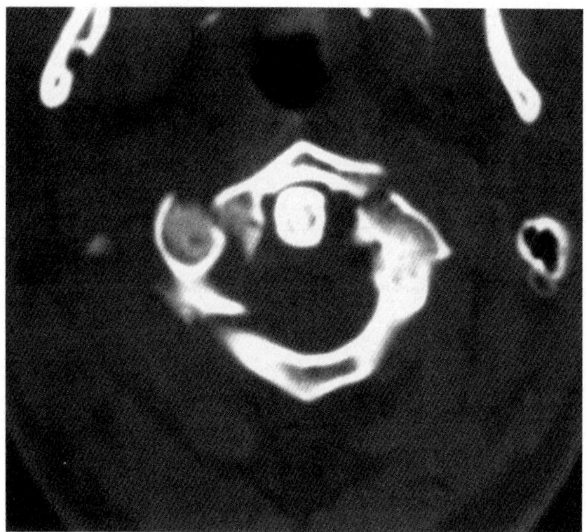

Fig. 3-96 Axial computed tomographic (CT) image with multiple breaks in the ring of C1 (Jefferson fracture) due to axial compression.

### Axial Compression Injuries and Image Features (4% of spinal injuries)

- Jefferson fractures (see Fig. 3-96)
- Burst fractures in lower cervical spine (Fig. 3-85)
- Vertical body fractures
- Occipital condyle fractures

## Suggested Reading

Bagley LJ. Imaging of cervical spine trauma. *Radiol Clin North Am.* 2006;44:1–12.

Berquist TH. *Imaging of orthopaedic trauma*, 2nd ed. New York: Raven Press; 1992:93–206.

Daffner RH, Brown RR, Goldberg AL. A new classification for cervical vertebral injuries: Influence of CT. *Skeletal Radiol.* 2000;29:125–132.

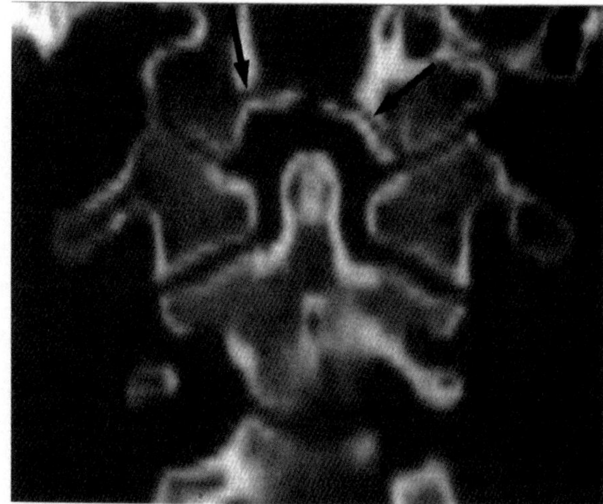



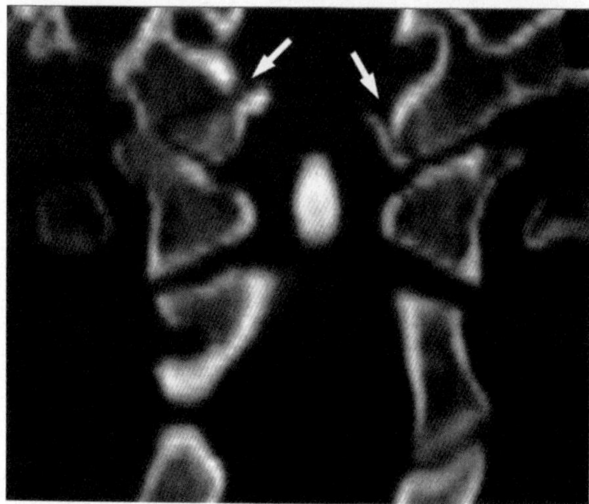



Fig. 3-97 Type III occipital condyle fractures. **A:** Coronal computed tomography (CT) shows avulsion of the anterior rim of the foramen magnum (*arrows*) which extends into the occipital condyles (*arrows* in **B**). (From Hanson JA, Deliganis AV, Baxter AB, et al. Radiologic and clinical spectrum of occipital condyle fractures: Retrospective review of 107 consecutive fractures in 95 patients. *Am J Roentgenol.* 2002;178:1261–1268.)

### Management of Cervical Spine Injuries

The goals of management of cervical spine injuries are to provide stability, achieve anatomic reduction, decompress neural structures, and avoid complications. Treatment options vary depending on the extent of injury, stability, and anatomic location. For purposes of discussion upper (occipital condyles to C2) and lower (C3-7) cervical spine injuries and their associated complications will be reviewed separately.

#### Occipital Condyles to C2

**Occipital condyle fractures** (see Fig. 3-97)

- Associated with high-velocity trauma
- Associated with instability through C1-2
- Anderson and Montesano Classification
  - **Type I**—impaction due to axial load, stable (3% of injuries)
  - **Type II**—fracture extends into foramen magnum (22% of injuries)
  - **Type III**—avulsion, with ligament injury, may be unstable (75% of injuries)
- Associated cervical spine fractures in 32%

**Atlantooccipital dislocations** (Fig. 3-87)

- Rare, often fatal injury more common in children and adolescents
- Dislocations are classified as Type I anterior dislocations, Type II distraction separation (Fig. 3-87), and Type III posterior dislocation
- Associated intracranial injuries increase fatality rates

**Rotary subluxation/fixation C1-2** (see Fig. 3-98)

- Associated with trauma, dental procedures, and infections
- Fielding and Hawkins classification

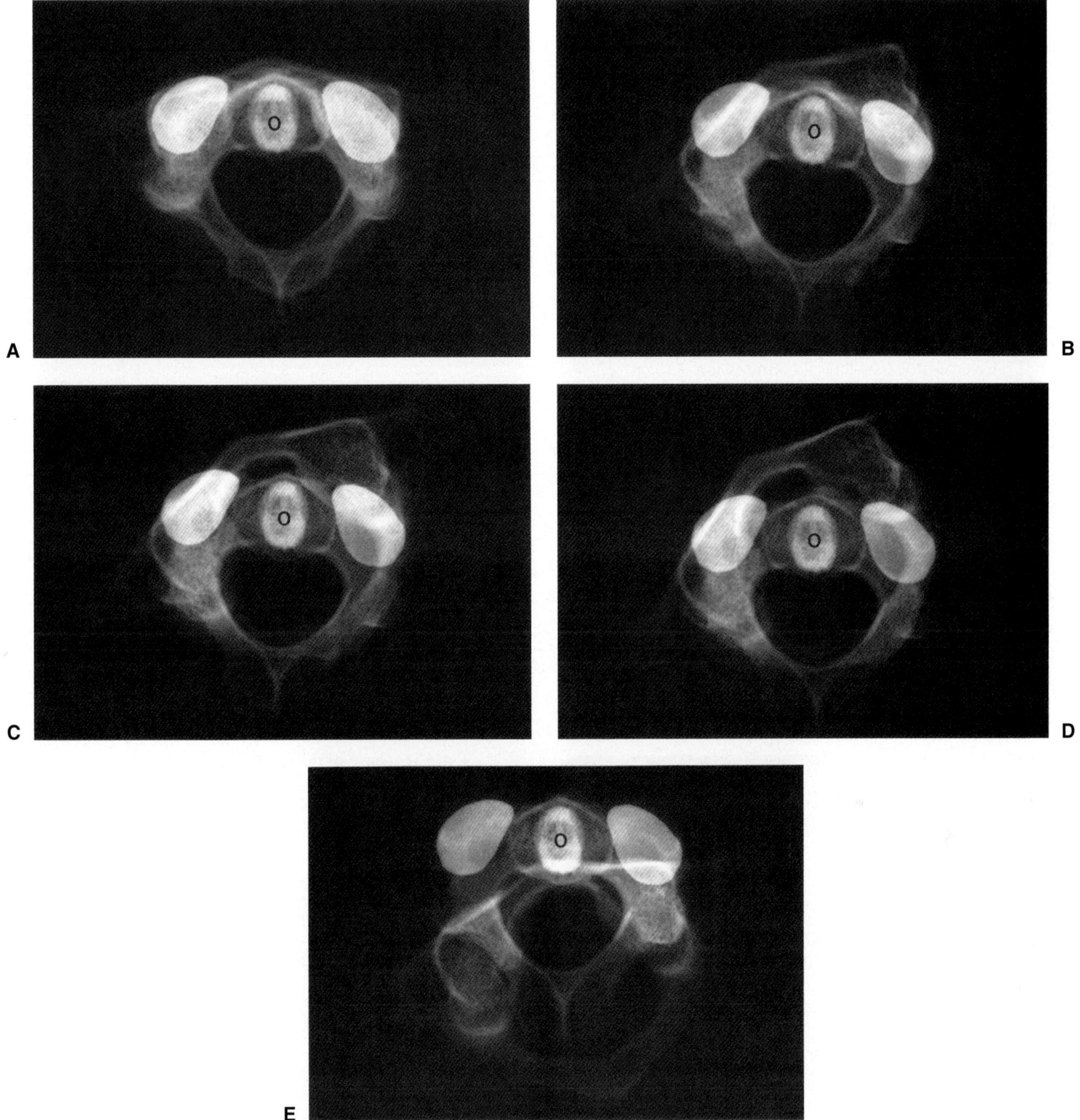


Fig. 3-98 Fielding and Hawkins classification for rotary fixation. Opaque markers placed on the C2 facets, odontoid-0. A: Normal C1-2 relationship. B: Type I—rotary fixation without subluxation of C1 on the odontoid. C: Type II—rotary fixation with 3- to 5-mm subluxation of C1 on the odontoid. D: Type III—rotary fixation with >5 mm subluxation of C1 on the odontoid. E: Type IV—rotary fixation with posterior displacement (deficient dens required). (From Berquist TH. *Imaging of orthopaedic trauma*, 2nd ed. New York: Raven Press; 1992.)

**Type I**—rotary fixation without anterior subluxation of C1 on the odontoid; transverse ligament intact (Fig. 3-96B)
**Type II**—rotary fixation with 3- to 5-mm subluxation (Fig. 3-96C)
**Type III**—rotary fixation with >5-mm subluxation (Fig. 3-96D)
**Type IV**—rotary fixation with posterior subluxation (Fig. 3-96E)

## C1 fractures

- Account for 4% of cervical spine fractures
- Anterior arch (see Fig. 3-92)—hyperextension
- Posterior arch—compressive hyperextension
- Lateral mass—vertical compression
- Transverse process—lateral compression
- Jefferson fractures—axial compression (Fig. 3-96)
- Associated injuries—hanged man's fractures 15%, C7 fractures 25%
- Generally no neurologic complications at C1

## C2 fractures

- Account for 15% to 25% of spinal injuries
- Odontoid—hyperflexion, hyperextension, shearing injuries (Figs. 3-80 and 3-88)
- Pedicles—hyperextension (Fig. 3-94)
- Vertebral body—hyperextension (see Fig. 3-99)
- Lamina—hyperextension
- Facets—lateral compression, rotation/compression

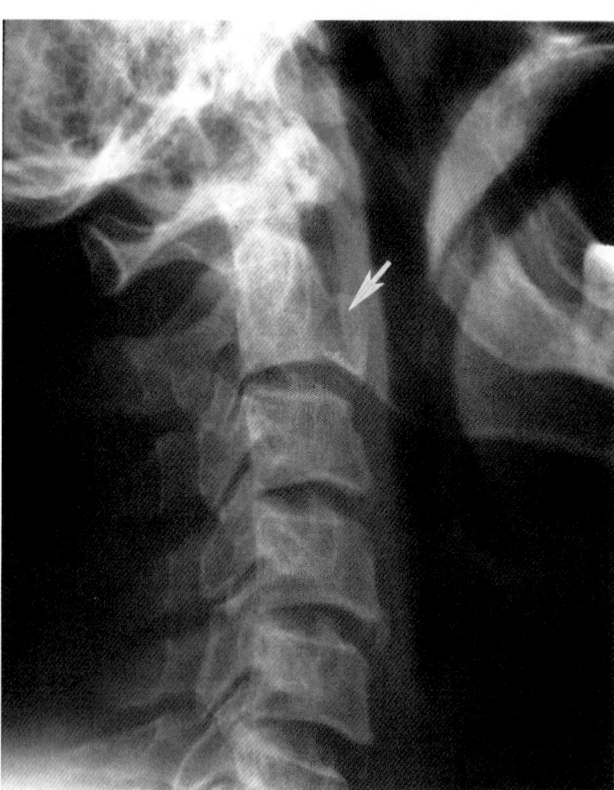

Fig. 3-99 Lateral radiograph demonstrating an anterior C2 body fracture (*arrow*).

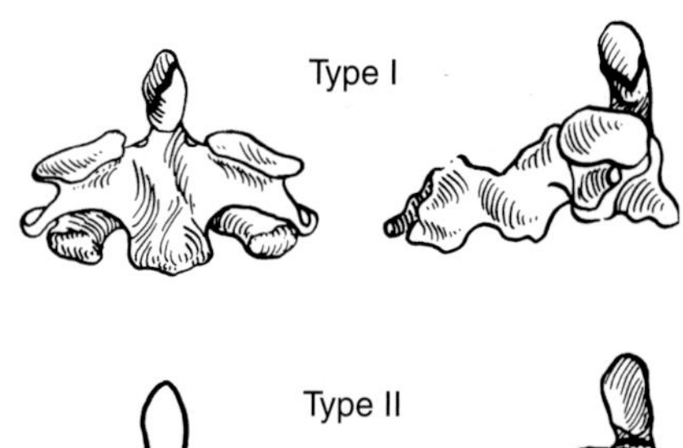


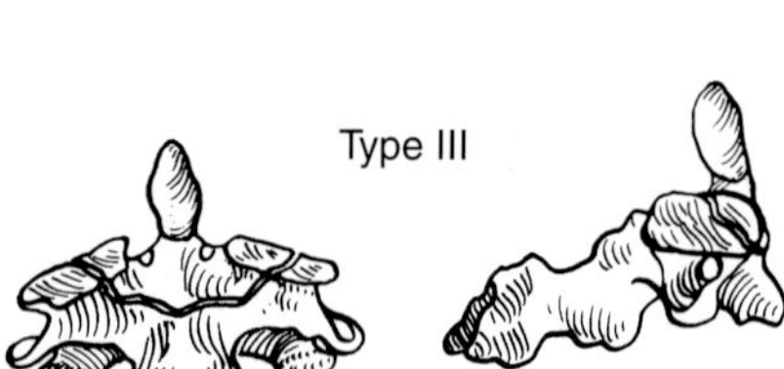


Type III

Fig. 3-100 Illustration of the Anderson-D'Alonzo classification for odontoid fractures. Type I—odontoid tip, type II—odontoid base, type III—extends into body below the accessory ligament and vascular entry point.

## Odontoid fractures

- Six percent of cervical spine fractures
- Anderson-D'Alonzo classification (see Fig. 3-100)
  **Type I**—odontoid tip (see Fig. 3-101)
  **Type II**—base of odontoid (Fig. 3-88)
  **Type III**—involving body below entry of accessory ligament (Fig. 3-80)

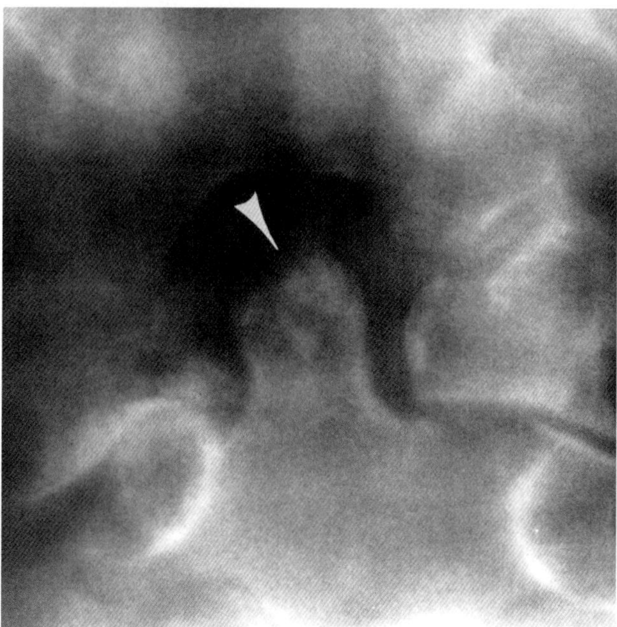

Fig. 3-101 Open-mouth odontoid view demonstrating a type I fracture (*arrowhead*).

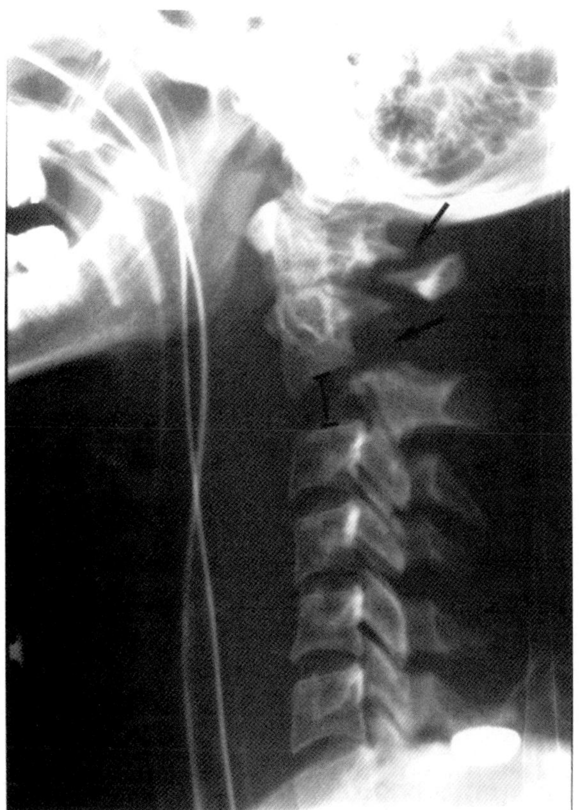

Fig. 3-102 Hyperextension injury with marked distraction of the C2 disc space (anterior lines) and fractures of the posterior arches of C1 and C2 (*arrows*).

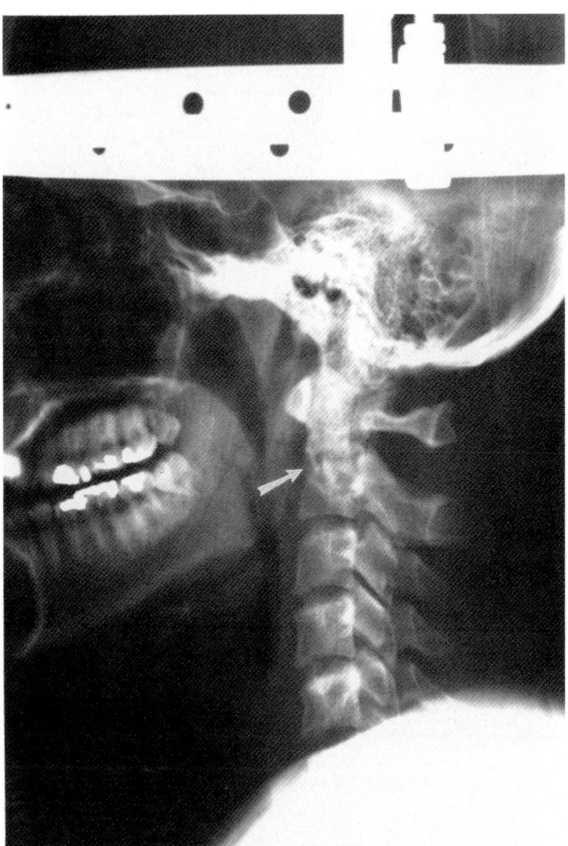

Fig. 3-103 Type III odontoid fracture (*arrow*) with minimal displacement treated with halo immobilization.

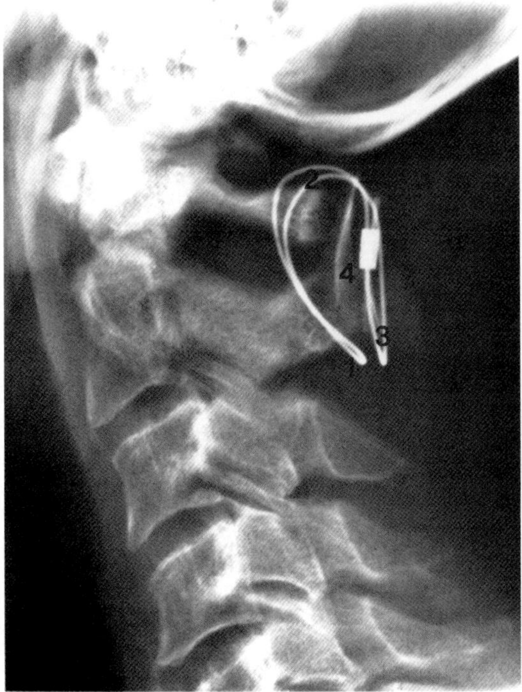


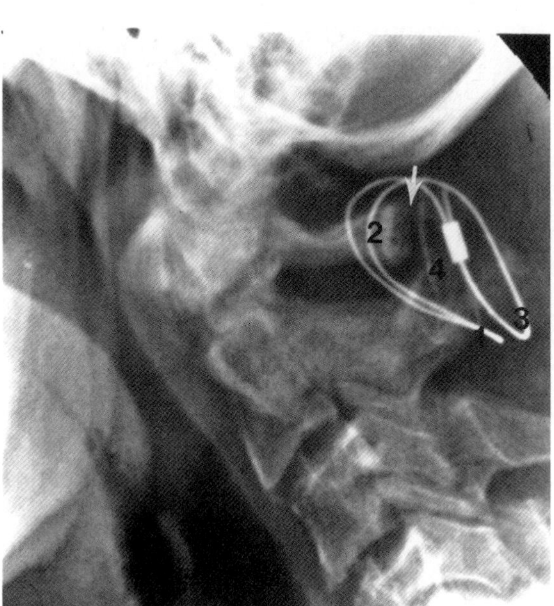


Fig. 3-104 Bone graft and cable fusion C1-2. Cable extends around the spinous process of C2 (*1*), around the arch of C1 (*2*), and back over the spinous process of C2 (*3*) with bone graft (*4*) linking the spinous processes. Neutral (**A**) and flexion (**B**) images show no disc space angulation or subluxation. However, the bone graft moves away from C1 (*arrow*) indicating nonunion proximally.

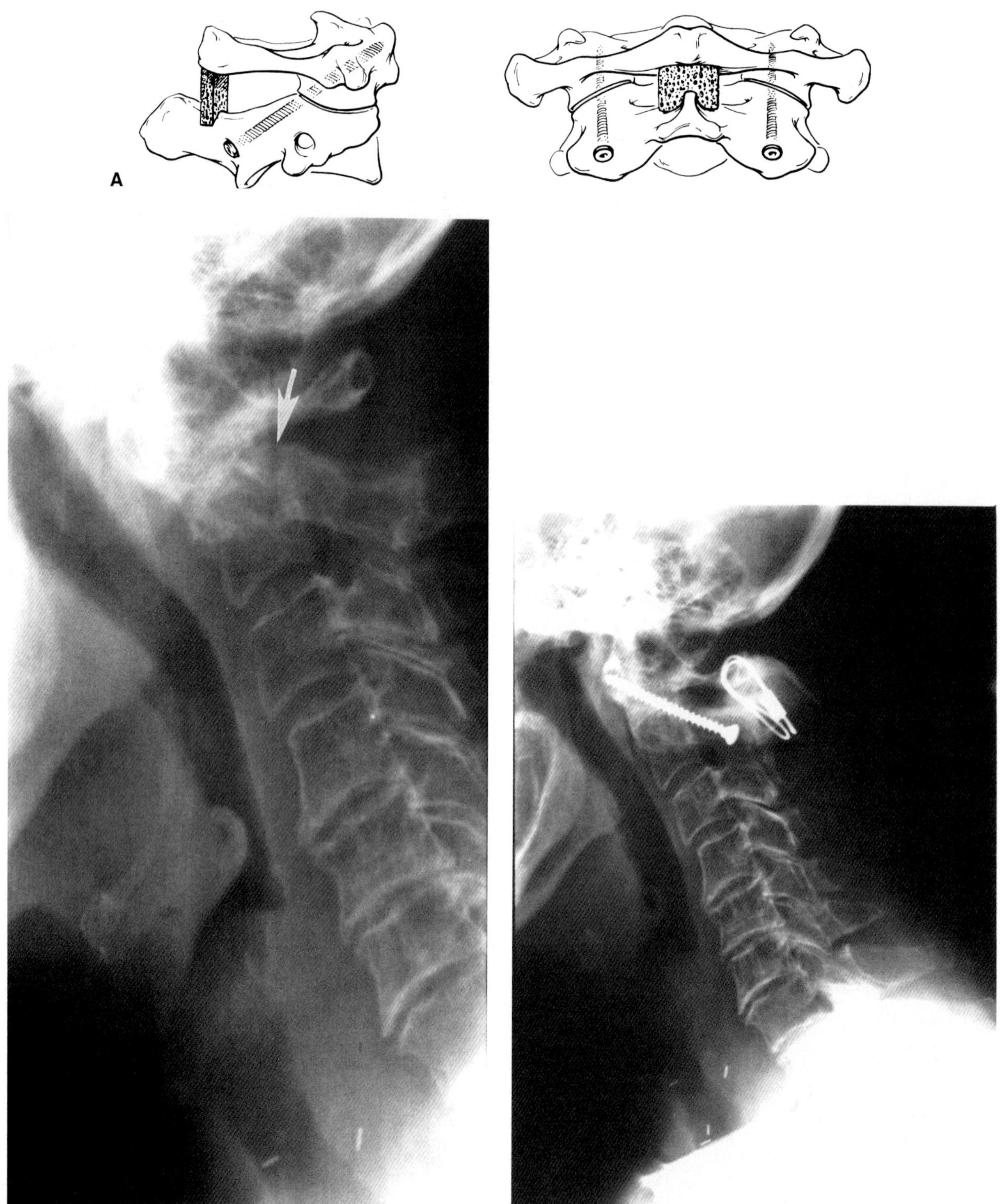


Fig. 3-105 A: Illustration of transarticular screw and posterior bone graft fixation. B: Lateral radiograph demonstrating an undisplaced Hanged man's fracture treated with (C) transarticular screws and posterior bone graft with cable fixation.

- **Type I**—8% of odontoid fractures, complications unusual
- **Type II**—59% of odontoid fractures, 20% neurologic complications, nonunion occurs in 54% to 72%, 100% if displaced >5 mm
- **Type III**—33% of odontoid fractures; neurologic complications less common; nonunion uncommon unless displaced >5 mm

### Hanged man's fractures

- Six percent of cervical spine injuries; hyperextension mechanism of injury
- Associated cervical spine fractures in 15% (see Fig. 3-102), T1-4 fractures in 10% of patients
- Transient neurologic complications in 10%

Injuries from the occipital condyles to C2 may be treated with halo fixation for more stable injuries or occipital spinal fusion for unstable injuries. For example, minimally displaced Type III odontoid fractures may be managed with halo fixation (see Fig. 3-103). Type II odontoid fractures (high incidence of nonunion), occipitoatlantal dislocations, C1-2 subluxations, and Hanged man's fractures generally require surgical fusion. Fusion can be accomplished with multiple approaches including bone grafting with wire or cable fixation (see Fig. 3-104); transarticular screws (see Fig. 3-105); Luque rectangles with wire fixation (see Fig. 3-106); plate and screw fixation; and more recently, modular universal posterior fixation systems that provide more flexibility using screws, rods, crosslinks, and plates.

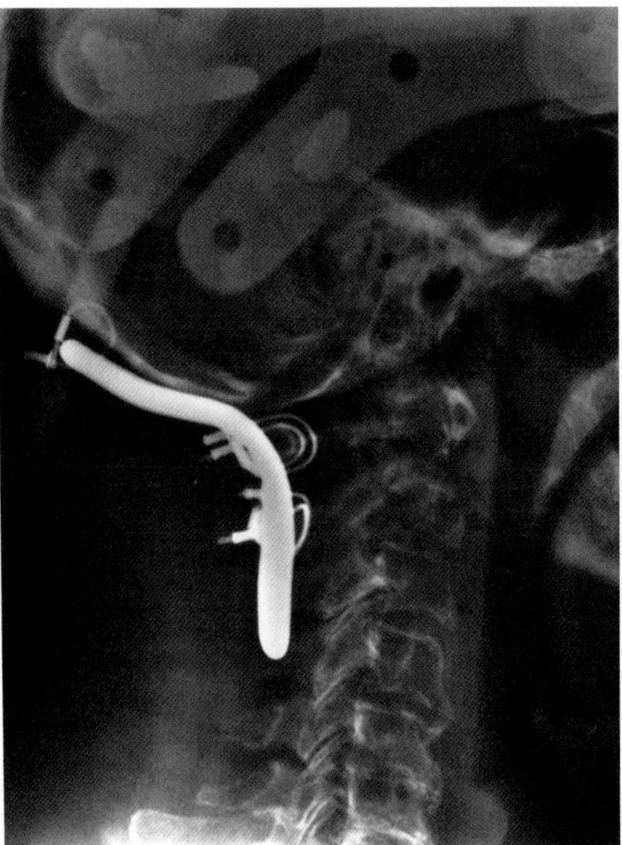

Fig. 3-106 Lateral radiograph after Luque rectangle and wire fusion from the occiput to C2 for a complex C2 body fracture.

## Suggested Reading

Berquist TH. *Imaging of orthopaedic trauma*, 2nd ed. New York: Raven Press; 1992:93–206.

Daffner RH, Brown RR, Goldberg AL. A new classification for cervical vertebral injuries: Influence of CT. *Skeletal Radiol.* 2000;29:125–132.

Deliganis AV, Baxter AB, Hanson JA, et al. Radiologic spectrum of craniocervical distraction injuries. *Radiographics.* 2000;20:S237–S250.

Hosalkar HS, Cain EL, Horn D, et al. Traumatic atlantooccipital dislocation in children. *J Bone Joint Surg.* 2005;87A: 2480–2488.

Stock GH, Vaccaro AR, Brown AK, et al. Contemporary posterior occipital fixation. *J Bone Joint Surg.* 2006;88A:1642–1649.

### Lower Cervical Spine (C3-7)

Lower cervical spine injuries account for 70% to 80% of cervical spine injuries. Most fractures occur at the C5-7 levels. In a Mayo Clinic series of 420 patients, the injuries were distributed as follows:

**Location of lower cervical spine injuries***

- Vertebral arch 42%
- Vertebral body 31%
- Disc 27%
- Posterior ligaments 22%
- Anterior ligaments 4%

* Multiple injuries result in total >100%

Combination injuries with involvement of the thoracic and lumbar spine occurred in 15% of patients. Therefore, if an injury is identified in the cervical spine the entire spine should be imaged.

Management of lower cervical spine injuries depends on neurologic involvement, stability, and position of fracture fragments. Neural decompression may be achieved by realignment; however, in some cases removal of fragments from the spinal canal or posterior decompression with laminectomy may be required. Most stable lesions can be treated with external support. These injuries would include spinous process fractures, mild compression fractures, and isolated transverse process, lateral mass or uncinate process fractures. Care must be taken not to overlook associated fractures or spinous process fractures that enter the spinolaminar line (see Fig. 3-107). These injuries are more apt to extend into the lamia or spinal canal and have associated posterior ligament injuries that can lead to instability and delayed neurologic complications.

Unstable or major injuries include posterior ligament tears with or without locked or perched facets, teardrop fractures, burst fractures, and two-column hyperextension sprains. Fixation may include posterior, anterior, or combined instrumentation. Halo fixation is used for postoperative support.

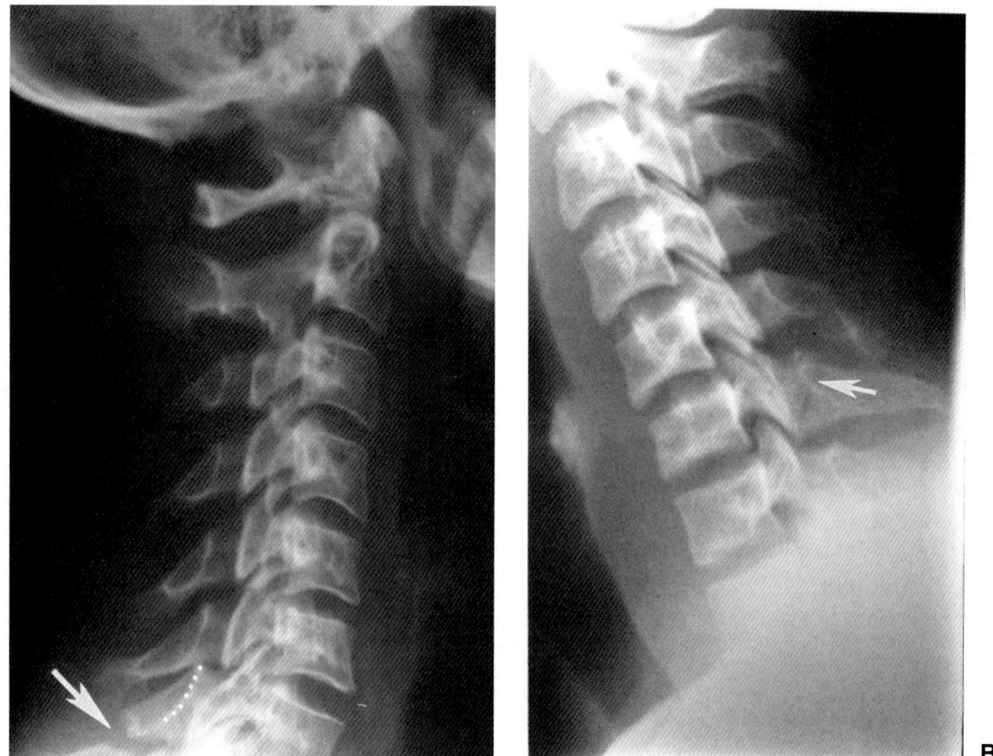

Fig. 3-107 A: Lateral radiograph of the cervical spine demonstrating the typical spinous process fracture (*arrow*) without extension into the spinolaminar line (*broken lines*). B: Lateral radiograph demonstrating spinous process fractures at C4-6. The fracture at C6 enters the lamina (*arrow*).

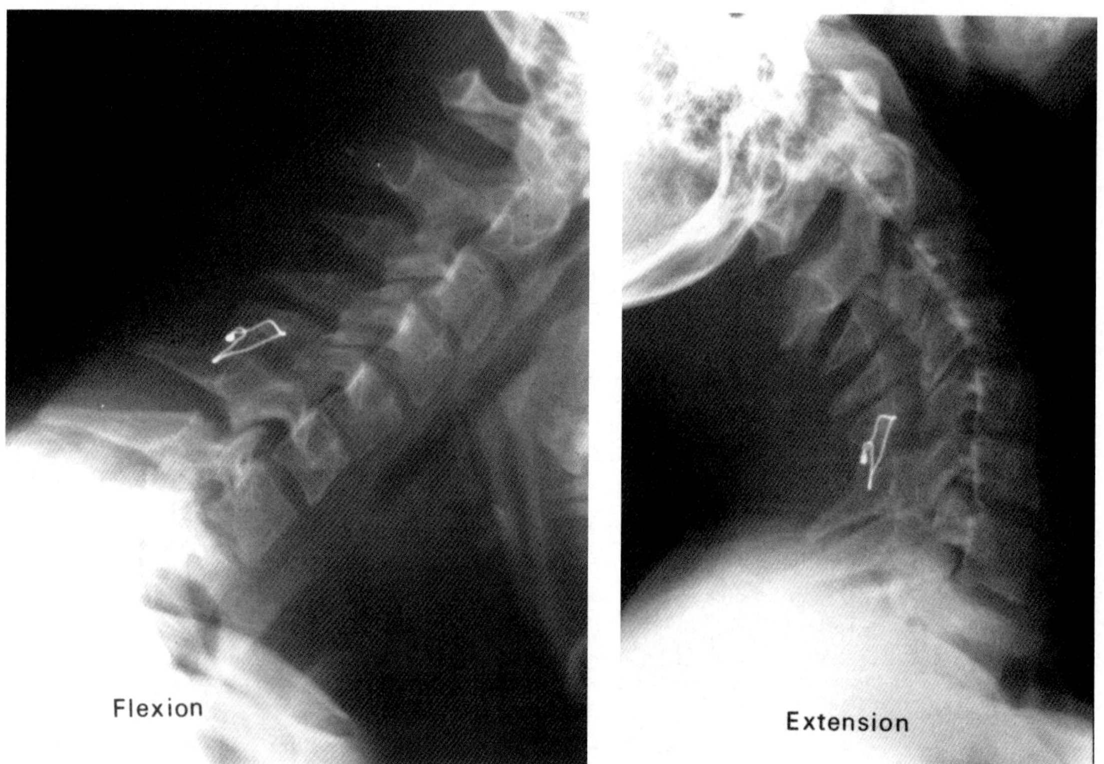


Fig. 3-108 Posterior ligament tear treated with wire and bone graft fixation. Flexion (A) and extension (B) images demonstrate solid fusion posteriorly with no motion at the C5-6 level.

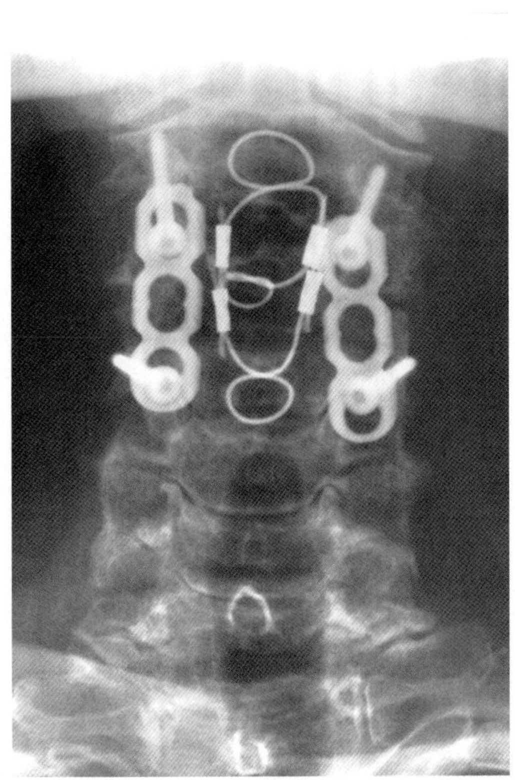

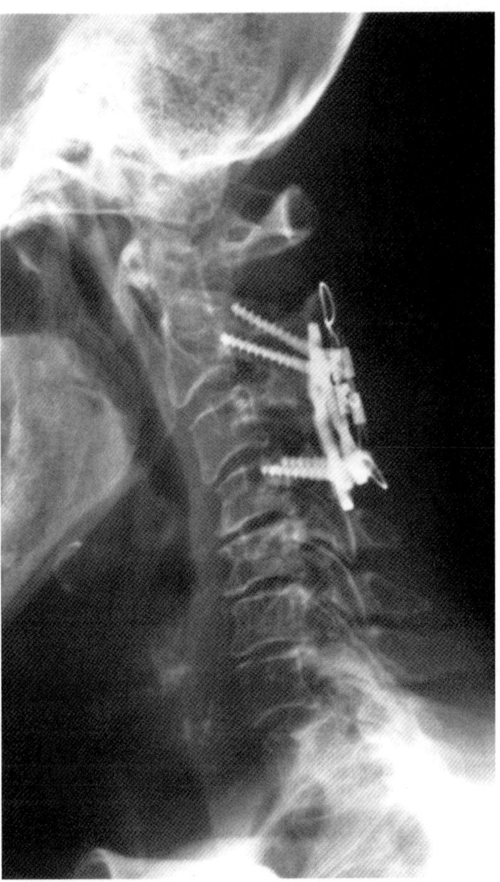

A B

Fig. 3-109 Anteroposterior (AP) (A) and lateral (B) radiographs following posterior plate and lateral mass screw fixation with cable spinous process fixation for complex C2-3 injury.

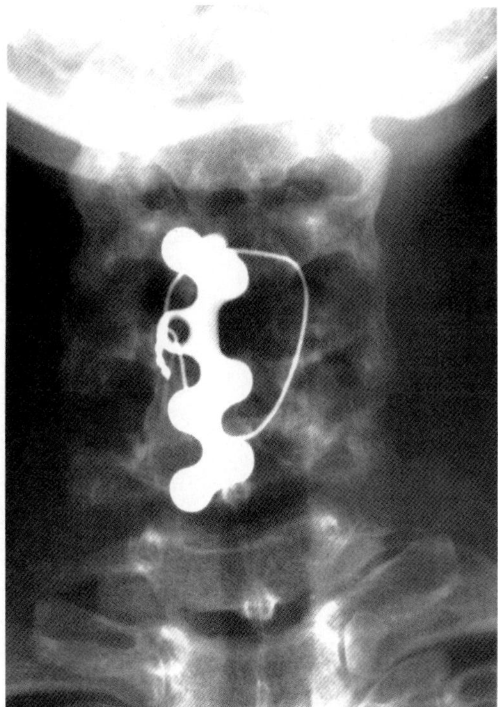

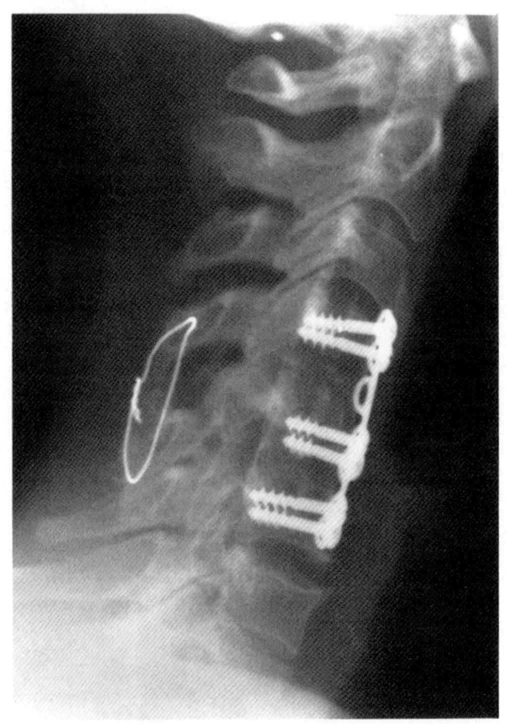

A B

Fig. 3-110 Anteroposterior (AP) (A) and lateral (B) radiographs following combined instrumentation with anterior plate and screw fusion C4-6 and posterior wire and bone graft fusion. Fusion is solid.

**Posterior instrumentation**

- Posterior wire or cable spinous process fixation with or without bone graft for ligament injuries (see Fig. 3-108)
- Rod or plate and screw fixation (see Fig. 3-109)
- Hook plates for discoligamentous instability

**Anterior instrumentation**

- Following anterior ligament injury or anterior decompression
- Plate and screw fixation typically used with disc grafts

**Combined instrumentation**

- Complex injuries with bone loss
- Loss of posterior soft tissue support (see Fig. 3-110)

## Suggested Reading

Abumi K, Itoh H, Taneichi H, et al. Transpedicular screw fixation for traumatice lesions of the middle and lower cervical spine: Description of the techniques and preliminary report. *J Spinal Disord*. 1194;7:19–28.

Aebi M, Zuber K, Marchesi D. Treatment of cervical spine injuries with anterior plating. Indications, techniques and results. *Spine*. 1991;16:S38–S45.

Cabanela ME, Ebersold MJ. Anterior plate stabilization for bursting teardrop fractures of the cervical spine. *Spine*. 1988;13:888–891.

Daffner RH, Brown RR, Goldberg AL. A new classification for cervical vertebral injuries: Influence of CT. *Skeletal Radiol*. 2000;29:125–132.

Lifeso RM, Colucci MA. Anterior fusion for rotationally unstable cervical spine fractures. *Spine*. 2000;25:2028–2034.

Matar LD, Helms CA, Richardson MJ. "Spinolaminar breach": An important sign in cervical spinous process fractures. *Skeletal Radiol*. 2000;29:75–80.

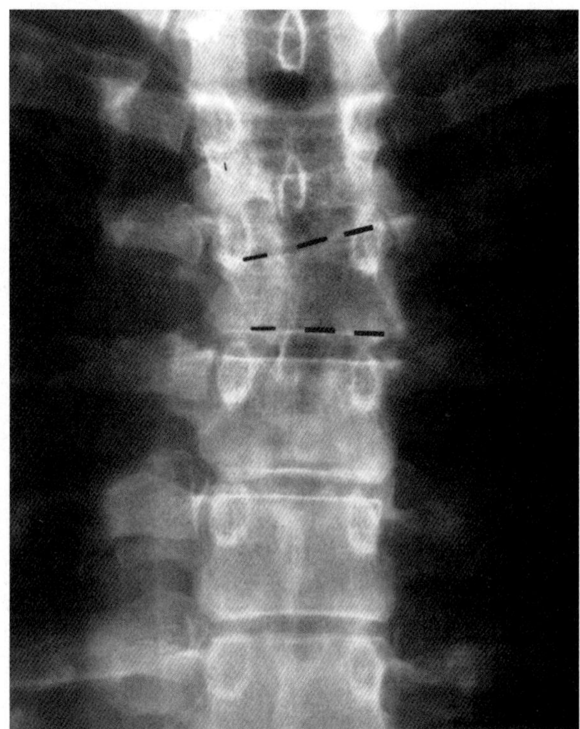

Fig. 3-111 Anteroposterior (AP) radiograph of the thoracic spine. There is asymmetric height of T4 due to lateral compression.

## Thoracolumbar Spine Trauma

Differences in anatomy have an impact on classification, diagnosis, and management of thoracic and lumbar spine injuries. There is normally a slight kyphotic curve in the thoracic spine. This is in contrast to the cervical and lumbar spine where there is normally a lordotic curve. The spinal canal is circular and smaller in the thoracic spine compared to the larger more triangular configuration in the lumbar spine. As one progresses inferiorly, the vertebral bodies increase in size and the discs increase in height resulting in an increasing resistance to axial loading.

Because of differences in range of motion, transition of the facet joints, and other anatomic factors, the thoracolumbar junction is most susceptible to injury. Up to 66% of injuries occur between T12 and L2.

### Imaging of Thoracolumbar Spine Injuries

Imaging of the thoracic and lumbar spine in suspected trauma is performed similar to the cervical spine. Radiographs or CR images in the AP and lateral projections are still useful for screening in many cases. Multichannel CT is increasingly used

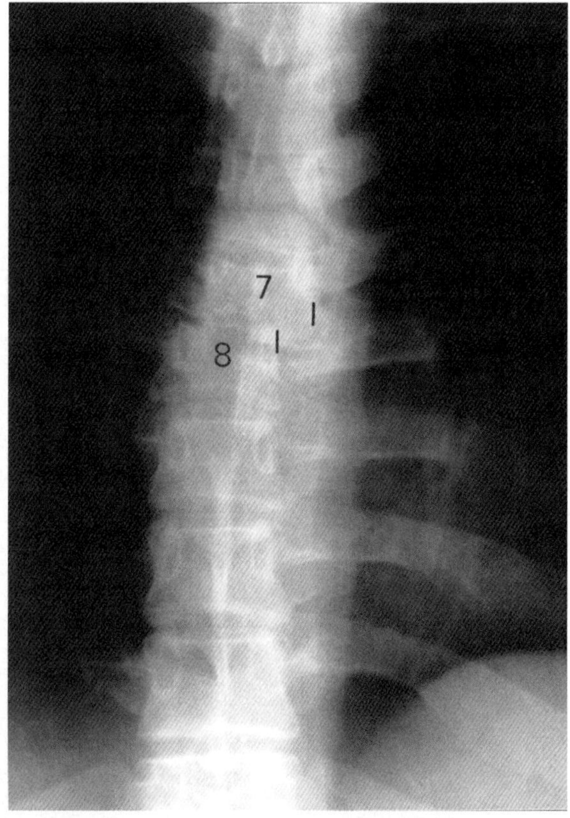


Fig. 3-112 Anteroposterior (AP) radiograph of the thoracic spine demonstrating translation of T7 on T8 (*vertical lines* mark the vertebral margins).

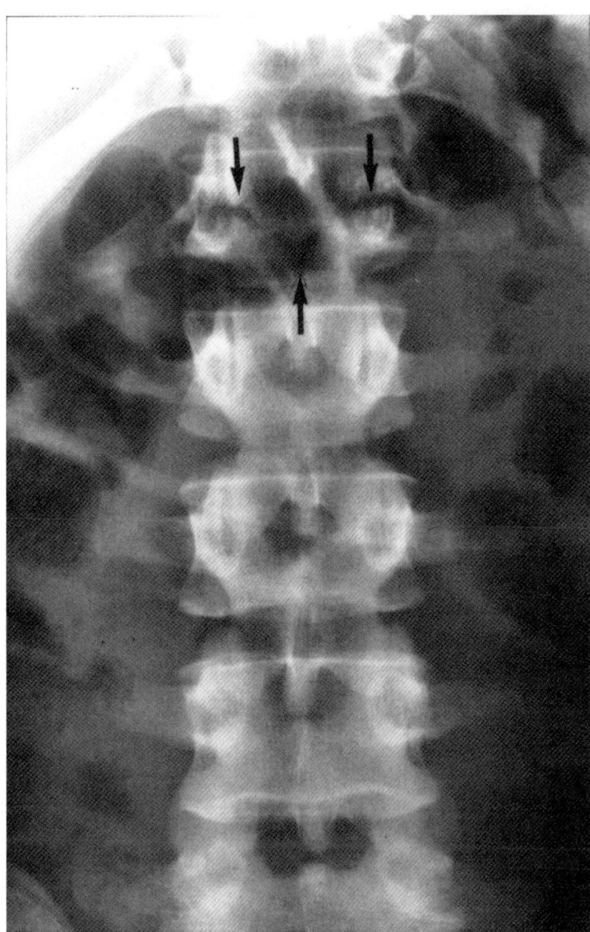

Fig. 3-113 Anteroposterior (AP) radiograph of the lumbar spine demonstrating a fracture (*arrows*) through the posterior elements due to a Chance fracture (flexion-distraction injury).

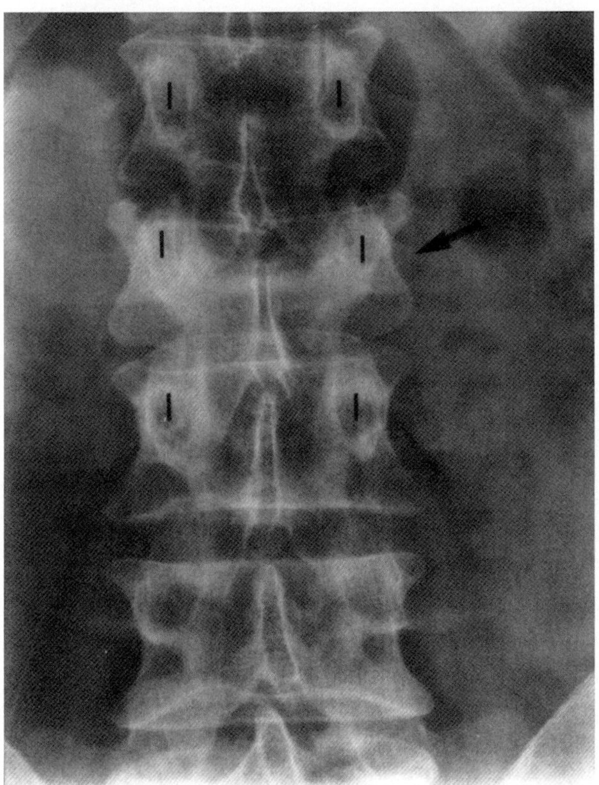

Fig. 3-114 Anteroposterior (AP) radiograph of the lumbar spine with widening of the interpedicular distance at L2 (*arrow*) due to a burst fracture.

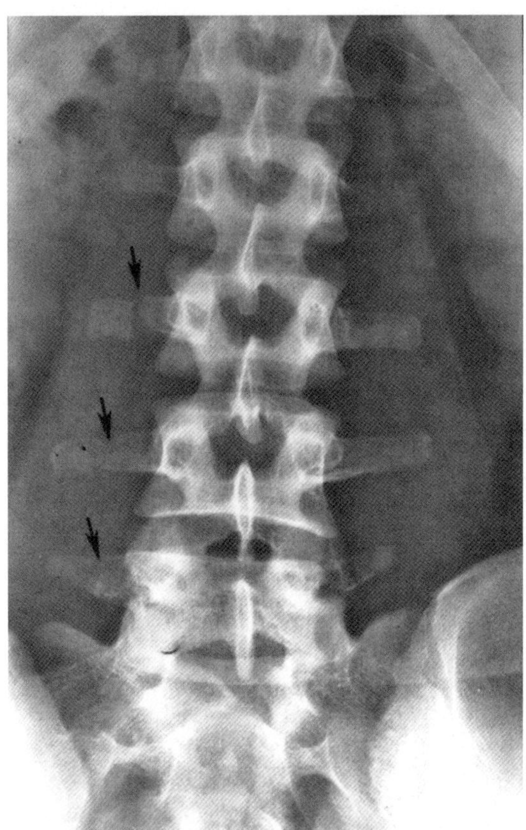

Fig. 3-115 Anteroposterior (AP) radiograph of the lumbar spine demonstrating multiple transverse process fractures (*arrows*).

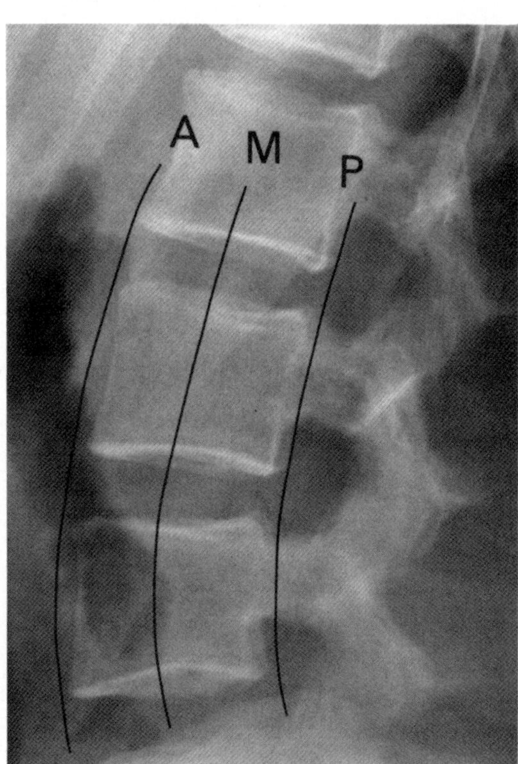


Fig. 3-116 Lateral radiograph of the lumbar spine demonstrating the three-column approach described by Denis. Anterior column—anterior longitudinal ligament plus anterior half of the vertebral body and disc. Middle column—posterior half of the disc and vertebral body plus the posterior longitudinal ligament. Posterior column—posterior bony arch, ligamentum flavum, facet capsules, intraspinous and supraspinous ligaments. A, anterior; M, middle; P, posterior.

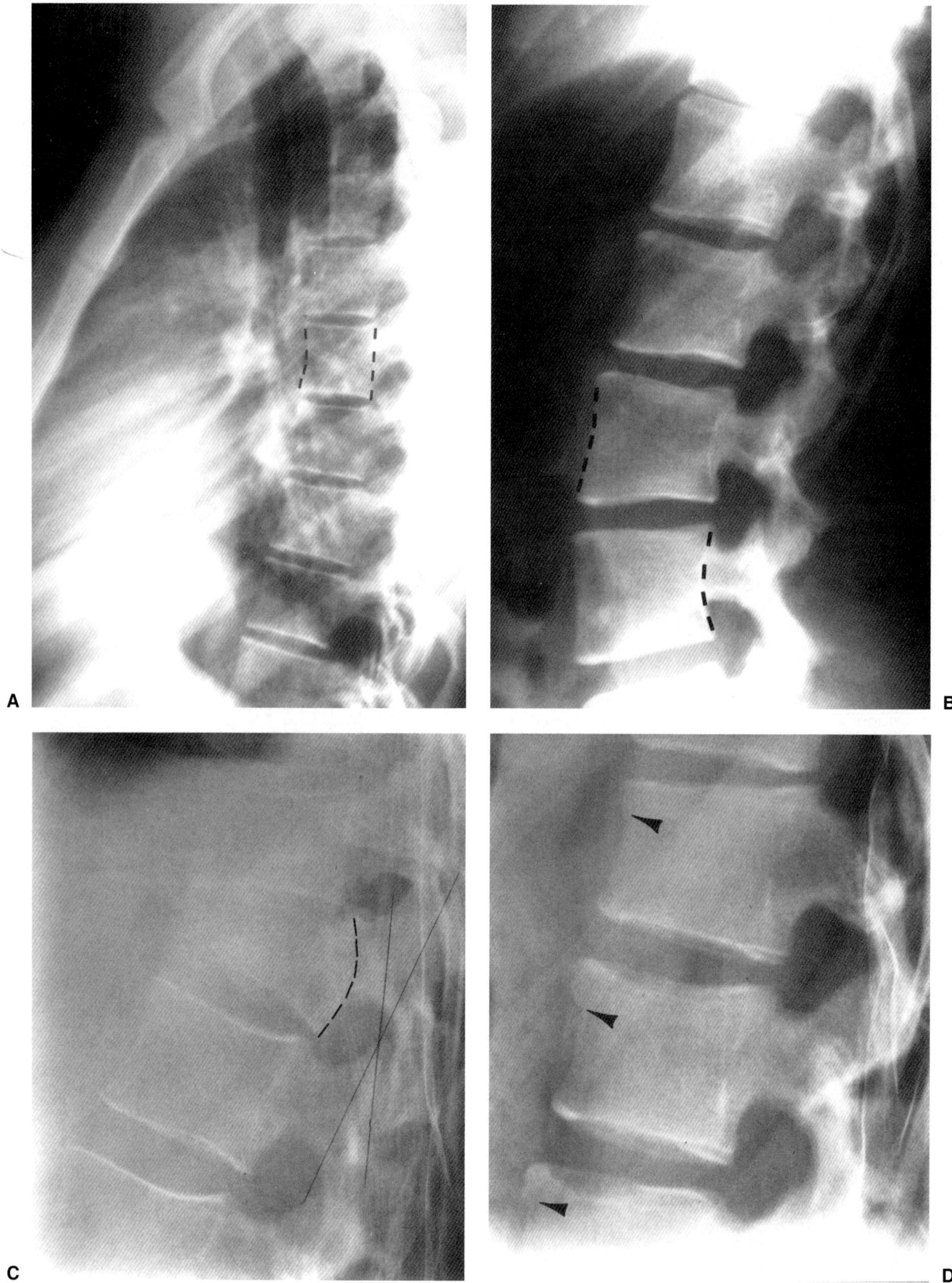


Fig. 3-117 Normal contour of the thoracic (A) and lumbar (B) vertebrae. The thoracic vertebrae are slightly concave anteriorly and straight posteriorly. The lumbar vertebrae are nearly straight anteriorly and concave posteriorly (*broken lines*). C: Lateral radiograph demonstrating a convex appearance (*broken lines*) due to a burst fracture. D: Lateral radiograph demonstrating subtle buckling of the anterior cortex (*arrowheads*) due to multilevel compression fractures.

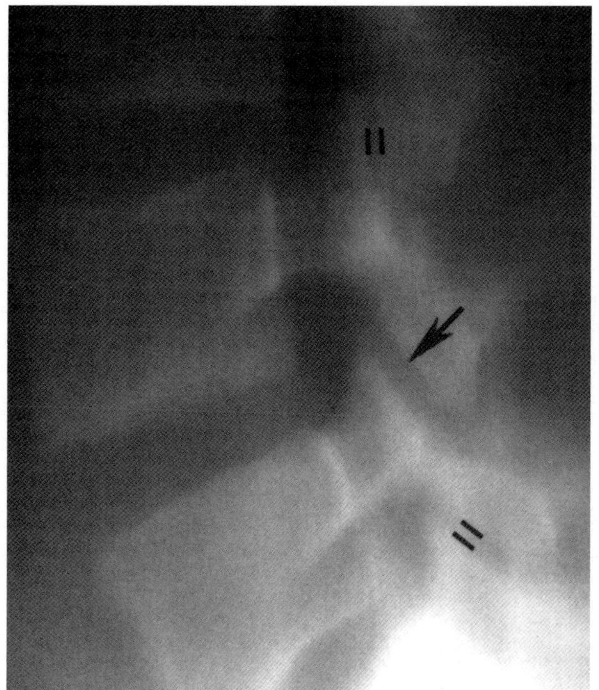

Fig. 3-118 Lateral radiograph demonstrating widening of the facet joint due to a rotation injury.

for screening, especially in patients with multitrauma. Data on these two modalities is similar to that provided in the preceding text for the cervical spine. Multichannel CT is reported to be 99.3% accurate for detecting thoracolumbar fractures.

| IMAGING TECHNIQUE | SENSITIVITY T SPINE (%) | SENSITIVITY L SPINE (%) |
|---|---|---|
| Radiography | 64 | 69 |
| Multichannel CT | 97 | 95 |

RADIOGRAPHS

## AP view

- Vertebral height should be uniform (see Fig. 3-111)
- Normal alignment (see Fig. 3-112)
- Spinous processes midline
- Look for linear defects in the posterior elements (see Fig. 3-113)
- Assess pedicles and interpedicular distance (see Fig. 3-114)
- Evaluate transverse processes (see Fig. 3-115)

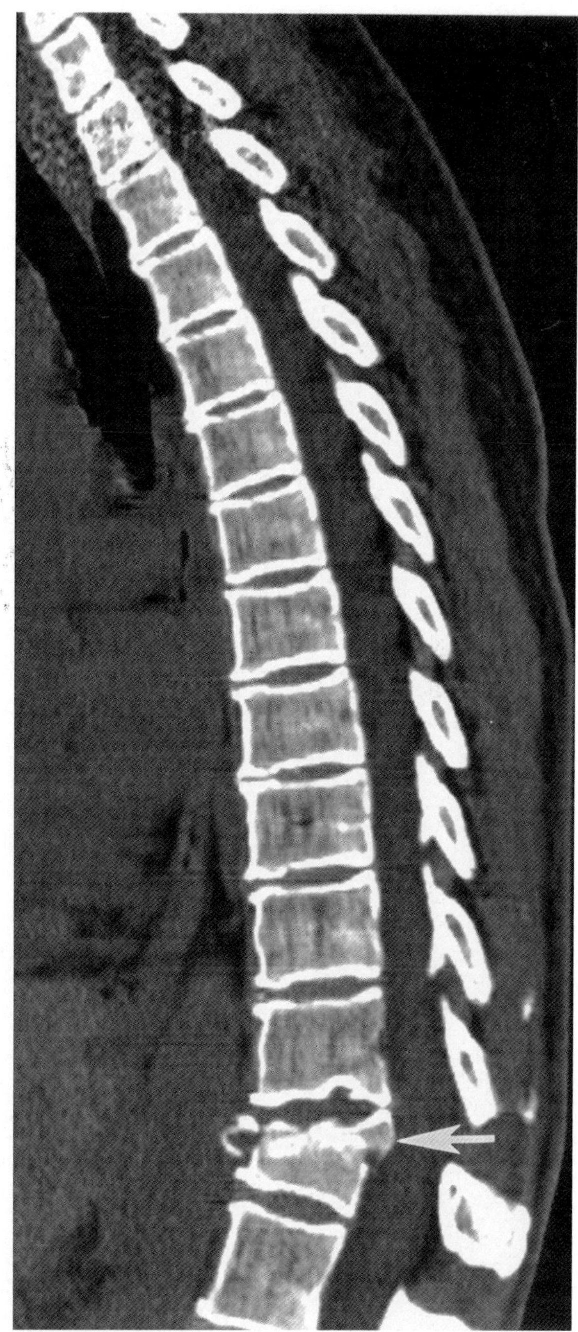


Fig. 3-119 Sagittal and coronal reformatted computed tomographic (CT) images demonstrating 50% compression of the vertebral body with a retropulsed fragment (*arrow*) and laterally displaced fragments (*arrowheads*).

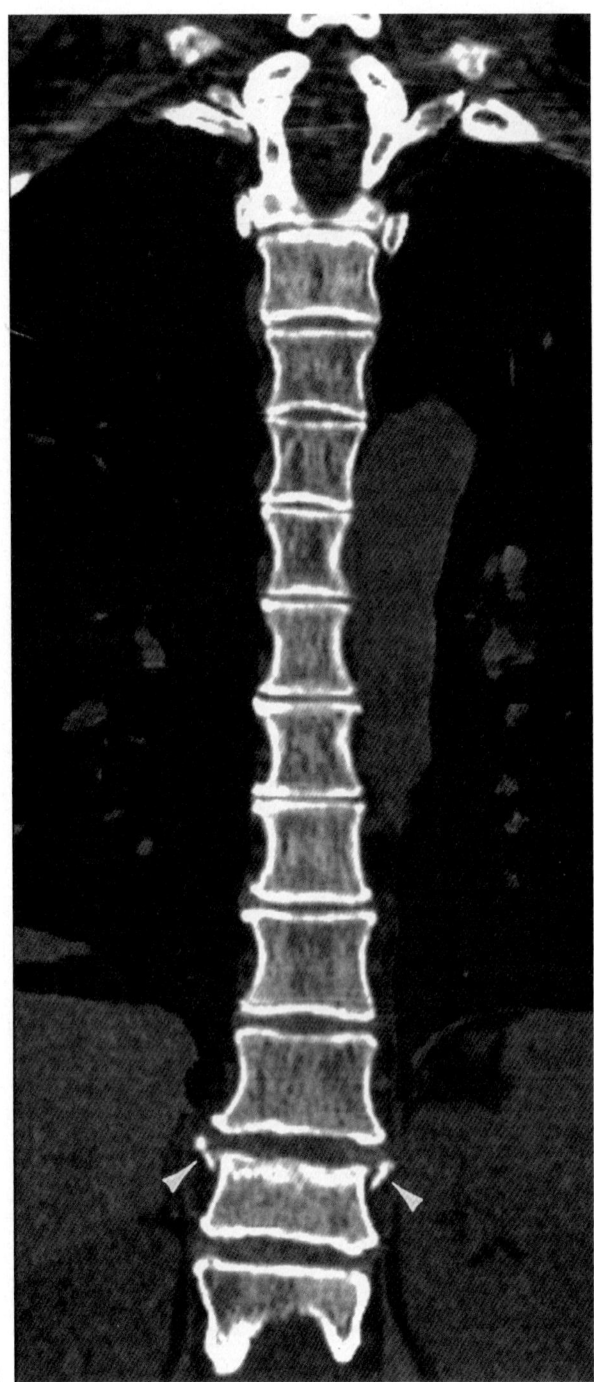

B

Fig. 3-119 *(Continued)*

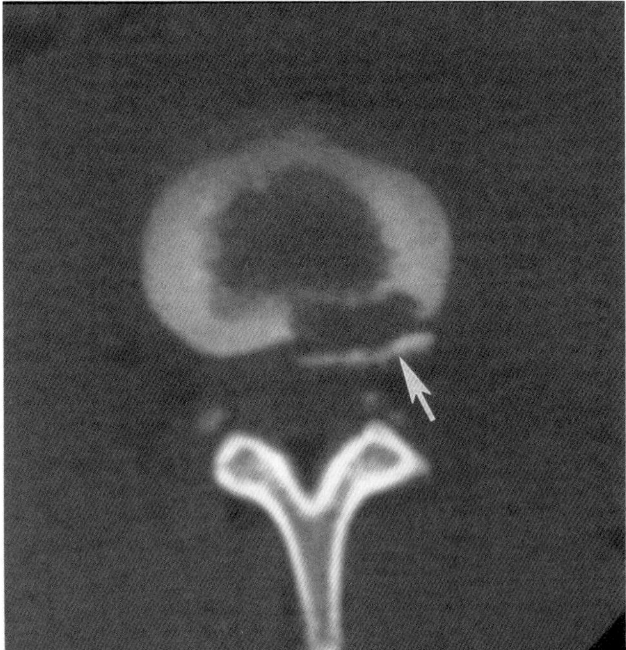

Fig. 3-120 Axial computed tomographic (CT) image demonstrating a posteriorly displaced marginal fragment (*arrow*).

**Lateral view**

- Use three-column approach to evaluate stability and the extent of injury (see Fig. 3-116)
- Upper thoracic spine often not well seen, add swimmer's view
- Evaluate normal vertebral contour (see Fig. 3-117)
- Symmetry of facet joints (see Fig. 3-118)

MULTICHANNEL COMPUTED TOMOGRAPHY

- Axial, coronal, and sagittal reformatted imxages (see Fig. 3-119)
- Evaluate alignment
- Disc space changes
- Vertebral height
- Presence and degree of spinal compromise due to posterior retropulsed cortex or fragments in the spinal canal (see Fig.3-120)

MAGNETIC RESONANCE IMAGING

- Suspected cord or nerve root injury
- Ligament injuries

## Suggested Reading

Bagley LJ. Imaging of spinal trauma. *Radiol Clin North Am.* 2006;44:1–12.

Brown CVR, Antevil JL, Sise MJ, et al. Spiral computed tomography for diagnosis of cervical, thoracic and lumbar spine fractures: Its time has come. *J Trauma.* 2005;58:890–896.

Grove CJ, Cassar-Pullicino VN, Tins BJ, et al. Chance-type flexion-distraction injuries to the thoracolumbar spine: MR imaging characteristics. *Radiology.* 2005;236:601–608.

Wintermark M, Mouhsine E, Theumann N, et al. Thoracolumbar spine fractures in patients who have sustained severe trauma: Depiction with multi-detector row CT. *Radiology.* 2003;227:681–689.

## Mechanism of Injury

Mechanisms of injury in the thoracic and lumbar spine are similar to the cervical spine. The thoracic spine is somewhat of an exception in that the rib cage decreases rotation injuries. Most thoracolumbar injuries are due to flexion forces associated with compression or in the lumbar spine rotation. Neurologic complications approach 71% with flexion torsion injuries. Common classification systems are listed in the subsequent text.

### Denis classification

- Three-column approach; one column may be stable; posterior- and middle-column involvement unstable
- Four categories of injury
  Compression, 31% of cases
  Burst, 41% of cases
  Seat-belt
  Fracture/dislocation

### AO (Arbeitsgemeinshaft fur Osteosynthesefragen)

- Three main categories with subtypes
  **Type A**—compression, 66% of cases
  **Type B**—distraction, 24% of cases
  **Type C**—fracture/dislocation, 10% of cases

### Frankel neurologic classification

- **Type A**—no motor or sensory activity below level of injury
- **Type B**—sensory intact, but no motor function below level of injury
- **Type C**—ineffective motor function
- **Type D**—motor function effective, but weak
- **Type E**—normal sensory and motor function

## Suggested Reading

Denis F. The three column spine and its significance in classification of acute thoracolumbar spinal injuries. *Spine.* 1983;8:817–831.

Frankel HL, Hancock DO, Hyslop G, et al. The value of postural reduction in the initial management of closed injuries of the spine with paraplegia and tetraplegia. *Paraplegia.* 1969;7:179–192.

Tsou PM, Wang J, Khoo L, et al. A thoracic and lumbar spine injury severity classification based upon neurologic function grade, spinal canal deformity and spinal biomechanical stability. *Spine J.* 2006;6:636–647.

Wood KB, Khanna G, Vaccaro AR, et al. Assessment of two thoracolumbar fracture classification systems as used by multiple surgeons. *J Bone Joint Surg.* 2005;87A:1423–1429.

## Management of Thoracolumbar Spine Fractures

Initially, the critical questions involve the extent of neurologic injury and stability. Complete injury at the T10 level or above usually indicates irreversible cord injury. Lesions below T10

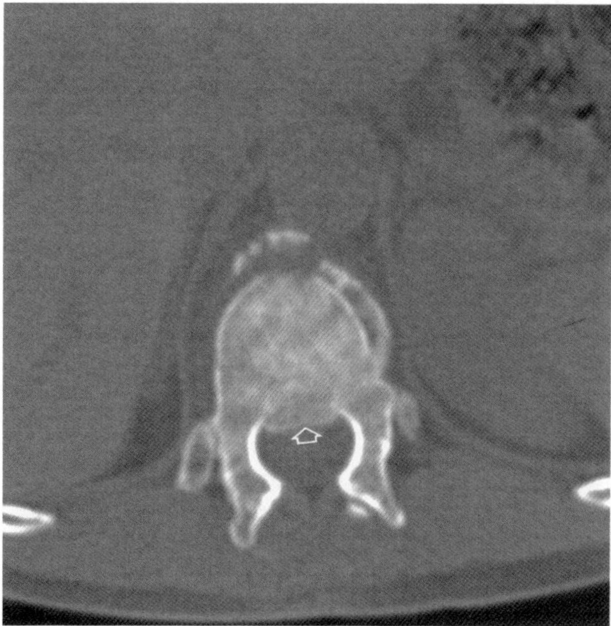

**Fig. 3-121** Axial computed tomographic (CT) image of the lower thoracic spine with a burst fracture and narrowing of the spinal canal.

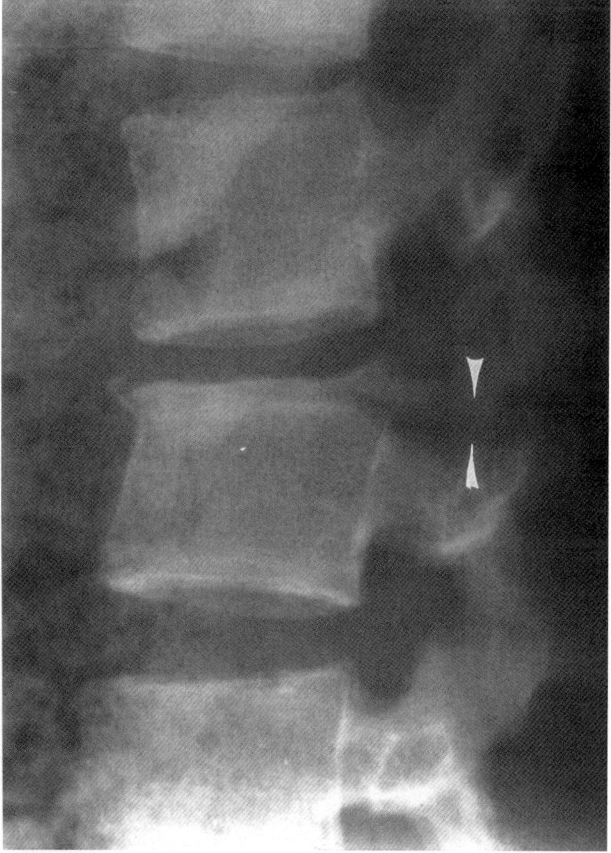

**Fig. 3-122** Lateral radiograph demonstrating an L1 Chance fracture with separation of the posterior arch (*arrowheads*) and two-column involvement.

may involve the cauda equina or nerve roots and have a better prognosis. Careful evaluation of imaging studies is useful to determine stability and the need to decompress neural structures due to displacement of osseous structures of fragments in the spinal canal. Anterior compression injuries with <40% loss of height and no posterior column involvement may be treated with external support. The goals of treatment are to decompress the spinal canal, improve deformity with relief of pain, maintain function, and achieve early ambulation when possible.

### Indications for surgical intervention

- Neural compression (see Fig. 3-121)
- Neurologic deterioration
- Disruption of the posterior ligaments (see Fig. 3-122)
- Failure to achieve correction with external means
- Vertebral compression >40% or multisegment involvement, which totals >50% (see Fig. 3-123)

Instrumentation approaches should preserve lumbar lordosis and reduce kyphotic deformity. In the lumbar spine, attempts

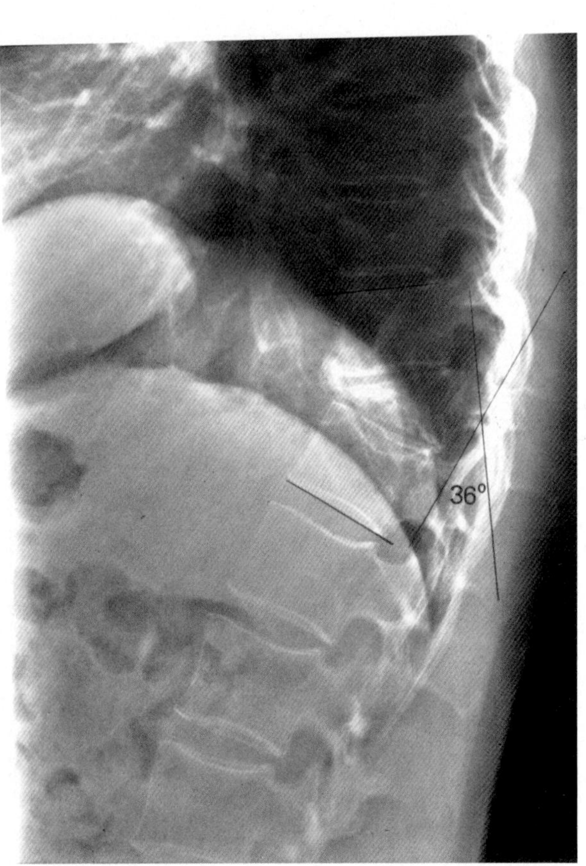


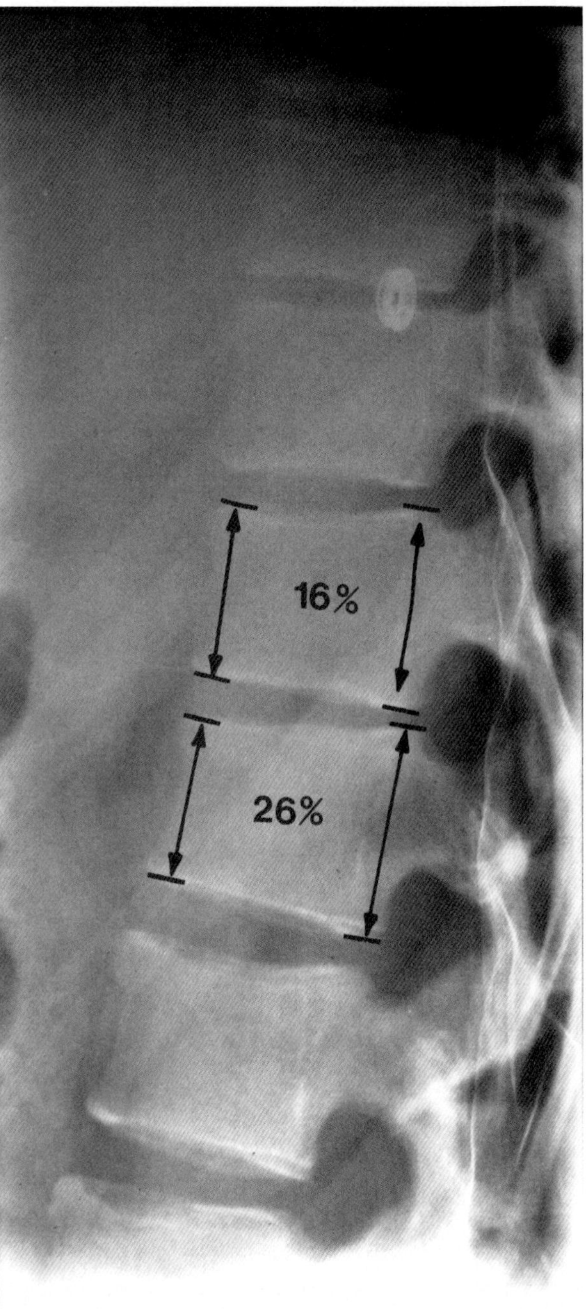


Fig. 3-123 Compression fractures. A: Lateral radiograph demonstrating marked compression of T12 with 36 degrees of kyphotic angulation. B: Mild compression of T12 (16%) and L1 (26%) for a combined 42%.

are made to fuse as few segments as possible to retain flexibility and prevent long-term low back pain.

### Posterior instrumentation

- Rods, pedicle screws, hooks, and sublaminar wires
- Locking hooks can be used to reduce displacement or pullout
- Systems similar to those described in the scoliosis section are used
- In the thoracic spine, fusion is usually extended two to three segments above and below the injury (see Fig. 3-124)

### Anterior instrumentation

- Used for hyperextension injuries or bone loss
- May require posterior procedure if posterior column not intact
- Systems include plate and screws, rods and screws, spacers, turnbuckle devices, and bone struts (see Figs. 3-125 and 3-126)

## Complications of Spinal Instrumentation for Trauma

Complications may be related to the initial injury, improper diagnosis, and management or related to instrumentation or the operative procedure. During the pretreatment phase, it is important for the radiologist and treating physician to communicate closely to optimize assessment of stability, extent of injury, and detection of associated injuries. Failure to identify unstable or combination injuries must be avoided to prevent patient deterioration. For example, up to 20% of patients

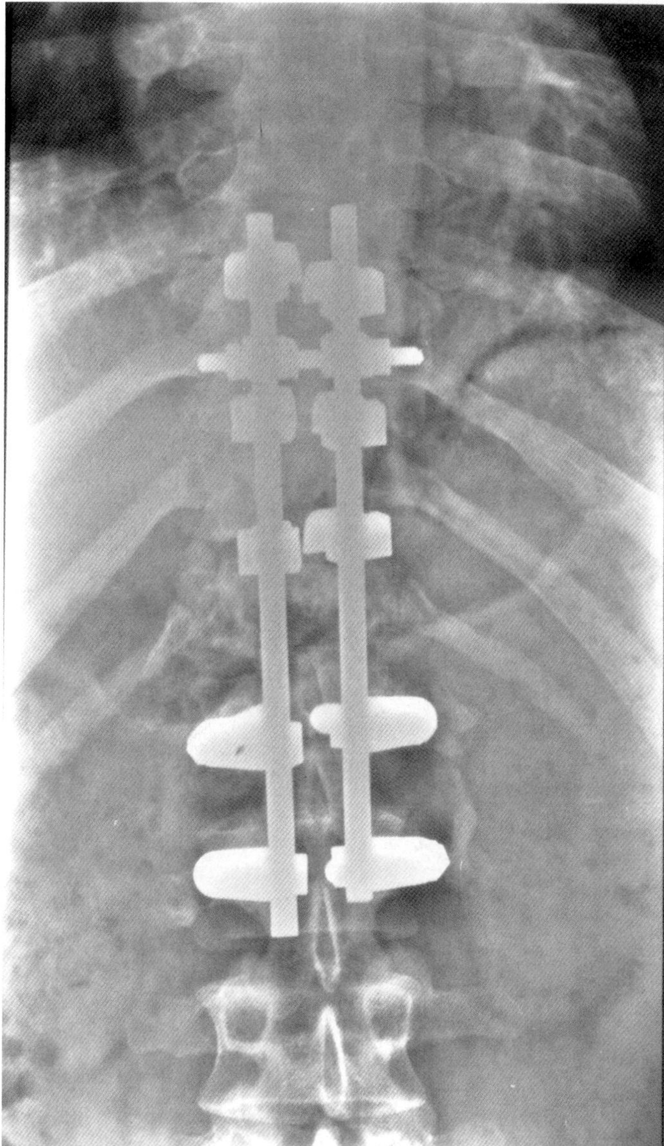


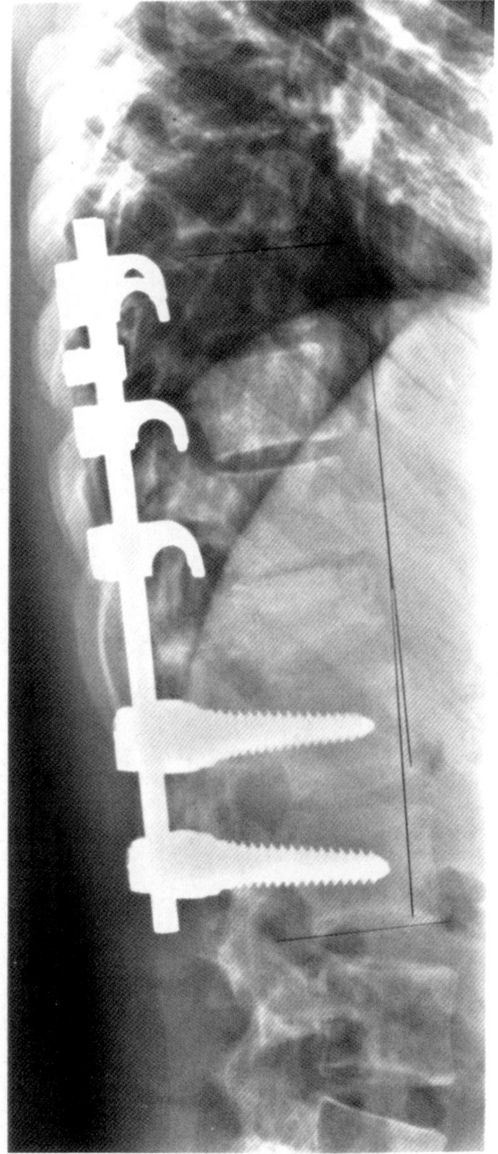


Fig. 3-124 Anteroposterior (AP) (A) and lateral (B) radiographs after ISOLA instrumentation with rods, hooks, and pedicle screws from T9 to L2 for compression fracture of T12. The kyphotic deformity has been reduced.

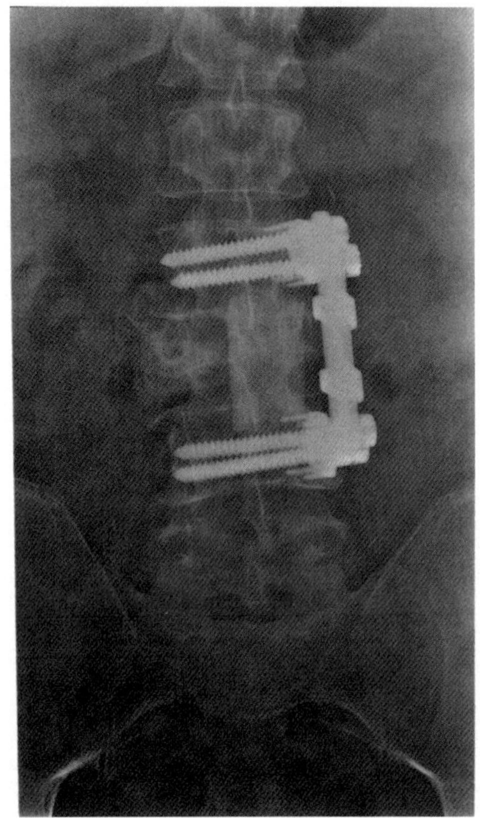

A

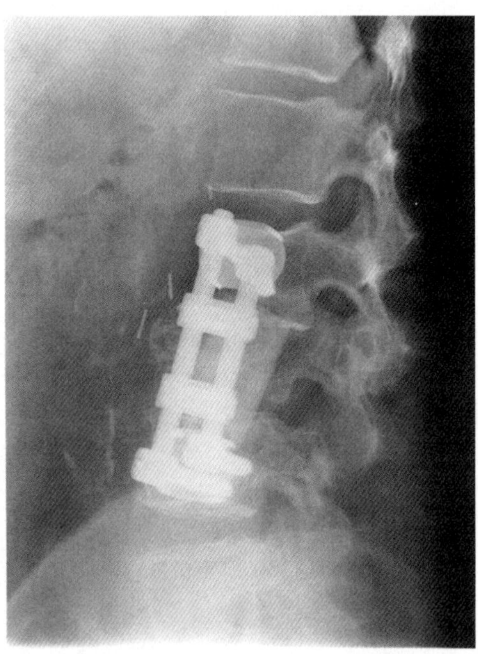

B

Fig. 3-125 Anteroposterior (AP) (A) and lateral (B) radiographs following anterior fusion with bone graft and Kaneda device for treatment of an L3 burst fracture.

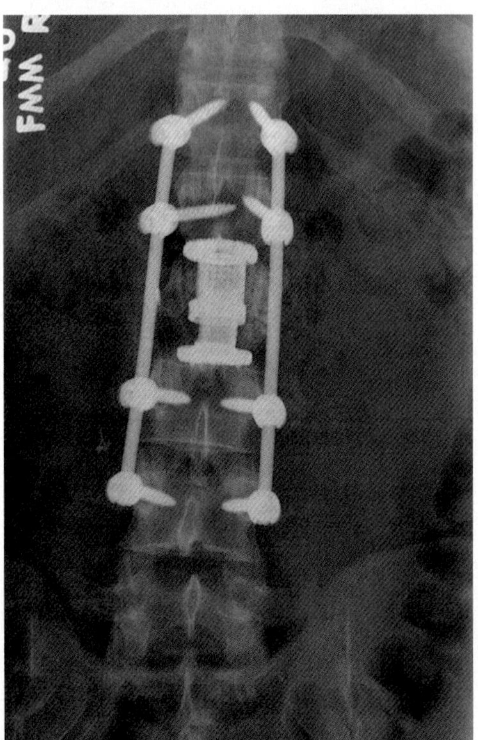

A

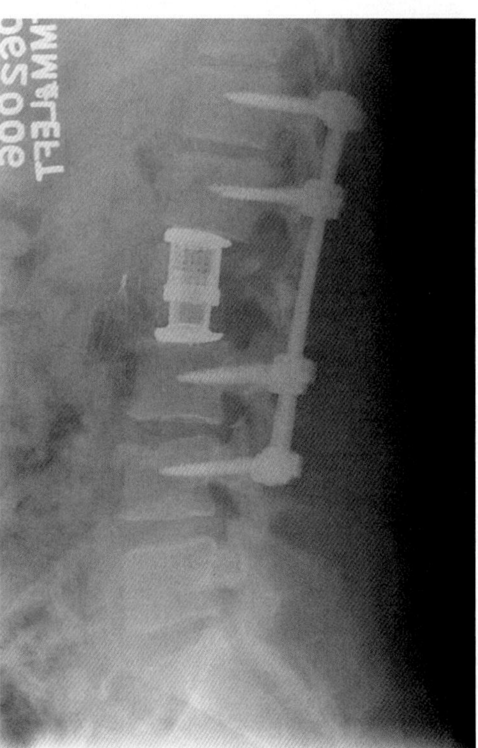

B

Fig. 3-126 Anteroposterior (AP) (A) and lateral (B) radiographs following combined anterior and posterior instrumentation for a complex fracture of L2. There is rod and pedicle screw fixation posteriorly with a turnbuckle spacer anteriorly. These devices can be turned to achieve the proper height. Note the anterior superior fracture of L4.

have combined upper and lower cervical spine injuries. Also, multisegment injuries (cervical, thoracic, and lumbar) occur in 15% to 20% of patients (see Fig. 3-127). Injuries associated with cervical spine fracture/dislocations were described earlier.

### Injuries associated with thoracolumbar fractures

- Multiple segment fractures, 15% to 20% (Fig. 3-127)
- Thoracic spine fracture/dislocations (Type C)
  Chest injuries, 50%
  Hemomediastinum, 20%
  Hemopneumothorax, 19%
  Other missed injuries, 22%
- **Chance fractures**— >40% have abdominal injuries (Fig. 3-127B)
  Bowel lacerations, 48%
  Mesenteric injuries, 38%
  Noncontiguous spine injuries, 33% (Fig. 3-127A)

Proper procedure and implant selection are also critical. For example, Luque rods and sublaminar wires do not counteract axial loading as effectively as hook or pedicle screws and rods (see Fig. 3-128). Following decompression, laminectomy instrumentation must be selected to prevent progressive kyphotic deformity and neurologic deficit (see Fig. 3-129).

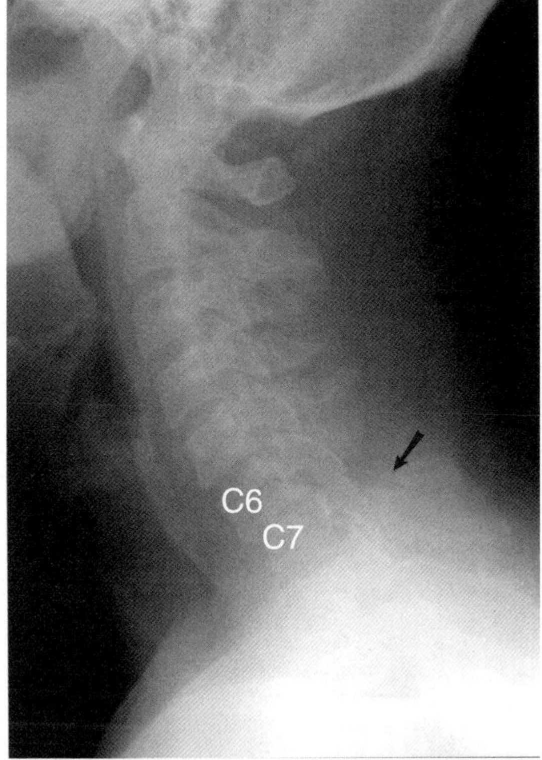


A

B

Fig. 3-127 Multisegment injury. A: Lateral radiograph of the cervical spine demonstrates subluxation of C6 on C7 with a displaced spinous process fracture (*arrow*). B: Lateral radiograph of the lumbar spine demonstrates a flexion-distraction injury (Chance fracture) of L1 with mild anterior compression (*arrow*) and splitting of the posterior elements (*arrowheads*). Chance fractures have a high incidence of associated abdominal injuries.

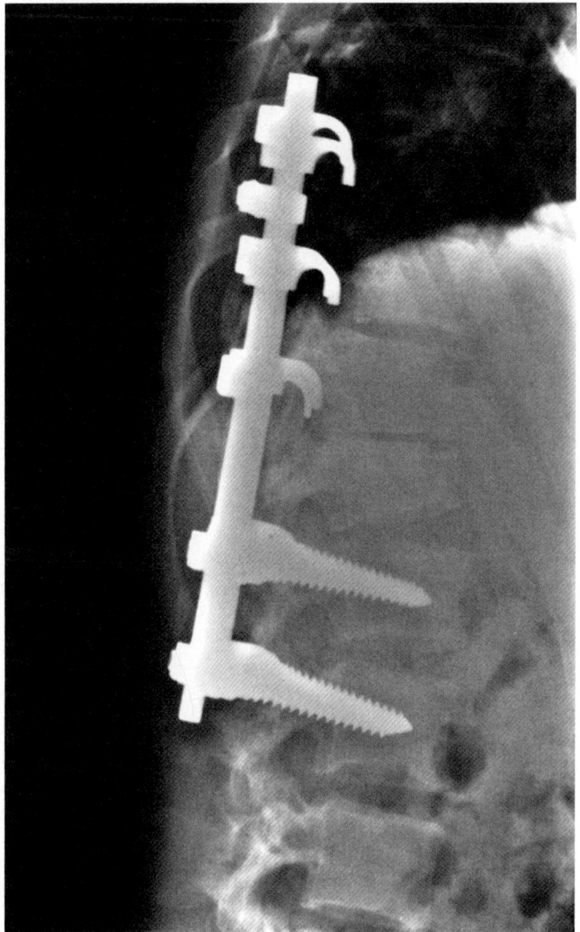

Fig. 3-128 Lateral radiograph demonstrating posterior instrumentation with rods, hooks, and pedicle screws for treatment of a T12 burst fracture.

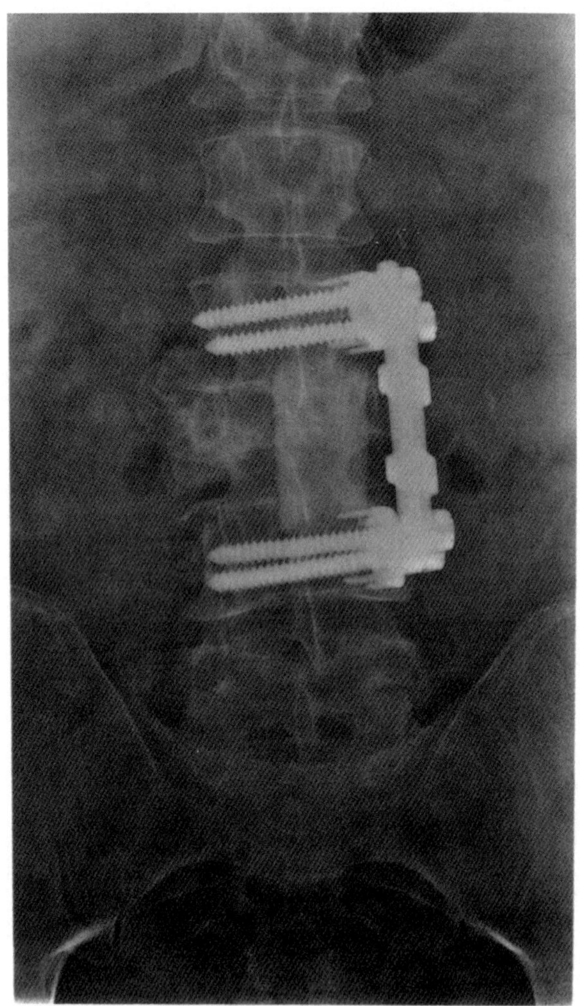

Fig. 3-129 Anteroposterior (AP) radiograph after laminectomy and fusion for an L3 burst fracture using a Kaneda device and bone strut anteriorly.

Complications and imaging approaches are similar to those described in Table 3-4.

## SUGGESTED READING


Berntein MP, Mirvis SE, Shanmuganathan K. Chance-type fractures of the thoracolumbar spine: Imaging analysis in 53 patients. *AJR Am J Roentgenol*. 2006;187:859–868.

Chang SD, Lee MJ, Munk PL, et al. MRI of spinal hardware: Comparison of conventional T1-weighted sequence with new metal artifact reduction sequence. *Skeletal Radiol*. 2001; 30:213–218.

Douglas-Akinwande AC, Buckwalter KA, Ryberg J, et al. Multidetector CT: Evaluating the spine in postoperative patients with orthopaedic hardware. *Radiographics*. 2006;26:S97–S110.

Groves CJ, Cassar-Pullicino VN, Tins PNM, et al. Chance-type flexion distraction injuries in the thoracolumbar spine: MR imaging characteristics. *Radiology*. 2005;236:601–608.

Vialle LR, Vialle E. Thoracic spine fractures. *Injury*. 2005;36: S-B65–S-B72.

# 4
# The Pelvis and Hips

## Introduction

This chapter will address clinical and imaging aspects of orthopaedic procedures in the pelvis and hips. Pelvic fractures, fracture/dislocations of the hip, intertrochanteric and subtrochanteric fractures, and treatment approaches will be reviewed in the first section. Joint replacement procedures will be discussed in the second section. This will include clinical indications, preoperative decisions and imaging, and imaging of joint replacement complications. The final section will review osteotomies of the pelvis and hips and hip arthrodeses.

### Trauma

Imaging plays an important role in detection, classification, and evaluation of complications related to fractures of the pelvis and hips and their treatment.

## Pelvic Fractures

Pelvic fractures account for only 2% to 3% of all skeletal injuries. Minor fractures occur more commonly in elderly patients. Most significant injuries (double breaks in the pelvic ring) more commonly occur with high-velocity trauma in younger individuals (50% younger than 50 years). Morbidity and mortality rates can be significant with more severe pelvic fractures.

### Fracture Classification

Multiple classification systems have been used over the years. Most based the classification on location, mechanism of injury, and stability.

**TILE CLASSIFICATION**

| CATEGORY | FRACTURE FEATURES |
|---|---|
| A | Stable injuries |
| A1 | Fracture does not involve the pelvic ring (avulsion, transverse sacral fractures) (see Fig. 4-1) |
| A2 | Stable minimally displaced isolated ring fractures (see Fig. 4-2 and also 4-1B) |
| B | Rotationally stable, vertically unstable |
| B1 | Open book fracture (diastasis of pubic symphysis +/− sacroiliac joints) (see Fig. 4-3) |
| B2 | Lateral compression: ipsilateral (pubic rami and ilium or sacroiliac joint) |
| B3 | Lateral compression: contralateral (bucket handle fracture) |
| C | Unstable rotationally and vertically |
| C1 | Unilateral |
| C2 | Bilateral |
| C3 | Associated acetabular fracture (see Fig. 4-4) |

**KEY AND CONWELL CLASSIFICATION**

| CLASS | PATIENTS (%) | DESCRIPTION |
|---|---|---|
| I | 25 | Isolated fracture not involving the pelvic ring (Fig. 4-1) |
| II | 36 | Single break in the pelvic ring (Figs. 4-1B and 4-2) |
| III | 16 | Double break in the pelvic ring (Fig. 4-3) |
| IV | 24 | Associated acetabular fracture (Fig. 4-4) |

YOUNG AND BURGESS CLASSIFICATION—BASED ON RADIOGRAPHIC PATTERNS

| CATEGORY | INCIDENCE (%) | RADIOGRAPHIC FEATURES |
|---|---|---|
| Lateral compression | 41–72 (see Fig. 4-5) | |
| Type I | | Oblique or horizontal pubic rami fractures with crush injury of ilium, sacrum, or sacroiliac joint, force directed posteriorly (Fig. 4-5A) |
| Type II | | Force directed anterolaterally, oblique or horizontal pubic rami fractures with diastasis of sacroiliac joints (IIA) or iliac wing fracture (IIB) (Fig. 4-5B) |
| Type III | | Anterolateral force with oblique or horizontal pubic rami fractures and diastasis of the sacroiliac ligaments bilaterally (IIIA) or sacroiliac ligaments and ipsilateral iliac wing fracture (IIIB) (Fig. 4-5C) |
| AP compression | 15–25 | Diastasis of pubic symphysis or vertical pubic rami fractures (see Fig. 4-6) |
| Type I | | Minimal diastasis or vertical pubic rami fractures (Fig. 4-6A) |
| Type II | | Wider diastasis or more displaced rami fractures (Fig. 4-6B) |
| Type III | | Wide diastasis of the symphysis and disruption of bilateral sacroiliac ligaments (same as Tile B1) (Figs. 4-3 and 4-6C) |
| Vertical shearing | 6 | Force transmitted vertically resulting in step off of fractures or the symphysis and sacroiliac joints (see Fig. 4-7) |
| Combination injuries | 14 | Combination of above injuries |

AP, anteroposterior.

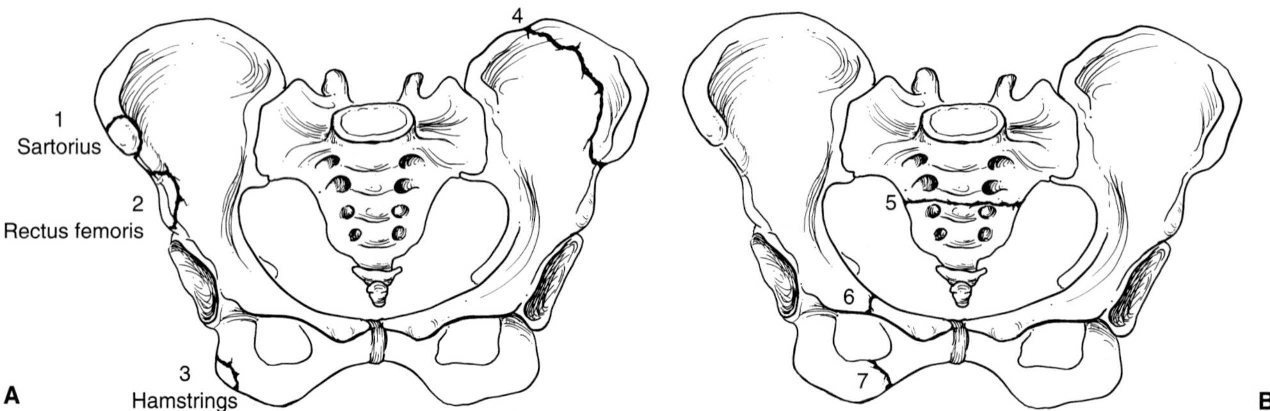


Fig. 4-1 Illustrations of stable pelvic fractures (Tile type A1, Key and Conwell class I). A: Avulsion fractures of the anterior superior iliac spine (*1*), anterior inferior iliac spine (*2*), ischial tuberosity (*3*), and isolated iliac wing (Duverney fracture) fracture. B: Illustration of isolated transverse sacral fracture (*5*) and isolated pubic rami fractures (*6* and *7*).

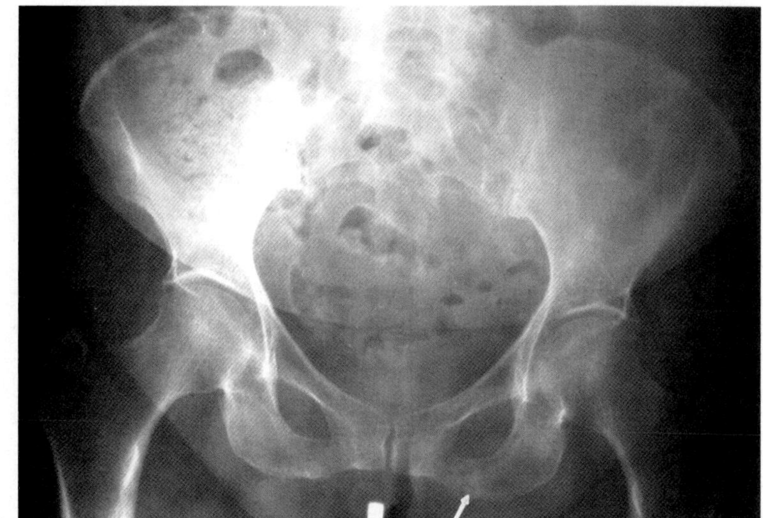

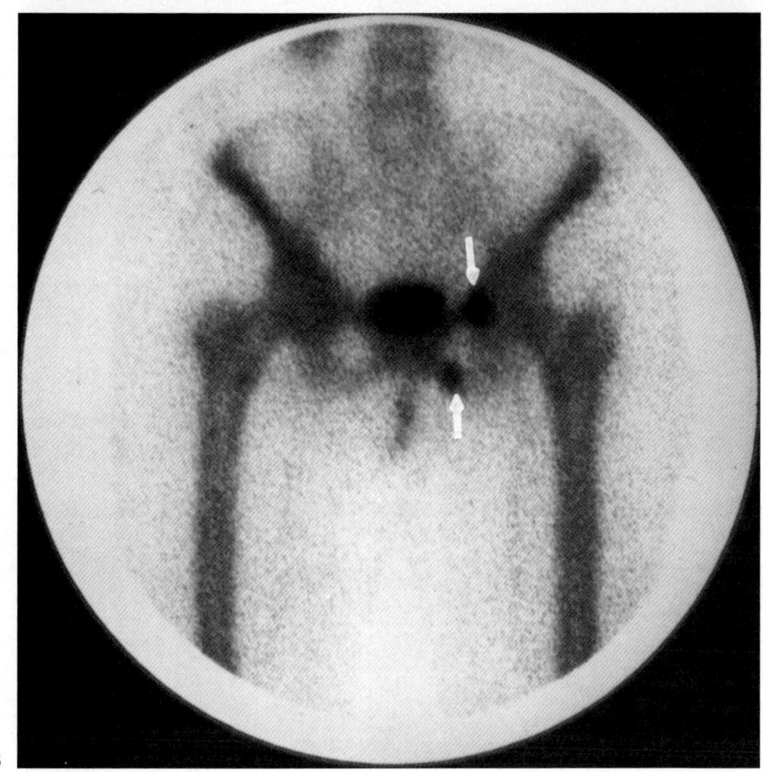

Fig. 4-2 Stable isolated pelvic ring fracture (Tile type A2, Key and Conwell class II). A: Anteroposterior (AP) radiograph demonstrates a subtle fracture (*arrow*) of the left inferior pubic ramus. B: Technetium 99m methylene diphosphonate (MDP) scan demonstrates undisplaced fractures (*arrows*) of both pubic rami.

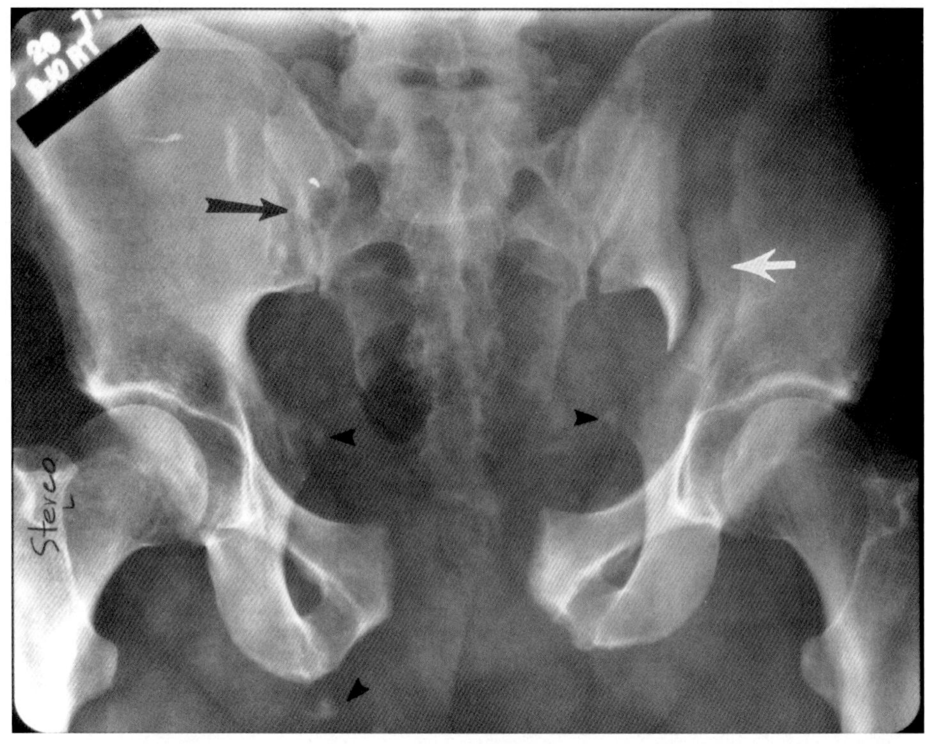


**Fig. 4-3** Open book fracture (Tile type B1, Key and Conwell class III, Young and Burgess antero-posterior [AP] compression type III). AP radiograph demonstrating wide diastasis of the pubic symphysis with widening of the right sacroiliac joint (*black arrow*) and a displaced left ilium fracture (*white arrow*). There are multiple avulsion fractures (*black arrowheads*).

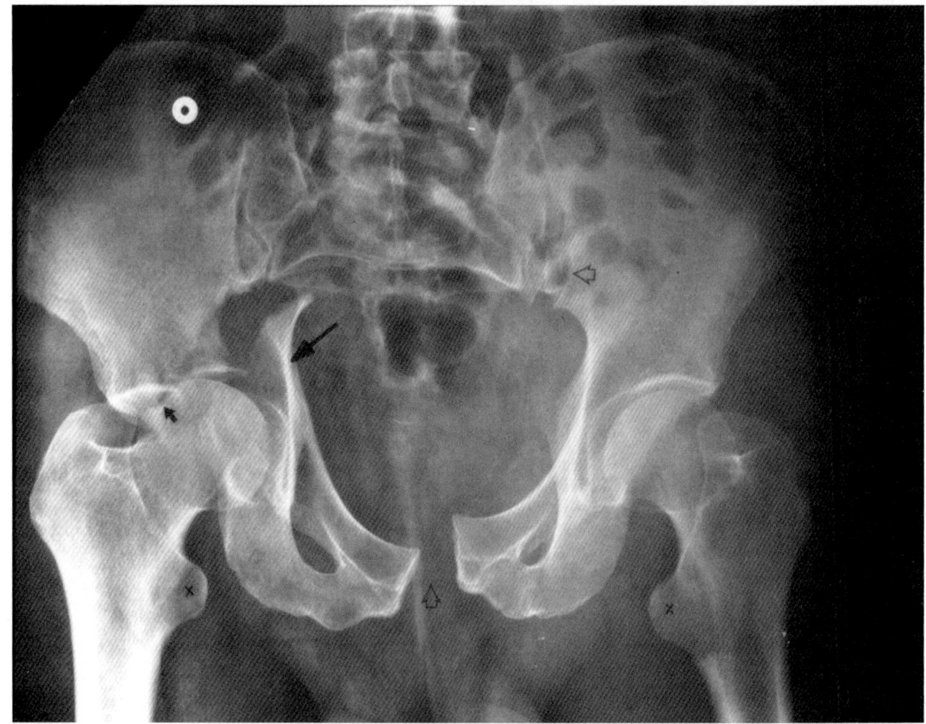

**Fig. 4-4** Double break in the pelvic ring with associated acetabular fracture (Tile type C3, Key and Conwell class IV, Young and Burgess combination injury). Anteroposterior (AP) radiograph of the pelvis demonstrates diastasis of the pubic symphysis and left sacroiliac joint (*open arrows*) with a step off indicating vertical shearing in addition to a displaced acetabular fracture (*arrows*) due to associated lateral compression.

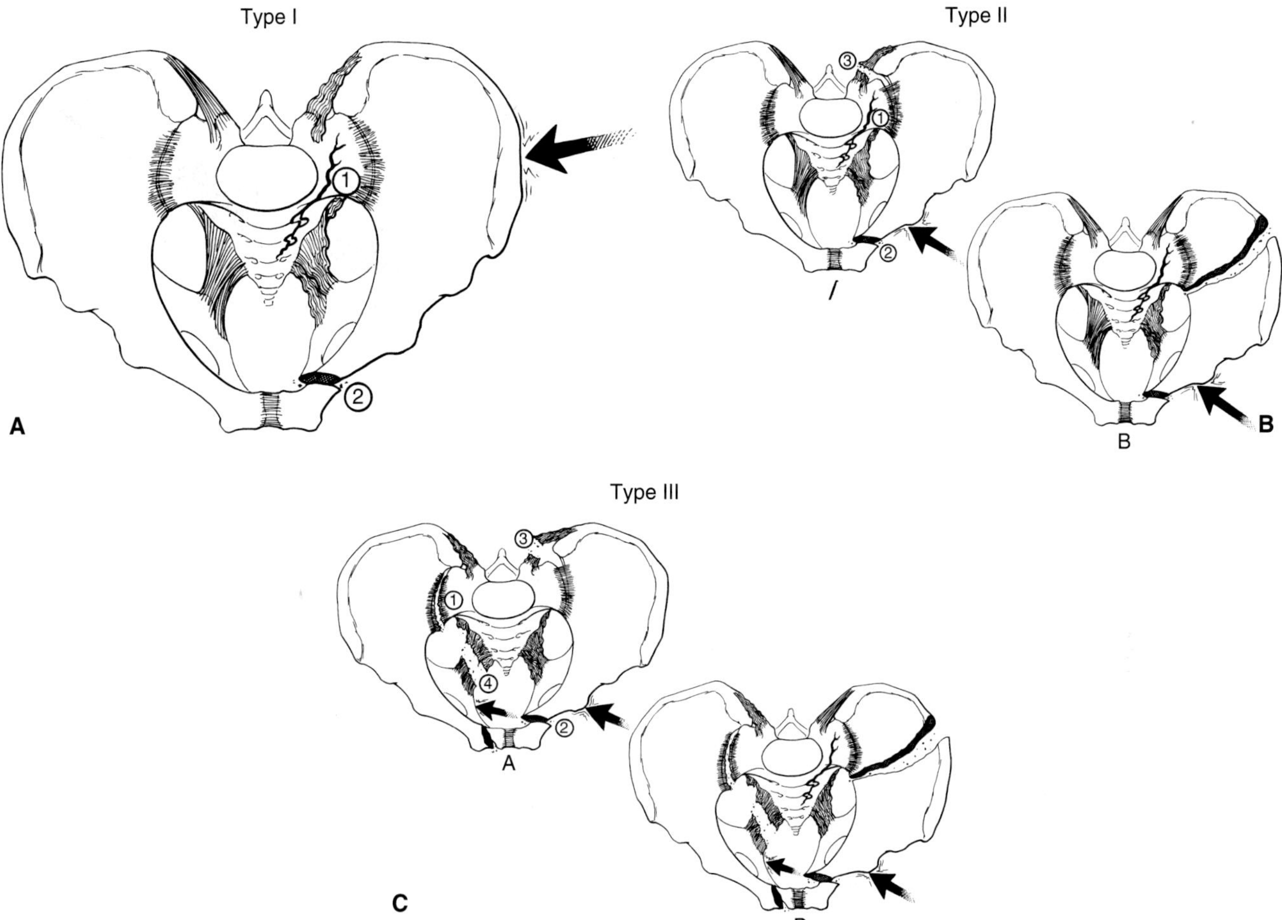


Fig. 4-5 Young and Burgess lateral compression injuries (41% to 72% of pelvic fractures). A: Type I—force applied to the posterior ilium resulting in a crush injury to the ilium, sacrum or sacroiliac joint (*1*), and oblique or horizontal pubic rami fracture (*2*). B: Type II—force is applied more anteriorly resulting in fracture or sacroiliac joint diastasis (*1*), horizontal pubic rami fracture (*2*), and posterior ligament injury (*3*) in type IIA or iliac wing fracture with the other associated injuries in type IIB. C: Type III—anterolateral force is applied resulting in diastasis of the contralateral sacroiliac joint (*1*), oblique or horizontal pubic rami fracture (*2*), disruption of both sacroiliac and associated posterior ligaments (*1*, *3*, and *4*) in type IIIA or with associated iliac wing fracture in type IIIB.

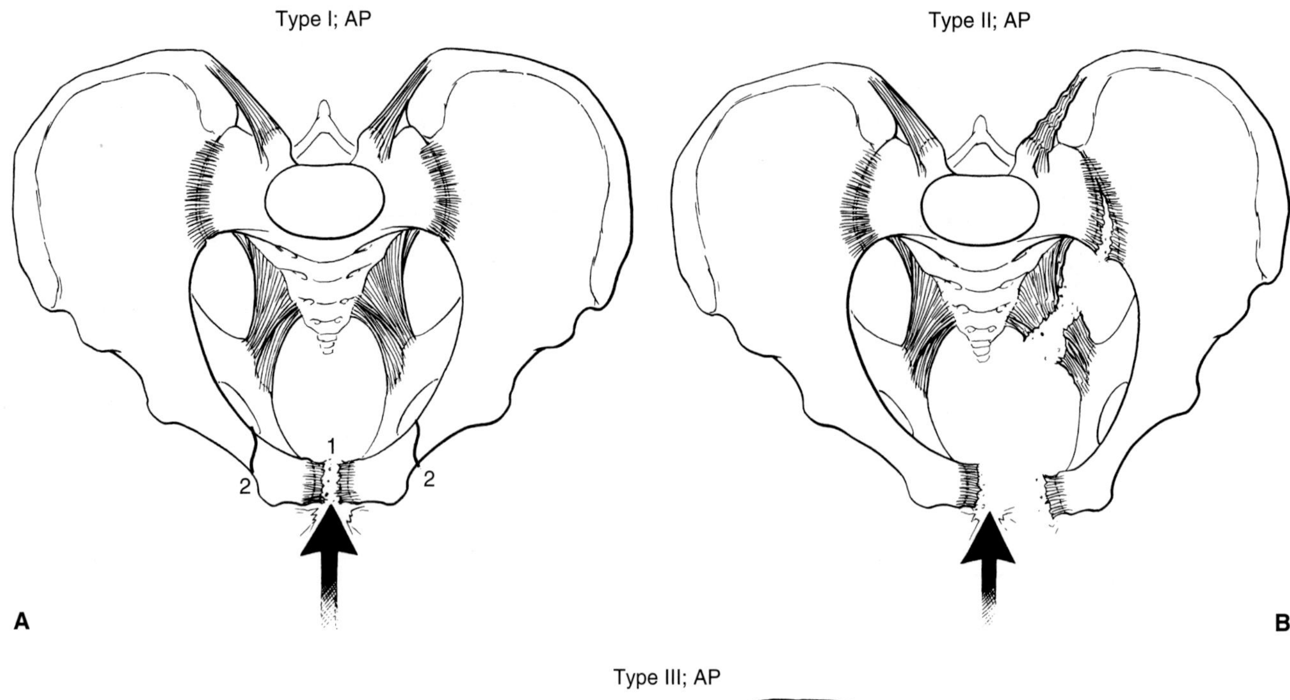


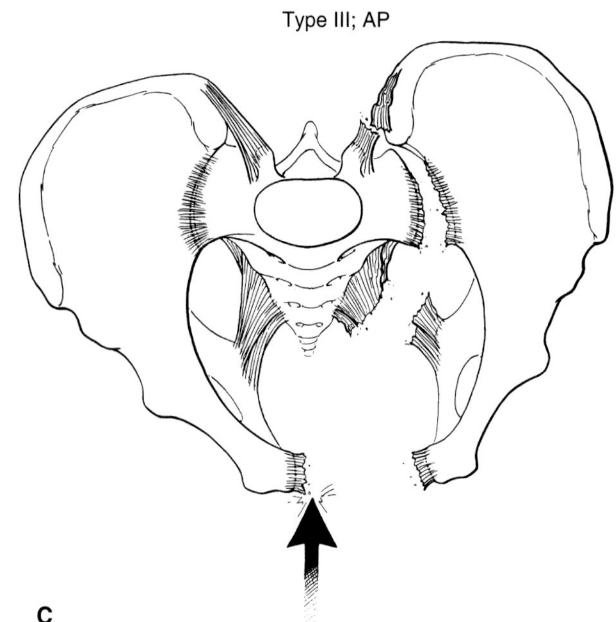


**Fig. 4-6** Young and Burgess anteroposterior (AP) compression injuries (15% to 25% of pelvic fractures). **A:** Type I—force directed anteriorly (*large arrow*) with minimal diastasis of the pubic symphysis (*1*) or vertical pubic rami fractures (*2*). **B:** Type II—force directed anteriorly (*large arrow*) with wider diastasis of the pubic symphysis or more displaced vertical pubic rami fractures. **C:** Type III—force directed anteriorly (*large arrow*) resulting in wide diastasis of the pubic symphysis or displaced vertically oriented pubic rami fracture and disruption of the sacroiliac ligaments (see Fig. 4-3).

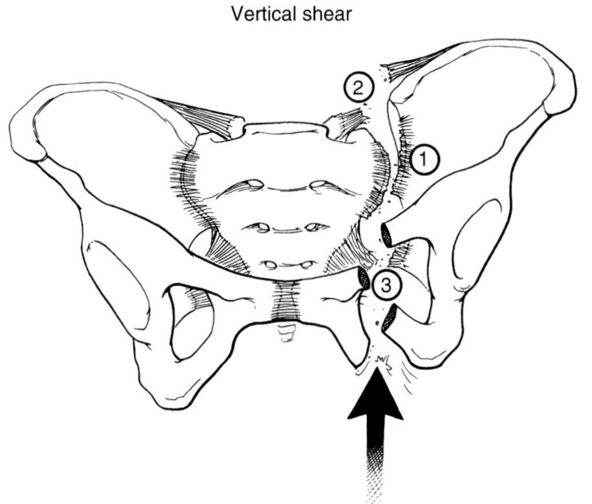


Fig. 4-7 Vertical shearing injuries (6% of pelvic fractures). Force directed vertically resulting in unilateral or contralateral disruption of the sacroiliac joint (*1*) and ligaments (*2*) and vertical displaced pubic rami fracture (*3*).

## Suggested Reading

Key JA, Conwell HE. *Management of fractures, dislocations and sprains*. St. Louis: Mosby; 1951.

Tile M. Pelvic ring fractures. *J Bone Joint Surg*. 1988;70B:1–12.

Young JWR, Burgess AR. *Radiologic management of pelvic ring fractures*. Baltimore: Urban & Schwarzenberg; 1987.

### Imaging of Pelvic Fractures

In high-risk trauma patients, an anteroposterior (AP) radiograph of the pelvis is obtained usually followed by computed tomography (CT). However, additional radiographic views and procedures may be required depending on clinical findings and hemodynamic status of the patient.

**Radiographs**

- AP view of the pelvis and hips—detect most anterior fractures, may miss up to 50% of posterior fractures (Fig. 4-3)
- Inlet and outlet views—tube is angled 40 degrees to the feet (inlet view) and 40 degrees to the head for females and 25 degrees for males (outlet view); improves detection and position of fracture fragments anteriorly and posteriorly
- Additional radiographs, especially of the lower extremity, may be required as 65% of patients have associated fractures beyond the pelvis

**Computed tomography:** Thin sections with reformatting and three-dimensional (3-D) reconstructions as necessary; intravenous contrast may be useful but can obscure hemorrhage if angiography is required to detect and treat bleeding vessels (see Fig. 4-8).

**Urethrograms:** Performed by placing a catheter carefully under fluoroscopic guidance while gently injecting contrast medium in patients with suspected urethral or bladder rupture

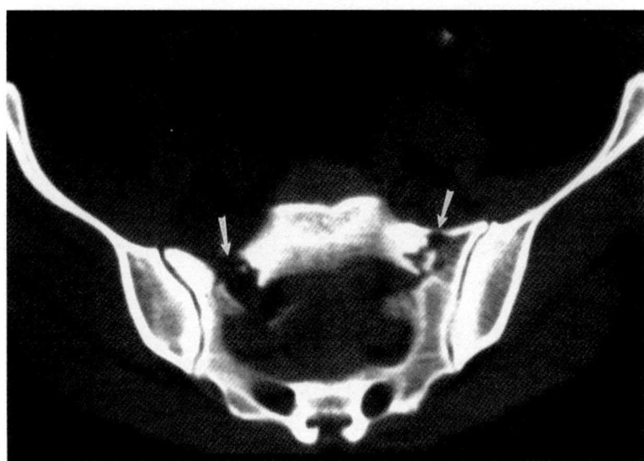

Fig. 4-8 Axial computed tomographic (CT) image demonstrating bilateral sacral fractures (*arrows*) not clearly demonstrated on radiographs.

**Angiography:** Identify bleeding vessels; embolization as required

## Suggested Reading

Burgess AR, Eastridge BJ, Young JW, et al. Pelvic ring disruptions: Effective classification protocols. *J Trauma*. 1990;30: 848–856.

Resnick CS, Stackhouse DJ, Shanmuganathan K, et al. Diagnosis of pelvic fracture trauma: Efficacy of plain radiographs. *AJR Am J Roentgenol*. 1992;158:109–112.

Young JW. Pelvic injuries. *Semin Musculoskelet Radiol*. 1998;2: 83–104.

### Treatment Options

Treatment options vary with the severity of the injury, presence of distant injuries, and the hemodynamic status of the patient. Minor fractures (avulsion fractures, fractures not involving the pelvic ring) may be treated conservatively (Fig. 4-1). These injuries are rarely associated with significant complications. More complex injuries are approached more aggressively and vary with the patient status. Significant pelvic hemorrhage (71% of patients have significant blood loss) is a common problem and must be addressed immediately. Blood loss and associated injuries create a high morbidity and significant mortality. The overall mortality rate varies from 6% to 22% with 39% of deaths related to uncontrolled hemorrhage. Hemorrhage may be controlled with pressure garments, angiography and embolization, external fixation, or open surgical procedures. This discussion will focus on orthopaedic options. Stability of the injury is critical in planning management. A stable lesion is one that will not undergo further deformity under normal physiologic forces. Examples would include Tile type A and Key and Conwell class I and II fractures. Tile type B fractures are vertically stable, but rotationally unstable. Tile type C fractures are vertically, posteriorly, and rotationally unstable.

### External Fixation

External fixation should be considered early in patients with unstable fractures, especially if the patient is hypotensive. Anterior fixation and stabilization can be achieved with external fixation (see Fig. 4-9). However, it is not unusual to require additional posterior internal fixation at a later date to stabilize the posterior complex and sacroiliac joints. When possible, fixation frames should not be placed so as to reduce access for emergency surgical laparotomy.

#### Indications for external fixation

- Decrease pelvic volume for hemorrhage control
- Fracture reduction and stabilization
- Other injuries that prevent internal fixation

### Internal Fixation

Conservative treatment with slings and external fixation may be suitable in the acute setting while patients are being stabilized. However, these methods may not be sufficient for treatment of unstable injuries.

#### Indications for internal fixation

- Posterior sacroiliac disruptions (Fig. 4-9D)
- Failed closed reduction
- Residual deformity after external fixation
- Acetabular fractures
- Certain open wounds
- Vertically unstable fractures

Surgical intervention can be performed in the first several days in patients with stable injuries. Patients with instability and hypotension may require more immediate intervention. Posterior stabilization can be accomplished with threaded rods and bolts with washers (Fig. 4-9D). Plate and screw fixation may also be employed. Anterior stabilization can be achieved with external or internal fixation. Diastasis of the symphysis >2 cm can be stabilized with plate and screw fixation (see Fig. 4-10). When vertical shearing injury has occurred, multiple plates are required to achieve stable fixation (Fig. 4-10C). Acetabular fractures will be discussed in the next section.

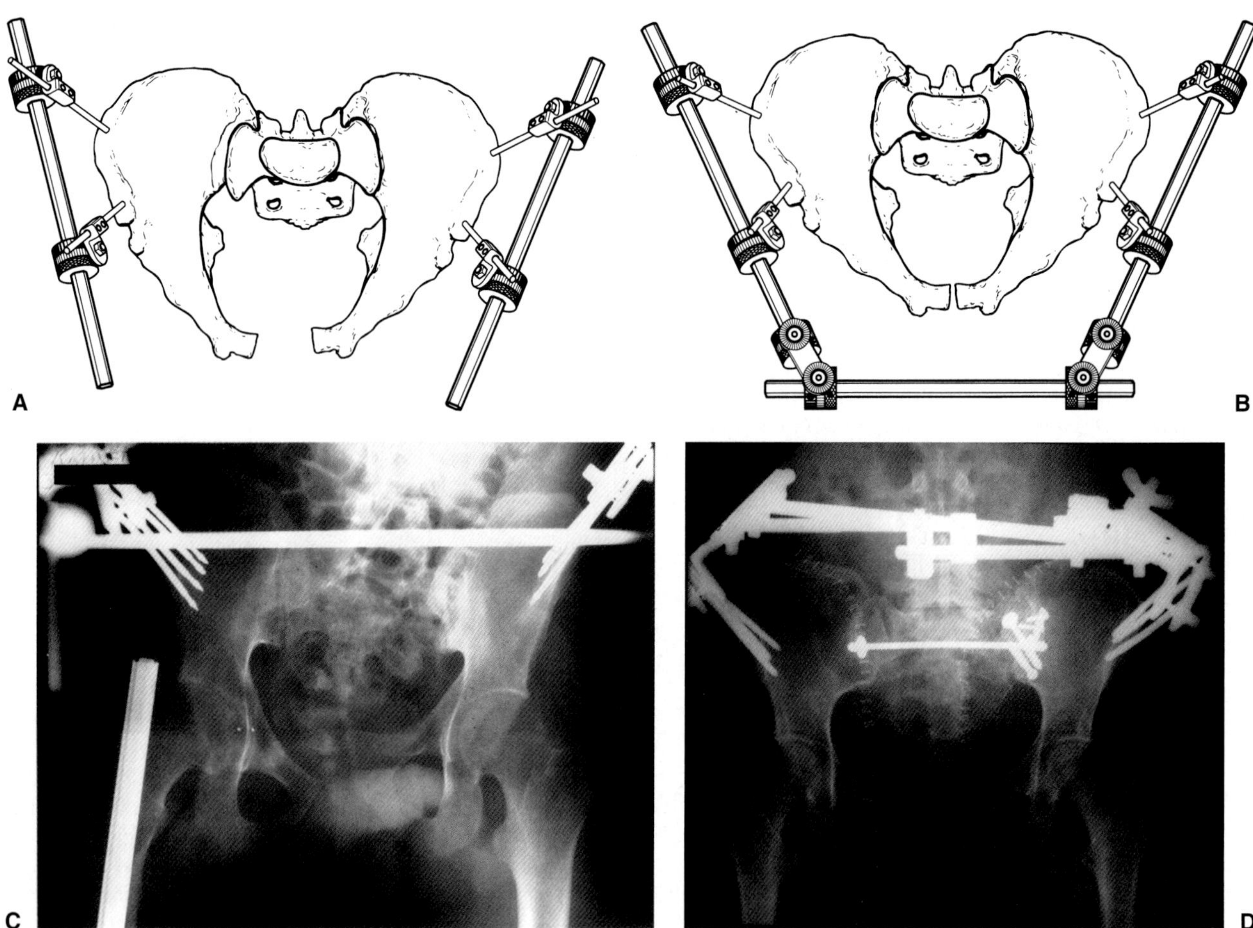


Fig. 4-9 External fixation. Illustrations of Hex-Fix external fixation with Steinman pins and rods attached anteriorly (A) and compression rod linkage (B) for anterior stability. (Courtesy of Smith and Nephew Richards, Memphis, TN.) C: Radiograph demonstrating a vertical shear injury with step off of the pubic symphysis and anterior external fixator in place. D: Radiograph demonstrating anterior external fixation with internal fixation of both sacroiliac joints. Posterior stabilization could not be accomplished with anterior external fixation alone.

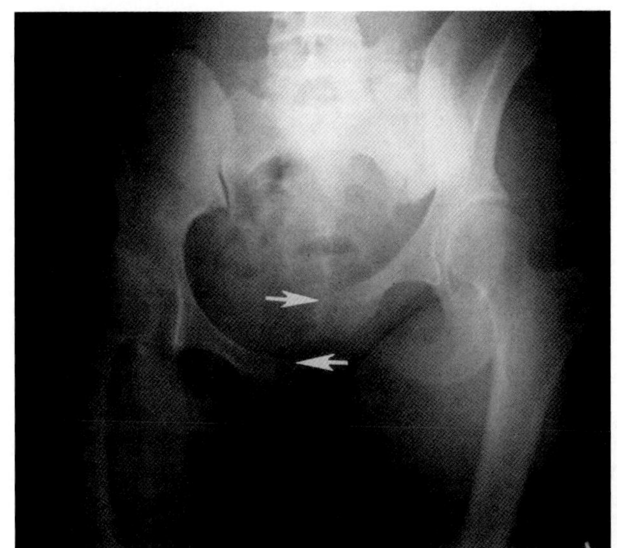
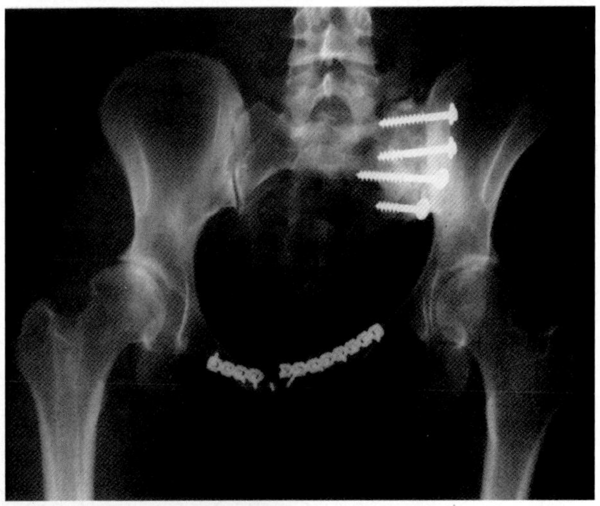
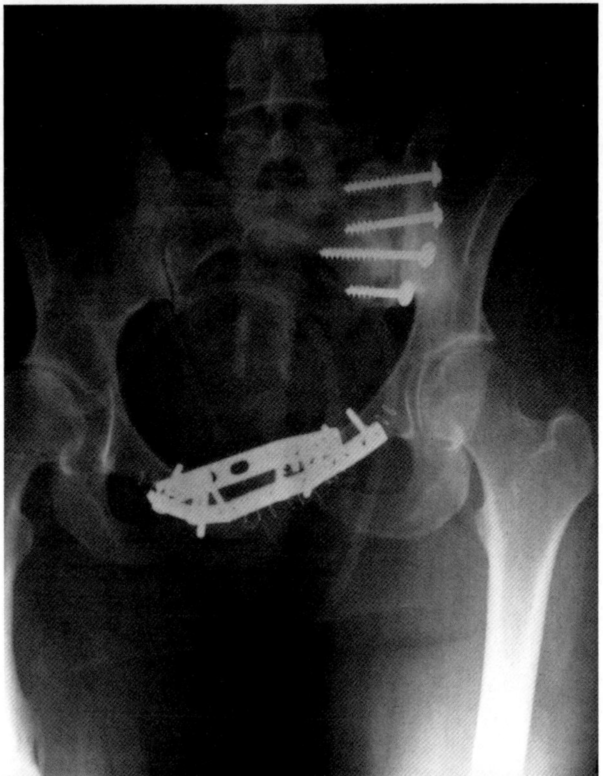

Fig. 4-10 A: Unstable vertical shearing injury with step off of the pubic symphysis (*arrows*) and left sacroiliac joint. B: Internal fixation of the left sacroiliac joint was accomplished with cancellous screws and washers and there is reconstruction plate and screw fixation of the symphysis. The anterior plate fractured. Therefore, reoperation with two plates (C) was performed to achieve stability.

## SUGGESTED READING

Failinger S, McGanity PL. Unstable fractures of the pelvic ring. *J Bone Joint Surg.* 1992;74A:781–791.

Hill RM, Robinson CM, Keating JF. Fractures of the pelvic rami. Epidemiology and five-year survival. *J Bone Joint Surg.* 2001;83B:1141–1144.

Matta JM, Saucedo T. Internal fixation of pelvic ring fractures. *Clin Orthop.* 1989;242:83–97.

Tile M. Pelvic fractures: Operative versus non-operative treatment. *Orthop Clin North Am.* 1980;11:423–464.

### Complications

Complications may be related to the pelvic trauma, associated injuries, or the surgical procedure. The most common and significant complication associated with pelvic fractures is hemorrhage. In the Mayo clinic series, transfusion of up to 10 units of blood was required in 71% of patients with double breaks in the pelvic ring. Mortality rates in this group were 22%. Hemorrhage can be controlled with pressure garments, external fixation systems, angiography with embolization of bleeding vessels, or rarely open surgical intervention (see Fig. 4-11). In recent years, the mortality rate has improved (6% compared to 22% in years past) with 39% of these deaths related to pelvic

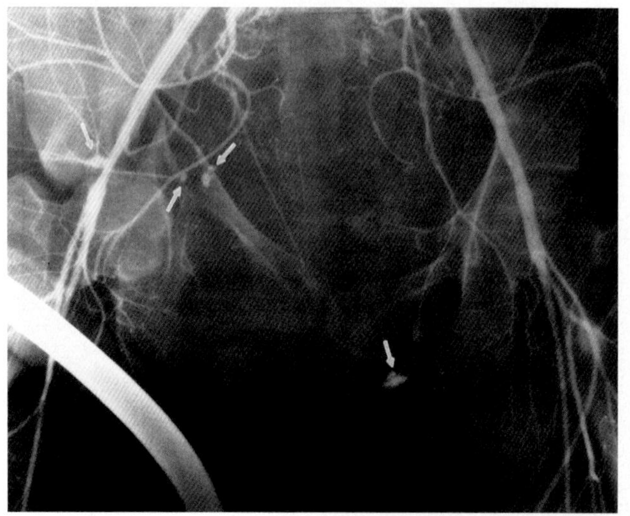


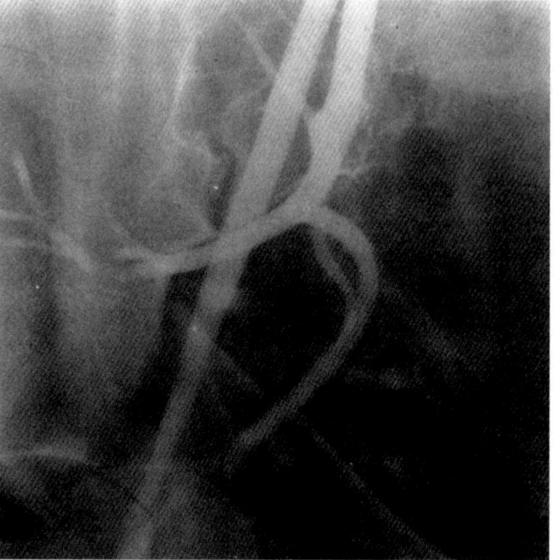


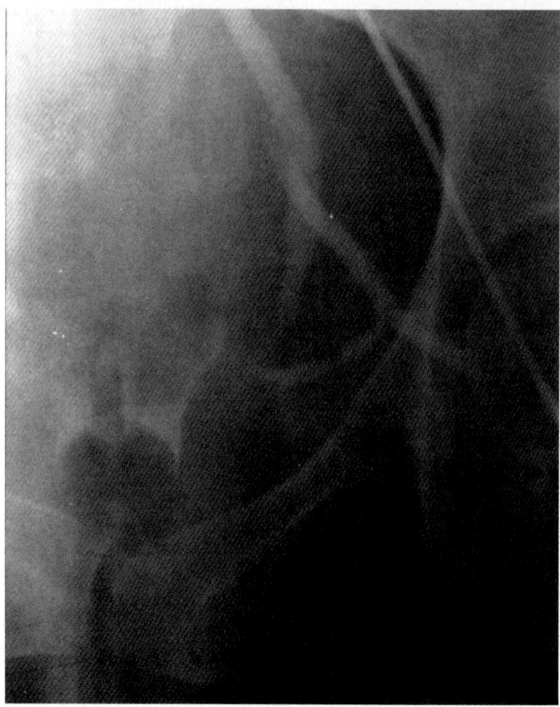


Fig. 4-11 Anteroposterior (AP) compression injury with displaced pubic rami fractures and hemodynamic instability. Angiogram (A) demonstrates bleeding sites bilaterally (*arrows*). Following embolization the bleeding sites have been occluded (B and C).

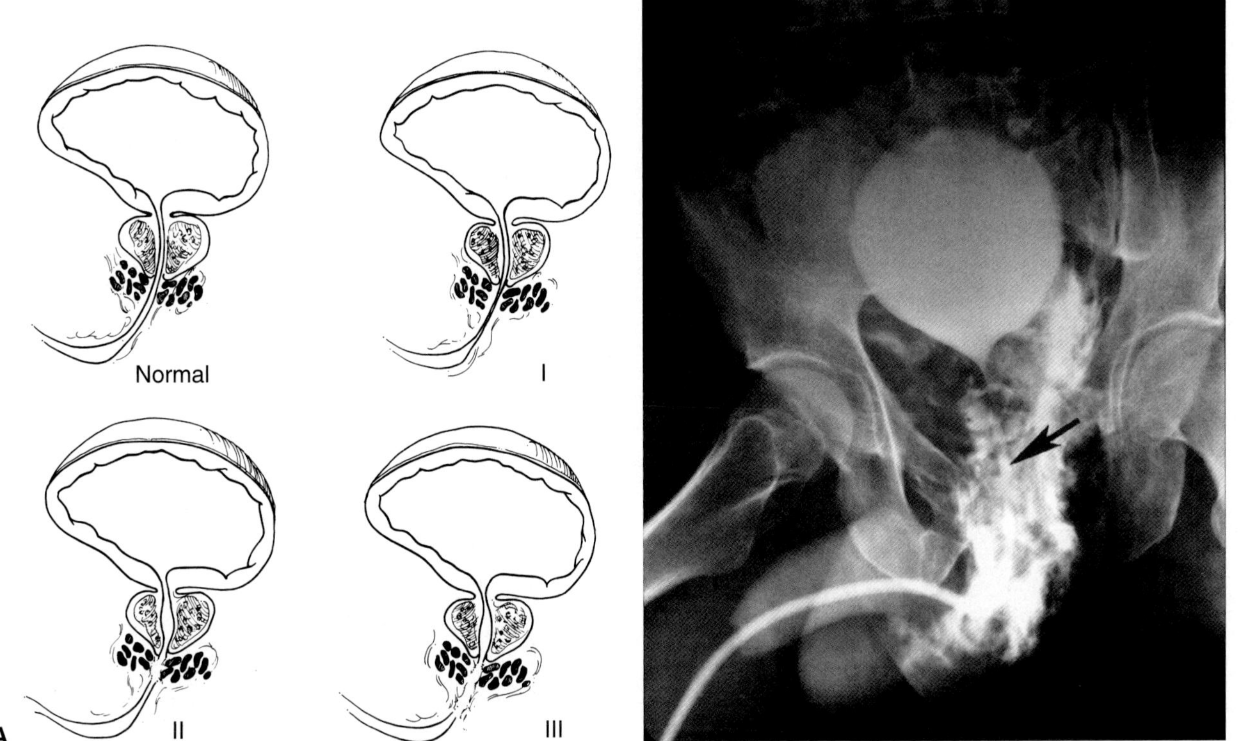


Fig. 4-12 A: Illustration of the normal male urethral anatomy and tears in the urethra. Type I—stretching of the urethra due to pelvic hematoma, type II—urethral tear above the urogenital diaphragm, type III—urethral tear below the urogenital diaphragm. B: Large urethral tear above and below the urogenital diaphragm. Note the catheter position (*arrow*) which was slowly advanced using fluoroscopic guidance in order to prevent further injury.

hemorrhage. The remaining deaths were related to associated head trauma (31%) or multiorgan failure (30%).

Genitourinary injuries occur in 19% to 30% of fractures and are most often seen following AP trauma with pubic rami fractures or vertical shearing injuries. Urethral injuries (see Fig. 4-12) are most common (males > females), followed by the bladder (see Figs. 4-13 and 4-14), vagina, and kidney. A carefully performed urethrogram and cystogram is still a useful approach for diagnosis and management (Figs. 4-13 and 4-14). Local neurologic injuries, primarily to the sacral plexus, occur in up to 21% of patients with sacral or sacroiliac joint involvement. Vaginal and rectal injuries occur less frequently. However, the latter may result in an infected hematoma, which results in significant morbidity and increased mortality (~50%).

Injuries to the gastrointestinal tract (7%), liver (7%), spleen (10%), and mesentery (4%) also occur. In our series, 11% of patients had associated head, chest, or abdominal injuries. Associated fractures occur in 48% to 65% of patients. Table 4-1 summarizes complications and imaging approaches for complex pelvic fractures.

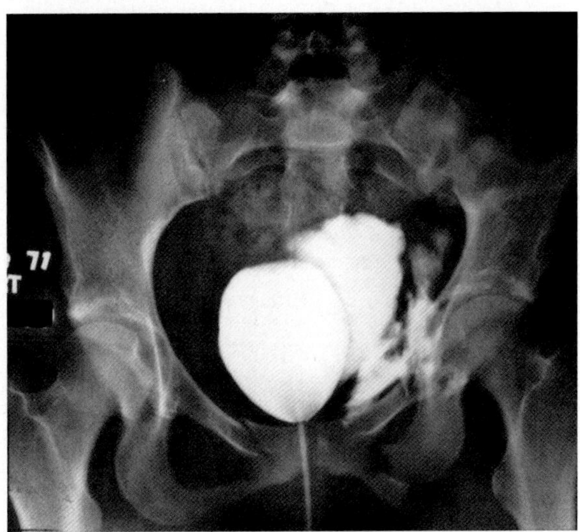

Fig. 4-13 Cystogram demonstrating extravasation of contrast from the bladder due to extraperitoneal rupture following an anteroposterior (AP) compression injury with pubic rami fractures.

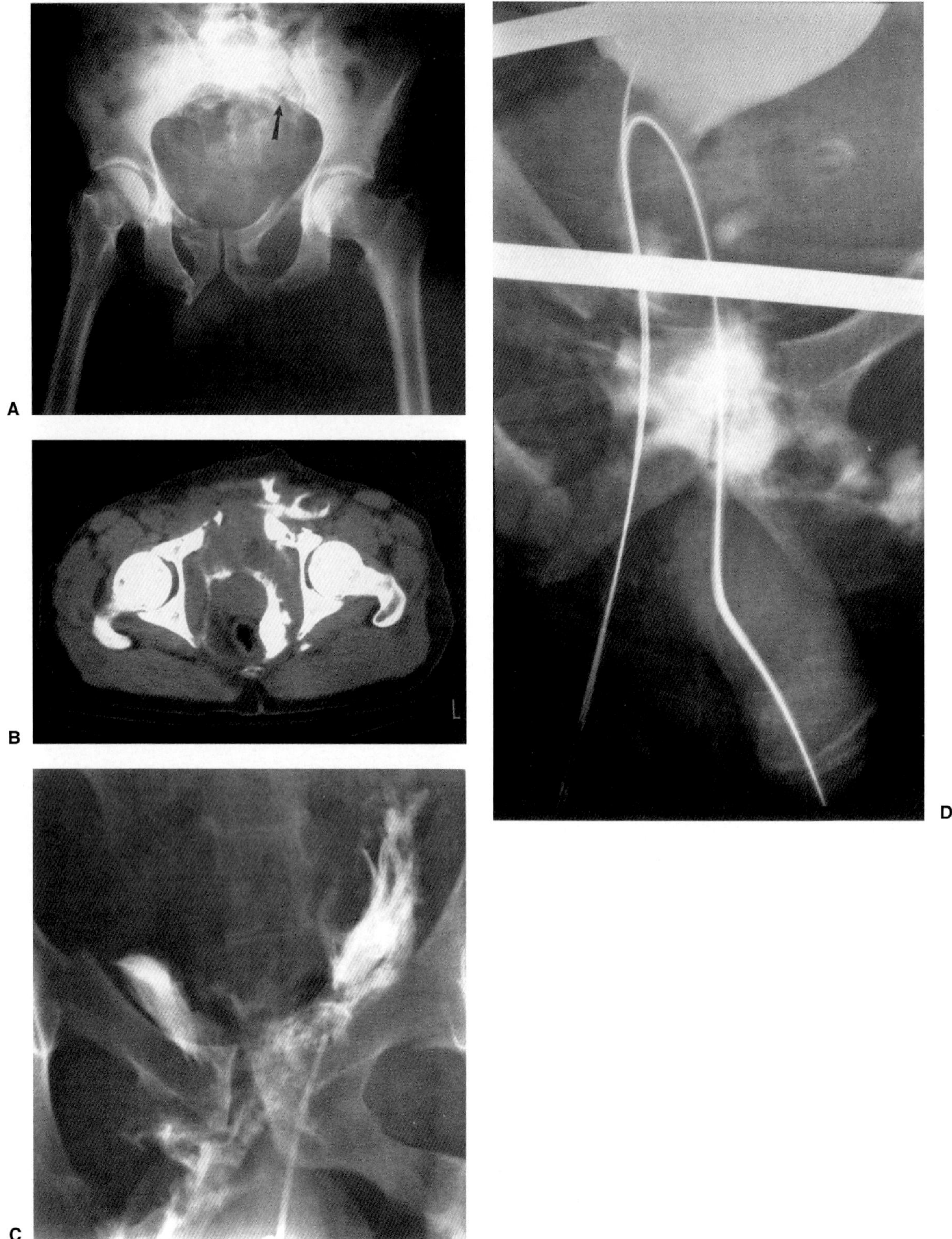

Fig. 4-14 Anteroposterior (AP) compression injury with bladder and urethral injuries. A: AP radiograph demonstrates vertical pubic rami fractures with a subtle posterior sacral fracture (*arrow*). B: Computed tomography with intravenous contrast demonstrates extravasation of contrast from the bladder and into the pelvis and anterior soft tissues. C: A Foley catheter was placed without fluoroscopic guidance and was improperly placed in the pelvis with contrast extravasation that is obviously not in the bladder. D: Using a guide wire and suprapubic approach the catheter was successfully placed.

**Table 4-1**

**COMPLICATIONS RELATED TO COMPLEX PELVIC FRACTURES**

| COMPLICATION | IMAGING APPROACHES |
|---|---|
| Primary pelvic fractures | |
| Hemorrhage (71%–75%) | Angiography/embolization (Fig. 4-11) |
| Urethral injury (15%–19%) | Retrograde urethrogram (Fig. 4-12) |
| Bladder (10%–25%) | Retrograde urethrogram followed by cystogram (Fig. 4-13) |
| Neurologic (21%) | CT or MRI |
| Associated injuries | |
| Head | CT initially, MRI as required |
| Chest | Radiographs/CT |
| Abdominal | CT |
| Orthopaedic | |
| Associated fractures (48–65%) | Radiographs/CT as indicated (Fig. 4-15) |
| Delayed or nonunion | Radiographs/CT |
| Instability (pubic symphysis or sacroiliac) | Standing, alternate weight-bearing images |
| AVN femoral head | MRI |
| Implant failure | Serial radiographs (Fig. 4-10) |
| Infection | |
| Pin tract | Fluoroscopically positioned images/CT |
| Deep infection | Radionuclide scans/CT or MRI |

CT, computed tomography; MRI, magnetic resonance imaging; AVN, avascular necrosis.

## Suggested Reading

Berquist TH, Lewallen DG, McComb BL. The pelvis and hips. In: Berquist TH, ed. *Imaging atlas of orthopaedic appliances and prostheses*. New York: Raven Press; 1995:217–352.

Hill RM, Robinson CM, Keating JF. Fractures of the pelvic rami. Epidemiology and five-year survival. *J Bone Joint Surg.* 2001;83B:1141–1144.

Perez JV, Hughes PMD, Bowers SK. Angiographic embolization in pelvic fracture. *Injury* 1998;29:191–197.

### Acetabular Fractures

Acetabular fractures account for 24% of pelvic injuries. Fractures of the acetabulum may be simple or complex. The latter have complications similar to complex pelvic fractures. The acetabulum is anatomically similar to an inverted "Y" with anterior and posterior columns. The type of fracture is related to the position of the femur or femoral head when the force is applied to these structures and extends into the acetabulum. The position of the femur at the time of injury dictates the type and extent of fracture (see Figs. 4-15 and 4-16).

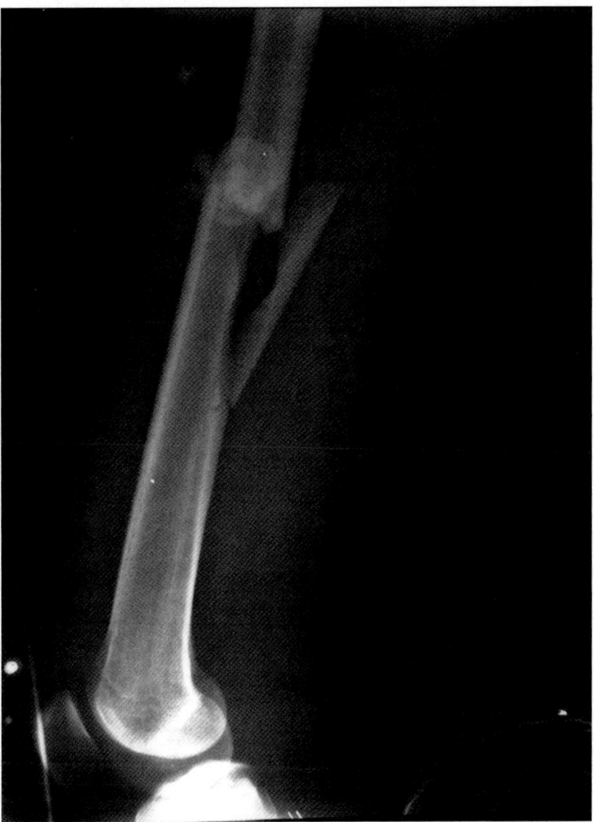

**Fig. 4-15** Radiograph of the femur demonstrating a comminuted midshaft fracture in a patient with a complex pelvic fracture.

#### Fracture Classification

There are multiple classification systems for acetabular fractures. These include the Tile, Judet and Letournel, AO

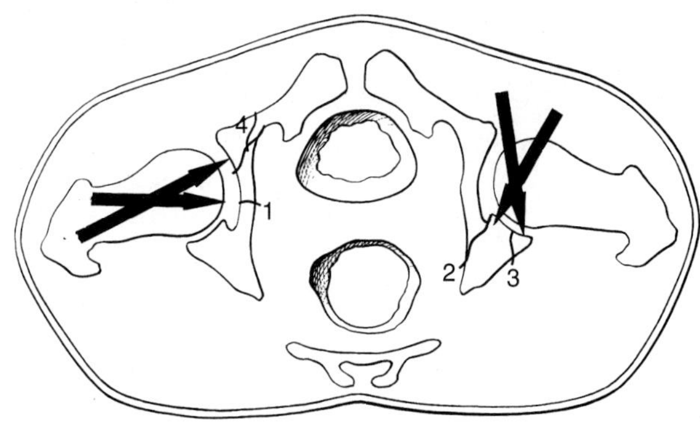


**Fig. 4-16** Illustration of force direction of the femur (*large arrows*) in relation to type and extent of acetabular fractures. *1*—central fracture; *2*—posterior wall or column; *3*—posterior rim; *4*—anterior wall.

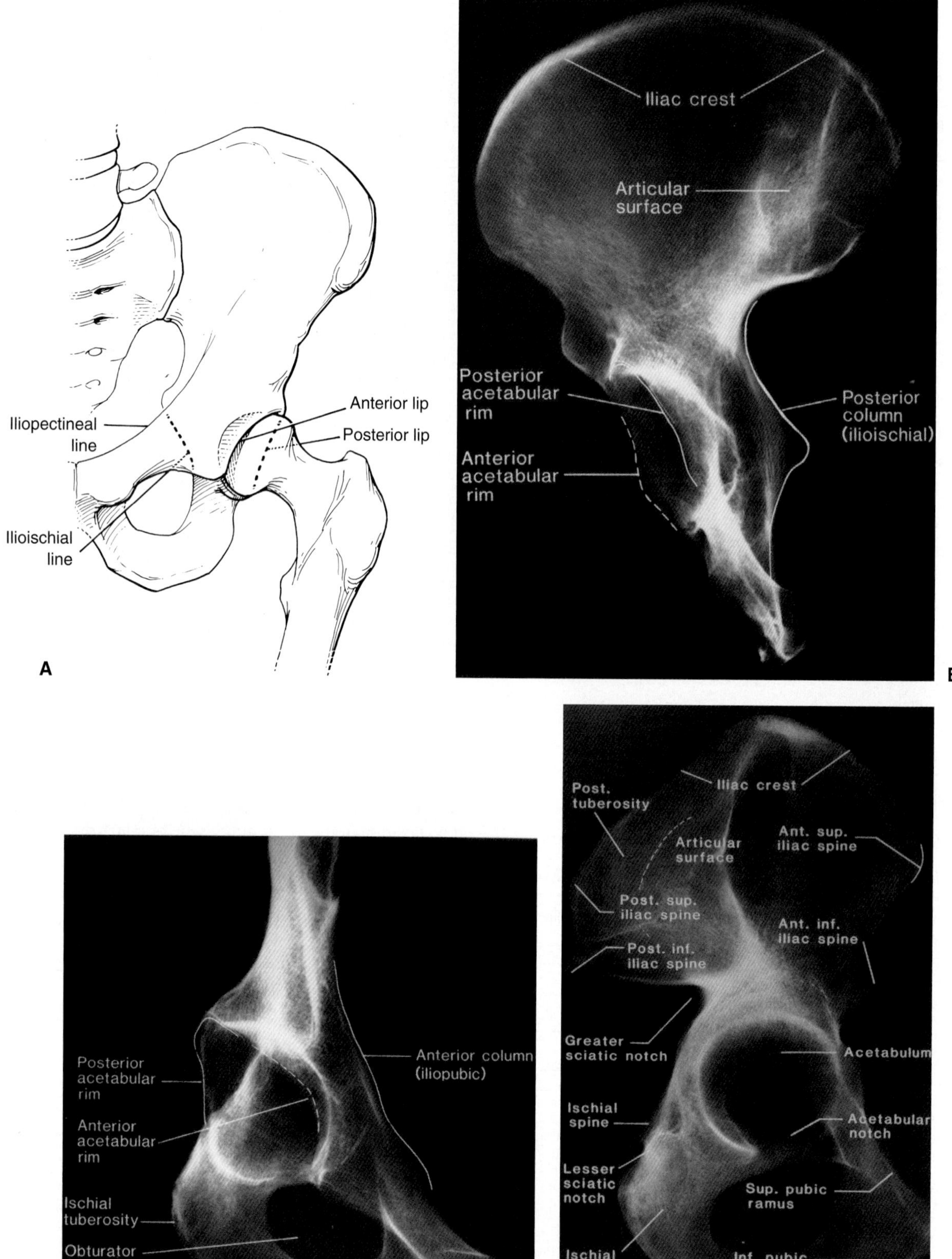


Fig. 4-17 A: Illustration of the anterior and posterior acetabular margins and iliopectineal line (anterior column) and ilioischial line (posterior column). Specimen radiographs in the posterior oblique (posterior Judet view) (B), anterior oblique (anterior Judet view) (C), and sagittal plane (D) demonstrating the acetabular margins and anterior and posterior columns.

(Arbeitsgemeinschaft fur Osteosynthesefragen), ATO (Orthopaedic Trauma Association), and more recently a CT classification system proposed by Harris et al. Classification systems are based on the extent of injury and provide guidance for fracture management. The anatomy of the acetabulum can be accurately depicted on radiographs and CT (see Fig. 4-17). As noted earlier, the acetabulum comprises three osseous structures that form an anterior and posterior column. The anterior column is larger extending inferiorly from the iliac wing to the superior pubic ramus. The posterior column begins at the sciatic notch and extends inferiorly to the ischium. Different fracture patterns are summarized in the classification systems discussed in the subsequent text.

### LETOURNEL AND JUDET CLASSIFICATION—TEN BASIC PATTERNS DIVIDED INTO ELEMENTARY AND ASSOCIATED PATTERNS

| ELEMENTARY FRACTURES | ASSOCIATED FRACTURES |
|---|---|
| Posterior wall | Posterior column + posterior wall (AO: A1, A2; see Fig. 4-18A) |
| Posterior column | Transverse + posterior wall (A): B1-2; Fig. 4-18B) |
| Anterior wall | Anterior column + posterior hemitransverse (AO: A3-1, A3-2; Fig. 4-18A) |
| Anterior column | T-shaped (AO: B2; Fig. 4-18B) |
| Transverse | Both columns (AO B1-1; Fig. 4-18B) |

### ARBEITSGEMEINSCHAFT FUR OSTEOSYNTHESEFRAGEN CLASSIFICATION SYSTEM

| TYPE | DESCRIPTION |
|---|---|
| Type A (Fig. 4-18A) | |
| A1 | Posterior wall fracture |
| A2 | Posterior column fracture |
| A3.1 | Anterior wall fracture |
| A3.2 | Anterior column fracture |
| Type B (Fig. 4-18B) | |
| B1.1 | Transverse |
| B1.2 | Transverse with posterior wall fracture |
| B2 | T fracture |
| B3 | Anterior column with posterior transverse fracture |
| Type C (Fig. 4-18C) | |
| C1 | Both columns with fracture extending to iliac crest |
| C2 | Anterior column extends to anterior inferior iliac spine |
| C3 | Both columns with fracture extending to the sacroiliac joint |

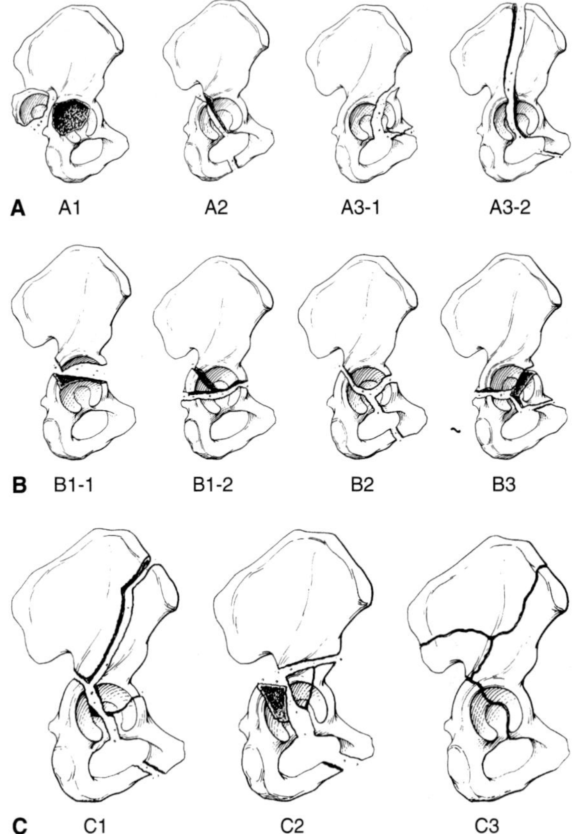


**Fig. 4-18** AO (Arbeitsgemeinschaft fur Osteosynthesefragen) fracture pattern classification. **A:** Type A—*A1*-posterior wall; *A2*-posterior column; *A3-1*-anterior wall; *A3-2*-anterior column. **B:** Type B—*B1-1*-transverse; *B1-2*-transverse with posterior wall fragment; *B2*-"T" fracture; *B3*-anterior column with posterior wall fracture. **C:** Type C—*C1*-both columns with fracture extending to iliac crest; *C2*-anterior column extending to anterior inferior iliac spine; *C3*-both columns with fracture extending to sacroiliac joint.

### COMPUTED TOMOGRAPHIC CLASSIFICATION SYSTEM: HARRIS, COUPE, LEE, AND TROTSCHER

| CATEGORY | FRACTURE DESCRIPTION |
|---|---|
| Type 0 | Wall fractures only |
| Type I | Acetabular fracture involving only one column (anterior or posterior) |
| Type II | Involves both columns (horizontal or T) |
| Type IIA | Limited to acetabulum with no extension |
| Type IIB | Involves both columns with superior extension |
| Type IIC | Involves both columns with inferior extension |
| Type IID | Both columns with inferior and superior extension |
| Type III | Floating acetabulum: articular surface not attached anteriorly or posteriorly |

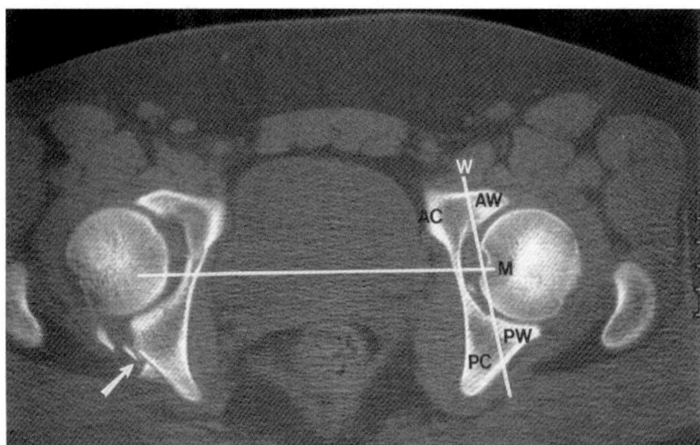


Fig. 4-19 Computed tomographic (CT) classification by Harris, Coupe, Lee, and Trotscher. Axial CT image demonstrating a posterior wall fracture on the left with multiple small fragments (*arrow*). Vertical line (*M*) separates the anterior (*AC*) and posterior (*PC*) columns. Line (*W*) through the lunar articulating surface defines and anterior (*AW*) and posterior (*PW*) walls. Therefore the fracture on the left would be a posterior wall fracture or type 0.

Two-column fractures, transverse fractures with posterior wall involvement, and posterior wall fractures account for 66% of acetabular fractures. T and transverse fractures are the next two most common injuries. These five patterns account for 90% of acetabular fractures (see Fig. 4-19).

## Suggested Reading

Durkee NJ, Jacobson J, Jamadar D, et al. Classification of common acetabular fractures: Radiographic and CT appearances. *AJR Am J Roentgenol.* 2006;187:915–925.

Harris JH, Coupe KJ, Lee JS, et al. Acetabular fractures revisited: 2. A new CT based classification. *AJR Am J Roentgenol.* 2004;182:1367–1375.

Letournel E, Judet R. *Fractures of the acetabulum*, 2nd ed. Hiedelberg, Germany: Springer-Verlag, New York; 1993.

Tile M, Kellam J, Joyce M. Fractures of the acetabulum: Classification, management protocols and results of treatment. *J Bone Joint Surg.* 1985;67B:324–335.

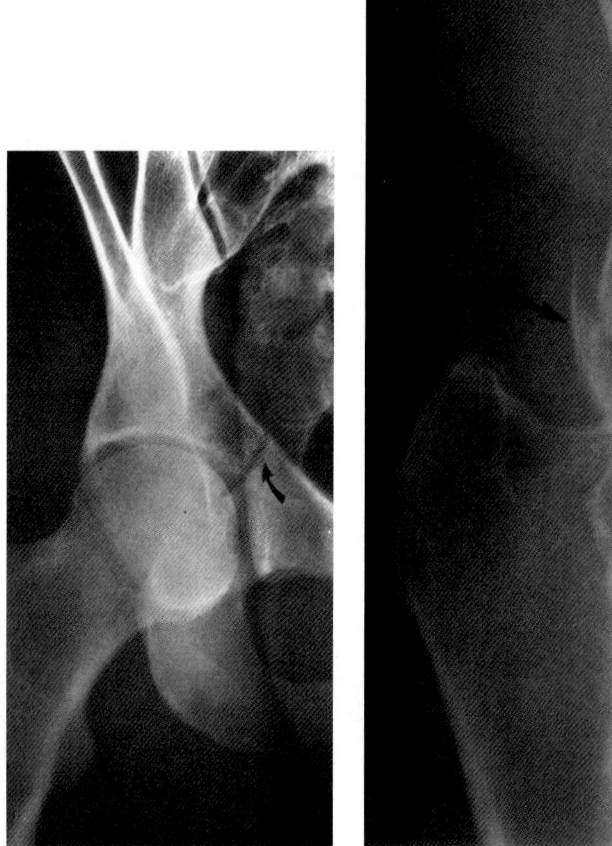


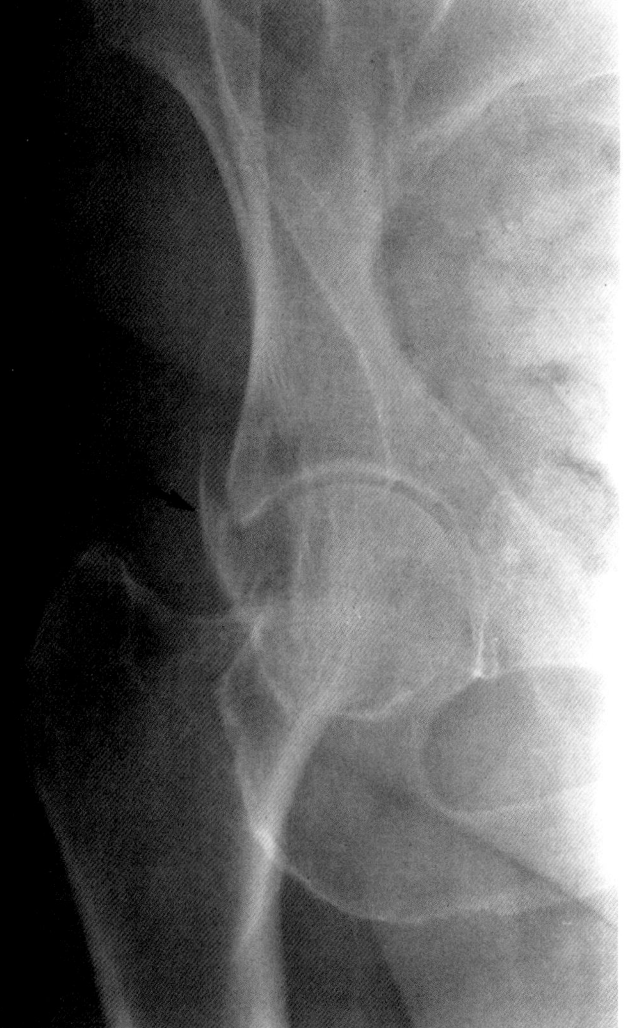


Fig. 4-20 Anterior oblique Judet views demonstrating an undisplaced central acetabular fracture (*curved arrow* in A) and posterior wall fracture (*arrow* in B).

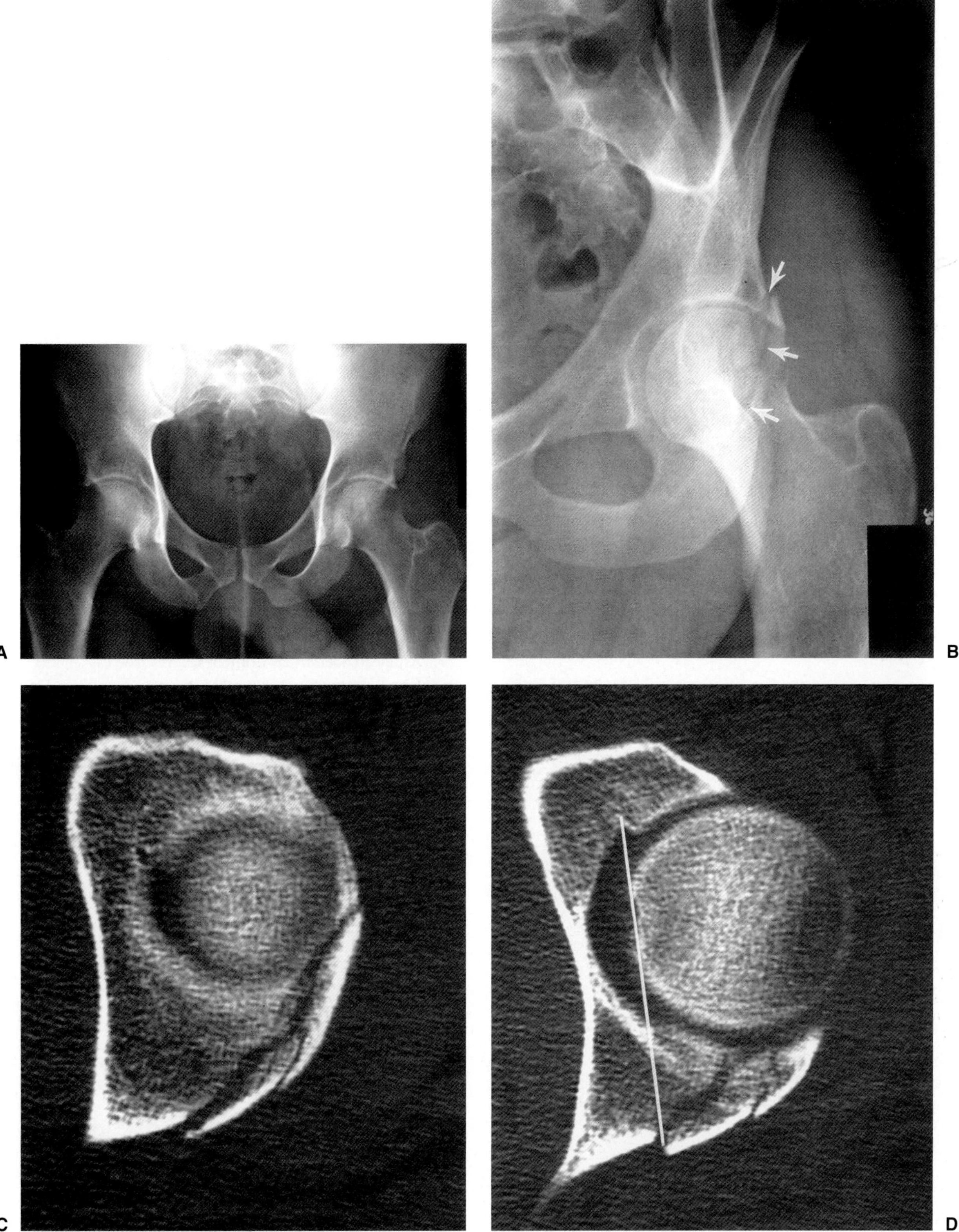


Fig. 4-21 Posterior wall and column fracture. A: Anteroposterior (AP) radiograph of the pelvis does not clearly demonstrate the fracture. B: Anterior Judet view demonstrates a posterior fracture extending along the rim (*arrows*). Computed tomographic (CT) images (C and D) demonstrate comminution of the posterior wall with extension into the posterior column (line in D). AO type A1-2, Harris type I. E: AP radiograph following internal fixation with reconstruction plate and screws.

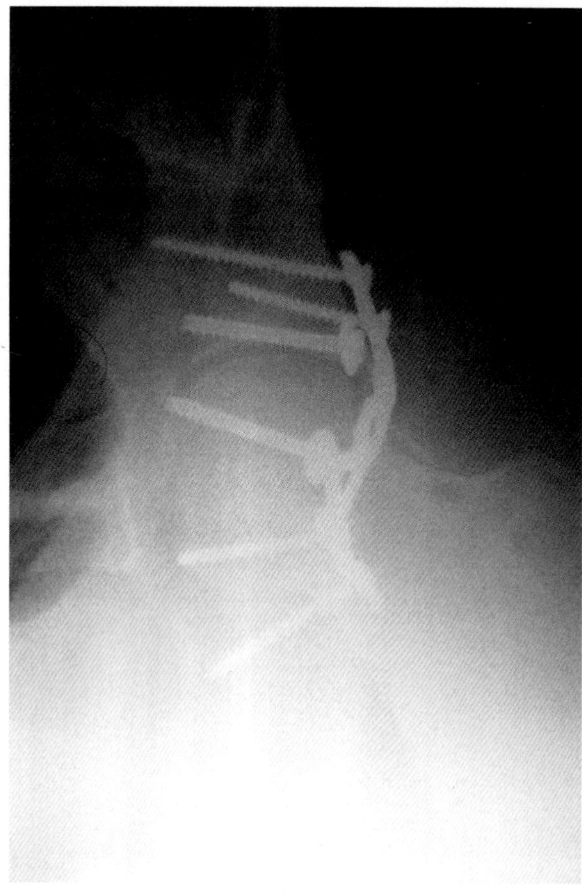


Fig. 4-21 *(Continued)*

## Imaging of Acetabular Fractures

Imaging of acetabular fractures has traditionally been accomplished with screening radiographs. AP views of the hip along with Judet views (45 degrees anterior and posterior rotation of the involved side) should be obtained (Figs. 4-17 and 4-18). Up to 30% of undisplaced fractures are overlooked without Judet views (see Fig. 4-20). Currently, CT is most commonly obtained following AP radiographs to fully evaluate the extent of involvement (see Fig. 4-21). Coronal and sagittal reformatted images are useful to effectively classify the injury. 3-D reconstructions can also be obtained (see Fig. 4-22).

## Treatment Options

The goals for treatment of acetabular fractures are to reestablish the articular anatomy and preserve joint function. Treatment is based on fracture pattern, patient status, and associated injuries. Patient age, weight, and activity status must also be considered. Minimally displaced fractures (2 to 5 mm), even if the dome is involved, can be managed conservatively. In some cases, displaced fractures can be treated with external fixation or percutaneous screw placement techniques. These approaches reduce blood loss, infection rates, and neurovascular complications. However, the standard for treatment of displaced fractures is open reduction and internal fixation.

### Indications for internal fixation

Unstable posterior fragment (Fig. 4-21)
Displaced acetabular dome fractures (see Fig. 4-23)
High T fractures
Displaced two-column fractures (see Fig. 4-24)

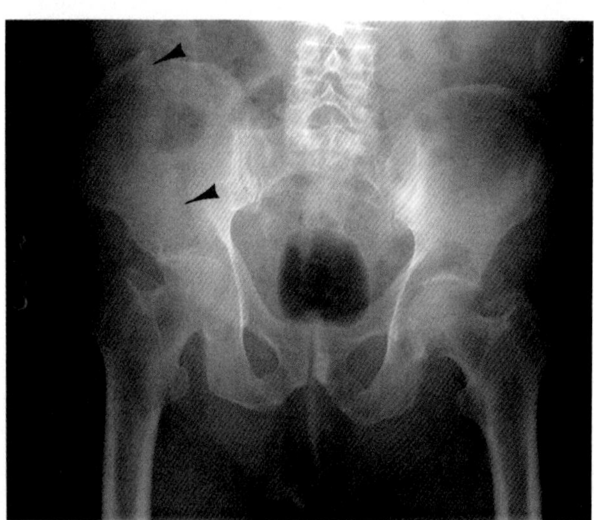


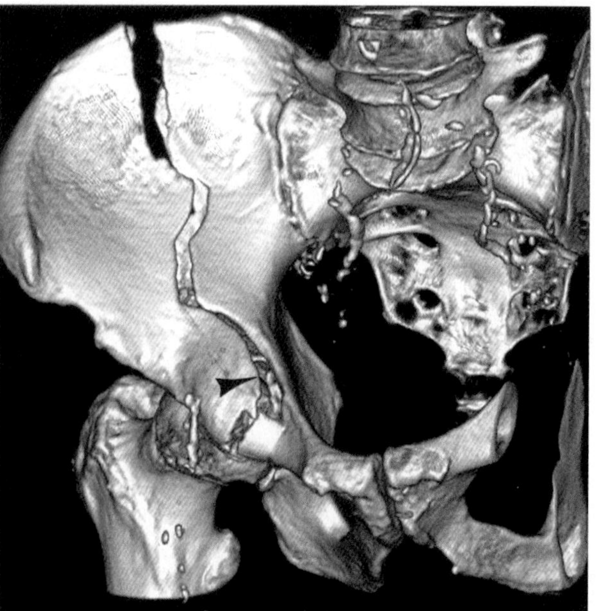


Fig. 4-22 Complex acetabular fracture. A: Anteroposterior (AP) radiograph demonstrates a fracture extending through the right ilium (*arrowheads*). The femoral head appears medially displaced, but a fracture line is not clearly defined. Oblique three-dimensional (3-D) images (B and C) clearly demonstrate the fracture in the ilium and the involvement of the acetabular dome and anterior column (*arrowheads*).

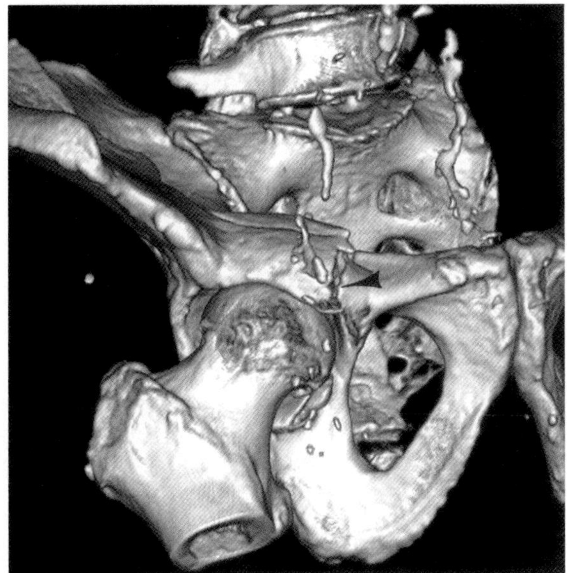


Fig. 4-22 (*Continued*)

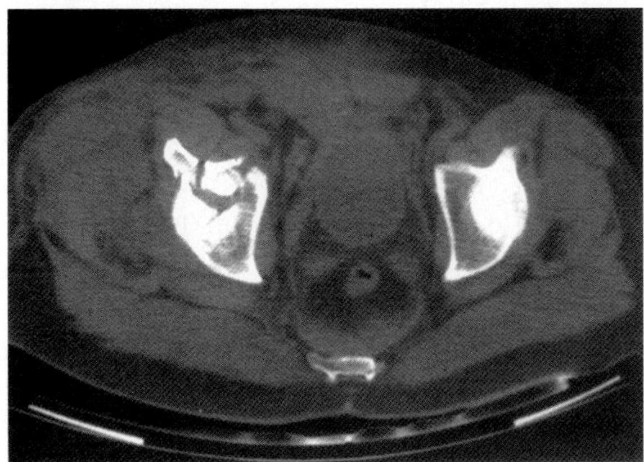

Fig. 4-23 Axial computed tomographic (CT) image demonstrating a displaced acetabular dome fracture.

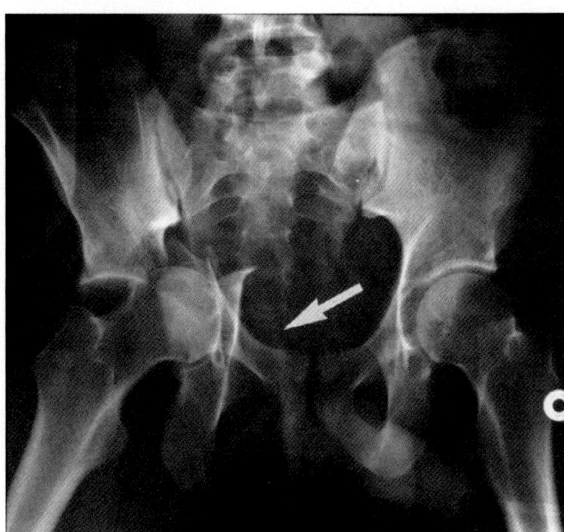

Fig. 4-24 Anteroposterior (AP) radiograph demonstrating a severely displaced two-column fracture (*arrow*).

Retained joint fragments
Femoral head or Garden III or IV neck fractures

Results following internal fixation are good to excellent in 80% to 90% of patients. Only approximately 8% of patients require reoperation, usually hip arthroplasty for secondary osteoarthritis.

## Suggested Reading


Crowl AC, Kahler DM. Closed reduction and percutaneous fixation of anterior column acetabular fractures. *Comput Aided Surg*. 2002;7:169–178.

Giannoudis PV, Grotz MRW, Papakostidis C, et al. Operative treatment of displaced pelvic fractures of the acetabulum: A META-analysis. *J Bone Joint Surg*. 2005;87B:2–9.

Judet R, Judet J, Letournel RE. Fractures of the acetabulum: Classification and surgical approaches to open reduction. *J Bone Joint Surg*. 1964;46A:1615–1647.

Matta J, Merritt PO. Displaced acetabular fractures. *Clin Orthop*. 1988;230:83–97.

Starr AJ, Reinert CM, Jones AL. Percutaneous fixation of the columns of the acetabulum: A new technique. *J Orthop Trauma*. 1998;12:51–58.


### Complications

Complications of displaced acetabular fractures are similar in many ways to complex pelvic fractures (unstable, double

**Table 4-2**

**ACETABULAR FRACTURE COMPLICATIONS AND IMAGING APPROACHES**

| COMPLICATIONS | IMAGING APPROACHES |
|---|---|
| Local complications | |
| Osteoarthritis (26–37%) | Serial radiographs |
| Nerve palsy (5–16%) | MRI or CT |
| Heterotopic ossification (25%) | Serial radiographs, CT |
| Avascular necrosis (6–10%) | Serial radiographs, MRI |
| Infection (4) | Radionuclide scans, MRI |
| Implant failure | Serial radiographs |
| Distant complications | |
| Extremity fractures (40%) | Radiographs |
| Head injuries (22%) | CT, MRI |
| Chest injuries (12%) | CT |
| Abdominal injuries (8%) | CT |
| DVT/PE (4–8%) | Ultrasound, CT, venography |

CT, computed tomography; MRI, magnetic resonance imaging; DVT, deep venous thrombosis; PE, pulmonary embolism.

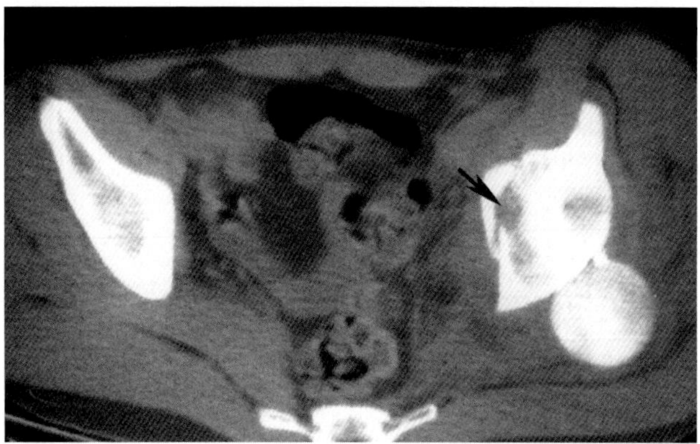

**Fig. 4-25** Axial computed tomographic (CT) image in a patient with acetabular fracture (*arrow*) and posterior dislocation of the femoral head compressing the sciatic nerve.

breaks in the pelvic ring). These include hemorrhage, local neurovascular and genitourinary injuries, extremity fractures (40%), as well as distant injuries to the abdomen (8%), chest (12%), and head (22%). The author will focus on complications more frequently related to acetabular fractures. Table 4-2 summarizes complications and imaging approaches.

The most common long-term complication is osteoarthritis of the hip on the involved side, which occurs in 26% to 37% of patients and may require hip arthroplasty. Post-traumatic nerve palsies are common (5% to 16%) and most often involve the sciatic nerve, but the femoral nerve may also be affected. Patients with associated posterior dislocation of the femoral head have sciatic nerve injury in 40% of cases (see Fig. 4-25).

The incidence of heterotopic ossifications (HOs) varies from 3% to 69%. In a large series of 23 articles, the average incidence was 26%. Avascular necrosis (AVN) of the femoral head occurs in approximately 6% to 10% of all cases, but the incidence increases when posterior dislocation of the femoral head occurs. Local infection occurs in 4% of cases and deep venous thrombosis or pulmonary embolus in 4% to 8%. Revision surgery is necessary in 8% of patients treated with open reduction and internal fixation.

## Suggested Reading


Giannoudis PV, Grotz MRW, Papakostidis C, et al. Operative treatment of displaced pelvic fractures of the acetabulum: A META-analysis. *J Bone Joint Surg*. 2005;87B: 2–9.

Issack PS, Toro JB, Buly RL, et al. Sciatic nerve release following fracture and reconstruction surgery of the acetabulum. *J Bone Joint Surg*. 2007;89A:1432–1437.

Kaempffe FA, Bone LB, Border JR. Open reduction and internal fixation of acetabular fractures: Heterotopic ossification and other complications of treatment. *J Orthop Trauma*. 1991;5: 439–445.

Matta JM, Merritt PO. Displaced acetabular fractures. *Clin Orthop*. 1988;230:83–97.


## Dislocations and Fracture/Dislocations of the Hip

Dislocations of the hip account for only 5% of all dislocations. High-velocity trauma such as motor vehicle accidents, motorcycle accidents, and fall from significant heights are the major mechanisms of injury. Because of the severity of trauma, multiple injuries are present in 75% of cases. Dislocations may be anterior, central, or posterior. As central dislocations (Fig. 4-24) occur with acetabular fractures described in the preceding text, the author will focus on anterior and posterior dislocations.

### Posterior Dislocations

Posterior dislocations of the hip are seven to ten times more common than anterior dislocations. The injury occurs when force is applied to the knee or foot with the hip in the flexed position. Associated posterior acetabular rim or posterior column fractures are common. The degree of involvement of the posterior acetabulum is related to the position of the femur at the time of injury (see Fig. 4-26, also Fig. 4-16). The more abducted the femur, the larger the fragment.

**Classification:** Thompson and Epstein with modification

- **Type IA**—dislocation with or without minor rim fracture
- **Type IB**—dislocation with simple posterior wall fracture, which becomes trapped in the joint with reduction (Fig. 4-26)
- **Type IIA**—dislocation with simple posterior wall fracture
- **Type IIB**—same as IIA with associated acetabular floor fracture
- **Type IIIA**—dislocation with comminution of posterior wall
- **Type IIIB**—same as IIIA with associated transverse acetabular fracture
- **Type IV**—dislocation with associated fracture of the femoral head or neck (see Fig. 4-27)

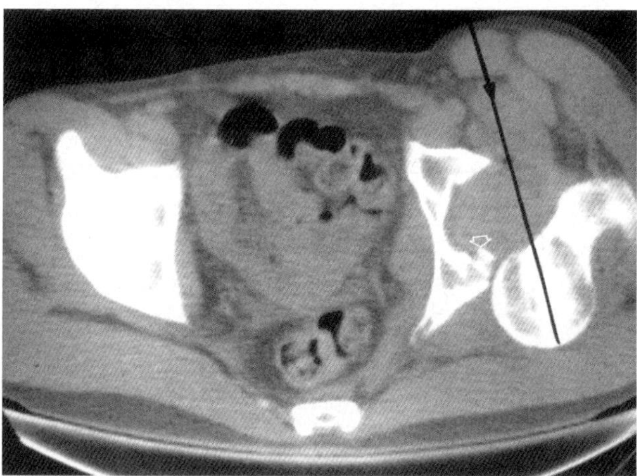

**Fig. 4-26** Axial computed tomographic (CT) image following posterior dislocation of the hip demonstrating the direction of the femoral displacement (*line with arrow*) and the actetabular rim fracture (*open arrow*) (Thompson and Epstein type IB).

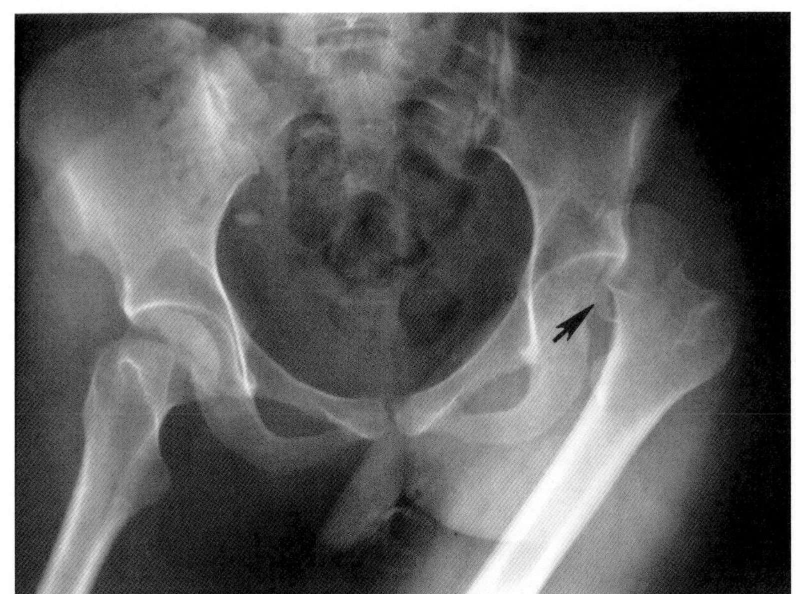


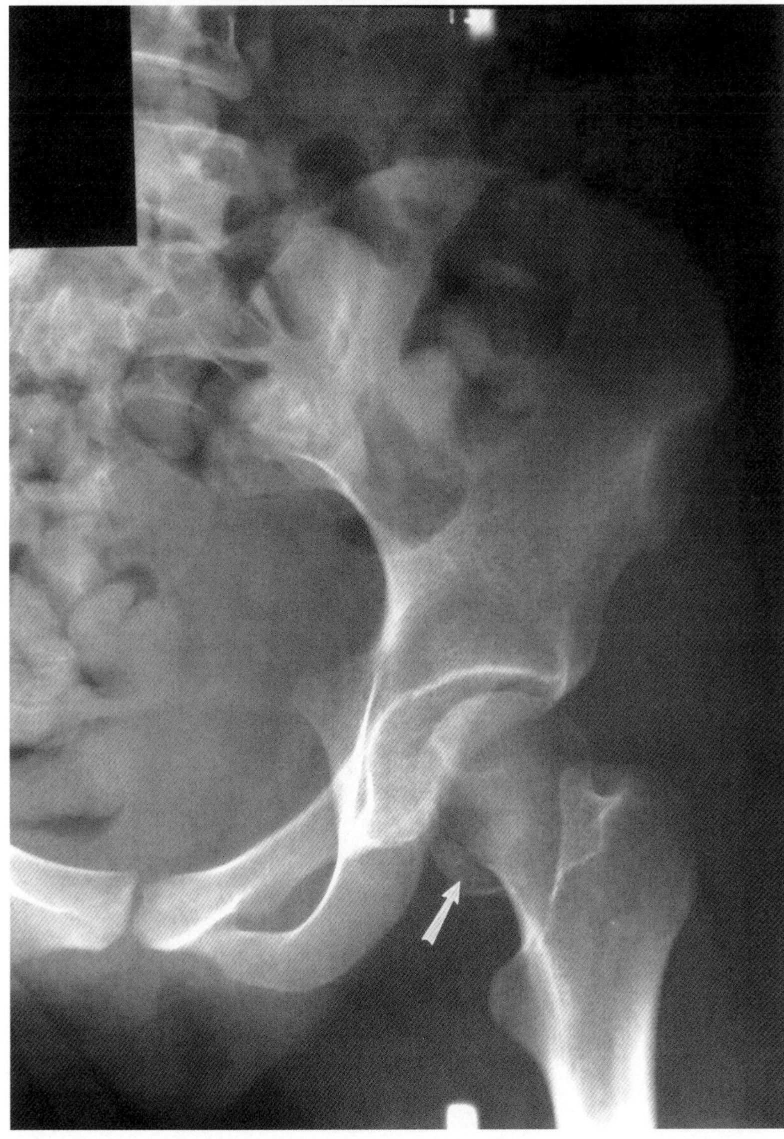


**Fig. 4-27** A: Anteroposterior (AP) radiograph demonstrating a Thompson and Epstein type IV fracture with posterior dislocation and a fracture of the femoral head (*arrow*). B: The fracture is more obvious (*arrow*) post reduction. Computed tomography (CT) is required for complete evaluation.

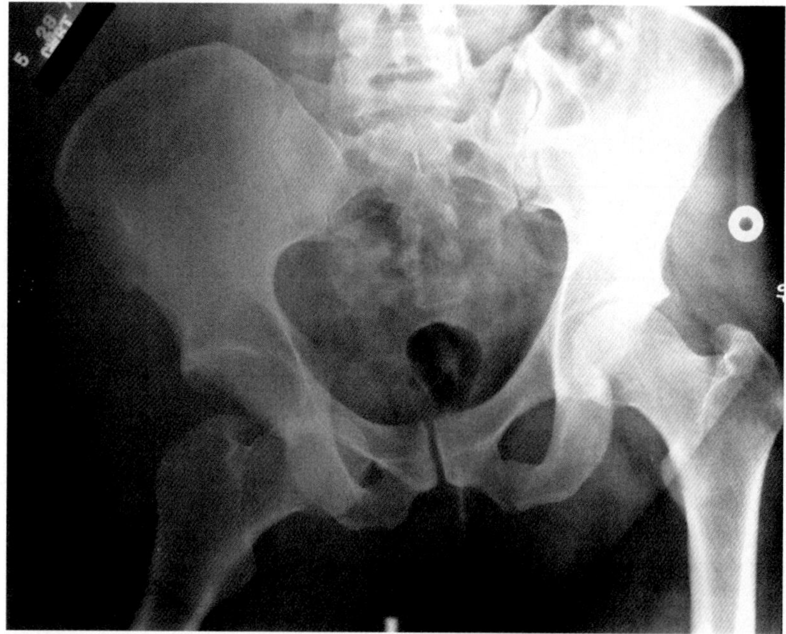

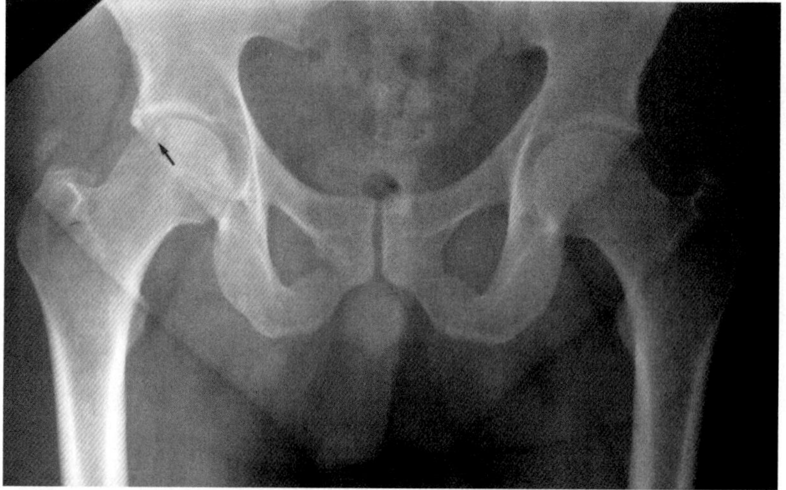

**Fig. 4-28** Anterior dislocation. **A:** Anteroposterior (AP) radiograph demonstrates an anterior dislocation with the femoral head overlying the obturator foramen (Epstein type IIB). **B:** Following reduction the impacted fracture of the femoral head (*arrow*) is more clearly seen.

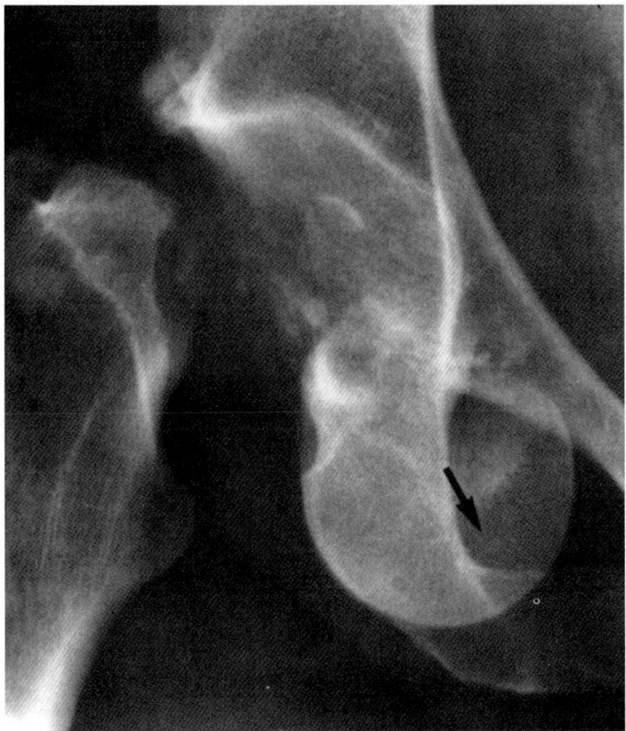

Fig. 4-29 Anterior dislocation of the femoral head (*arrow*) with comminuted femoral neck fracture (Epstein type IIIB).

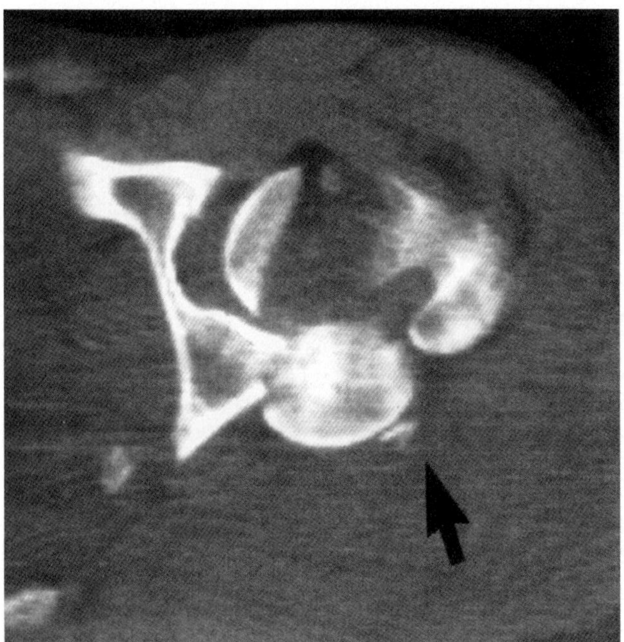

Fig. 4-30 Posterior dislocation with comminution of the femoral head and a large posterior fragment (*arrow*).

### Anterior Dislocations

Anterior dislocations account for 10% to 14% of hip dislocations (see Fig. 4-28). The injury occurs with forced abduction and external rotation of the hip. Associated fractures of the femoral head occur in 70% to 75% of cases. Both shearing osteochondral and impacted fractures of the superolateral femoral head are common (Fig. 4-28).

**Classification:** Epstein classification

- **Type IA**—superior dislocation with femoral head in pubic or supraspinous position, no associated fracture
- **Type IB**—same as IA with associated femoral head or neck fracture
- **Type IIA**—inferior dislocation with head over the obturator foramen, no associated fracture
- **Type IIB**—same as IIA with associated femoral head or neck fracture (see Fig. 4-29)
- **Type IIC**—same as IIA with associated acetabular fracture (see Fig. 4-30)

## Suggested Reading

Epstein H. Traumatic dislocation of the hip. *Clin Orthop.* 1973;92:116–142.

Epstein H. Posterior fracture-dislocations of the hip. *J Bone Joint Surg.* 1974;56A:1103–1127.

Erb RE, Steele JR, Nance PE, et al. Traumatic anterior dislocation of the hip: Spectrum of plain film and CT findings. *AJR Am J Roentgenol.* 1995;165:1215–1219.

Selvey DM, Siboto GM. Classification of posterior fracture dislocation of the hip joint: A modification of the Thompsen Epstein classification. *Injury.* 2001;32:217–219.

### Imaging of Hip Dislocations

Radiographs in the AP, lateral, and Judet positions clearly demonstrate the position of the femoral head as well as the anterior and posterior columns and central acetabulum (Figs. 4-28 and 4-29). In most cases, CT is required to completely evaluate the injury and associated changes to the femoral head, neck, and acetabulum (Fig. 4-30). CT is especially important after reduction to evaluate the acetabulum and identify fragments in the joint space (Fig. 4-26).

## Suggested Reading

Erb RE, Steele JR, Nance PE, et al. Traumatic anterior dislocation of the hip: Spectrum of plain film and CT findings. *AJR Am J Roentgenol.* 1995;165:1215–1219.

Richardson P, Young JWR, Porter D. CT detection of cortical fracture of the femoral head associated with posterior hip dislocations. *AJR Am J Roentgenol.* 1990;155:93–94.

### Treatment Options

As soon as possible, dislocations without associated fractures should be reduced using closed techniques. The incidence of AVN of the femoral head is high if the dislocation is not reduced in the first 6 to 12 hours, specifically posterior dislocations. Conservative management can be used until soft tissue healing has occurred.

When there are associated fractures, management varies depending on the degree of injury to the femoral head, neck, or acetabulum. Open reduction and internal fixation is indicated if more than one third of the femoral head is fractured or if there are any significantly displaced fragments that involve the weight-bearing surface or prevent joint congruency (Fig. 4-30). Smaller posterior acetabular fractures may be ignored. Larger or comminuted fragments must be reduced to maintain stability of the joint. Reconstruction plates and screws are typically used in this setting.

Treatment of associated femoral neck fractures is more complicated. This will be discussed more fully in the next section.

## SUGGESTED READING

Ghormley RK, Sullivan R. Traumatic dislocations of the hip. *Am J Surg.* 1953;85:298–301.

Yang EC, Cornwall R. Initial treatment of traumatic hip dislocations in the adult. *Clin Orthop.* 2000;377:24–31.

Yang R-S, Tsuang Y-H, Hang Y-S, et al. Traumatic dislocations of the hip. *Clin Orthop.* 1991;265:218–227.

### Complications

Complications associated with fracture dislocations of the hip along with imaging approaches are summarized in Table 4-3.

**Table 4-3**

COMPLICATIONS OF FRACTURE/DISLOCATIONS OF THE HIP

| COMPLICATION | IMAGING APPROACHES |
|---|---|
| Osteoarthritis (23–35%) | Serial radiographs |
| Avascular necrosis (5–26%) | Serial radiographs, MRI |
| Sciatic nerve injury (10–17%) | CT, MRI |
| Infection (2–4%) | Radionuclide scans, MRI |
| Myositis ossificans | CT |
| Redislocation | Serial radiographs, CT |
| Implant failure | Serial radiographs |

MRI, magnetic resonance imaging; CT, computed tomography.

Early reduction is critical regardless of the type of dislocation. The incidence of AVN of the femoral head is 5% to 26%, but results are uniformly poor if the dislocation is not reduced within 48 hours. The incidence of AVN of the femoral head is slightly less (8%) with anterior dislocations.

Sciatic nerve injury occurs in 10% to 17% of patients with posterior dislocations (see Fig. 4-26). Prompt reduction is necessary when sciatic nerve injury is suspected. Associated fractures beyond the femoral head, neck, and acetabulum are also not uncommon.

Post-traumatic arthritis occurs in 23%. The incidence is higher (35%) in patients treated with closed reduction or when there are associated acetabular fractures. Less common complications include myositis ossificans and redislocation. As with acetabular and pelvic fractures, deep venous thrombosis and pulmonary emboli may occur during the hospital phase of treatment.

## SUGGESTED READING

Berquist TH, Lewallen DG, McComb BL. The pelvis and hips. In: Berquist TH, ed. *Imaging atlas of orthopaedic appliances and prostheses*. New York: Raven Press; 1995:217–352.

Erb RE, Steele JR, Nance PE, et al. Traumatic anterior dislocation of the hip: Spectrum of plain film and CT findings. *AJR Am J Roentgenol.* 1995;165:1215–1219.

Hillyard RF, Fox J. Sciatic nerve injuries associated with traumatic posterior dislocations. *Am J Emerg Med.* 2003;21: 545–548.

### Femoral Neck Fractures

Femoral neck fractures occur most commonly in elderly patients. They are more common in females than males. Bone mineral density is commonly low resulting in fractures with minimal trauma such as a simple fall. Hip fractures are rare in children accounting for only 1% of pediatric fractures. Unlike adults, the injury is usually related to high-velocity trauma. When hip fractures occur, the femoral neck is the most common site of fracture (40% to 50% of hip fractures).

Femoral neck fractures may be subcapital, transcervical, or basicervical (see Fig. 4-31). Fractures may be complete or incomplete. Stress and insufficiency fractures of the femoral neck are common in young athletes and elderly patients, respectively.

**Classification:** Garden classification based on degree of displacement

- **Stage I**—incomplete involving the lateral cortex with intact medial trabeculae
- **Stage II**—complete, but undisplaced (see Fig. 4-32)
- **Stage III**—complete and partially displaced (see Fig. 4-33)
- **Stage IV**—complete and completely displaced

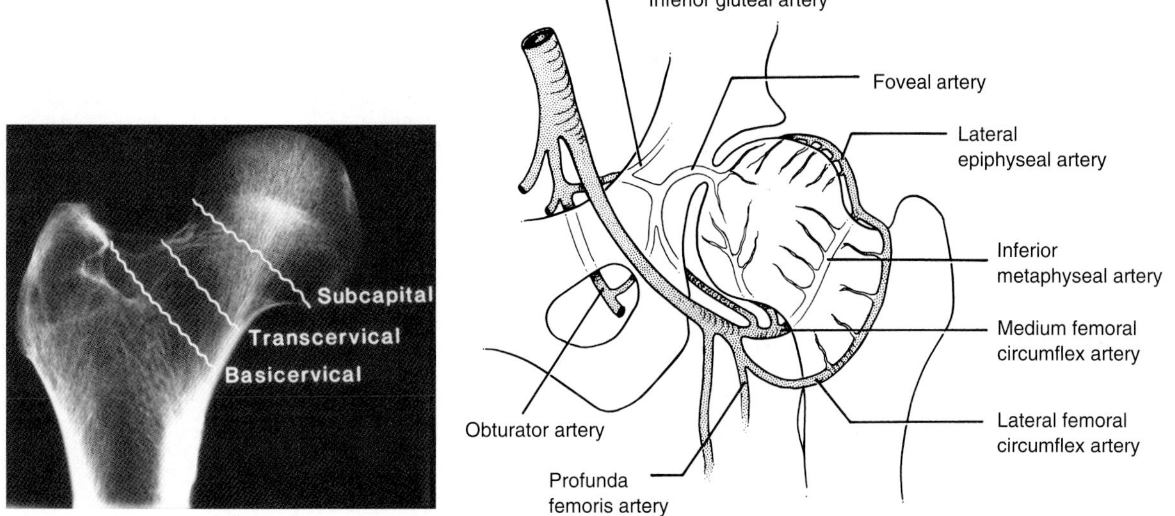


Fig. 4-31 A: Specimen radiograph demonstrating the locations of femoral neck fractures. B: Illustration of the vascular supply to the femoral head demonstrating the increased risk for avascular necrosis with femoral neck fractures compared to intertrochanteric fractures.

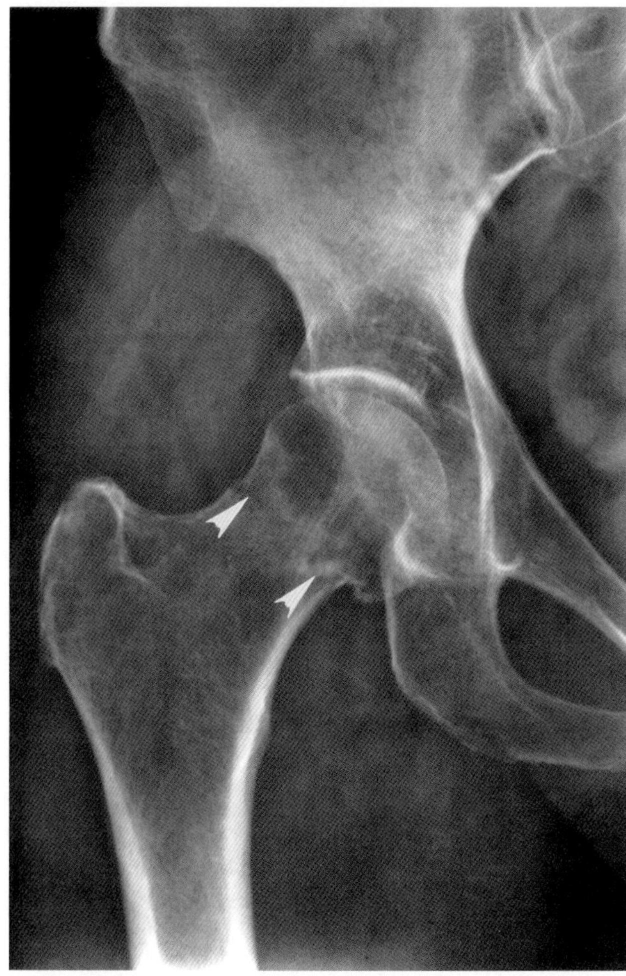

Fig. 4-32 Anteroposterior (AP) radiograph demonstrating a complete, but undisplaced femoral neck fracture (*arrowheads*) (Garden stage II).

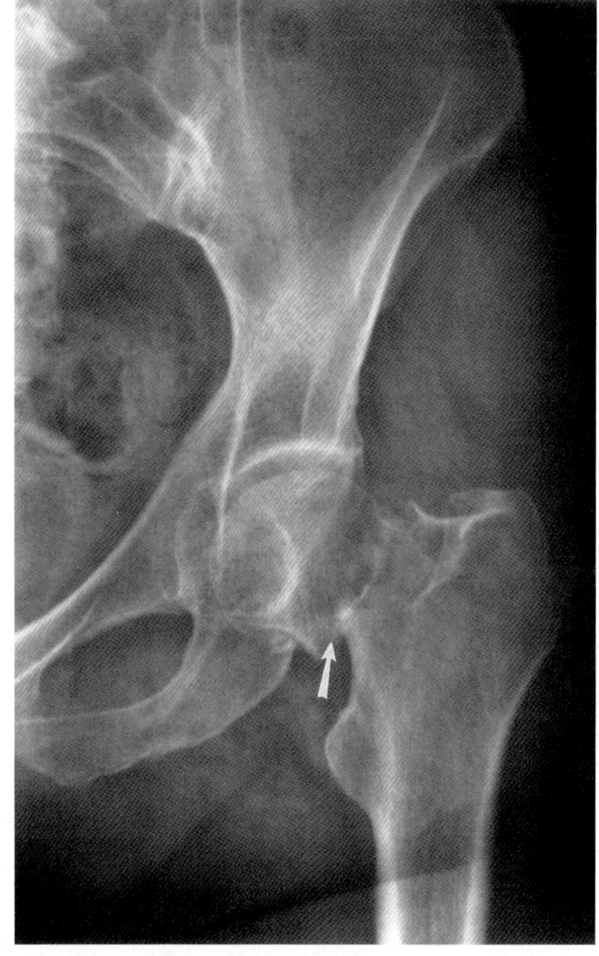


Fig. 4-33 A: Anteroposterior (AP) radiograph of the hip demonstrating a displaced (*arrow*) (Garden stage III) fracture. B: AP radiograph following bipolar hip replacement preserving the acetabulum and acetabular cartilage.

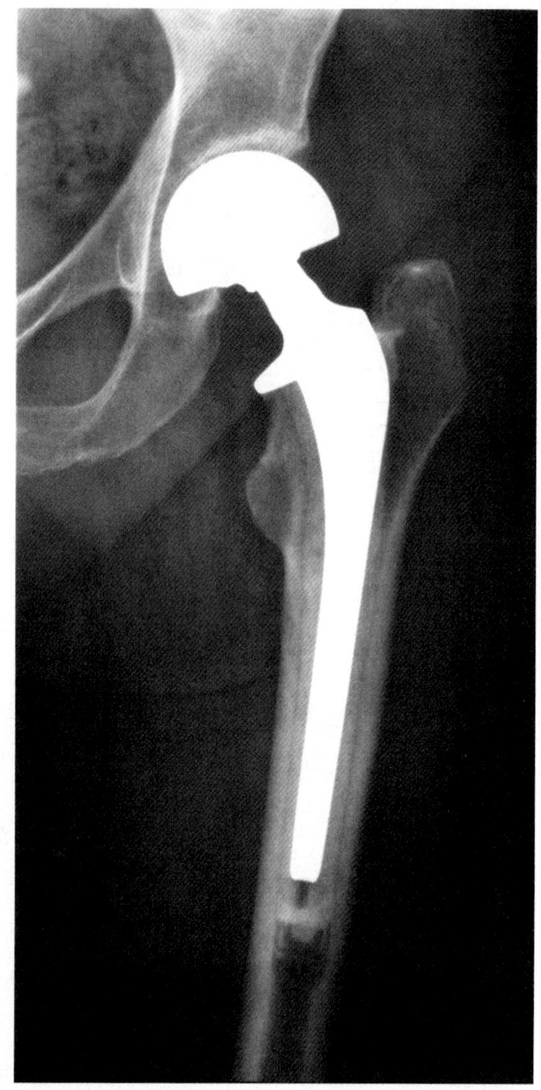


Fig. 4-33 *(Continued)*

For treatment purposes, many simply combine I and II (undisplaced) (Fig. 4-32) and III and IV (displaced) (Fig. 4-33).

## Suggested Reading

Beaty JH. Fractures of the hip in children. *Orthop Clin North Am*. 2006;37:223–232.

Garden RS. Reduction and fixation of subcapital fractures of the femur. *Orthop Clin North Am*. 1974;5:683–712.

Schmidt AH, Swiontkowski MF. Femoral neck fractures. *Orthop Clin North Am*. 2002;33:97–111.

### Preoperative Imaging

Imaging of patients with suspected femoral neck fractures begins with screening AP and lateral radiographs (Figs. 4-32 and 4-33). Care must be taken not to mistake overlying osteophytes for a fracture line. Subtle fractures may not be obvious on radiographs. In the past, radionuclide scans with Technetium Tc 99m methylene diphosphonate (MDP) were obtained (see Fig. 4-34). However, in the acute setting, scans can provide false-negative results. Scans are positive in 80% of patients in 24 hours and in 95% after 72 hours. Currently, magnetic resonance imaging (MRI) is often used as this technique is extremely sensitive in the acute setting. Either T1-weighted or short T1 inversion recovery (STIR) sequences can be used in the coronal plane for screening (see Fig. 4-35). This is more cost effective than a full examination. The examination is tailored such that additional image planes and sequences are obtained if necessary.

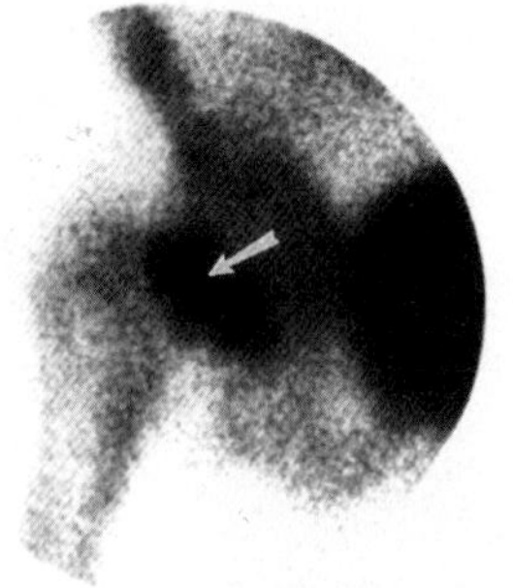
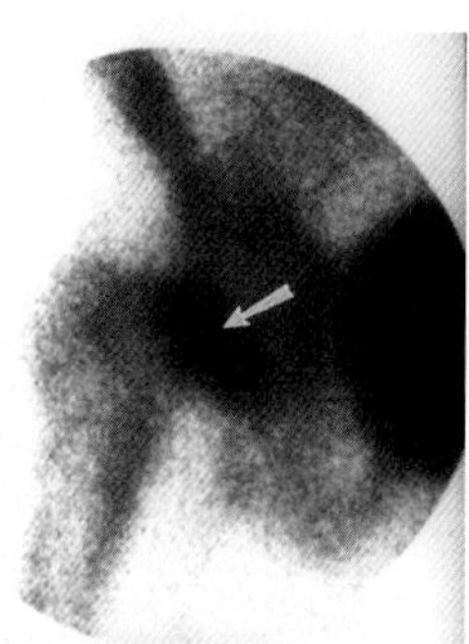

Fig. 4-34 Radionuclide scan demonstrating linear increased tracer in the femoral neck 72 hours following a fall due to a stage I femoral neck fracture.

## Suggested Reading

Bogost GA, Lizerbram EK, Crues JV III. MR imaging in evaluation of suspected hip fracture: Frequency of unsuspected bone and soft tissue injury. *Radiology*. 1995;197:263–267.

Quinn SF, McCarthy JL. Prospective evaluation of patients with suspected hip fracture and indeterminate radiographs: Use of T1-weighted MR images. *Radiology*. 1993;187:469–471.

Rizzo PE, Gould ES, Lyden JP, et al. Diagnosis of occult fractures about the hip. *J Bone Joint Surg*. 1993;75A:395–401.

### Treatment Options

Treatment of femoral neck fractures depends on stability of the fracture, patient status (age, activity, weight, and general health factors), and patient compliance. Stable fractures include incomplete stress or insufficiency fractures and Garden stage I and II injuries. Garden stage III and IV fractures are unstable and have a high incidence of AVN of the femoral head. When there is comminution of the posterior femoral neck, management is even more difficult.

**GARDEN STAGE I AND II** Conservative treatment can be used in selected situations. However, pinning of hip fractures in children and stage I and II fractures is usually performed due to patient compliance and to prevent complete fractures or displacement from occurring. Fixation is accomplished with cannulated, Hagie, or Knowles pins (see Fig. 4-36). Dynamic hip screws or sliding nails can also be used. However, these approaches may displace an otherwise impacted or stable injury.

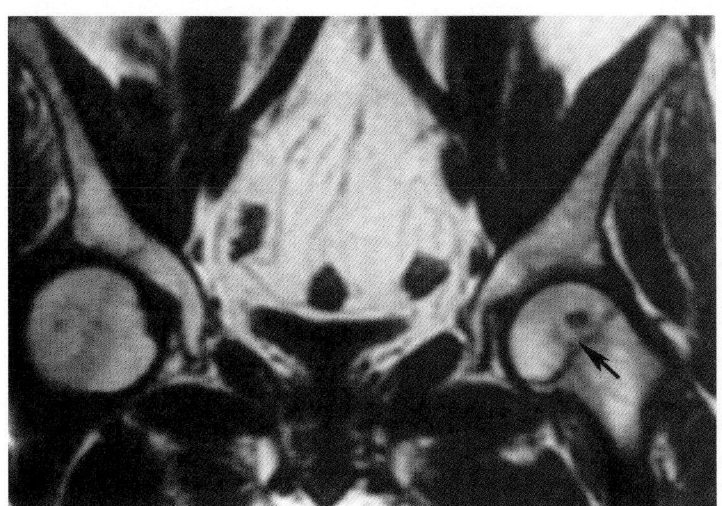

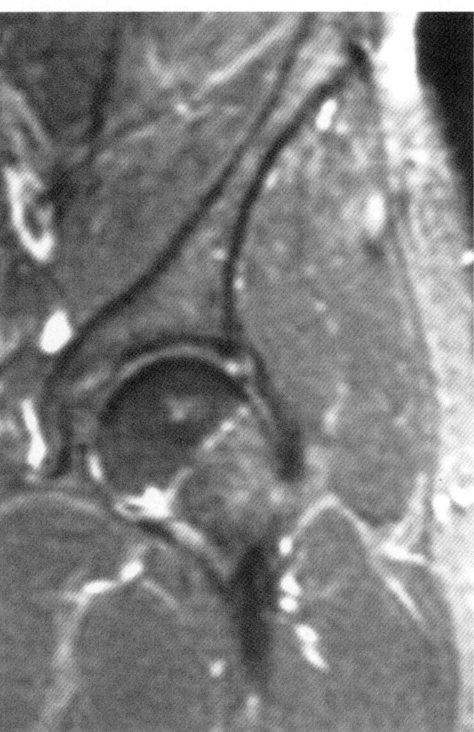

Fig. 4-35 A: Coronal T1-weighted image of the hips demonstrating a femoral neck fracture on the left (*arrow*). B: Postcontrast T1-weighted image shows decreased flow with low signal intensity in the femoral head compared to the remaining osseous structures.

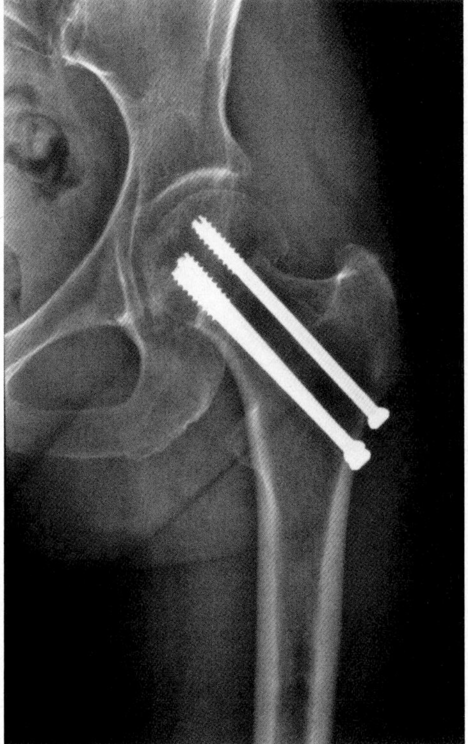

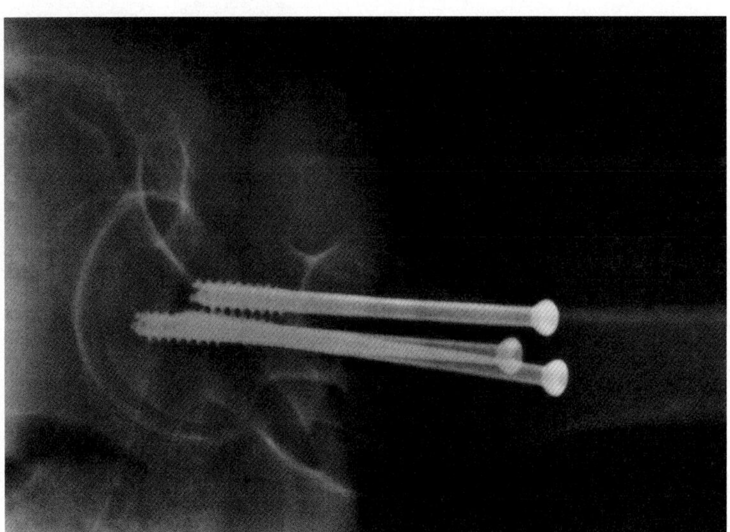

Fig. 4-36 Anteroposterior (AP) (A) and lateral (B) radiographs of a Garden II fracture treated with cannulated hip pins. The central cannulated portion allows the pin to be placed over a K-wire. This feature is obvious on radiographs.

**Fig. 4-37** A: Anteroposterior (AP) radiograph of the pelvis and hips demonstrating a displaced Garden stage III fracture of the right femoral neck. In this case, the patient was treated with an uncemented total hip replacement (B).

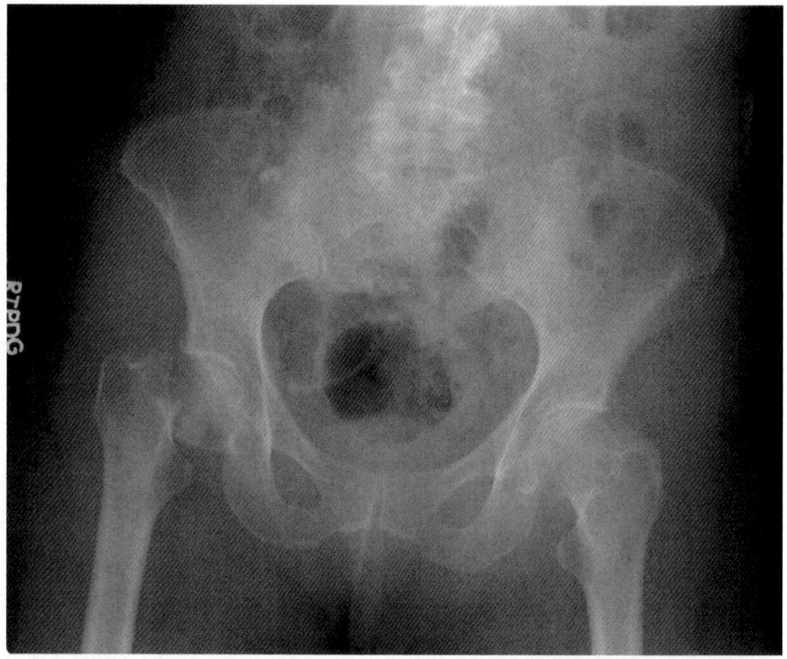

A

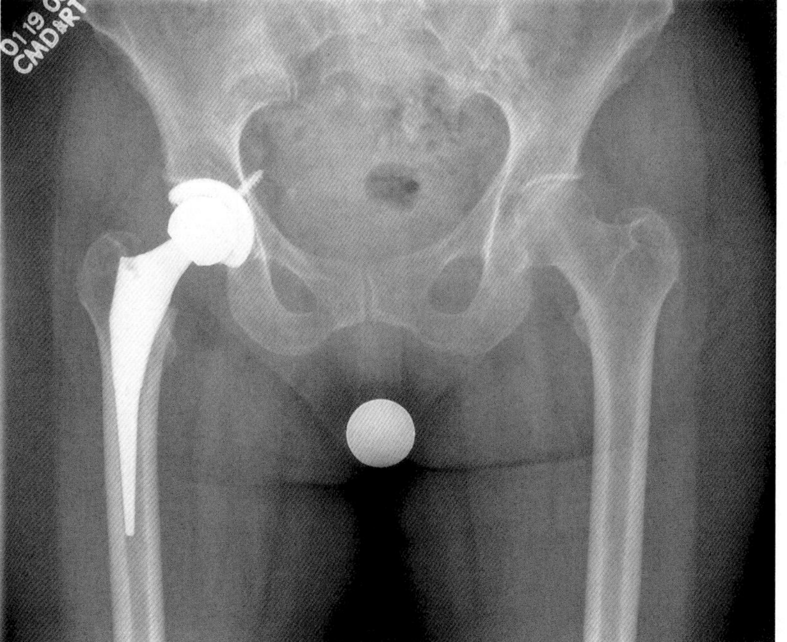

B

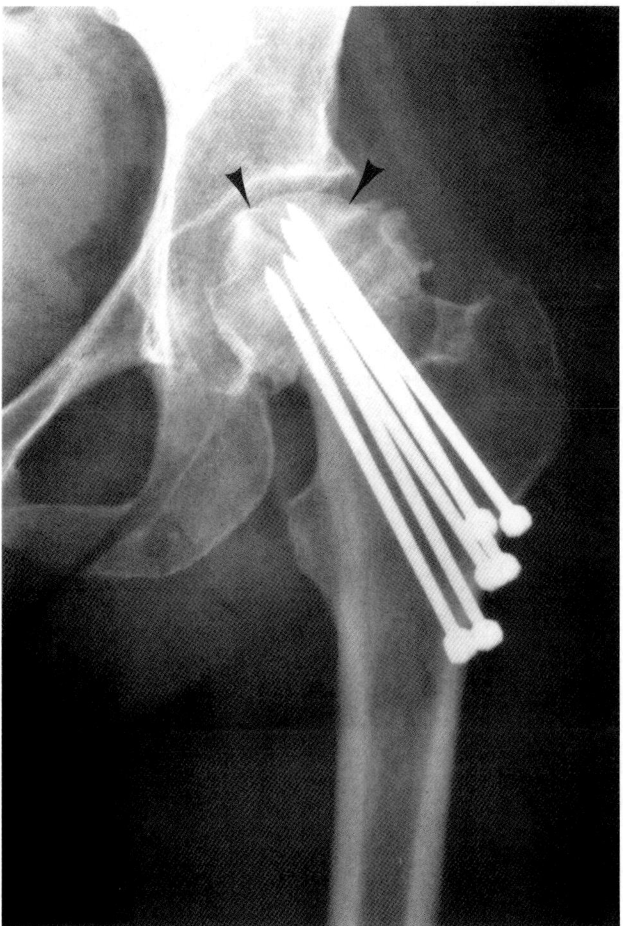

Fig. 4-38 Anteroposterior (AP) radiograph following pinning of a left femoral neck fracture. There is sclerosis and collapse (*arrowheads*) of the femoral head due to avascular necrosis.

GARDEN STAGE III AND IV Treatment options for these unstable fractures include reduction and internal fixation, hemiarthroplasty with bipolar implants (Fig. 4-33), and total hip arthroplasty (see Fig. 4-37). Simple pin fixation described earlier is generally inadequate with a 14% incidence of nonunion. The high incidence of AVN leads to use of hemiarthroplasty commonly in these patients.

### Indications for hemiarthroplasty

Garden III or IV in patients older than 75 years
Debilitated patients
Pathologic fractures
Fractures with femoral head dislocation
Failed internal fixation
Poor patient compliance

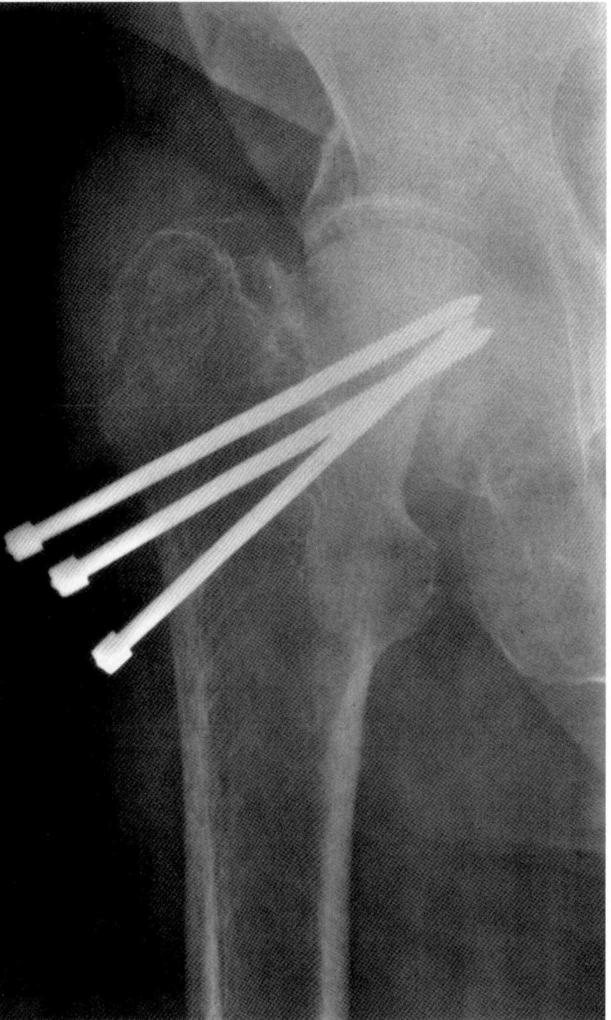

Fig. 4-39 Radiograph of the hip following pinning of a right femoral neck fracture. The femoral head is collapsed and sclerotic due to avascular necrosis (AVN) and the pins have backed out.

## Complications

Complications related to femoral neck fractures depend on the stage and viability of the femoral head (Fig. 4-35). Mortality rates approach 20% in elderly patients during the year following the injury. The most significant complications are AVN of the femoral head and nonunion. Other complications include malunion, infection, deep venous thrombosis, and pulmonary emboli.

AVN is most common with Garden stage III and IV adult fractures and similarly in children with displaced fractures (90%). Serial radiographs may demonstrate changes (see Fig. 4-38). Depending on the type of metal and implant, MRI is more sensitive and specific.

Nonunion occurs in 20% to 30% of displaced adult fractures treated with internal fixation (see Fig. 4-39). Hence, along with the incidence of AVN, the reason arthroplasty is so commonly selected. Nonunion is most easily evaluated with reformatted CT imaging. Other complications can be imaged similar to examples in Table 4-2 and 4-3.

## SUGGESTED READING


Beaty JH. Fractures of the hip in children. *Orthop Clin North Am.* 2006;37:223–232.

Schmidt AH, Swiontkowski MF. Femoral neck fractures. *Orthop Clin North Am.* 2002;33:97–111.


## Trochanteric Fractures

There are three basic fracture categories including avulsion fractures of the lesser and greater trochanters, intertrochanteric, and subtrochanteric fractures.

### Intertrochanteric Fractures

Intertrochanteric fractures are extracapsular and therefore there are fewer problems with nonunion and AVN compared to femoral neck fractures. Fractures may be simple and follow the intertrochanteric line or comminuted with significant displacement. Fractures are most common in the elderly related to falls or other minor trauma. There are multiple classifications systems including Evans, Jensen modification of Evans, and the Orthopaedic Trauma Association classification. Most use the Jensen modification of the Evans classification.

**Classification:** Evans with Jensen modification (see Fig. 4-40)

- **Type 1**—undisplaced two-part fracture; stable (Fig. 4-40A)
- **Type 2**—displaced two-part fracture (Fig. 4-40A)
- **Type 3**—three-part fracture; displaced greater trochanter (Fig. 4-40B)
- **Type 4**—three-part fracture; displaced calcar and lesser trochanter (Fig. 4-40B)
- **Type 5**—four-part fracture with medial and posterior cortex fractures (Fig. 4-40B)

### Subtrochanteric Fractures

Subtrochanteric fractures account for 10% to 30% of hip fractures. The subtrochanteric region is an area from the lesser trochanter to 5 cm distally in the cortical region of the femur. Subtrochanteric fractures occur in the elderly due to falls or minor trauma and in the younger population related to high-velocity trauma. Fractures involve the femur below the lesser trochanter, but they frequently extend distally and proximally into the intertrochanteric region. Healing is cortical resulting in a slow consolidation process. Also, forces transmitted through this region present a significant treatment challenge. Several classification systems have been used, but there is no universally accepted system. The Russell-Taylor classification is based on involvement of the greater trochanter and piriformis fossa (type II) and noninvolvement of these

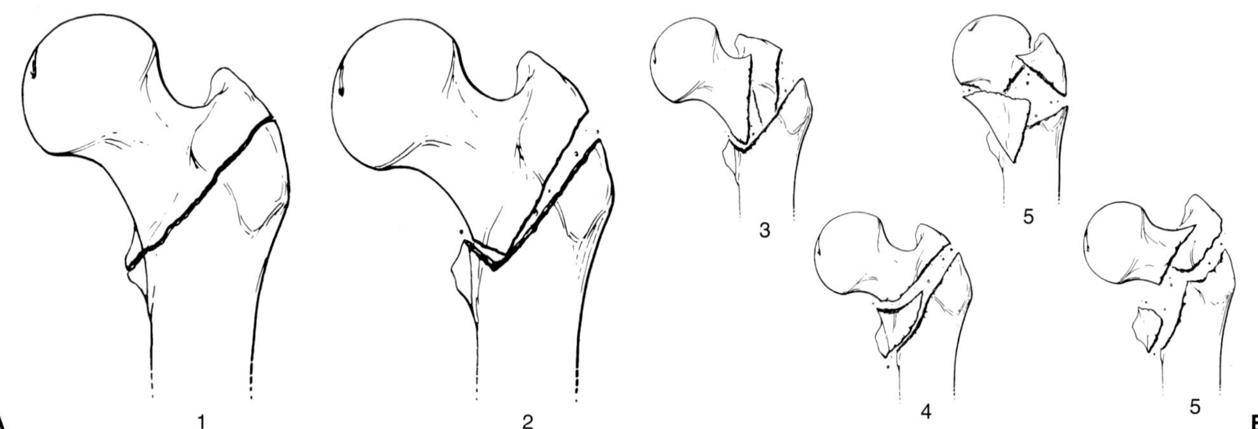


**Fig. 4-40** Evans classification with Jensen modification. **A:** Illustration of type *1*—undisplaced two-part and type *2*—displaced two-part. **B:** Illustration of type *3*—three-part fracture with displaced greater trochanter, type *4*—three-part fracture with displaced calcar and lesser trochanter, type *5*—four-part fractures with medial and posterior cortex fractures.

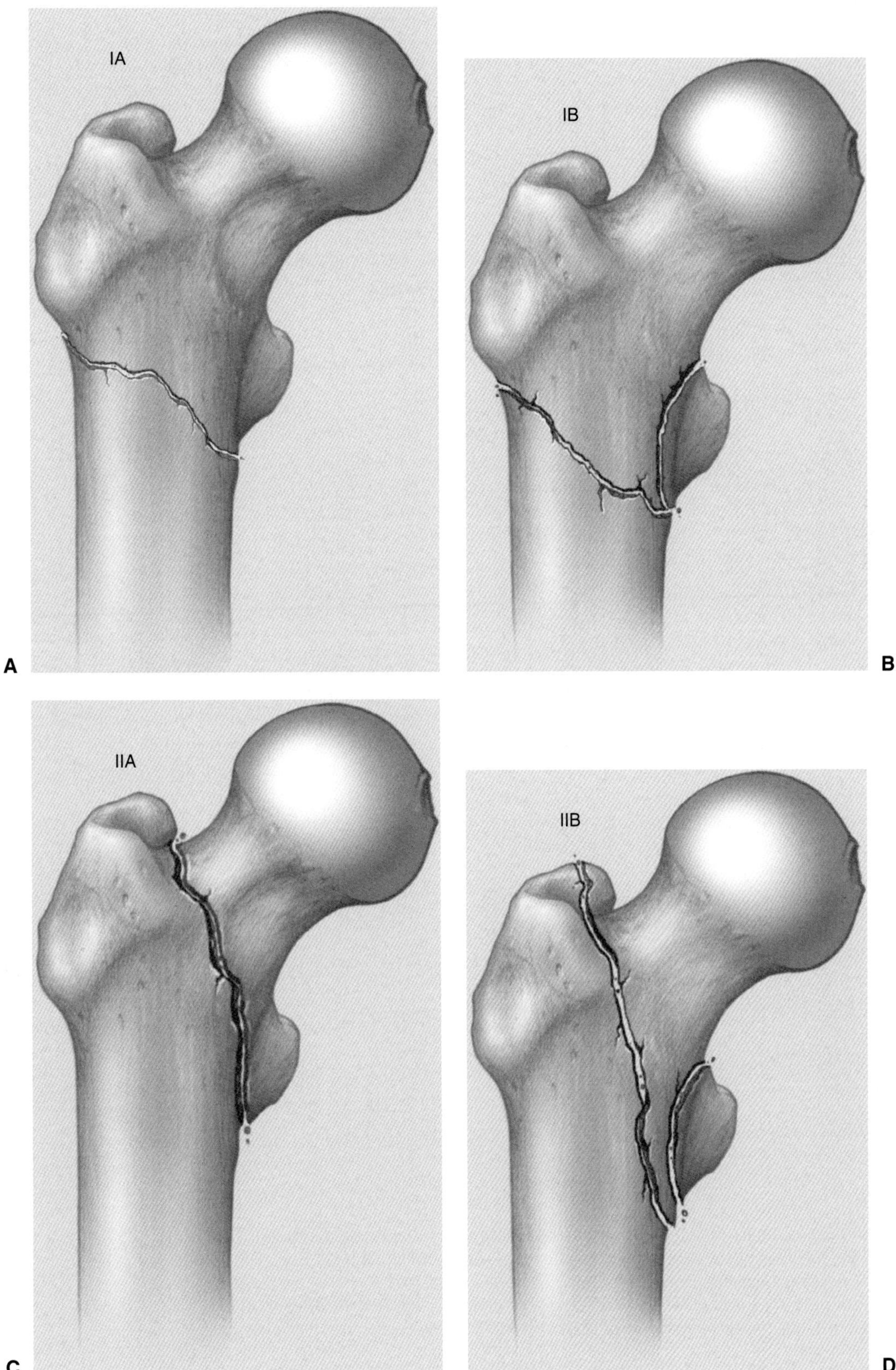


**Fig. 4-41** Russell-Taylor classification. Type I injuries do not enter the piriformis fossa. **A:** Type IA—spare the lesser trochanter. **B:** Type IB—comminution involving the lesser trochanter and posteromedial femoral cortex. Type II injuries involve the piriformis fossa. **C:** Type IIA—single fracture line extending into the piriformis fossa. **D:** Type IIB—comminuted with piriformis fossa, lesser trochanter, and posteromedial cortex involvement.

areas (type I) (see Fig. 4-41). The Seinsheimer classification is summarized in the subsequent text.

**Seinsheimer classification** (see Fig. 4-42)

- **Type I:** Any undisplaced (<2 mm) fracture
- **Type II:** Two-part fractures
  - A—transverse subtrochanteric
  - B—spiral subtrochanteric
  - C—spiral fracture with lesser trochanter involved
- **Type III:** Three-part fractures
  - A—spiral three part with displaced lesser trochanter
  - B—spiral three part with lateral butterfly fragment
- **Type IV:** Four or more fragments
- **Type V:** Subtrochanteric fracture that extends to greater trochanter

## Avulsion Fractures

Avulsion fractures of the greater and lesser trochanter are uncommon. Greater trochanteric avulsion occurs with abrupt contraction of the gluteal muscle. These injuries are more common in elderly patients with osteopenia. Lesser trochanteric avulsions occur in younger individuals due to abrupt iliopsoas contractions.

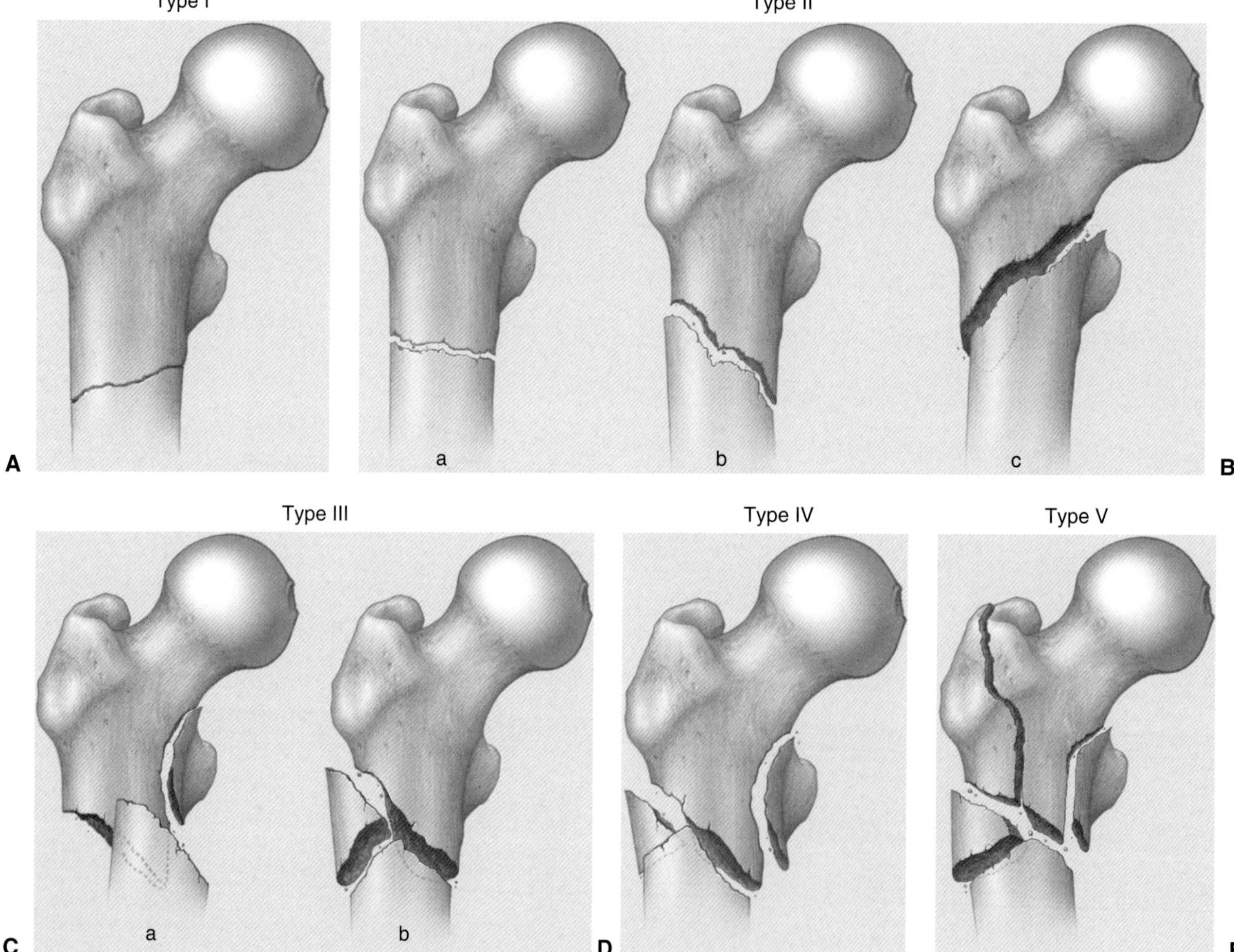


Fig. 4-42 Seinsheimer classification. A: Type I—any fracture with <2 mm displacement. B: Type II—two-part fractures: *a*-transverse subtrochanteric, *b*-spiral subtrochanteris, *c*-spiral subtrochanteric with lesser trochanteric involvement. C: Type III—three-part fractures: *a*-spiral three-part fracture with lesser trochanter displaced, *b*-spiral three-part fracture with lateral butterfly fragment. D: Type IV—four or more fragments. E: Type V—subtrochanteric fracture that extends into the greater trochanter.

## Suggested Reading

Beaty JH. Fractures of the hip in children. *Orthop Clin North Am*. 2006;37:223–232.

Bedi A, Le TT. Subtrochanteric fractures of the femur. *Orthop Clin North Am*. 2004;35:473–483.

Jensen JS. Classification of trochanteric fractures. *Acta Orthop Scand*. 1980;51:803–810.

Russell TA, Taylor JC. Subtrochanteric fractures of the femur. In: Browner BD, Jupiter JB, Levine AM, eds. *Skeletal trauma*, 2nd ed. Philadelphia: WB Saunders; 1992:1883–1895.

Seinsheimer F. Subtrochanteric fractures of the femur. *J Bone Joint Surg*. 1978;60A:300–306.

### Imaging of Trochanteric Fractures

In most cases, trochanteric fractures can be properly identified and classified with AP and lateral radiographs of the hip (see Figs. 4-43 to 4-45). Subtle or incomplete fractures may be undetectable unless MRI is obtained. More complex injuries should be evaluated with CT for optimal operative planning.

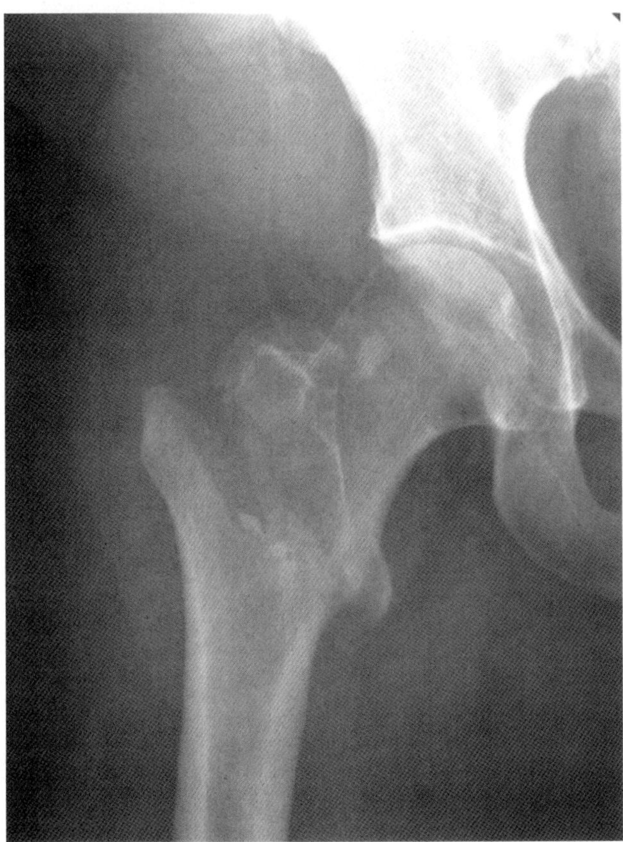

**Fig. 4-43** Anteroposterior (AP) radiograph of a type 2-displaced two-part fracture.

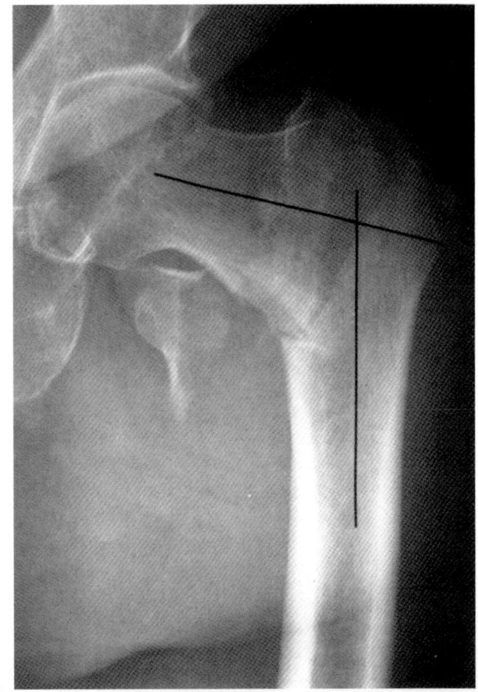


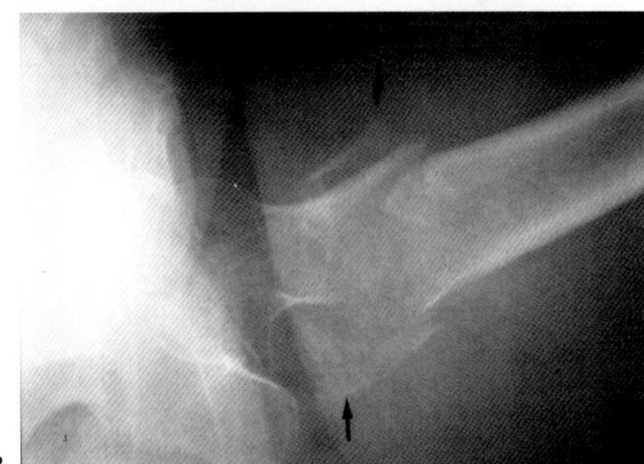


**Fig. 4-44** Displaced four-part fracture—type 5. Anteroposterior (AP) (**A**) and lateral (**B**) radiographs demonstrate a four-part fracture with varus angulation (*lines* in **A**) and displaced lesser and greater trochanteric fragments (*arrows*).

## Suggested Reading

Schultz E, Miller TE, Boruchov D, et al. Incomplete intertrochanteric fractures: Imaging features and clinical management. *Radiology* 1999;211:237–240.

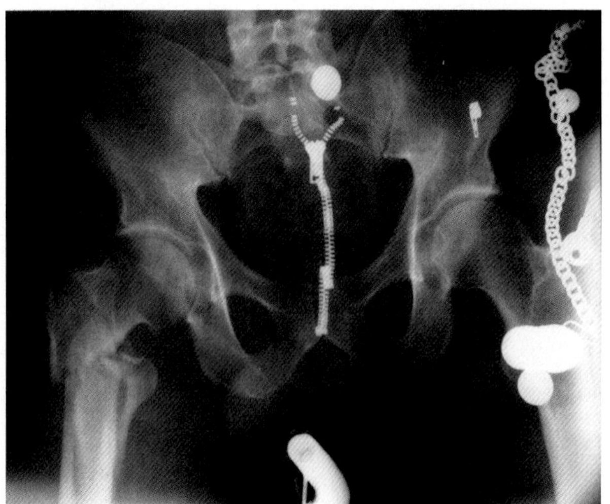

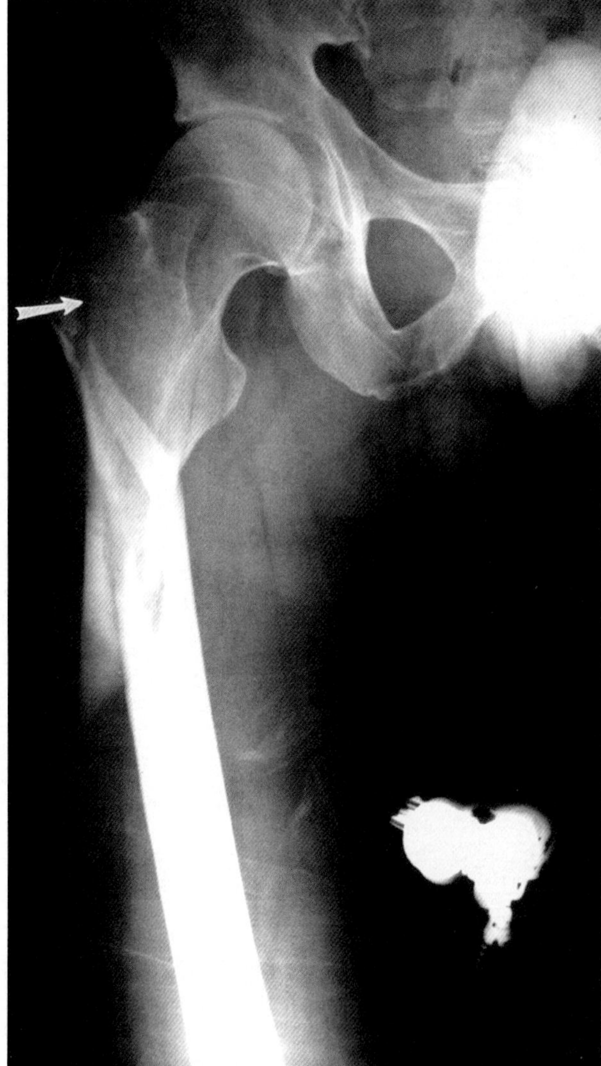

Fig. 4-45 Subtrochanteric fractures. Type IV Seinsheimer (A) and type V (B) with extension into the greater trochanter (*arrow*).

### Treatment Options

Treatment of avulsion injuries of the lesser and greater trochanters is usually conservative. Internal fixation may be necessary if the fragment is displaced >2 cm. Intertrochanteric fractures, whether displaced or undisplaced, typically require internal fixation. Anatomic reduction in which the posterior and medial cortices are brought back into contact is important to achieve stability and prevent varus and posterior deformities. A dynamic hip screw and side plate are most commonly used in this setting (see Fig. 4-46). Oversliding of the screw can lead to limb shortening and medialization of the distal fragment. Therefore, other options may also be used (see Fig. 4-47). Short intramedullary nails improve load transfer and the sliding hip screw still allows for fracture fragments to impact (see Fig. 4-48). External fixation and joint prostheses may also be used. However, these approaches are much less common than the dynamic hip screw and side plate or intramedullary nail.

Subtrochanteric fractures are more complex. Intramedullary nails (Fig. 4-48), fixed-angle devices (blade plates), and dynamic hip screws with longer side plates may be used (see Fig. 4-49). Intramedullary nails may be preferred for fractures that spare the piriformis fossa (Russell-Taylor type I). Fixed-angle blade plates and dynamic screw and plate fixation are effective options when fractures involve the piriformis fossa and greater trochanter. External fixation is not commonly used, but may be advantageous for open fractures.

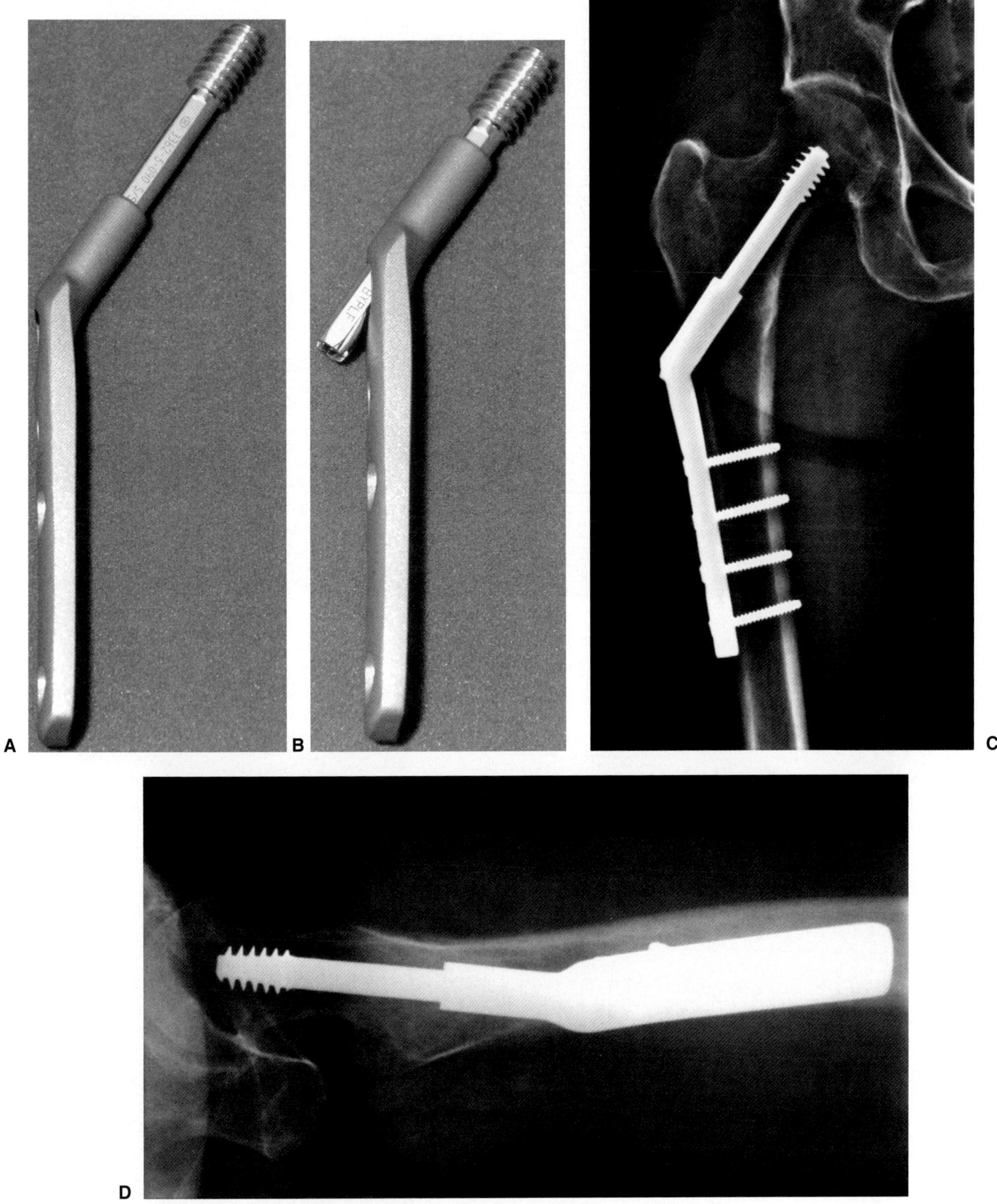


Fig. 4-46 Dynamic hip screw fixation. Image of dynamic hip screw (A) and with screw impacted into the barrel of the side plate (B). (Courtesy of Stryker Orthopaedics, Mahwah, New Jersey.) Anteroposterior (AP) (C) and lateral (D) radiographs of a healed two-part fracture with dynamic hip screw and four-hole side plate for fixation.

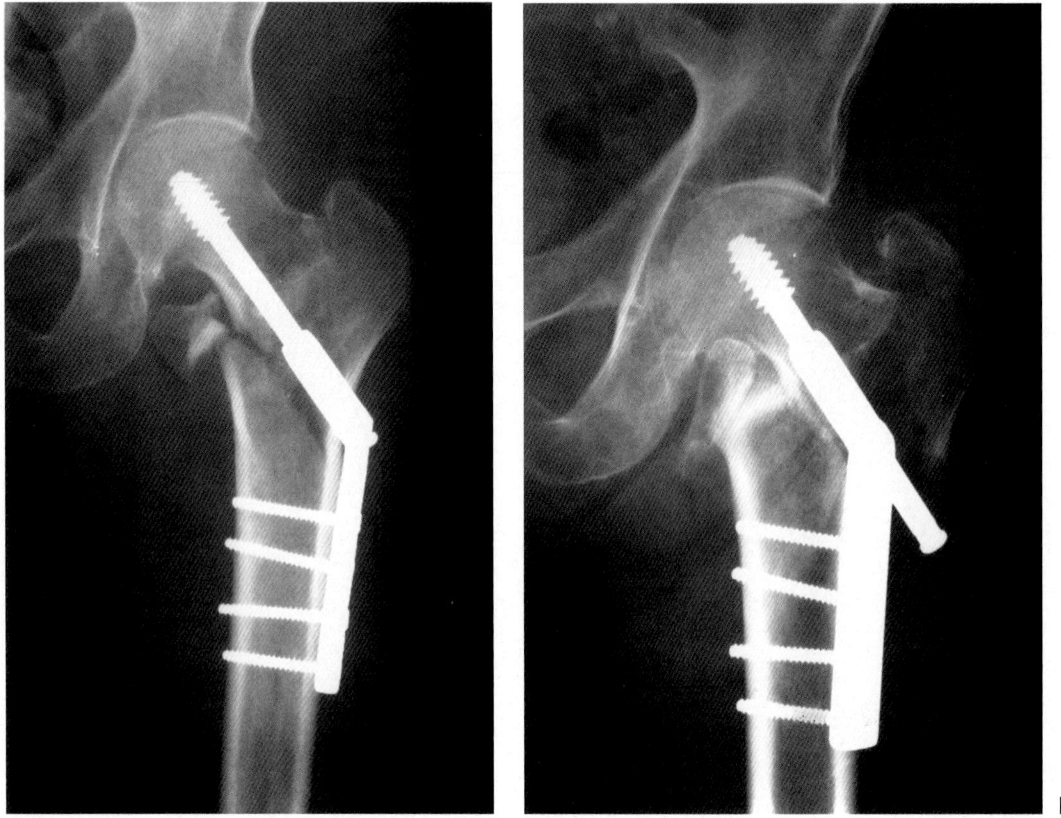

Fig. 4-47 Failed dynamic hip screw with medialization of the distal fragment. Anteroposterior (AP) radiographs following implantation (A) and 2 months later (B) demonstration marked lateral displacement of the screw in the barrel and shortening with medialization of the distal fragment.

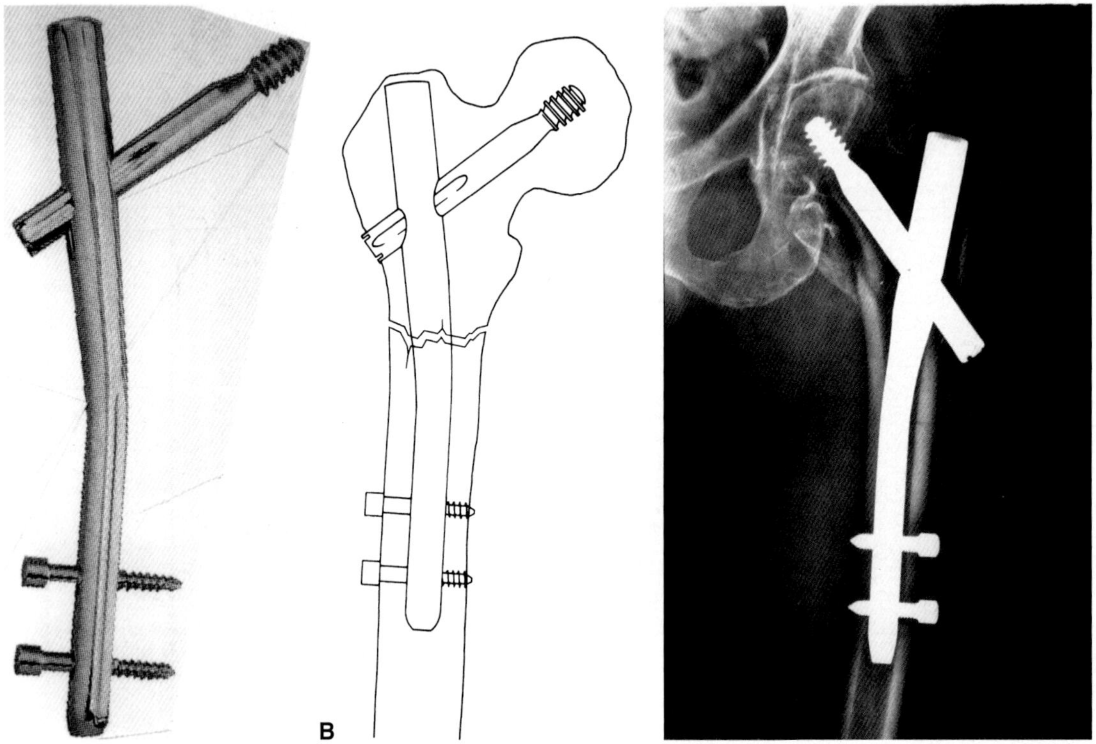

Fig. 4-48 Short intramedullary nail fixation. Photo (A) and illustration (B) of a Gamma locking nail. (Courtesy of Stryker Howmedica Osteonics, Allendale, New Jersey.) Anteroposterior (AP) (C) and lateral (D) radiographs of Gamma nail fixation of a trochanteric/subtrochanteric fracture.

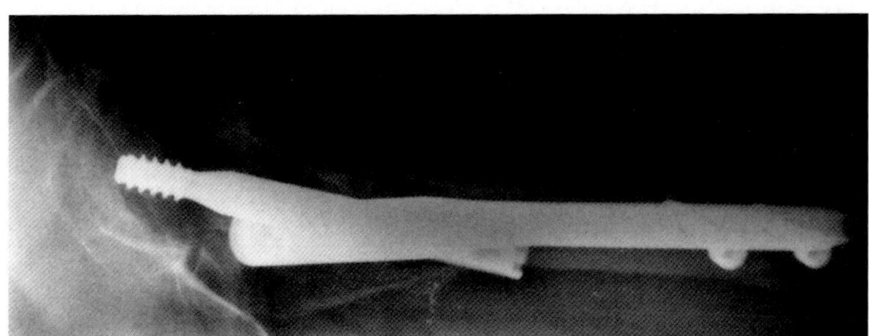

D

Fig. 4-48 (*Continued*)

## Suggested Reading

Bedi A, Le TT. Subtrochanteric fractures of the femur. *Orthop Clin North Am*. 2004;35:473–483.

Boyd AD, Wilber JH. Patterns and complications of femur fractures below the hip in patients over 65 years of age. *J Orthop Trauma*. 1992;6:167–174.

Larrson S, Friberg S, Hansson LI. Trochanteric fractures. Mobility, complications and management of 607 cases treated with sliding screw technique. *Clin Orthop*. 1990;260:232–241.

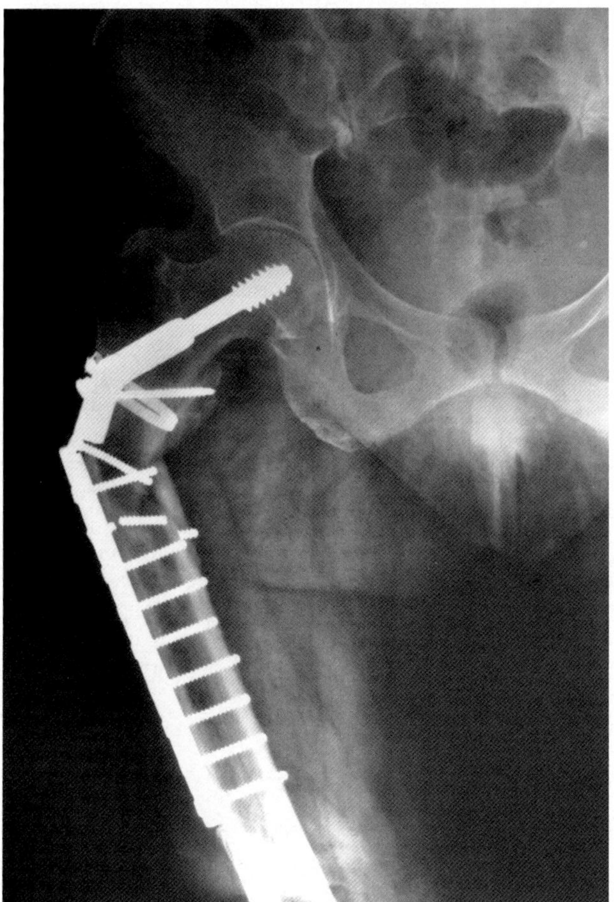

Fig. 4-49 Subtrochanteric fracture internally fixed with dynamic hip screw and long side plate. The fixation plate has fractured with varus deformity at the fracture site.

### Complications

Complications associated with trochanteric and subtrochanteric fractures may be related to the injury or fixation method used. Common complications include loss of fixation, which occurs in 15% to 20% (Figs. 4-47 and 4-49). This is particularly common

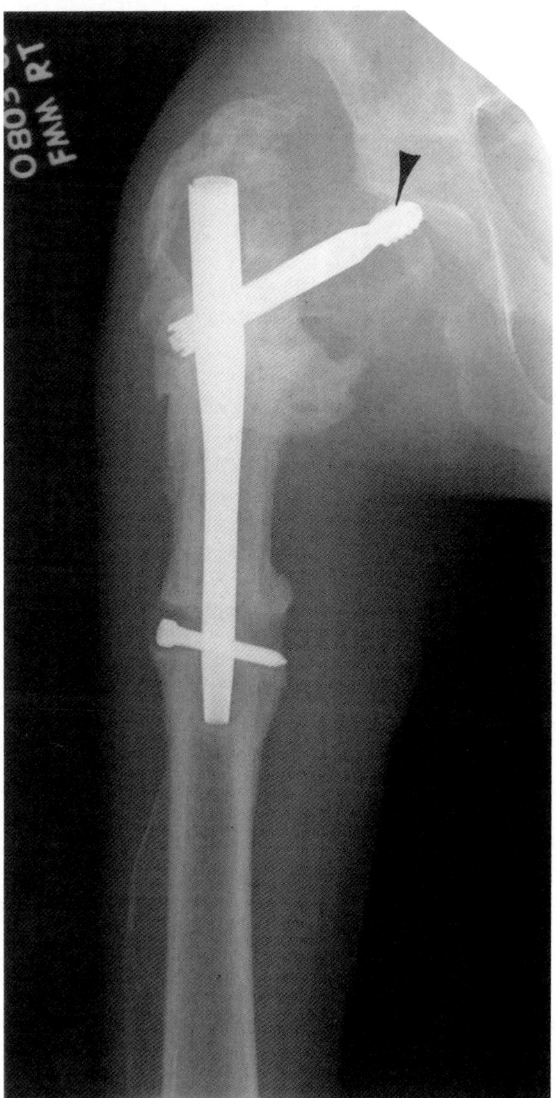


Fig. 4-50 Failed fixation with short intramedullary locking nail. There is breakthrough and avascular necrosis of the femoral head (*arrowhead*) and obvious loosening about the locking screw.

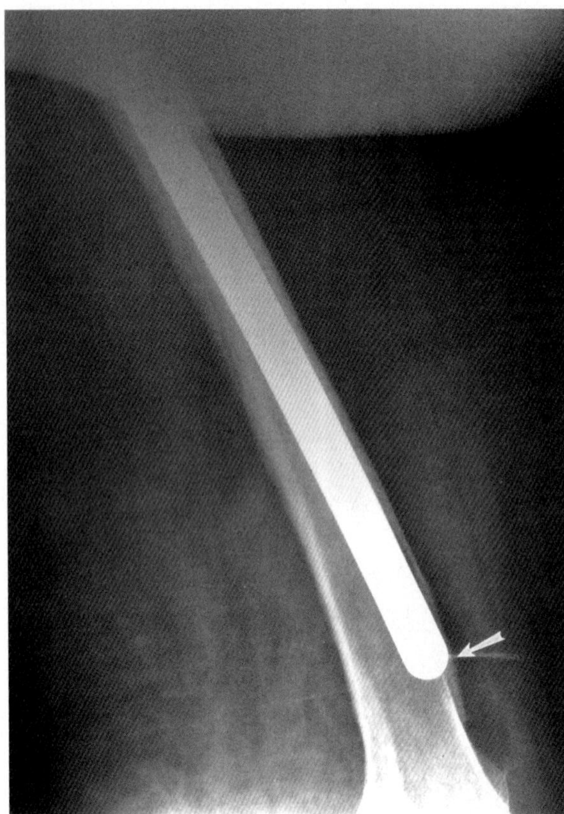

Fig. 4-51 Lateral radiograph of the distal femur demonstrating breakthrough of the anterior cortex (*arrow*) by a long intramedullary nail.

with unstable fracture patterns and is usually characterized by progressive varus collapse. Depending on the patient status, this may be accepted, revised, or hip arthroplasty may be performed. Serial radiographs are usually diagnostic.

Delayed union or nonunion are more common with subtrochanteric fractures but also occur with other unstable fracture patterns. Diagnosis of nonunion can be made confidently at 6 months in patients with pain, loss of fixation, abnormal callus, and persistent fracture line. CT is preferred to evaluate union and the status of callus organization.

Additional complications include hardware failure (see Fig. 4-50) and periprosthetic fractures. The latter are most common with short large-diameter intramedullary nails. Long intramedullary nails may erode through the anterior femoral cortex at the distal tip (see Fig. 4-51). Again, serial radiographs provide the needed information to evaluate these complications.

AVN is rare with trochanteric fractures. Laceration of the superficial femoral artery can occur with displaced lesser trochanteric fractures.

## Suggested Reading

Beaty JH. Fractures of the hip in children. *Orthop Clin North Am*. 2006;37:223–232.

Bedi A, Le TT. Subtrochanteric femur fractures. *Orthop Clin North Am*. 2004;35:473–483.

Haidukewych GJ, Berry DJ. Hip arthroplasty for salvage of failed treatment of intertrochanteric hip fractures. *J Bone Joint Surg*. 2003;85A:899–904.

# Hip Arthroplasty

Hip arthroplasty procedures have progressed dramatically in the last 30 years providing valuable data for development of joint replacements in other articulations. Approximately 200,000 total hip replacements, 100,000 partial replacements, and 36,000 revision hip arthroplasties are performed each year. Sixty percent of patients are older than 65 years at the time of the initial hip replacement procedure. This section will focus on patient selection, indications, implant options, and pre- and postoperative imaging for patient selection and evaluation of potential complications.

## Patient Selection

Hip replacement arthroplasty is an elective procedure that is most frequently performed on patients older than 60 years. Modifications or bone preservation procedures may be performed on younger patients in certain situations. Patient selection is based on clinical evaluation, image features, and careful evaluation of risk versus benefits of the procedure. Up to 75% of patients have at least one associated disease process that increases comorbidity. Advanced age and comorbidities are associated with inferior outcomes and increased postoperative complications. Active infection, paralysis, and significant neuromuscular dysfunction are contraindications for joint replacement.

The goals of hip replacement procedures are to improve function and activity and reduce pain. The most common indications are osteoarthritis, rheumatoid arthritis, AVN, and congenital or post-traumatic deformities. Certain neoplasms may also be managed in this manner. Patients older than 65 years are considered for joint replacement when pain interferes with activity or sleep and has not improved after appropriate trials of conservative treatment. Younger patients are usually given a longer period of conservative therapy or considered for bone-preserving approaches, such as resurfacing procedures or osteotomy. Implant survival rates are significantly higher for replacement procedures in older patients.

Clinical scoring systems are used in addition to image features to assist with decision making and compare postarthroplasty improvement with the baseline data. The Harris Hip Score is a commonly used clinical system. Patients with severe pain are given $<10$ points. Functional categories include stair climbing, walking, daily activities, and need for support (cane or crutches).

| HARRIS HIP SCORE | |
|---|---|
| Pain | 0–44 points |
| Function | 0–47 points |
| Deformity | 0–4 points |
| Range of motion | 0–5 points |

## Suggested Reading

Berquist TH. Imaging of joint replacement procedures. *Radiol Clin North Am.* 2006;44:419–437.

Soderman P, Malchau H. Is the Harris Hip Score system useful to study outcomes of total hip replacement. *Clin Orthop.* 2001;384:189–197.

Zhan C, Kaczmarek R, Loyo-Berrios N, et al. Incidence and short-term outcomes of primary and revision hip replacement in the United States. *J Bone Joint Surg Am.* 2007:89:526–533.

## Preoperative Imaging

Standard radiographs include an AP view of the pelvis and AP and lateral views of the hip and upper femur with magnification markers on each image. This allows use of electronic or hard copy templates (see Fig. 4-52) to accurately measure component size before selection and insertion of components. The length of femur included in the image may have to be increased in the case of prior surgery or fracture. The patient should be positioned with the patellae anterior and toes touching on the AP views to assure consistency in the position of the femoral head and neck. Radiographs should be evaluated for multiple features.

### Radiographic assessment

- Bone stock
- Diffuse idiopathic skeletal hyperostosis (DISH)
- Previous surgery
- Calcar deficiency
- Trochanteric abnormalities
- Femoral canal
- Acetabulum

### Radiographic measurements

Ischial tuberosity line: leg length discrepancy, baseline for acetabular angle (see Fig. 4-53)

Ilioischial line (Koler): acetabular protrusio (Fig. 4-53)

Acetabular angle: femoral head coverage (Fig. 4-53)

Femoral neck angle: normal 135 degrees (see Fig. 4-54)

Femoral offset: perpendicular distance from the center of the femoral head to a line along the center of the femoral shaft (Fig. 4-54)

Additional studies may be required in certain situations. In patients who have undergone prior surgery, especially in the acetabulum, or when revision procedures are indicated, CT is useful to evaluate bone stock and osteolysis (see Fig. 4-55). MRI may be indicated in younger patients to evaluate articular cartilage or AVN. In some cases, preoperative diagnostic anesthetic injections of the hip, facets, and sacroiliac joints may be warranted to confirm the source of pain.

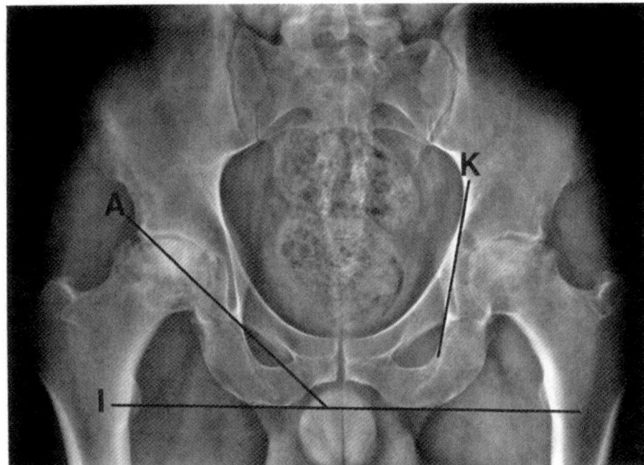


Fig. 4-53 Anteroposterior (AP) radiograph demonstrating bilateral stage IV avascular necrosis. Preoperative measurements made on this image include *I*—ischial tuberosity line drawn along the ischial margins; the intersection of the lesser trochanters indicates slight limb length discrepancy. *K*—Kohler (ilioischial) line; demonstrates no protrusion. *A*—acetabular angle formed by a line along the margins intersecting the ischial tuberosity line.

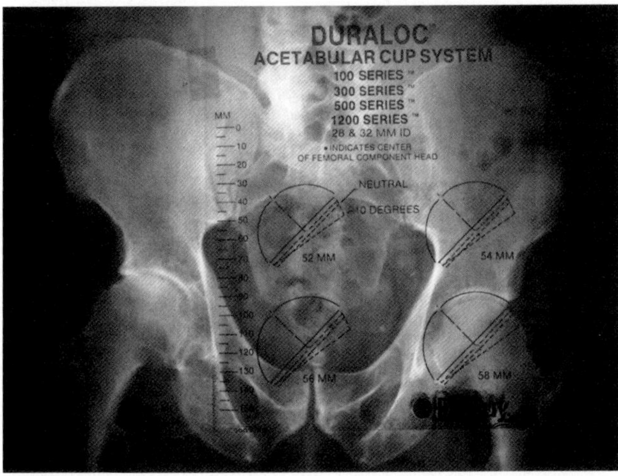


Fig. 4-52 Anteroposterior (AP) radiograph with acetabular templates in place for selection of the appropriate component size.

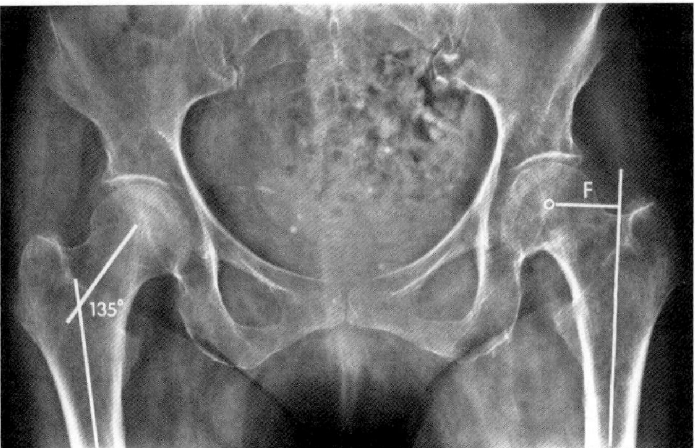


Fig. 4-54 Anteroposterior (AP) radiograph demonstrating the normal femoral neck angle (135 degrees) on the right and femoral offset measured by the distance from the center of the femoral head to a line along the shaft (*F*).

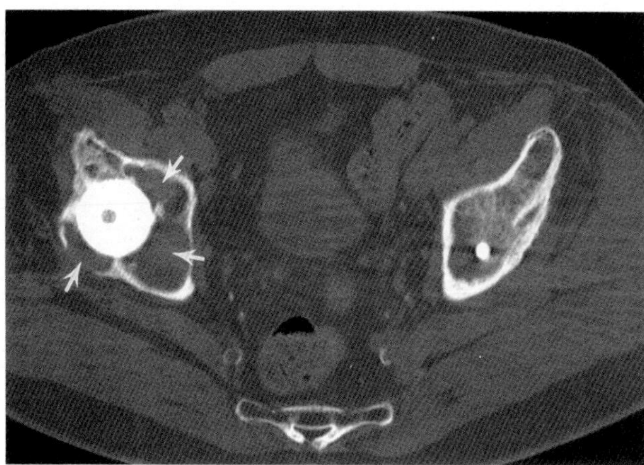

Fig. 4-55 Axial computed tomographic (CT) image obtained before revision hip replacement demonstrating extensive acetabular osteolysis (*arrows*).

## Suggested Reading

Berquist TH. Imaging of joint replacement procedures. *Radiol Clin North Am*. 2006;44:418–437.

Berquist TH, Lewallen DG, McComb BL. The pelvis and hips. In: Berquist TH, ed. *Imaging atlas of orthopaedic appliances and prostheses*. New York: Raven Press; 1995:217–352.

### Component Selection

Hip prostheses have evolved considerably over the years. There are numerous configurations for total or partial replacement procedures. Components are configured from metal alloys, ultra–high molecular weight polyethylene (UHMWPE), and ceramic materials. Components are designed to provide low friction, strength, and minimal local and systemic effects. Ceramic components have smooth hard surfaces to facilitate smooth articulation (see Fig. 4-56). These components are selectively used in younger patients in whom long-term wear is a greater concern. Currently, most components are modular to allow flexibility in head size, acetabular structure, and femoral stem design. Components are designed to be used with or without cement (press fit or ingrowth). Components designed for bone ingrowth have different types of coating including hydroxyapatite or calcium phosphate (see Fig. 4-57).

The choice of implant depends on indications, anatomy, bone stock, patient age, weight, activity, and, of course, the surgeon's preference. Unipolar, resurfacing, bipolar, and total joint replacement systems may be selected.

**Unipolar:** Unipolar implants consist of either a femoral stem with fixed head or modular head with no acetabular component (see Fig. 4-58). These implants are used in patients with hip, femoral neck, or head fractures with normal acetabulae. Over time, articular cartilage wears down resulting in osteoarthritic changes.

**Bipolar implants:** Bipolar implants have a cup over the femoral head. However, the cup is not attached to the acetabulum and typically covers more of the head than acetabular components used in total joint replacement (see Fig. 4-59). This allows motion of the cup on the head and also against the acetabulum, which over time wears down the acetabular cartilage. Bipolar implants are commonly used in patients with AVN and normal acetabular cartilage and in patients with Garden III and IV femoral neck fractures. Implants have been reported to survive up to 15 years.

**Resurfacing implants:** Resurfacing arthroplasty is primarily designed for bone preservation in younger patients. The femoral head and acetabulum may be resurfaced (see Fig. 4-60). Resurfacing of the femoral head alone may be used in patients with AVN or other femoral head abnormalities and a normal acetabulum. The femoral neck and canal are preserved for later revision. The resurfaced head is also more similar to the native

A

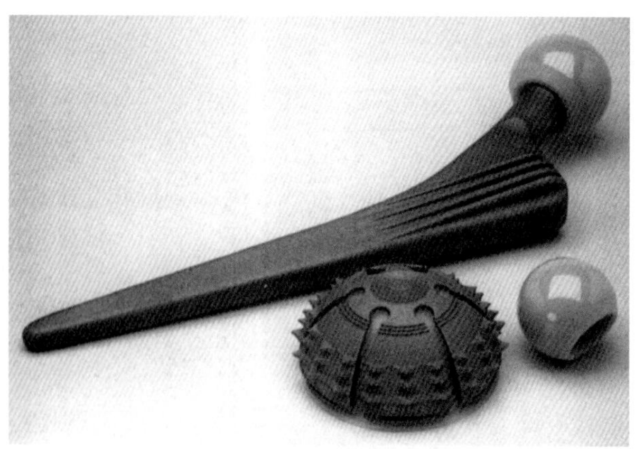

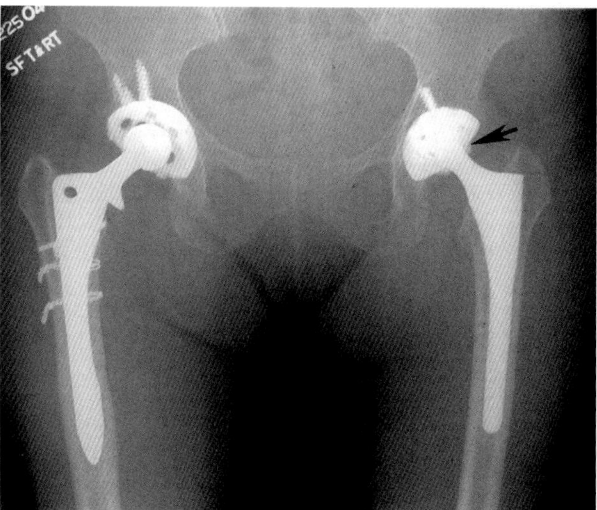



B

Fig. 4-56 A: Total joint replacement system with titanium alloy acetabular and femoral components and a ceramic head. (Courtesy of Protek AG, Berne, Switzerland.) B: Anteroposterior (AP) radiograph of bilateral uncemented total joint replacements with a metal modular head on the right and a lower density ceramic head on the left (*arrow*).

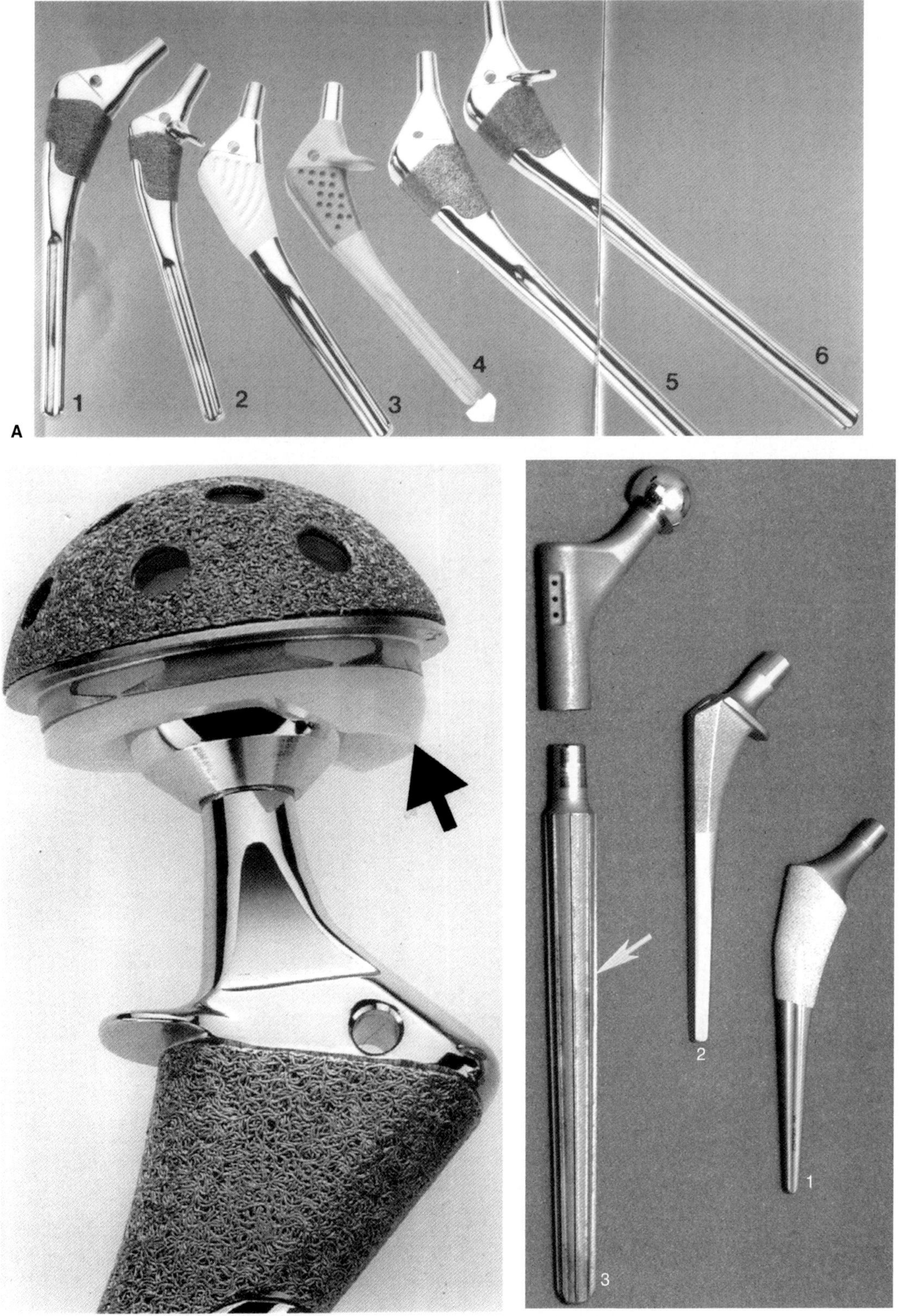


Fig. 4-57 A: Femoral components. *1*—Anatomic porous coated with no collar; *2* —similar to *1*, but with a collar; *3*— no collar with hydroxyapatite proximal surface; *4*—polymethyl methacrylate proximal surface with distal centralizer; *5*—anatomic with long stem; *6*—anatomic with long stem and collar. B: Porous-coated proximal femoral component and acetabular cup with augmented (*arrow*) polyethylene liner. (Courtesy of Zimmer, Warsaw, Indiana.) C: Conventional femoral components (*1* and *2*) with different proximal coatings and revision system with modular insert (*arrow*, *3*). (Courtesy of Stryker Orthopaedics, Mahwah, New Jersey.)

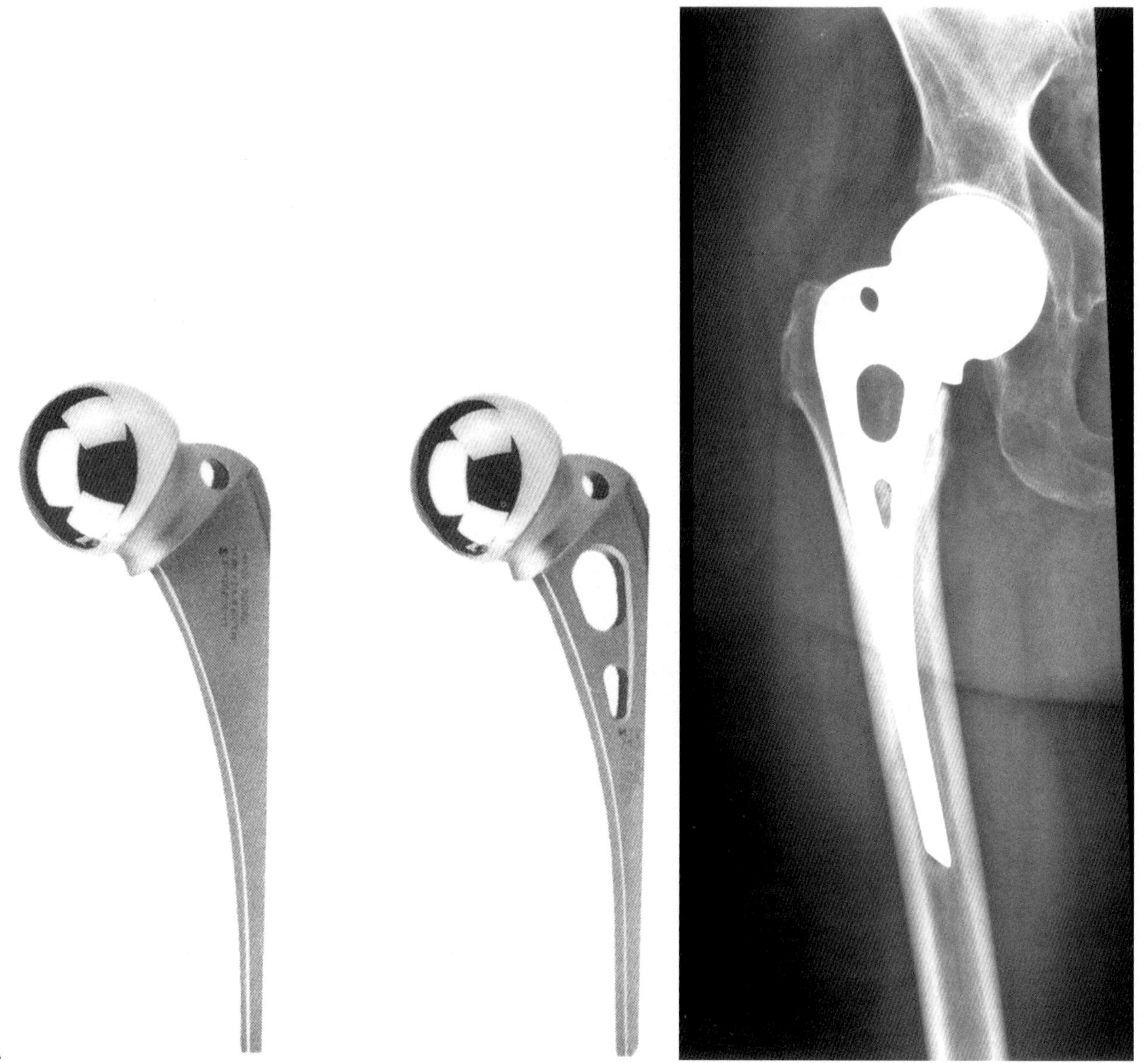


Fig. 4-58 A: Moore unipolar prostheses with solid (*left*) and fenestrated (*right*) stems. Components of cobalt-chromium-molybdenum alloys. (Courtesy of Zimmer, Warsaw, Indiana.) B: Anteroposterior (AP) radiograph of a fenestrated Moore prosthesis.

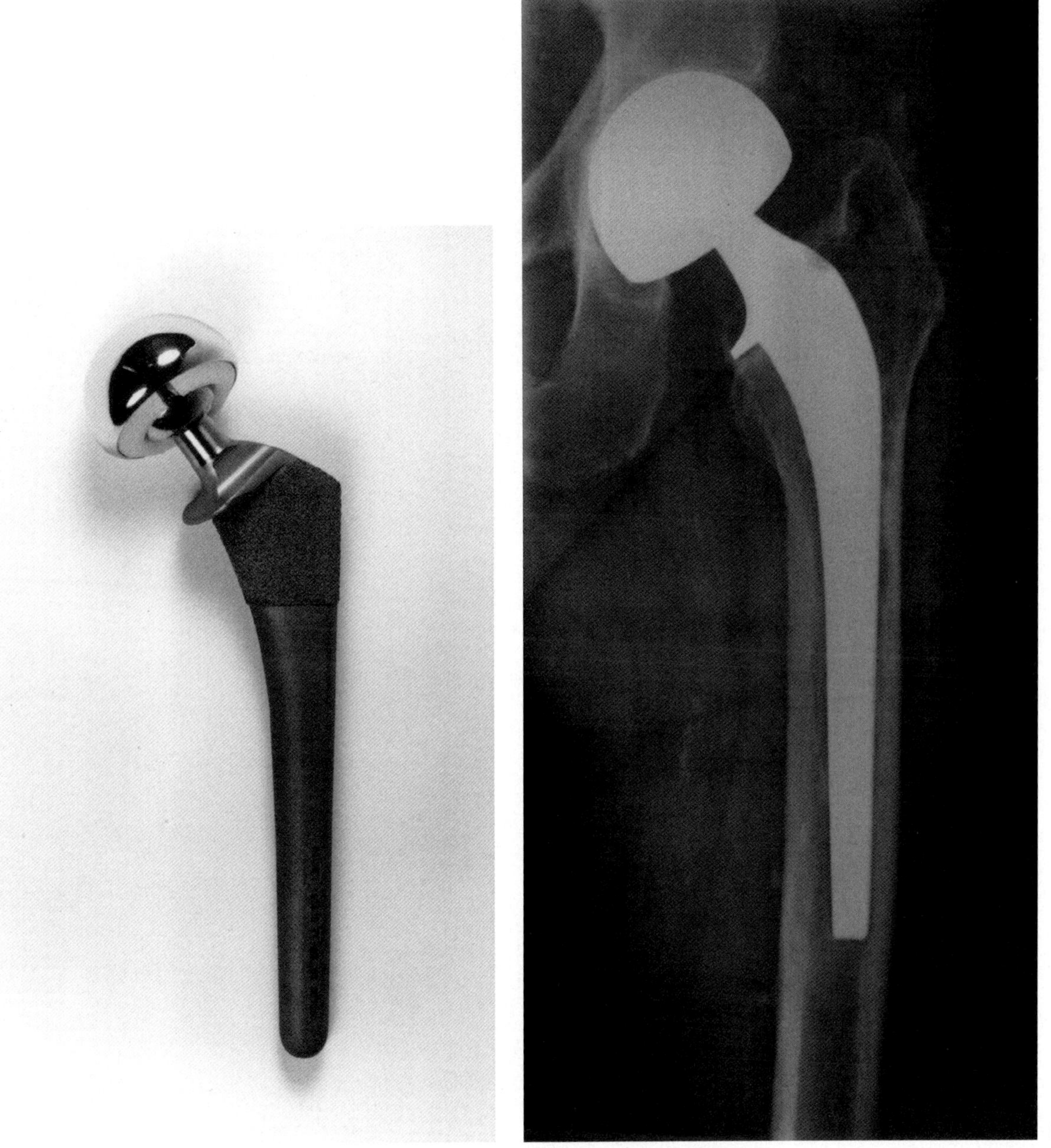


Fig. 4-59 A: Bipolar hip implants with porous-coated proximal femoral stem. (Courtesy of Biomet, Warsaw, Indiana.) B: Radiograph of a bipolar hip implant. Note there are no acetabular screws, no cement, and the cup covers more of the femoral head than a total joint replacement (compare Fig. 4-56B).

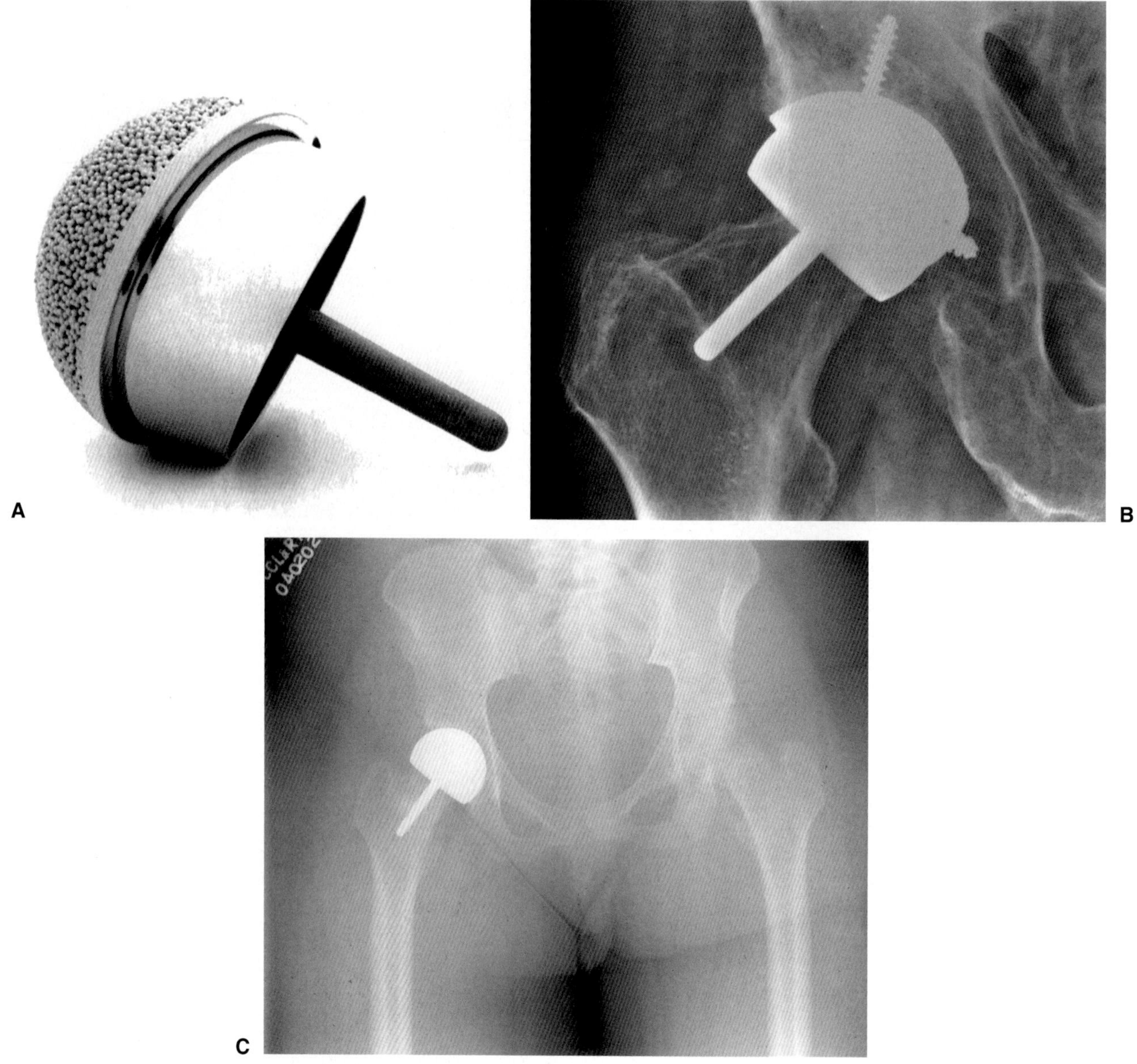

Fig. 4-60 Resurfacing hip arthroplasty. A: Illustration of a Birmingham Hip System with porous-coated acetabular component. (Courtesy of Smith and Nephew, Memphis, Tennessee.) Radiographs of different uncemented femoral and acetabular resurfacing implants (B) and a femoral head (C) resurfacing implant.

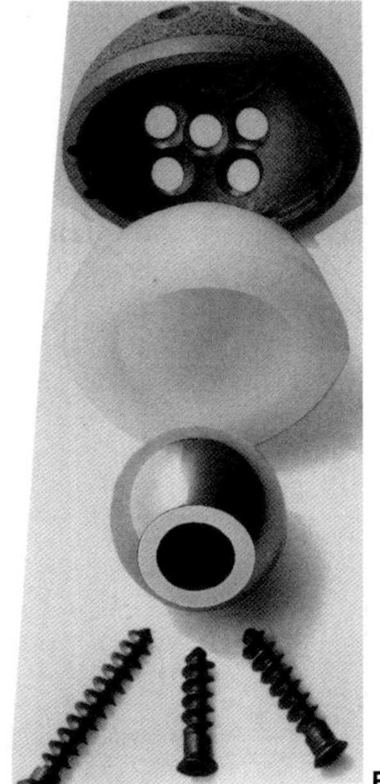

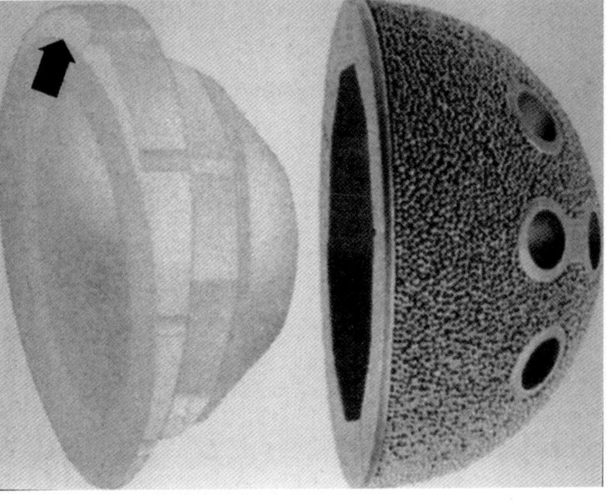

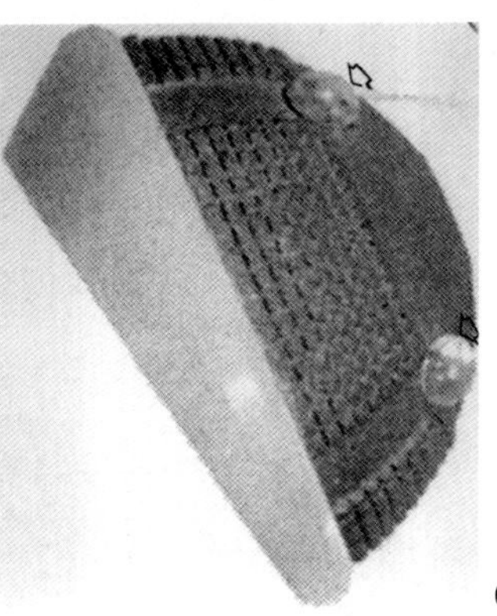

Fig. 4-61 Acetabular components. A: Titanium acetabular cup with polyethylene liner, modular head, and anchor screws. B: Porous-coated acetabular cup with polyethylene liner with exaggerated upper margin (*arrow*). (Courtesy Stryker, Howmedica, Osteonics, Allendale, New Jersey.) C: Acetabular cup with polyethylene spacers (*open arrows*) designed to be used with cement and spacers provide more uniform cement technique.

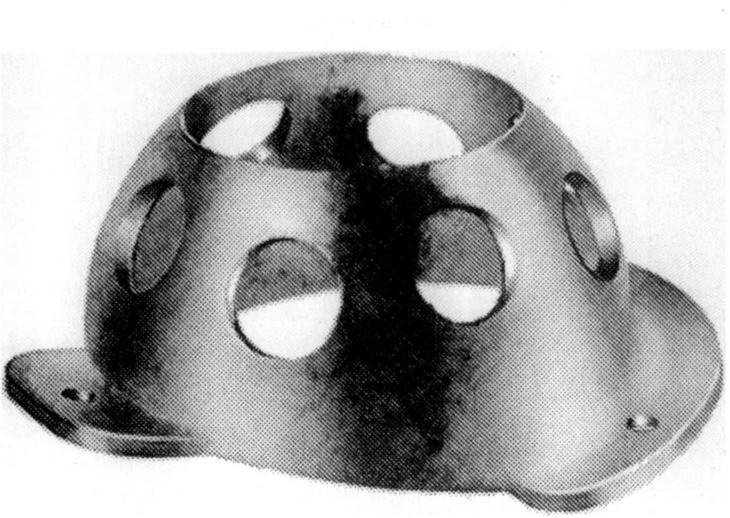

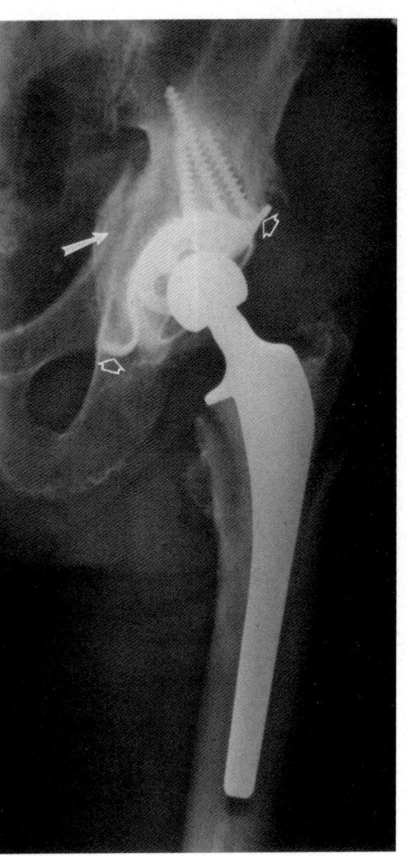

Fig. 4-62 Protrusio shell. A: Protrusio shell for acetabular reinforcement. B: Radiograph demonstrating an old acetabular fracture with bone graft (*arrow*). The acetabular component is placed in the protrusio shell (*open arrows*).

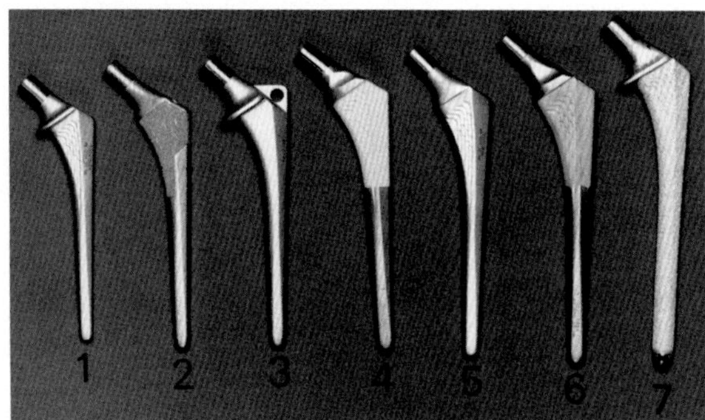


Fig. 4-63 Seven different femoral components with (*1, 3, 7*) and without collars (*2, 4, 5, 6*) and with differing segments and types of porous coating. (Courtesy of Stryker, Howmedica, Osteonics, Allendale, New Jersey.)

femoral head, thereby reducing the incidence of dislocation compared to total joint replacement. Both surfaces can also be replaced. However, there tend to be more problems with wear debris.

**Total joint replacement:** Total joint replacement involves placing femoral and acetabular components. The acetabular component may be press fit, cemented, or anchored with cancellous screws (see Fig. 4-61). Protrusio shells and other support devices may be required in patients with inadequate acetabular bone stock (see Fig. 4-62). Femoral components vary in length, may be selected with or without a collar, and can be positioned with or without cement (see Fig. 4-63). It is not uncommon to use cement with the femoral component and not the acetabular component (see Fig. 4-64). There are also special femoral designs for use in patients with bone deficiency in the proximal femur (see Fig. 4-65).

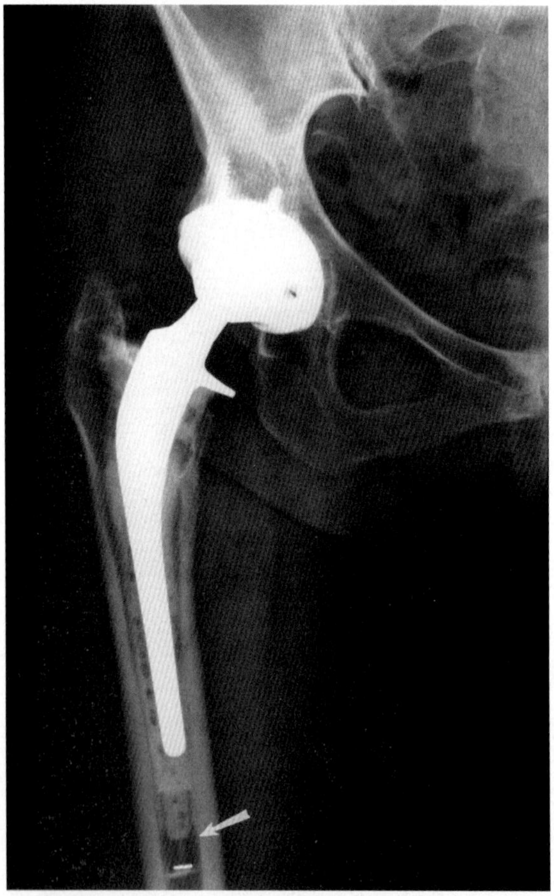

Fig. 4-64 Radiograph demonstrating a hybrid system with cemented femoral component and uncemented acetabular component. There is a cement restrictor distally (*arrow*) to assist in placing a uniform cement mantle about the component.

## Suggested Reading

Firestone DE, Callaghan JJ, Liu SS, et al. Total hip arthroplasty with cemented, polished, collared femoral stem and a cementless acetabular component. *J Bone Joint Surg.* 2007;89A:126–132.

Howie DW, McGee MA, Costi K, et al. Metal-on-metal resurfacing versus total hip replacement–the value of a randomized clinical trial. *Orthop Clin North Am.* 2005;36:195–201.

Lestrange NR. Bipolar arthroplasty for 496 hip fractures. *Clin Orthop.* 1990;251:7–19.

## Postoperative Imaging and Complications

It is essential to understand the normal appearance of hip implants in order to properly evaluate potential complications related to joint replacement procedures.

### Normal Radiographic Appearance

Regardless of the system implanted, there are basic positioning parameters and measurements that can serve as a baseline to follow up patients with hip implants. The femoral and acetabular components will be discussed separately.

**Normal femoral component:** Whether unipolar, bipolar, or part of a total joint replacement the position of the femoral component can be viewed similarly. The femoral component can be cemented or uncemented (ingrowth or press fit). The stem should be in neural or slight valgus position in relation to the femoral shaft. When placed in varus position (tip directed laterally) there is a predisposition to loosening (see Fig. 4-66). The femoral component can be divided into zones on the AP and lateral radiographs (see Fig. 4-67). This system is used to describe findings related to loosening or other complications. One should evaluate the component-bone (uncemented) or bone–cement and component–cement (cemented components) interfaces in each zone. A cement restrictor is used with cemented components to assist in providing a more uniform cement mantle around the component (Fig. 4-64). If an osteotomy is performed during implant placement, the greater trochanter is reattached using cerclage wires or a cable-claw system (see Fig. 4-68). Radiographs should include about 5 cm beyond the component tip for complete evaluation.

**Normal acetabular component:** The acetabular component is positioned such that it is angled approximately 45 degrees to the ischial tuberosity line on the AP radiograph (range 35 to 55 degrees) (see Fig. 4-69) and antiverted 10 to 20 degrees on the lateral radiograph (Fig. 4-67B). It is divided into three zones on the AP radiograph for evaluation purposes (Fig. 4-69). Baseline measurements are important in following potential complications related to the acetabular component. Also, the femoral head should be symmetrically positioned. Depth of the femoral head in the acetabular component may vary with the thickness of polyethylene liner and size of the modular head. Constrained liners may extend beyond the margin of

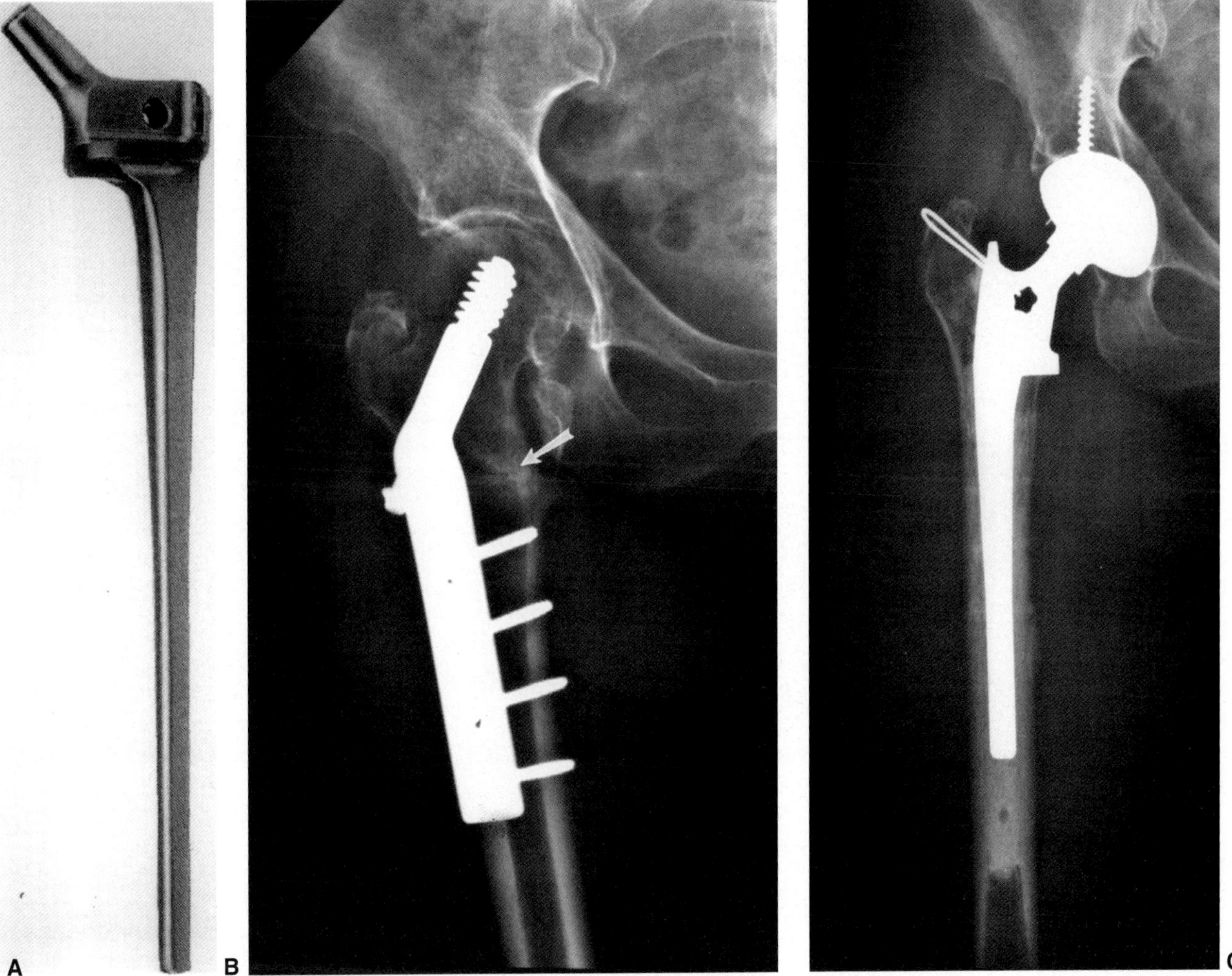

Fig. 4-65 Specific femoral stem designs. Photo (A) of a calcar replacement stem for medial bone loss. (A-Courtesy of Zimmer, Warsaw, Indiana.) B: Failed dynamic hip screw fixation of an intertrochanteric fracture. Radiograph shows sclerosis along the medial fracture line due to nonunion (*arrow*). C: The hip was revised using a cemented calcar femoral component and uncemented acetabular component. D: S-ROM femoral component with modular femoral sleeves designed for proximal femoral deficiency. (Courtesy Joint Medical Products, Stamford, Connecticut.) E: Radiograph of an S-ROM system.

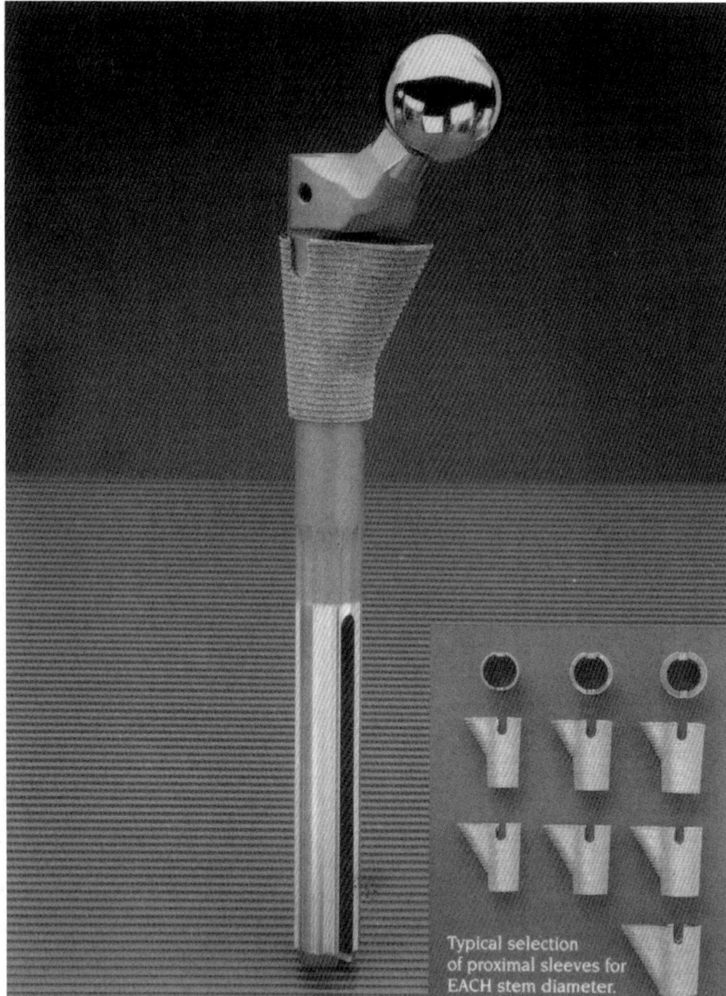


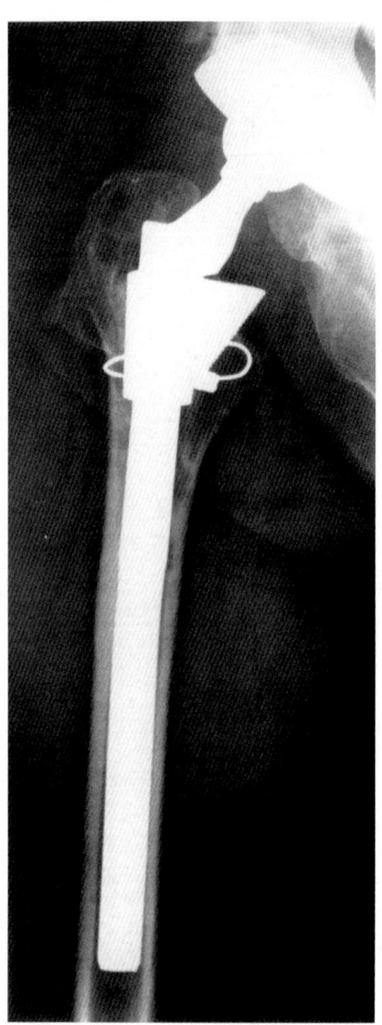


Fig. 4-65 *(Continued)*

the acetabular metal shell. In patients with unipolar or bipolar implants, there is no acetabular component. In this setting, the acetabular cartilage thickness (joint space) should be evaluated on follow-up images.

## Complications

Complications following hip arthroplasty can usually be evaluated with serial radiographs. Additional studies may be required in specific situations described in the following text (see Table 4-4). Although ultrasound and MRI have been used in some settings, these modalities are not frequently used for evaluation of joint replacement complications.

**Loosening:** Loosening is one of the most common complications following hip replacement. Loosening occurs in 6% to 18% of femoral components and 6% to 28% of acetabular components (see Fig. 4-70). It is the most common reason for revision surgery. Serial radiographs may be diagnostic. In more subtle cases, subtraction arthrograms may be useful for confirmation (see Fig. 4-71). Radionuclide studies and positron emission tomography (PET) may also be useful if performed >1 year after surgery.

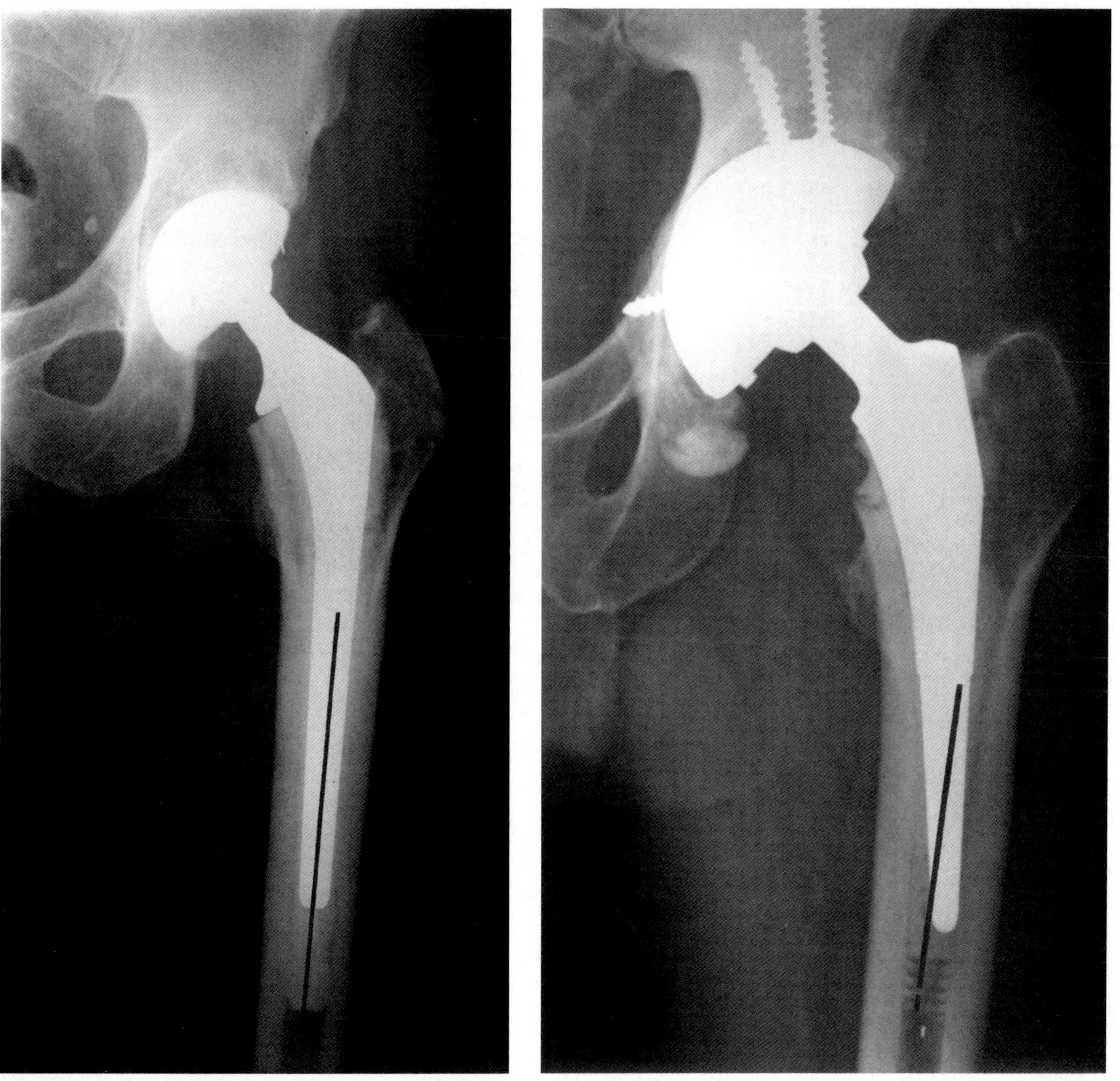


Fig. 4-66 Normal femoral component position. A: Cemented femoral component aligned with the femoral shaft (*line*). B: Cemented femoral component in slight varus position with the tip directed lateral to the line of the shaft.

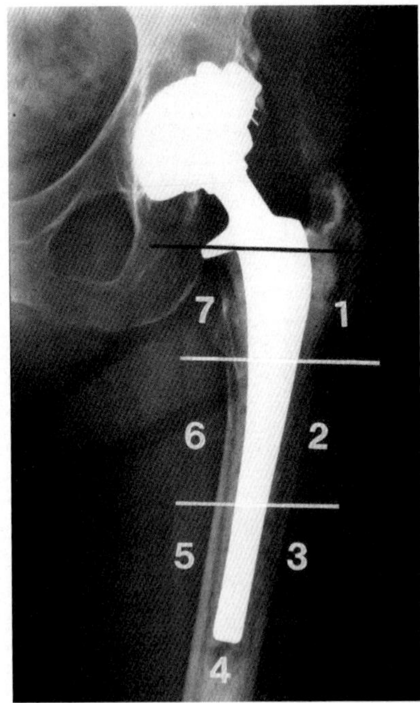


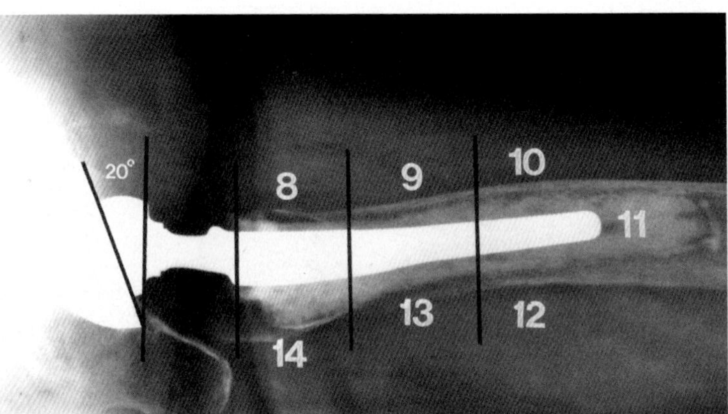


Fig. 4-67 Anteroposterior (AP) (A) and lateral (B) radiographs demonstrating the zones used to evaluate the femoral component. The acetabular component is usually anteverted approximately 20 degrees on the lateral view.

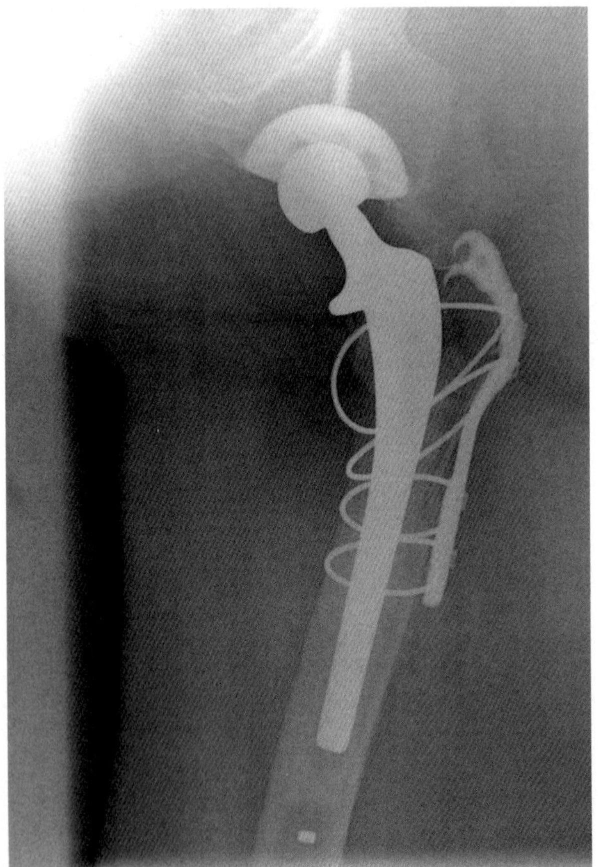

Fig. 4-68 Radiograph demonstrating a hip arthroplasty with a Zimmer cable-claw system for trochanteric fixation.

## Component Loosening

RADIOGRAPHIC FEATURES

### Femoral component cemented

Lucent zones at bone–cement or metal–cement interface >2 mm (see Fig. 4-72)

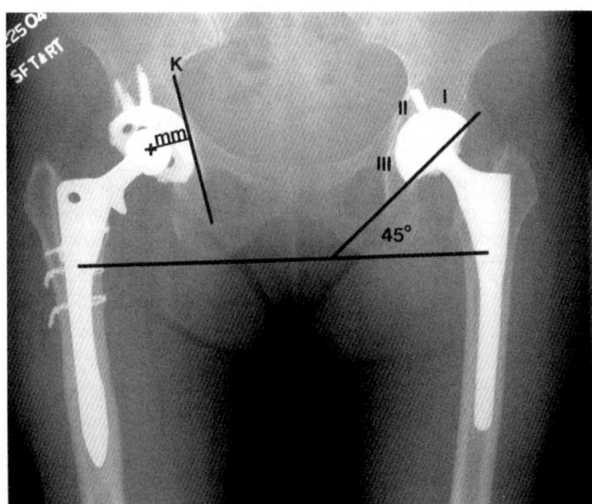


Fig. 4-69 Normal acetabular component features. There are three zones numbered lateral to medial (*I* to *III*). The acetabular component should be angled (ischial tuberosity line and a line along the component margin) approximately 45 degrees, range 35 to 55 degrees. Kohler line (*K*) can be used to measure medial migration of the femoral head or acetabulum by measuring a perpendicular distance (mm) to Kohler line from either margin, in this case the femoral head distance (+).

**Table 4-4**

**HIP REPLACEMENT COMPLICATIONS AND IMAGING APPROACHES**

| COMPLICATION (INCIDENCE %) | IMAGING APPROACHES |
|---|---|
| Loosening | |
| Acetabular (6–28) | Serial radiographs, CT, subtraction arthrography |
| Femoral (6–18) | |
| Deep Infection (2–3) | Serial radiographs, radionuclide scans PET, joint aspiration and arthrogram |
| Dislocation (3–7) | Serial radiographs |
| Osteolysis (5–9) | Serial radiographs, CT |
| Pseudobursae (43) | Subtraction arthrograms |
| Periprosthetic fractures (1–2) | Serial radiographs |
| Heterotopic ossification (8–90) | Serial radiographs, CT |

PET, positron emission tomography; CT, computed tomography.

Progressive widening or irregularity of lucent zone
Component migration, especially varus (Fig. 4-71)
Cement fracture (Fig. 4-72)
Stem fracture
Subsidence (see Fig. 4-73)

### Femoral component uncemented

Lucent zones at metal–bone interface >2 mm or progressing or new 1 mm lucency >2 years after surgery (see Fig. 4-74)
Progressive subsidence (Fig. 4-74)
Migration >2 degrees (Fig. 4-74)
Shedding of beads or porous coating material (see Fig. 4-75)

### Acetabular component cemented

Lucent zone >2 mm, especially in zone II (see Fig. 4-76 and also 4-71)
Progressive widening of lucent zones
Cement fracture (see Fig. 4-77)
Migration or acetabular protrusio (see Fig. 4-78)
Component fracture

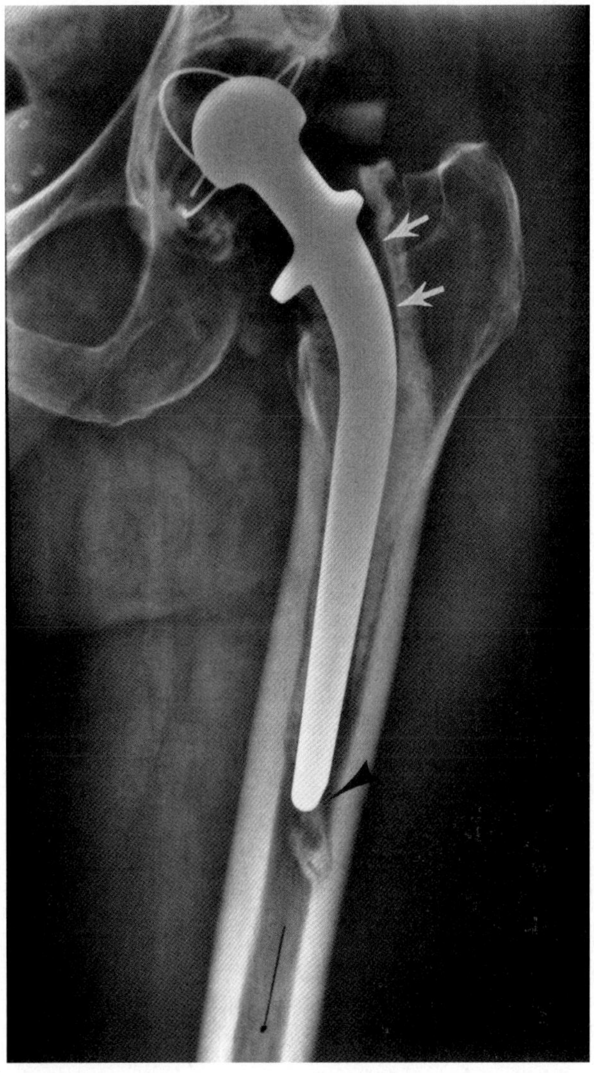

Fig. 4-70 Loosening of the femoral component in a patient with cemented implants. There is varus migration with a wide lucent zone (*arrows*) in zone 1 and lateral position of the tip of the stem with cement fracture (*arrowhead*).

### Acetabular component uncemented

Lucent zones >2 mm or progressing
Component migration (Fig. 4-78)
Bead or porous coating shedding

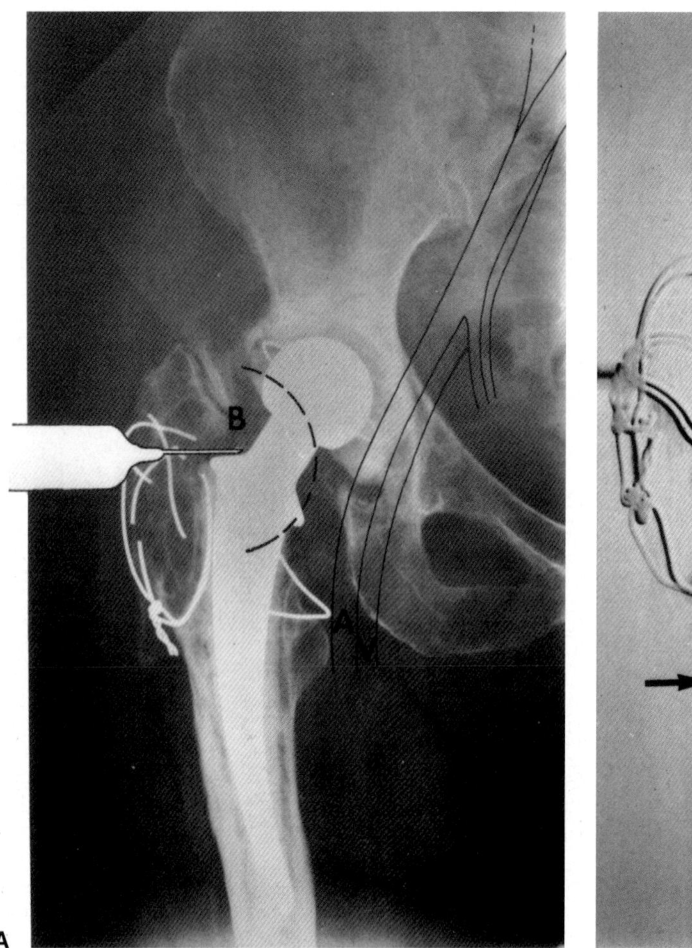


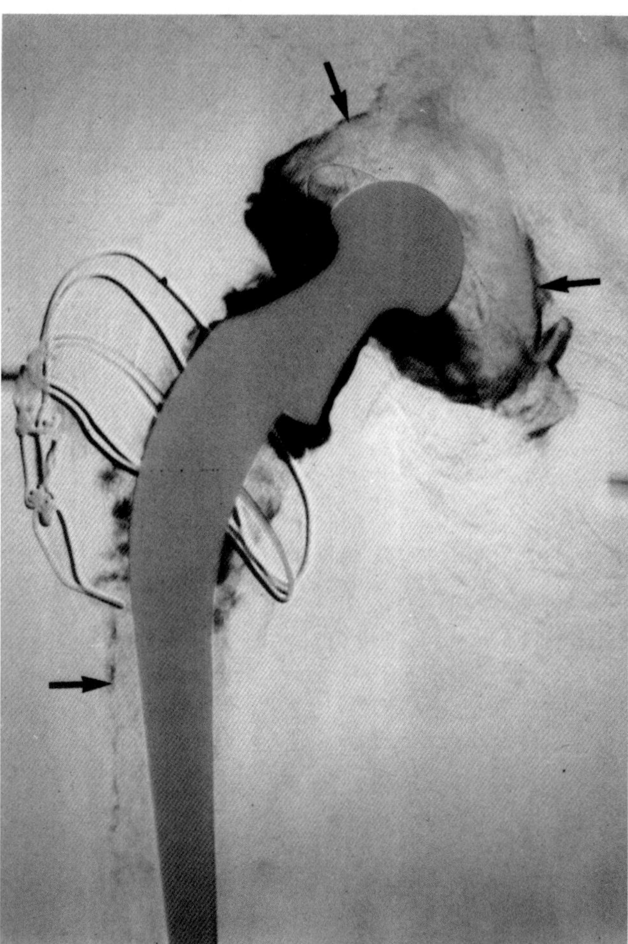

**Fig. 4-71** **A:** Illustration of the vascular anatomy and injection site for digital subtraction arthrography. Advantages of subtraction arthrography include anesthetic injection to confirm the source of pain, capsular anatomy can be defined, and fluid can be aspirated for culture. The injection should be continued until the joint is distended or lymphatic filling is noted. **B:** Subtraction arthrogram demonstrating contrast at the bone–cement interface (*arrow*) extending into zone III of the femoral component and in zones I and III of the acetabular component due to loosening of both components. Note the contrast at the interface is thick and irregular and clearly exceeds 2 mm.

**Infection:** Infection occurs in 2% to 3% of hip replacements. Signs of loosening are invariably present (Fig. 4-77). Osteolysis may also be evident. Features on serial radiographs may be helpful. However, subtraction arthrography, preceded by joint aspiration and culture, is very useful to identify the organism and image features are also useful. Localization of the organism is not always possible (28% to 92% accuracy). However, arthrographic demonstration of fistulae with irregular pseudocapsules and outpouchings is more common with infection compared to loosening alone (see Fig. 4-79). Radionuclide studies can be useful for confirming infection. Multiple approaches have been used including three-phase bone scans with Tc 99m MDP, technetium-labeled white blood cells, antigranulocyte antibody–labeled technetium, indium In 111–labeled white

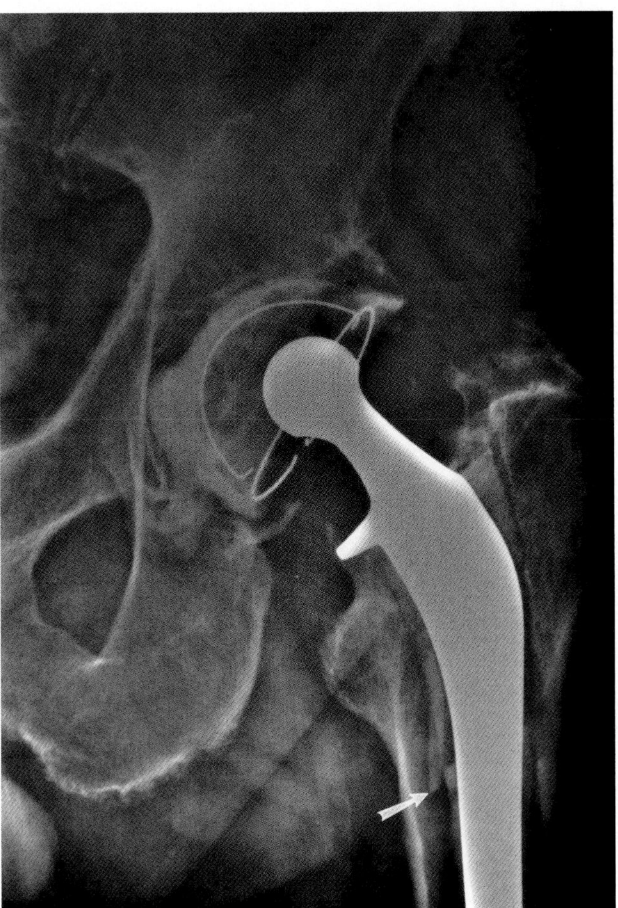

Fig. 4-72 Loose femoral component. Lucency at the bone–cement interface and cement fracture medially (*arrow*). There is also irregular lucency about the bone–cement interface of the acetabular component due to loosening.

blood cells, and more recently, F-18 fluorodeoxyglucose PET imaging. Technetium-labeled white blood cells disassociate at a rate of 5% to 7% per hour following injection. This results in significant unwanted background activity. PET studies report sensitivities of 92% and specificities in the 97% range (see Fig. 4-80). In 111-labeled white blood cells remain the gold standard in physician practice. Sensitivity ranges from 84% to 96% with specificity exceeding 96%.

Documented infection requires component removal and placement of temporary antibiotic impregnated implants before later revision surgery (see Fig. 4-81).

## Infection

### Radiographic features

- Signs of loosening (Fig. 4-77)
- Irregular lucency at bone–cement or metal–bone interfaces
- Osteolysis or areas of bone destruction
- Periosteal reaction

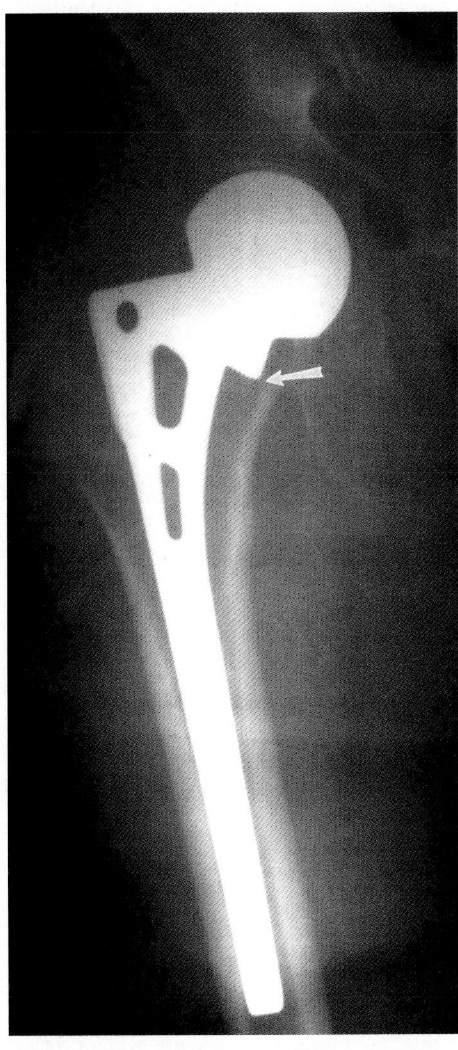


Fig. 4-73 Subsidence. Unipolar implant following placement (A) and 1 year later (B) demonstrating subsidence (*curved arrow*) with the component well below the calcar.

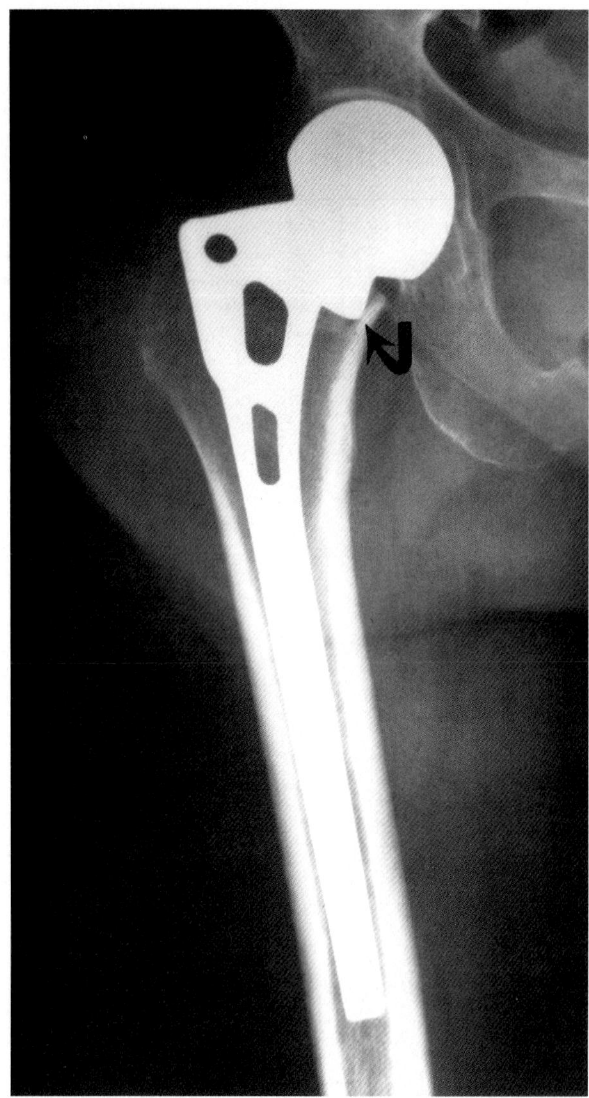


Fig. 4-73 *(Continued)*

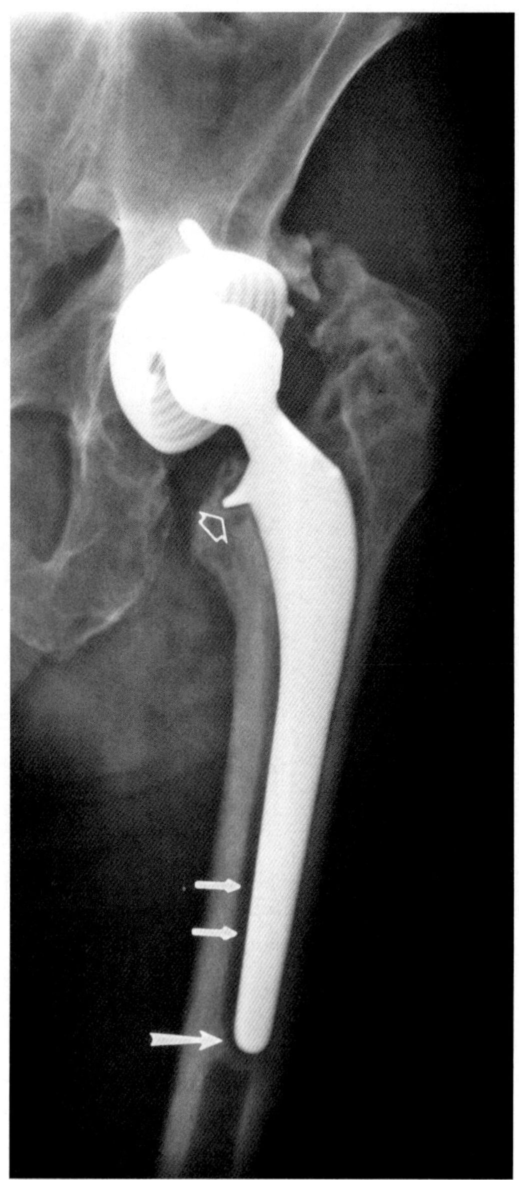

Fig. 4-74 Loose uncemented femoral component. Anteroposterior (AP) radiograph demonstrates lateral displacement of the femoral tip (*arrow*) with lucency along the distal stem (*small arrows*) and chronic subsidence (*open arrow*).

**Osteolysis:** Osteolysis occurs in 5% to 9% of patients. Geographic lucent areas, unlike lucent lines, develop about the components related to cement, metal, or polyethylene particles that induce a histiocytic inflammatory response (particle disease). Osteolysis is usually evident on radiographs. However, CT with coronal and sagittal reformatting is routinely performed to grade the extent of bone loss before revision surgery (see Fig. 4-82). Revision and bone grafting may be required depending on the extent of bone loss. Other image features of osteolysis include asymmetry of the femoral head due to polyethylene wear or liner dislocation (see Fig. 4-83), metal fragments (see Fig. 4-84), or cement fragments in the joint or about the components. Polyethylene wear is a slower progressive process compared to liner dislocation, which occurs more quickly on serial images and the degree of asymmetry in position of the femoral head is more dramatic with liner dislocation (Fig. 4-83).

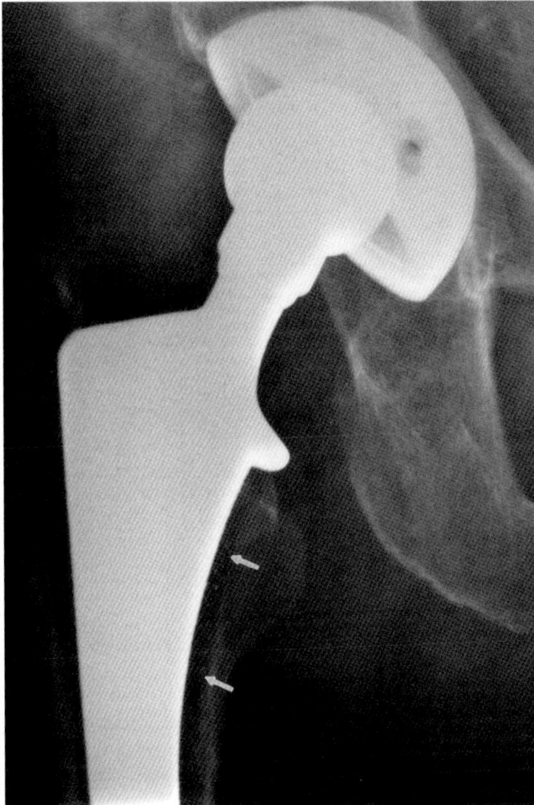

Fig. 4-75 Loose uncemented femoral component. Anteroposterior (AP) radiograph demonstrates multiple bead fragments medially (*arrows*) due to loosening.

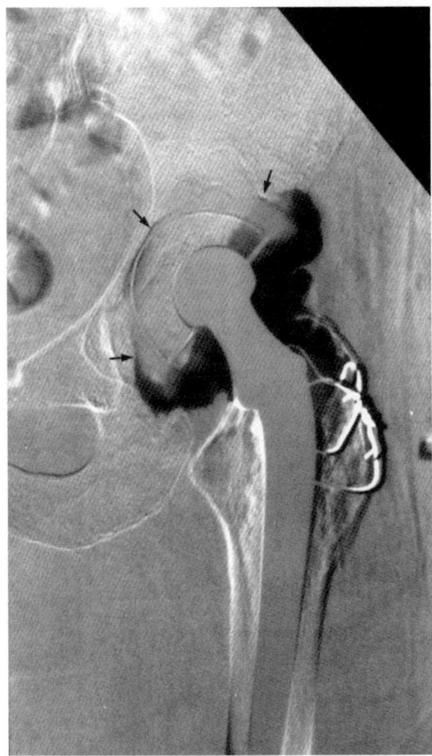

Fig. 4-76 Loose acetabular component. Subtraction arthrogram demonstrates contrast at the bone–cement interface in all three zones (*arrows*).

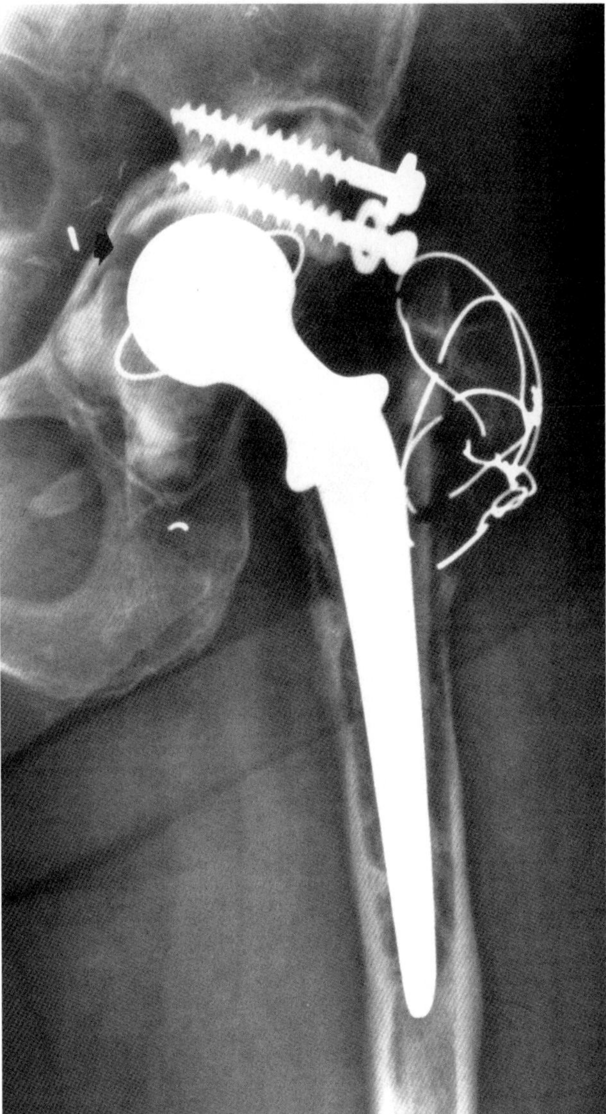

Fig. 4-77 Grossly loose acetabular component with cement fracture (*black arrow*). There is also irregular lucency about the femoral component due to loosening and infection.

**Pseudobursae:** Formation of pseudobursae or outpouchings from the pseudocapsule following joint replacement is common. Up to 43% of patients develop these bursae (see Fig. 4-85). Typical locations include the superior acetabular region, along the greater trochanter and lesser trochanter. These bursae may be painful, but have a smooth appearance unlike the more irregular outpouchings seen with infection. Diagnosis and definition is most easily accomplished with subtraction arthrography, although MRI, CT, or ultrasound can also demonstrate these fluid collections.

**Dislocations:** Dislocation of the femoral component occurs in 3% to 7% of patients. This is the second most common indication for revision arthroplasty. Most dislocations occur in the early postoperative period during the initial weight bearing. However, dislocations may also occur later. There are a number of situations that make patients more prone to dislocation. Dislocation is easily diagnosed on radiographs (see Fig. 4-86).

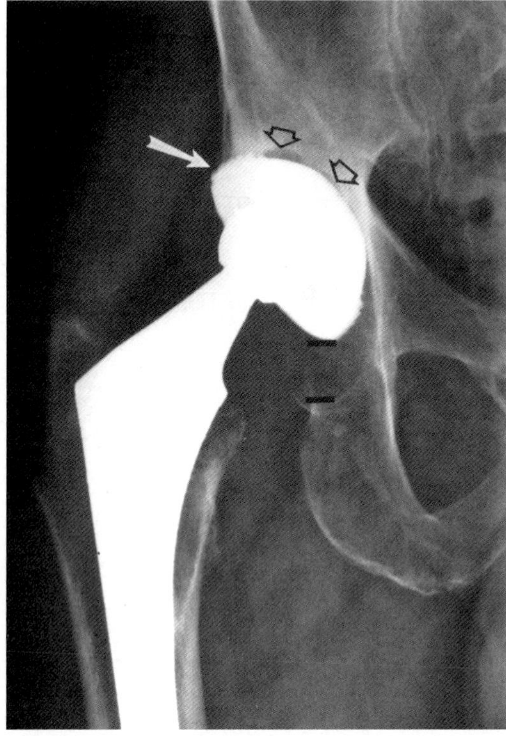

Fig. 4-78 Uncemented right hip arthroplasty. There is sclerosis and lucency (*open arrows*) about the acetabular component with superior migration (*arrow*) and the prior position noted with *black lines*.

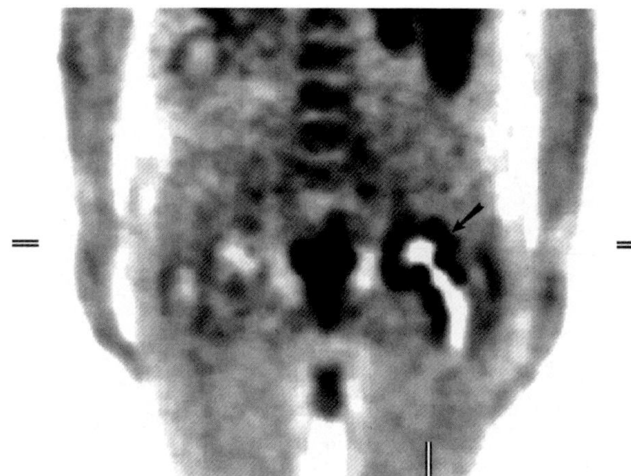

Fig. 4-80 Positron emission tomographic (PET) scan demonstrating increased uptake about the acetabular and proximal femoral components (*arrow*) in a patient with an infected hip arthroplasty.

## Femoral Head Dislocations

### Etiologic factors

- Smaller modular heads
- Posterior surgical approach
- Older patients
- Greater trochanteric avulsion
- Poor component position (see Fig. 4-87)

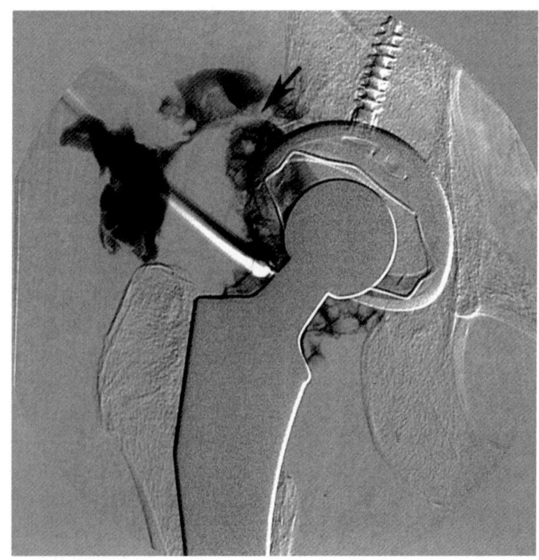



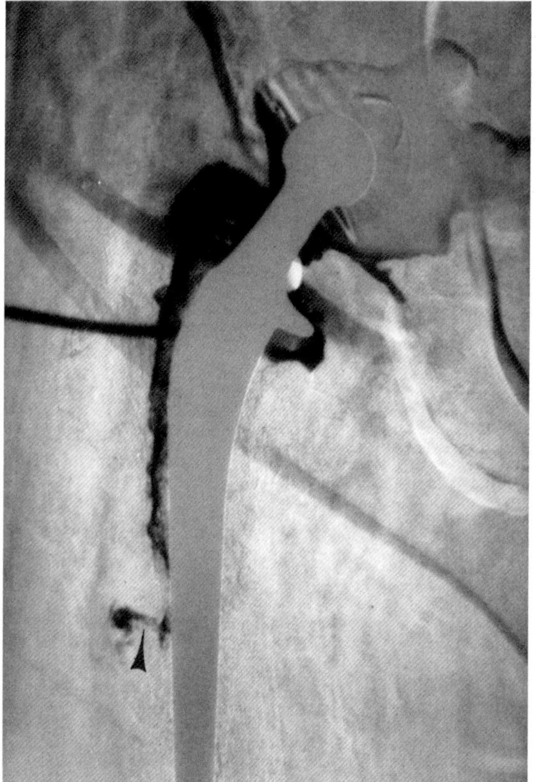



Fig. 4-79 Infection. Subtraction arthrograms on two different patients demonstrate a fistula from the acetabular margin (*arrow* in A) filling an irregular pocket laterally. B: Irregular contrast extending along the femoral component laterally with a distal fistula (*arrowhead*).

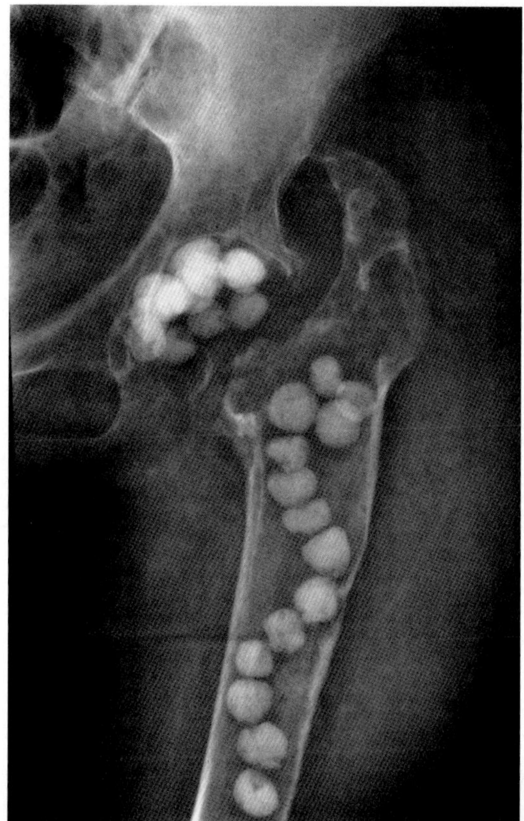

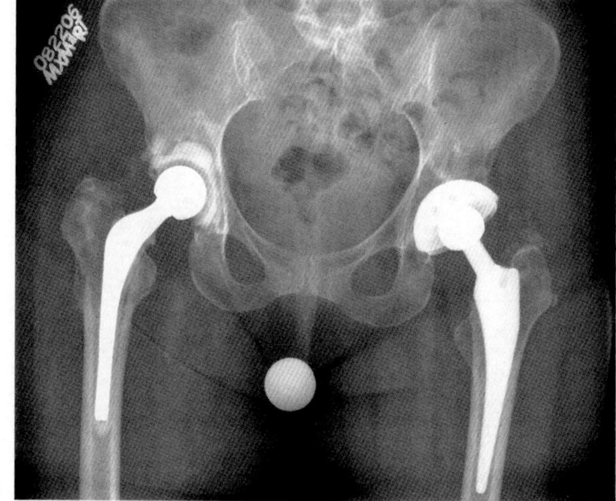

Fig. 4-81 Implant removal for infection. A: Girdlestone procedure with removal of the femoral and acetabular components and antibiotic methyl methacrylate beads placed in the medullary canal and joint to treat the infection. B: Infected right hip arthroplasty treated with a temporary PROSTOLAC (prosthesis with acrylate-loaded antibiotic cement) implant.

**Periprosthetic fractures:** Periprosthetic fractures are uncommon, occurring in 1% to 2% of patients. Fractures may occur during implant placement (see Fig. 4-88) or later in the course of follow-up. Delayed fractures are most common at the tip of the femoral component (see Fig. 4-89). Fractures that occur during surgery due to implant placement and reaming tend to involve the proximal femur (Fig. 4-88). Intraoperative fractures are more common with uncemented components (5%) and revision implants (7.8%).

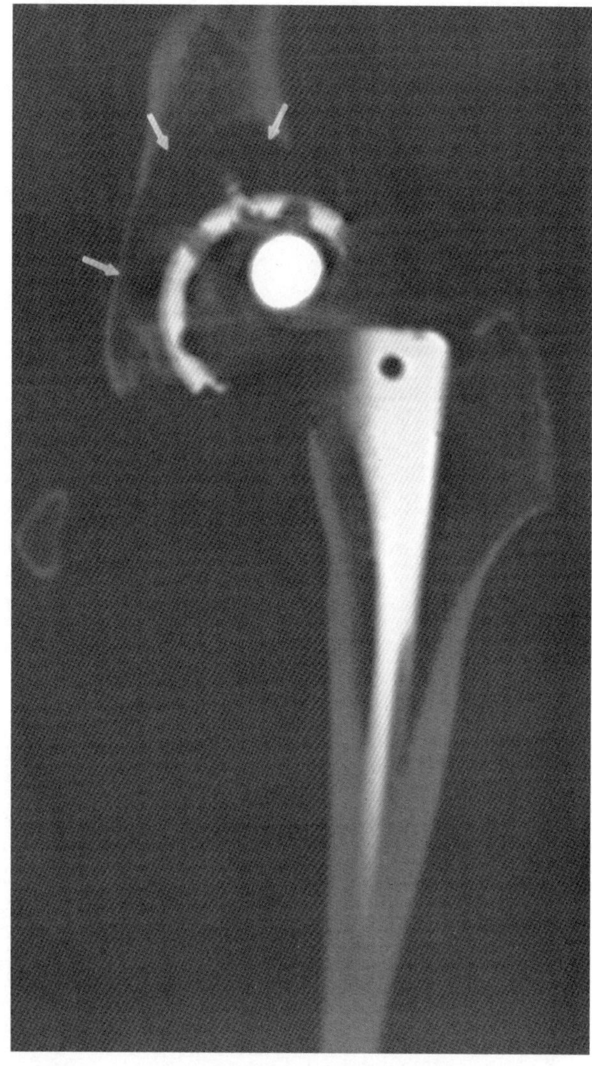

Fig. 4-82 Coronal (A) and sagittal (B) computed tomographic (CT) images demonstrate extensive acetabular osteolysis (*arrows*) with marked asymmetry in position of the femoral head due to polyethylene wear.

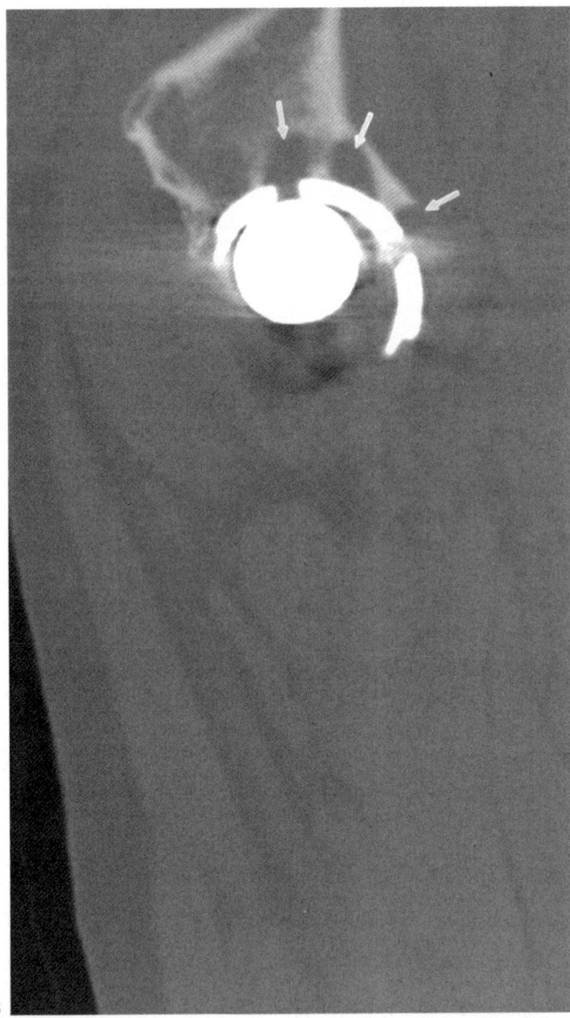

B

Fig. 4-82 *(Continued)*

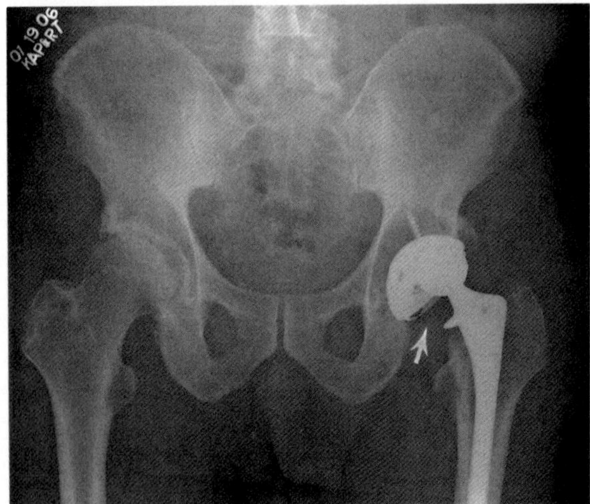

Fig. 4-83 Anteroposterior (AP) radiograph demonstrating marked displacement of the femoral head due to liner dislocation. The lucent liner can be seen inferiorly (*arrow*).

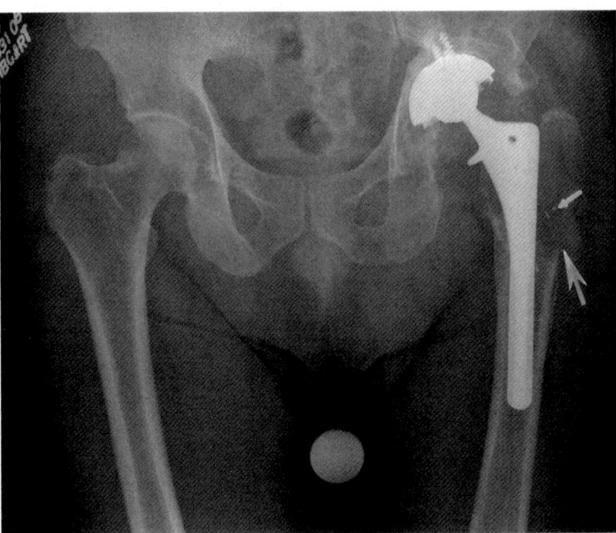

Fig. 4-84 Osteolysis with loosening of the femoral component and metal fragments from the porous-coated stem (*arrow*) laterally. There is also a pathologic fracture of the femur (*large white arrow*).

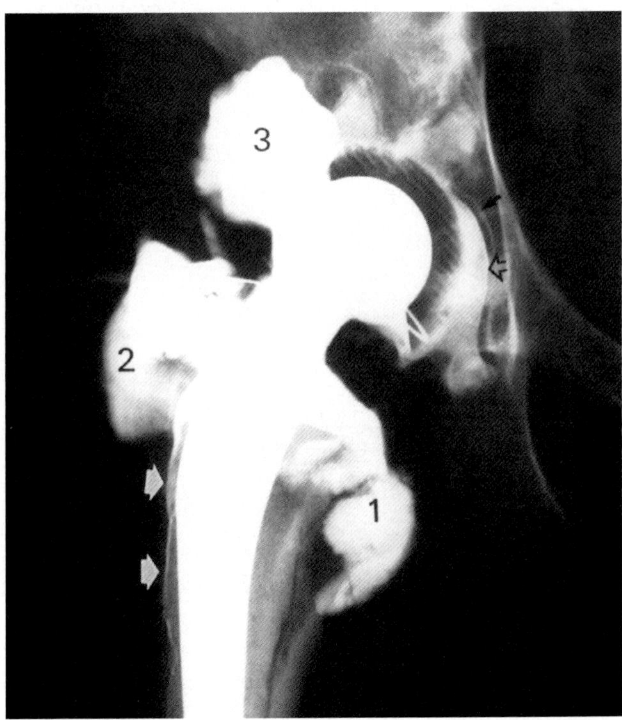


Fig. 4-85 Pseudobursae. Arthrogram demonstrating three pseudobursae at the lesser trochanter (*1*), greater trochanter (*2*), and acetabular margin (*3*). There is also contrast extending along the bone–cement interface of the femoral component (*large white arrows*) due to loosening. *Small black arrow* demonstrates contrast about zones II and III (*open arrow*) of the acetabular component due to loosening.

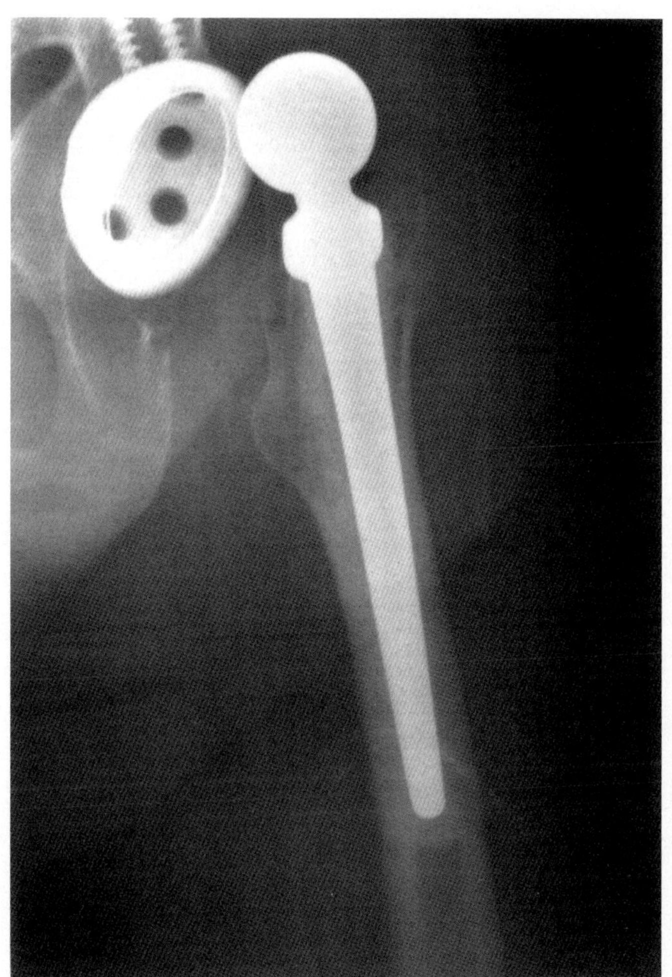


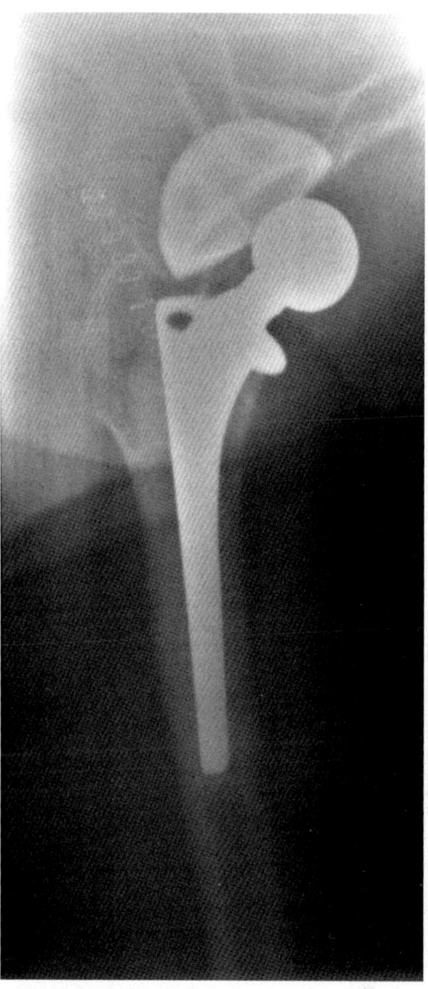


Fig. 4-86 Dislocation. Anteroposterior (AP) (A) and lateral (B) radiographs several days after weight bearing (note skin staples still present in B) demonstrating dislocation of the femoral component.

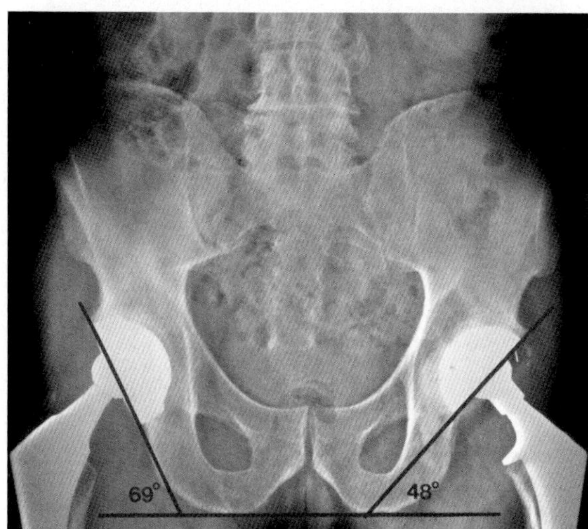


Fig. 4-87 Bilateral total joint replacements. The normal acetabular angle should be approximately 45 degrees (range 35 to 55 degrees). The component on the left is angled 48 degrees and the component on the right is too steeply angled at 69 degrees.

**Implant failure:** Implant failure may occur with the acetabular or femoral component. The acetabular liner may wear over time resulting in asymmetric position of the femoral head (Fig. 4-82). Liners may also dislocate, which results in more severe superior position of the femoral head occurring in a short period of time compared to wear (Fig. 4-83). Acetabular component fracture is unusual although fractures in the femoral stem do occur (see Fig. 4-90).

**Heterotopic ossification:** HO is common (8% to 90%) following joint replacement procedures (see Fig. 4-91). The incidence is increased in males, patients older than 65 years, and patients with spondyloarthropathies or DISH. Preoperative anti-inflammatory medications or low-dose radiation therapy may reduce HO in higher-risk patients. Serial radiographs are adequate for diagnosis and classification. HO is graded based on the extent of periarticular involvement. Grade I HO includes bone formation extending approximately 5 mm along the capsular margin. By dividing the periarticular region into four segments it is simple to report the extent of involvement as grade I, grade II (2 of 4 quadrants), or grade IV (ankylosis) (Fig. 4-91). CT may be useful if intervention or revision surgery is required.

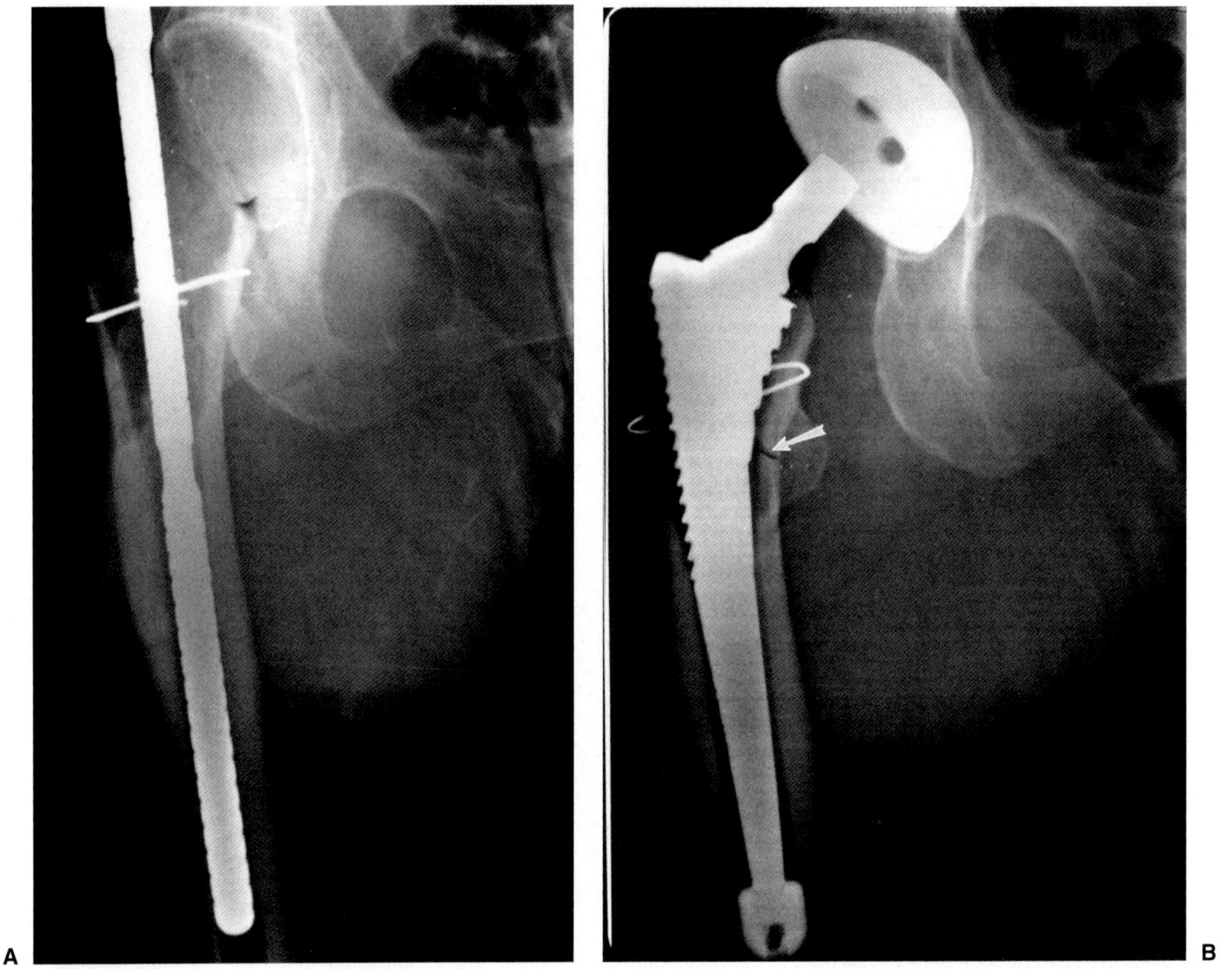

Fig. 4-88 Preparing for femoral component insertion with reaming (A) and broach (B). Note that a fracture has occurred medially (*arrow*).

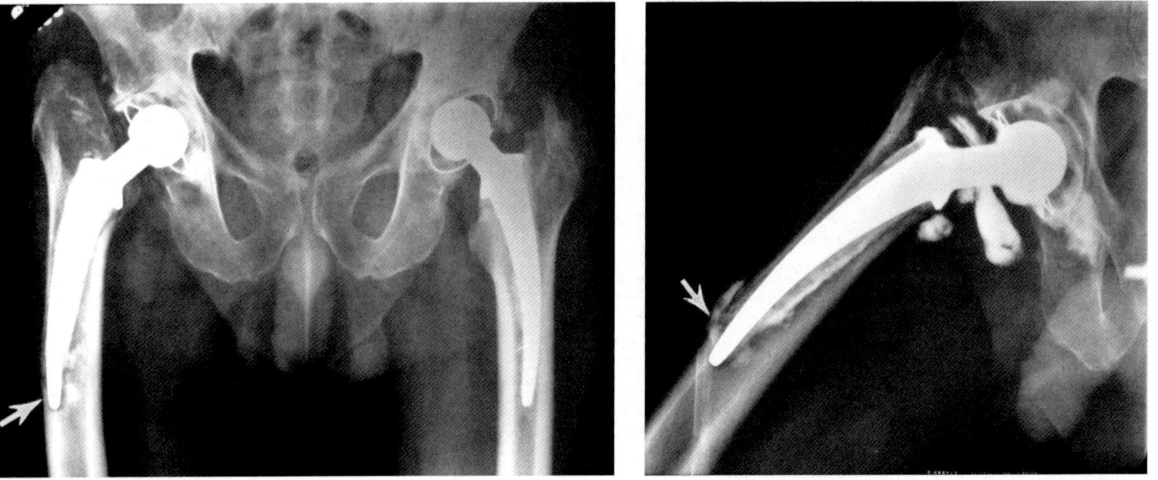

Fig. 4-89 Fracture at the tip of the femoral component. A: Anteroposterior (AP) radiograph of the pelvis and hips in a patient with bilateral total hip replacements. The right femoral component has migrated into varus position and there is marked thinning and irregularity of the cortex laterally (*arrow*). Both components are loose. Is this an incomplete fracture? B: An arthrogram demonstrates loosening with contrast about both components at the bone–cement interface. There is contrast extending through the cortex at the tip of the femoral stem (*arrow*) due to an incomplete fracture. Revision with a longer stem femoral component will be indicated to prevent a complete displaced femoral fracture.

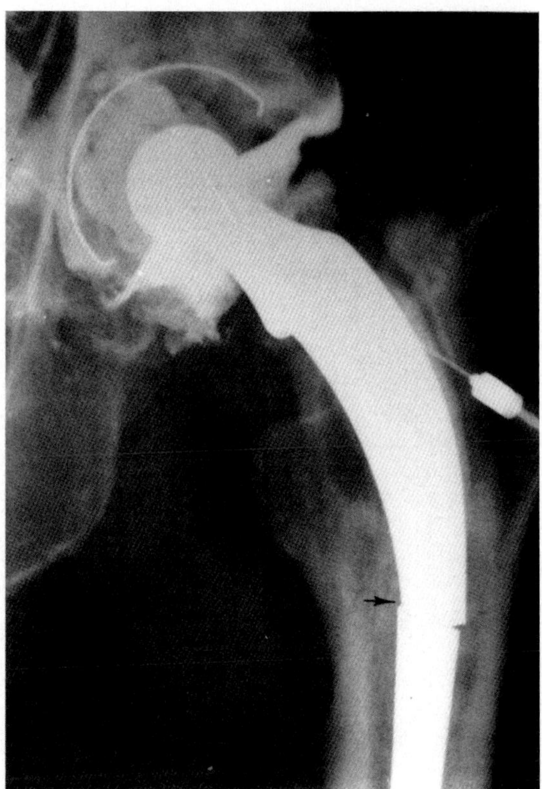

Fig. 4-90 Arthrogram in a patient with a fracture (*arrow*) of the femoral component.

## Suggested Reading


Bauer TW, Parvizi J, Kobayashi N, et al. Diagnosis of periprosthetic infection. *J Bone Joint Surg*. 2006;88A:869–882.

Berquist TH. Imaging of joint replacement procedures. *Radiol Clin North Am*. 2006;44:419–437.

Buckwalter KA, Parr JA, Choplin RH, et al. Multichannel CT imaging of orthopaedic hardware and implants. *Semin Musculoskelet Radiol*. 2006;10:86–97.

Gratz S, Renner JJM, Boerman OC. $^{99m}$Tc-HMPAO-labeled autogenous versus heterogenous leukocytes for imaging of infection. *J Nucl Med*. 2002;43:918–924.

Kalicke T, Risse JH, Arens S, et al. Fluorine-18 fluorodeoxyglucose PET in infectious bone diseases. *Eur J Nucl Med*. 2000;27:524–528.

Miller TT. Imaging of hip arthroplasty. *Semin Musculoskelet Radiol*. 2006;10:30–46.

Naraghi AM, White LM. Magnetic resonance imaging of joint replacements. *Semin Musculoskelet Radiol*. 2006;10:98–106.

Sofka CM. Current applications of advanced cross-sectional imaging techniques in evaluating the painful arthroplasty. *Skeletal Radiol*. 2007;36:183–193.

Termaat MF, Raijmakers PGHM, Scholten HJ, et al. The accuracy of diagnostic imaging for assessment of chronic osteomyelitis: A systematic review and meta-analysis. *J Bone Joint Surg*. 2005;87A:2464–2471.


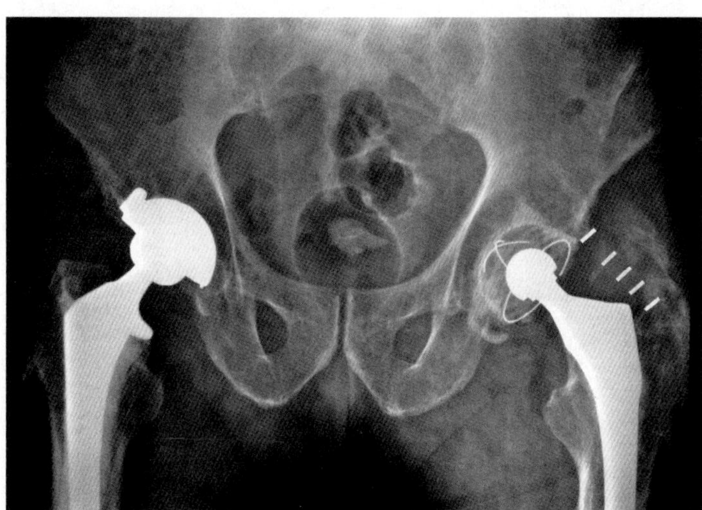

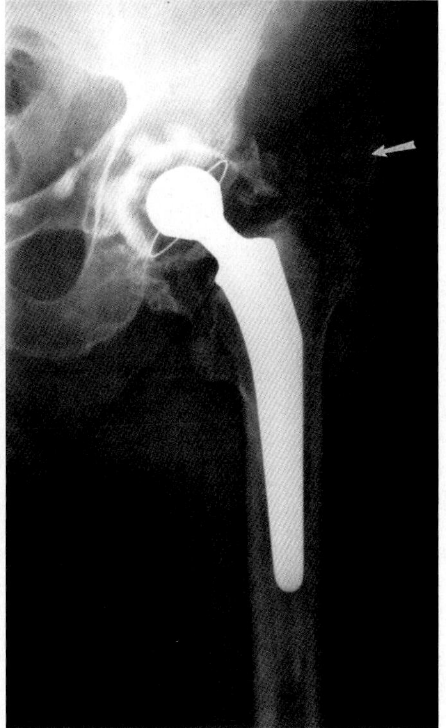

A B

Fig. 4-91 Heterotopic ossification. A: Bilateral total joint replacements with heterotopic ossification on the left in three of four zones (*lines*) and one zone on the left or grade III and grade I, respectively. B: Anteroposterior (AP) radiograph of the left hip demonstrating heterotopic ossification medially, laterally, and in the gluteal muscles (*arrow*).

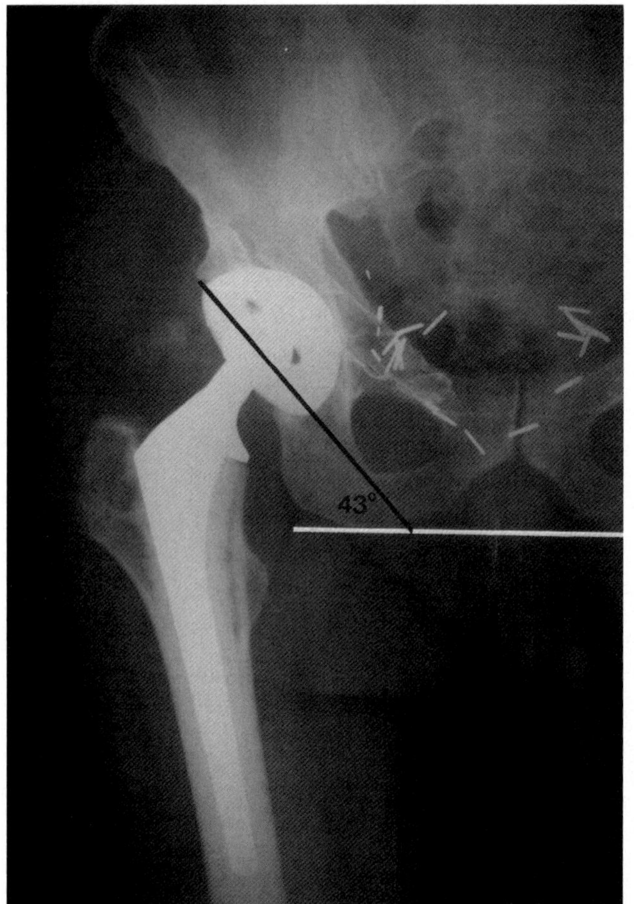


A

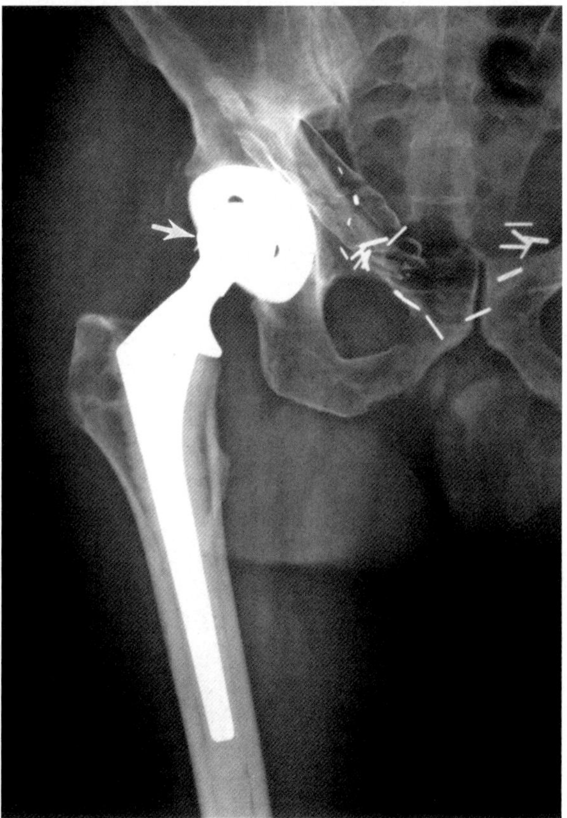

C

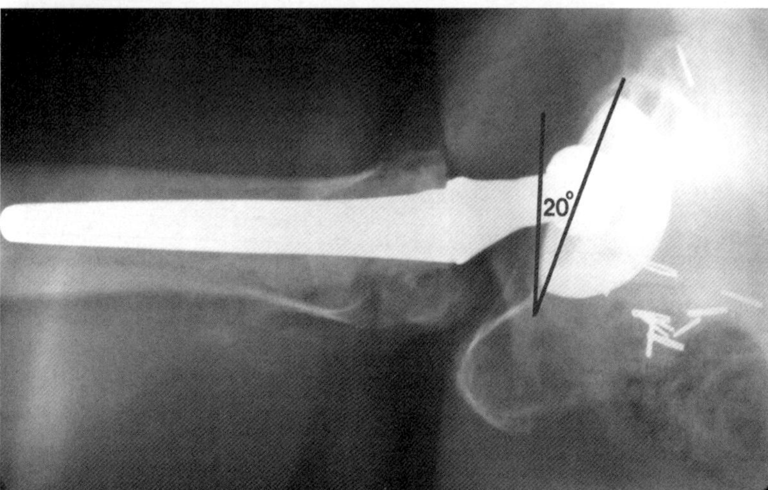


B

Fig. 4-92 Patient with right total joint replacement and chronic posterior dislocations. Anteroposterior (AP) (A) and lateral (B) radiographs demonstrate a hybrid (cemented femoral and uncemented acetabular) hip replacement with the acetabular angle measuring 43 degrees on the AP view (A) (range 35 to 55 degrees) and 20 degrees on the lateral view. At surgery the hip could be easily dislocated, but the acetabular component was well fixed and in good position. Therefore, the acetabular liner was replaced and a new, larger modular head (*arrow*) put in place. The changes are subtle radiographically, but if one compares A with C the change in head configuration is obvious.

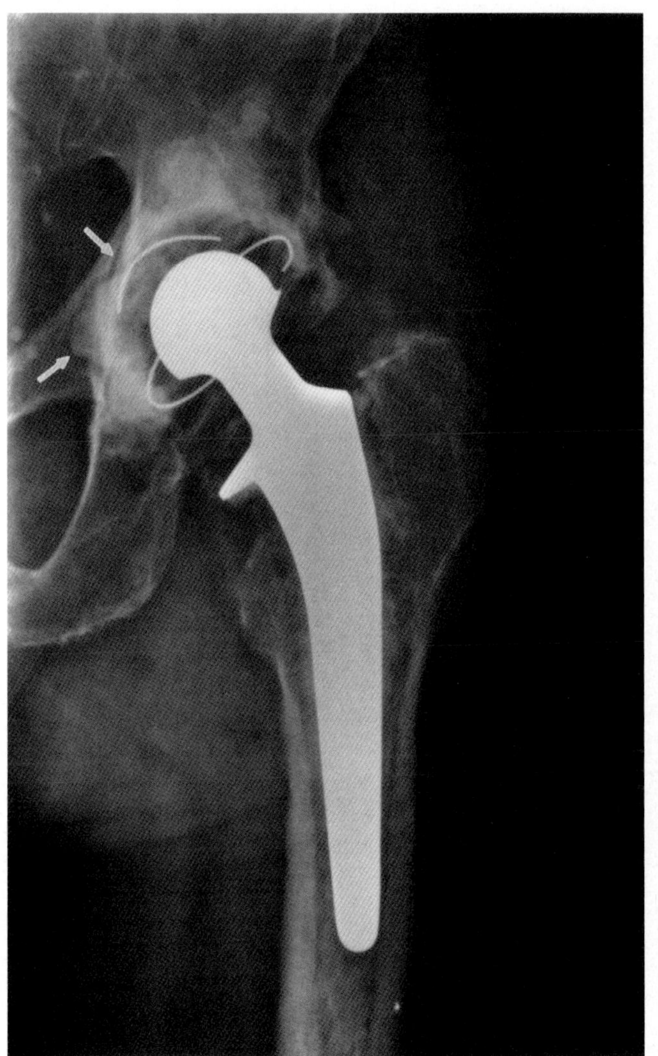


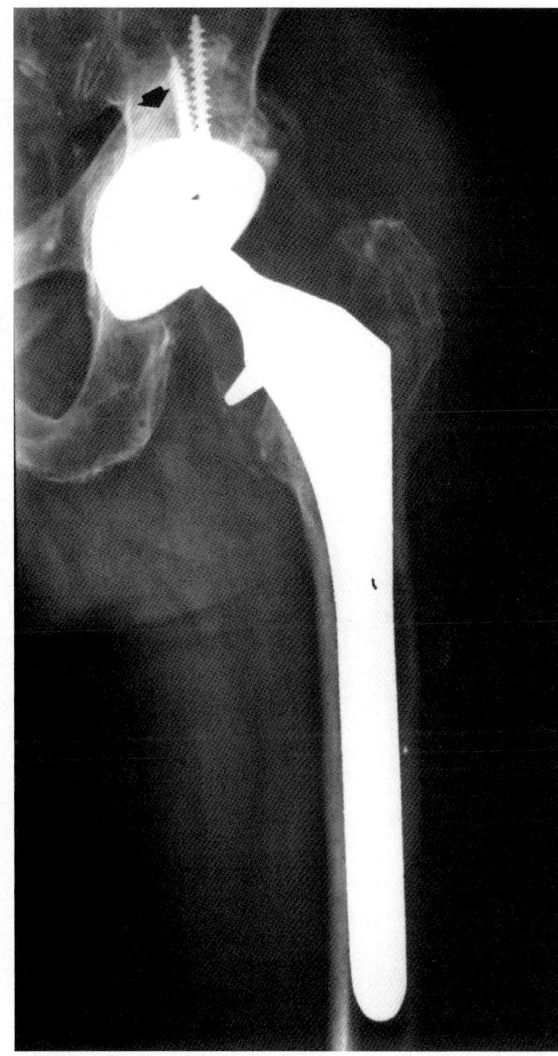


Fig. 4-93 Anteroposterior (AP) (A) radiograph of a failed left hip arthroplasty with cemented components. There are obvious lucent lines (*arrows*) in zones II and III about the acetabular component and the femoral component is in varus position with lucency at the bone–cement interface. The implants were revised with an uncemented longer stem femoral component with allograft and a large allograft in the acetabular region (*arrow*) with acetabular anchor screws.

## Revision Arthroplasty

Revision hip arthroplasty is a common procedure, which consumed 19% of Medicare hip replacement expenditures between 1997 and 2003. The impact is expected to increase by 137% by 2030. The primary indications for revision hip arthroplasty are loosening, dislocation, and infection in that order. Problems with cement removal when components are cemented and bone loss can present significant problems with revision. CT is commonly performed in patients considered for revision to evaluate bone stock and the degree of osteolysis (Fig. 4-82).

### Acetabular Components

Revision of acetabular components may be as simple as liner replacement. The modular head can also be changed in size to conform to the new liner and cup (see Fig. 4-92). However, in many cases, bone grafting, protrusion shells, or special revision systems are required due to acetabular bone loss (see Fig. 4-93).

### Femoral Components

Femoral component replacement can be equally challenging depending on the type and length of the primary system and whether cement was used. When bone defects are present, a longer stem that extends at least several centimeters beyond the defect should be used (Fig. 4-93). In some cases, cortical on-lay bone grafts are required due to diminished bone stock or cortical thinning (see Fig. 4-94). Special components including modular calcar replacement stems or special proximal sleeves may improve fit and stability.

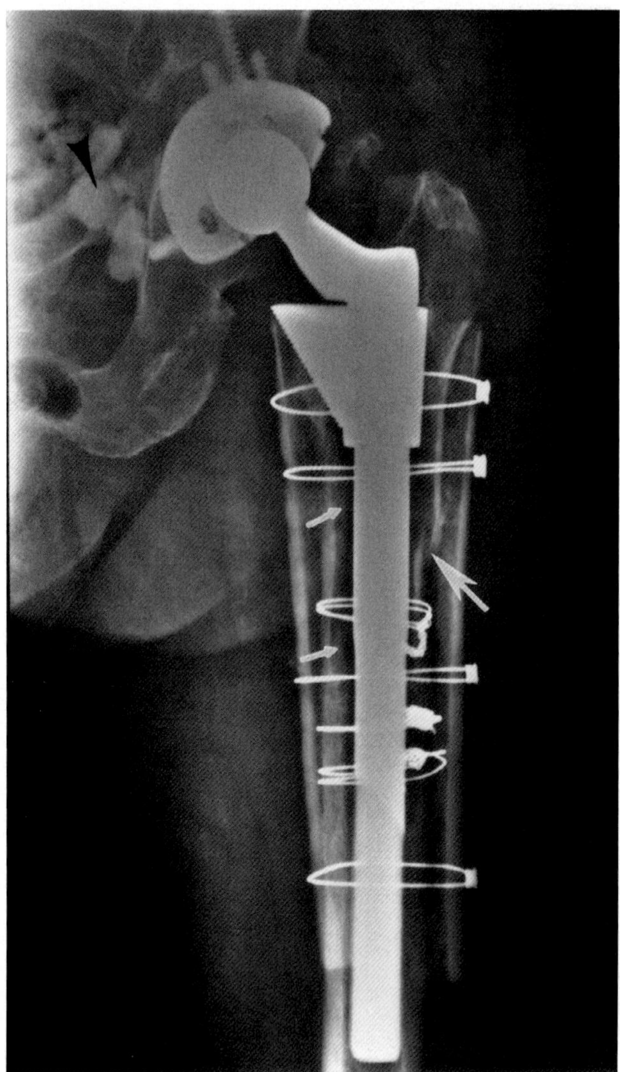

Fig. 4-94 Failed hip replacement revised with a new uncemented acetabular component. Note cement remnants from the prior component (*arrowhead*). There was significant osteolysis (*small white arrows*) about the old component and a lateral femoral fracture (*large white arrow*). A longer femoral stem with an S-ROM system was placed with cortical on-lay bone graft for femoral support. Bone grafts were secured with Dall-miles cables.

## Suggested Reading

Kurtz S, Ong K, Lau E, et al. Projections of primary and revision hip and knee arthroplasty in the United States from 2005–2030. *J Bone Joint Surg.*2007;89A:780–785.

Sotereanos N, Sewecke J, Raukar GJ, et al. Revision total hip arthroplasty with custom cementless stem with cross-locking screws. *J Bone Joint Surg.*2006;88A:1079–1084.

# Arthrodeses and Osteotomies

Arthrodesis (fusion) and several types of osteotomy are used for treatment of conditions in the hip in children and adults.

## Arthrodesis

Hip arthrodesis was initially performed in the late 1800s and early 1900s to treat conditions such as tuberculosis. At that time, nonunion and pseudarthrosis were common (15% to 30%). Newer techniques have greatly improved the success rates with hip arthrodesis.

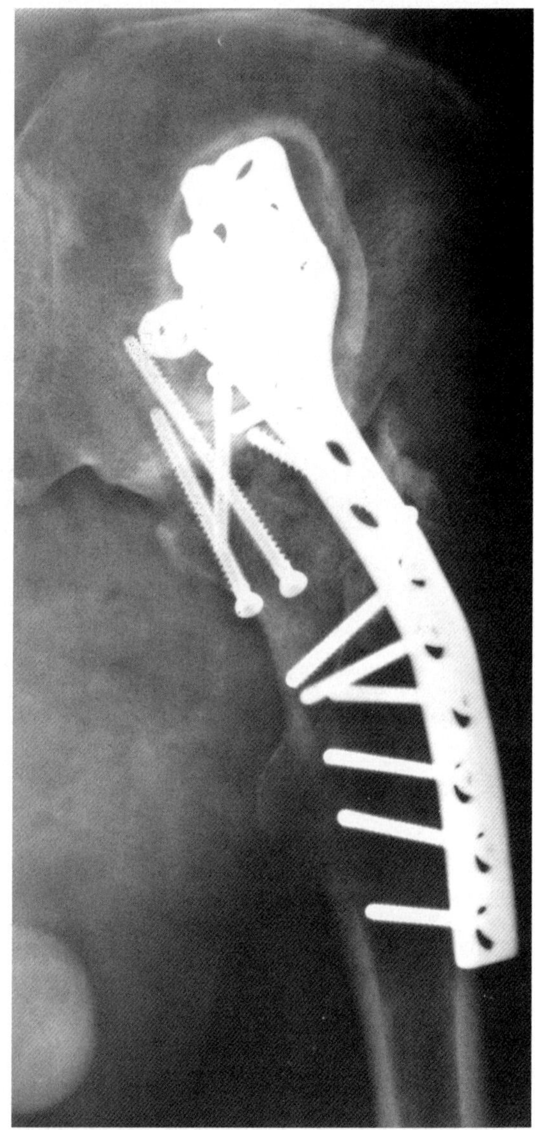

Fig. 4-95 Hip arthrodesis with cobra head plate and screws. Anteroposterior (AP) radiograph demonstrates lucency about the plate with no union at the fusion site.

Arthrodesis is best suited for young active patients with monoarticular disease, usually related to trauma or infection. This procedure remains an alternative to joint replacement in younger patients due to failure rates and the potential for multiple revisions if joint replacement is used. Hips are usually fused in 30 degrees of flexion, 0 to 5 degrees of abduction, and 10 to 15 degrees of external rotation. In children, the angles of flexion and adduction increase, which may require a second corrective procedure.

## Preoperative Imaging

Preoperative imaging is accomplished with AP and lateral radiographs. CT of the involved hip is useful to assess bone stock. In some cases, CT or MRI of both hips may be indicated to assure monoarticular involvement.

## Treatment Options

There are numerous treatment options including intra-articular, extra-articular, and combined approaches. Blade plates, cobra head plates (see Fig. 4-95), threaded pins, and compression screws (see Fig. 4-96) may be used for fixation.

## Complications

Complications include nonunion or pseudarthrosis (Fig. 4-96), deep infection, pain in the ipsilateral knee, contralateral hip, and low back pain. New techniques have reduced the incidence of nonunion to 10%. Joint pain in the knee on the operated side, contralateral hip, and back occurs in 60% of patients. Imaging of patients with suspected nonunion is most easily accomplished with CT. However, radionuclide scans may also be useful if surgery has been performed at least a year before the study.

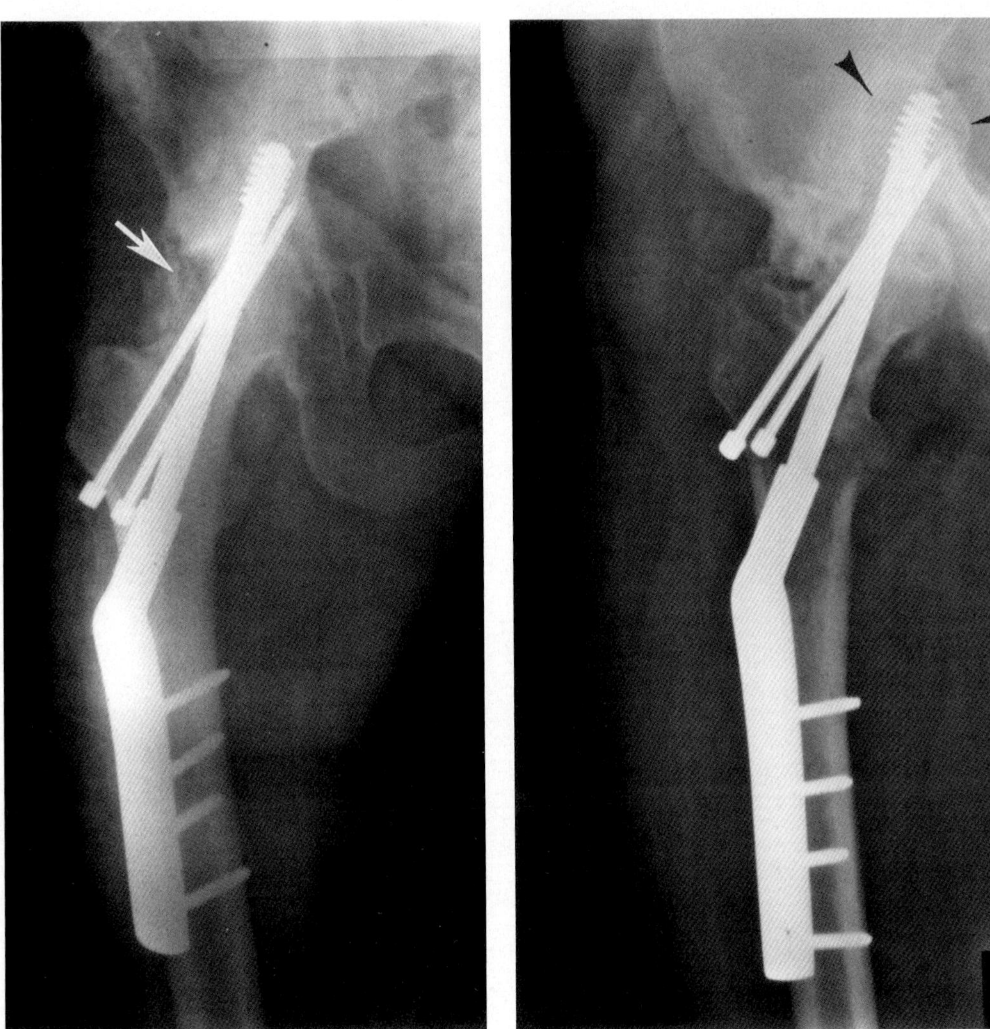


Fig. 4-96 A: Anteroposterior (AP) radiograph following a right hip arthrodesis with dynamic hip screw, two Knowles pins and bone graft (*arrow*). B: Radiograph 6 months later demonstrates loosening and migration of the screw into the acetabulum (*arrowheads*) and an irregular joint space due to failed fusion.

Radionuclide scans with indium- or technetium-labeled white blood cells or antigranulocyte antibodies can be used when infection is suspected. Fused hips can later be converted to hip arthroplasty.

## SUGGESTED READING

Beaule PE, Matta JM, Mast JW. Hip arthrodesis: Current indications and techniques. *J Am Acad Orthop Surg*. 2002;10: 249–258.

Joshi AB, Markovic L, Hardinge K, et al. Conversion of fused hip to total hip arthroplasty. *J Bone Joint Surg*. 2002;84A: 1335–1341.

### Osteotomies

Osteotomies of the hip are performed to improve femoral head coverage, change the weight-bearing surface of the femoral head (see Fig. 4-97), and correct femoral rotation or anteversion deformities. In young adults, this approach can improve symptoms and later be converted to joint replacement. In children, pelvic or acetabular osteotomies are

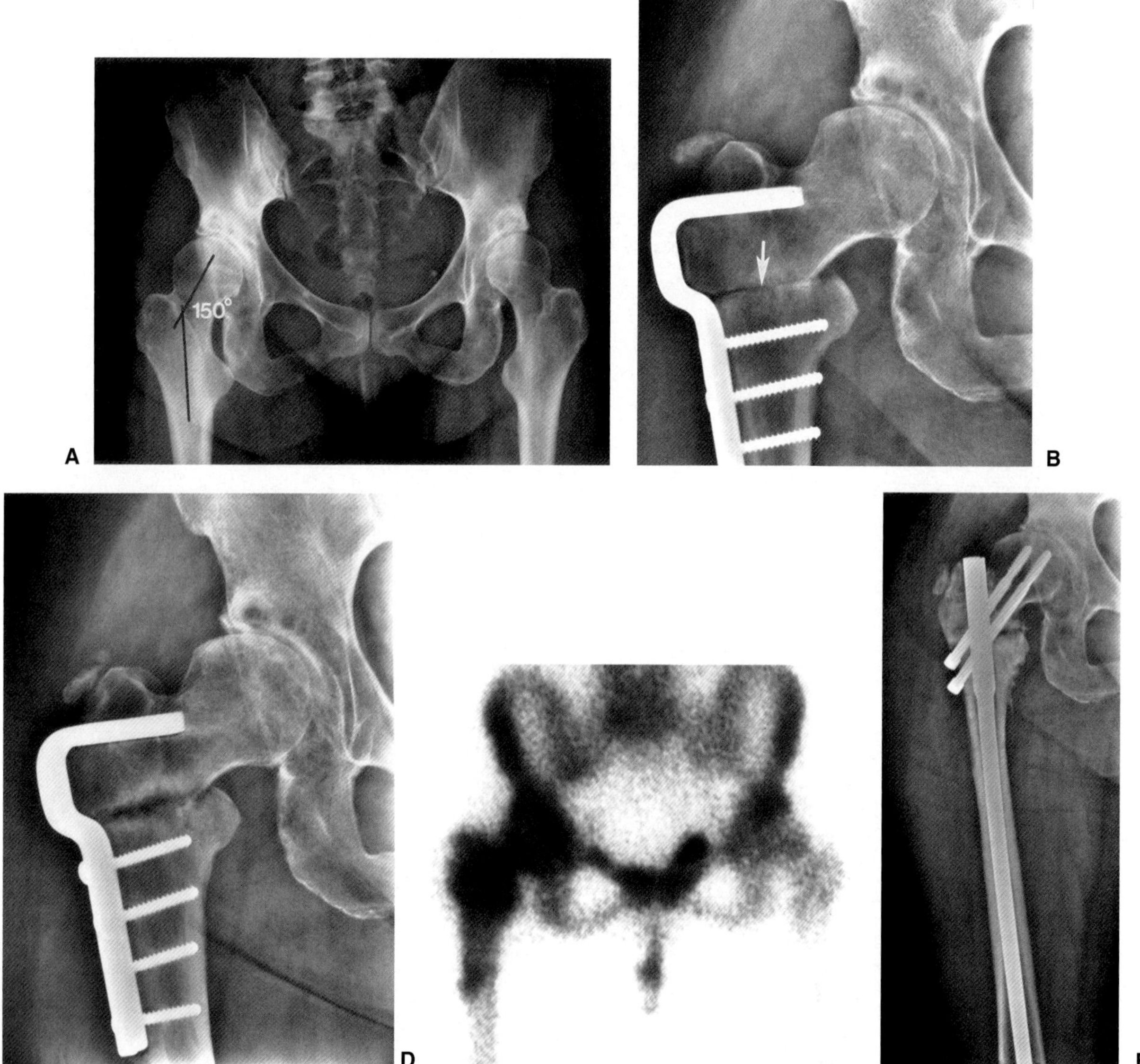


**Fig. 4-97** Varus osteotomy. **A:** Anteroposterior (AP) radiograph demonstrates bilateral coxa valga with increased femoral neck angles (normal 135 degrees, in this case 150 degrees), degenerative joint space narrowing and subchondral cysts. **B:** A varus osteotomy (*arrow*) was performed with a 90-degree blade plate and screws for fixation. **C:** Three months later there is widening of the fracture line with marginal sclerosis indicating delayed union. **D:** Radionuclide bone scan at 1 year demonstrates intense uptake due to nonunion. **E:** The blade plate was removed and replaced with a long intramedullary locking nail and bone graft.

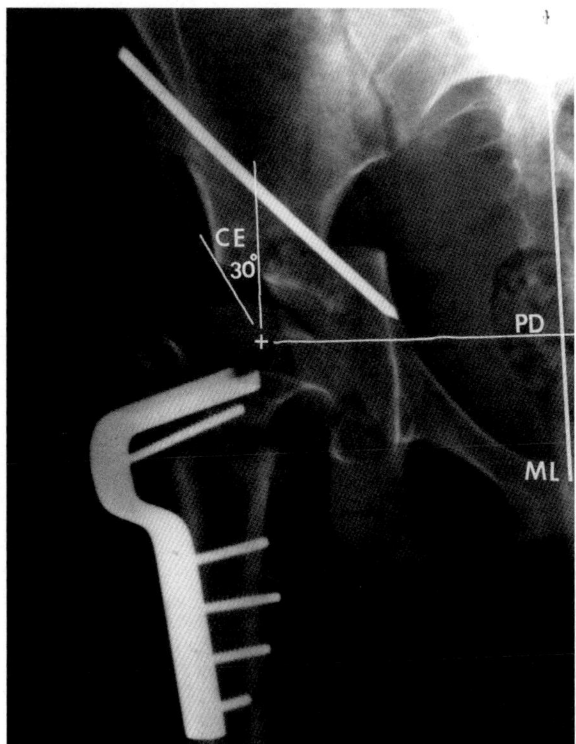


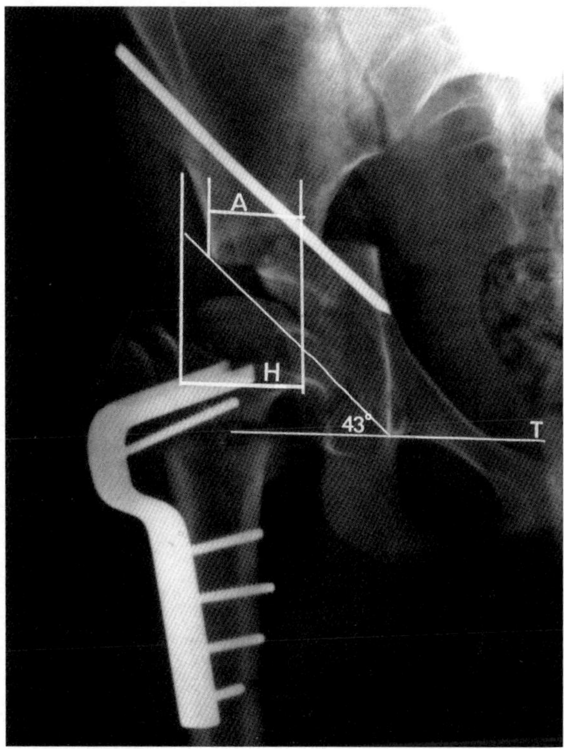


**Fig. 4-98** Salter osteotomy with pin fixation and varus femoral osteotomy with 90-degree blade plate and screw fixation. **A:** Anteroposterior (AP) radiograph demonstrates the midline (*vertical white line* from the S1 to the pubic symphysis-*ML*). The perpendicular distance (*PD*) is the distance from the midline to the center of the femoral head. The Wiberg center-edge (*CE*) angle is 30 degrees. **B:** The same patient with additional measurement used to evaluate osteotomies. Acetabular angle measured by a line along the teardrops bilaterally (*T*) and a line along the acetabular margin, in this case 43 degrees. The acetabular head index: width of the head covered (*A*) divided by the width of the head (*H*) ×100%. In this case the index is 70%.

most often performed for developmental dysplasia of the hip or Legg-Perthes disease. Several techniques have been used depending on the age and extent of correction required.

**Pemberton osteotomy:** This procedure is designed for children 18 months to 10 years of age. The osteotomy is placed at the cove above the acetabulum and uses the triradiate cartilage to rotate the acetabular roof anteriorly and laterally.

**Salter osteotomy:** This approach is designed for children 18 months to 6 years of age. The osteotomy is extended from the sciatic notch to the anterior inferior iliac spine. The fragments and a triangular bone graft are fixed with a K-wire or Steinman pin (see Fig. 4-98).

**Chiari osteotomy:** This approach is designed for children older than 6 years. A transverse iliac osteotomy is performed shifting the inferior innominate bone medially to improve coverage of the femoral head.

## Preoperative Imaging

Preoperative imaging varies with the condition. AP, frog leg oblique, and lateral radiographs may be diagnostic. Evaluation of the acetabulum and labrum may require arthrography or MRI. MRI is particularly useful to evaluate the unossified femoral epiphysis or degree of AVN (see Fig. 4-99).

Radiographs are used pre- and postoperatively to provide certain measurements.

**Midline:** Vertical line from the S1 spinous process to the pubic symphysis (Fig. 4-98A)

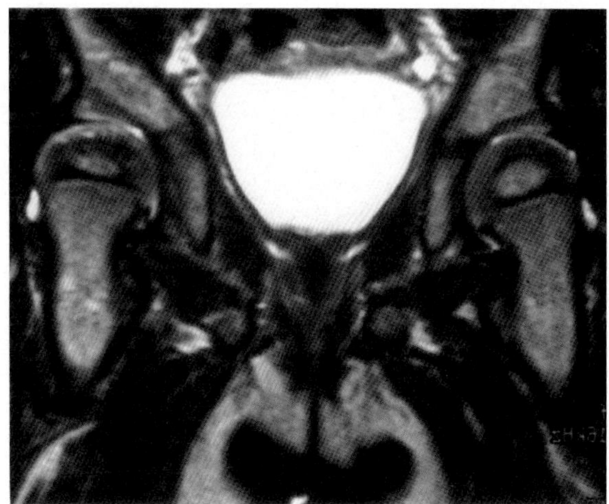

**Fig. 4-99** Coronal T1-weighted magnetic resonance (MR) image demonstrating the partially ossified epiphyses in a patient with developmental dysplasia of the hip on the right.

**Perpendicular distance:** Distance from the midline to the center of the femoral head (PD) (Fig. 4-98A)

**Wiberg angle:** Angle formed by a vertical line to the center of the femoral head and a line from the center of the femoral head to the acetabular margin (CE); the greater the coverage the larger the angle (Fig. 4-98A)

**Acetabular angle:** Teardrop line to acetabular margin (Fig. 4-98B)

**Acetabular head index:** Distance from the medial margin of the femoral head to the acetabulum divided by the transverse width of the femoral head (Fig. 4-98B)

### Complications

Complications are similar to those described in the preceding text. Nonunion (Fig. 4-97), deep infection, AVN, and implant failure may occur. Serial radiographs are useful to consider these complications. MRI is optimal for evaluation of AVN depending on the position of the metal implants. The same approaches described with arthrodesis can be used for nonunion and infection.

## Suggested Reading

Clohisy JC, Nunley RM, Curry MC, et al. Periacetabular osteotomy for the treatment of acetabular dysplasia associated with major aspherical femoral head deformities. *J Bone Joint Surg*. 2007;89A:1417–1423.

Hasegawa Y, Iwase T, Kitamura S, et al. Eccentric rotational osteotomy for acetabular dysplasia: Follow-up of one hundred and thirty-two hips for five to ten years. *J Bone Joint Surg*. 2002;84A:404–410.

Pogliacomi F, Stark A, Vaienti E, et al. Periacetabular osteotomy of the hip: Ilioinguinal approach. *Acta Biomed Ateneo Parmense*. 2003;74:38–46.

Steel HH. Triple osteotomy of the innominate bone. *J Bone Joint Surg*. 1973;55A:343–350.

Sutherland DJ, Moore M. Clinical and radiographic outcome of patients treated with double innominate osteotomy for congenital hip dysplasia. *J Pediatr Orthop*. 1991;11:143–148.

# 5 The Femoral Shaft

The femur is the longest, largest, and strongest osseous structure in the body. Because of its length, width, and weight-bearing role, it must tolerate extremes of axial loading in addition to angular and rotational stresses. The femur is surrounded by large muscle groups and an extensive vascular supply. Therefore, the major problem following fracture is not healing, but maintaining length and alignment. Fractures of the femoral head, neck, and trochanteric region were included in Chapter 4. Distal femoral and intercondylar fractures will be reviewed in Chapter 6. Limb-saving procedures for neoplastic processes will be discussed in Chapter 14.

## Trauma

Femoral shaft fractures are usually associated with high-velocity trauma such as motor vehicle accidents (90%). The incidence (2% of all skeletal fractures) is similar for adults and children. In children and adolescents the incidence is three times higher in males than females. A significant number (70%) of fractures in children younger than 3 years of age are related to nonaccidental trauma (child abuse). In patients with hip or knee arthroplasty, fractures tend to occur at the tip of the femoral components.

Associated injuries are common. Proximal shaft fractures may be associated with pelvic, femoral neck (5% to 6%), trochanteric fractures, and hip dislocations. Distal shaft fractures are more often associated with knee or tibial fractures and ligament or meniscal injuries in the knee.

Most femoral fractures involve the middle third of the diaphysis. Classification and radiographic description are based on segment involvement, rotation, angulation, and shortening. Fractures may be closed (soft tissues intact) or open (penetrating wound or fragment extrusion).

### Fracture classification: Winquist/Hansen

**Type I:** Small comminuted fragment, >50% cortical contact by main fragments (see Fig. 5-1)
**Type II:** Larger comminuted fragment, >50% cortical contact by main fragments (see Fig. 5-2)
**Type III:** Larger comminuted fragment, with <50% cortical contact by major fragments (see Fig. 5-3)
**Type IV:** Severely comminuted with no cortical contact of main fragments (see Fig. 5-4)
**Segmental transverse:** Comminuted segmental transverse fractures (see Fig. 5-5)
Segmental oblique and comminuted (see Fig. 5-6)
Spiral mid-shaft fracture (see Fig. 5-7)
Proximal transverse fracture (see Fig. 5-8)
Proximal oblique fracture (see Fig. 5-9)
Proximal comminuted fracture (see Fig. 5-10)
Distal transverse fracture (see Fig. 5-11)
Distal oblique fracture (see Fig. 5-12)
Distal comminuted fracture (see Fig. 5-13)

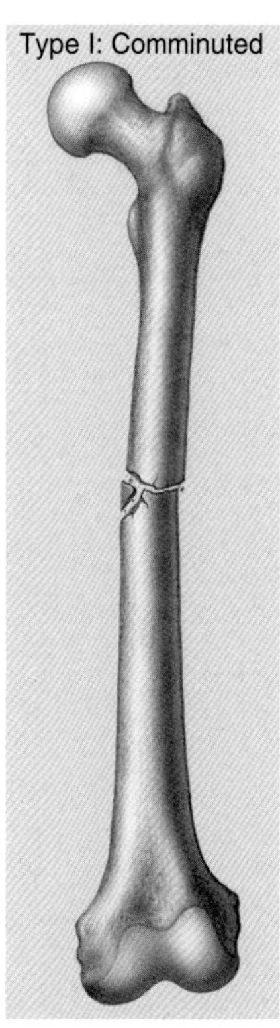


Fig. 5-1 Type I fracture: small comminuted fragment with >50% cortical contact of main fragments.

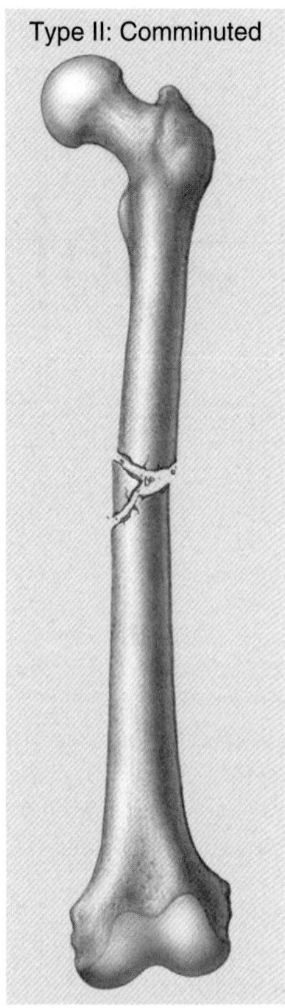


Fig. 5-2 Type II fracture: larger comminuted fragment with >50% cortical contact of main fragments.

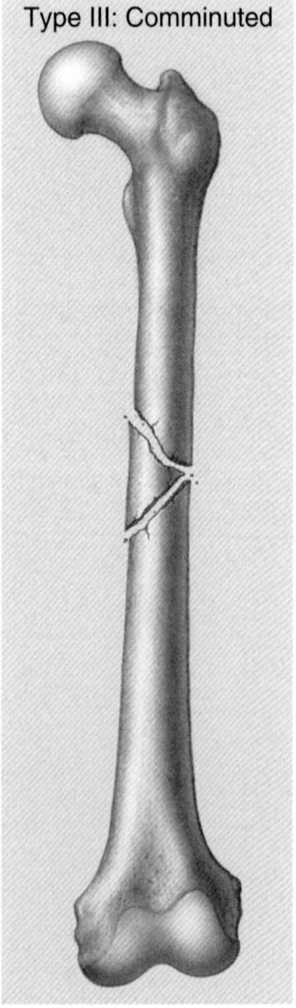


Fig. 5-3 Type III fracture: <50% cortical contact.

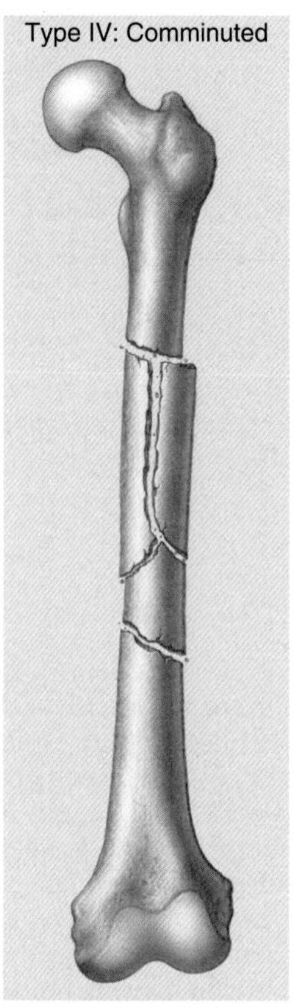


Fig. 5-4 Type IV fracture: severely comminuted with no cortical contact.

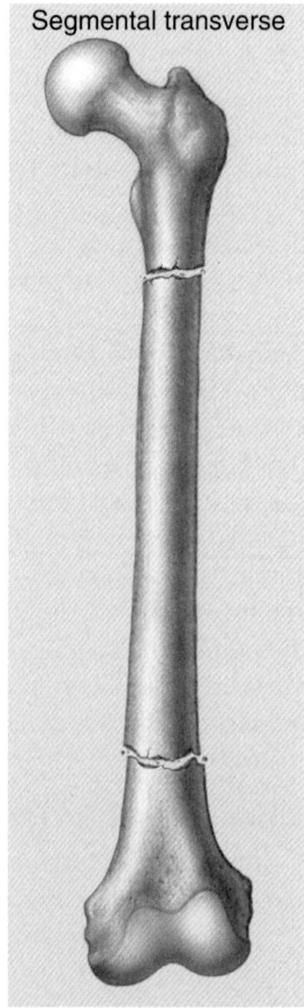


Fig. 5-5 Comminuted segmental transverse fractures.

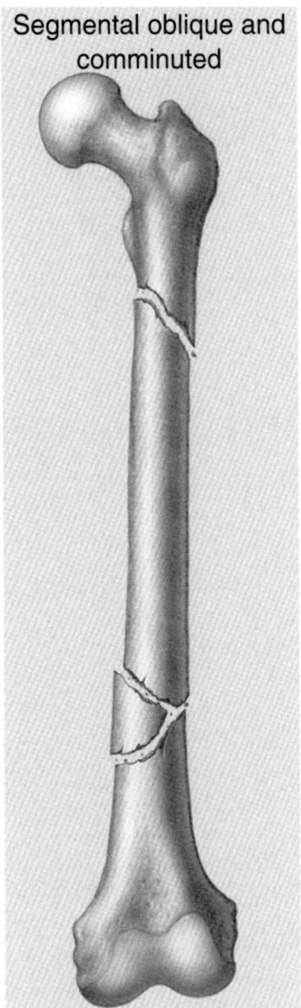


Fig. 5-6 Segmental oblique and comminuted fractures.

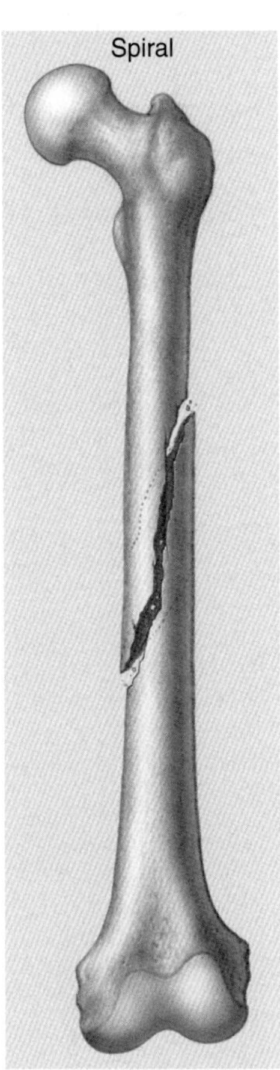


Fig. 5-7 Mid-shaft spiral fractures.

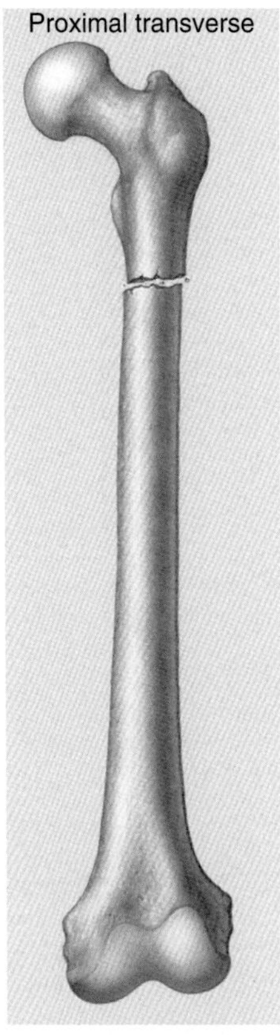


Fig. 5-8 Proximal transverse fractures.

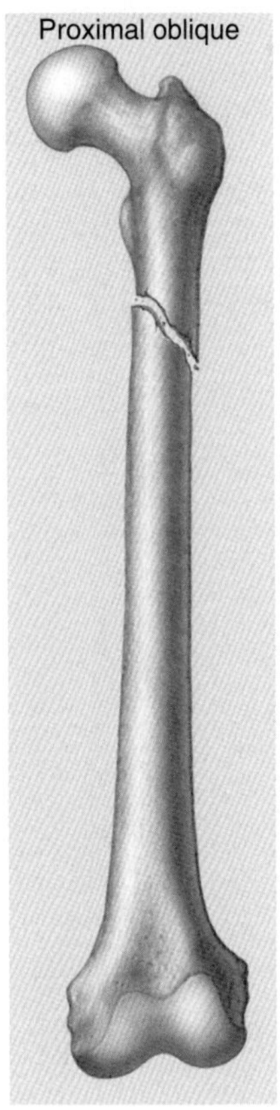


Fig. 5-9 Proximal oblique fractures.

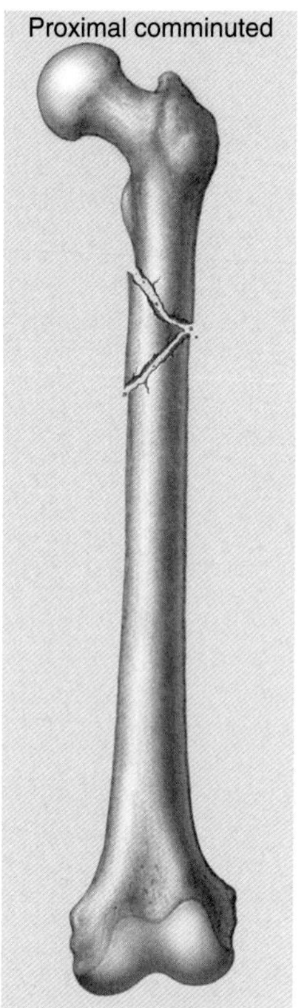


Fig. 5-10 Proximal comminuted fractures.

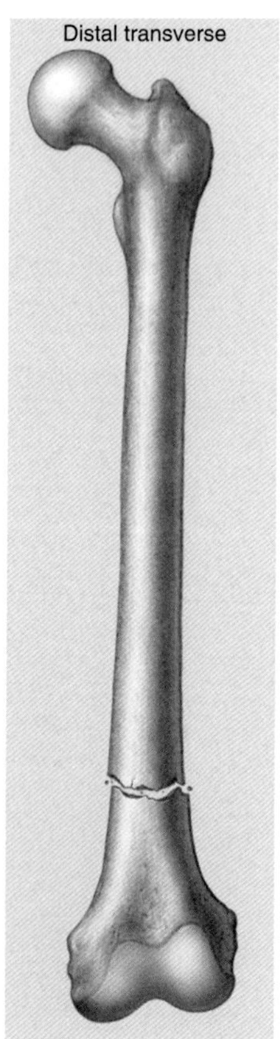


Fig. 5-11 Distal transverse fractures.

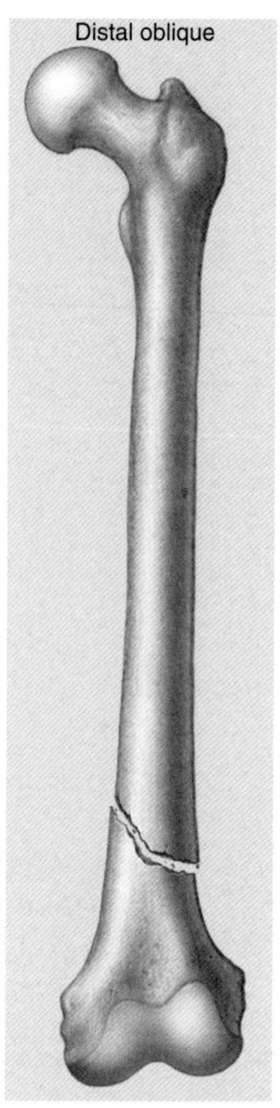


Fig. 5-12 Distal oblique fractures.

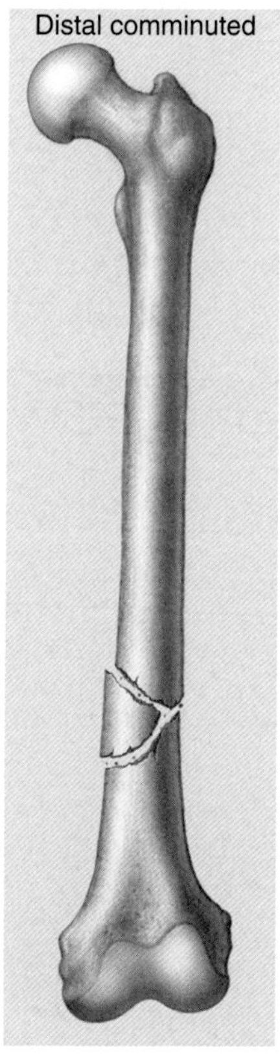


Fig. 5-13 Distal comminuted fractures.

**Open fracture classification: Gustilo/Anderson**

**Type I:** Wound clean and <1 cm

**Type II:** Wound >1 cm without extensive soft tissue damage

**Type IIIA:** Extensive soft tissue wound (≥10 cm), periosteum intact

**Type IIIB:** More severe with periosteal stripping, bone exposure, and extensive contamination

**Type IIIC:** A and B plus arterial injury requiring vascular repair

## SUGGESTED READING


Beaty JH. Operative treatment of femoral shaft fractures in children and adolescents. *Clin Orthop*. 2005;434:114–122.

Gustilo RB, Anderson JT. Prevention of infection in treatment of 1025 open fractures of the long bones. Retrospective and prospective analysis. *J Bone Joint Surg*. 1976;58A:543–548.

Winquist RA, Hansen ST, Clawson DK. Closed intramedullary nailing of femoral fractures. *J Bone Joint Surg*. 1984;66A:529–539.

Winquist RA, Hansen ST, Clawson DK. Closed intramedullary nailing of femoral fractures: A report of 520 cases. *J Bone Joint Surg*. 2001;83A:1912.


# Preoperative Imaging

Standard radiographs (computed radiographic [CR] images) of the femur include anteroposterior (AP) and lateral views. The hip and knee should be included in the images due to frequently associated involvement of the hip and knee (see Fig. 5-14). These projections provide the necessary data for fracture classification and evaluation of shortening, angulation, and rotation. Associated femoral neck fractures (occurring in 5% to 6% of femoral shaft fractures) should be excluded.

Computed tomography (CT) may be required to more fully evaluate fragment position and callus formation. Magnetic resonance imaging (MRI) may be useful in patients with suspected vascular injury or compartment syndrome. Conventional angiography is still a useful tool to demonstrate small vessel detail in patients with vascular injury.

## SUGGESTED READING


Berquist TH, Broderson MP. The femoral shaft. In: Berquist TH, ed. *Imaging atlas of orthopaedic appliances and prostheses*. New York: Raven Press; 1995:353–397.


# Treatment Options

Treatment goals for femoral shaft fractures include the following:

- Preserve vascular supply
- Restore position and alignment
- Maintain length; <1.5 cm of shortening
- Restore apposition
- Restore function
- Prevent infection

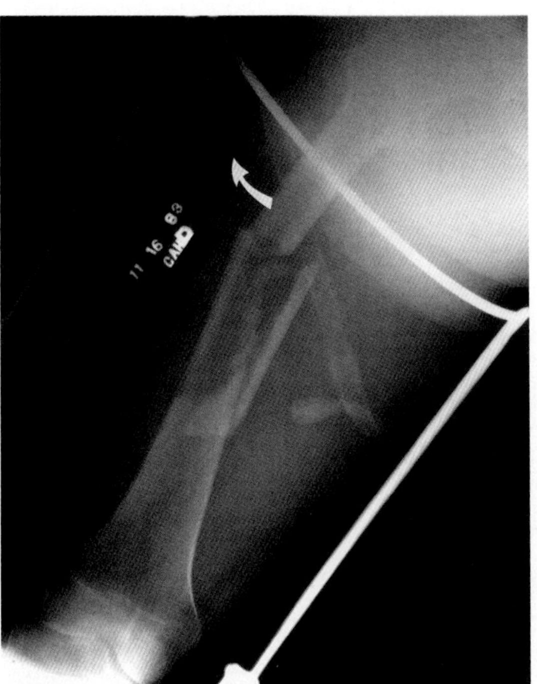


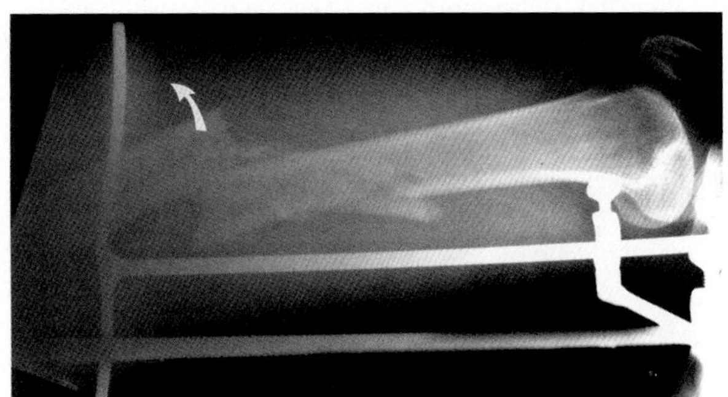


Fig. 5-14 Anteroposterior (AP) (A) and lateral (B) radiographs of a type IV femoral shaft fracture. The proximal fragment is flexed and abducted (*curved arrows*) by the gluteal muscles, external rotators, and iliopsoas muscle.

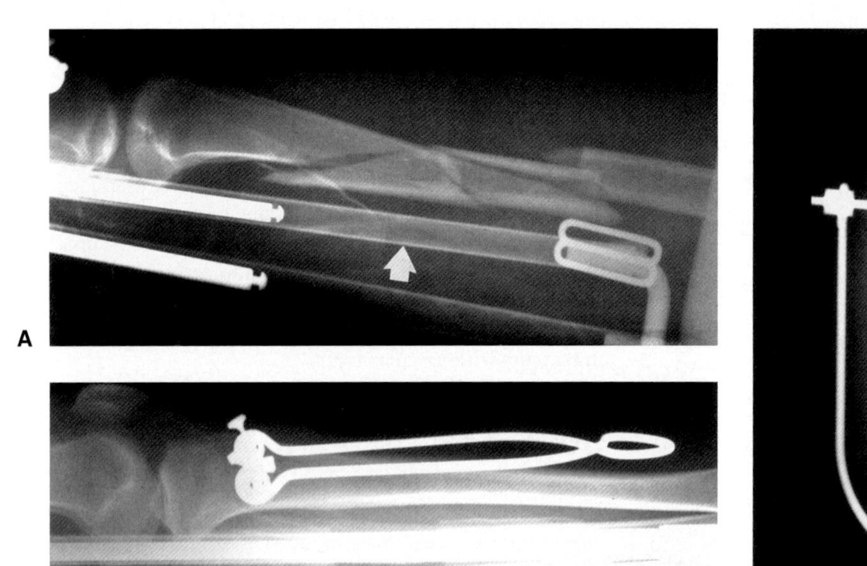
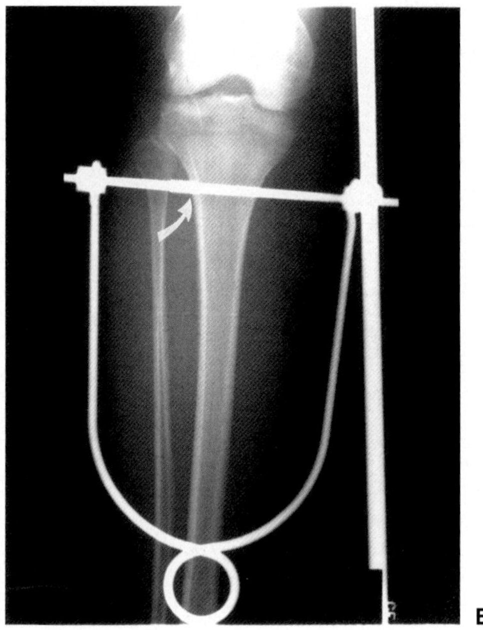

Fig. 5-15 Traction for a Winquist type IV fracture. Lateral radiograph (A) shows a comminuted mid-shaft fracture. Note the high support of the traction device (*arrow*) is radiolucent throughout most of its length. Anteroposterior (AP) (B) and lateral (C) radiographs show the partially threaded Steinman pin (*curver arrow in C*) with the treads just entering the cortex. The pin is parallel to the articular surface of the knee to allow uniform traction. The traction pin is held in a Bohler holder.

Fracture management varies with the patient age and presence of other injuries (multiple traumas).

## Traction

Skeletal traction is useful in early treatment when surgery must be delayed due to other injuries and in children from infancy to 10 years of age before application of a spica cast (see definitions in Chapter 2). Traction is the treatment of choice for highly comminuted fractures when fixation or immobilization cannot be achieved. The goal of early traction is to restore length in the first 24 hours. After this period of time hematoma begins to form and organize about the fracture.

Traction is usually accomplished using a K-wire or threaded Steinman pin in the upper tibia (see Fig. 5-15). Steinman pins are larger and may cause more soft tissue damage while K-wires tend to cut through bone over time. Tibial traction is contraindicated with associated ligament injuries to the knee. In this setting, distal femoral traction can be used (see Fig. 5-16). This allows more direct force to be applied to the fracture. Femoral traction may cause scarring in the vastus medialis and lateralis muscles. Calcaneal traction should be avoided due to the high risk of infection.

### Types of Traction

#### Thomas splint

Half ring to hold the traction pin with thigh sling to prevent soft tissue injury and a Pearson attachment (Fig. 5-15 and see Fig. 5-17).

#### Newfold roller attachment

Steinman pins in plaster to allow early knee motion with traction applied to plaster.

#### 90–90 traction

Both the hip and knee flexed 90 degrees with vertical traction on femur. Used with proximal or subtrochanteric fractures to reduce flexion of the proximal fragment.

#### Perkins traction

Traction pin in the tibia with traction applied to two pulleys at the end of the bed (~20 lb for adults)

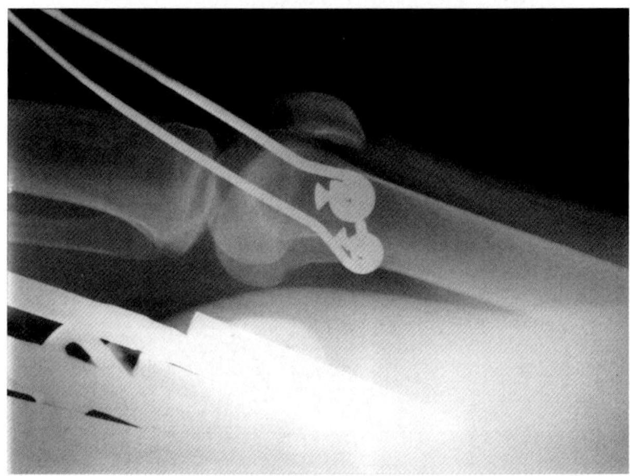

Fig. 5-16 Lateral radiograph demonstrating a traction pin in the distal femur.

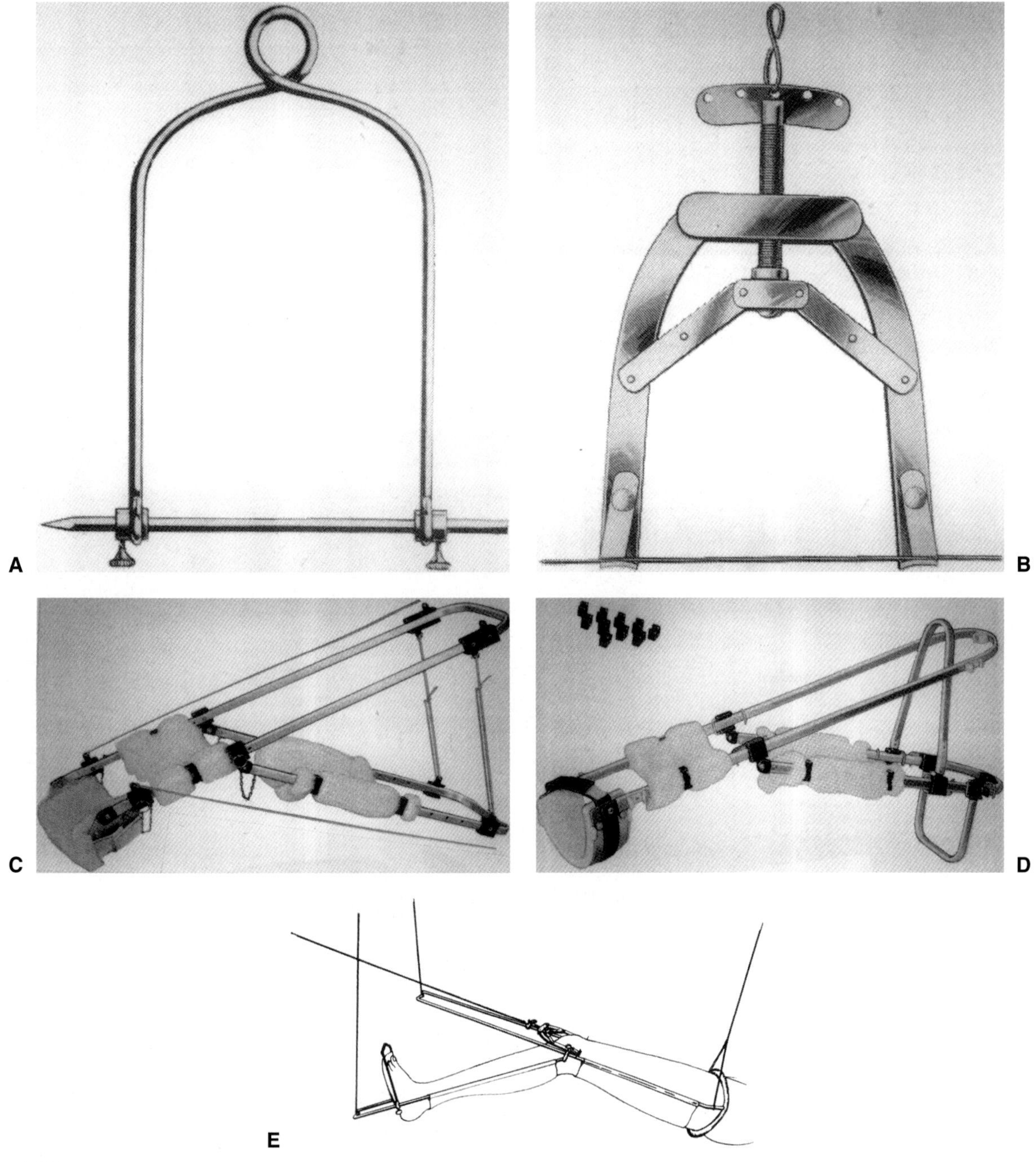


Fig. 5-17 Traction devices. A: Bohler Steinman pin holder with an unthreaded Steinman pin. B: K-wire tractor. C: Brady suspension device for femur and lower extremity fractures. D: Radiolucent Thomas splint with Pearson attachment. E: Illustration of a Thomas splint with Pearson attachment.

## Traction Advantages

Early reduction for complex injuries
Alternative to early surgery

## Traction Disadvantages

Requires frequent radiographs to check fracture fragment position
Increased incident of nonunion, delayed union (30%), shortening, and malunion
Loss of knee motion
Pin tract infections
Prolonged immobilization and bed rest increases medical complications

## Suggested Reading

Beaty JH. Operative treatment of femoral shaft fractures in children and adolescents. *Clin Orthop*. 2005;434:114–122.

Bucholz RW, Jones A. Current concepts review: Fractures of the shaft of the femur. *J Bone Joint Surg*. 1991;73A:1561–1566.

Buxton RA. The use of Perkins traction in treatment of femoral shaft fractures. *J Bone Joint Surg*. 1981;63B:362–366.

Whittle AP, Wood GW. Fractures of the lower extremity. In: Canale ST. *Campbell's operative orthopaedics*, 10th ed. St. Louis: Mosby; 2003:2669–2724.

## Cast-Brace Fixation

This technique is used following traction for open fractures, distal third shaft fractures, and comminuted fractures (see Fig. 5-18). This approach is contraindicated for proximal third fractures and transverse fractures. The cast provides a

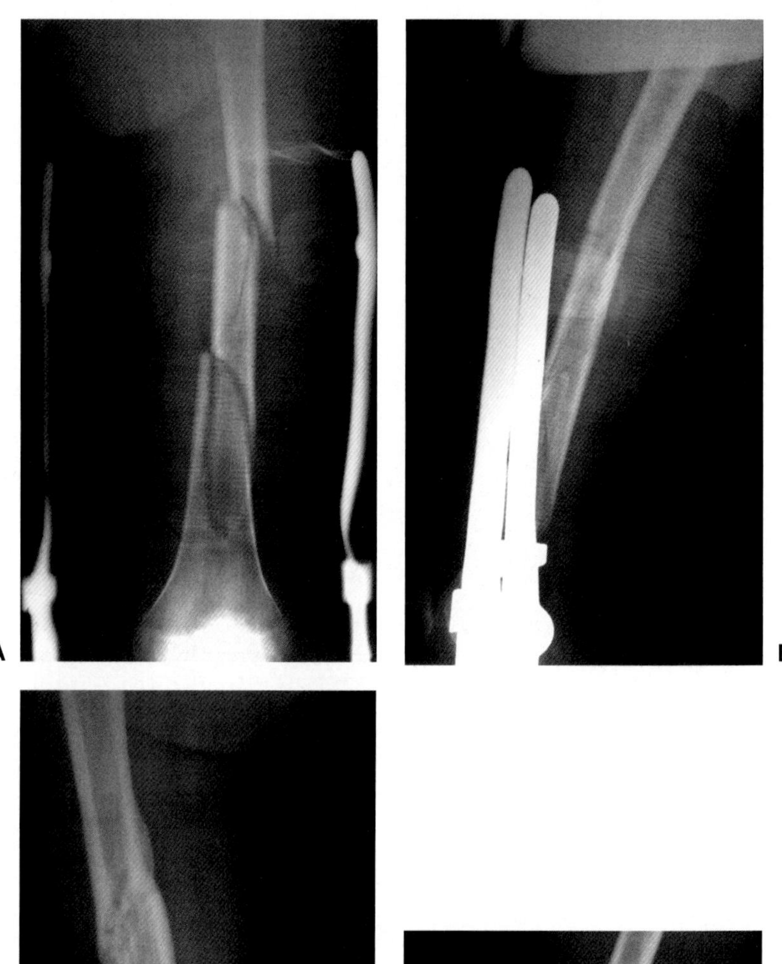

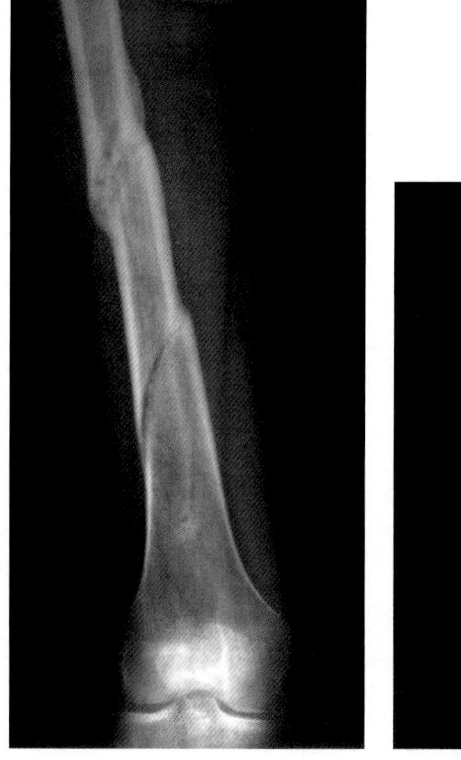

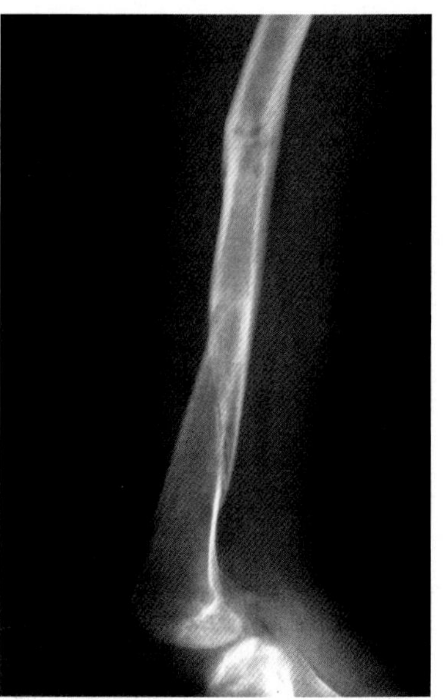

**Fig. 5-18** Segmental fracture of the femur seen on anteroposterior (AP) (**A**) and lateral (**B**) radiographs with cast-brace immobilization. AP (**C**) and lateral (**D**) radiographs 5 months later after healing.

supporting capsule about the thigh musculature providing a stabilizing effect on the fractures.

**Advantages**

Early mobilization
Improved muscle function
Avoids surgical complications
Reduced knee stiffness

**Disadvantages**

More prone to shortening and rotation

## SUGGESTED READING


Hardy AE. Treatment of femoral fractures with cast-brace application and early mobilization. *J Bone Joint Surg.* 1983;65A:56–64.

Whittle AP, Wood GW. Fractures of the lower extremity. In: Canale ST. *Campbell's operative orthopaedics*, 10th ed. St. Louis: Mosby; 2003:2669–2724.


## External Fixation

External fixation was introduced in the mid-20th century as an option to cast immobilization and internal fixation. Steinman pins in plaster (see Fig. 5-19), unilateral, ring, or hybrid external fixation systems may be selected. The advantages of external fixation include less disruption of soft tissues, preservation of blood supply, wound access for open fractures, ongoing fracture manipulation, and early ambulation. Unilateral fixation systems allow the extremity to remain functional while providing the ability to manipulate fracture fragments into the desired position and then maintain stability (see Fig. 5-20). Ring fixators use pins, wires, or both. Newer systems with reduced diameter increase the frame stiffness significantly. The classic ring fixator is the Ilizarov system (see Fig. 5-21) which has more recently been integrated with the Taylor Spatial Frame (TSF) by Smith and Nephew, Memphis, Tennessee (see Fig. 5-22). The new frame is designed for more complex axial, sagittal, and rotational deformities. The TSF system is composed of rods, struts, and rings. Variations include full rings, open rings, and arches. Full rings provide the most stability.

External fixation systems can be modified (dynamization) at the appropriate time to increase the load at the fracture site to increase callus stability. The frames can be removed when there is radiographic evidence of healing and the bone can tolerate unsupported weight.

## Internal Fixation

Internal fixation is commonly used to treat femoral shaft fractures. Multiple approaches can be used including flexible intramedullary nails, locking intramedullary nails, and plate and screw fixation.

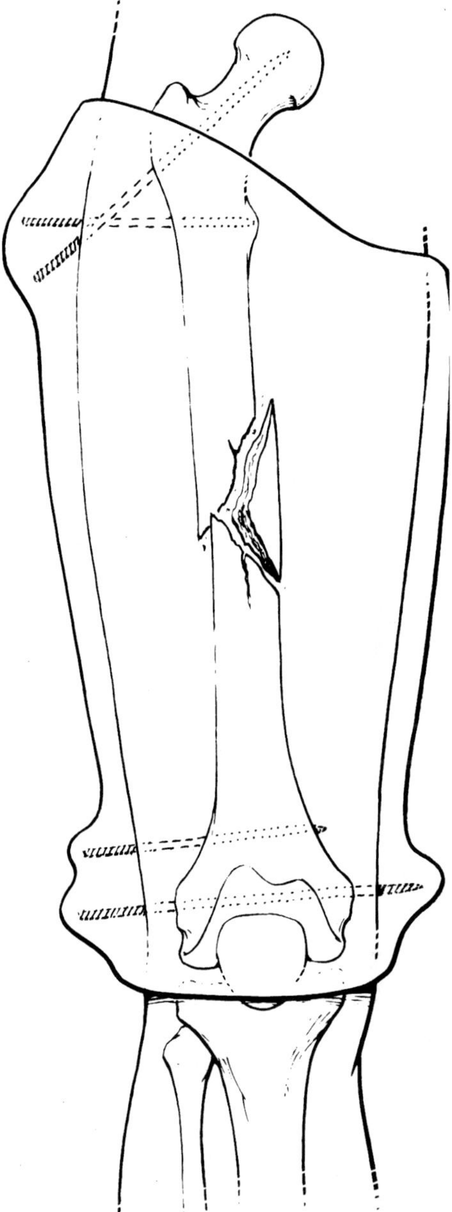

**Fig. 5-19** Illustration of external fixation using Steinman pins in plaster for a comminuted mid-shaft fracture of the femur.

### Intramedullary Fixation

Intramedullary nails were introduced by Kuntscher in 1940 but did not gain popularity in the United States until the 1970s. Intramedullary nails may be introduced using a proximal (antegrade) or distal (retrograde) femoral approach depending on the type of injury. Standard, flexible, and interlocking (static or dynamic) nails are available.

### Flexible Intramedullary Nails

Flexible intramedullary nails include Ender, Nancy, and Rush nails. The latter is uncommonly used in the femur. These devices can be used in children and adolescents to reduce

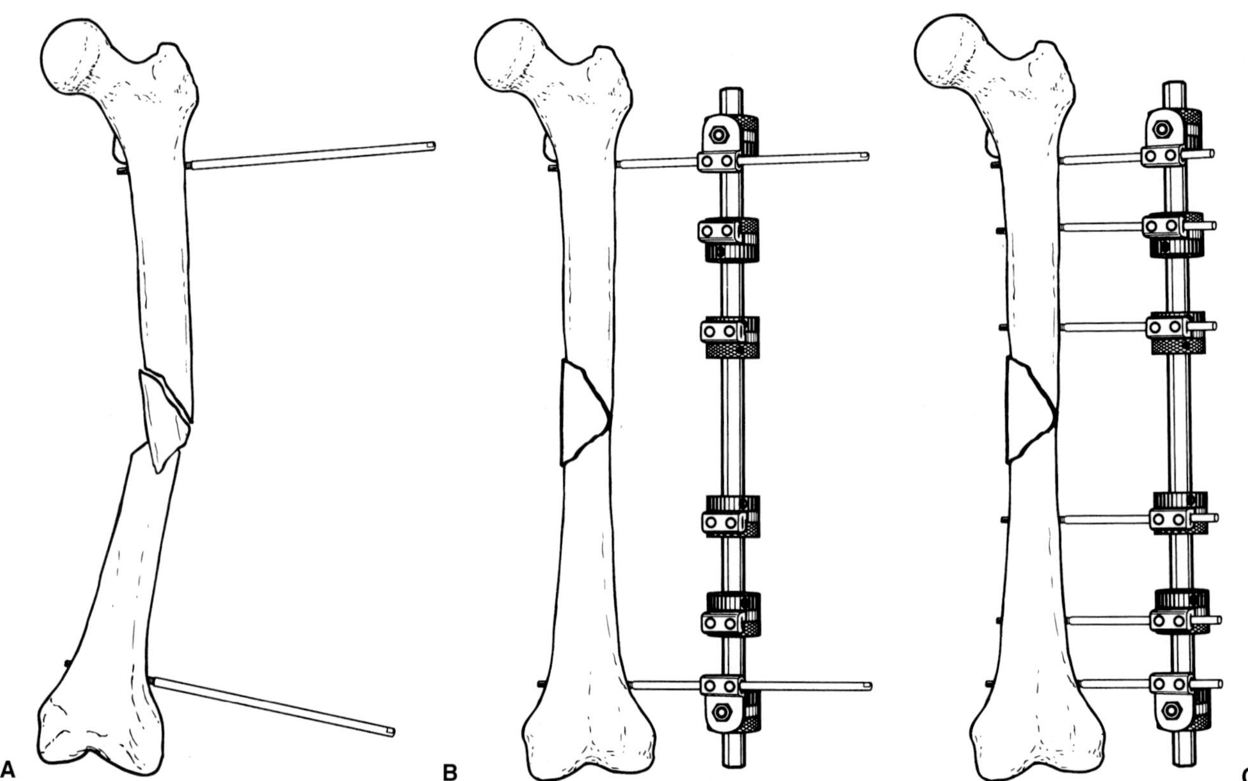


Fig. 5-20 Unilateral external fixator. Illustration (A) of external fixation pins proximal and distal to the fracture used to reduce the fracture with attachment of the pins to the fixation rod (B) and additional pins added for stability (C). (Courtesy Smith and Nephew Richards, Memphis, Tennessee.)

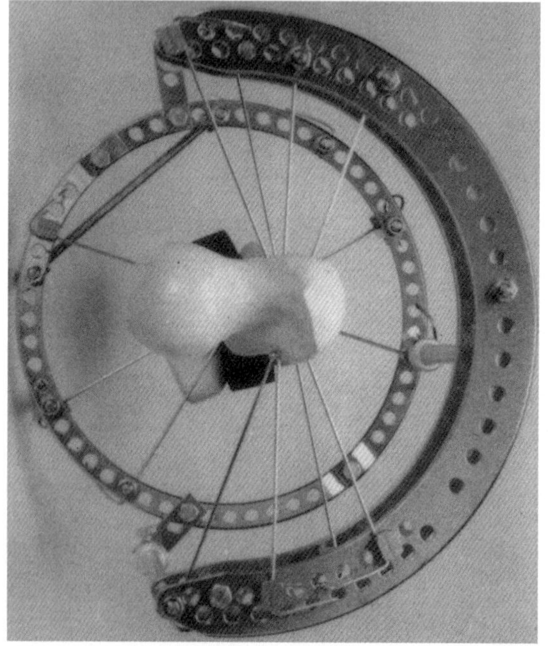


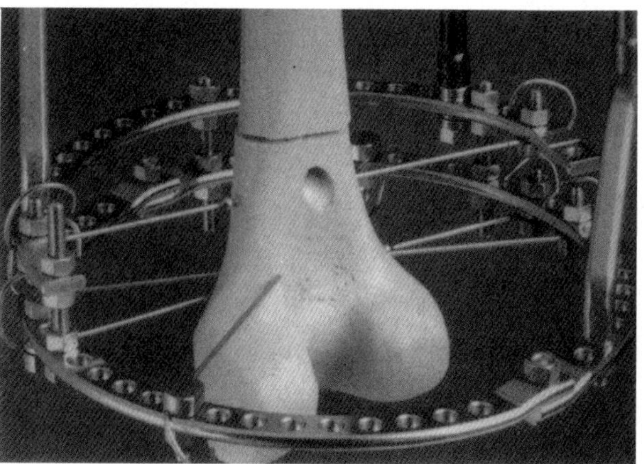


Fig. 5-21 Ilizarov system seen from above (A), distally (B) and the entire femur (C). D: New standard circular frame. (Courtesy Smith and Nephew Richards, Memphis, Tennessee.)

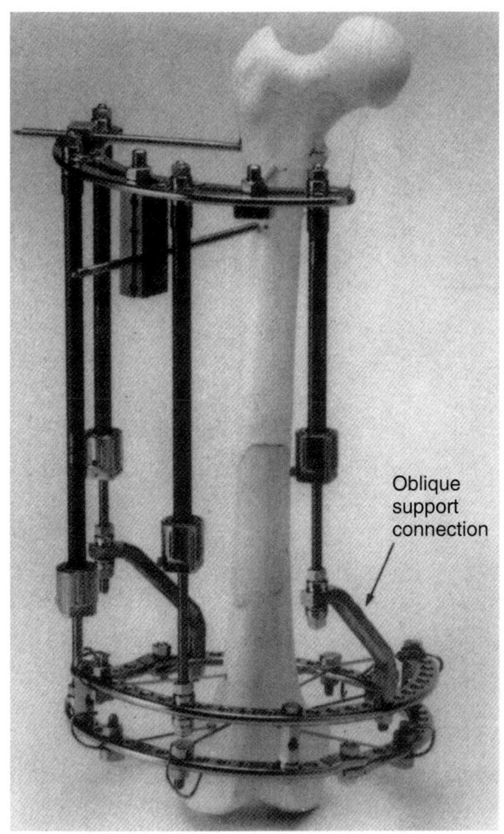


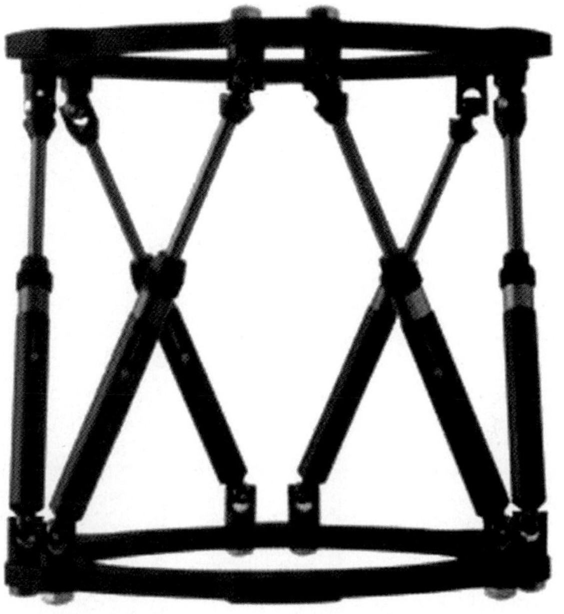


Fig. 5-21 *(Continued)*

hospital stays and allow early ambulation. In younger individuals this technique can avoid the proximal and distal physes so that growth plate complications can be avoided. The approach is similar in children and adults. Radiographs are used to measure the length of the femur and diameter of the medullary canal. One nail is inserted for each 5 mm of diameter of the medullary canal. Nails can be prebent to match the configuration of the femoral canal. Nails are typically inserted in a retrograde manner for mid and proximal third fractures and antegrade insertion for distal fractures (see Fig. 5-23). In adults, this technique is best suited for fractures with good cortical contact and minimal comminution. In children, the technique is most often employed for patients 6 to 10 years of age with axial length stable fractures.

## Locking Intramedullary Nails

Standard intramedullary nails are less commonly used now. These fixation devices may require reaming of the medullary canal before insertion. When used, the largest diameter nail to fit the canal is selected to reduce rotational deformities. Figures 5-24 and 5-25 demonstrate standard intramedullary nails.

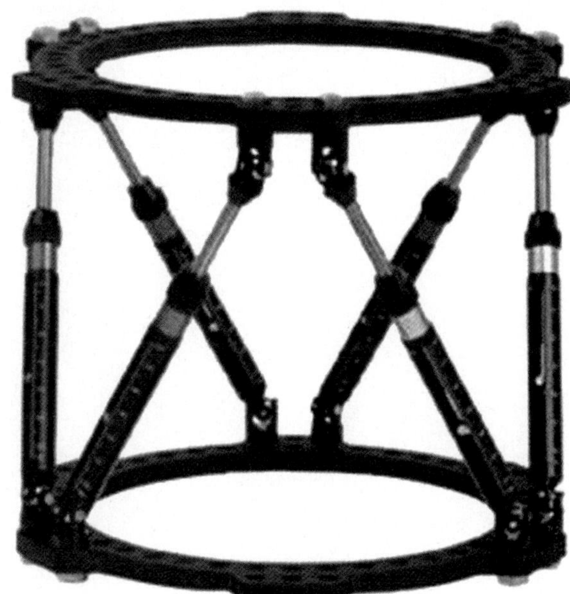

Fig. 5-22 Illustration of the Taylor Spatial Frame. (Courtesy Smith and Nephew Richards, Memphis Tennessee.)

Locked intramedullary nails can be used in adults and older adolescents. There are multiple configurations, but all follow the same principles. Nails may be static (screws at both ends) or dynamic (fixation at one end) (see Fig. 5-26). The latter may be a conversion from the static configuration to increase fracture impaction (see Fig. 5-27). Locking intramedullary nails can be used with any of the fracture configurations (Fig. 5-1 through 5-13). Locking nails provide excellent axial and rotational stabilization. They also allow for early mobilization and reduced risk of loss of range of motion in the hip and knee. Nails may be inserted in an antegrade or retrograde manner. The latter is more often used for distal femoral fractures in which case shorter nails may be used (see Fig. 5-28).

## Plate and Screw Fixation

Plate fixation is useful in certain settings (see Figs. 5-29 and 5-30). However, this technique has been largely replaced by

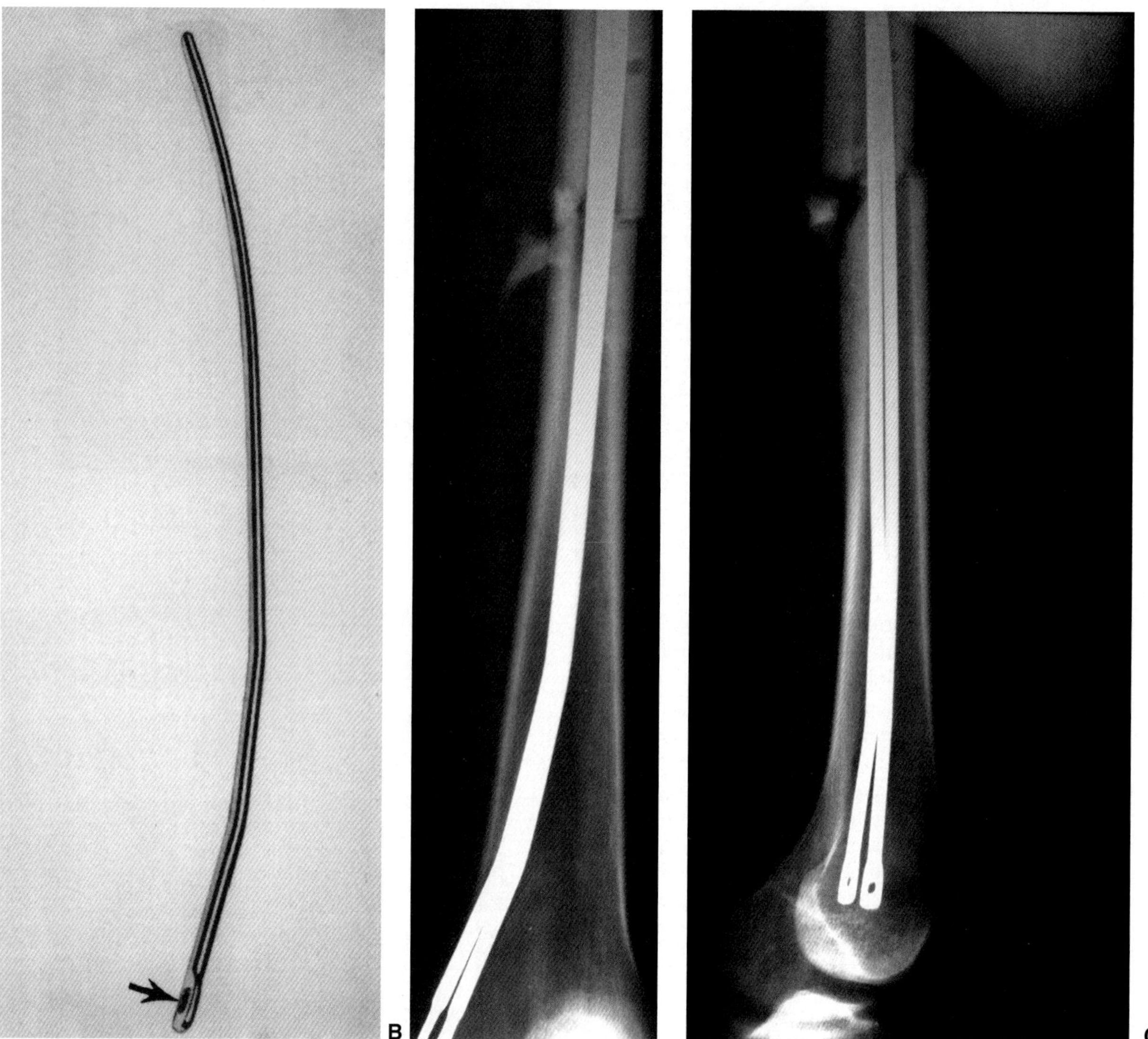

Fig. 5-23 Ender nails for fixation of a mid-shaft fracture (Winquist/Hansen type II). A: Prebent Ender nail with distal hole (*arrow*) for sutures. Anteroposterior (AP) (B) and lateral (C) radiographs following placement of two Ender nails. AP (D) and lateral (E) radiographs following healing of the fracture.

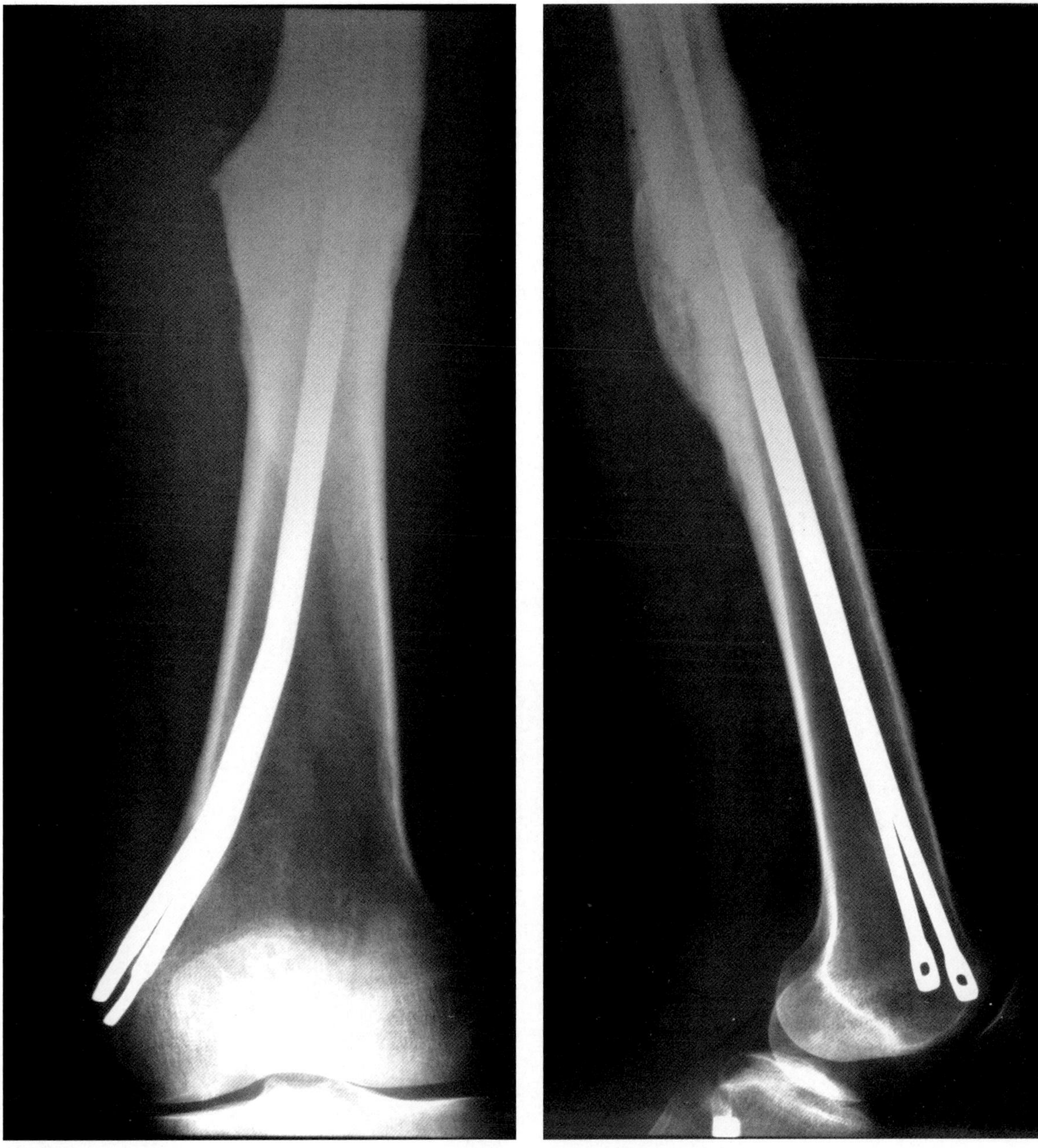


Fig. 5-23 *(Continued)*

intramedullary nailing. Previously, dynamic compression plates were used to achieve anatomic reduction (Fig. 5-29). This was an open procedure that put blood supply at risk during bone exposure. The closely applied compression plate put the periosteal vascular supply at risk. Currently, less invasive stabilization systems (LISS) are available that preserve vascular supply and require less invasive approaches (see Fig. 5-31). Bridge plates are useful for comminuted fractures. These long plates require fewer screws and may be used in adolescents and adults.

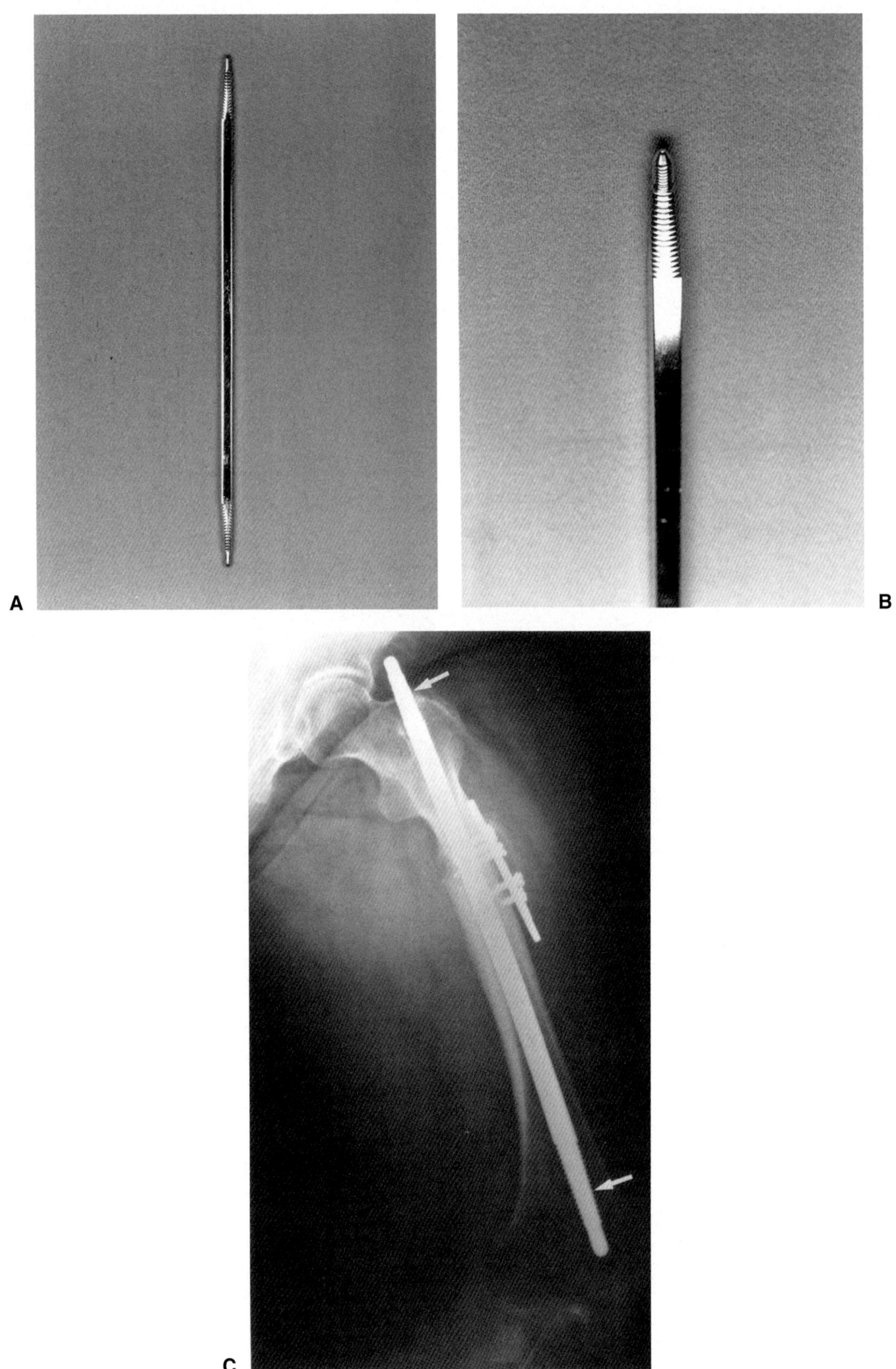


Fig. 5-24 Schneider nail with threaded ends (A) and close-up view of tip (B). Radiograph (C) of an ununited fracture with a Schneider nail (*arrows mark threaded ends*) and failed side plate for fixation.

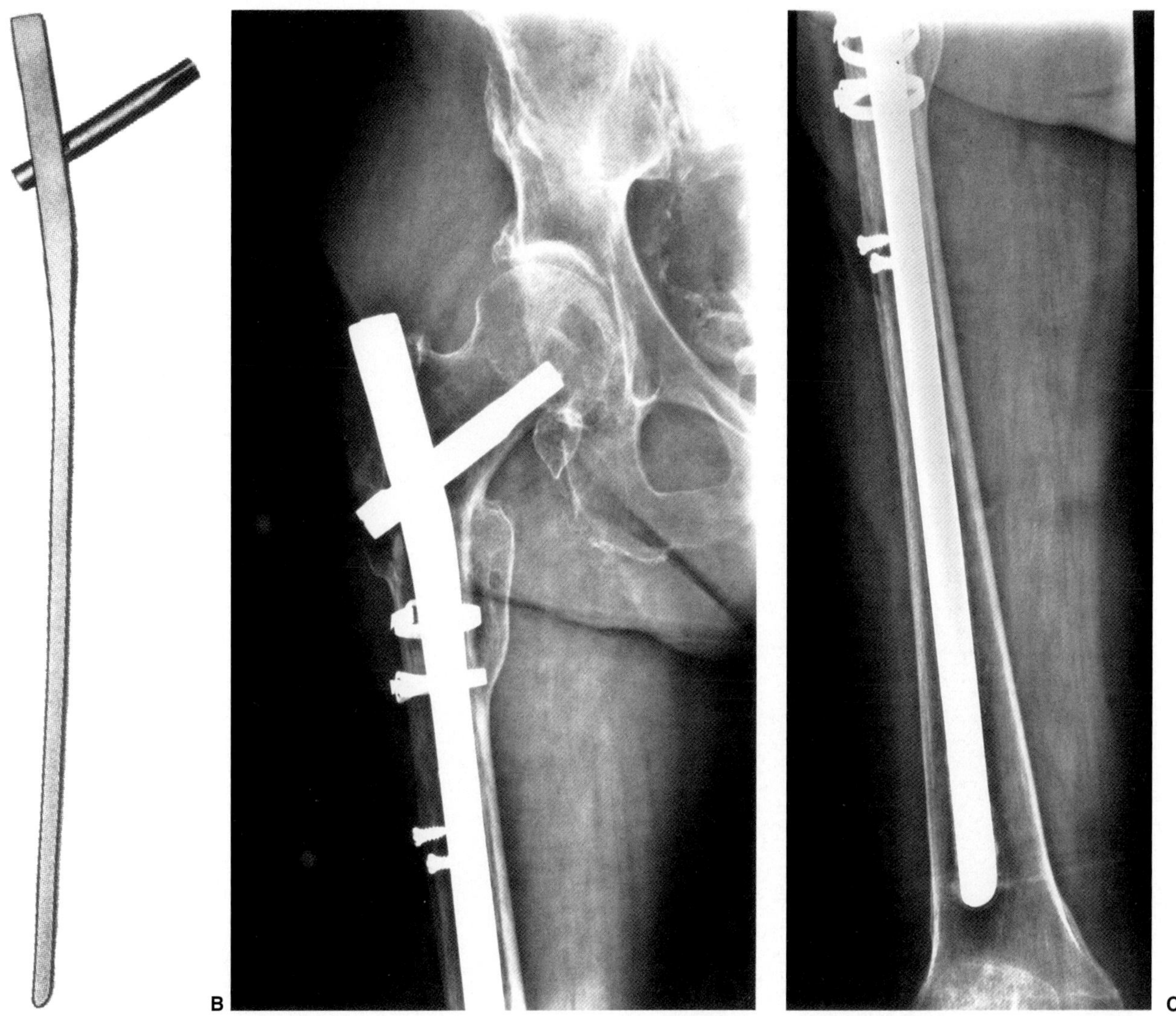


Fig. 5-25 A: Zickel nail (Courtesy of Howmedica, Rutherford, New Jersey). Radiographs of the upper (B) and lower (C) femur demonstrating a healed proximal fracture with Zickel fixation.

## Suggested Reading

Acharya KN, Rao MR. Retrograde nailing for distal third femoral shaft fractures: A prospective study. *J Orthop Surg.* 2006;14:253–258.

Beaty JH. Operative treatment of femoral shaft fractures in children and adolescents. *Clin Orthop.* 2005;434:114–122.

Fragomen AT, Rozbruch SR. The mechanics of external fixation. *HSS Journal.* 2007;3:13–29.

Ho CA, Skaggs DL, Tang CW, et al. Use of flexible intramedullary nails in pediatric femur fractures. *J Pediatr Orthop.* 2006;26:497–504.

Kubiak EN, Fulkerson E, Strauss E, et al. The evolution of locked plates. *J Bone Joint Surg.* 2006;88A:189–200.

Moed BR, Watson JT. Retrograde intramedullary nailing without reaming of fractures of the femoral shaft in multiply injured patients. *J Bone Joint Surg.* 1995;77A:1520–1528.

Winquist RA, Hansen ST, Clawson DK. Closed intramedullary nailing of femoral fractures. *J Bone Joint Surg.* 1984;66A:529–539.

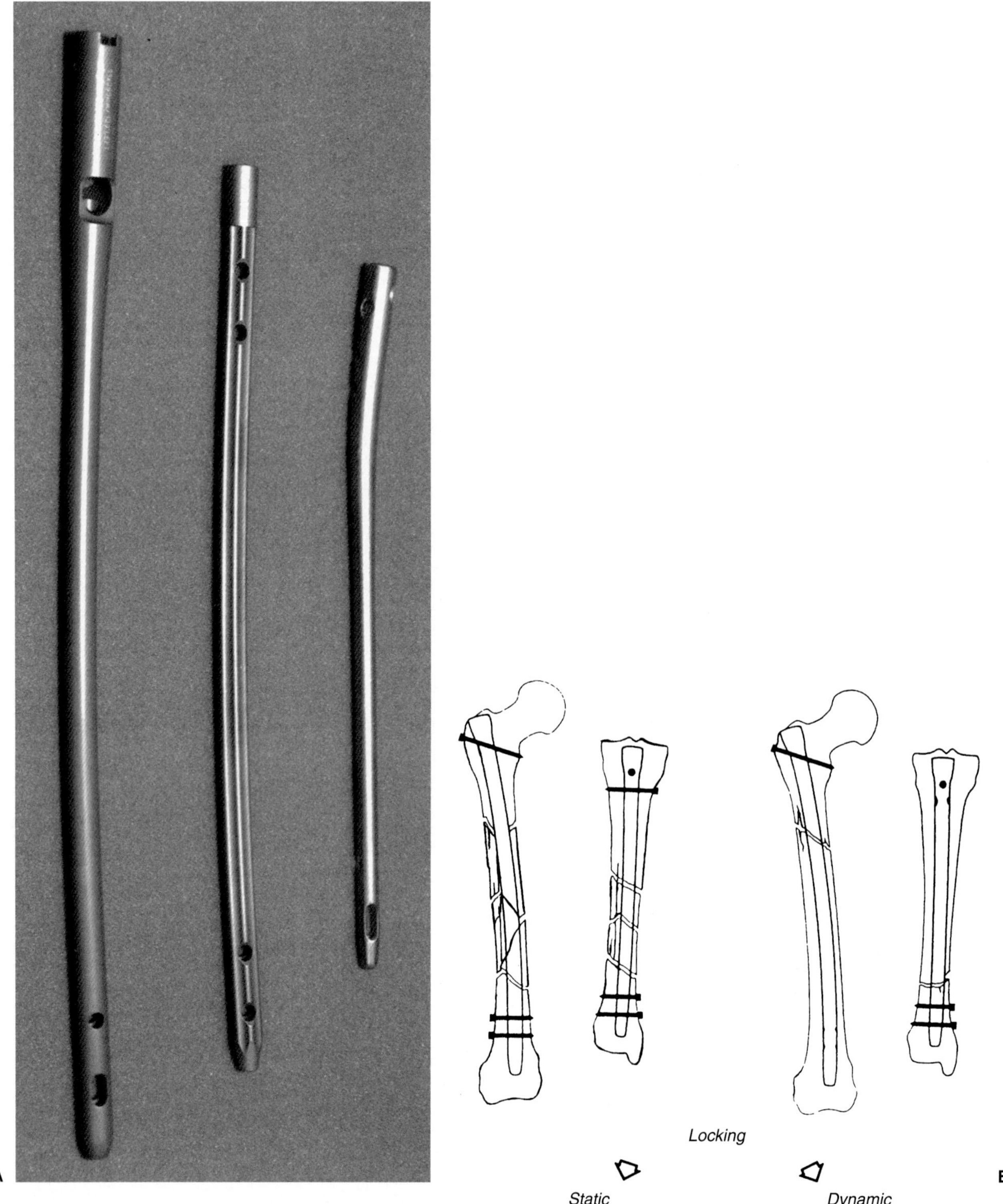


Fig. 5-26 A: Stryker intramedullary nails with screw holes at both ends for static or dynamic configuration. (Courtesy of Stryker Orthopaedics, Mahwah, New Jersey.) B: Illustration of locking nails in the femurs and tibia. Static configuration has screws proximally and distally while dynamic configuration has screws at only one end.

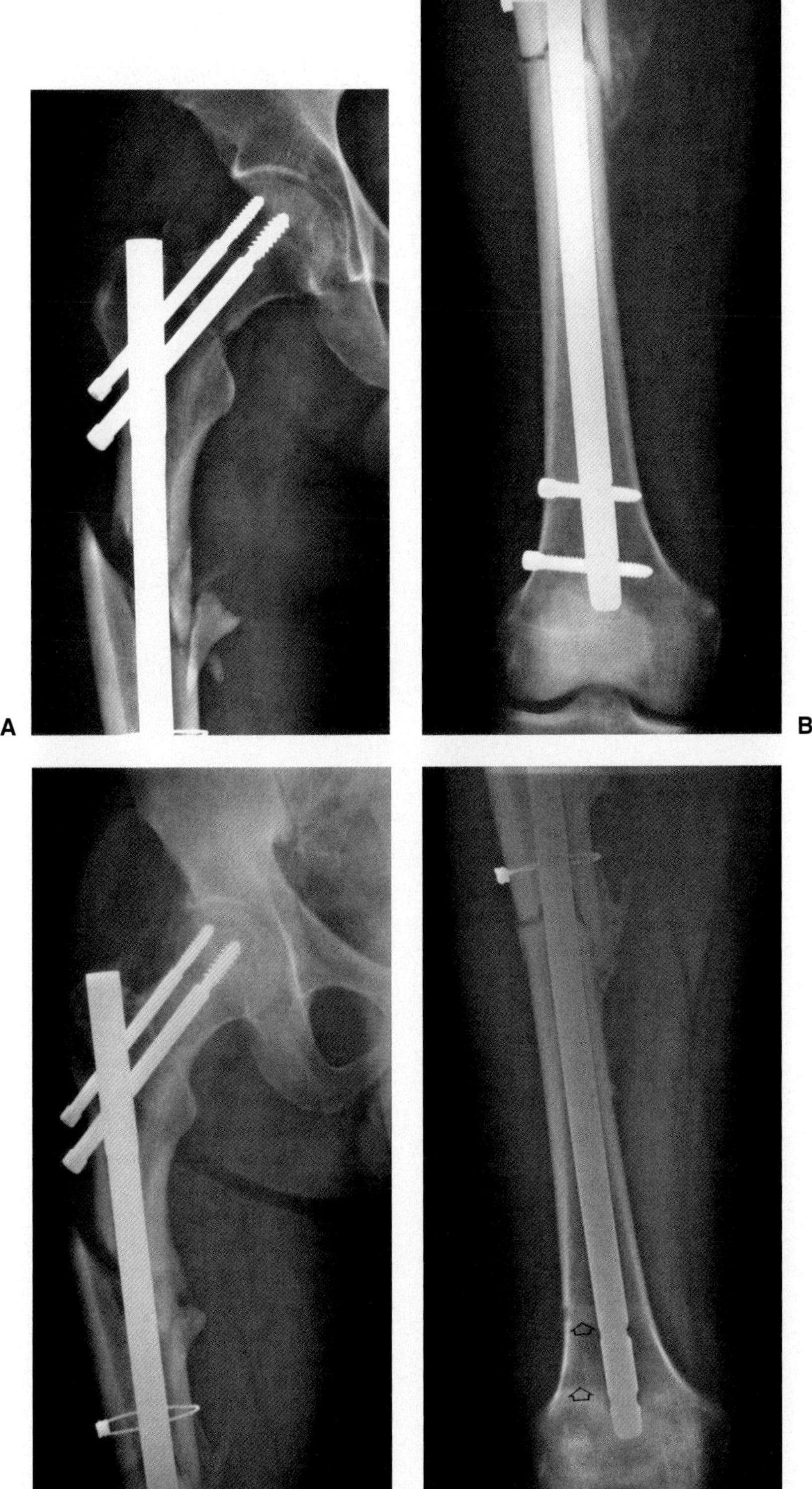


Fig. 5-27 Conversion of static to dynamic configuration. Anteroposterior (AP) radiographs of the femur (**A** and **B**) demonstrate femoral neck lag screws proximally and distal screws for fixation of a comminuted femoral fracture. There is a single Dall-Miles cable (*arrow*). Following conversion to dynamic configuration (**C** and **D**) the distal screws have been removed. The proximal fracture is more impacted and the screw holes in the nail have moved distally compared to the original screw tracts (*open arrows*).

A 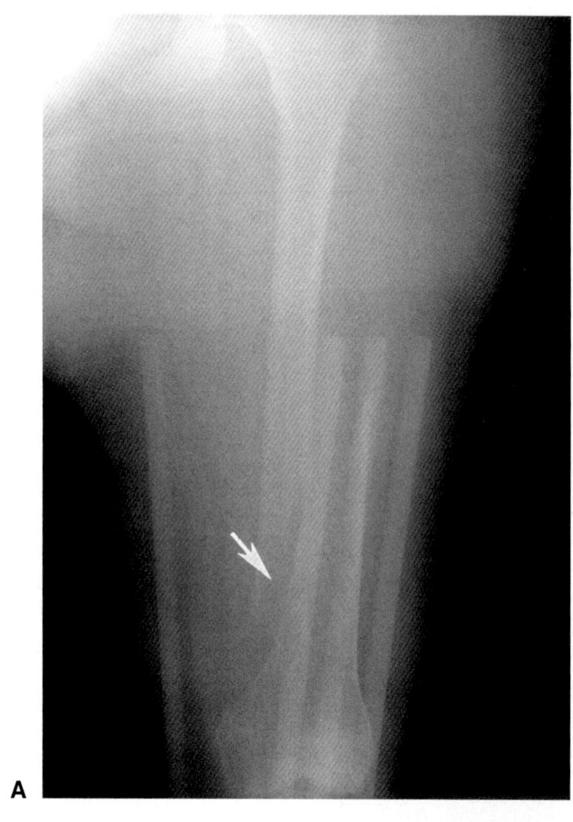

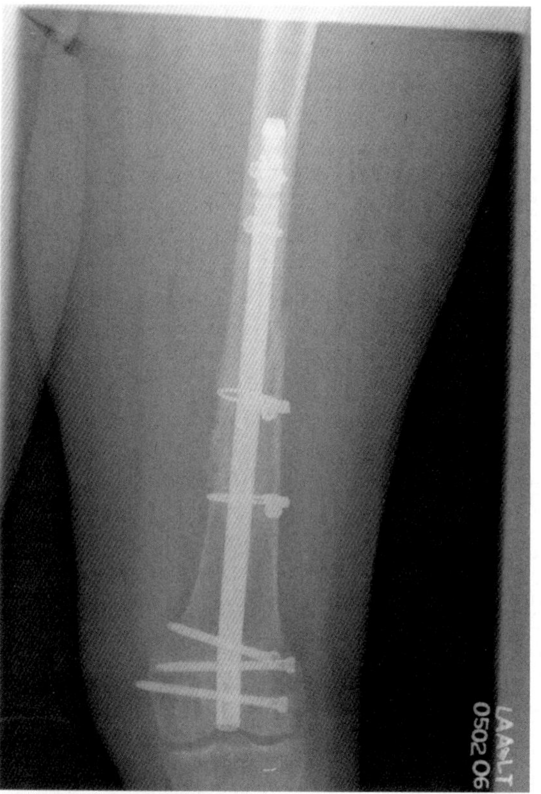 B

C 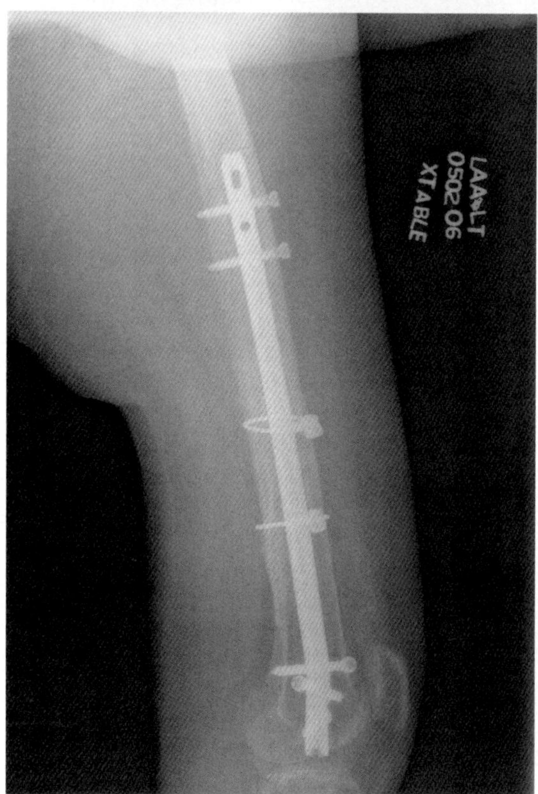

Fig. 5-28 A: Radiograph demonstrating an oblique overriding fracture of the distal femur (*arrow*). Anteroposterior (AP) (B) and lateral (C) radiographs demonstrate a locking intramedullary nail inserted distally with Dall-Miles cable support. The fracture is healed.

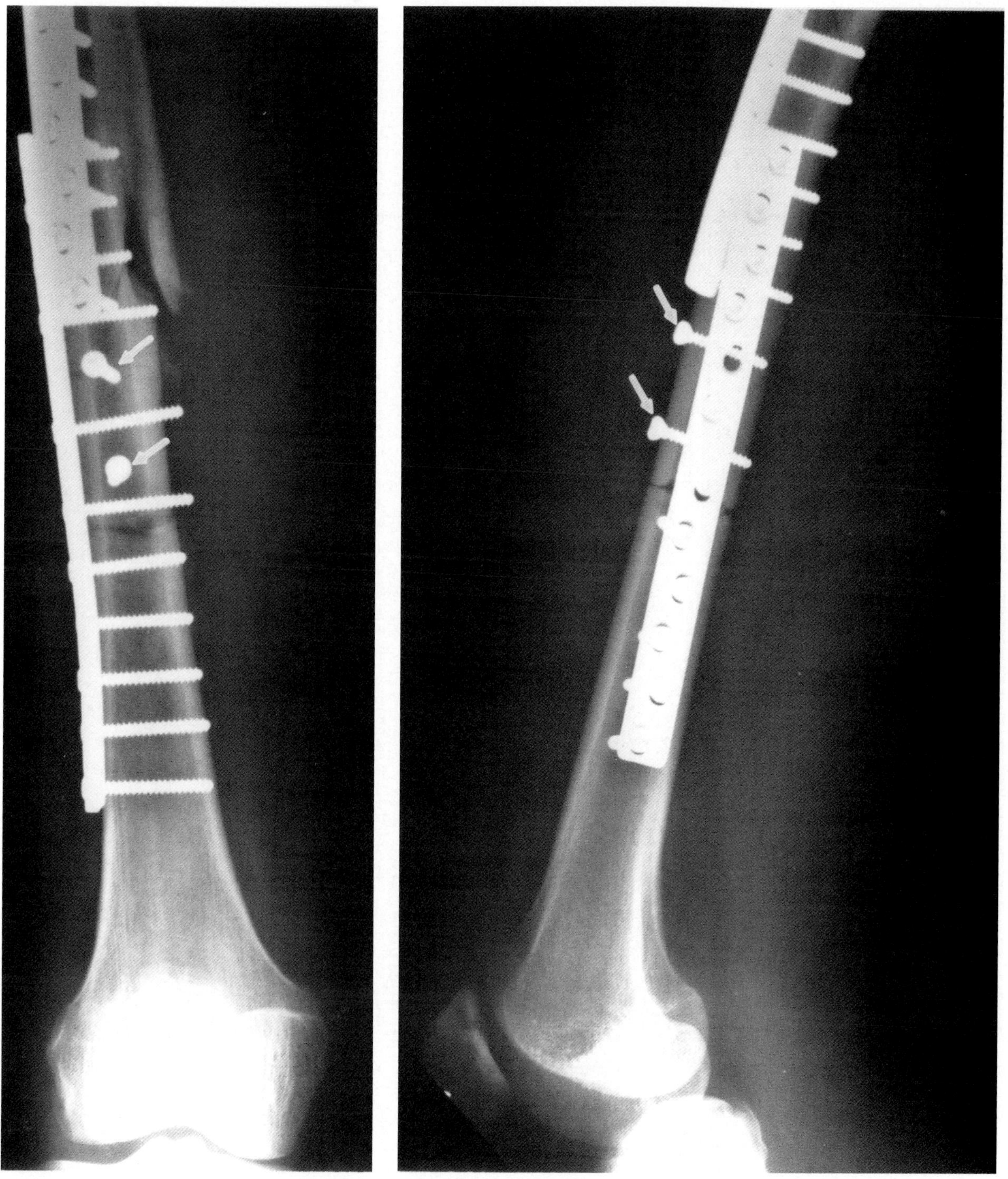


Fig. 5-29 Anteroposterior (AP) (A) and lateral (B) radiographs following fixation of a complex femoral fracture with two dynamic compression plates and cortical screws. There are also two interfragmentary screws (*arrows*).

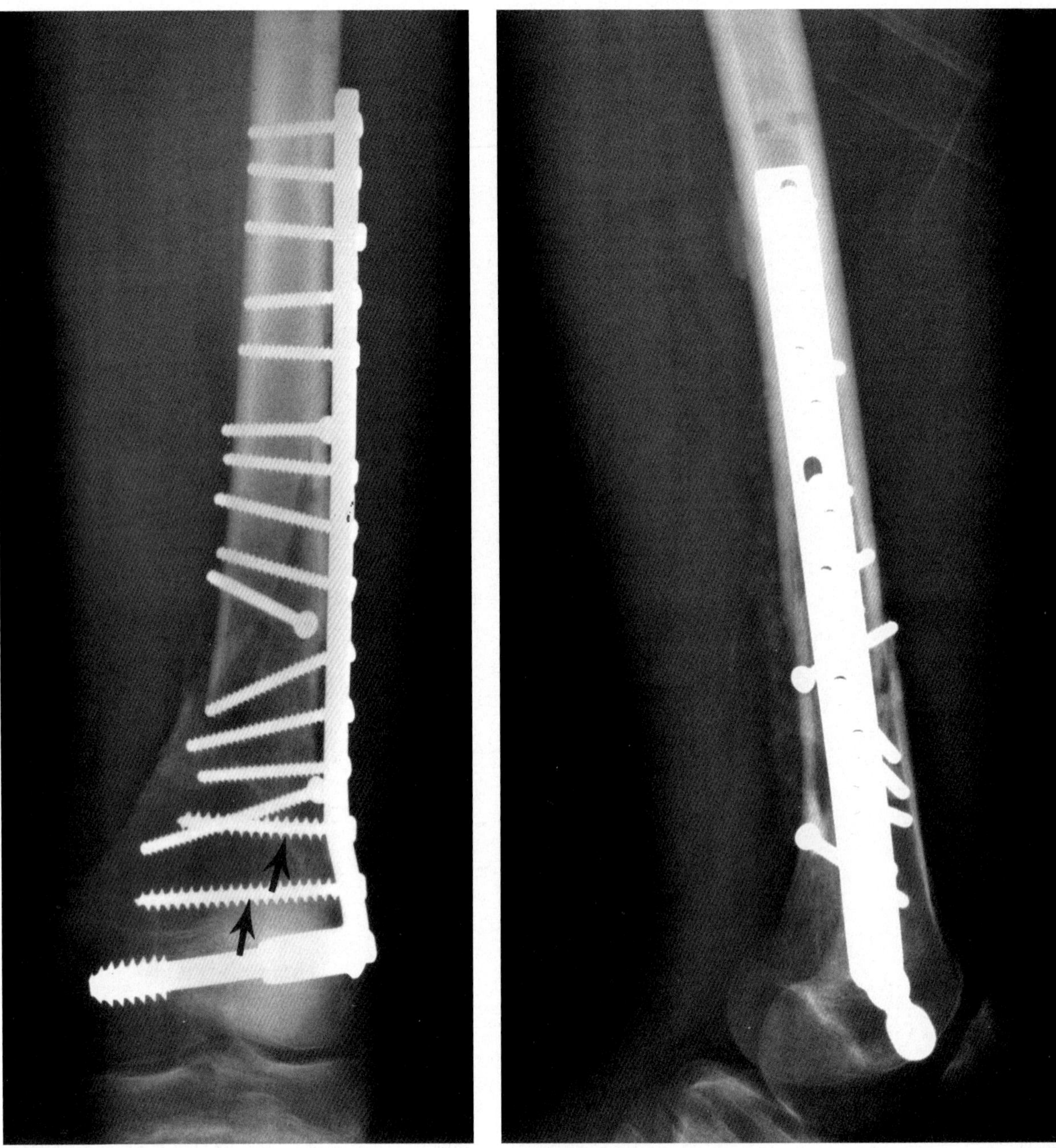



Fig. 5-30 Anteroposterior (AP) (A) and lateral (B) radiographs following fixation with a dynamic condylar screw and long 15-hole side plate. There are fully threaded cancellous screws distally (*arrows*) and several interfragmentary screws.

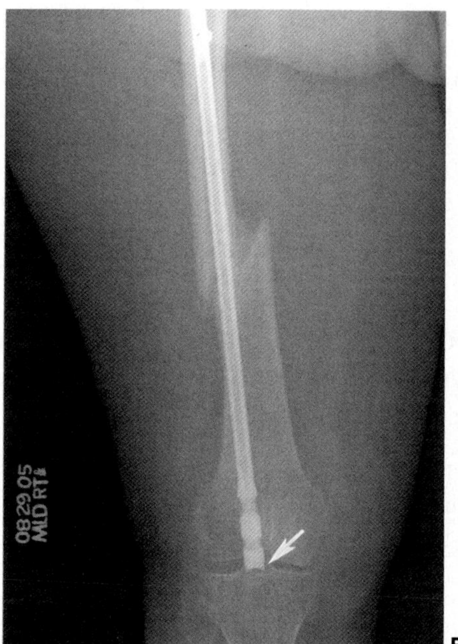


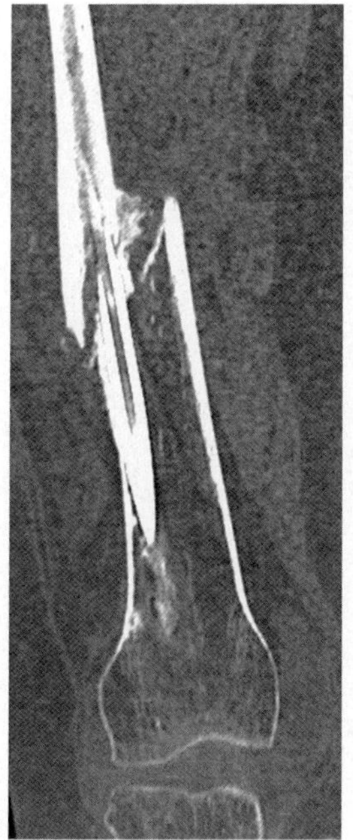


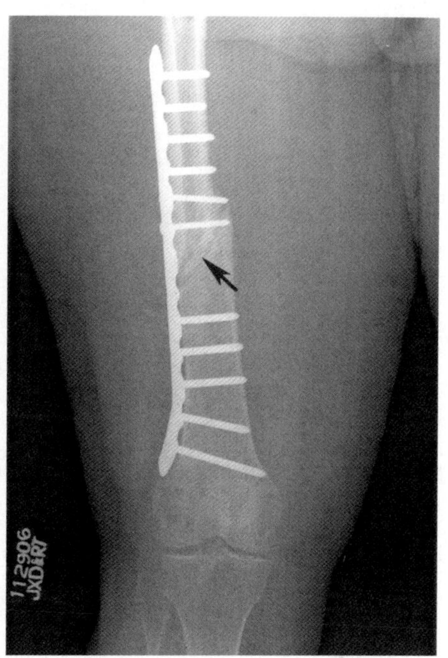


Fig. 5-31 Failed intramedullary nail. **A:** Anteroposterior (AP) radiograph demonstrates pulling out of the retrograde intramedullary nail with erosion (*arrow*) into the tibia. Reformatted computed tomography (CT) image (**B**) demonstrates sclerosis along the fracture line and poor callus formation. The nail was removed and the fracture site grafted (*arrow*) with fixation using an less invasive stabilization systems (LISS) plate and screws.

## Leg Length Discrepancy

Length discrepancy in the lower extremity is a common problem with numerous causes (see Table 5-1). The tibia and femur have primary diaphyseal and secondary epiphyseal ossification centers. The femur contributes 54% and the tibia 46% of overall growth potential. A determination of whether intervention is indicated depends upon multiple factors (see Table 5-2). Minimal differences in leg length are not unusual. Differences of up to 2 cm can be treated conservatively. Length differences of ≤5 cm in children can be treated by epiphysodesis of the opposite extremity. More significant deformities require leg lengthening procedures.

**Table 5-1**

| CAUSE OF LEG LENGTH DISCREPANCY |
|---|
| Congenital |
| Focal femoral deficiency |
| Congenitally short femur |
| Developmental dysplasia of the hip |
| Paralysis |
| Infection |
| Trauma |
| Shortening |
| Physeal Injury |
| Malunion, overriding |
| Diaphyseal growth acceleration |
| Neoplasms |
| Bone diseases |
| Osteogenesis imperfecta |
| Fibrous dysplasia |

### Preoperative Imaging

Preoperative imaging can be accomplished with standing radiographs, scanograms, CT, and MRI (see Fig. 5-32). CT in the lateral and coronal planes may be preferable in patients with rotational deformities. Recent studies have compared radiographic scanograms with CT and MRI. Although all three techniques provided good results, radiographs varied 0.52 mm, CT 0.68 mm, and MRI 2.9 mm when compared to direct caliper measurements. The technique selected should be used consistently pre- and postoperatively to assure validity of measurements.

**Table 5-2**

| CONSIDERATIONS FOR OPERATIVE INTERVENTION |
|---|
| Cause |
| Degree of length discrepancy |
| Age/sex |
| Anticipated growth potential |
| Patient requirements |

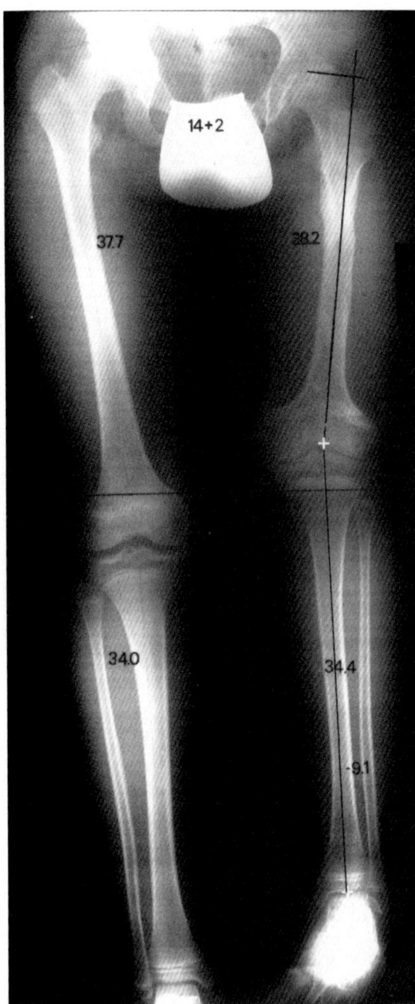


Fig. 5-32 Scanogram for leg length discrepancy. Anteroposterior (AP) full-length radiograph with posttraumatic shortening of the left femur. Lines are drawn along the femoral shaft with endpoints at a perpendicular line to the top of the femoral head and distally the femoral notch. The left femur measures 28.2 and the right 37.7 cm for a difference of 9.5 cm.

Demonstrating serial measurement change on scanograms or lack of progression is important in determining whether discrepancy can be corrected. Length discrepancies of >2 and <18 cm can be considered for reconstructive procedures (see Fig. 5-32).

## Suggested Reading

Aaron A, Weinstein D, Thickman D, et al. Comparison of orthoroentgenography and computed tomography in measurement of limb-length discrepancy. *J Bone Joint Surg.* 1992;74A:897–902.

Cooke TDV, Scudamore RA, Bryant JT, et al. A quantitative approach to radiography of the lower limb. *J Bone Joint Surg.* 1991;73B:715–720.

Harris I, Hatfield A, Walton J, et al. Assessing leg length discrepancy after femoral fracture: Clinical examination or computed tomography. *ANZ J Surg.* 2005;75:319–321.

Leitzes AH, Potter HG, Amaral T, et al. Reliability and accuracy of MRI scanogram in evaluation of limb-length discrepancy. *J Pediatr Orthop.* 2005;25:747–749.

Sabharwal S, Zhao C, McKeon JT, et al. Computed radiographic measurement of limb-length discrepancy. *J Bone Joint Surg.* 2006;88A:2243–2251.

### Treatment Options

#### Epiphysodesis/Epiphyseal Plate Stapling

This technique is designed to cause physeal growth arrest. The distal femur or proximal tibia and fibular epiphyses are most often used. If successful, the opposite extremity will continue to grow, reducing leg length discrepancy. This procedure is usually reserved for discrepancy of 5 cm or less.

#### Femoral Shaft Shortening or Lengthening

Femoral shortening or lengthening can be used to reduce the discrepancy. In the former, a segment of bone is resected and the bone ends drawn together and internally or externally fixed. Leg lengthening can be accomplished using several approaches. Following an osteotomy the bone fragments can be distracted in increments of 1.5 mm per day using external fixation systems described earlier until the desired result is achieved. Radiographs are used to follow the changes and adjust external fixation devices. Bone graft is then placed in the gap created. The femur is plated until healing occurs (see Fig. 5-33). Another approach is callus distraction. An osteotomy is performed and using an external fixator the gap is distracted using four 0.25-mm adjustments (1 mm per day). Distraction is continued until the desired length is attained. The fixation device is left in place until solid union is obtained (see Fig. 5-34).

## Suggested Reading

Dahl MT. Limb length discrepancy. *Pediatr Clin North Am.* 1996;43:849–865.

Dahl MT, Fischer DA. Lower extremity lengthening by Wagner's method and by callus distraction. *Orthop Clin North Am.* 1991;22:643–649.

### Complications

Complications associated with fracture fixation and treatment of leg length discrepancy can be similar, specifically related to external fixation systems. However, for discussion purposes they will be considered separately.

### Trauma

Complications related to trauma may be associated with extent of injury (osseous, soft tissue, open wound, etc.), type of treatment or fixation, and associated distant injuries or systemic complications. Fractures unite successfully with antegrade

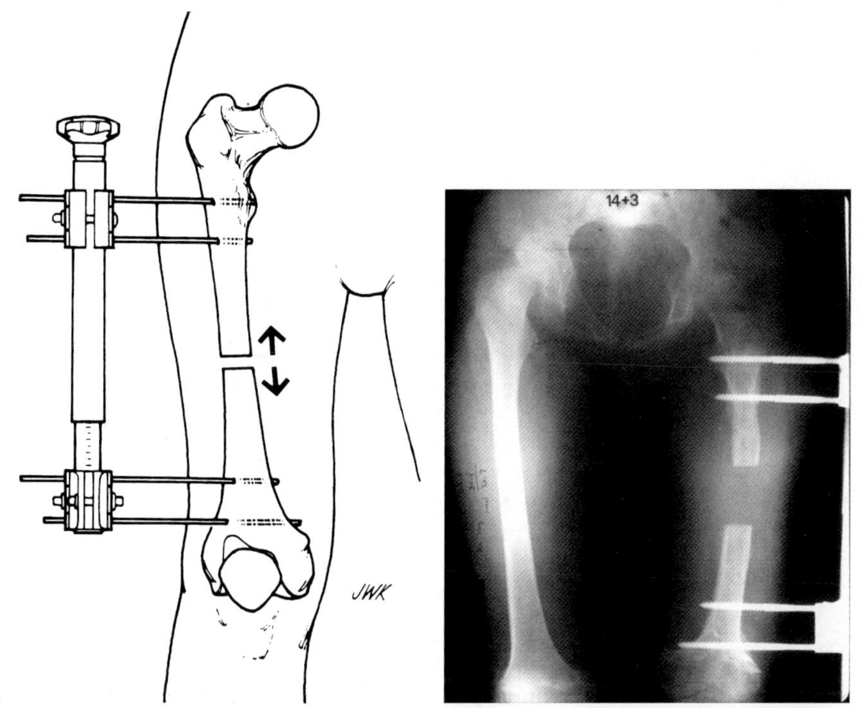


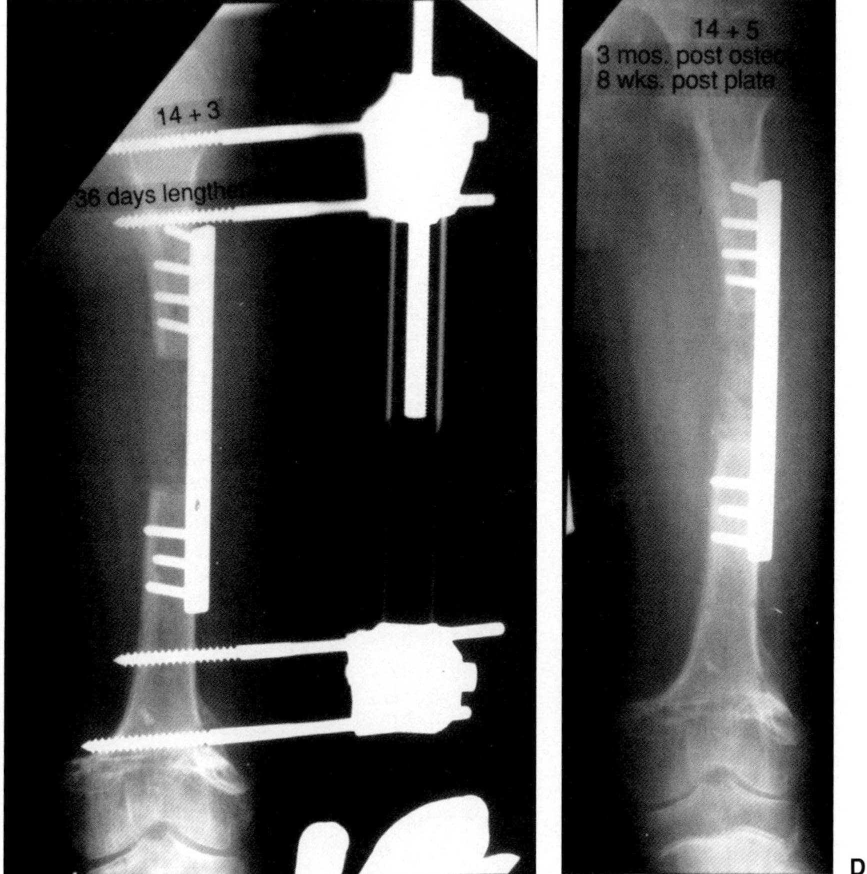


**Fig. 5-33** A: Illustration of osteotomy with Wagner apparatus to increase distraction gradually (*arrows*). B: Radiograph after desired length has been obtained. Three months later, a bridge plate is placed (C) and bone graft positioned in the gap. The external fixator can then be removed (D).

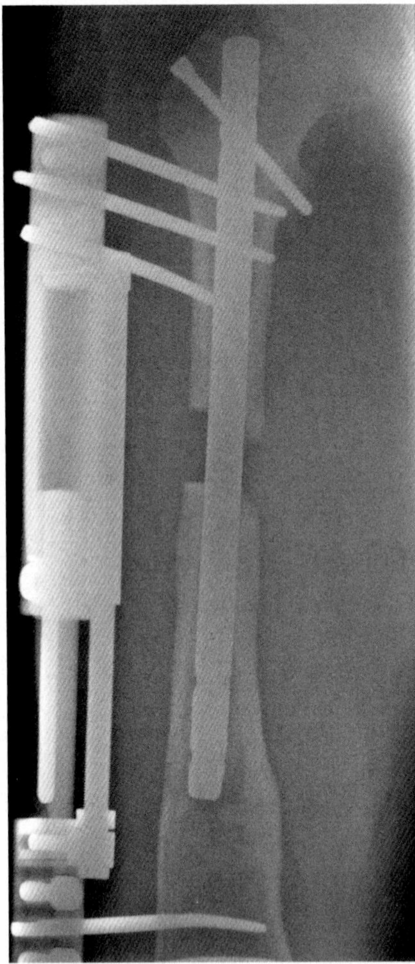

Fig. 5-34 Anteroposterior (AP) radiograph after shortening with prior internal fixation. An osteotomy has been performed and femoral lengthening performed using an Orthofix fixator.

intramedullary locking nails in 97% of cases and in 93% when retrograde locking nails are used. In some cases, the distal screws are removed (dynamic status) to improve healing (Fig. 5-27). Delayed union is usually defined as nonhealing 6 months after injury (Fig. 5-31). Nonunion occurs more commonly with less rigid forms of fixation. This is also the case with malunion and angular or rotational deformities. Angulation in the sagittal plane of 4 to 31 degrees (mean 17.8 degrees) and lateral angulation in the frontal plane are not uncommon with conservative or nonoperative treatment. However, shortening and rotation may also occur in up to 8% of patients treated with locking intramedullary nails (see Fig. 5-35). Serial radiographs may be adequate for evaluation of position and union. However, CT with metal artifact reduction techniques is superior to evaluate callus formation and the degree of union (Fig. 5-31).

Associated fractures must be defined as well as knee injuries, especially if traction is considered. Patients with femoral shaft fractures may have distant injuries and up to 6% have associated but often subtle femoral neck fractures (Fig. 5-35). Patients treated with locking intramedullary nails may have knee stiffness and decreased range of motion, specifically with retrograde nails. Anterior knee pain may be associated with the original injury or quadriceps atrophy. Refracture is unusual with internal fixation. However, the incidence is reported to be 2% to 21% with external fixation. Refracture may occur at the original fracture site or adjacent to the fixation site due to stress risers created in the unprotected portion of the femur. Refracture at the original fracture site correlates with the amount of callus and cortices involved. This is most effectively evaluated with CT.

Deep infection may be related to the extent of injury or treatment (see Fig. 5-36). Infection occurs in 24% of patients with Gustilo type III fractures (open fracture with significant soft tissue injury). Pin tract infection is the number one complication in patients treated with external fixation. Local wound care and oral antibiotics are usually successful in these cases.

Instrument failure may be related to rod, plate, or screw fractures (see Fig. 5-37). Rod fractures occur more commonly with severely comminuted fractures or when the rod diameter selected is too small for the medullary canal. Rod fractures also

**Table 5-3**

**FEMORAL SHAFT FRACTURE COMPLICATIONS**

| COMPLICATION | IMAGING APPROACHES |
|---|---|
| **Local complications** | |
| Osseous | |
| Refracture | Serial radiographs (Fig. 5-37) |
| Nonunion | Serial radiographs, CT (see Fig. 5-40) |
| Malunion | Serial radiographs |
| Delayed union | Serial radiographs, CT (Fig. 5-31) |
| Associated fractures | Radiographs (Fig. 5-37) |
| Avascular necrosis | Radiographs, MRI |
| Leg length discrepancy | Scanograms |
| Infection | |
| Pin tract | Serial radiographs |
| Deep infection | Serial radiographs, radionuclide scans, CT, MRI (Fig. 5-36) |
| Instrument failure | Serial radiographs (see Fig. 5-41) |
| Soft tissue injuries | |
| Compartment syndrome | MRI |
| Venous thrombosis | Ultrasound, venograms |
| Arterial injury | Angiography |
| Neural injury | MRI (Fig. 5-38) |
| Knee injuries | Flexion/extension, stress views, MRI |
| **Systemic complications** | |
| Distant fractures | Radiographs, CT |
| Fat/pulmonary emboli | Lung scans, CT |
| Pneumonia | Radiographs |
| Head injuries | CT, MRI |
| Abdominal injuries | CT |

CT, computed tomography; MRI, magnetic resonance imaging.

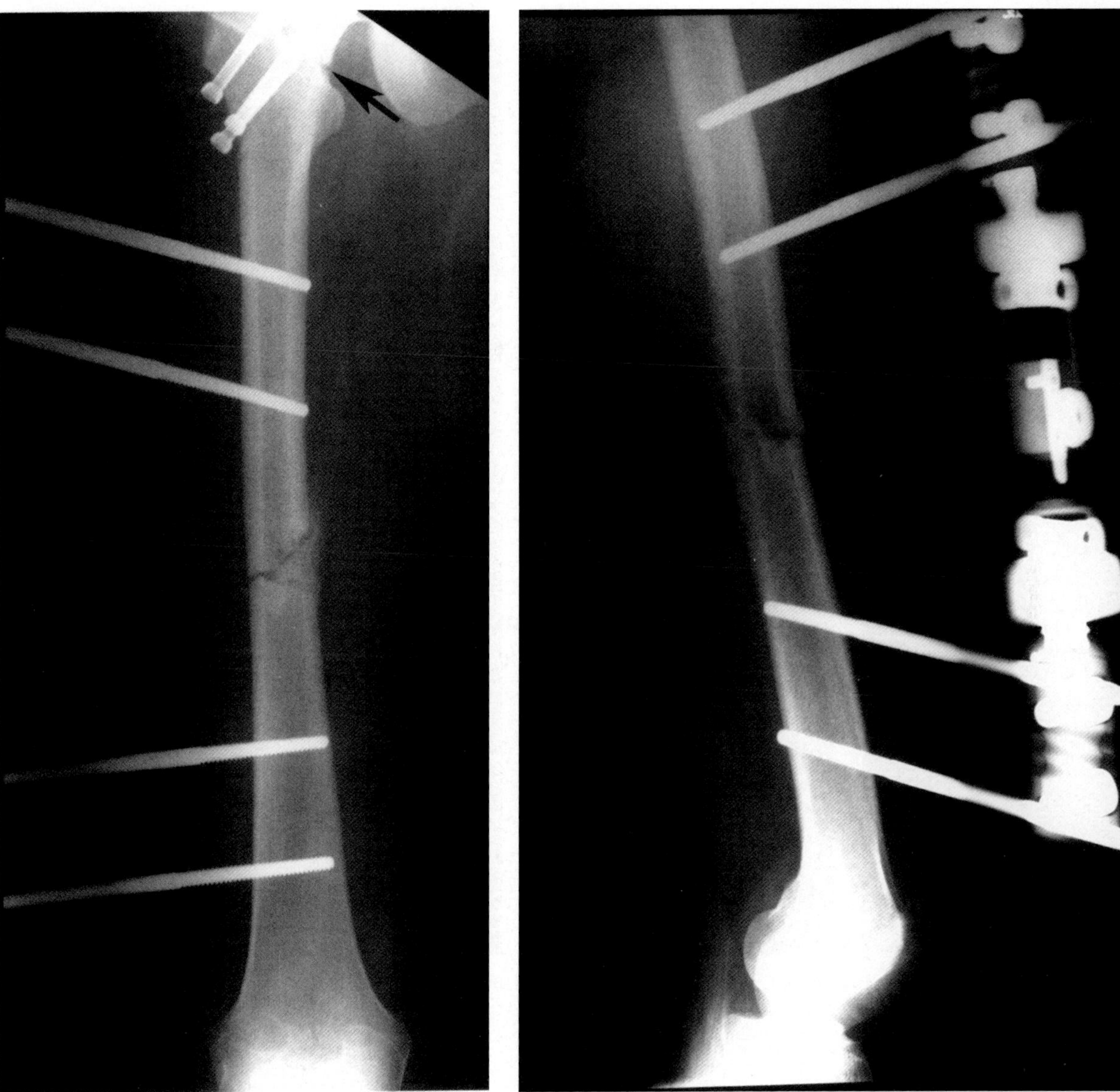


Fig. 5-35 Anteroposterior (AP) (A) and lateral (B) radiographs in a patient with a Winquist/Hansen type II femoral shaft fracture and associated femoral neck fracture (*arrow in A*). The femoral neck was treated with three cannulated hip pins and the femoral shaft with external fixation.

occur more commonly when the fracture extends to within 5 cm of the distal locking screw holes.

Soft tissue complications may be related to the original injury or treatment approach. Knee injury related to retrograde nailing was noted earlier. Quadriceps scarring may also be seen with femoral traction. External fixation pins may cause similar problems. Other soft tissue complications include compartment syndrome, deep venous thrombosis, and arterial and neural injury (see Fig. 5-38). Soft tissue symptoms may also develop related to screws projecting too far into the soft tissues. It is also not unusual for heterotopic ossification to develop over the proximal end on an antegrade intramedullary nail (see Fig. 5-39).

Avascular necrosis of the femoral head may occur related to the original injury or an antegrade intramedullary nail. In adolescents, the nail entry point near the greater trochanter may cut off flow in the medial circumflex artery which is critical to vascular supply at this age. The incidence of avascular necrosis is reported to be approximately 2%.

Systemic complications occur most commonly with multisystem trauma, with treatment delays, and prolonged immobilization. The frequent use of intramedullary nails has resulted in early mobilization and reduction in these complications. Table 5-3 summarizes complications and imaging approaches.

## Complications of Leg Length Discrepancy

The complications discussed in the preceding text may also be associated with procedures to treat leg length discrepancy. However, there are some differences and the incidence

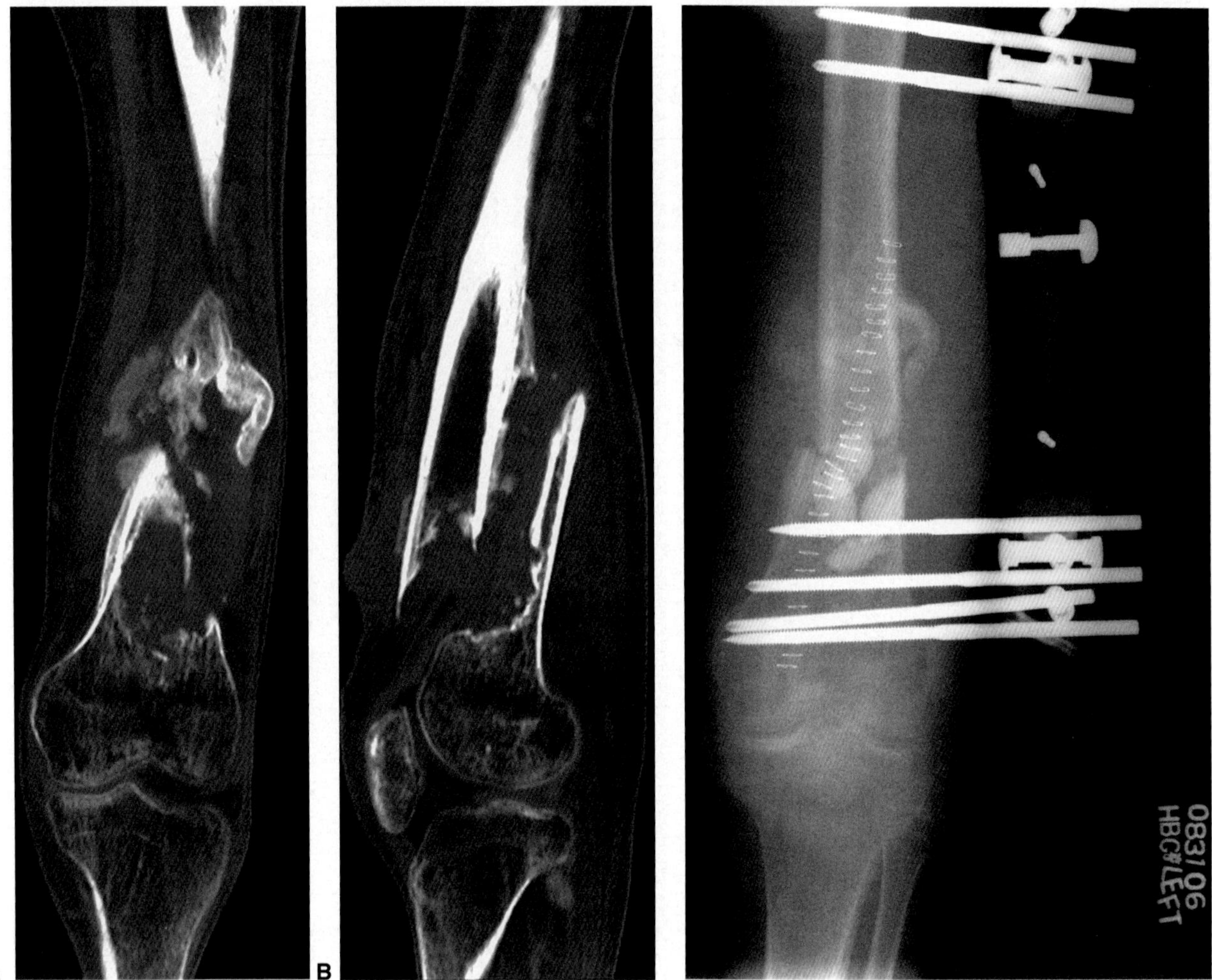


Fig. 5-36 Deep infection with nonunion. Coronal (A) and sagittal (B) computed tomography (CT) images demonstrate bone destruction at the fracture site with nonunion. Anteroposterior (AP) radiograph (C) after external fixation and implanting antibiotic methyl methacrylate beads.

Table 5-4

LEG LENGTHENING COMPLICATIONS

| COMPLICATION | WAGNER (%) | CALLOTASIS (%) | IMAGING APPROACHES |
|---|---|---|---|
| Pin tract infection | 22 | 2–10 | Serial radiographs |
| Deep infections | 7 | 2 | Serial radiographs, radionuclide scans, MRI |
| Nonunion | 10 | 1 | Serial radiographs, CT |
| Malunion | 22 | 1–3 | Serial radiographs, CT |
| Compartment syndrome | 3 | 0 | MRI |
| Implant failure | 2 | 0 | Serial radiographs |
| Late fracture | 11 | 3 | Serial radiographs |

MRI, magnetic resonance imaging; CT, computed tomography.

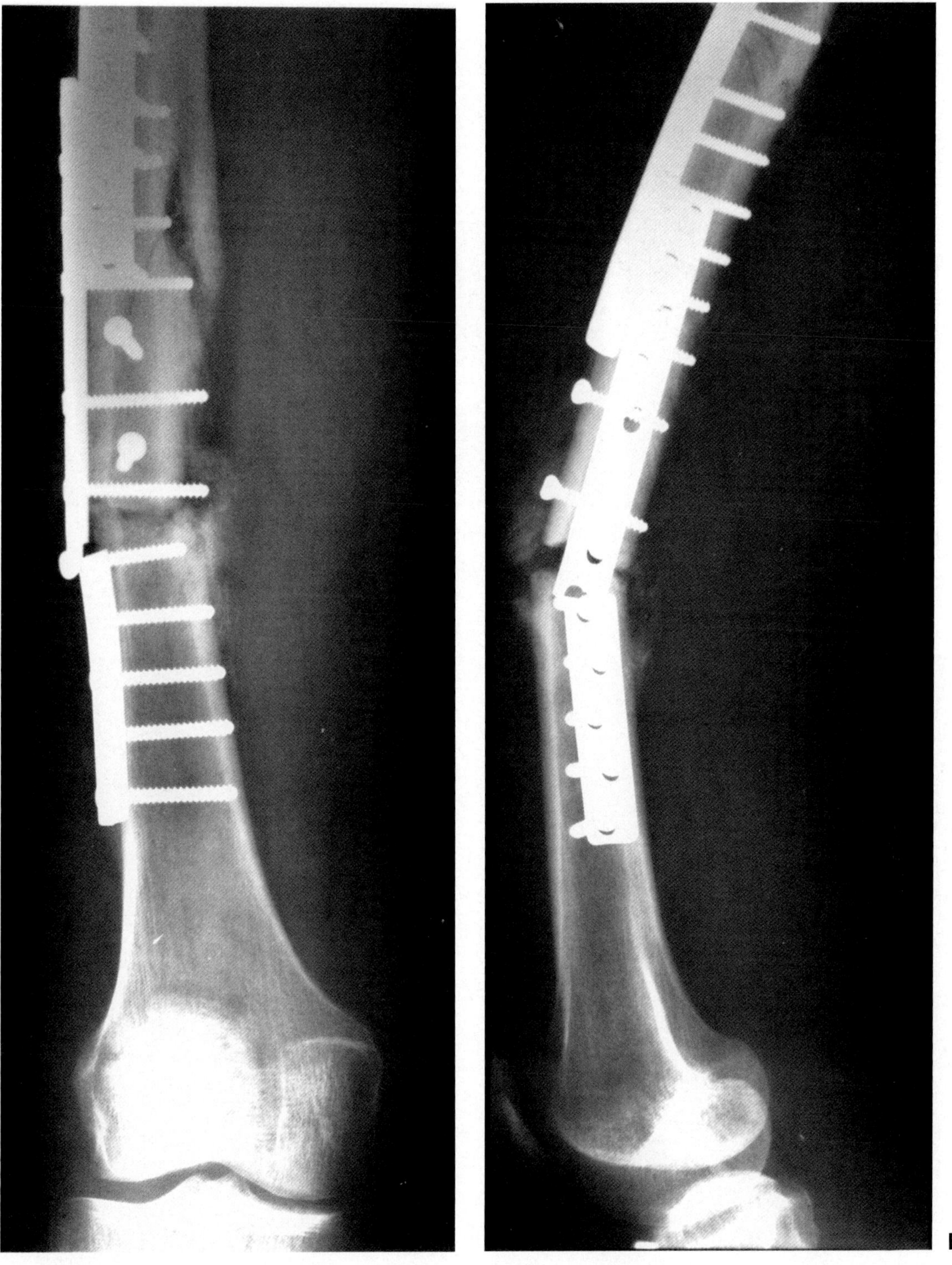


Fig. 5-37 Anteroposterior (AP) (A) and lateral (B) radiographs following fracture of the dynamic compression plate at the fifth screw hole from the end of the plate and refracture through the existing callus.

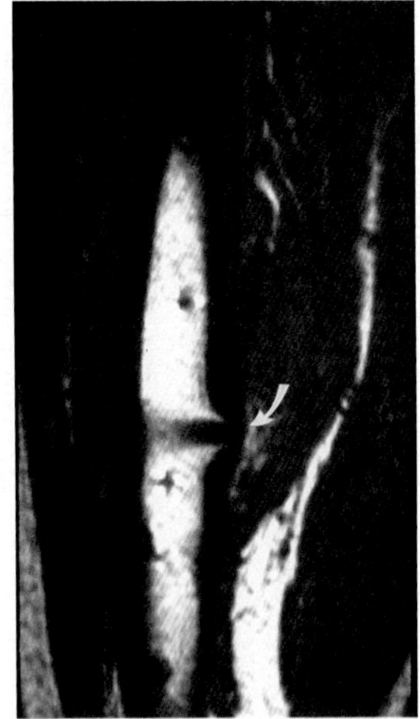


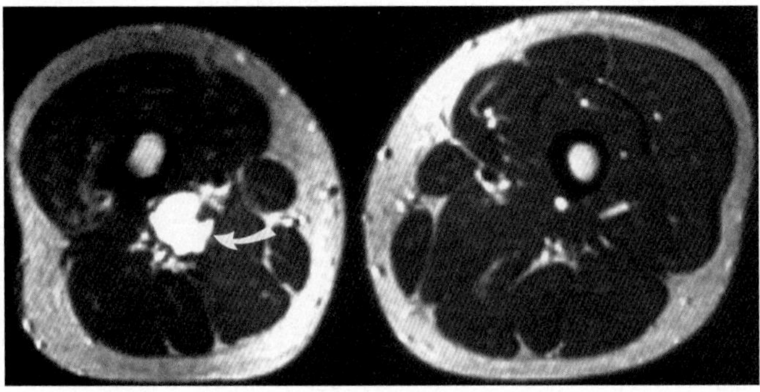


**Fig. 5-38** Plate and screws were removed due to persistent thigh pain. Sagittal T1-weighted image demonstrates cortical deformity near the screw tract (*curved arrow*). Axial T2-weighted image demonstrates a well defined high signal intensity lesion (*curved arrow*) due to a post-traumatic neuroma.

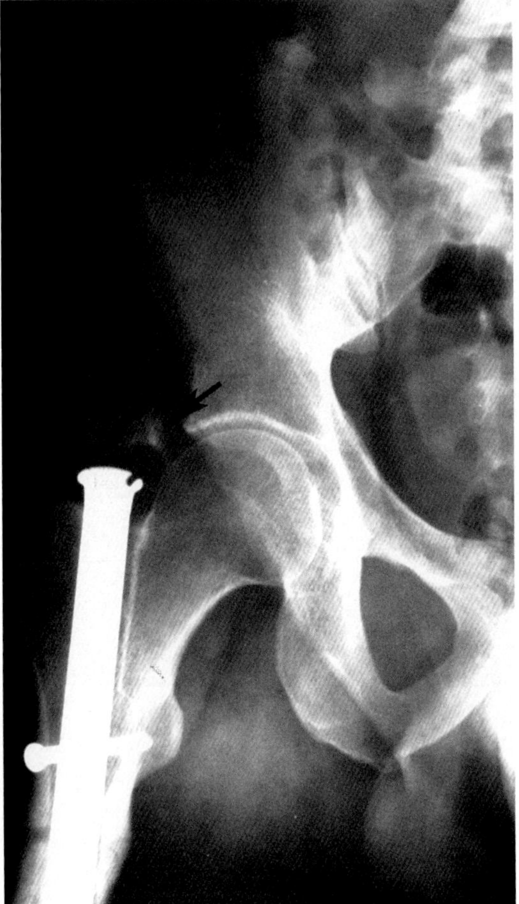

**Fig. 5-39** Anteroposterior (AP) radiograph with intramedullary nail in place. There is heterotopic ossification over the proximal nail (*arrow*).

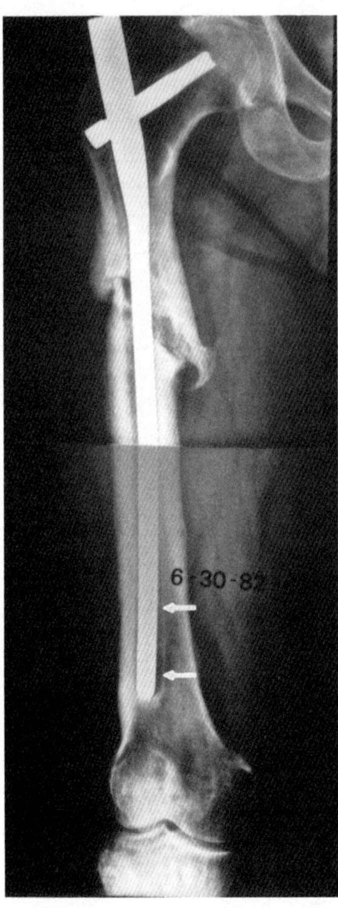

**Fig. 5-40** Anteroposterior (AP) radiograph following Zickel nail fixation of a proximal femoral shaft fracture. There is lucency about the nail (*arrows*) due to motion and hypertrophic nonunion at the fracture site.

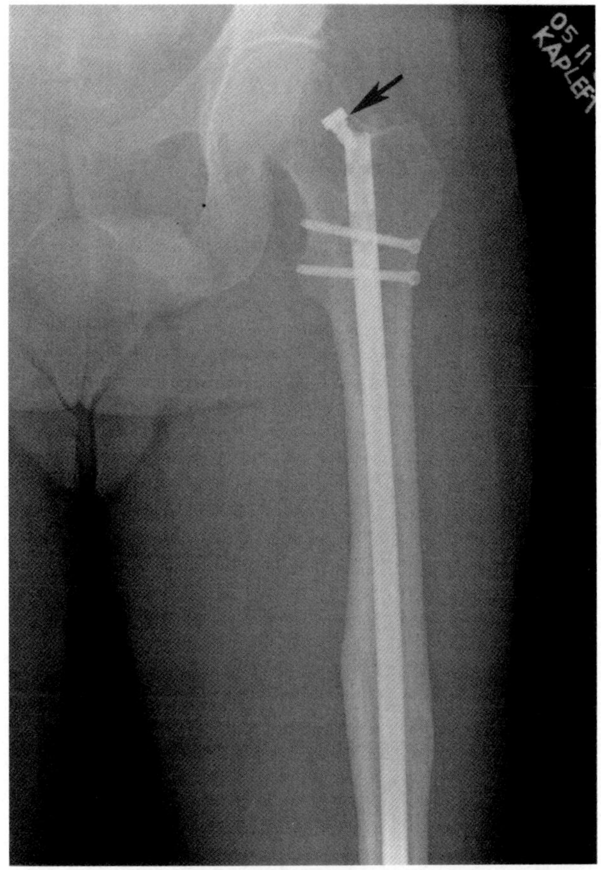


A

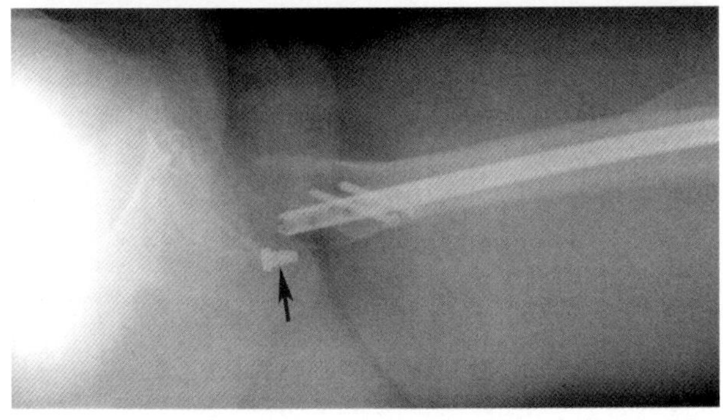

B

Fig. 5-41 Anteroposterior (AP) (A) and lateral (B) radiographs following intramedullary nail placement and healing of a mid-femoral fracture. The nail cap (*arrow*) has displaced posteriorly.

of complications is much higher. Complications have been reported in 29% to 81% of cases, although many are minor in nature. Pin tract infection is the most common complication followed by pin loosening. Skin slough at the osteotomy site, fractures, and angular deformities may also occur. Table 5-4 summarizes complications and imaging approaches for the Wagner technique (gradual distraction then bone grafting) and callotasis (microdistraction with callus forming at the osteotomy site).

## Suggested Reading

Acharya KN, Rao MR. Retrograde nailing for distal third femoral shaft fractures: A prospective study. *J Orthop Surg*. 2006;14:253–258.

Beaty JH. Operative treatment of femoral shaft fractures in children and adolescents. *Clin Orthop*. 2005;434:114–122.

Dahl MT, Fischer DA. Lower extremity lengthening by Wagner's method and callus distraction. *Orthop Clin North Am*. 1991;22:643–649.

Elridge JC, Bell DF. Problems with substantial limb-lengthening. *Orthop Clin North Am*. 1991;22:625–631.

Fragomen AT, Rozbruch SR. The mechanics of external fixation. *HSS Journal*. 2007;3:13–29.

Harris I, Hatfield A, Walton J. Assessing leg length discrepancy after femoral fracture: Clinical examination or computed tomography? *ANZ J Surg*. 2005;75:319–321.

Ho CA, Skaggs DL, Tang CW, et al. Use of flexible intramedullary nails in pediatric femur fractures. *J Pediatr Orthop*. 2006;26:497–504.

Thometz JG, Lamdan R. Osteonecrosis of the femoral head after intramedullary nailing of a fracture of the femoral shaft in an adolescent. *J Bone Joint Surg*. 1995;77A:1423–1426.

# 6 The Knee

The anatomy of the knee is complex. Osseous, cartilaginous, and passive and dynamic restraints must be preserved to ensure optimal function. To this end, numerous orthopaedic devices and prostheses have been designed to maintain a knee that is functional and pain-free. This chapter will review orthopaedic devices and imaging techniques for trauma, joint replacement, and other common surgical procedures about the knee.

## Trauma

### Preoperative Imaging

Imaging of the knee in patients with suspected trauma is different from certain other indications. Patients may not be able to tolerate special views. Therefore, anteroposterior (AP), lateral, and both oblique views (see Fig. 6-1) are routinely obtained. The lateral view (Fig. 6-1E and F) should be obtained using cross-table lateral technique because a lipohemarthrosis may be the only indication of a subtle intra-articular fracture. Standing views are not usually required. Additional views, such as the notch or patellar views, should be considered if the patient can tolerate the necessary positioning. These views are useful for detection of patellar fracture or alignment abnormalities and osteochondral injuries.

When indicated, computed tomography (CT) is useful to further evaluate suspected fractures or fragment position (see Fig. 6-2). Magnetic resonance imaging (MRI) is also able to detect subtle osseous injuries as well as evaluate the articular cartilage (see Fig. 6-3) and soft tissue supporting structures.

### Suggested Reading


Berquist TH. Osseous and myotendinous injuries about the knee. *Magn Reson Imaging Clin N Am*. 2007;15:25–38.

Mui LW, Engelsohn E, Umans H. Comparison of CT and MRI in patients with tibial plateau fractures: Can CT findings predict ligament tear or meniscal injury? *Skeletal Radiol*. 2007; 36:145–151.


### Supracondylar Fractures of the Femur

Supracondylar fractures of the femur are fractures involving the distal 9 to 15 cm, as measured from the articular surface of the femoral condyles. These fractures are relatively uncommon, accounting for only 7% of femoral fractures. Fractures may be impacted, undisplaced, comminuted, and involve the articular surface of the femur. Associated injuries of the tibial plateau, proximal tibia, proximal femur, and soft tissues of the knee are common. Approximately 5% to 10% of supracondylar fractures are open injuries, usually anterior and proximal to the patella.

The mechanism of injury is usually varus or valgus stress with associated axial or rotary forces. Injuries are usually related to high-velocity trauma such as motor vehicle accidents in younger patients or due to more minor trauma in the elderly. There are multiple classification systems based on extra-articular, one or more condyle involvement, the plane of the fracture, and the degree of comminution.

**Classification: Orthopaedic Trauma Association** (see Fig. 6-4)

- **Type A:** Extra-articular, simple, or comminuted
  - A1—simple (Fig. 6-4A)
  - A2—metaphyseal, wedge (Fig. 6-4B)
  - A3—metaphyseal, complex
- **Type B:** Partial articular, one condyle involved (Fig. 6-4C)
  - B1—lateral condyle, sagittal fracture line
  - B2—medial condyle, sagittal fracture line
  - B3—frontal coronal fracture line
- **Type C:** Complete articular, both condyles involved with "T" or "Y" pattern, or comminuted
  - C1—both condyles, simple (Fig. 6-4D)
  - C2—both condyles, multiple metaphyseal fragments (Fig. 6-4E)
  - C3—both condyles, all segments comminuted

### Suggested Reading


Schatzker J. Fractures of the distal femur revisited. *Clin Orthop*. 1998;347:43–56.

Orthopaedic Trauma Association Committee on Coding and Classifications. Fractures and dislocations compendium. *J Orthop Trauma*. 1996;10(Suppl 1):41–45.

## Treatment Options

The goals for treatment are to restore alignment and articular anatomy. Both closed and open techniques may be employed depending on the patient status (i.e., other injuries) and the type of fracture. Reduction may be difficult to maintain due to muscle forces acting on the fragments.

**Traction:** Traction is a useful temporary approach to comminuted fractures or when patient status will not allow primary definitive fixation. Single or double traction pins may be used. A single pin can be placed in the proximal tibia with the option of a second pin in the distal femoral fragment (see Fig. 6-5). The latter can add problems such as quadriceps scarring.

**External Fixation:** As noted in previous chapters, external fixation is particularly useful in multitrauma patients, with complex fractures and when there are open wounds that require easy wound access. Fractures that are considered for external fixation fall into the above-mentioned categories and are typically complex nonarticular (OTA A3), and complex bicondylar (OTA C3). Unilateral, ring, or hybrid fixators can be used (see Fig. 6-6). Mean healing time is 4 months. Secondary procedures are required in approximately 20% of cases (Fig. 6-6B and C).

**Internal Fixation:** Internal fixation can be accomplished using multiple approaches. The type of fracture pattern, other injuries, and surgical preference dictate the approach selected. Extra-articular fractures (OTA type A) and fractures with condylar fragmentation (OTA type C3) can be treated with blade plates or dynamic condylar screws (see Figs. 6-7 and 6-8). Antigrade or retrograde intramedullary locking nails may also be used. In recent years, use of less invasive stabilization system (LISS) plates has become more popular. These plates have screws with threaded heads to lock them to the plate at a fixed angle (see Chapter 2) analogous to external fixation. The

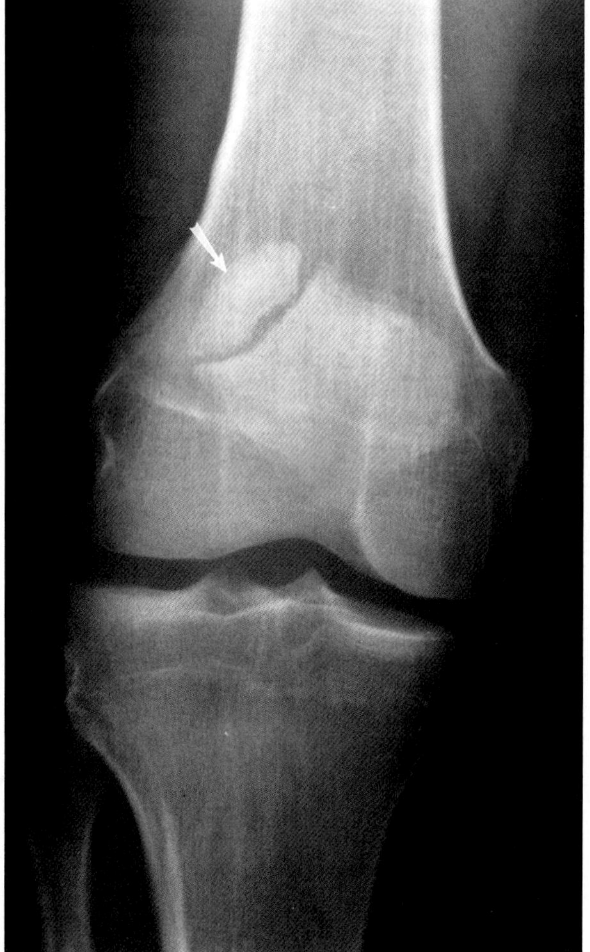


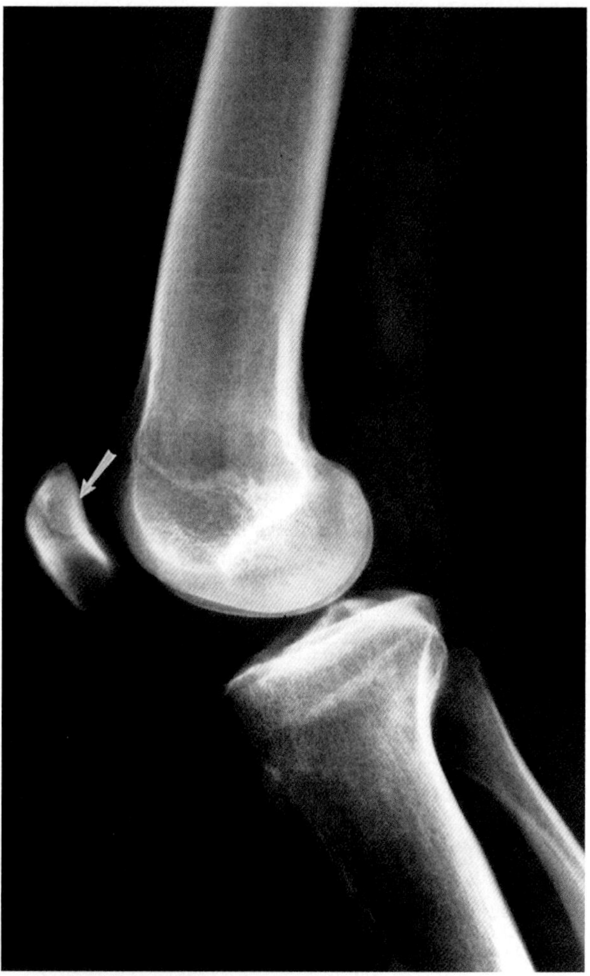


**Fig. 6-1** Routine views of the knee. Anteroposterior (AP) (**A**) and lateral (**B**) radiographs of the knee demonstrating a bipartite patella (*arrow*). Oblique views are obtained in internal (**C**) and external rotation (**D**). These views may detect subtle injuries not identified on AP and lateral views. Note the femoral condyle fracture (*arrows*) on the external oblique radiograph. The normal lateral view may demonstrate an effusion (**E**) (*arrow*), but a cross table lateral view (**F**) is more useful and can demonstrate a lipohemarthrosis (*arrows*).

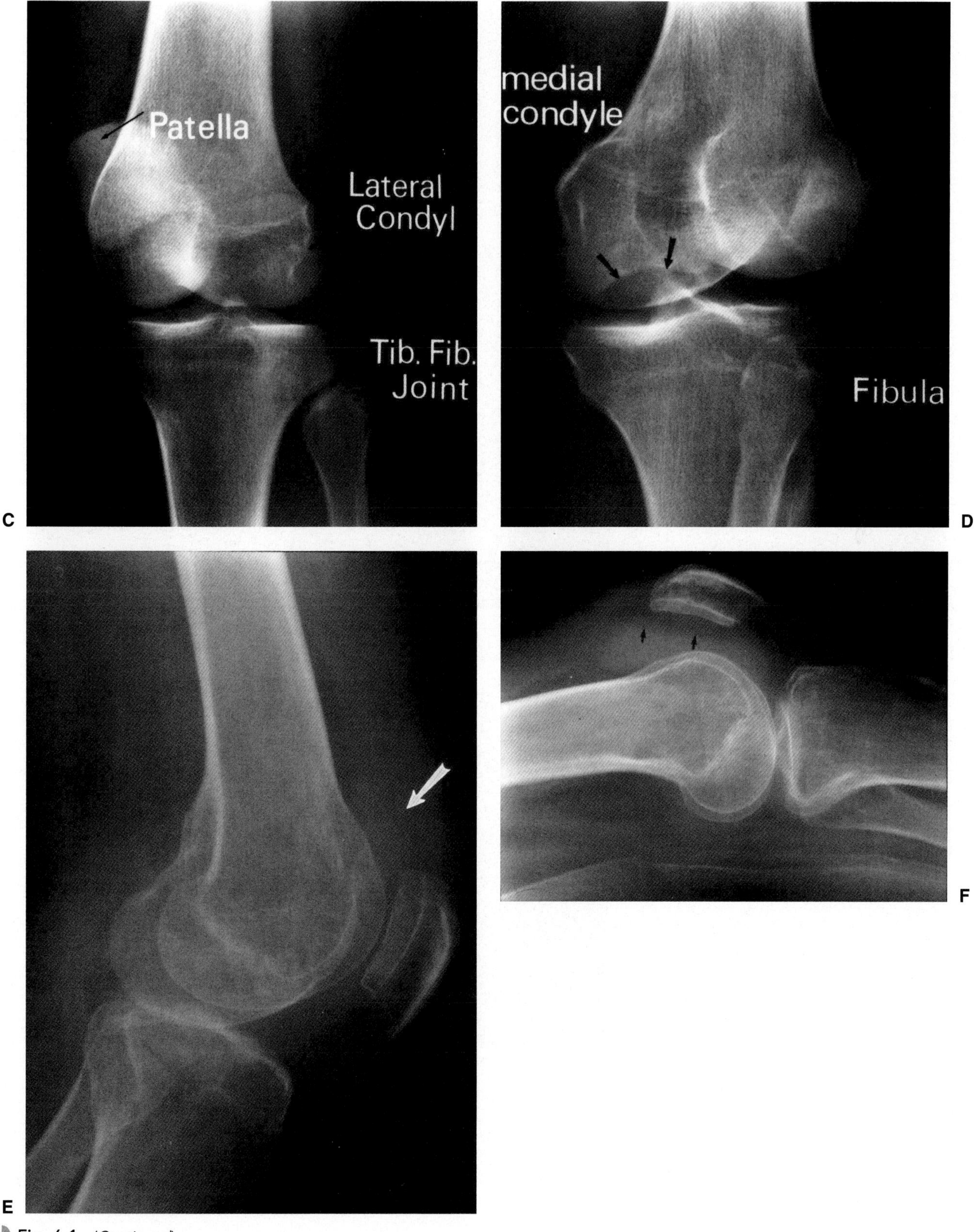


Fig. 6-1 (*Continued*)

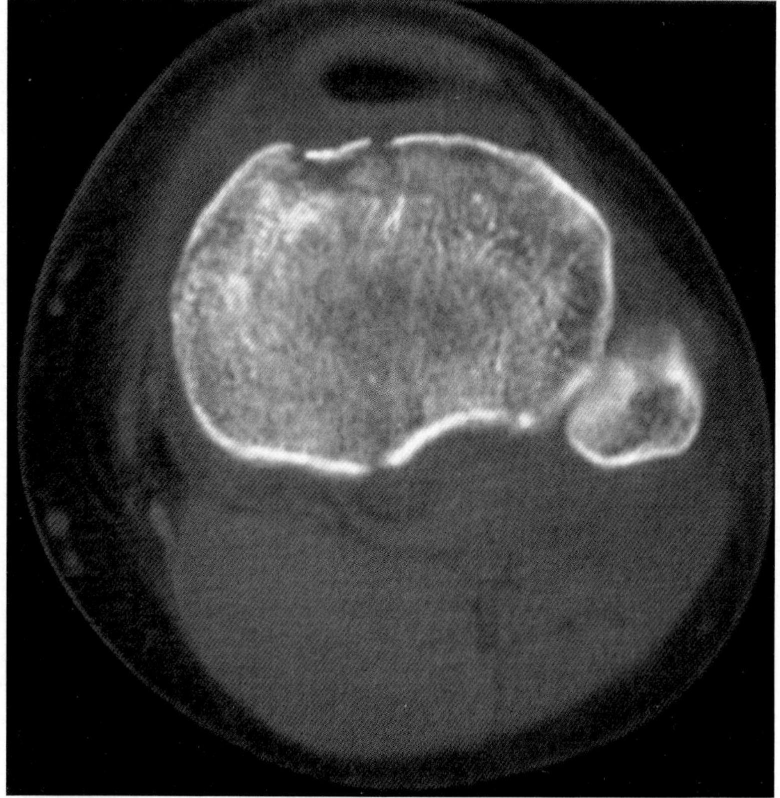

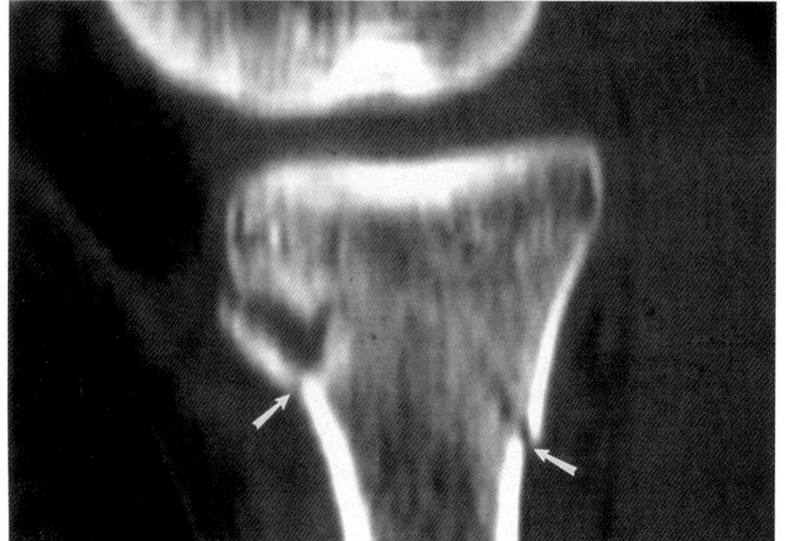

**Fig. 6-2** Axial (**A**) and sagittal reformatted (**B**) computed tomographic (CT) images demonstrating a tibial plateau fracture with metaphyseal involvement (*arrows*).

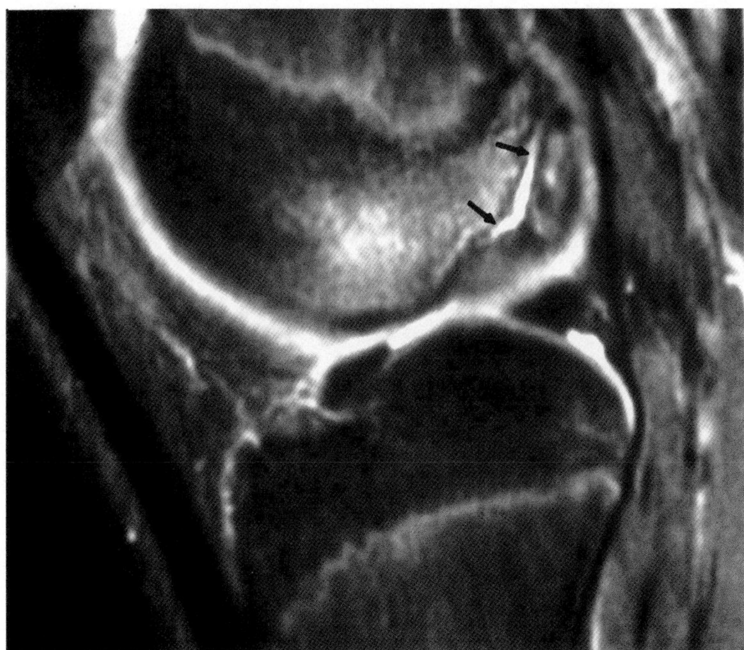

Fig. 6-3 Sagittal T2-weighted magnetic resonance (MR) image demonstrating a separated osteochondral fragment posteriorly (*arrows*).

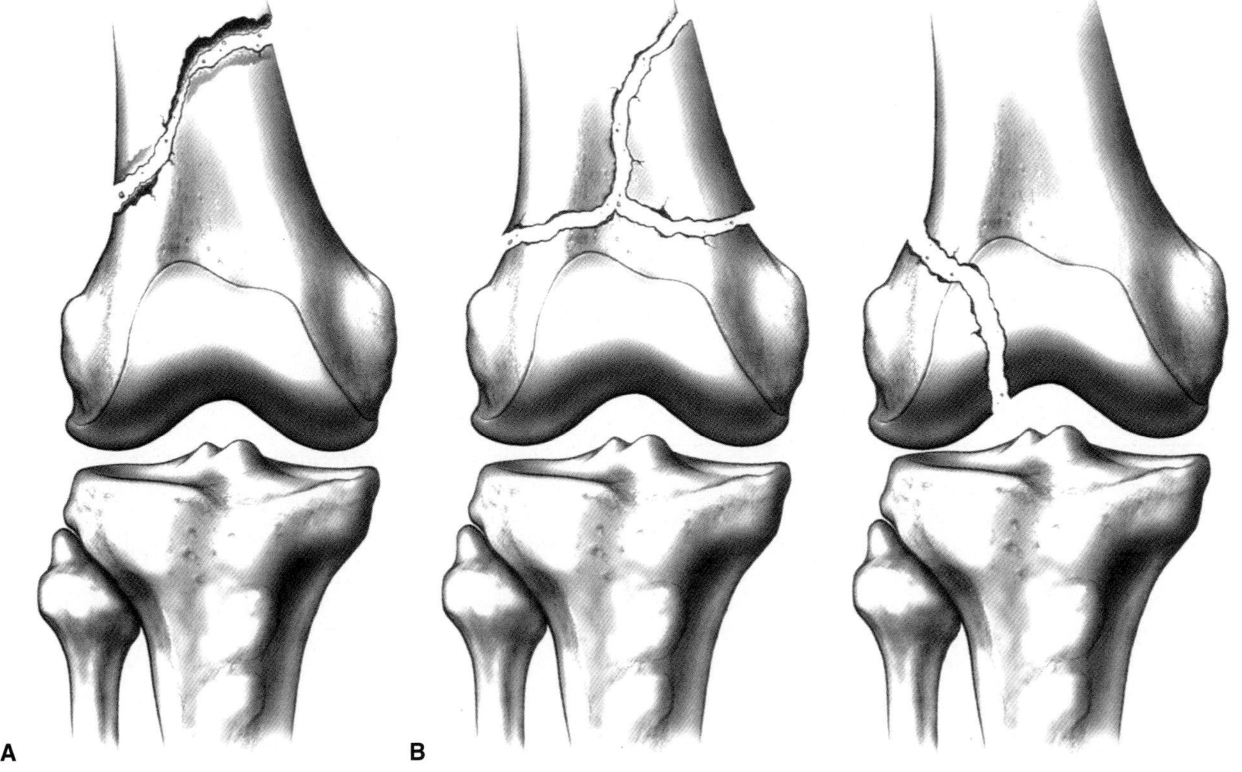


Fig. 6-4 Orthopaedic Trauma Association classification for supracondylar fractures. A: Simple extra-articular type A1. B: More complex extra-articular, in this case a metaphyseal wedge or type A2. C: Partial articular or unicondylar, in this case involving the lateral condyle or type B1. D: Complete or bicondylar type C1. E: Complete bicondylar with metaphyseal comminution or type C2.

Fig. 6-4 (*Continued*)

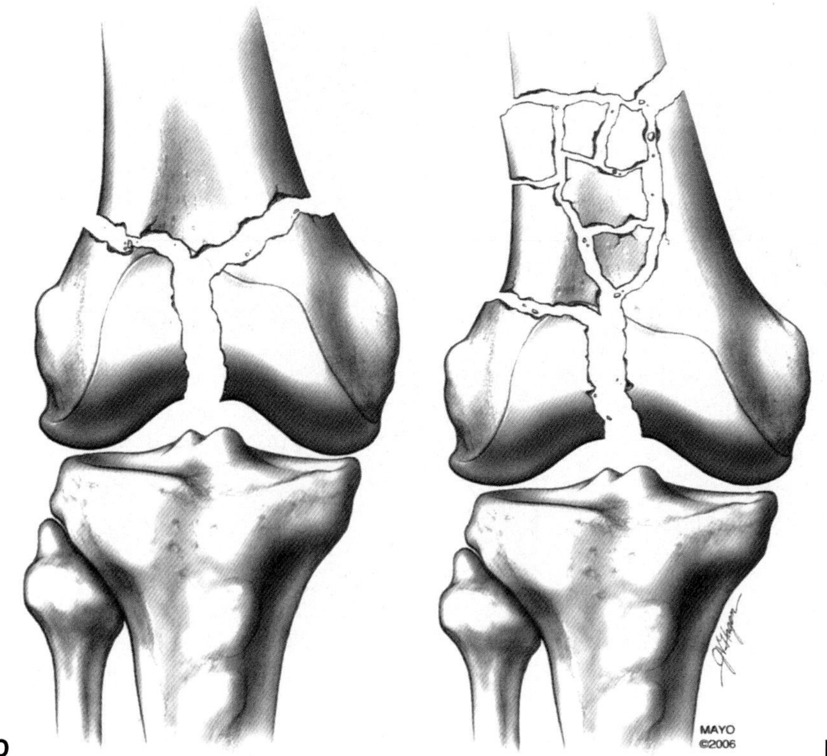


D Complete articular (bicondylar) — articular simple and metaphyseal simple (a T or Y fracture pattern)

E Complete articular (bicondylar) — articular simple and metaphyseal multifragmentary

construct does not need to contact the bone and can be placed with less invasion of the soft tissue envelope preserving the blood supply (see Fig. 6-9). This system is particularly useful in patients with periprosthetic fractures. In some situations, custom knee prostheses are employed for complex distal femoral fractures.

## Suggested Reading

Arazi M, Memik R, Ogun TC, et al. Ilizarov external fixation for severely comminuted supracondylar and intercondylar fractures of the distal femur. *J Bone Joint Surg*. 2001;83B:663–667.

Davila J, Malkani A, Paiso JM. Supracondylar distal femoral fracture nonunions treated with megaprosthesis in the elderly: A report of two cases. *J Orthop Trauma*. 2001;15:574–578.

Helfet DL, Lorich DG. Retrograde intramedullary nailing of supracondylar fractures. *Clin Orthop*. 1998;350: 80–84.

Schultz M, Muller M, Krettek C, et al. Minimally invasive fracture stabilization of distal femoral fractures with the LISS: A prospective multicenter study. *Injury*. 2001; 32(Suppl 3):48–54.

### Patellar Fractures

Patellar fractures account for approximately 1% of all skeletal fractures in both adults and children. They most commonly occur between 20 and 50 years of age and males outnumber females 2:1. The superficial position places the patella at risk for direct trauma. Direct trauma compresses the patella against the femoral condyle resulting in more cartilage damage and comminution although there is less displacement of fragments compared to indirect trauma. Indirect trauma, such as rapid flexion against a contracted quadriceps mechanism, results in less comminution, but greater displacement. In fact most indirect patellar fractures are transverse.

Patellar fractures are classified on the basis of radiographic configuration (see Fig. 6-10). Most fractures are transverse (50% to 80%), comminuted fractures account for 30% to 35%, and vertical 12% to 17% of patellar fractures. Osteochondral fractures may occur with patellar dislocations (see Fig. 6-11). There is often an associated bone bruise of the femoral condyle. Less frequently patellar fractures may follow total knee replacement (0.68%) (see Fig. 6-12) or anterior cruciate ligament (ACL) repairs. The latter are due to stress risers in the patella when patellar tendon graft with bone from the patella and tibial tuberosity (see Fig. 6-13) is used for the ligament graft. Open fractures occur with 7% of patellar fractures and have a more guarded prognosis.

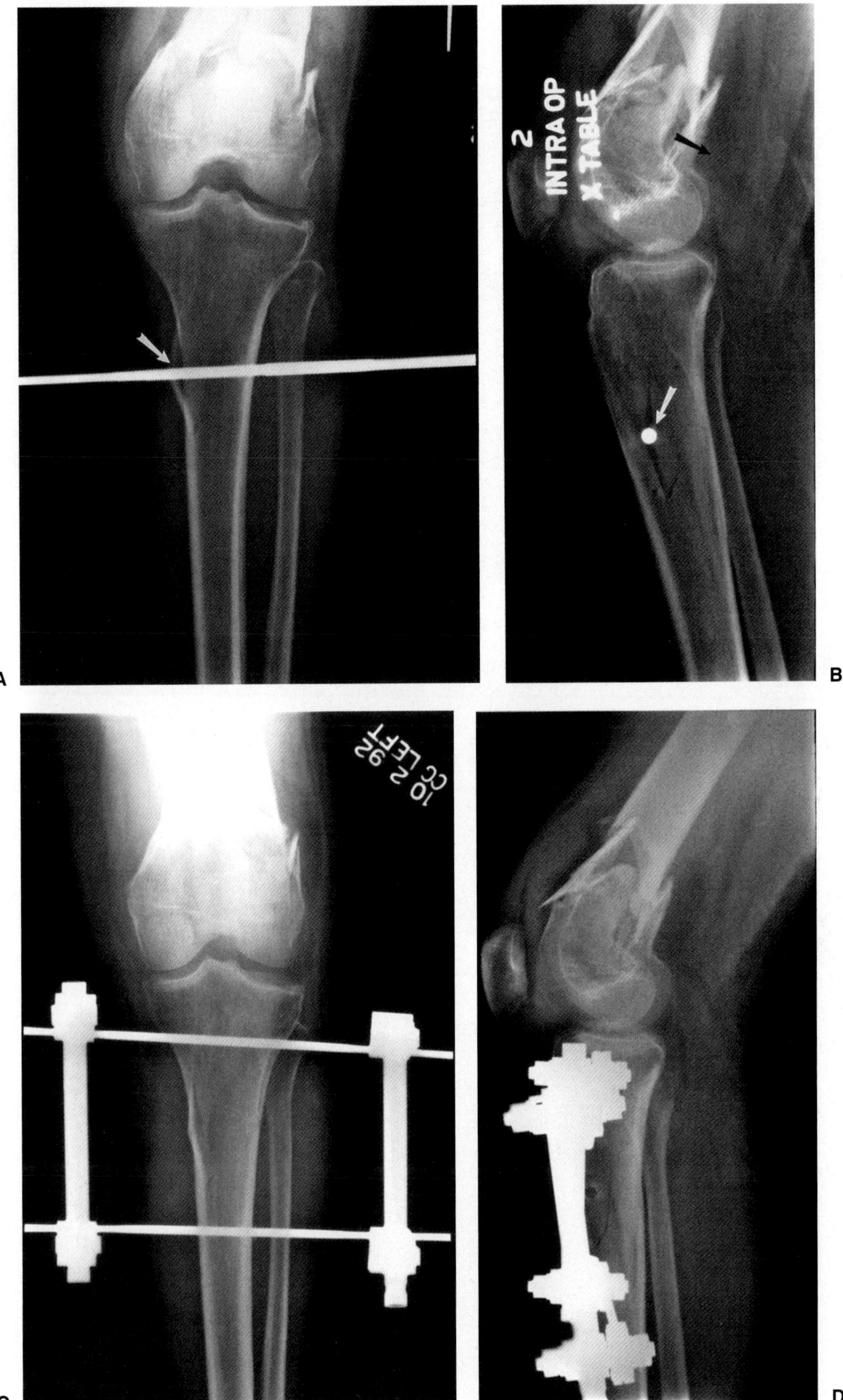


Fig. 6-5 Severely comminuted distal femoral fracture (OTA type A3, extra-articular complex). Anteroposterior (AP) (A) and lateral (B) radiographs obtained during pin placement show the complex fracture with posterior displacement of the distal fragment due to gastrocnemius muscle forces (*arrow* in B). The traction pin fractured the opposite cortex (*white arrow*) requiring replacement with double pins above and below the fracture site demonstrated on AP (C) and lateral (D) radiographs. AP (E) and lateral (F) radiographs in traction. This was later converted to a hinged cast brace (G). At 1-year follow-up the fracture has healed (H) with shortening and angular deformity. OTA, Orthopaedic Trauma Association.

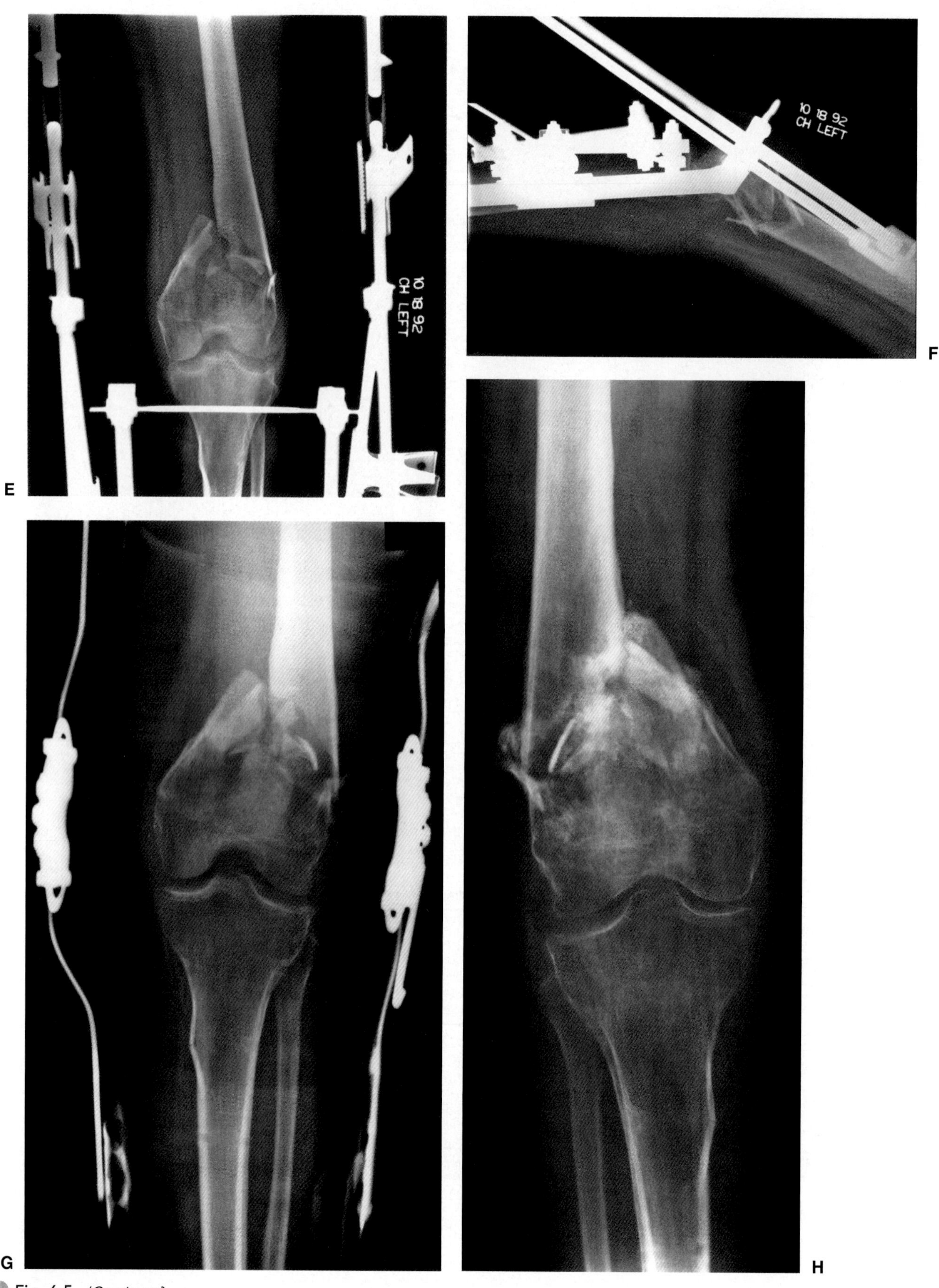


Fig. 6-5 *(Continued)*

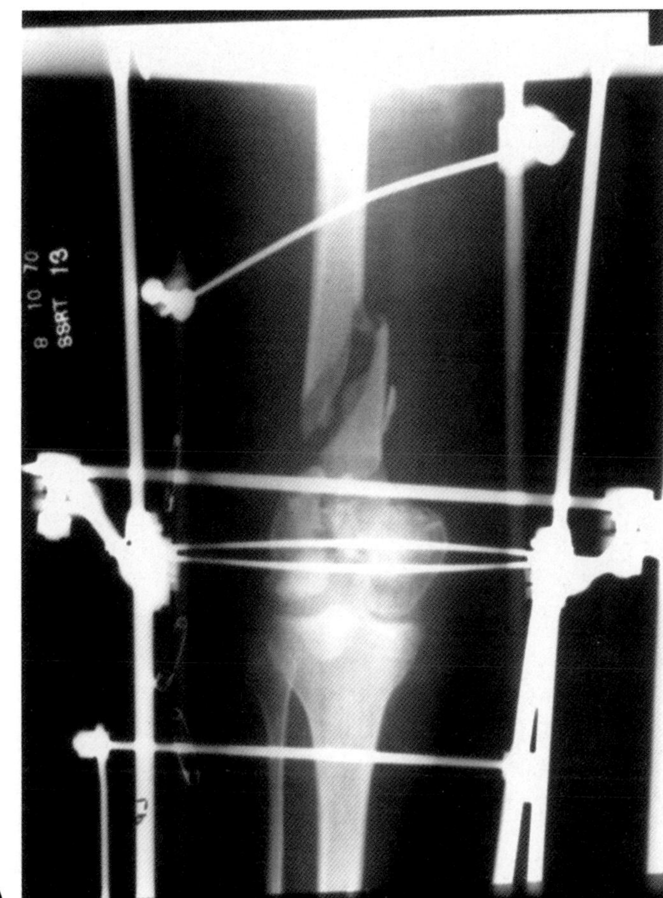

A

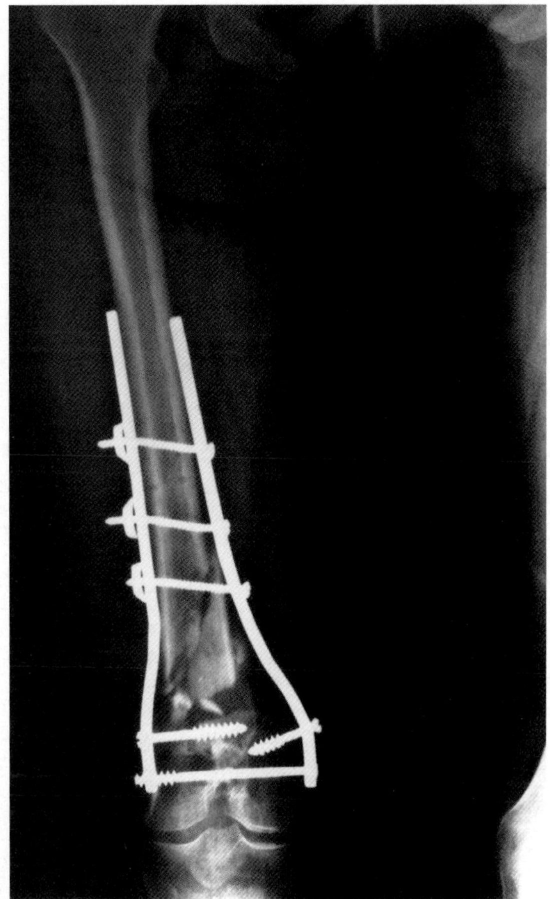
B

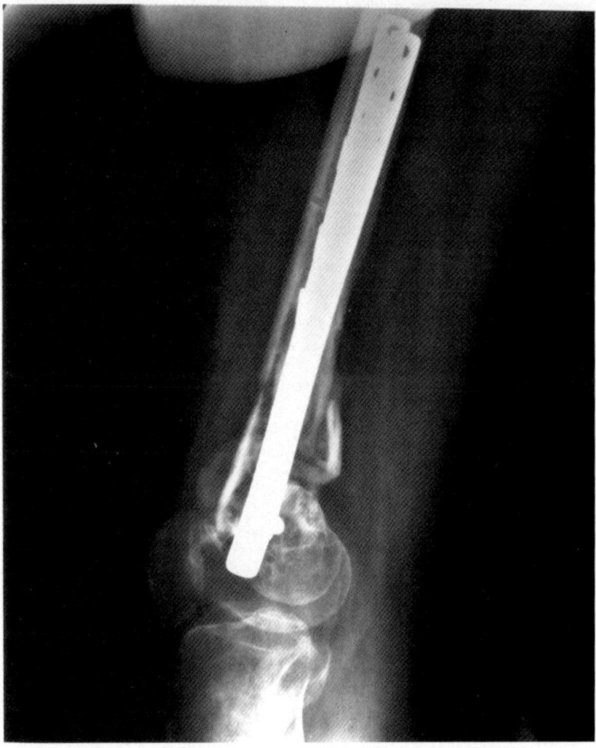
C

Fig. 6-6 A: Anteroposterior (AP) radiograph of a complex (OTA C3) fracture treated with hybrid external fixation. This was eventually treated with open reduction and internal fixation using bilateral plates and screws with locking bolts (B and C). OTA, Orthopaedic Trauma Association.

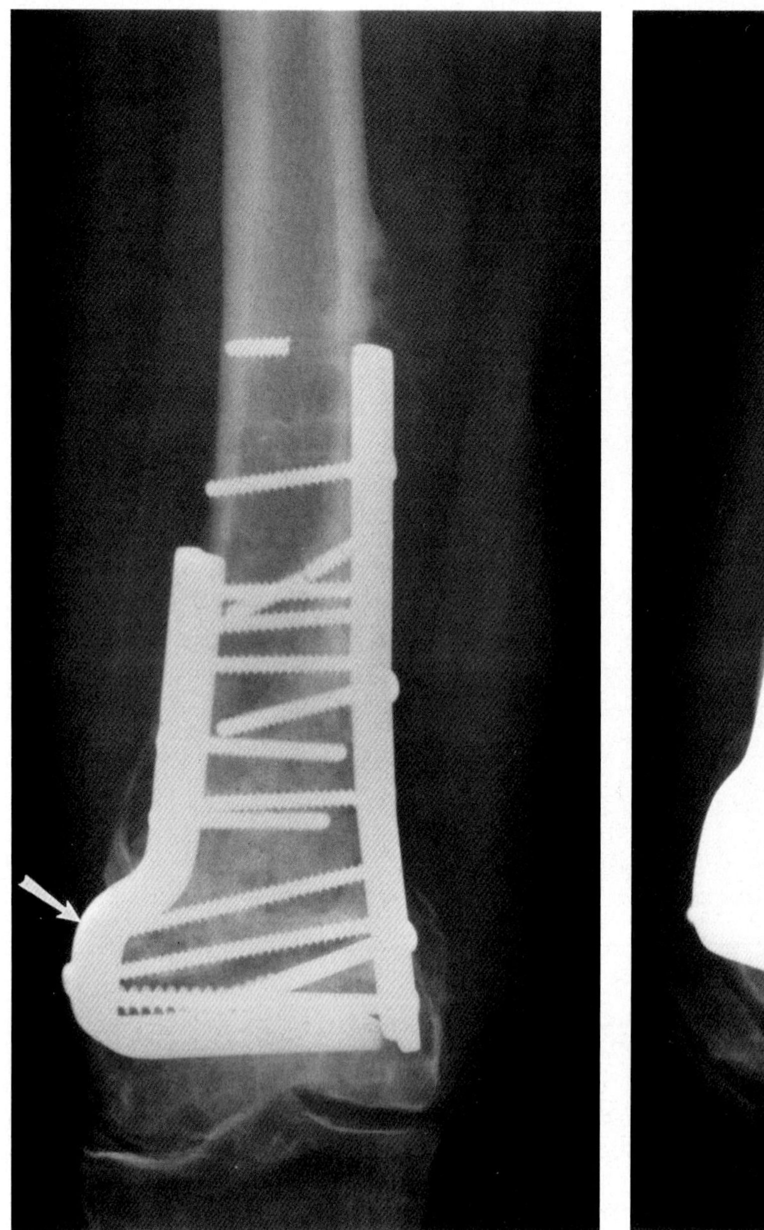


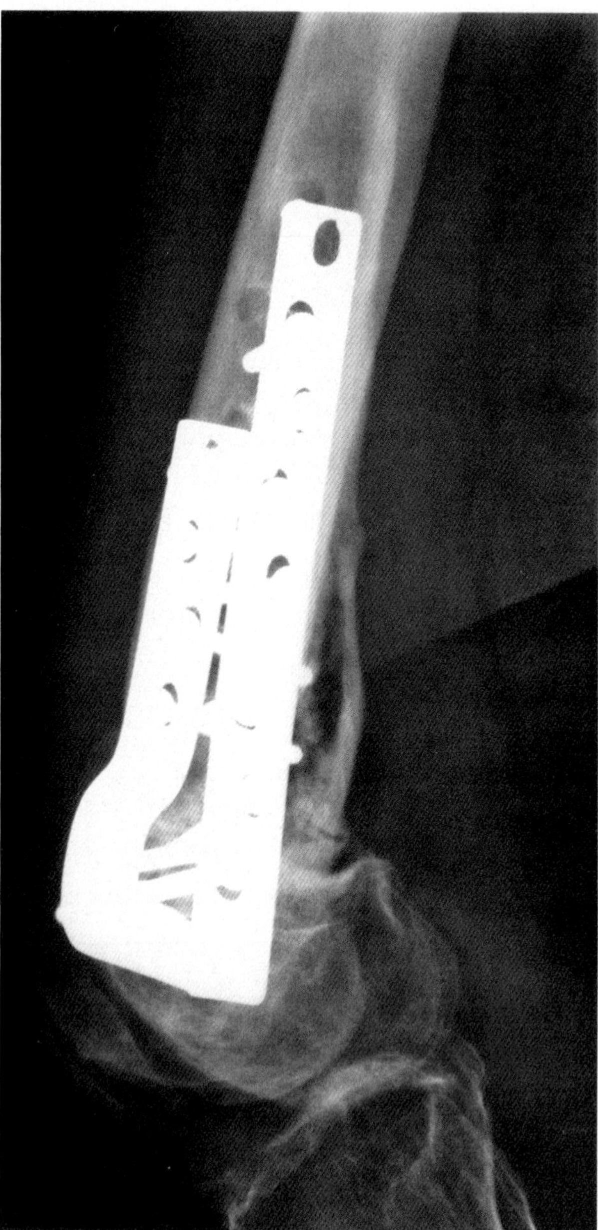


Fig. 6-7 Anteroposterior (AP) (A) and lateral (B) radiographs demonstrating a complex distal femoral fracture treated with open reduction and internal fixation using a dynamic compression plate and blade plate (*arrow*). The compression plate has been revised with proximal screw remnants and fractures.

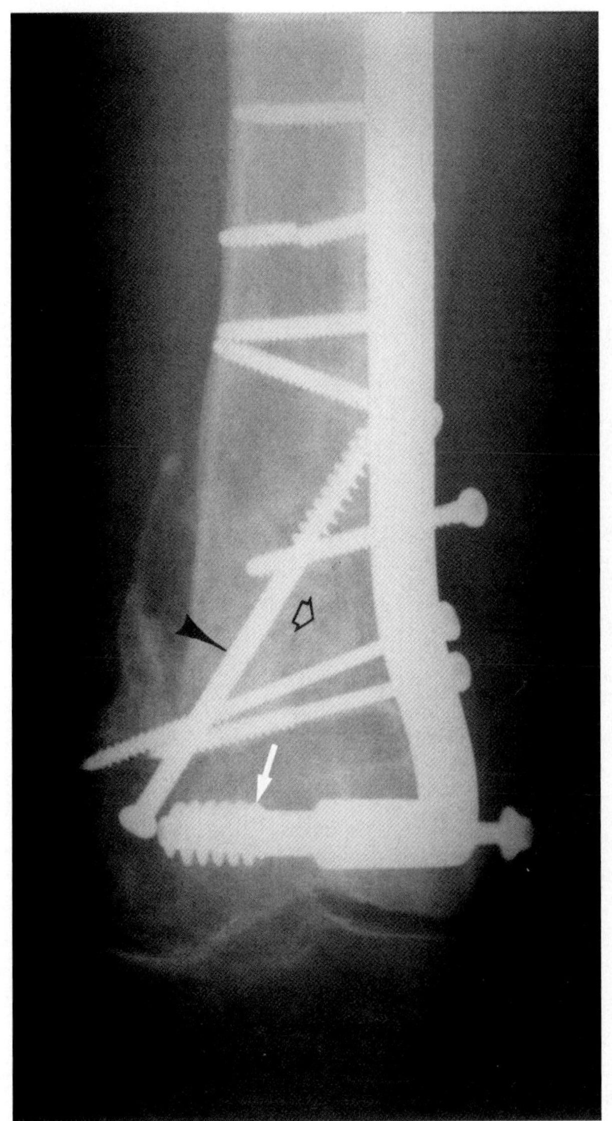


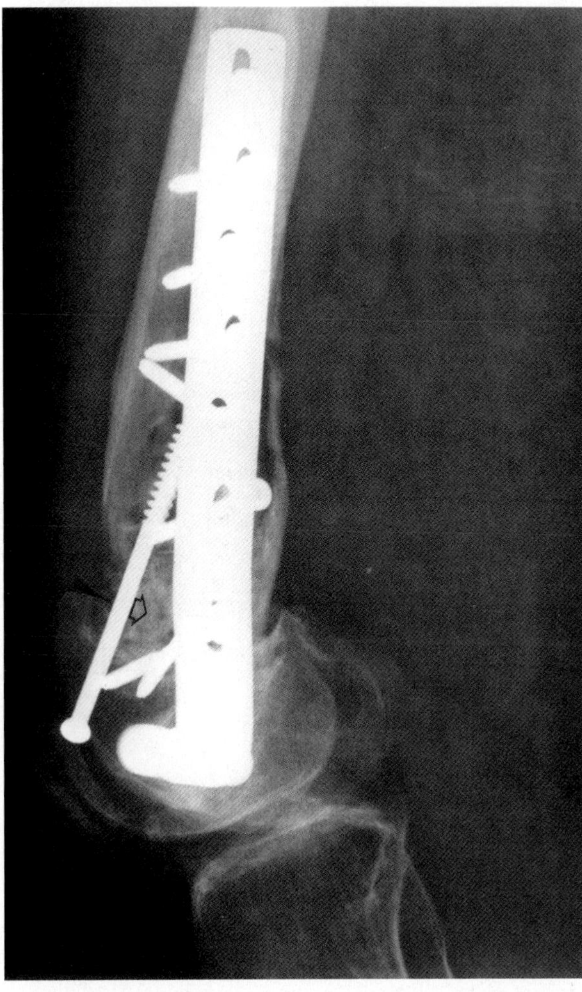


Fig. 6-8 Anteroposterior (AP) (A) and lateral (B) radiographs demonstrating internal fixation with a dynamic condylar screw (*white arrow*). There is also bone graft (*open arrow*) and a lag screw (*black arrowhead*).

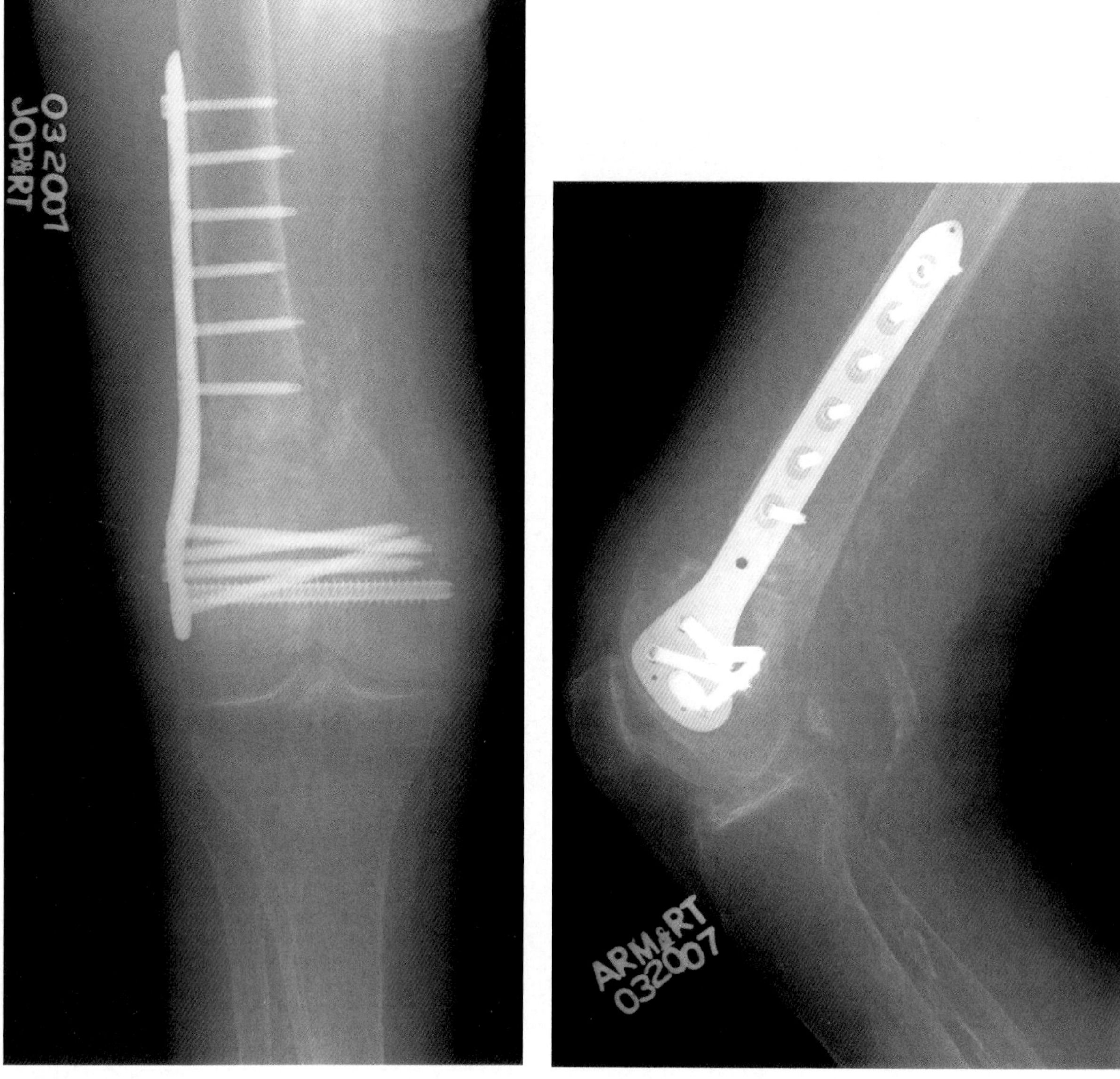

Fig. 6-9 Anteroposterior (AP) (A) and lateral (B) radiographs in an elderly patient with a complex distal femoral fracture with metaphyseal comminution and intra-articular involvement (OTA type C2) treated with an less invasive stabilization system (LISS) plate and screws.

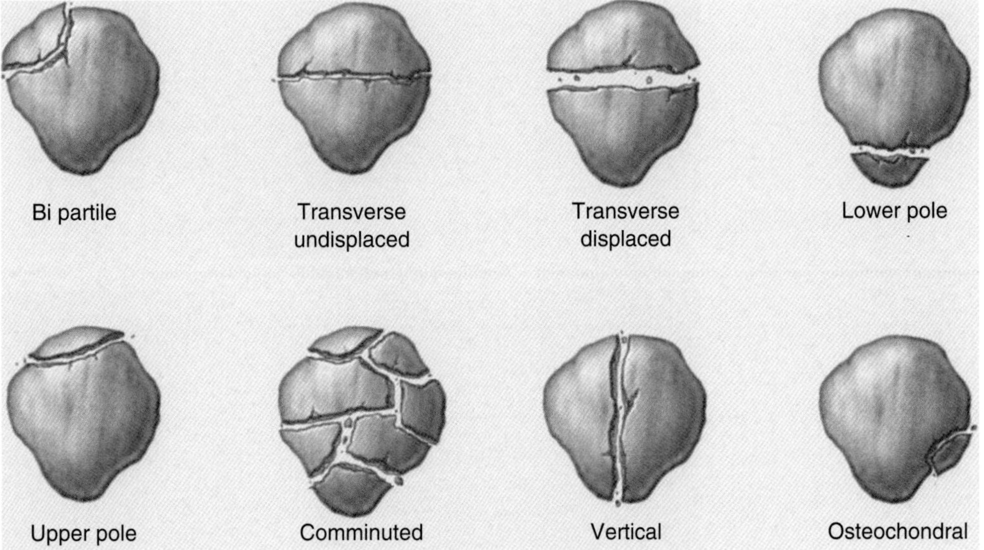


**Fig. 6-10** Illustration of the different types of patella fracture including the bipartite patella, which is a normal variant.

Imaging can be accomplished with AP, lateral, and patellar (Merchant) views. Bipartite patellae are frequently bilateral and should not be confused with a fracture (Figs. 6-10 and 6-1). MRI is useful to fully evaluate osteochondral lesions (Fig. 6-11) and associated soft tissue injuries.

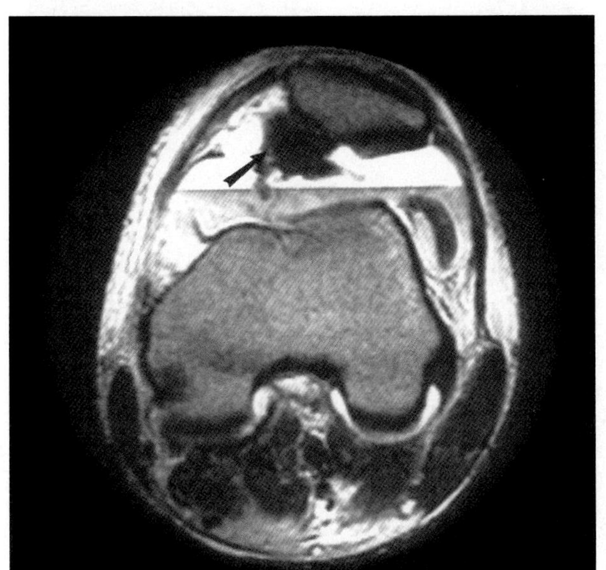

**Fig. 6-11** Osteochondral fracture following patellar dislocation and relocation. Axial T2-weighted magnetic resonance (MR) image demonstrates a lipohemarthrosis and large osteochondral fracture (*arrow*) of the patella.

## SUGGESTED READING

Carpenter JE, Arbor A, Kasman R. Fractures of the patella. *J Bone Joint Surg*. 1993;75A:1550–1560.

Ortigera CJ, Berry DJ. Patellar fracture after total knee arthroplasty. *J Bone Joint Surg*. 2002;84A:532–540.

Sonin AH, Fitzgerald SW, Bresler ME, et al. MR imaging appearance of the extensor mechanism of the knee: functional anatomy and injury patterns. *Radiographics*. 1995;15:367–382.

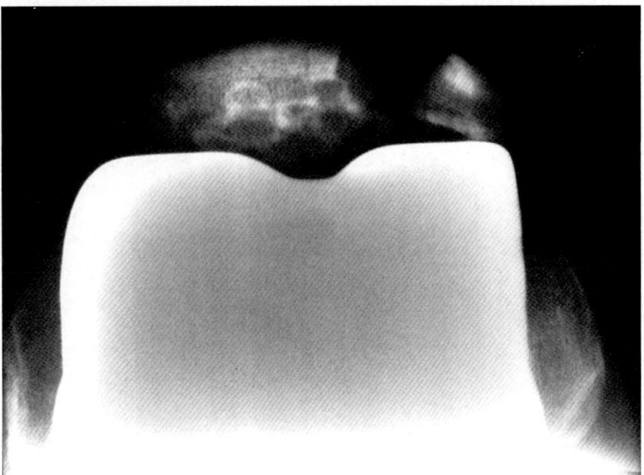

**Fig. 6-12** Patellar fracture following total knee replacement. Merchant view demonstrating a displaced lateral patellar fracture.

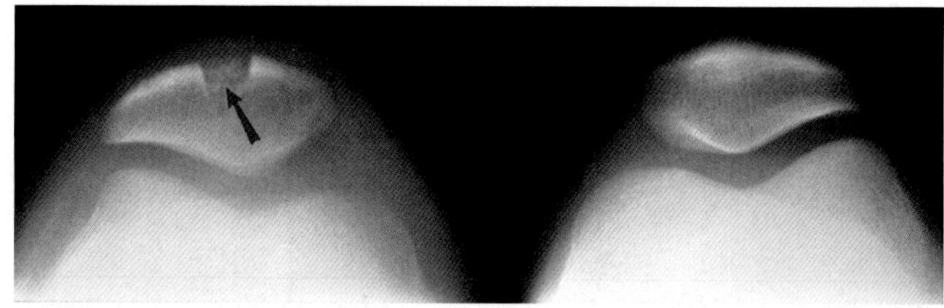

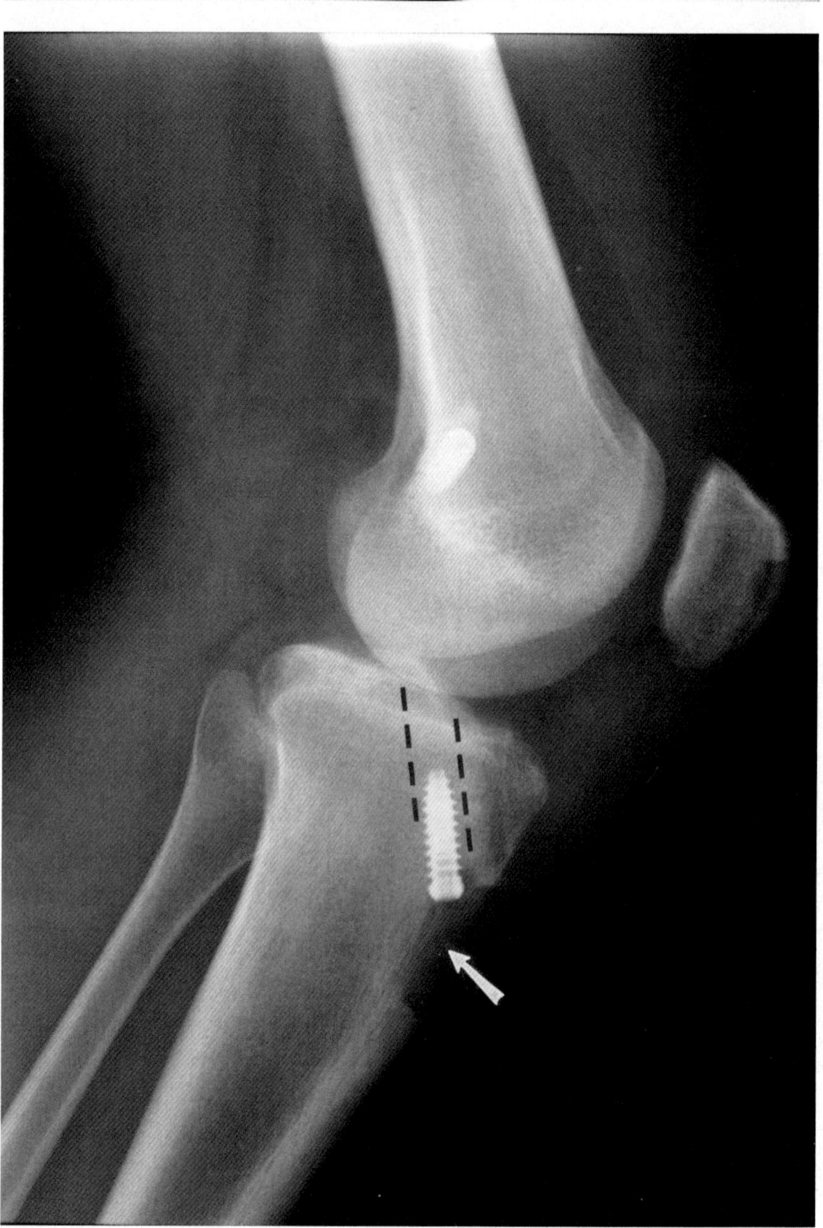

**Fig. 6-13** Anteroposterior (AP) (**A**) and lateral (**B**) radiographs following anterior cruciate ligament (ACL) repair with donor sites in the tibial plateau (*arrow* in **B**) and patella (*arrow* in **A**). This places the patella at increased risk for fracture.

## Treatment Options

Treatment of patellar fractures should achieve the goals of anatomic reduction with realignment of the articular surface and restoration of soft tissue, specifically the retinacula and extensor mechanism. Undisplaced fractures (≤2 mm) with minimal articular irregularity (≤2 mm) may be treated in a cylinder cast (see Chapter 2) for 4 to 6 weeks. Displaced fractures (≥2 mm articular deformity and ≥3 mm of separation) (see Fig. 6-14) should be treated with open reduction and internal fixation. Typically, tension band and K-wires (see Fig. 6-15) or

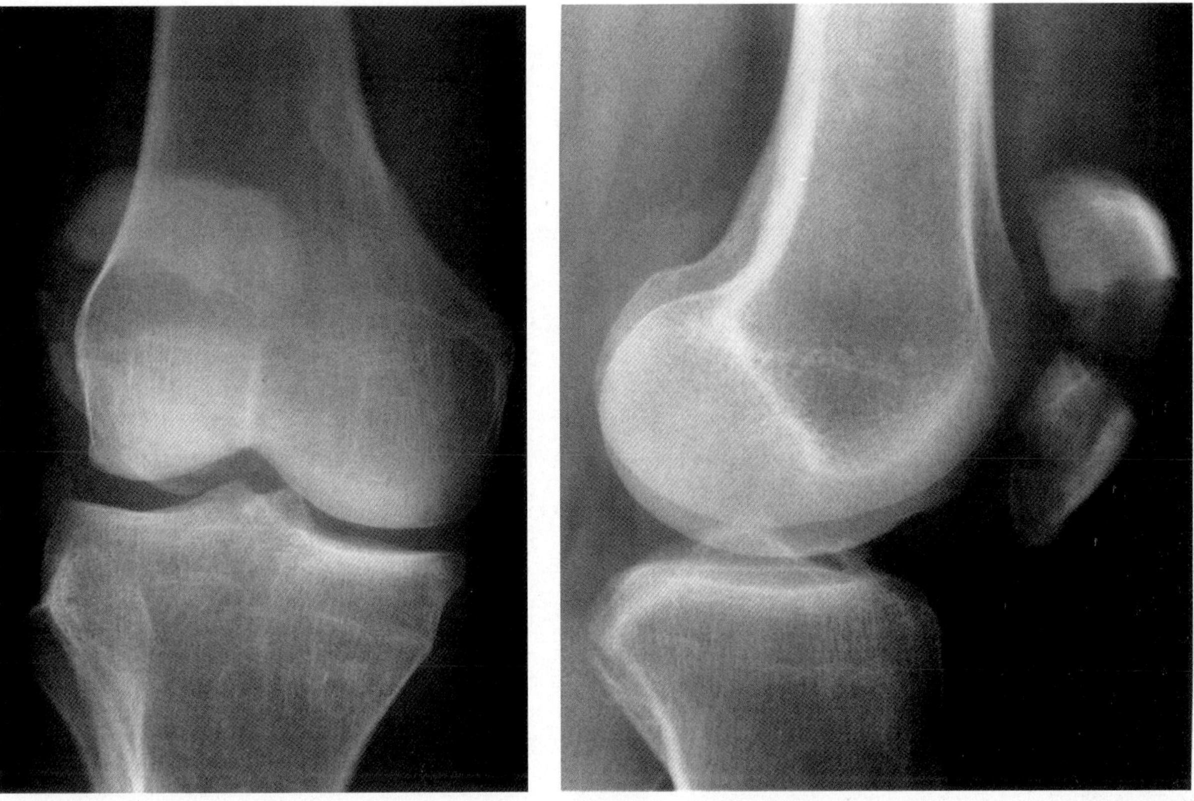

Fig. 6-14 Anteroposterior (AP) (A) and lateral (B) radiographs demonstrating a comminuted displaced patellar fracture.

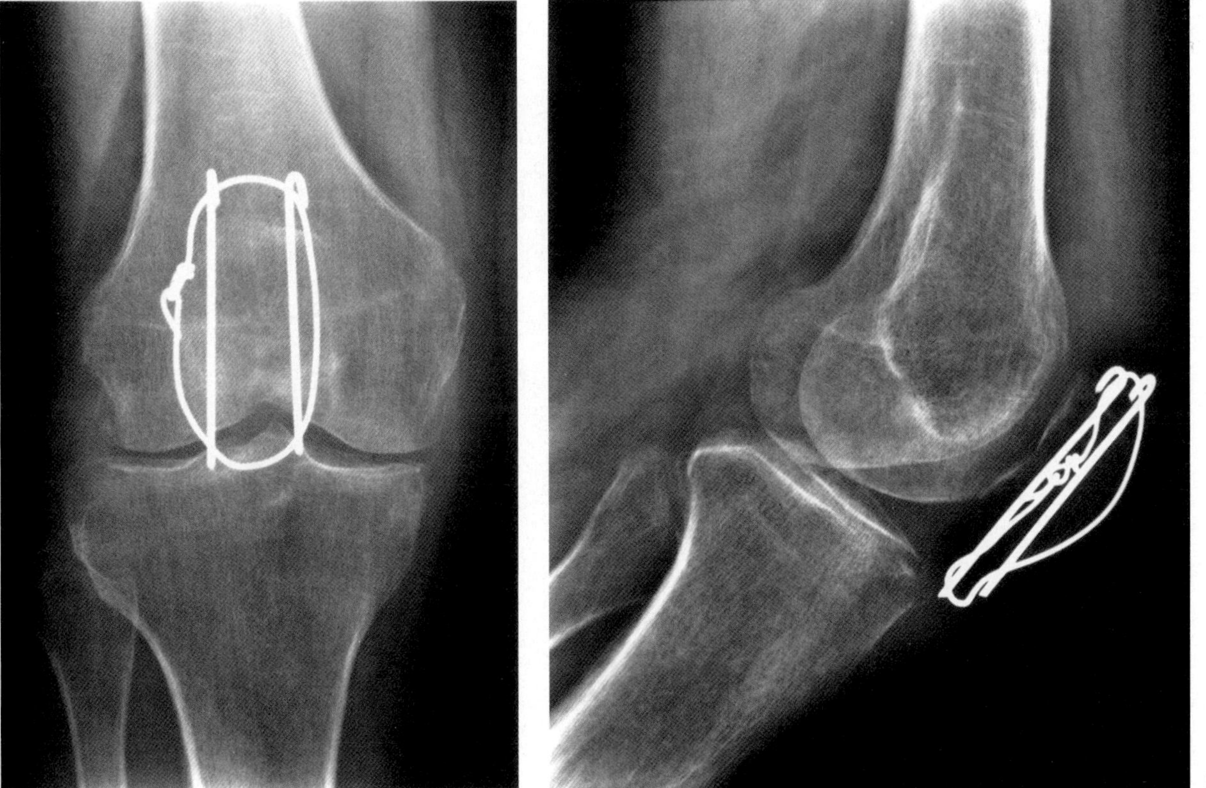

Fig. 6-15 Anteroposterior (AP) (A) and lateral (B) radiographs demonstrating reduction of the patellar fracture with two K-wires and tension band technique. There is minimal articular deformity.

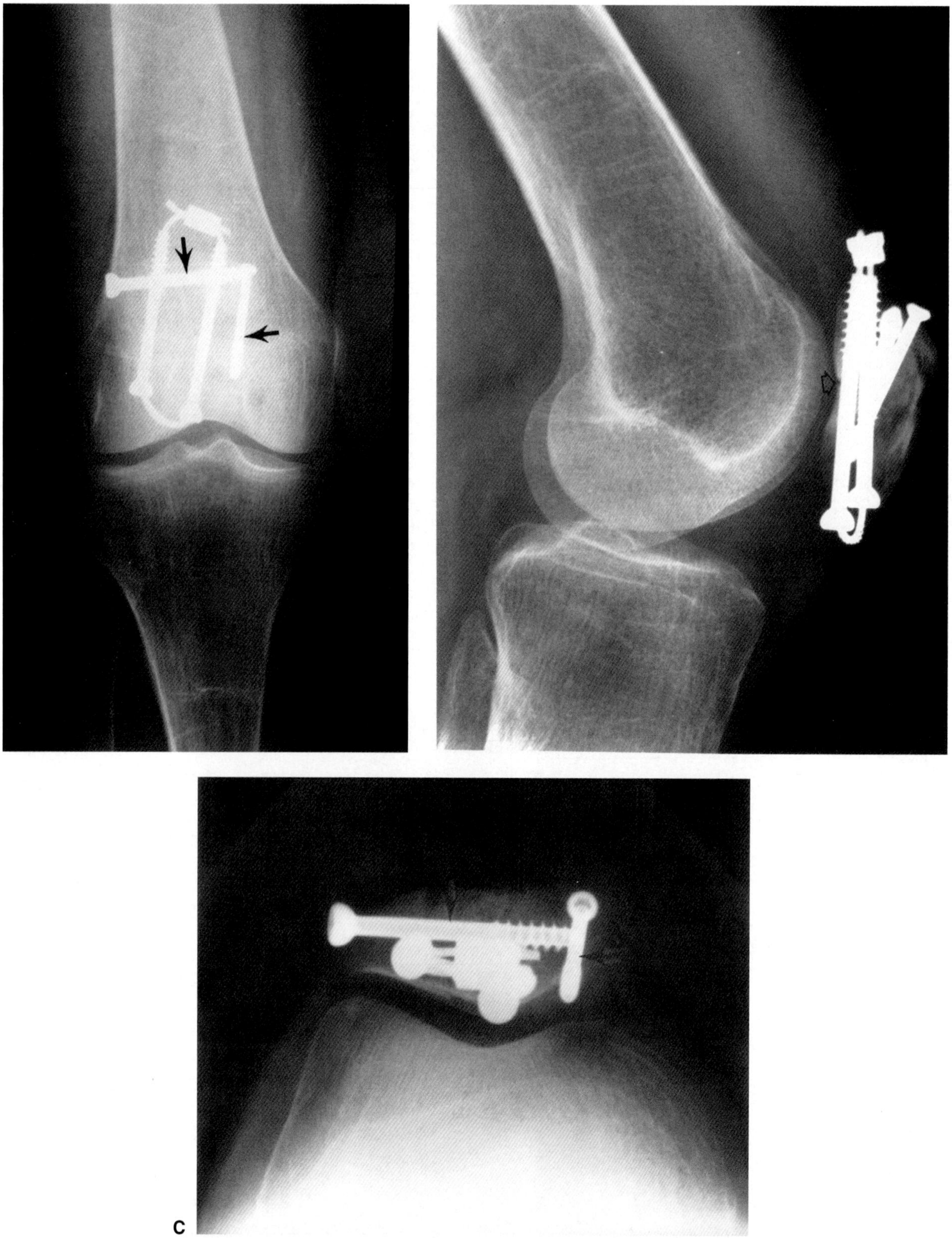

A

B

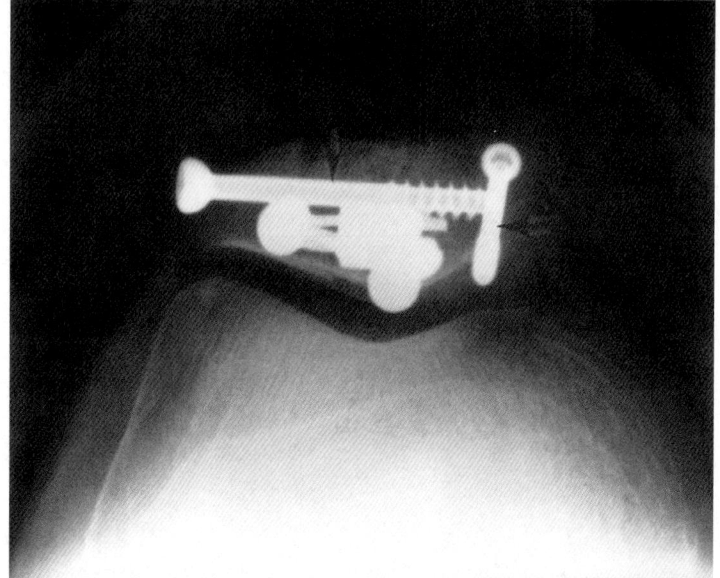

C

Fig. 6-16 Anteroposterior (AP) (A), lateral (B), and Merchant (C) radiographs demonstrate fixation of a comminuted patellar fracture with two cannulated screws and a threaded Dall-Miles cable. There are also two cannulated interfragmentary screws (*arrows*). There is slight residual articular separation (*open arrow* in B).

cannulated screws with wires or cables (see Fig. 6-16) are used. For comminuted fractures portions or the entire patella may have to be removed.

## Suggested Reading


Carpenter JE, Arbor A, Kasman R. Fractures of the patella. *J Bone Joint Surg*. 1993;75:1550–1560.

Ray JM, Hendrix J. Incidence, mechanism of injury, and treatment of fractures of the patella in children. *J Trauma*. 1992;32:464–467.


## Proximal Tibial Fractures

Fractures of the proximal tibia in adults may involve the articular surface (osteochondral, tibial eminence, plateau) metaphysis or tuberosity without articular involvement. In children and adolescents, fractures more frequently involve the tuberosity, tibial eminence, or physis. The latter are uncommon and account for <5% of physeal fractures.

### Tibial Condyle/Plateau Fractures

Tibial condyle fractures result from significant falls or high-velocity trauma. Vertical compression forces may lead to T- or

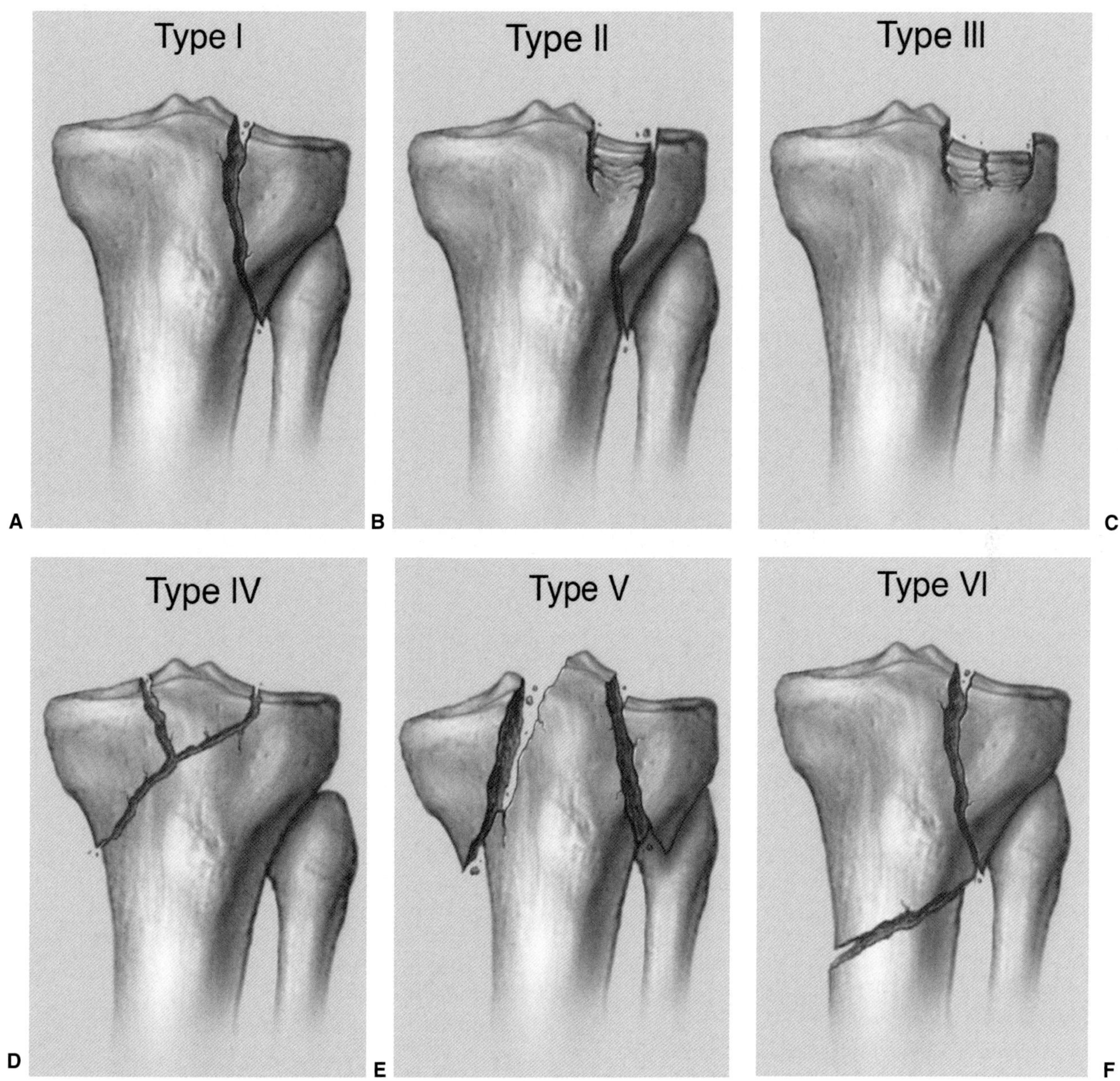


**Fig. 6-17** Schatzker classification. **A:** Type I—pure lateral plateau split. **B:** Type II—lateral split with depressed plateau. **C:** Type III—central depression alone. **D:** Type IV—medial plateau with lateral extension. **E:** Type V—both plateaus with displacement. **F:** Type VI—lateral split with metaphyseal fracture.

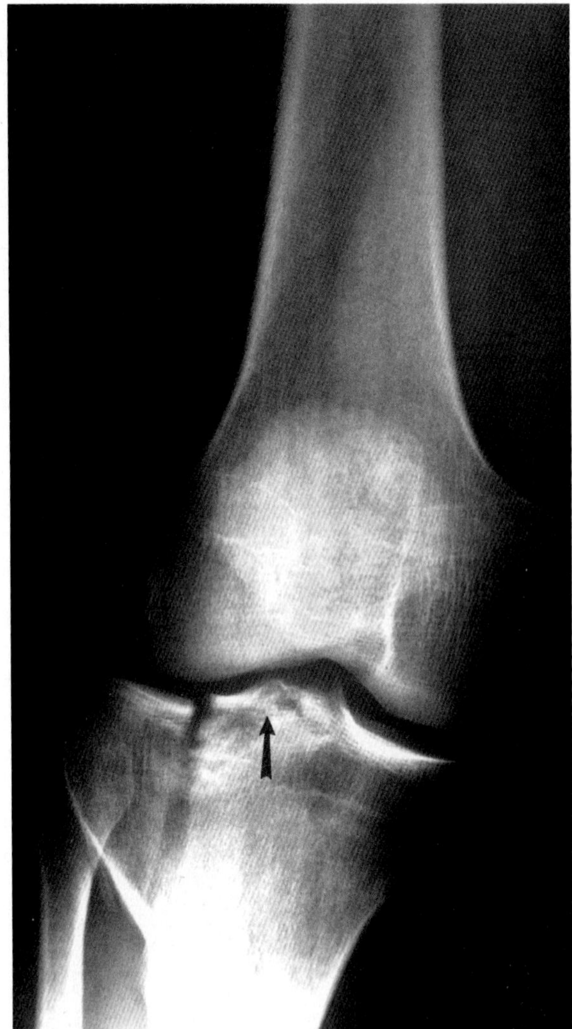

Fig. 6-18 Schatzker type II or OTA type B1.3. Anteroposterior (AP) radiograph demonstrating a lateral plateau split with slight separation and depression and involvement (*arrow*) of the tibial eminence.

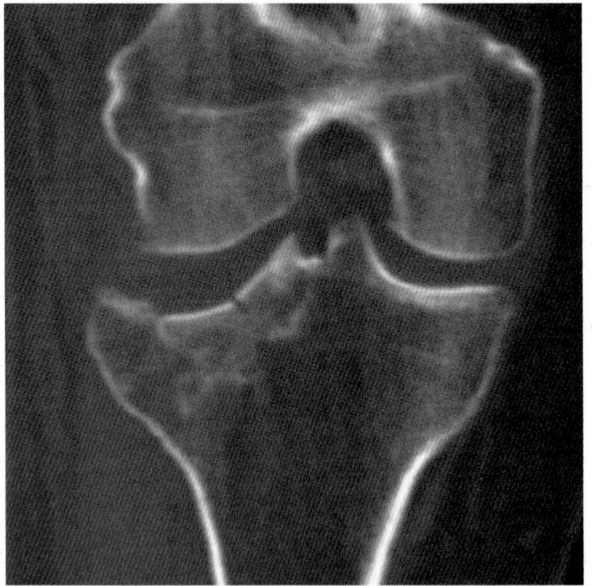

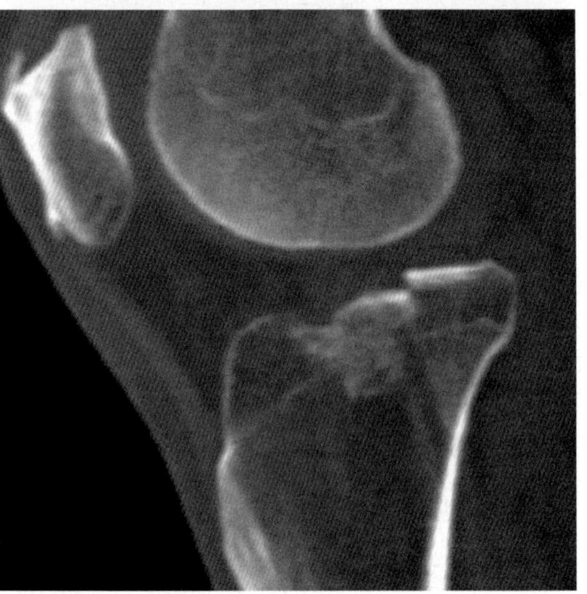

Fig. 6-19 Simple partial depression of the lateral plateau in an elderly female demonstrated on coronal (**A**) and sagittal (**B**) reformatted computed tomographic (CT) images.

Y-fracture configurations. Varus or valgus forces involve the medial or lateral plateaus, respectively. Internal derangement is common. Rotational forces are also often part of the injury pattern causing a variety of fracture patterns.

**Classifications:** Multiple fracture classifications have been used for these injuries beginning with the Hohl Classification in the 1960s and followed by the Schatzker, Moore, Honkonen, and Orthopaedic Trauma Association (OTA) in 1996. Classifications are based on radiographic features. The most commonly used patterns are the Schatzker and OTA classifications. These are summarized in the subsequent text.

**Schatzker classification:** (see Fig. 6-17)

- **Type I:** Lateral plateau split (common in young adults)
- **Type II:** Lateral plateau split with depressed fragment, medial collateral ligament (MCL) injury (see Fig. 6-18)
- **Type III:** Lateral depression only (common in older patients), no instability, may treat conservatively (see Fig. 6-19)
- **Type IV:** Medial split often involving tibia eminence, associated neurovascular injury
- **Type V:** Bicondylar with severe soft tissue injury
- **Type VI:** Metaphyseal/diaphyseal dissociation, associated compartment syndrome

**OTA classification:** (see Fig. 6-20)

- **Type A1:** Extra-articular avulsion (Fig. 6-20A)
  - A1.1—fibular head avulsion
  - A1.2—tibial tuberosity avulsion
  - A1.3—cruciate insertion avulsion
- **Type A2:** Extra-articular, simple metaphyseal fracture (Fig. 6-20B)
  - A2.1—oblique fracture in frontal plane

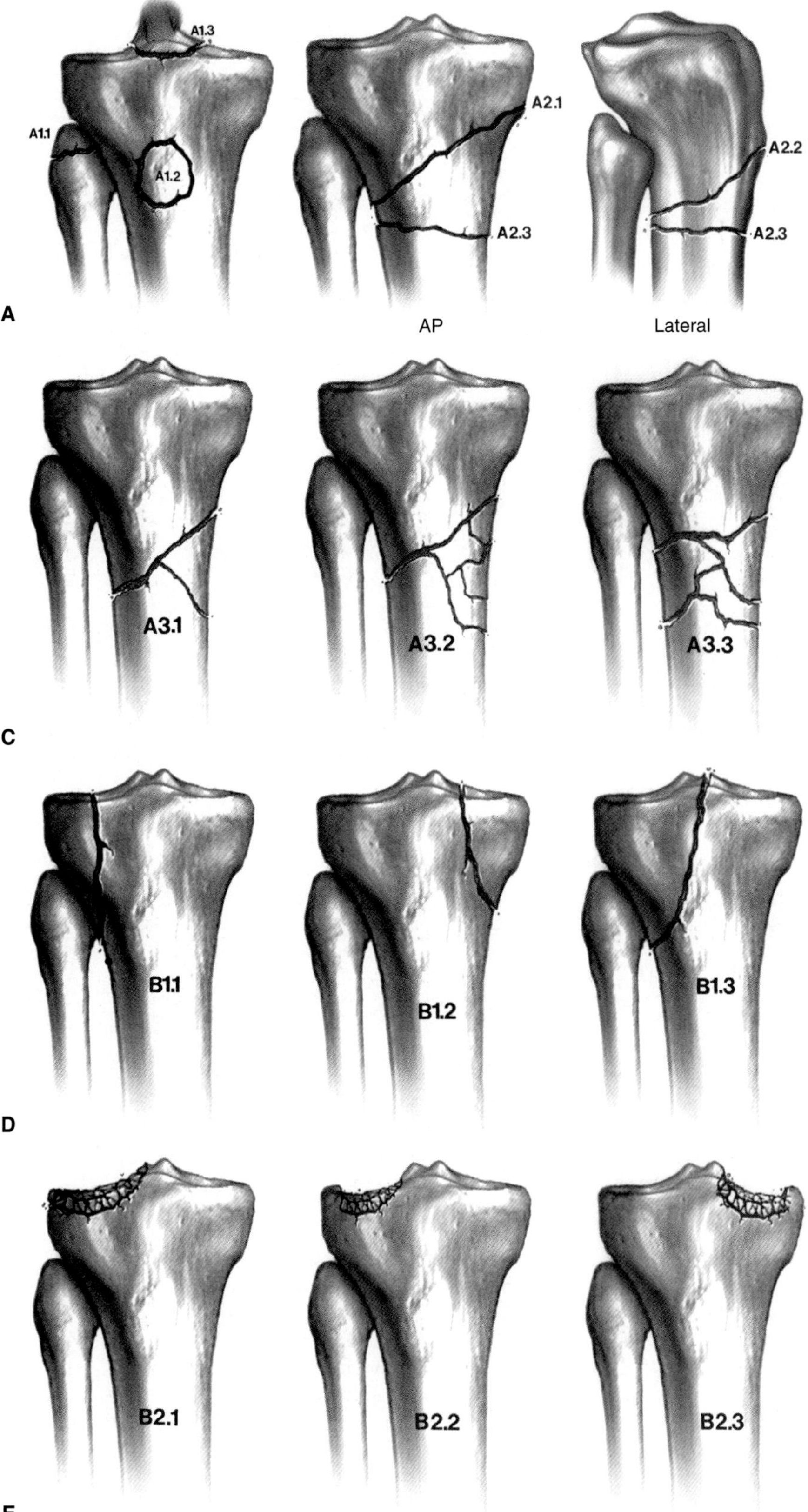


**Fig. 6-20** Orthopaedic Trauma Association classification. **A:** Type A1—avulsion injuries. *A1.1*—fibular head avulsion, *A1.2*—tibial tuberosity avulsion, *A1.3*—cruciate avulsion. **B:** Type A2—metaphyseal extra-articular. *A2.1*—oblique frontal plane, *A2.2*—oblique sagittal plane, *A2.3*—transverse. **C:** Type A3—extra-articular comminuted. *A3.1*—intact wedge, *A3.2*—fragmented wedge, *A3.3*—complex. **D:** Type B1—partial articular, pure split. *B1.1*—lateral split, *B1.2*—medial split, *B1.3*—split involving tibial spines. **E:** Type B2—pure depression. *B2.1*—total lateral depression, *B2.2*—limited depression, *B2.3*—medial depression. **F:** Type C1—complete articular. *C1.1*—slight displacement, *C1.2*—one condyle displaced (*arrow*), *C1.3*—both condyles displaced (*arrows*). **G:** Type C2—simple articular, metaphysis complex. *C2.1*—intact wedge, *C2.2*—comminuted wedge, *C2.3*—metaphysis complex. **H:** Type C3—complex articular and metaphysis. *C3.1*—lateral complex, *C3.2*—medial complex, *C3.3*—both medial and lateral complex.

Fig. 6-20 *(Continued)*

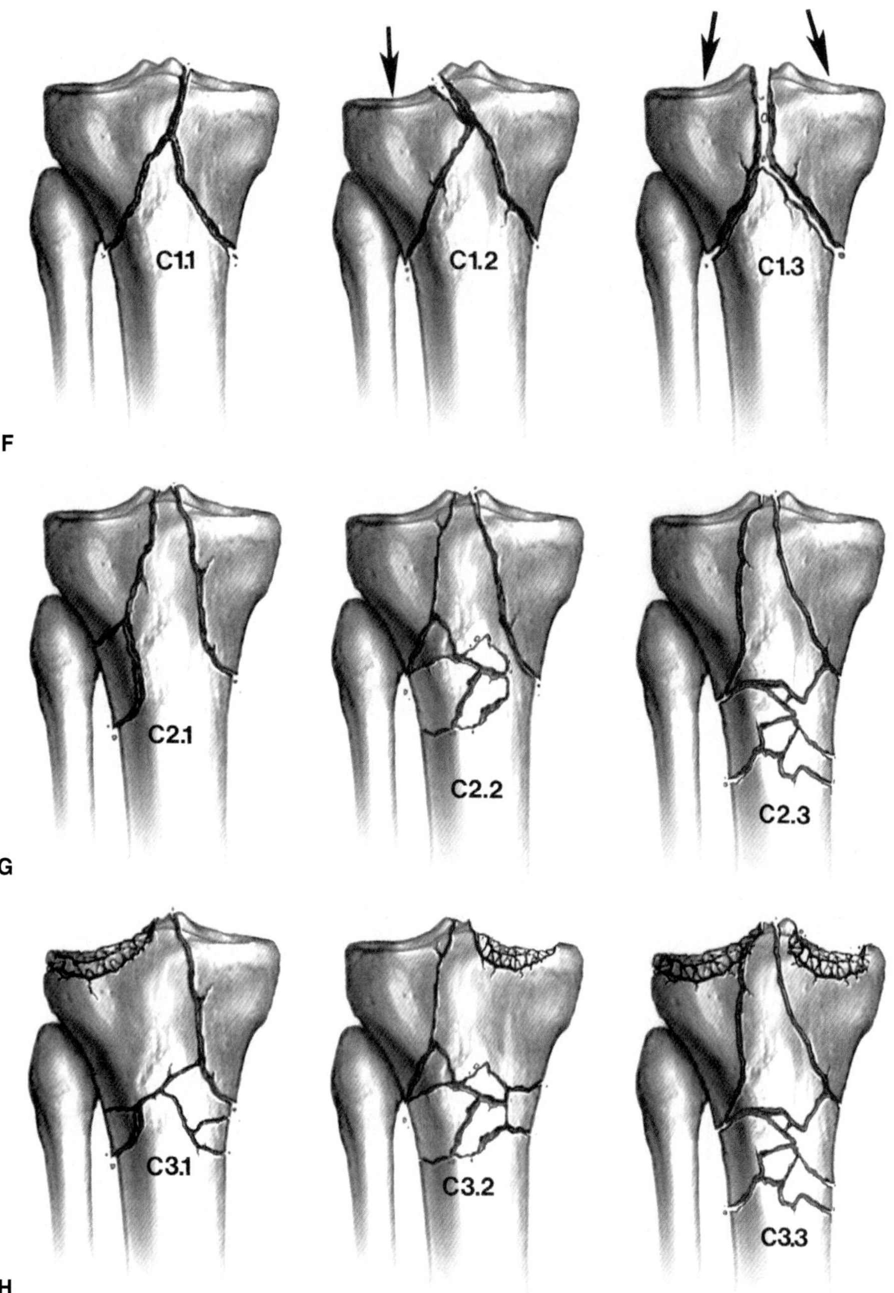


A2.2—oblique fracture in sagittal plane
A2.3—transverse fracture

**Type A3:** Extra-articular comminuted (Fig. 6-20C)
A3.1—intact wedge fracture
A3.2—fragmented wedge fracture
A3.3—complex fracture

**Type B1:** Partial articular, split fracture (Fig. 6-20D)
B1.1—lateral split
B1.2—medial split
B1.3—medial or lateral involving tibia eminence (Fig. 6-18)

**Type B2:** Partial articular, pure depression (Fig. 6-20E)
B2.1—lateral total articular surface
B2.2—lateral but limited (Fig. 6-19)
B2.3—medial depression

**Type C1:** Complete articular with simple metaphyseal fracture (Fig. 6-20F)
C1.1—slight displacement
C1.2—one condyle displaced
C1.3—both condyles displaced

**Type C2:** Complete simple articular with comminuted metaphysic (Fig. 6-20G)
C2.1—intact wedge
C2.2—comminuted wedge
C2.3—complex metaphysic

**Type C3:** Complex articular, complex metaphysic (Fig. 6-20H)
C3.1—complex lateral plateau

C3.2—complex medial plateau
C3.3—complex both plateaus

The significant factors regarding these classifications is the degree of depression or displacement of the articular surface and secondary injuries associated with the categories of injury. A split fracture of the medial plateau (Schatzker IV or OTA B1.2) is associated with vascular injury and peroneal nerve palsy. Schatzker types V and VI or OTA type C fractures involve both condyles, and with tibial fragmentation there is an increased risk for compartment syndrome and soft tissue injury. Obviously, more complex fractures are much more difficult to manage surgically. These concepts will be discussed more fully under treatment options.

## Suggested Reading

Barei DP, Nork SE, Mills WJ, et al. Functional outcomes of severe bicondylar tibial plateau fractures treated with dual incisions and medial and lateral plates. *J Bone Joint Surg*. 2006; 88A:1713–1721.

Martin J, Marsh JL, Nepola JV, et al. Radiographic fracture assessments: Which ones can we reliably make. *J Orthop Trauma*. 2000;14:379–385.

Orthopaedic Trauma Association Committee on Coding and Classifications. Fractures and dislocations compendium. *J Orthop Trauma*. 1996;10(Suppl 1):41–45.

Schatzker J, McBroom R, Bruce D. The tibial plateau fracture: The Toronto experience 1968–1975. *Clin Orthop*. 1979;138: 94–104.

### Preoperative Imaging

AP, lateral, and oblique images will usually define the complex fracture of the tibial condyles. A cross-table lateral image may demonstrate a lipohemarthrosis, which may be the only finding in subtle intra-articular fractures. In most cases, CT with reformatting in the coronal and sagittal planes and 3-D reconstructions provide the necessary data for treatment planning (see Fig. 6-21). MRI is useful to evaluate soft tissue injury. In fact, some would argue that MRI can accurately evaluate the extent of both osseous and soft tissue injuries (see Fig. 6-22). It is generally stated that depression of 5 to 8 mm and separation of ≥4 mm indicates the need for open reduction and internal fixation.

## Suggested Reading

Kode L, Lieberman JM, Motta AO, et al. Evaluation of plateau fractures: Efficacy of MR imaging compared with CT. *AJR Am J Roentgenol*. 1994;163:141–147.

### Treatment Options

Treatment of tibial condyle or plateau fractures depends on the extent of bone and soft tissue injury, patient age, activity status, and whether there are associated injuries. Minimally displaced fractures can be treated conservatively with cast immobilization or bracing. No weight bearing is permitted for 12 to 16 weeks. Schatzker type III or OTA B2 (simple central depression) fractures generally do not require internal fixation.

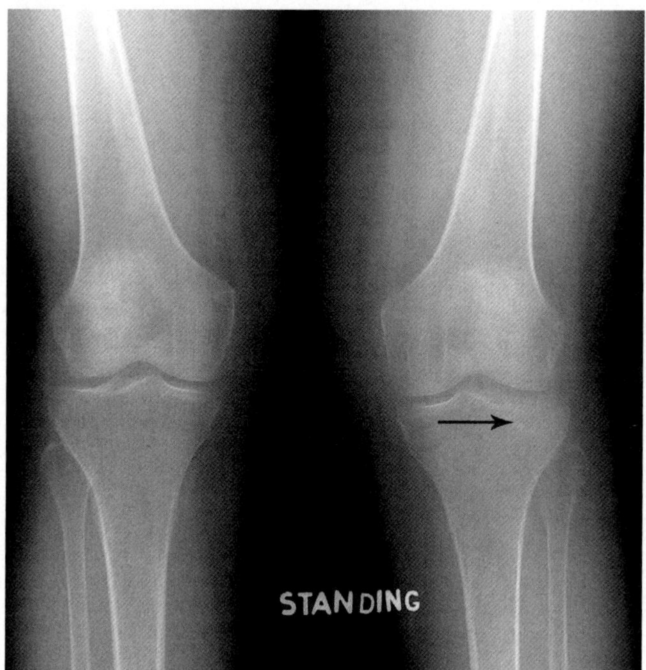


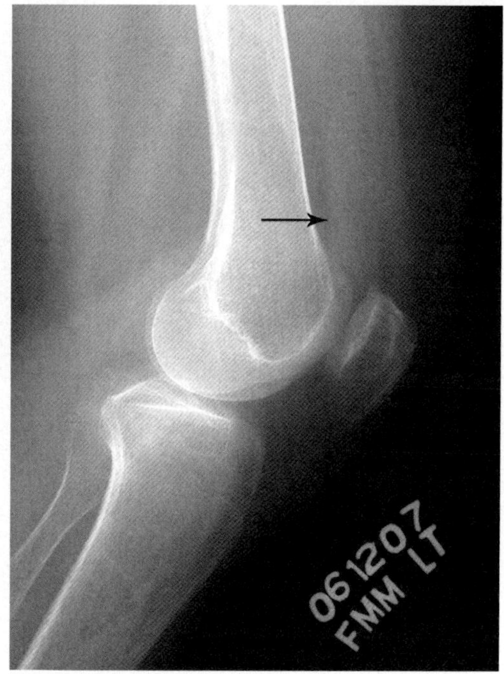


Fig. 6-21 Subtle depression of the lateral tibial plateau. Anteroposterior (AP) (A) and lateral (B) radiographs demonstrate a subtle lateral plateau fracture on the left in A (*arrow*) and a joint effusion on the lateral radiograph (*arrow* in B). Axial (C), coronal (D), and sagittal (E) reformatted computed tomographic (CT) images demonstrate a slightly displaced posterior plateau fracture clearly depicted on the 3-D image (F) (*arrow*).

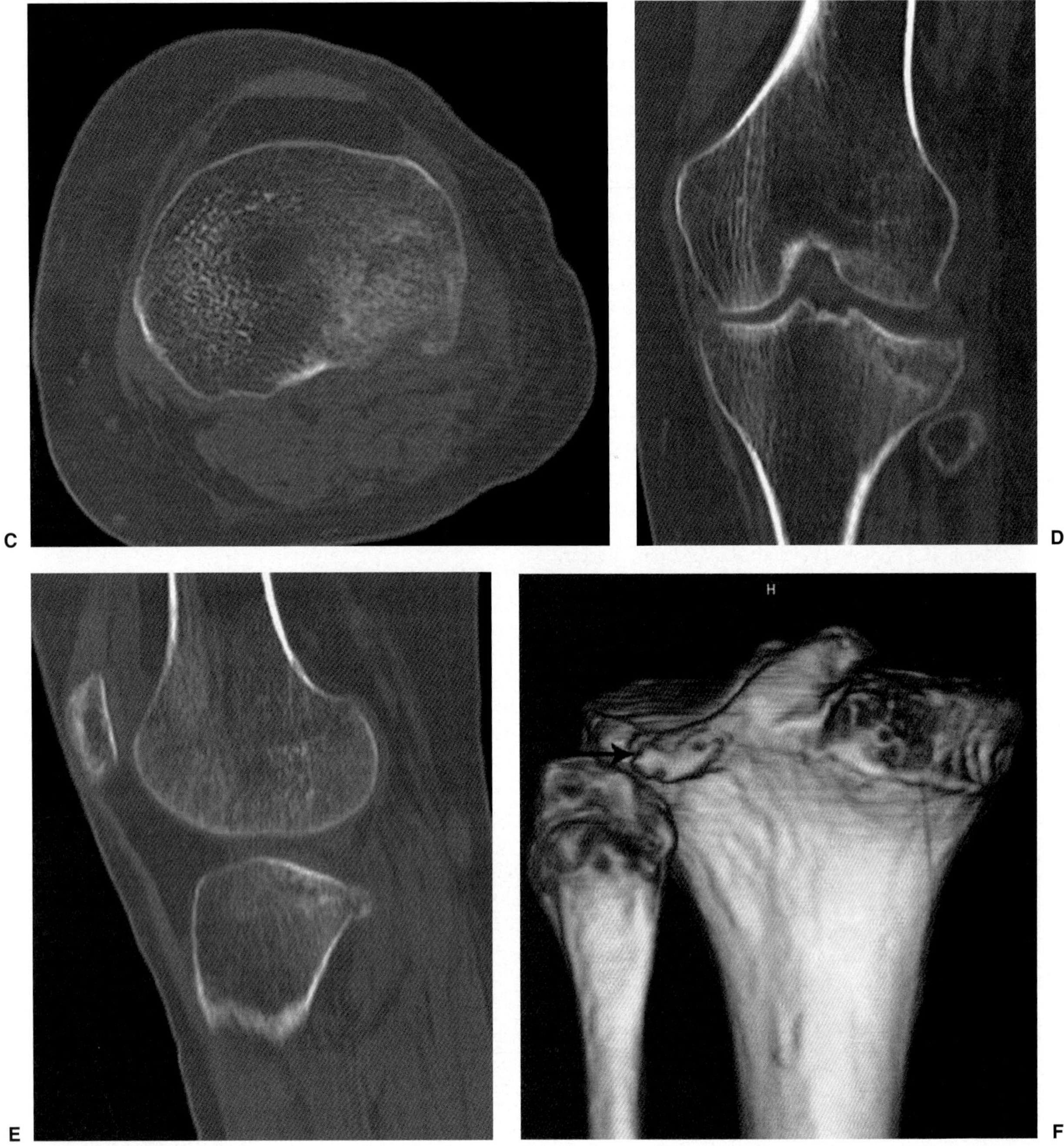


Fig. 6-21 *(Continued)*

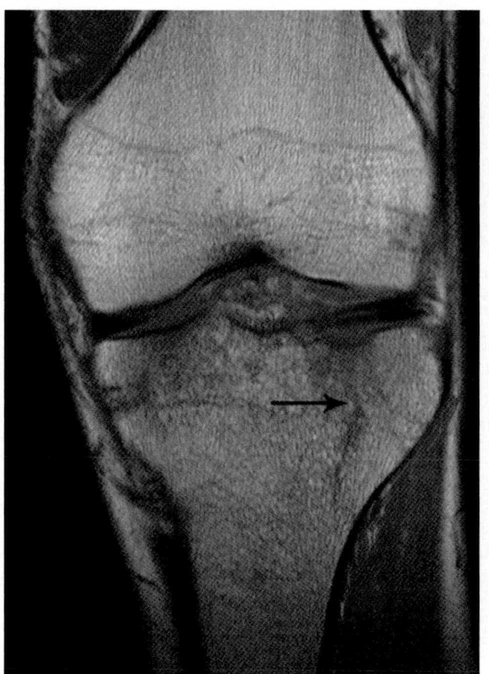
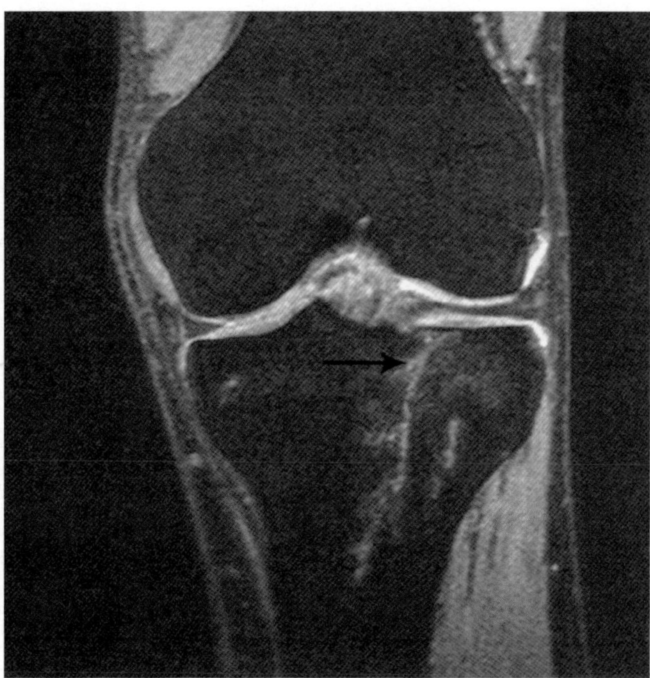

Fig. 6-22 Coronal T1-weighted (A) and dual echo steady state (DESS) (B) images demonstrating a subtle undisplaced plateau fracture (*arrow*).

**External Fixation:** Most unstable fractures are treated with internal fixation. However, bicondylar fractures (Schatzker types V and VI and OTA type C1 to 3) have been treated with external fixation using ring fixators. Soft tissue infection and wound necrosis are not unusual following internal fixation techniques. Comparison of external fixation and medial and lateral plate fixation had equal anatomic results. External fixation afforded a shorter hospital stay, less blood loss, and earlier ambulation.

**Internal Fixation:** Open reduction and fixation allows the depressed fragments to be elevated and reduction to be

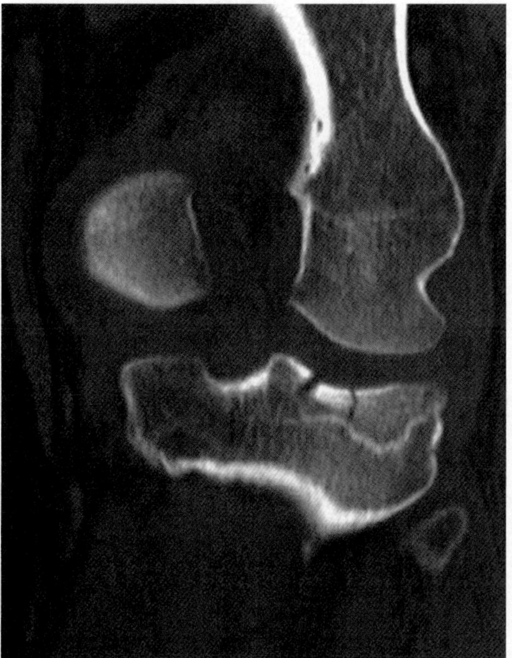
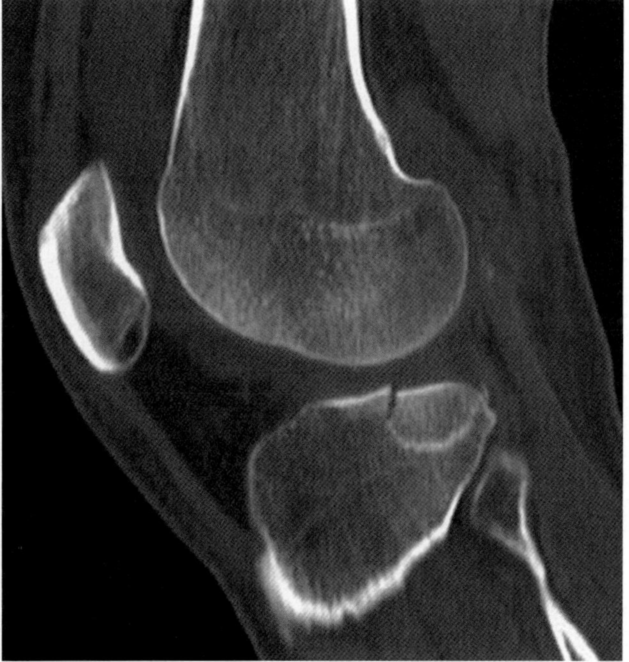

Fig. 6-23 Coronal (A) and sagittal (B) computed tomographic (CT) images demonstrate a minimally depressed plateau fracture without significant separation of the fragments. The fragments were elevated and reduction achieved with cannulated screws and washers as seen on anteroposterior (AP) (C) and lateral (D) radiographs.

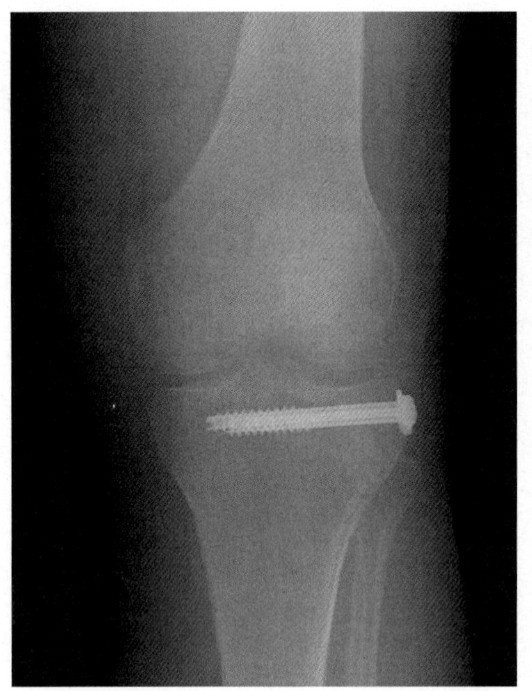

C

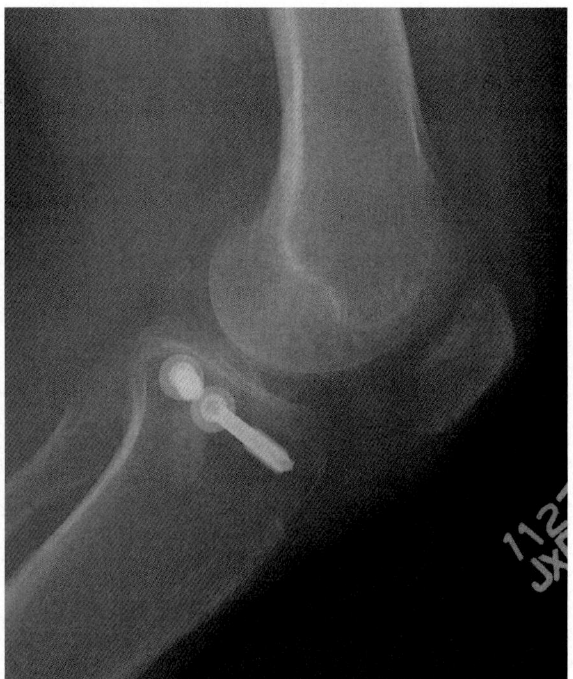

D

Fig. 6-23 (*Continued*)

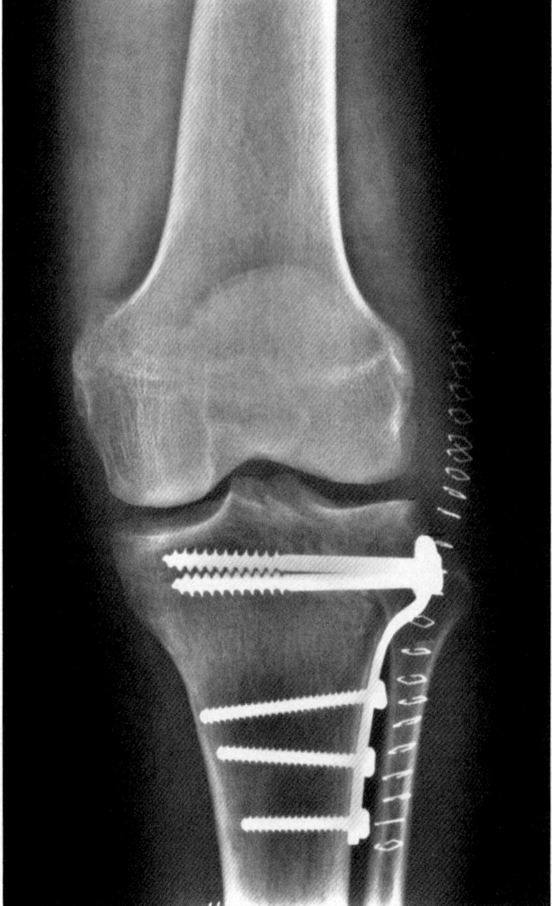

A

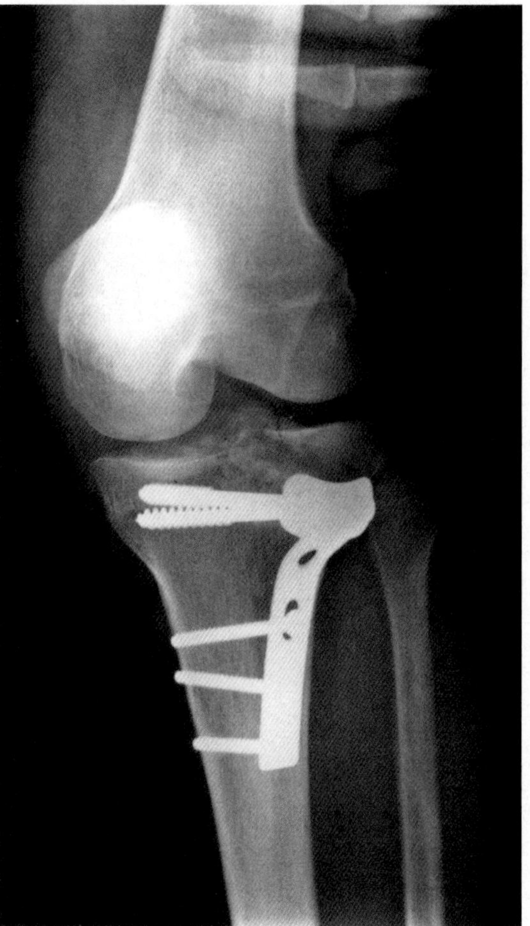

B

Fig. 6-24 Lateral plateau fracture that enters the eminence. Radiographs in the anteroposterior (AP) (A) and oblique (B) projections demonstrate reduction achieved with a T-buttress plate and screws.

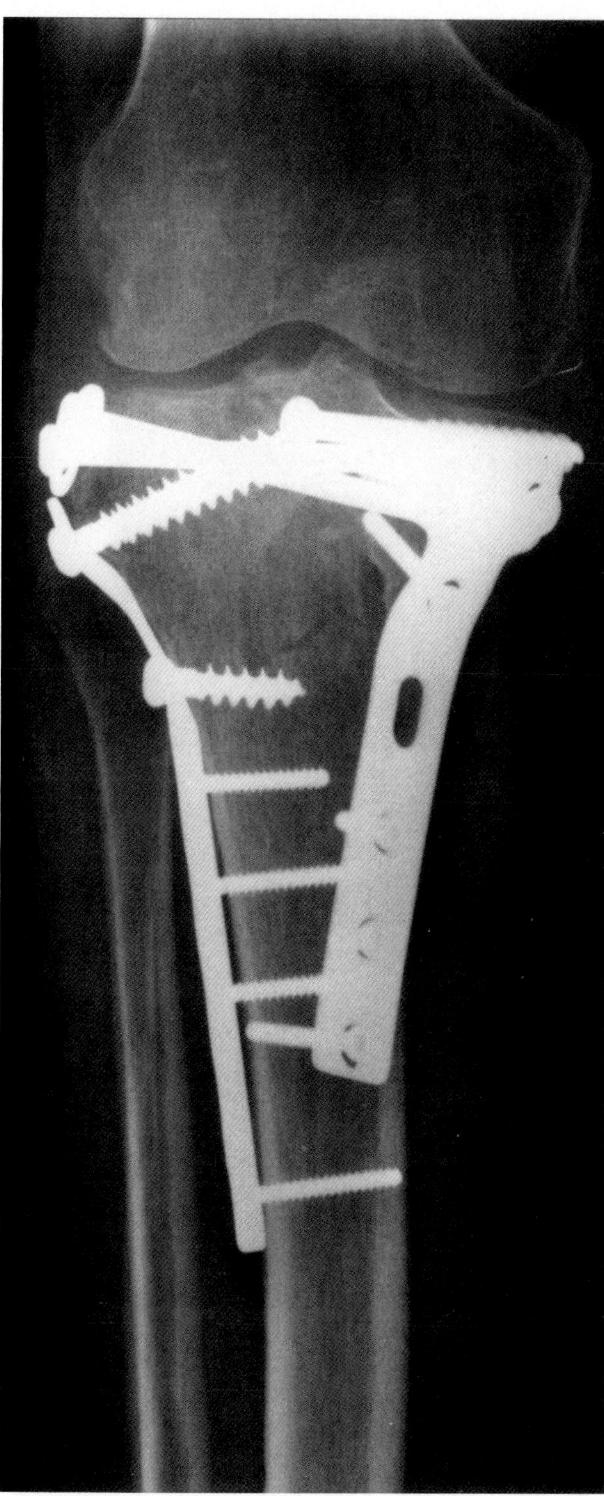

Fig. 6-25 Anteroposterior (AP) radiograph following reduction of a complex plateau and metaphyseal fracture with bilateral plate and screws and cancellous screws and washers laterally.

maintained with differing approaches depending on the degree of injury. For split fractures, cancellous screws and washers may be sufficient (see Fig. 6-23). Buttress plates can also be used (see Fig. 6-24). Bicondylar fractures (Schatzker type V and VI and OTA type C) usually require bilateral plates (see Fig. 6-25) and frequently bone graft (see Fig. 6-26) to achieve optimal results. Regardless of the surgical approach, early motion is important to restore function.

## Suggested Reading

Barie DP, Nork SE, Mills WJ, et al. Functional outcomes of severe bicondylar tibial plateau fractures treated with dual incisions and medial and lateral plates. *J Bone Joint Surg*. 2006; 88A:1713–1721.

Canadian Orthopaedic Trauma Society. Open reduction and internal fixation compared to circular fixator application for bicondylar tibial plateau fractures. *J Bone Joint Surg*. 2006;88A: 2613–2623.

Lachiewicz PF, Funcik T. Factors influencing the results of open reduction and internal fixation of tibial plateau fractures. *Clin Orthop*. 1990;259:210–215.

Waddell JP, Johnston DW, Neidre A. Fractures of the tibial plateau: A review of ninety-five patients and comparison of treatment methods. *J Trauma*. 1981;21:376–381.

### Miscellaneous Tibial Fractures

There are other, often more subtle, fractures about the knee. Some of these are included in the OTA type A1 category, which includes avulsion fractures of the tibial spine (see Fig. 6-27), fibular head, and tibial tuberosity (see Fig. 6-28, also Fig. 6-20). Tibial tuberosity fractures are classified into three simple categories (see Fig. 6-29). Type I fractures may be treated conservatively, whereas types II and III usually require fixation with a cancellous screw and washer.

**Tibial tuberosity fractures** (Fig. 6-29)

- **Type I:** Small avulsed fragments (39% of fractures)
- **Type II:** Anterior hinging of the entire tuberosity (18%)
- **Type III:** Tuberosity fracture extends into the joint space (43%)

Tibial eminence or spine fractures are similarly classified on the basis of the degree of displacement. Type I and II fractures can be treated conservatively, whereas type III fractures require surgical intervention.

**Tibial spine fractures** (see Fig. 6-30)

- **Type I:** Undisplaced (16% of fractures)
- **Type II:** Elevated anteriorly (39%)
- **Type III:** Displaced (45%)

A Segond fracture (see Chapter 2) is an avulsion at the insertion of the middle third of the capsular ligament on the

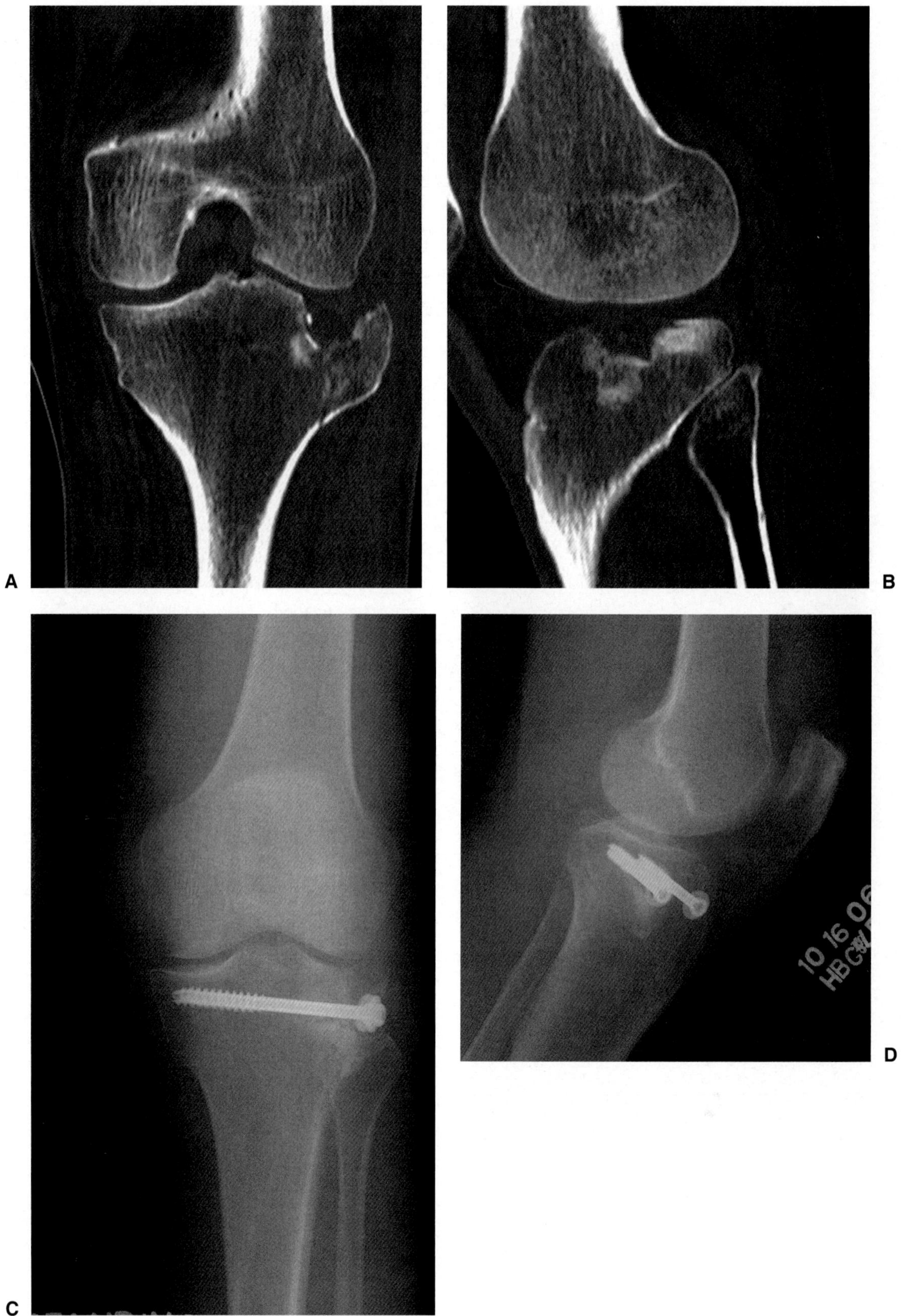


Fig. 6-26 Coronal (A) and sagittal (B) computed tomographic (CT) images demonstrating a lateral split fracture with marked depression. Reduction was accomplished (C and D) with bone graft and screws and washers.

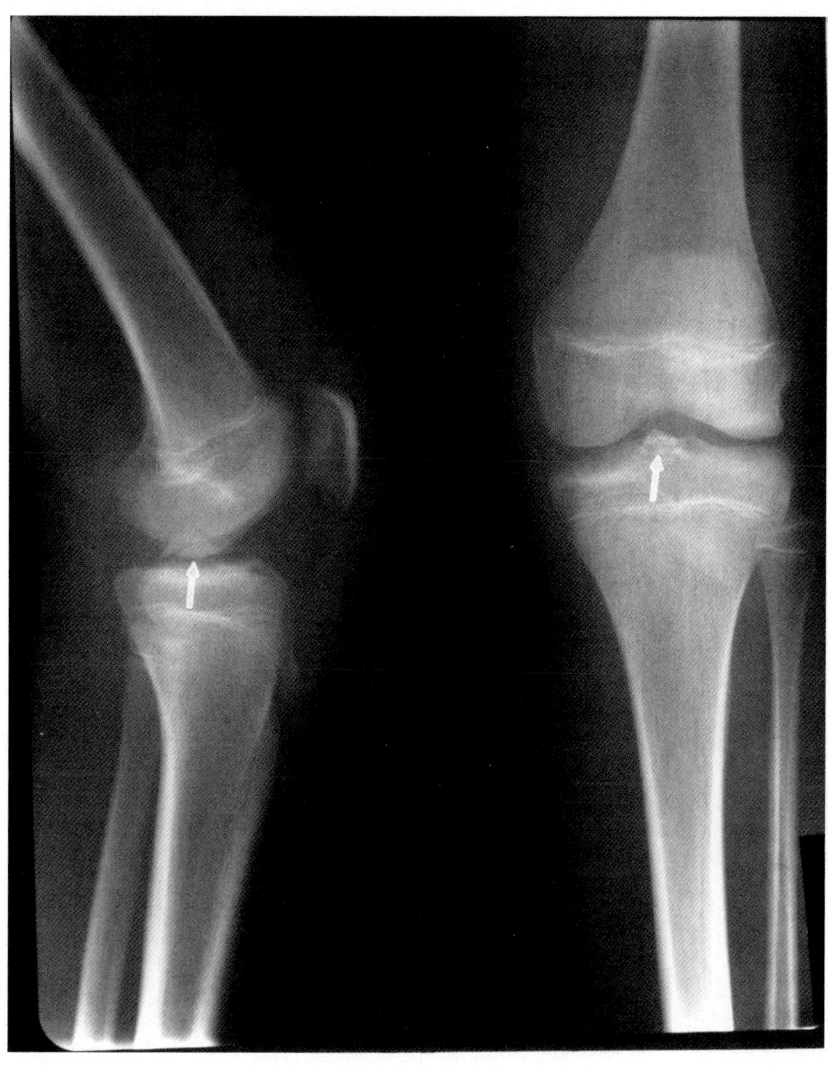

Fig. 6-27 Anteroposterior (AP) and lateral radiographs demonstrating an undisplaced (type I) tibial spine fracture (*arrow*).

proximal lateral tibia. This injury is frequently associated with ACL and meniscal tears (see Fig. 6-31). Bone bruises are also associated with ligament tears. Stress fractures may also occur in the proximal tibia and fibula.

Physeal fractures about the knee are uncommon. Fractures of the tibial physis account for only 0.5% to 3% of all physeal injuries. Femoral physeal fractures are slightly more common due to the ligament support about the knee. The ligaments extend below the tibial physis providing additional support, but attach to the femur just below the physis (see Figs. 6-32 and 6-33). Radiographic features may be subtle if the fracture is not displaced. MRI is preferred to detect and follow up physeal injuries (Fig. 6-33B).

## Suggested Reading

Berquist TH. Osseous and myotendinous injuries about the knee. *Magn Reson Imaging Clin N Am.* 2007;15:25–38.

Dezell PB, Schils JP, Recht MP. Subtle fractures about the knee: Innocuous-appearing yet indicative of internal derangement. *AJR Am J Roentgenol.* 1996;167:699–703.

### Ipsilateral Femoral and Tibial Fractures

Ipsilateral combined injuries of the tibia and femur present significant management issues. The injury has been termed *floating knee*. These fractures are usually related to high-velocity trauma, such as motor vehicle accidents. Local and distant injuries are common. Approximately 60% of fractures are open further complicating treatment approaches.

**Fraser classification:** (see Fig. 6-34)

- **Type I:** Shaft fracture without articular involvement (71% of injuries)
- **Type IIA:** Femoral fracture with tibial plateau fracture (16.5%)
- **Type IIB:** Femoral articular and tibial nonarticular fracture (4.5%)
- **Type IIC:** Both articular surfaces (8%)

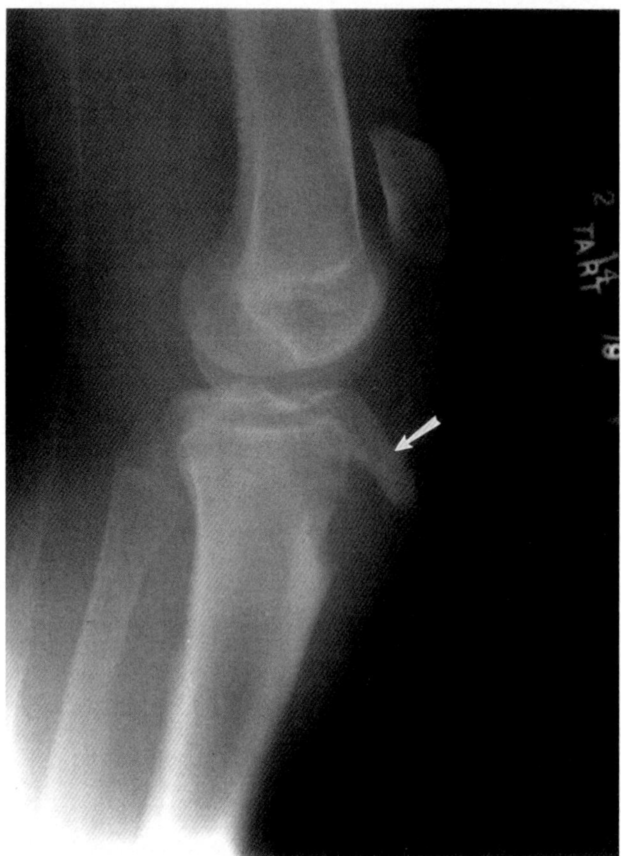

Fig. 6-28 Lateral radiograph demonstrating a tibial tuberosity avulsion (*arrow*) with the fracture extending into the joint space (type III).

Treatment usually requires internal fixation, though external fixation may be included especially when there are associated open wounds (see Fig. 6-35). See Chapter 5 for review of femoral treatment options.

## SUGGESTED READING

Fraser RD, Hunter GA, Waddel JP. Ipsilateral fracture of the femur and tibia. *J Bone Joint Surg*. 1978;60B:510–515.

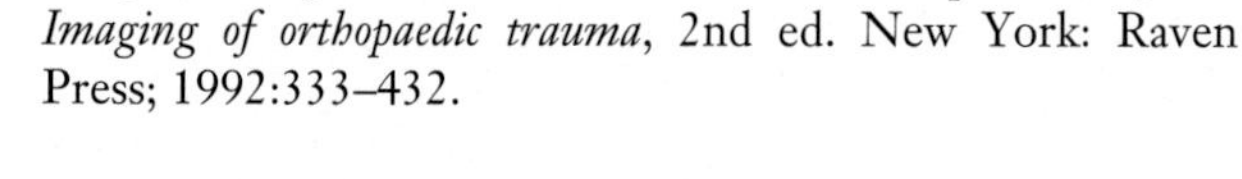

Rand JA, Berquist TH. The knee. In: Berquist TH, ed. *Imaging of orthopaedic trauma*, 2nd ed. New York: Raven Press; 1992:333–432.

## Soft Tissue Injuries

Soft tissue injuries about the knee may be associated with obvious or subtle (bone bruises) osseous fractures. This section will focus on those injuries that require some type of fixation device. The ACL is most often injured (39%). Injury may result from multiple mechanisms including forced valgus and external rotation, external rotation and hyperextension, internal rotation with extension, and forward displacement of the tibia. Most patients describe hearing a loud pop and are unable to bear weight. Up to 75% have an acute hemarthrosis. Also, 70% have other associated injuries including the MCL and posterior horn of the medial meniscus. When all three occur together it is termed *O'Donoghue's triad*. Combined ACL, MCL, and medial capsular tears account for 30% of soft tissue injuries about the knee. Lateral collateral ligament injuries occur in 19% and posterior cruciate ligament (PCL) tears in 5% of ligament injuries to the knee.

Imaging of patients with suspected soft tissue injury should begin with radiographs. Certain injuries may be evaluated with ultrasound or conventional/CT arthrography. However, in most cases MRI is the technique of choice to evaluate the ligaments, tendons, menisci, and articular cartilage. Following repair, baseline radiographs are important to evaluate the fixation devices and tunnels for ligament repair. A hyperextended cross-table lateral has been included to evaluate the position of the tibial tunnel compared to the condylar roof in patients with ACL repairs (see Fig. 6-36).

### Treatment Options

Treatment options for ligament repair include primary repair and reconstruction. With the former, the ligament is repaired by suturing the tear together. This approach may be most useful with ACL avulsions with the bone reattached to the tibia. In most cases reconstruction is preferred because results are superior. Autografts (patellar tendon, hamstring, or other tendon grafts), allografts, and synthetic materials have been used. Depending on the extent of repair the procedure can be done arthroscopically or as an open procedure. Grafts for the cruciate ligament are held in place with interference screws

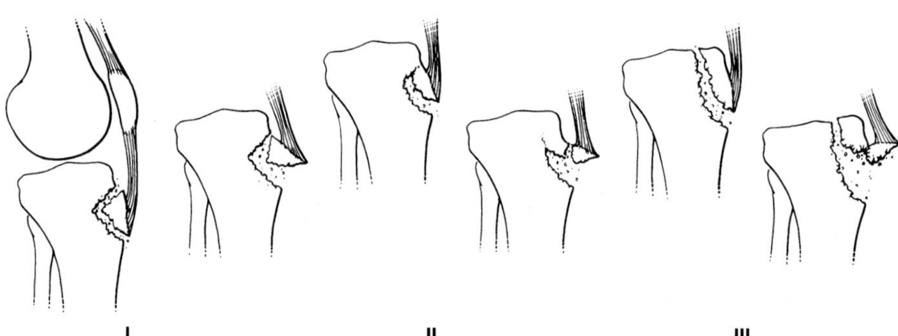


Fig. 6-29 Illustration of tibial tuberosity fractures. Type I—simple avulsion, type II—anterior hinging of the entire tuberosity, and type III—fracture extending into the joint space.

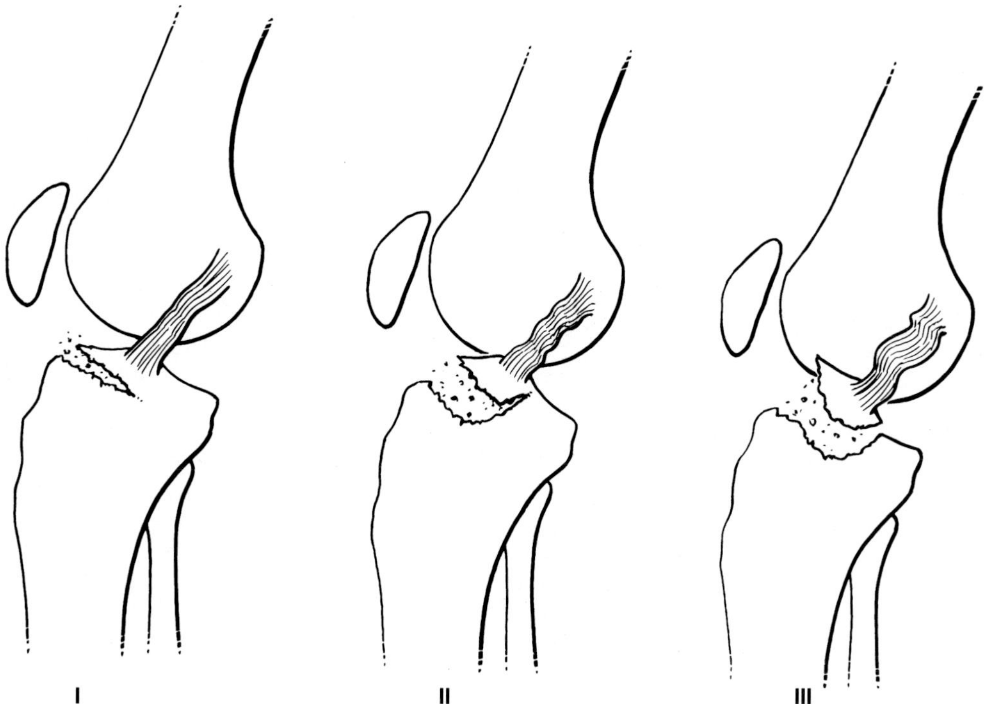


Fig. 6-30 Illustration of tibial eminence or spine fractures. Type I—undisplaced, type II—elevated anteriorly, and type III—displaced.

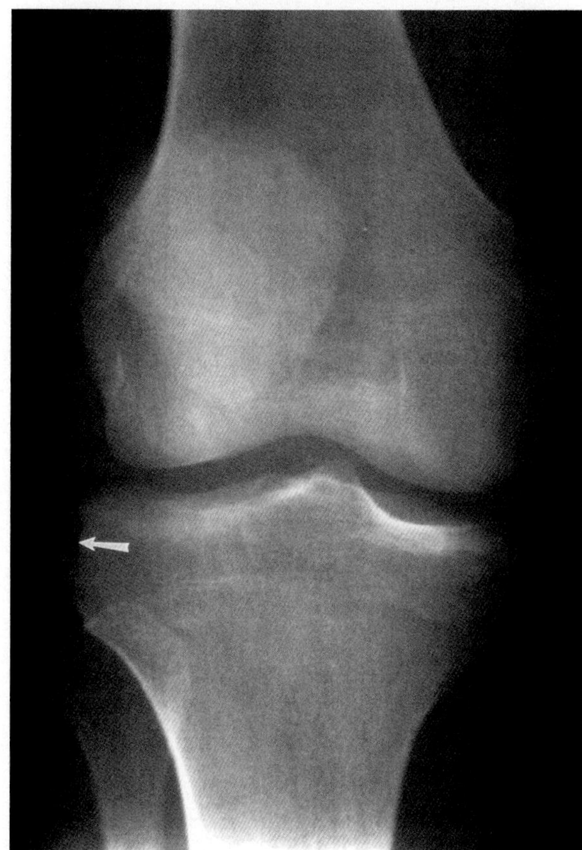

Fig. 6-31 Anteroposterior (AP) radiograph of the knee demonstrating the Segond fracture (*arrow*).

in most cases (see Fig. 6-37). However, staples, screws with variegated washers, and other fixation devices may also be used. It is important that the tunnels for cruciate repair are placed in isometric position (Fig. 6-36).

## Suggested Reading

Freedman KB, D'Amato MJ, Dedeff DD, et al. Arthroscopic anterior cruciate ligament reconstruction: A meta-analysis comparing patellar tendon and hamstring autografts. *Am J Sports Med.* 2003;31:2–11.

Manaster BJ, Remley K, Newman AP, et al. Knee ligament reconstruction: Plain film analysis. *AJR Am J Roentgenol.* 1988; 150:337–342.

Noyes FR, Barber-Westin SD. Reconstruction of the anterior cruciate ligament with human allograft: Comparison and early results. *J Bone Joint Surg.* 1996;78A:524–537.

### Postoperative Imaging and Complications

Complications and associated injuries vary with the nature of the fracture, mechanism of injury, and treatment approach. More significant injuries (comminuted fractures, fracture dislocations, ipsilateral femur, and tibia fractures) are more likely to have local or systemic complications.

Osseous complications include nonunion (see Fig. 6-38), malunion (see Fig. 6-39), deep infection, and implant failure (Figs. 6-38 and 6-40). The incidence varies with the specific fracture. Malunion is reported in 6% of supracondylar femur fractures. Complex tibial plateau fractures achieve satisfactory reduction in only approximately 55% of cases with

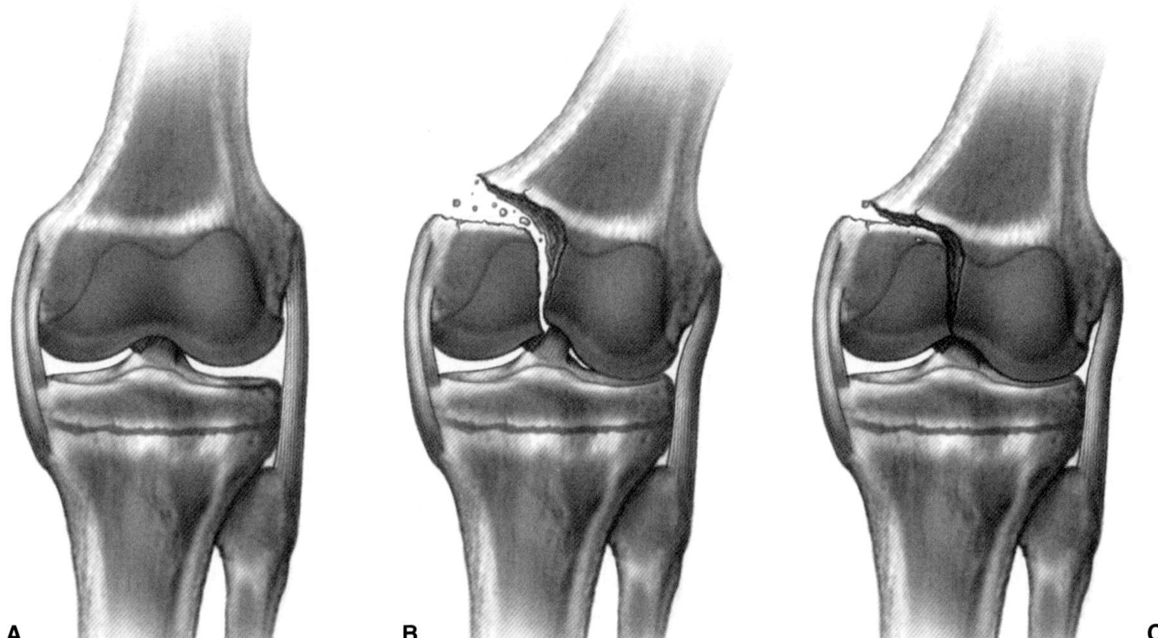

Fig. 6-32 Illustrations of the physeal and ligament anatomy of the knee. The ligaments extend beyond the tibial physis (A), but attach just below the femoral physis placing it at greater risk for fracture (B and C).

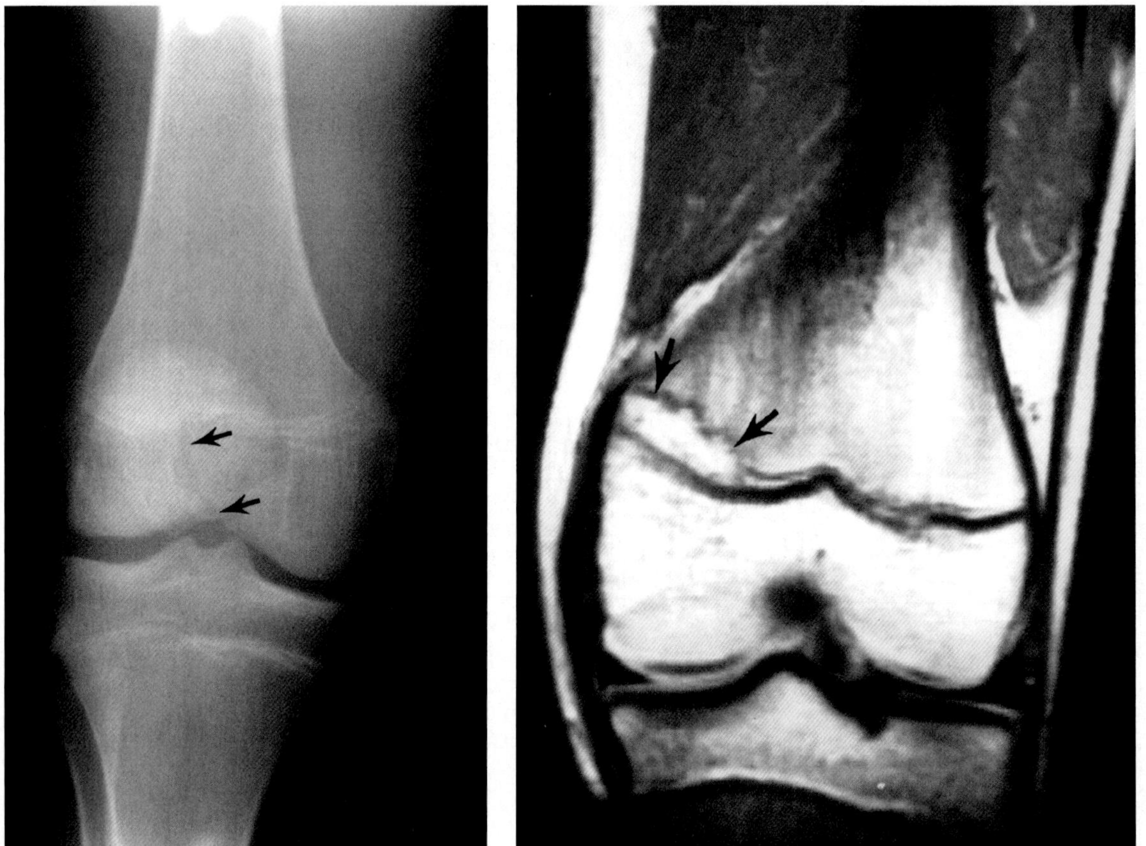

Fig. 6-33 Anteroposterior (AP) radiograph (A) shows a subtle Salter-Harris type III physeal fracture (*arrows*). Magnetic resonance (MR) is superior for demonstrating and evaluating the physes as seen on the coronal proton density image (B) demonstrating a partial femoral physis fracture (*arrows*).

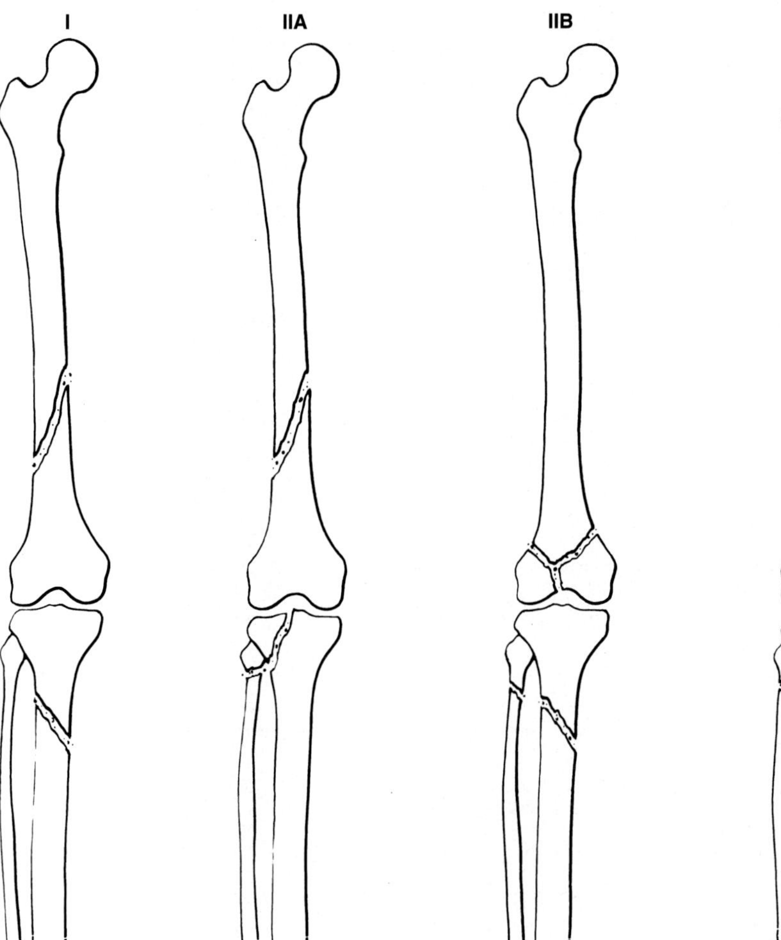


Fig. 6-34 Illustration of the Frazer classification for ipsilateral femoral and tibial fractures. Type I—shaft fractures without articular involvement, type IIA—femoral shaft and tibial plateau, type IIB—femoral articular and tibial nonarticular, and type IIC—both articular surfaces.

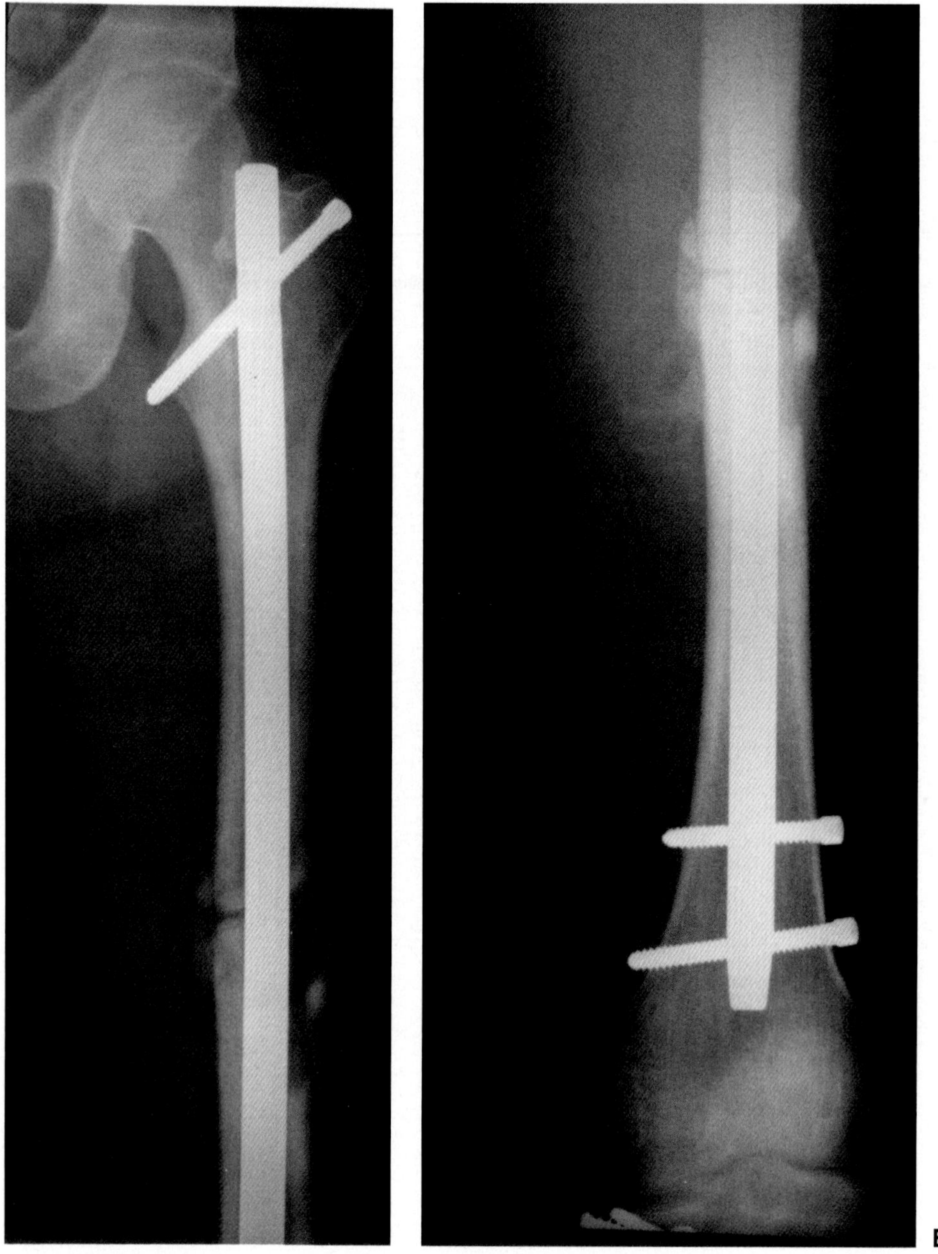


Fig. 6-35 Ipsilateral femoral and tibial fractures type IIA with femoral shaft and tibial plateau fractures. Anteroposterior (AP) (A and B) and lateral (C and D) radiographs demonstrate a static intramedullary nail for femoral fixation and buttress plate and cancellous screws and washers for fixation of the tibial plateau fracture.

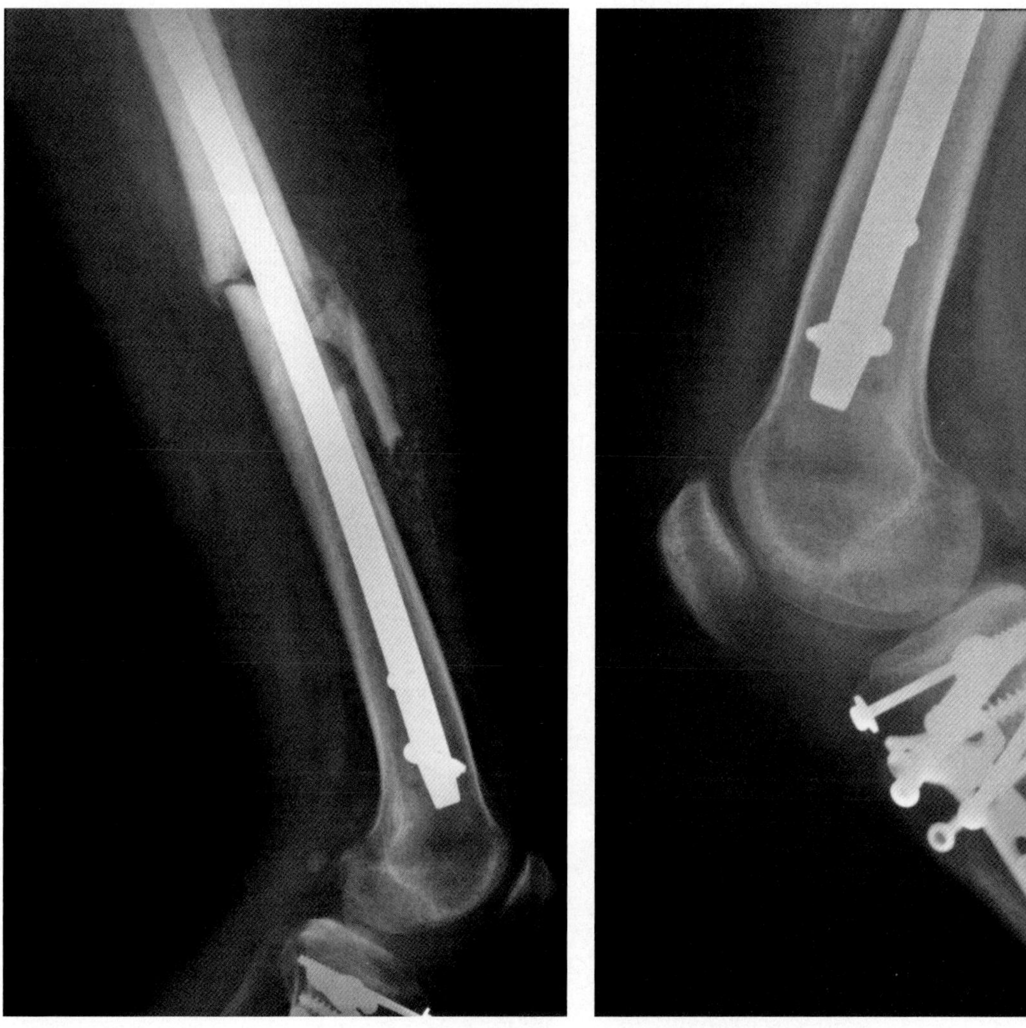


Fig. 6-35 (*Continued*)

residual articular deformities of 3 to 5 mm occurring in the remaining cases. This obviously results in early osteoarthritis (see Fig. 6-41). Deep infection occurs more frequently with open fractures. Up to 12% of complex tibial plateau fractures (Shatzker type V and VI and OTA type C) and 7% of patellar fractures are open. The incidence of deep infection is also increased with open reduction and internal fixation. The overall incidence of deep infection ranges from 5% to 17%. Pin tract infection seen with external fixation occurs in 21%. However, these infections usually respond to local treatment and oral antibiotics.

Articular deformity can occur with physeal, supracondylar, tibial plateau, and patellar fractures resulting in arthrosis, joint deformity, and reduced function. Associated articular and periarticular injuries are also an issue. Associated meniscal tears (55%) and ligament tears (68%) are common with complex tibial plateau fractures. Compartment syndrome is present in 10% of complex tibial plateau fractures. Deep venous thrombosis (DVT) occurs in 20% of patients. Other neurovascular injuries are also associated with complex intra-articular fractures in the knee. The peroneal nerve is most commonly involved. Table 6-1 summarizes complications and imaging approaches for fractures about the knee.

Complications related to ligament repair differ in some respects. Although implant failure and tunnel position can often be evaluated on serial radiographs including a hyperextended cross-table lateral projection, MRI is the primary method for evaluation of ligament reconstruction complications. In some cases, intravenous or intra-articular contrast may enhance the imaging evaluation of the graft. Metallic interference screws may cause some artifact but this can usually be overcome by proper selection of pulse sequences (see Chapter 1) (see Fig. 6-43). New biodegradable screws do not cause artifact on MR images. Graft impingement and arthrofibrosis (cyclops lesion) (see Fig. 6-44) are the most common causes for loss of extension. Infection is uncommon (0.5%), but this can also be evaluated with MRI. Table 6-2 summarizes complications of ligament reconstruction and imaging approaches.

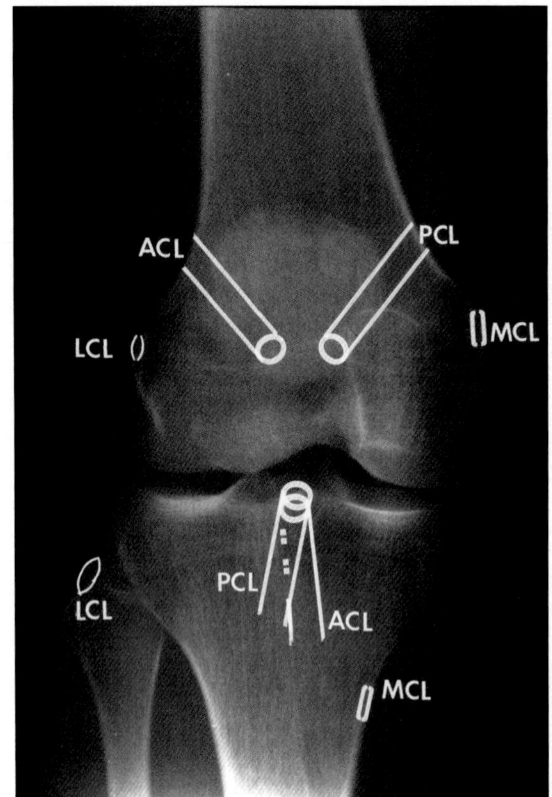


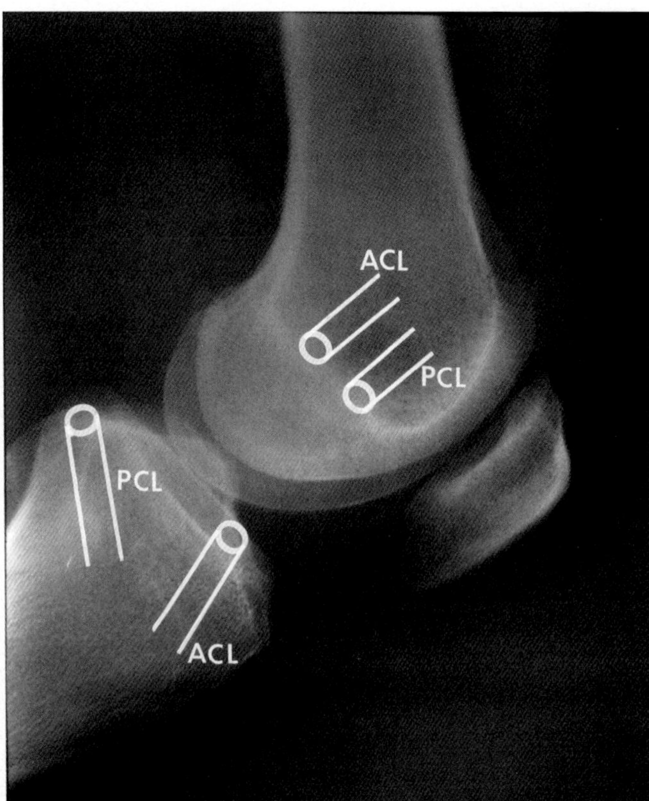


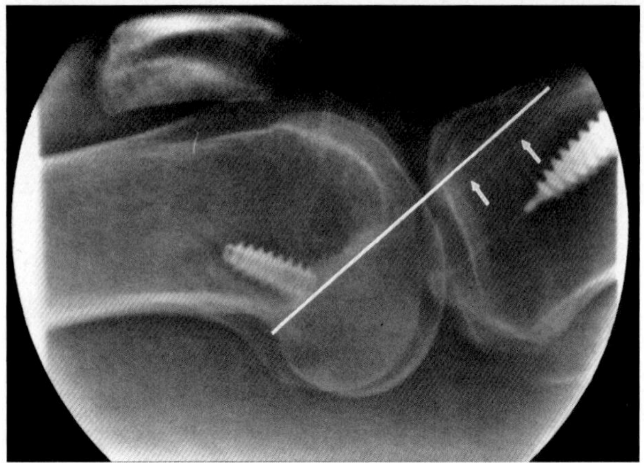


Fig. 6-36 Imaging evaluation of ligament repairs. Anteroposterior (AP) (A) and lateral (B) radiographs demonstrating the position of the femoral and tibial tunnels for anterior cruciate ligament (ACL) and posterior cruciate ligament (PCL) grafts. The sites of attachment for the medial collateral ligament (MCL) and lateral collateral ligament (LCL) are also demonstrated. (C) Hyperextended cross-table lateral radiograph demonstrates the normal position of the tibial tunnel for ACL repair (*arrows*) posterior to the intercondylar line (*white line*). If the tunnel is anterior to the condylar line it usually causes graft impingement.

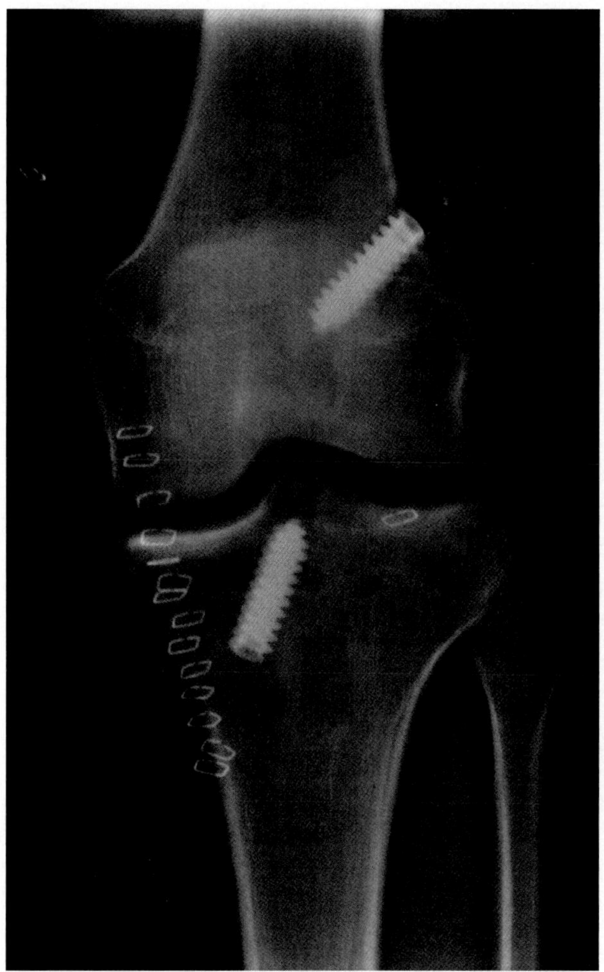


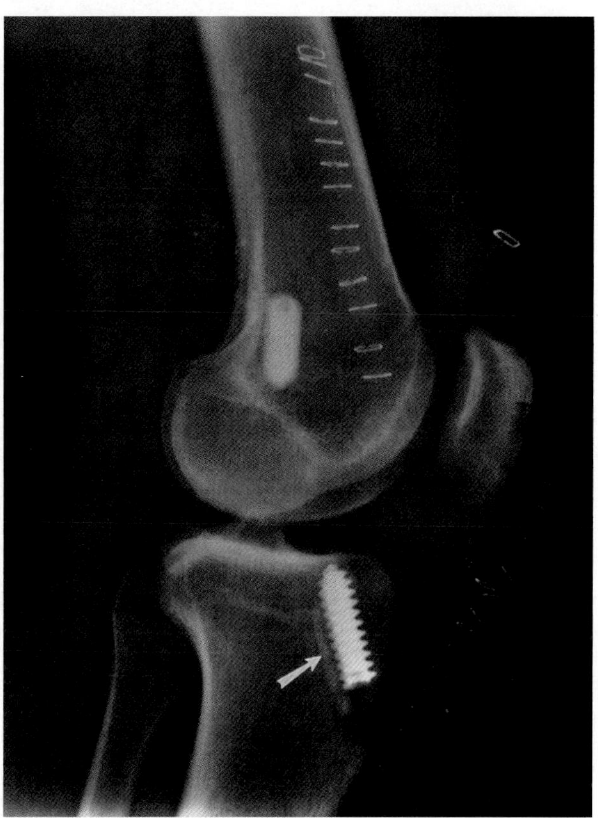


Fig. 6-37 Anterior cruciate ligament (ACL) repair. Anteroposterior (AP) (A) and lateral (B) radiographs demonstrate interference screws used to hold the bone plugs (*arrow* in B) in place in the femoral and tibial tunnels.

## Suggested Reading


Arazi M, Memik R, Ogun TC, et al. Ilizarov external fixation for severely comminuted supracondylar and intercondylar fractures of the distal femur. *J Bone Joint Surg*. 2001;83B:663–667.

Barei DP, Nork SE, Mills WJ, et al. Functional outcomes of severe bicondylar tibial plateau fractures treated with dual incisions and medial and lateral plates. *J Bone Joint Surg*. 2006;88A:1713–1721.

McCauley TR, Elfar A, Moore A, et al. MR arthrography of anterior cruciate reconstruction grafts. *AJR Am J Roentgenol*. 2003;181:1217–1223.

Pailo AF, Malavolta EA, Dos Santos ALG, et al. Patellar fractures: A decade of treatment at IOT-HC-FMUSP-Part I: Functional analysis. *Acta Orthop Bras*. 2005;13:221–225.


## Knee Arthroplasty

Knee arthroplasty was developed as an alternative to arthrodesis. Hemiarthroplasty with femoral resurfacing began in the 1930s, followed by use of metal components in the 1940s. Hinged prostheses (see Fig. 6-47) followed in the 1950s, but were ineffective because of high failure rates. Since that time there have been numerous improvements and continuous modifications are ongoing to design the most appropriate system for the patients' needs.

### Indications and Contraindications

Total knee replacement has increased at a rate of 10% per year since the 1980s, with more than 350,000 primary and 29,000 revision procedures in 2002 in the United States. It is critical for radiologists to thoroughly understand the indications, normal

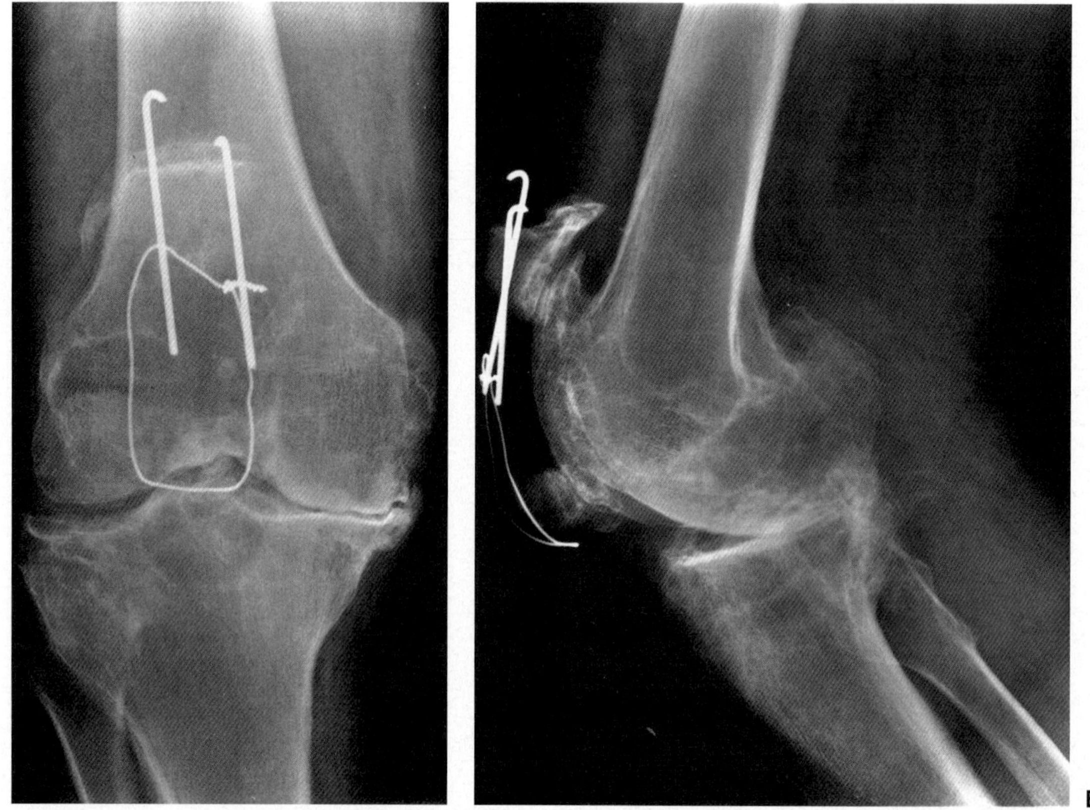

Fig. 6-38 Transverse patellar fracture with implant failure and nonunion. Anteroposterior (AP) (A) and lateral (B) radiographs demonstrate failure of the K-wire and tension band fixation with wide separation of the patellar fragments.

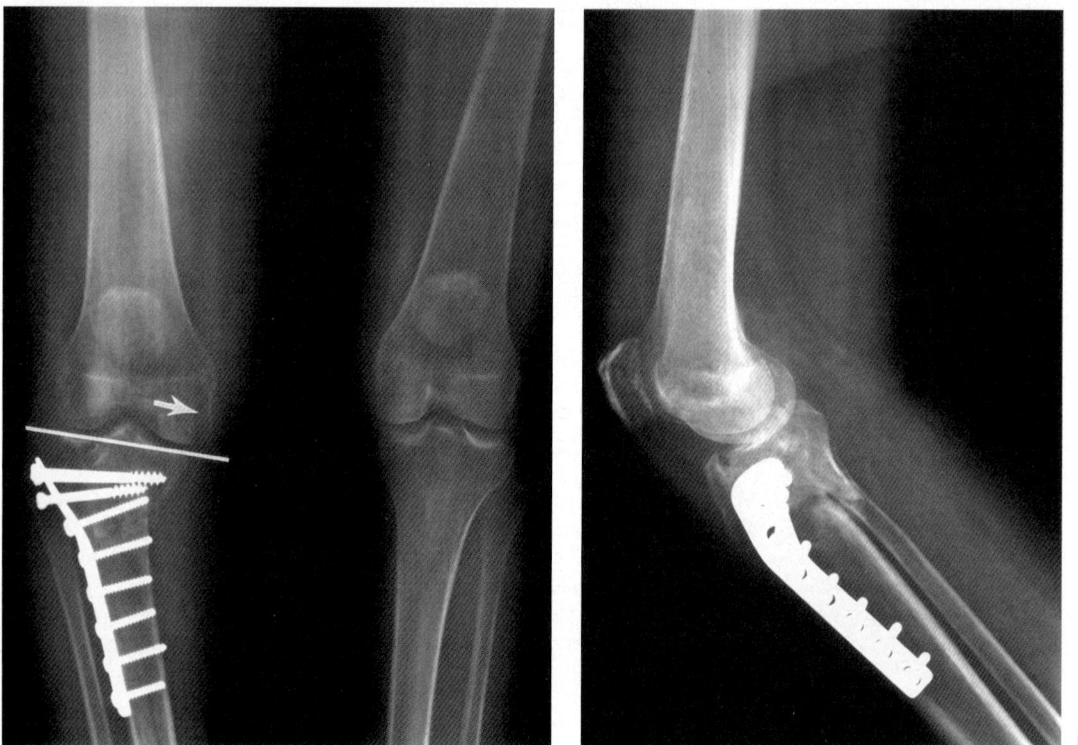

Fig. 6-39 Malunion. Anteroposterior (AP) standing (A) and lateral (B) radiographs demonstrate a complex tibial plateau fracture with collapse medially resulting in marked joint asymmetry (*line*) and medial femoral subluxation (*arrow*).

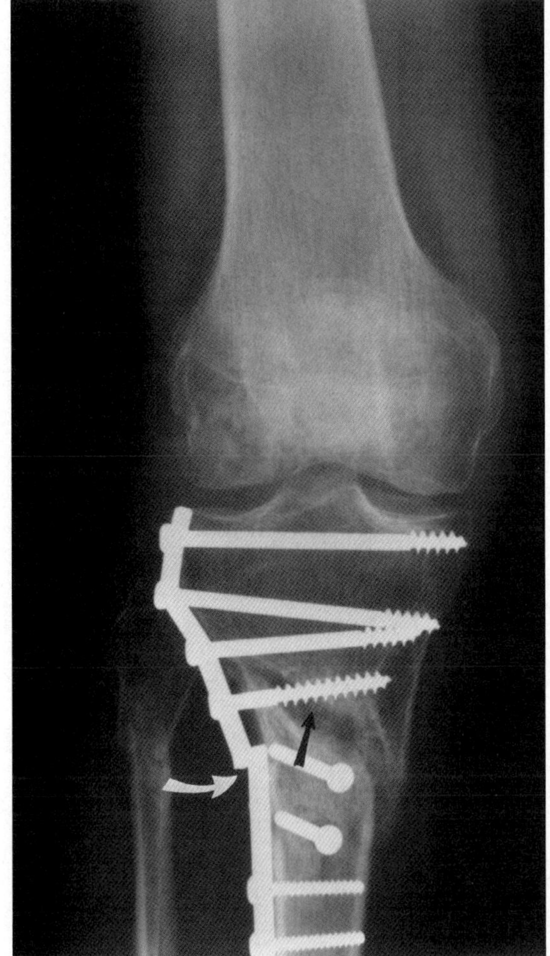


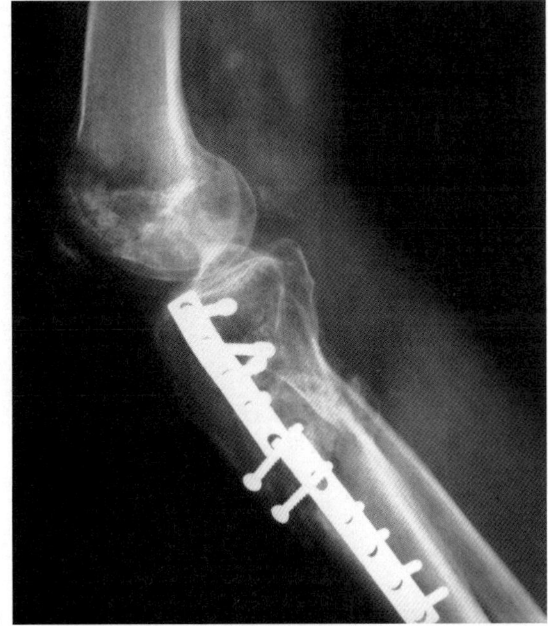


Fig. 6-40 Implant failure. Anteroposterior (AP) (A) and lateral (B) radiographs demonstrate a complex tibial fracture with bone loss (*black arrow*) centrally and fracture of the fixation plate (*curved white arrow*).

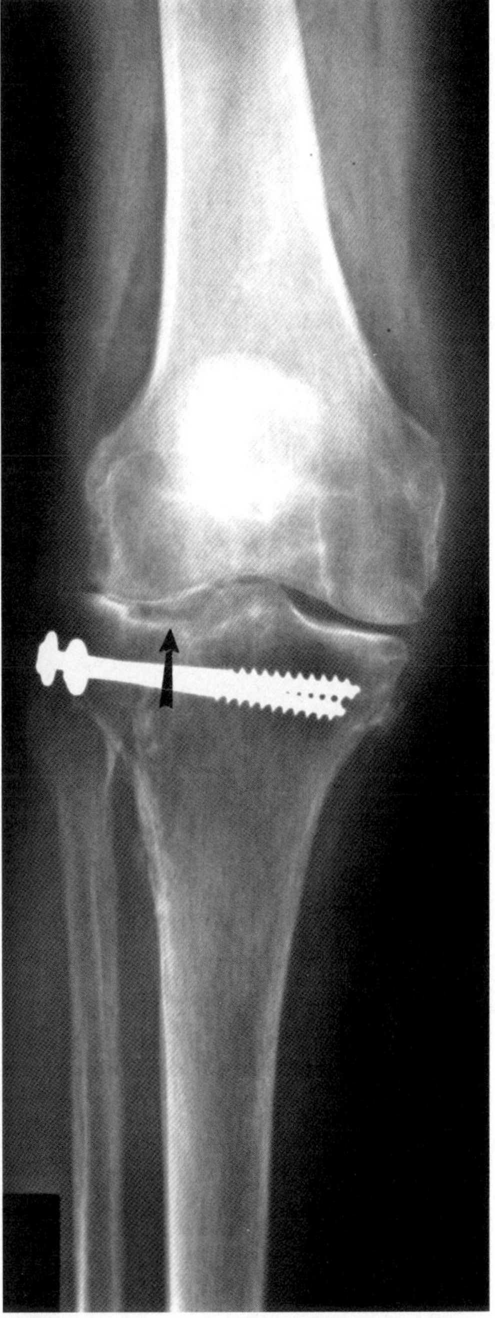

Fig. 6-41 Anteroposterior (AP) radiograph demonstrates incomplete elevation of a central depression fracture in the lateral plateau (*arrow*) leading to osteoarthritis.

appearances, and potential complications associated with knee replacement procedures.

The goals of knee replacement procedures are to relieve pain and improve range of motion, function, and stability. The most common indications are severe degenerative arthritis or advanced inflammatory arthropathies, such as rheumatoid arthritis. Knee arthroplasty is contraindicated in patients with neuropathic arthropathy or infection. Patients with excessive occupational or physical demands and markedly

**Fig. 6-42** Premature growth arrest following physeal fractures. **A:** Coronal fat-suppressed fast spin-echo T2-weighted image shows the normal high signal intensity of the tibial growth plate with a bony bar (*arrow*) in the mid tibia anteriorly. **B:** Sagittal proton density image in a different patient shows a bar involving >50% of the physis (*arrows*). Multiple image planes and T2 or T2* sequences are preferred to quantify the extent of premature fusion.

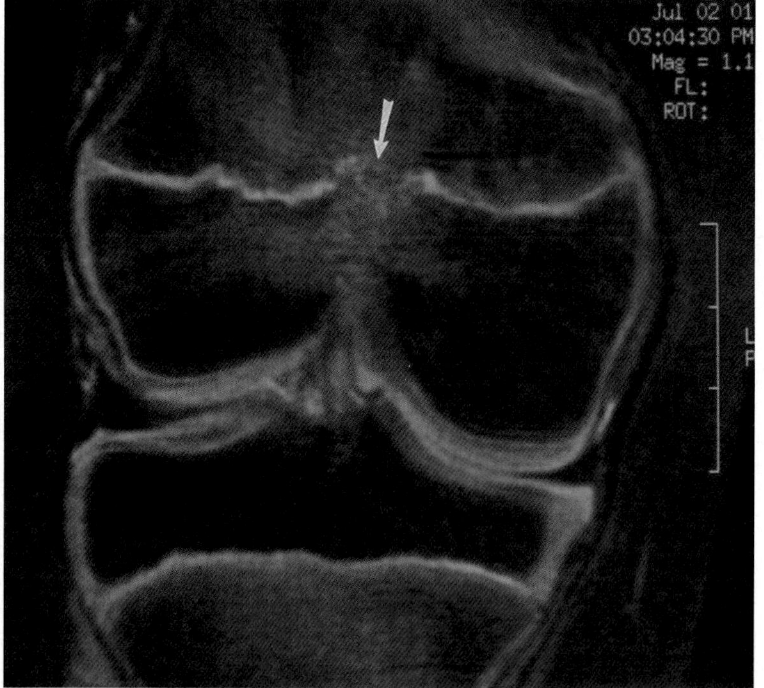


A

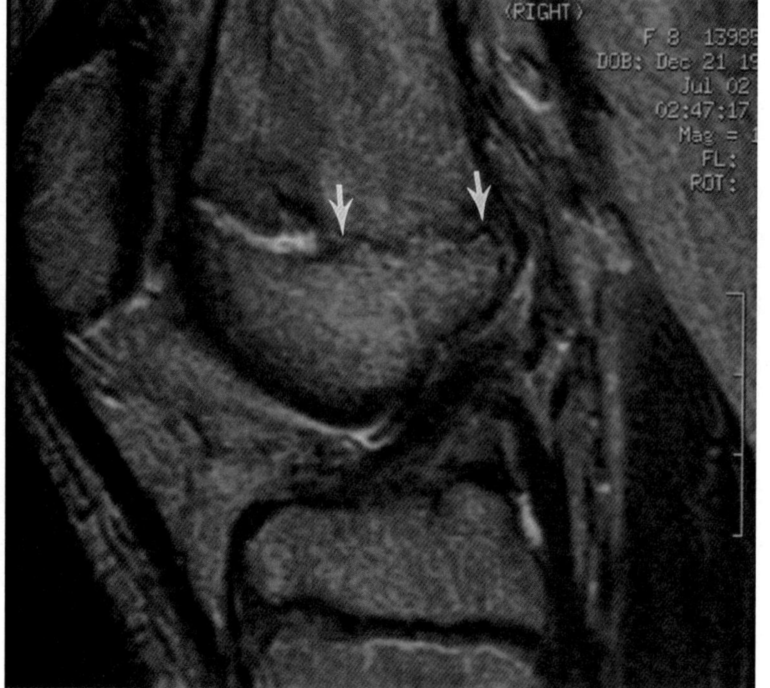


B

**Table 6-1**

**FRACTURE COMPLICATIONS AND IMAGING APPROACHES**

| COMPLICATIONS | IMAGING APPROACHES |
|---|---|
| Malunion | Serial radiographs, CT |
| Nonunion | Serial radiographs, CT |
| Physeal bars | MRI (Fig. 6-42) |
| Articular deformity | Serial radiographs, MRI |
| Infection | MRI, radionuclide scans |
| Menisci, ligaments | MRI, CT arthrography |
| Nerve injuries | MRI |
| Vascular injuries | Angiography |
| Venous thrombosis | Ultrasound, venography |

CT, computed tomography; MRI, magnetic resonance imaging.

obese patients are also poor candidates for knee replacement procedures. Custom prostheses are available for limb salvage procedures in patients with neoplasms about the knee (see Chapter 14).

Patient factors are important for appropriate selection of implants and timing of the procedure. Factors include age, gender, weight, activity levels, patient compliance, and expectations. When possible, joint replacement in the knee is reserved for patients older than 65 years. Typically, patients are considered candidates if pain interferes with sleep or activity and has not responded to conservative therapy over a 3- to 6-month time frame. Patients aged 55 years or younger are usually given longer periods of conservative therapy or alternative bone-sparing techniques are considered. Rand et al. reported implant survivals of 83% for patients younger than 55 years compared to 94% for patients older than 70 years at the time of primary knee replacement. Duffy et al. have reported survivals of 99% at 10 years and 95% at 15 years in patients younger than 55 years treated with total knee replacement. Most patients had rheumatoid arthritis.

## Suggested Reading

Berquist TH. Imaging of joint replacement procedures. *Radiol Clin North Am.* 2006;44:419–437.

Duffy GP, Trousdale RT, Stuart MJ. Total knee arthroplasty in patients 55 years old or younger, 10 and 17 year results. *Clin Orthop.* 1998;356:22–27.

Mahomed NN, Barrett J, Katz JN, et al. Epidemiology of total knee replacement in the United States medicare population. *J Bone Joint Surg.* 2005;87A:1222–1228.

Rand JA, Trousdale RT, Ilstrup DM, et al. Factors affecting the durability of primary total knee prostheses. *J Bone Joint Surg.* 2003;85A:259–265.

### Component Designs

Normal knee motion includes flexion-extension (hinge) along with sliding, rolling, and spinning motions. Spinning motion

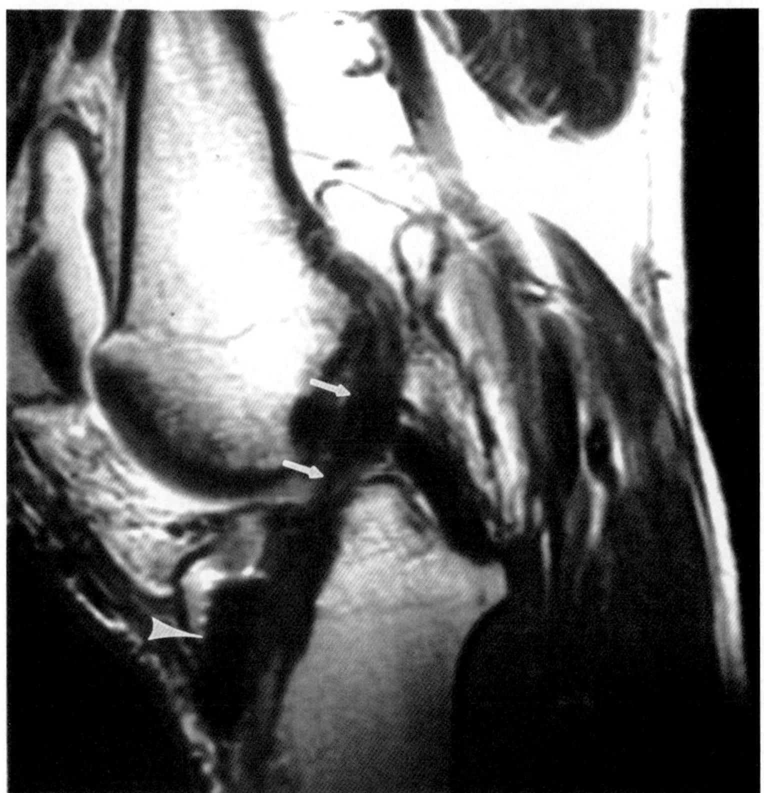

**Fig. 6-43** Sagittal proton density magnetic resonance (MR) image demonstrating an intact anterior cruciate ligament (ACL) graft (*arrows*) with little artifact from the tibial interference screw (*arrowhead*).

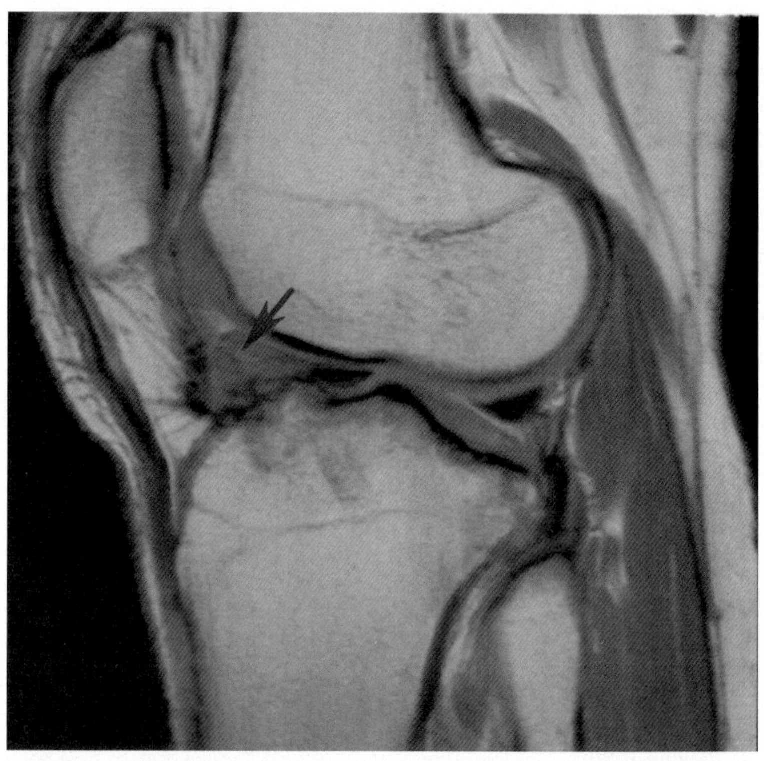

**Fig. 6-44** Sagittal T1-weighted magnetic resonance (MR) image demonstrating low signal fibrosis (*arrow*) due to a cyclops lesion.

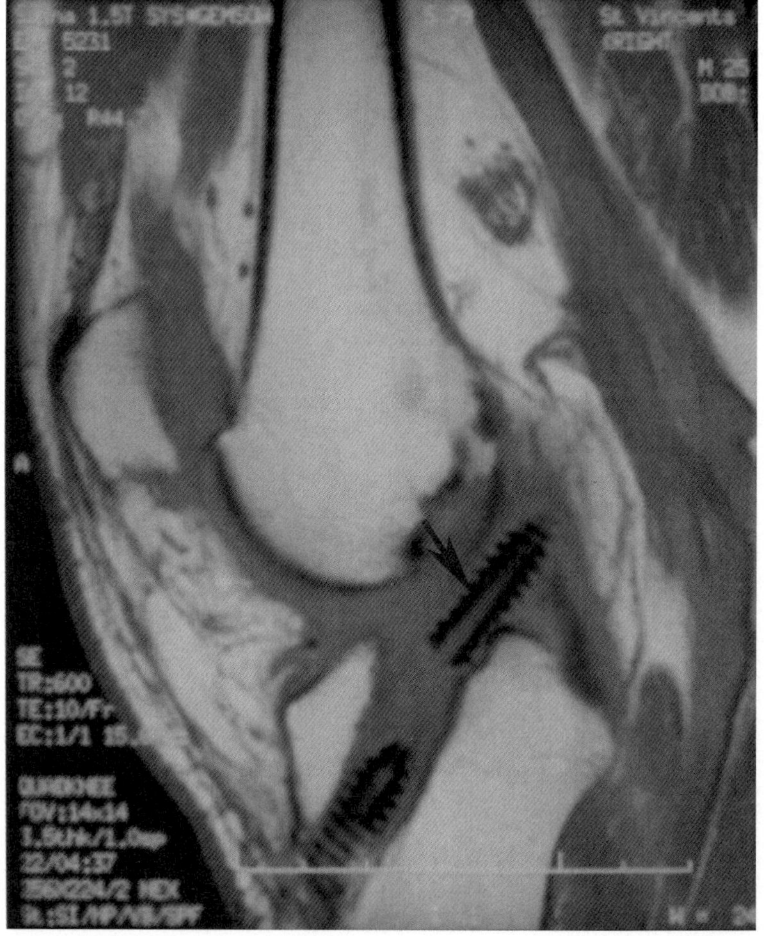


**Fig. 6-45** Sagittal T1-weighted image following anterior cruciate ligament (ACL) reconstruction with biodegradable interference screws. The femoral screw (*arrow*) has pulled back into the joint.

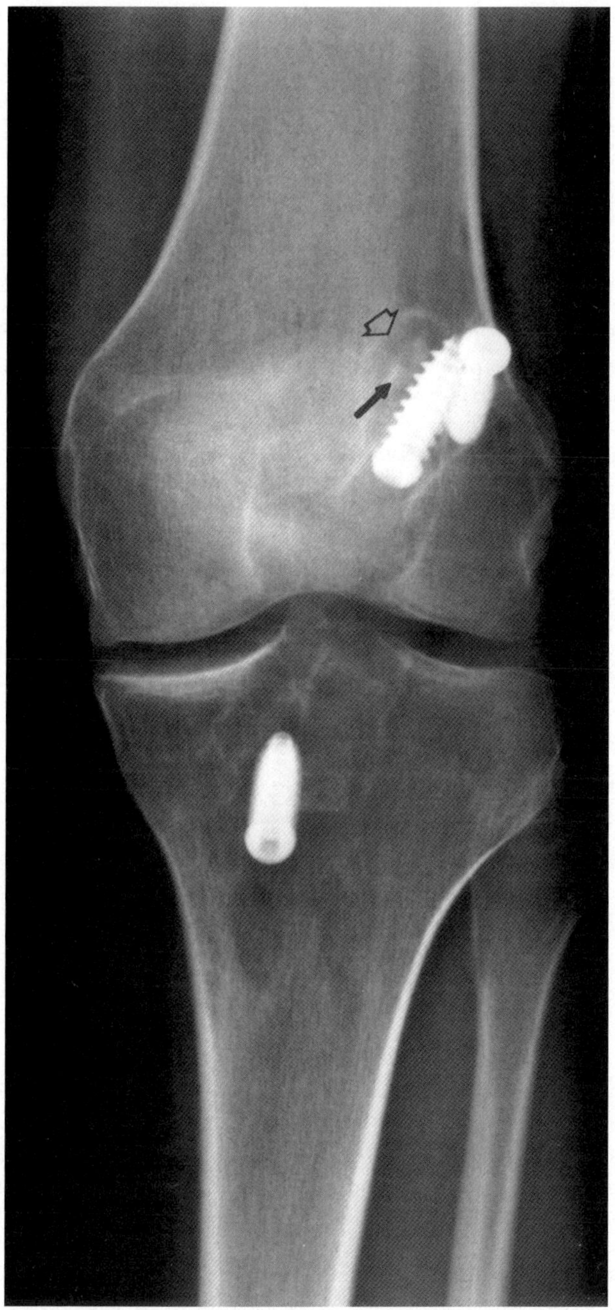

Fig. 6-46 Anteroposterior (AP) radiograph demonstrates fracture of the bone plug (*black arrow*) and lucency about the tunnel due to loosening (*open arrow*).

has no change in position of the contract point. Moderate wear and friction occur. With rolling motion, the areas of contact for the two surfaces are similar so the degree of wear and friction are the least.

Prosthetic components are designed to mimic certain knee motions, depending on the constraint of the prosthesis. Constraint refers to the stability afforded to the knee by the configuration of the components.

**Unconstrained:** This prosthesis is a resurfacing prosthesis that relies upon intact collateral and cruciate ligaments. The tibial components are flatter and relatively normal knee motion is maintained (see Fig. 6-48A).

**Table 6-2**

**LIGAMENT RECONSTRUCTION COMPLICATIONS AND IMAGING APPROACHES**

| COMPLICATIONS | IMAGING APPROACHES |
|---|---|
| Improper tunnel position | Radiographs, hyperextended cross-table lateral, MRI |
| Hardware failure | Serial radiographs, MRI (See Fig. 6-45) |
| Bone plug fracture | Radiographs, MRI (See Fig. 6-46) |
| Patellar fracture (stress riser) | Serial radiographs |
| Graft rupture | MRI |
| Graft impingement | Cross-table extended lateral, MRI |
| Cyclops lesions | MRI (Fig. 6-44) |
| Infection | MRI |

MRI, magnetic resonance imaging.

**Semiconstrained:** Semiconstrained prostheses add some stability by using a concave tibial polyethylene spacer. The ACL is sacrificed and the spacer configuration is selected to keep the collateral ligaments in proper tension. The PCL is preserved with the femoral component notched or open posteriorly (total condylar prosthesis, Fig. 6-48A and B and see Fig. 6-49). Posterior stabilized (PCL substituting) semiconstrained prostheses sacrifice both cruciate ligaments. The tibial component has a central post that articulates with a femoral cam which controls femoral roll back during flexion (see Fig. 6-50).

**Constrained:** Constrained prostheses are used in patients with inadequate soft tissue support, bone loss, or for revision arthroplasty. Constrained designs provide more stability, but transfer more forces to the bone resulting in more susceptibility to loosening and wear (see Fig. 6-51).

**Fixed bearing:** Fixed bearing is a tibial component where the polyethylene spacer is fixed to the tibial tray.

**Mobile bearing:** The tibial spacer is not fixed but can glide or rotate on the tibial tray during knee motion, theoretically reducing polyethylene wear (see Fig. 6-52).

Considerable research has been accomplished to establish the most useful configurations, metals, and polyethylene for knee implants. Metal alloys of cobalt-chromium, cobalt-chromium-molybdenum, zirconium, and titanium alloy are most often used currently. Polyethylene is ultra–high molecular weight for tibial spacers. Components have been designed to use with or without cement. Currently, most are cemented. Also, metal-backed patellar components are not commonly used currently because failure rates are higher than polyethylene alone.

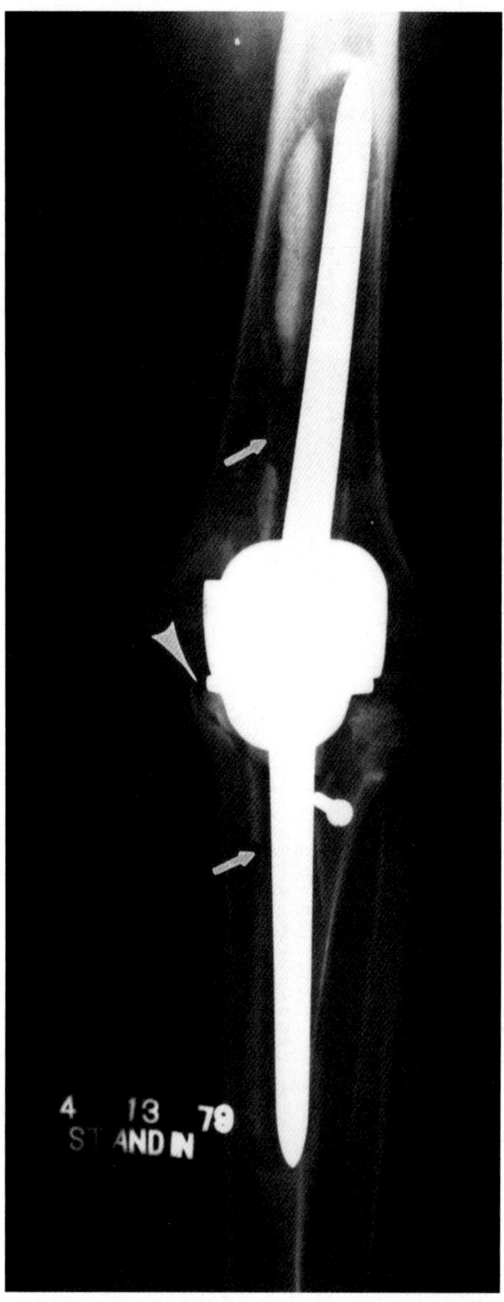


Fig. 6-47 Geupar metal on metal-hinged prostheses. Anteroposterior (AP) radiograph demonstrates cement fractures (*arrows*) about both the tibial and femoral stems with considerable lucency about the components and subsidence of the tibial component (*arrowhead*) due to gross loosening.

## Suggested Reading

Math KR, Zaidi SF, Petchprapa, C, et al. Imaging of total knee arthroplasty. *Semin Musculoskelet Radiol.* 2006;10:47–63.

Raphael B, Haims AH, Wu JS, et al. MRI comparison of periprosthetic structures around zirconium knee prostheses and cobalt-chrome prostheses. *AJR Am J Roentgenol.* 2006;186:1771–1777.

Rodricks DJ, Patil S, Pulido P, et al. Press-fit condylar design total knee arthroplasty: Fourteen to seventeen year follow-up. *J Bone Joint Surg.* 2007;89A:89–95.

Wood DJ, Smith AJ, Collopy D, et al. Patellar resurfacing in total knee arthroplasty. *J Bone Joint Surg.* 2002;84A:187–193.

### Preoperative Clinical Evaluation

As noted earlier, multiple factors related to patient status figure in decision making with regard to appropriateness and timing for knee replacement procedures. In addition, the Knee Society has developed a clinical scoring system that can be used to evaluate the patient preoperatively and postoperatively. The scoring system is divided into knee rating section and functional assessment. The knee rating section focuses on three essential parameters—pain, stability, and range of motion. A well-aligned knee with 125 degrees of motion, no pain, and negligible instability is awarded 100 points. The maximum score for stair climbing, walking, and normal activities is also 100 points. There are point deductions for decreased range of motion, instability, pain levels, use of walking assistance, such as canes and diminished function. Table 6-3 summarizes the categories and scores. There are more categories in each than demonstrated in the table.

## Suggested Reading

Insall JN, Dorr LD, Scott RD, et al. Rationale of the Knee Society clinical rating system. *Clin Orthop.* 1989;248:13–14.

Lingard EA, Wright RJ, Katz J, et al. Validity and responsiveness of the Knee Society clinical rating system in comparison with the SF-36 and WOMAC. *J Bone Joint Surg.* 2001;83A:1856–1864.

### Preoperative Imaging

Preoperative radiographs or computed radiographic (CR) images are important to evaluate alignment, joint spaces, bone stock, and soft tissue anatomy. The entire lower extremity is evaluated on the standing AP full-length radiograph. Both sides can be compared. AP, lateral, Merchant, and standing flexion views are routinely obtained. The last is taken with the knees flexed 45 degrees in the posteroanterior (PA) position and provides more tangential evaluation of the femorotibial joints.

Standing full-length images provide information regarding joint deformity in the hips, knees, and ankles as well as long bone deformities, leg length discrepancy, and fracture deformities. Multiple important measurements are made using this image (see Fig. 6-53). The mechanical axis is determined by extending a line from the center of the femoral head to the center of the talar dome. The line should pass through or near the center of the knee. The mechanical axis is generally 3 degrees off the vertical axis. The anatomic axis is the angle formed by lines drawn along the femur and tibia. The femorotibial angle is formed by a line down the center of both structures and is normally 5 to 7 degrees valgus.

In certain situations, MRI may be required to fully evaluate articular cartilage, especially if unicompartmental replacement

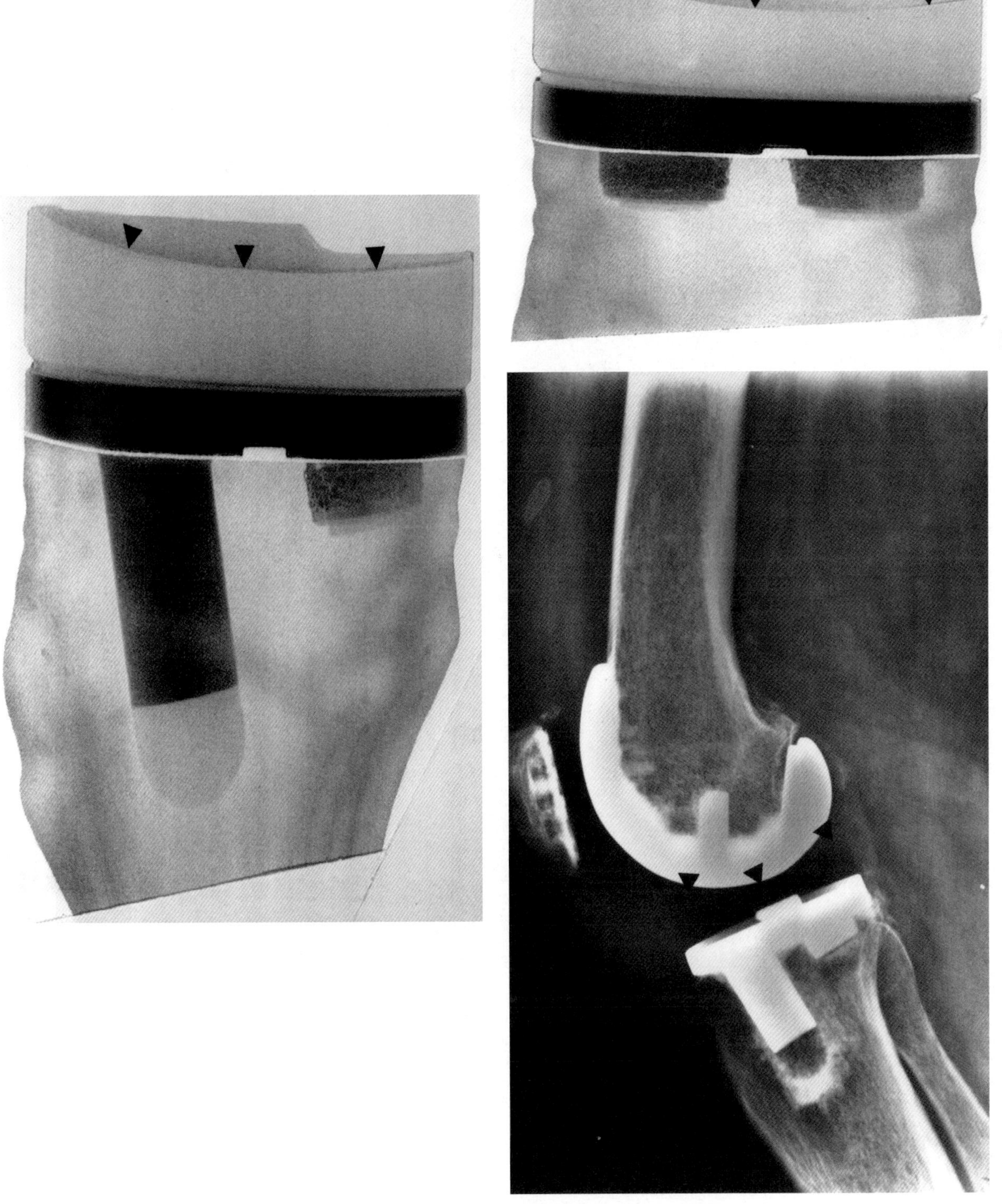


Fig. 6-48 Lateral illustrations of polyethylene tibial components (*arrowheads*) with a relatively flat surface (A) for minimal constraint and a more concave surface (B) providing more constraint with a condylar or posterior cruciate spearing femoral component (C). The lucent concave tibial tray is obvious (*arrowheads*) on the lateral radiograph. (A and B Courtesy of Zimmer, Warsaw, Indiana.)

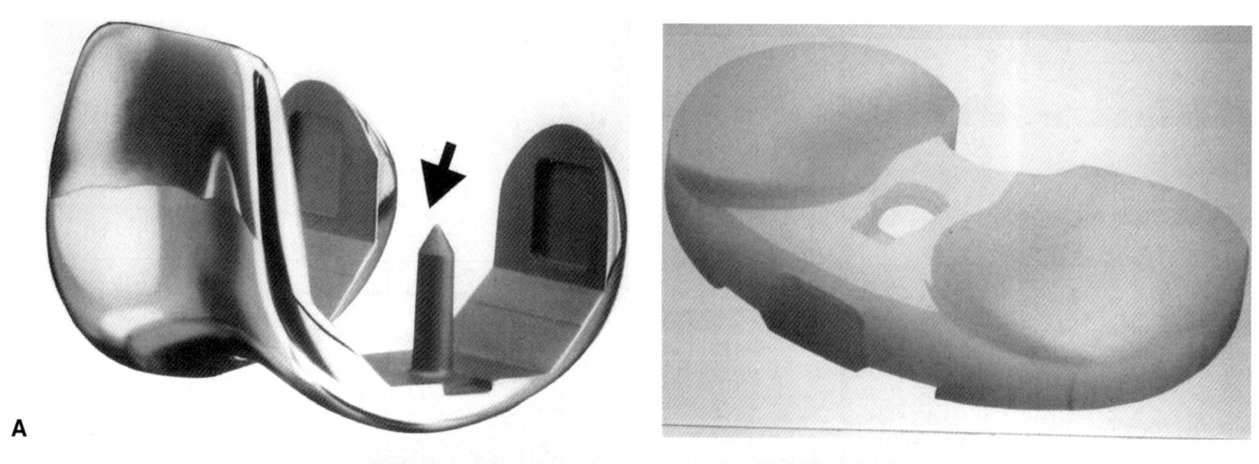

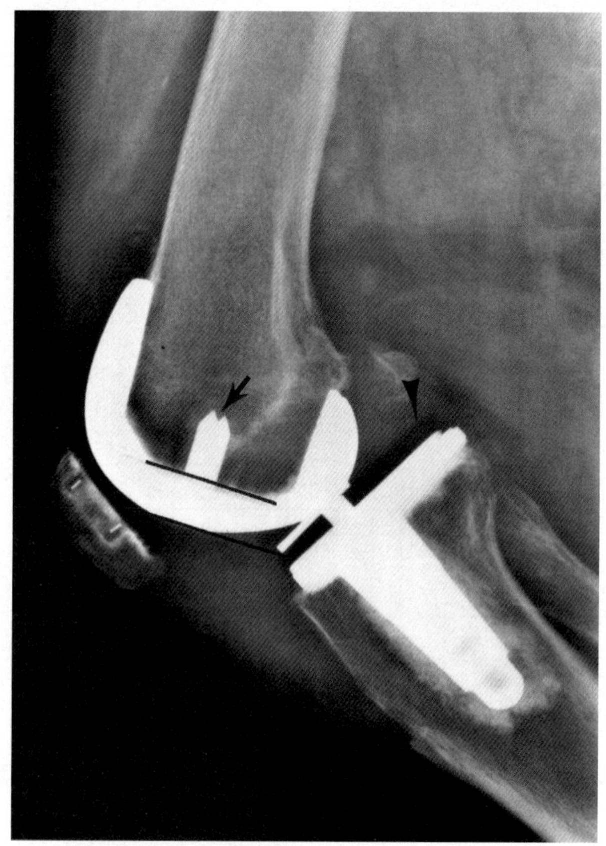

Fig. 6-49 Condylar knee replacement with posterior cruciate ligament (PCL) retention. A: Condylar femoral component with open back (*arrow*) for preservation of the PCL. B: Condylar tibial insert with no central post. C: Lateral radiograph demonstrating a condylar knee replacement. The metal posts (*arrow*) and thickness (*lines*) of the femoral component are characteristic of a condylar knee. Note also the flat polyethylene insert (*arrowhead*) for minimal constraint. (A and B Courtesy of DePuy, a Johnson and Johnson Company, Warsaw, Indiana.)

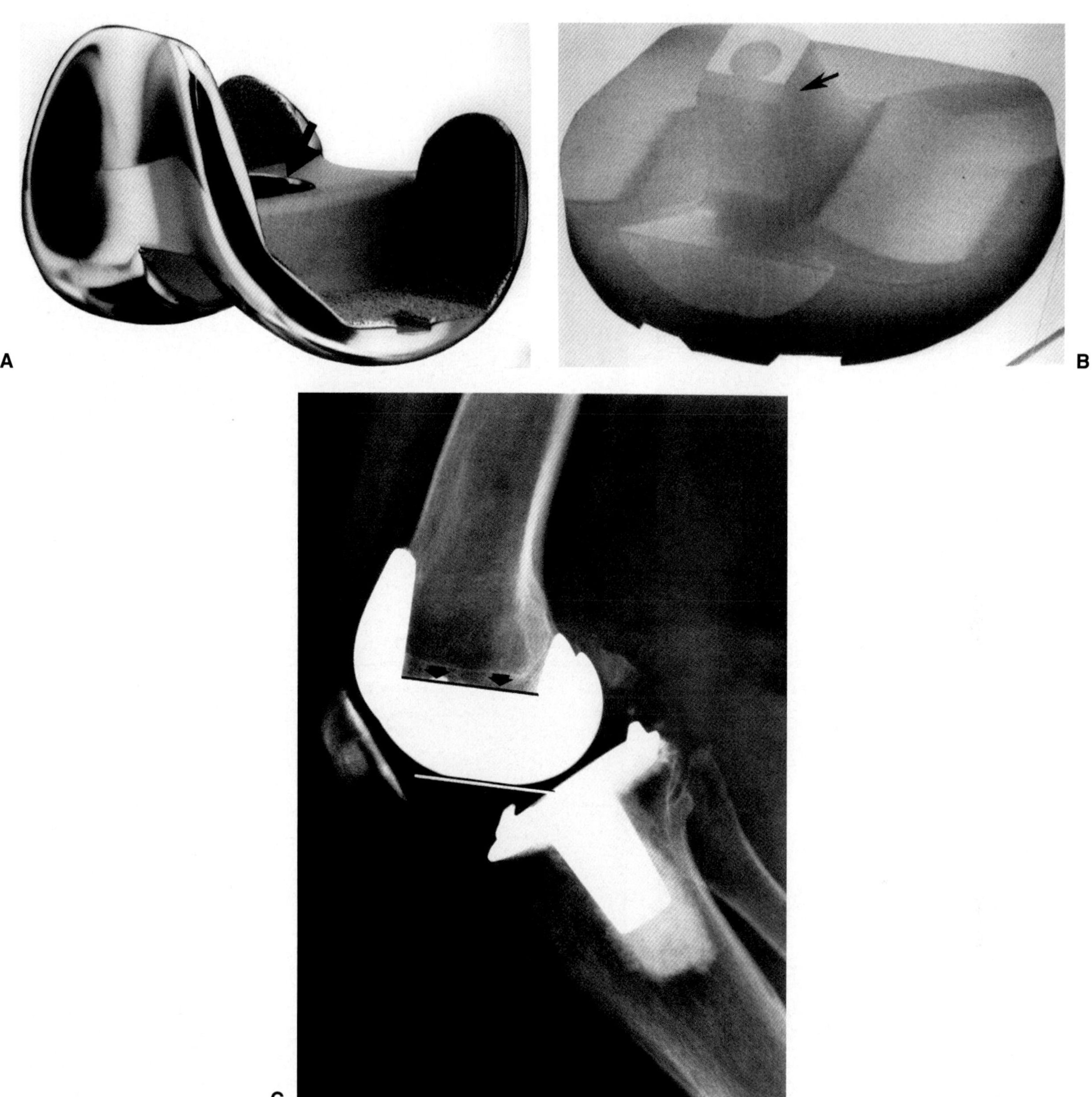


Fig. 6-50 Posterior stabilized knee replacement (posterior cruciate ligament [PCL] resected). A: Posterior stabilized femoral component with central box (*arrow*) for the tibial post. The back is not open as with the condylar design. B: Posterior stabilized tibial insert with a central post (*arrow*) to articulate with the femoral component. C: Lateral radiograph of a posterior stabilized knee replacement. Note the thicker, flat appearance of the femoral component (*arrows* and *lines*) compared to the condylar design (Fig. 6-49). (A and B Courtesy of DePuy, a Johnson and Johnson Company, Warsaw, Indiana.)

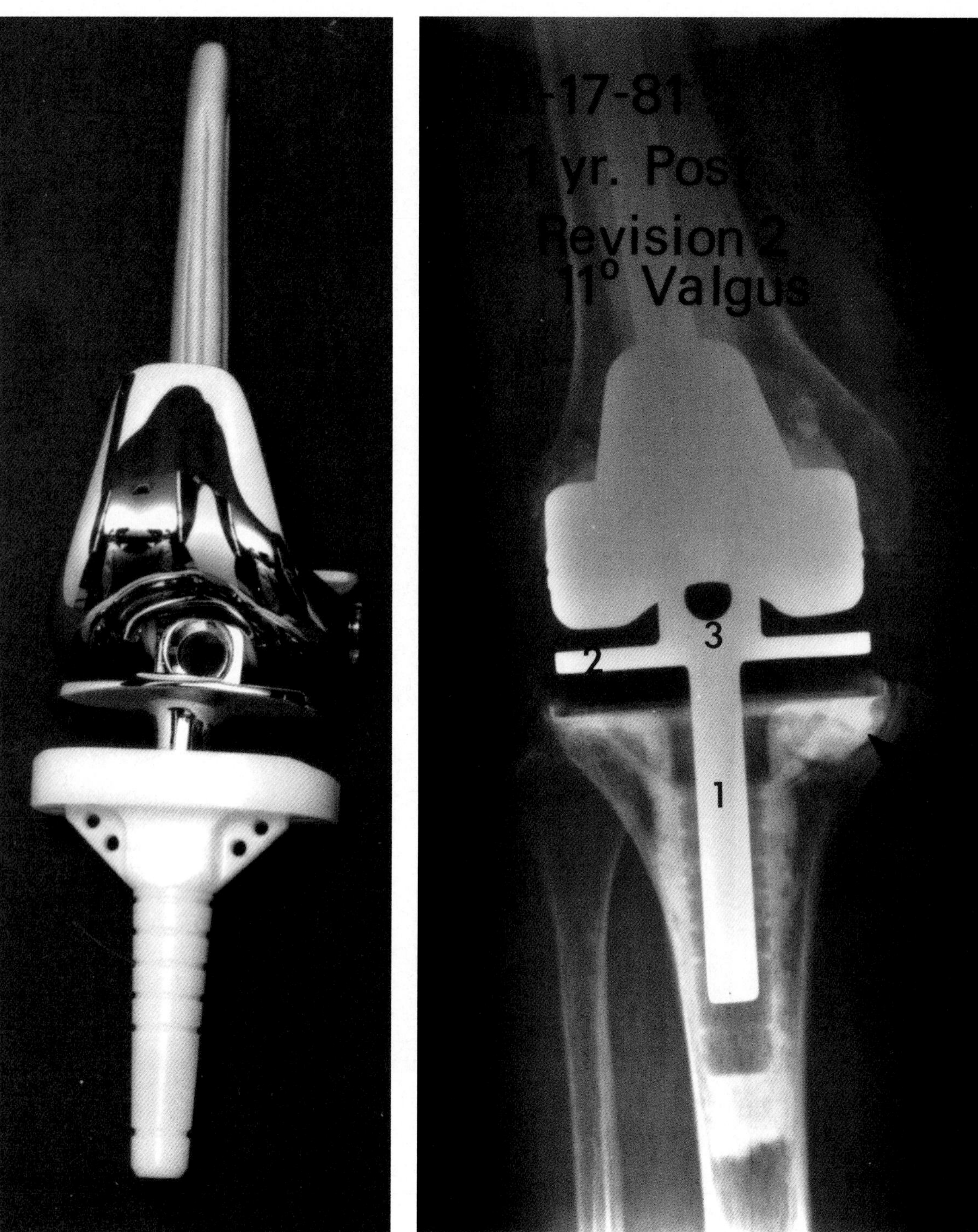


Fig. 6-51 Constrained prosthesis. **A:** Kinematic Rotating hinge knee replacement used primarily for revision. (Courtesy Howmedica, Rutherford, New Jersey.) Anteroposterior (AP) **(A)** and lateral **(B)** radiographs demonstrating a kinematic rotating hinge prosthesis. The tibial component has a large central stem (*1*), an elevated metal tray (*2*), and a posterior metal post with a central hole on the AP view (*3*). There are areas of lucency at the bone–cement interface (*arrowheads*). (From Rand JA, Berquist TH. The Knee. In: Berquist TH, ed. *Imaging of Orthopaedic Trauma and Surgery*. WB Saunders: Philadelphia; 1986:293–391.)

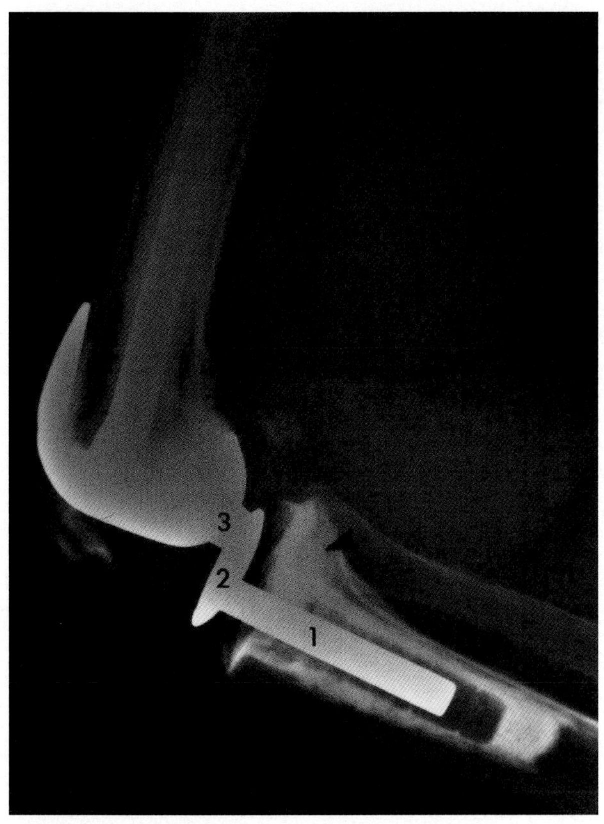


Fig. 6-51 *(Continued)*

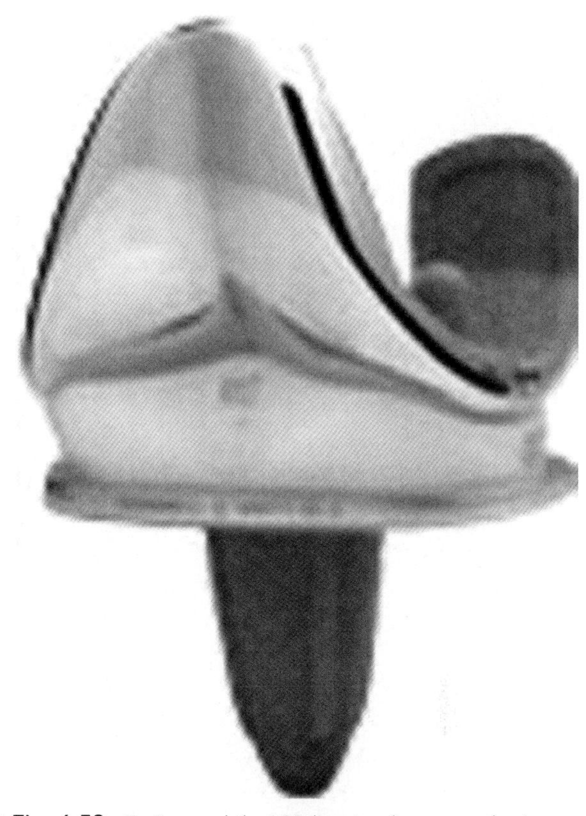

Fig. 6-52 DePuy mobile LCS bearing knee prosthesis. (Courtesy of DePuy, a Johnson and Johnson Company, Warsaw, Indiana.)

Table 6-3

KNEE SOCIETY CLINICAL SCORING SYSTEM

| PARAMETER | POINTS | FUNCTIONAL TASK | POINTS |
|---|---|---|---|
| Pain | | Walking | |
| None | 50 | Unlimited | 50 |
| Moderate | 25 | >10 blocks | 40 |
| Severe | 0 | 5–10 blocks | 20 |
| | | Housebound | 0 |
| Range of motion (maximum 25 points). 5 degrees = 1 point | | Stairs | |
| | | Normal | 50 |
| Stability | | Descend with railing | 15–40 |
| AP <5 mm | 10 | Unable to climb stairs | 0 |
| AP >10 mm | 0 | | |
| Medial–lateral <5 degrees | 15 | | |
| 6–9 degrees | 10 | | |
| 10–14 degrees | 5 | | |
| ≥15 degrees | 0 | | |

AP, anteroposterior.

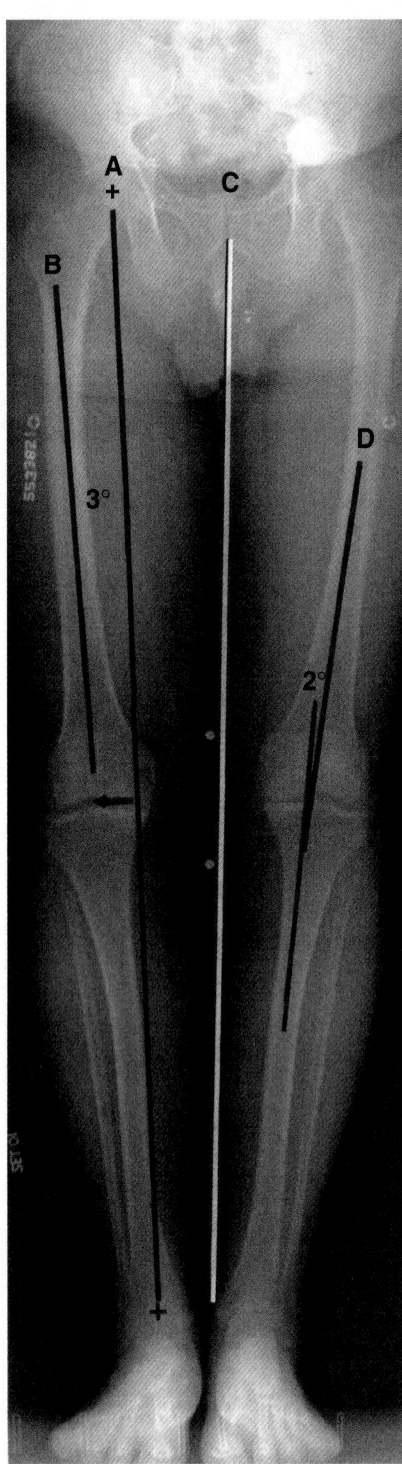


Fig. 6-53 Standing anteroposterior (AP) radiographs with measurements. *A*: Mechanical axis—a line from the center of the femoral head to the center of the ankle mortise should pass through or near the center of the knee. In this case there is medial compartment narrowing and the mechanical axis passes 3 cm medial (*arrow*) to the center of the knee. *B*: Mechanical axis of the femur—normally approximately 6 degrees valgus to the mechanical axis (*A*). In this case it is 3 degrees. *C*: Vertical axis—vertical line from the pubic symphysis. *D*: Femorotibial angle—angle formed by the axis of the femur and tibia, normally 5 to 7 degrees valgus. In this case, it is only 2 degrees.

is a consideration. MRI is also useful to evaluate subchondral bone changes (avascular necrosis [AVN], subchondral fracture) and soft tissue support. CT is useful to evaluate bone stock.

## Suggested Reading

Berquist TH. Imaging of joint replacement procedures. *Radiol Clin North Am.* 2006;44:419–437.

### Treatment Options

Treatment options for knee replacement include unicompartmental (usually medial compartment, uncommonly patellofemoral compartment), bicompartmental with femorotibial replacement, and total knee replacement with patellar resurfacing. The latter is most common. Currently, new minimally invasive (quadriceps sparing) surgical approaches reduce recovery time compared to conventional surgical approaches.

#### Unicompartmental Knee Replacement

Patients with isolated compartment disease may be treated with unicompartment arthroplasty. Isolated compartment arthropathy is less common but occurs in the medial compartment in 25%, patellofemoral compartment in 10%, and lateral compartment in 5% of patients. The medial compartment of the knee is most often replaced (see Fig. 6-54). This is an alternative tibial osteotomy. Medial compartment joint replacements were popular in Europe during the 1970s and 1980s, but decreased in number due to higher failure rates (see Fig. 6-55). New implants, increased experience, and improved results in the late 1990s in the United States generated new interest in this approach (see Fig. 6-56). Also, new minimally invasive surgical techniques allowed medial compartment replacement to reduce postoperative recovery time comparted to medial tibial osteotomy. New data for medial compartment arthroplasty documents 10-year survivals of 94% to 95%. The tibial component may be fixed or mobile bearing. The latter is technically more difficult to insert. The cruciate ligaments are both preserved.

**Indications**

Normal lateral and patellofemoral compartments
Early isolated medial compartment disease
Intact ACL and PCL
Good range of motion
Correctable varus deformity (see Fig. 6-57)

**Contraindications**

Multicompartment disease
Inflammatory polyarthropathies
Young very active patients
Chondrocalcinosis is a relative contraindication

Patellofemoral disorders are common and difficult to treat. In advanced cases patellectomy can be performed, but success rates are only approximately 50%. In recent years, patellofemoral joint replacement procedures have gained in

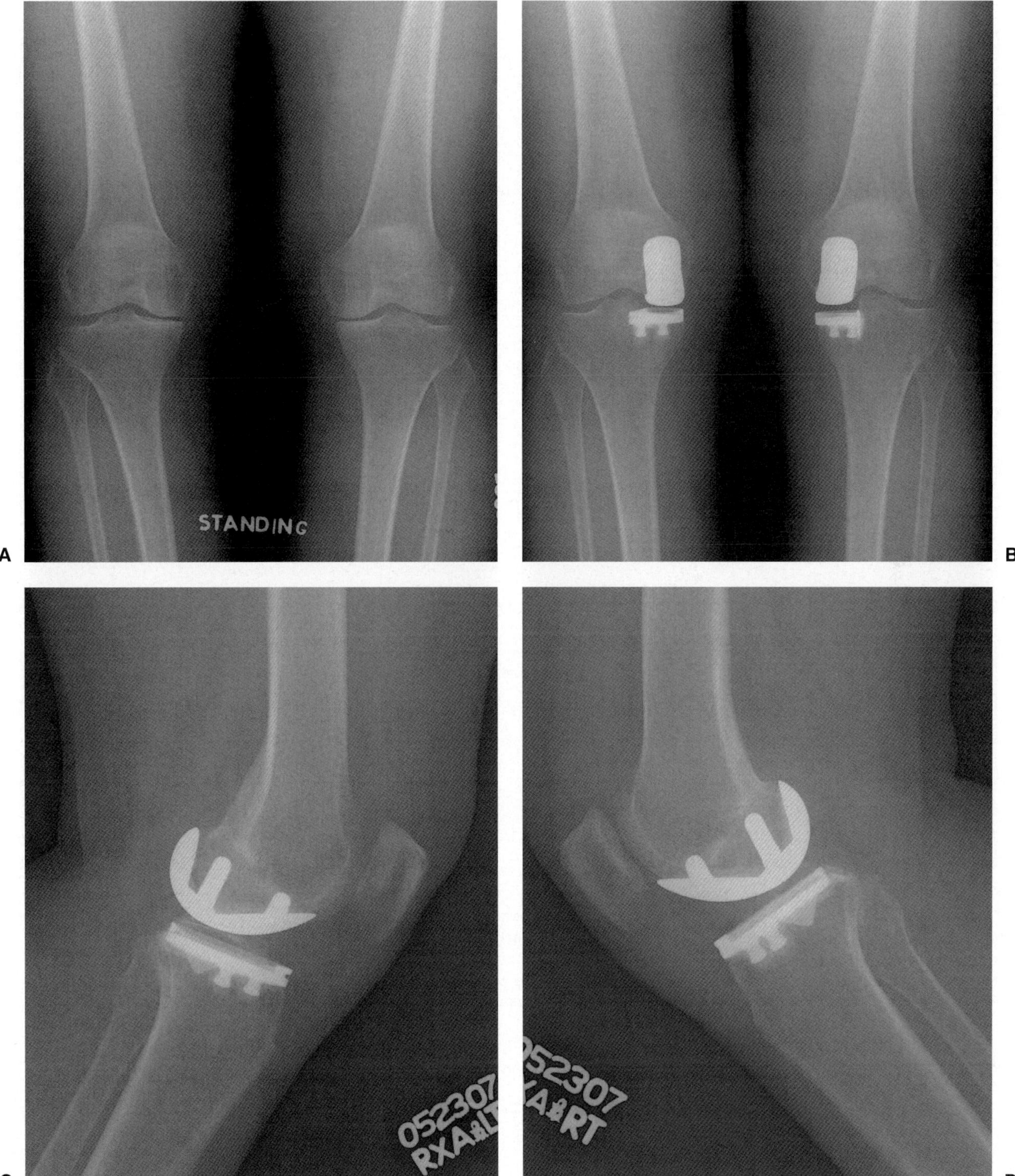


Fig. 6-54 Unicompartmental knee replacement. A: Standing radiographs demonstrate degenerative arthritis with joint space narrowing in both knees in a 50-year-old woman. Standing anteroposterior (AP) (B) and lateral radiographs (C and D) after medial compartment replacements bilaterally.

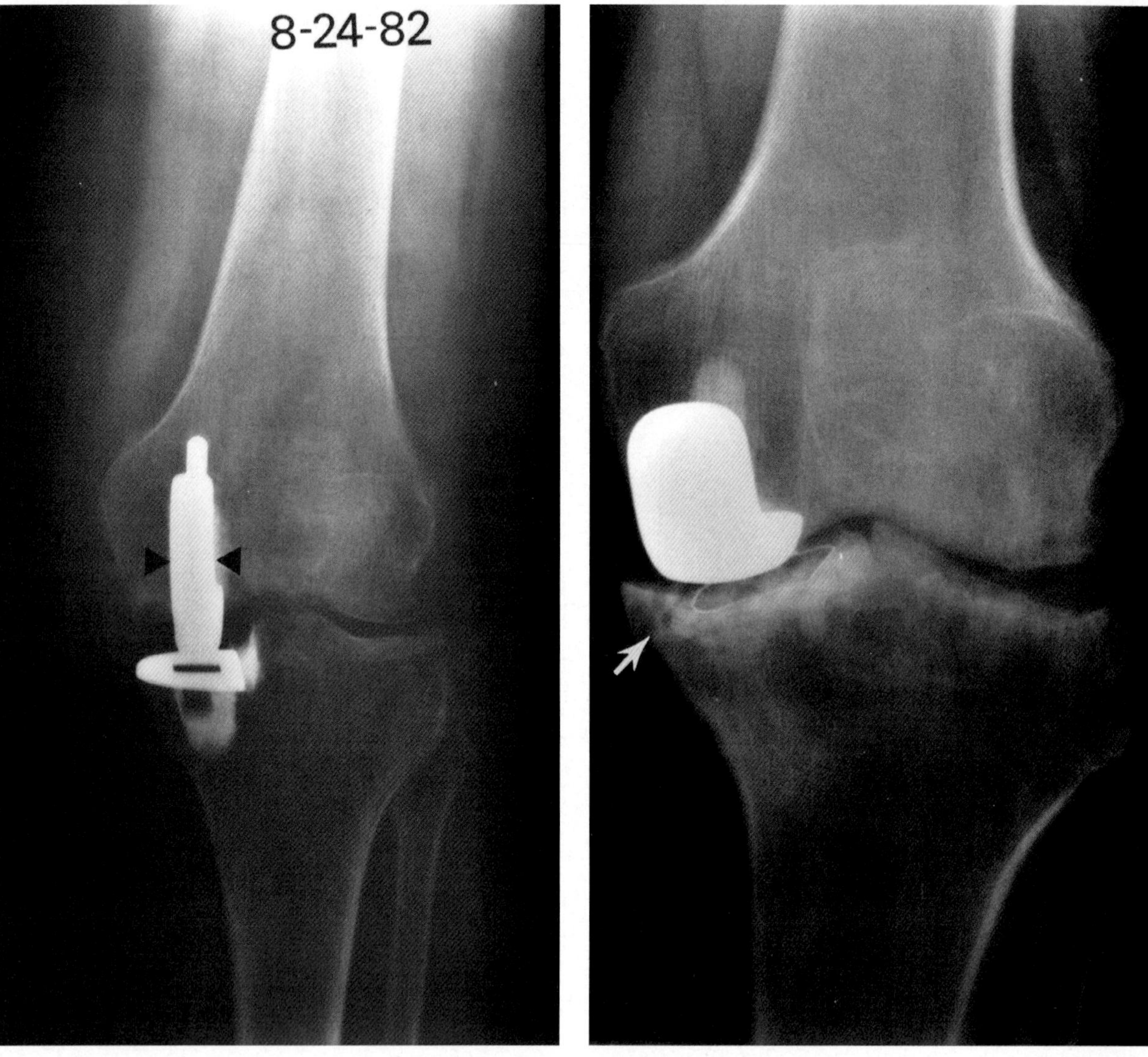


Fig. 6-55 Early unicompartmental implants. A: Anteroposterior (AP) radiograph of the knee in a patient with a polycentric medial compartment arthroplasty. Note the narrow width of the femoral component (*arrowheads*). The tibial component is metal backed. B: AP radiograph of a Marmor medial compartment arthroplasty with polyethylene tibial component, which has subsided and fractured the tibial margin (*arrow*). There is advanced arthropathy in the lateral compartment. Disease progression in the untreated compartments is a common cause for revision surgery.

utility and popularity (see Fig. 6-58). Patients must still be carefully selected. However, success rates have improved and the need to proceed to total knee replacement can be as low as 5% at 5-year follow-up.

## Indications

- Severe signs and symptoms correlating with radiographic features
- Grade III and IV chondromalacia
- Patellofemoral malalignment
- No flexion deformity
- No varus or valgus malalignment
- Essentially normal medial and lateral compartments

## Contraindications

- No attempt at other treatment methods
- Arthritis in the medial and lateral compartments (>grade I Kellgren-Lawrence)
- Systemic inflammatory arthropathy
- Patella infra
- Patellofemoral instability
- Infection

Because joint changes are essential for evaluation of unicompartmental joint replacement and also play a role in total knee replacement the Kellgren-Lawrence system is summarized in Table 6-4.

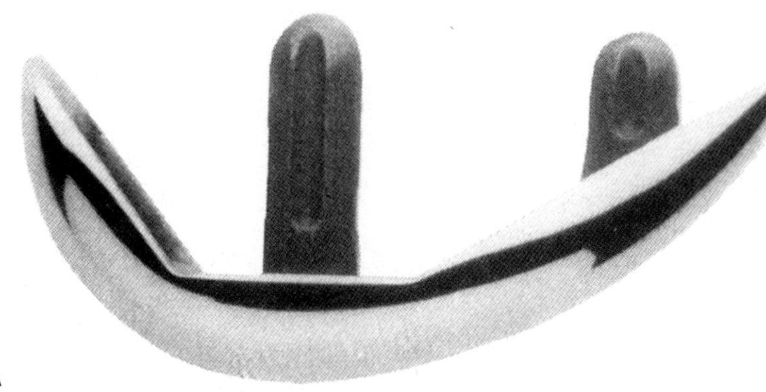

A

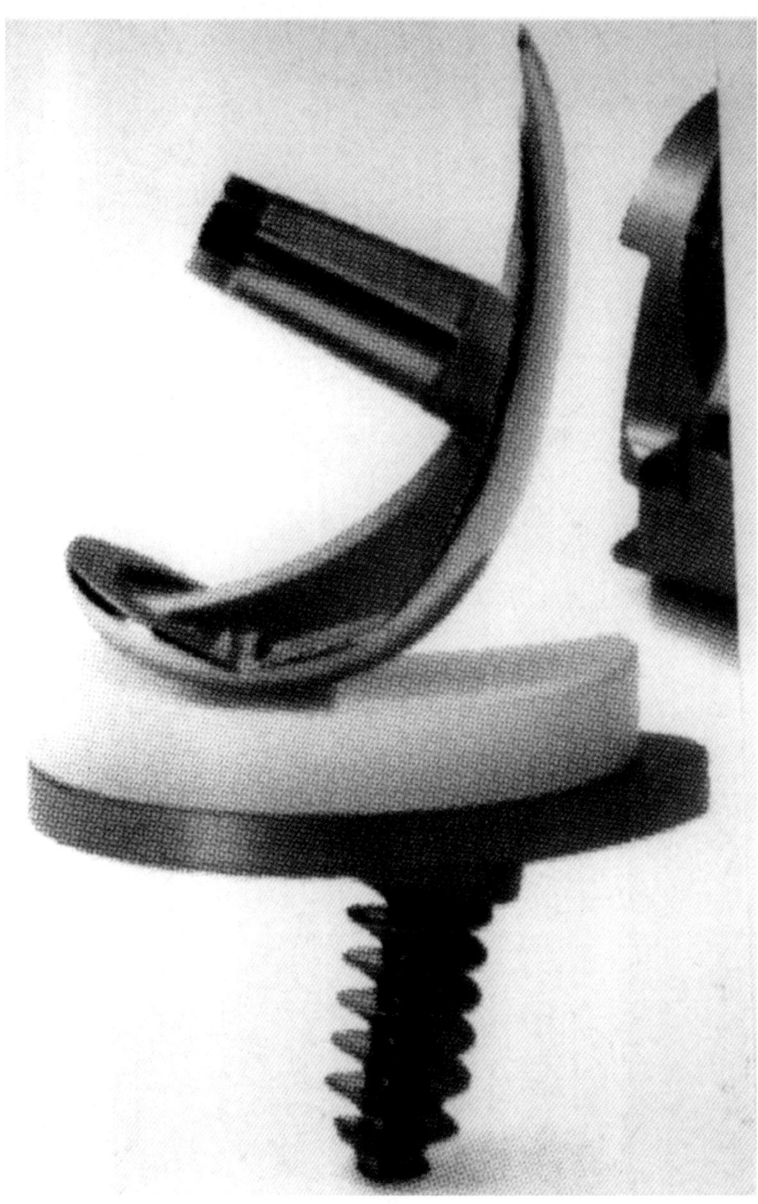

B

Fig. 6-56 Unicompartment implants. A: Zimmer Miller-Galante femoral component (cobalt-chromium-molybdenum alloy) (Courtesy of Zimmer, Warsaw, Indiana). B: Genesis medial compartment implant. (Courtesy of Smith and Nephew Richards, Memphis, Tennessee.)

**Fig. 6-57** Standing anteroposterior (AP) radiograph in a patient with isolated medial compartment narrowing and 6 degrees varus deformity.

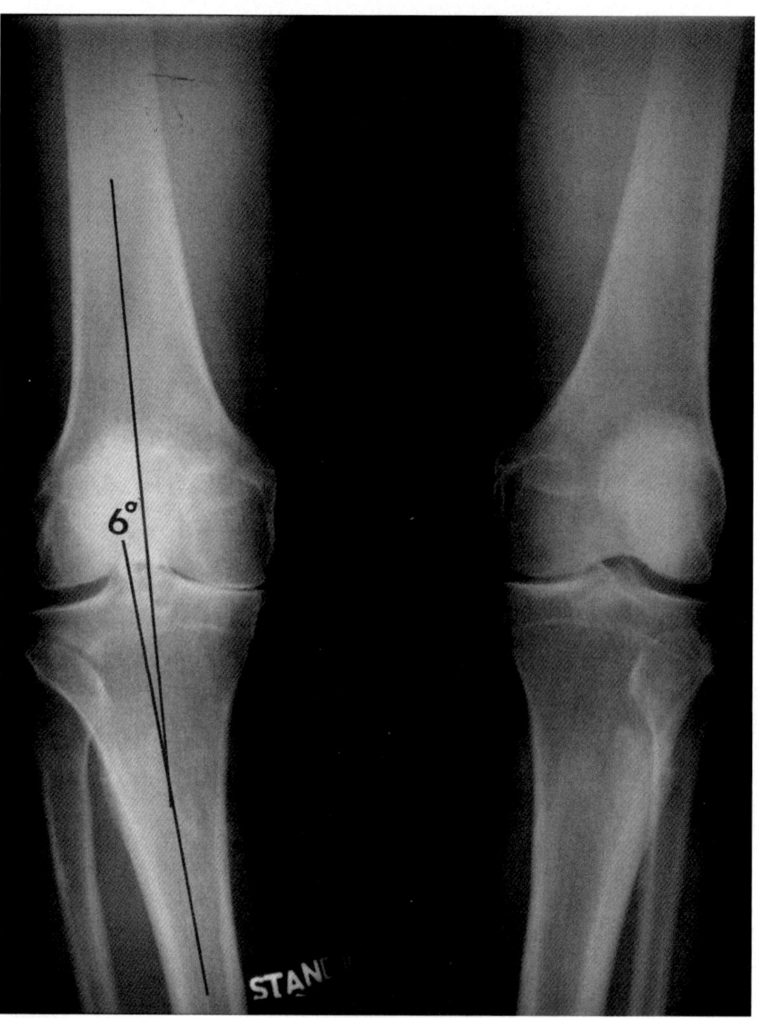


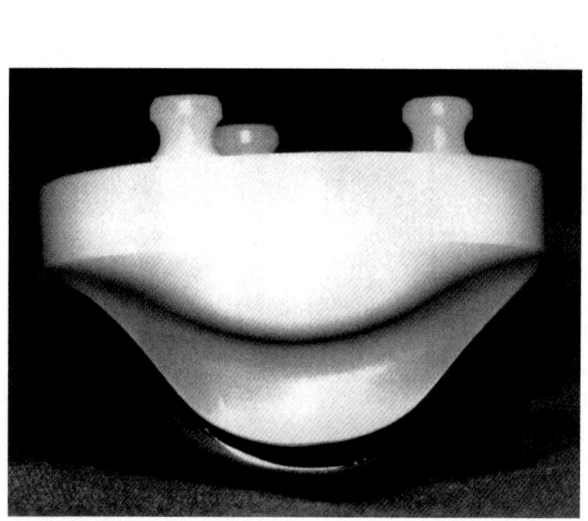
A

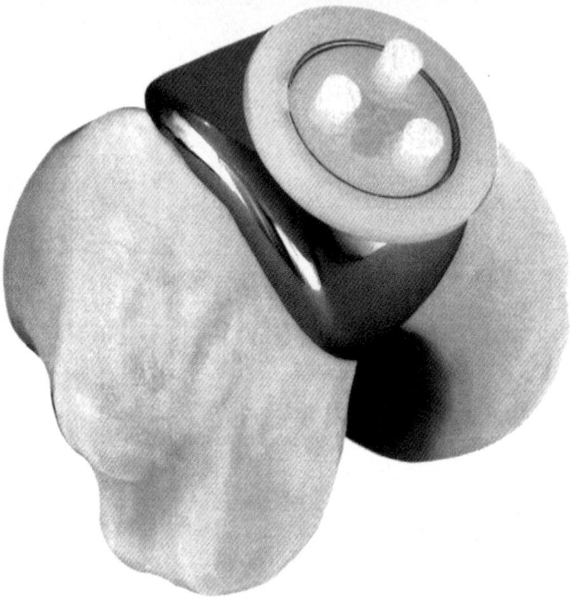
B

**Fig. 6-58** Patellofemoral implants. **A:** Natural-Knee II system (Courtesy of Zimmer, Warsaw, Indiana). **B:** KineMatch implant (Courtesy of Kinamed, Camarillo, California). Anteroposterior (AP) (**C**), lateral (**D**), and Merchant (**E**) views of the knee in a patient with a unicompartmental patellofemoral arthroplasty and bilateral patellar tendon transfers.

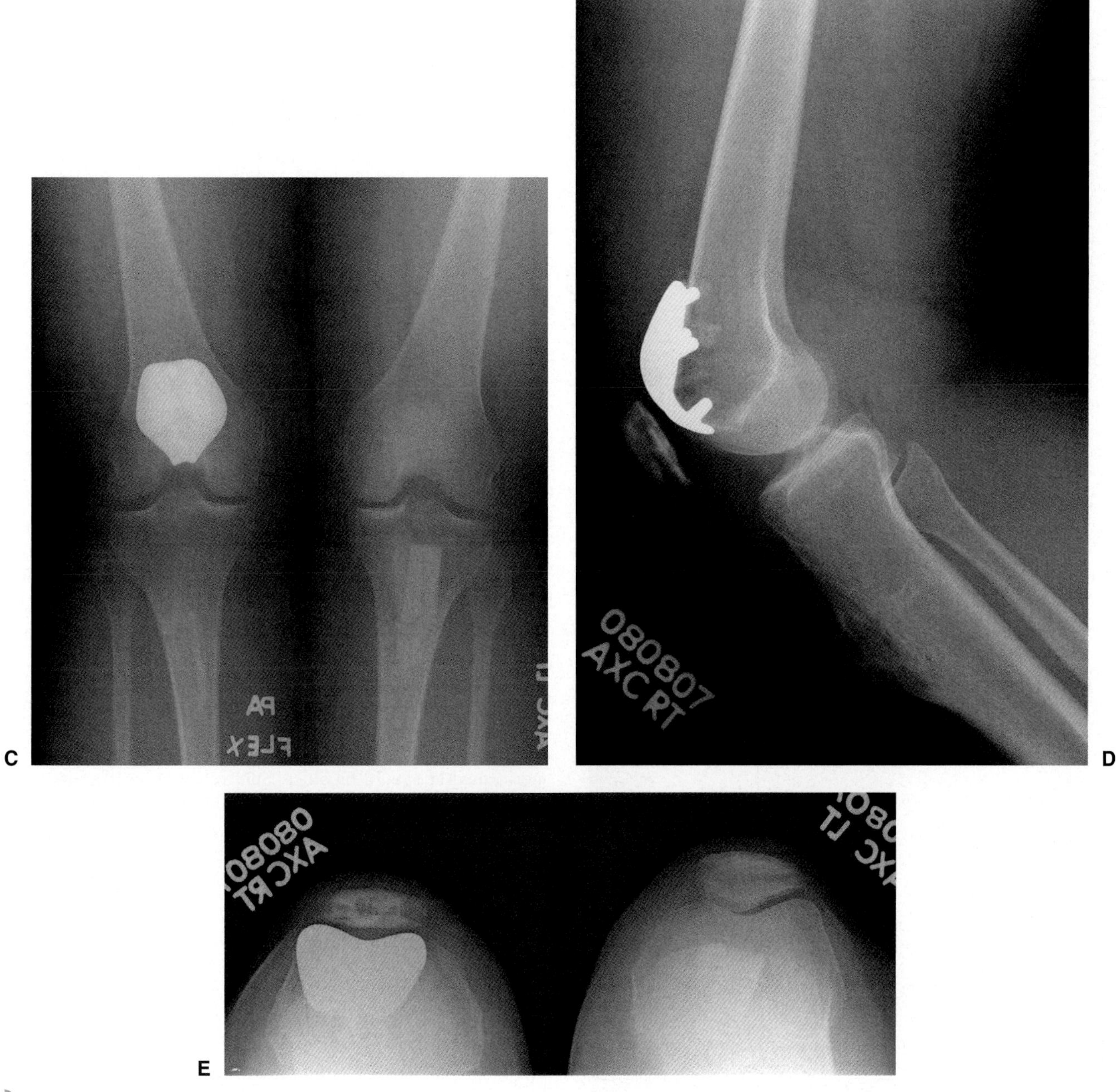


Fig. 6-58 *(Continued)*

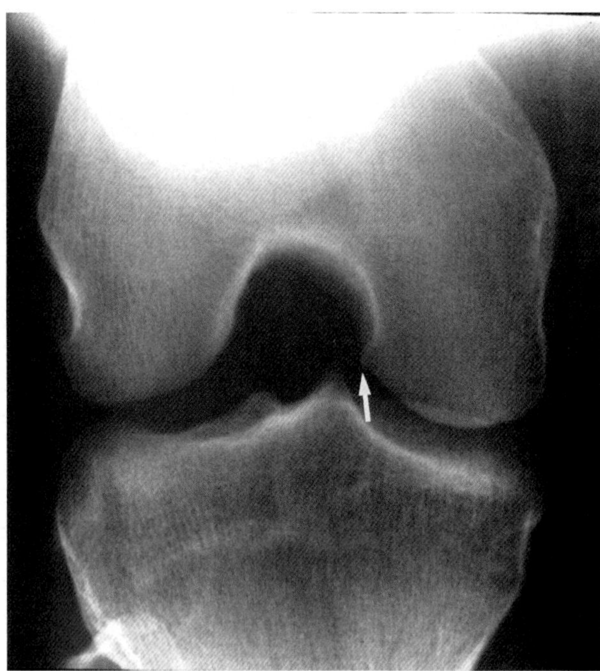

Fig. 6-59 Kellgren-Lawrence grade I. Notch view demonstrating a minimal osteophyte (*arrow*). The joint spaces were preserved.

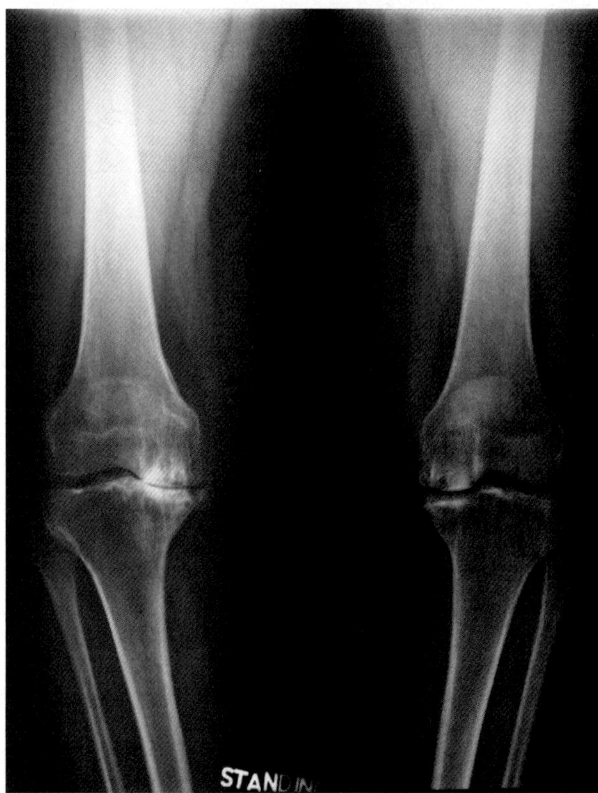


Fig. 6-60 Kellgren-Lawrence grade III on the left and IV on the right demonstrated on standing anteroposterior (AP) radiographs. On the left, there is joint space narrowing with marginal osteophytes and subchondral sclerosis. On the right, changes are more advanced with more bone sclerosis and subchondral cysts.

**Table 6-4**

KELLGREN-LAWRENCE CLASSIFICATION FOR OSTEOARTHRITIS

| GRADE | RADIOGRAPHIC FEATURES |
|---|---|
| 0 | Normal |
| I | No narrowing, minimal osteophytes (Fig. 6-59) |
| II | Definite osteophytes with minimal or no joint space narrowing |
| III | Definite narrowing, multiple moderate osteophytes, bone sclerosis, mild contour abnormalities (Fig. 6-60) |
| IV | Marked narrowing, large osteophytes, bone sclerosis, and deformities |

### Total Knee Replacement

Although tibial and femoral implants can be used alone, currently, most surgeons prefer total replacement with patellar resurfacing. The incidence of reoperation for anterior pain is reduced when patellar resurfacing is performed with the initial procedure. Survival rates for total knee replacement vary slightly with the type of implant and patient factors, such as weight, activity level, and systemic factors. However, implant survival rates are excellent, especially if the initial procedure is performed after 65 or 70 years of age. Survival was 83% at 10 years if performed at 55 years of age or less and 94% if performed at age 70 or older. Survival rates at 10 years were 90% for patients with osteoarthritis and 95% for patients with inflammatory arthritis. Patients with condylar (PCL retained) implants had component survival rates of 91% compared to 76% for posterior stabilized (PCL resected) implants. Cemented components survived in 92% at 10 years compared to only 61% for uncemented implants.

## Suggested Reading


Ackroyd CE. Medial compartment arthroplasty of the knee. *J Bone Joint Surg*. 2003;85B:937–942.

Ackroyd CE. Development and early results of a new patellofemoral arthroplasty. *Clin Orthop*. 2005;436:7–13.

Berger RA, Meneghini RM, Jacobs JJ, et al. Results of unicompartmental knee arthroplasty at a minimum of ten years of follow-up. *J Bone Joint Surg*. 2005;87A:999–1006.

Furnes O, Espehaug B, Lie SA, et al. Failure mechanisms after unicompartmental and tricompartmental primary knee replacement with cement. *J Bone Joint Surg*. 2007;89A: 519–525.

King J, Stamper DL, Schaad DC, et al. Minimally invasive total knee arthroplasty compared with traditional knee arthroplasty. *J Bone Joint Surg*. 2007;89A:1497–1503.

Leadbetter WB, Seyler TM, Ragland PS, et al. Indications, contraindications and pitfalls of patellofemoral arthroplasty. *J Bone Joint Surg*. 2006;88A:122–137.

Pakos EE, Ntzani EE, Trikalinos TA. Patellar resurfacing in total knee arthroplasty. A meta-analysis. *J Bone Joint Surg.* 2005;87A:1438–1476.

Rand JA, Troudale RT, Ilsrup DM, et al. Factors affecting the durability of primary total knee prostheses. *J Bone Joint Surg.* 2003;85A:259–265.

Wood DJ, Smith AJ, Collopy D, et al. Patellar resurfacing in total knee arthroplasty. *J Bone Joint Surg.* 2002;84A:187–193.

## Postoperative Imaging

Radiographs should be obtained immediately following surgery to evaluate component position and exclude obvious problems such as periprosthetic fractures. When the patient can tolerate a full radiographic evaluation AP, lateral, Merchant, and full length standing views are obtained, which can be compared with preoperative images. In the ideal situation, a fluoroscopically positioned series should be obtained to assure optimal alignment of the component interfaces (see Fig. 6-61). Each image will be described separately.

### Standing Anteroposterior View

The full-length standing AP radiograph (see Fig. 6-62A) is evaluated and compared to the preoperative image. The mechanical axis, femoral axis, femorotibial angles, and vertical axis are measured. The femorotibial angle should be 5 to 7 degrees valgus (Fig. 6-62A). The tibial tray should be at 90 degrees (±5 degrees) to the shaft with coverage of the bony surface (Fig. 6-62B). Overhang of the tray laterally is acceptable, but medial overhang may cause pes anserine bursitis. If the tibial tray is angled more than 95 degrees it is considered in valgus position and if <85 degrees in varus position. The angle of the femoral component to the femoral shaft should be 97 to 98 degrees (Fig. 6-62B). When evaluating lucent lines or osteolysis, the AP image is divided into zones similar to those used in the hip (Fig. 6-62C). The zones were formulated by the Knee Society.

### Lateral View

The angle of the tibial tray to the shaft on the lateral radiograph should also be 90 degrees. Slight variation is acceptable. When the component is angled at >90 degrees it is considered in extension and when <90 degrees it is in flexion. The femoral component should also be at 90 degrees to the femoral shaft. The patella should be 9 to 10 mm above the anterior margin of the tibial component (see Fig. 6-63A). The zones for the femoral and tibial component are also used on the lateral view. Zones 1 and 2 are reserved for the anterior flange and 3 and 4 for the posterior. The central stem or central area is zone 5 to 7 similar to the tibial component on the AP view. The tibial

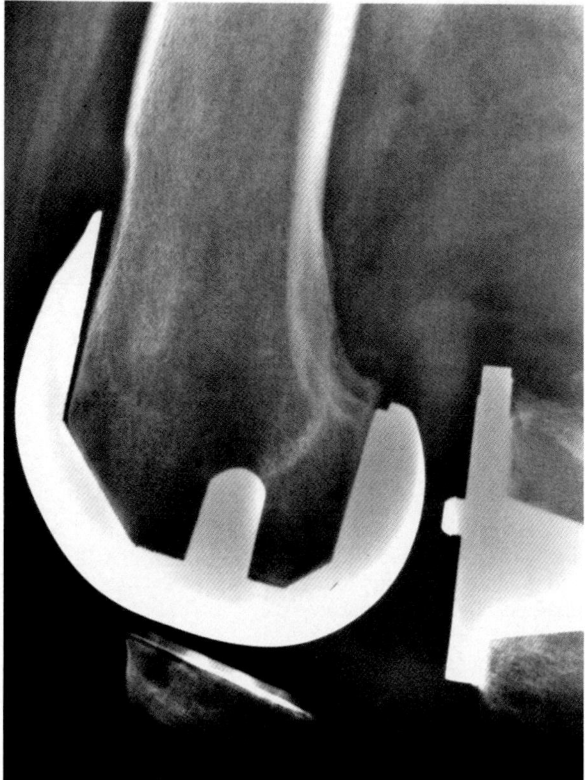


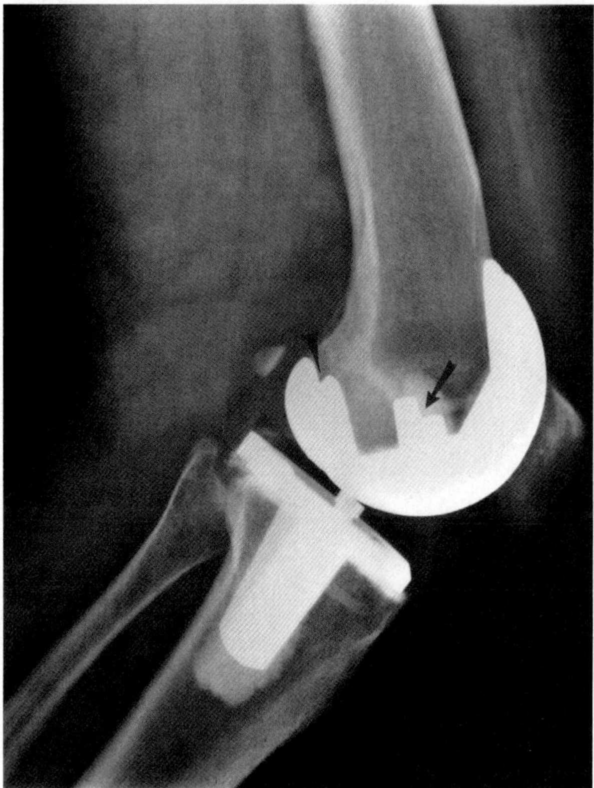


**Fig. 6-61** A: Fluoroscopically positioned lateral image in flexion clearly demonstrates the component interfaces with the patella, femur, and tibia. B: Conventionally positioned lateral with rotation of the femoral components showing overlap of the femoral component pegs (*arrow*) and condylar components (*arrowhead*). The tibial component interface is not well demonstrated and the patellar interface is not seen.

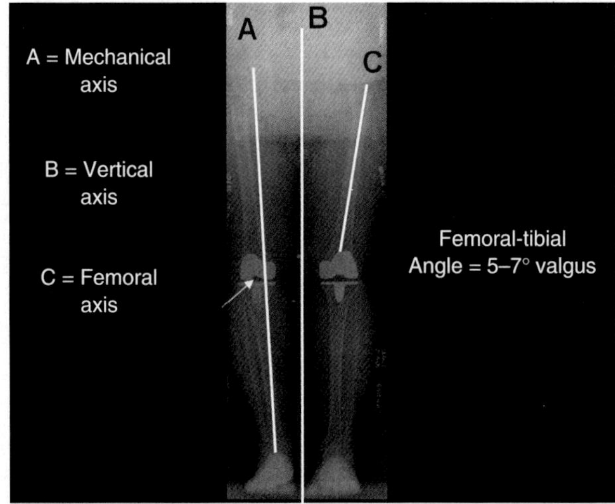


A

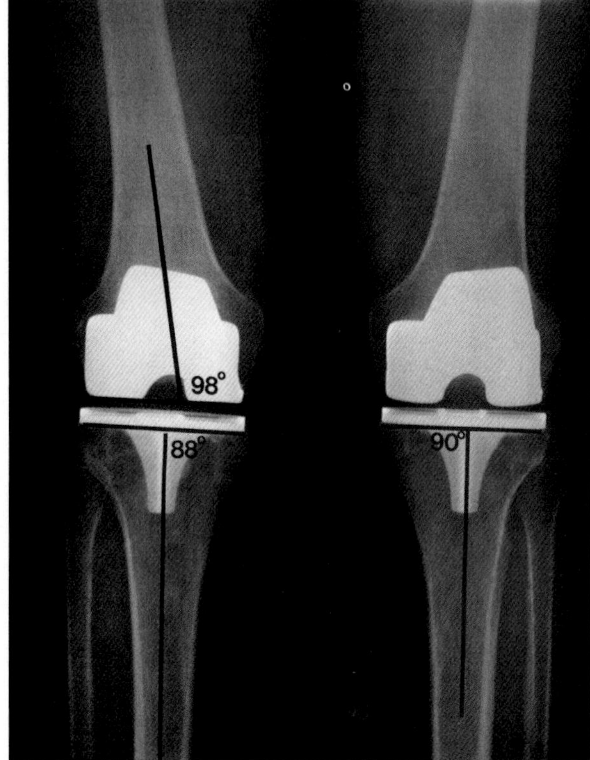


B

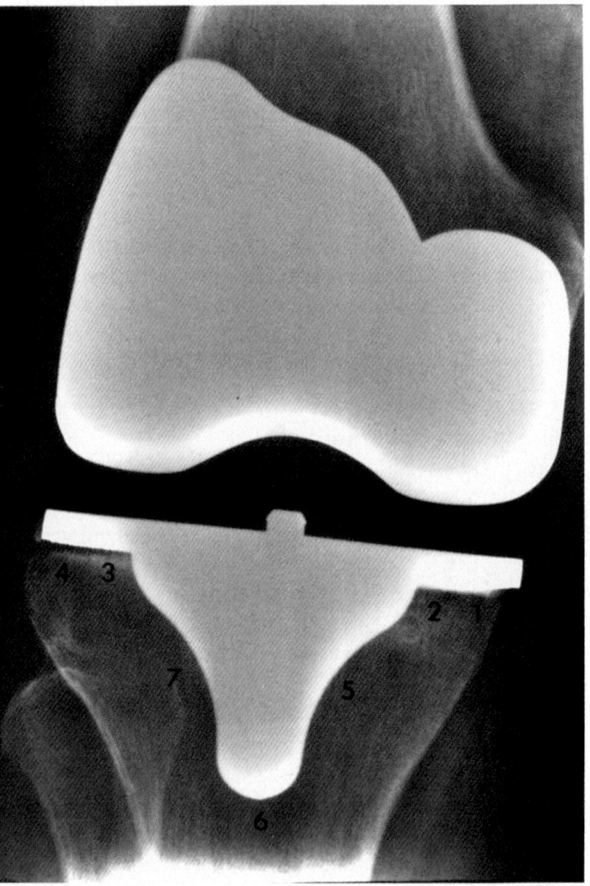


C

**Fig. 6-62** A: Full length standing anteroposterior (AP) radiograph following knee replacements. The mechanical axis on the right (*arrow*) is still slightly medially displaced. B: Standing AP radiograph demonstrating the position of the tibial tray in relation to the shaft. This should be at 90 degrees. The femoral angle should be approximately 98 degrees to the femoral shaft. The polyethylene spacers should provide symmetrical medial and lateral compartments although spacer width may vary from left to right. The tibial tray should cover the bony surface. Slight overhang laterally is acceptable. Medial overhang may result in pes anserine bursitis. C: Zones derived by the Knee Society with zones *1* and *2* for the medial plateau, *3* and *4* for the lateral plateau, and *5* to *7* reserved for the stem regardless of the length. If there are no stems the central zone is broken down in zone *5* to *7*. Zone *5* is medial and zone *7* is lateral. In this case there is lucency at the bone–cement interface in zones *3* and *4*.

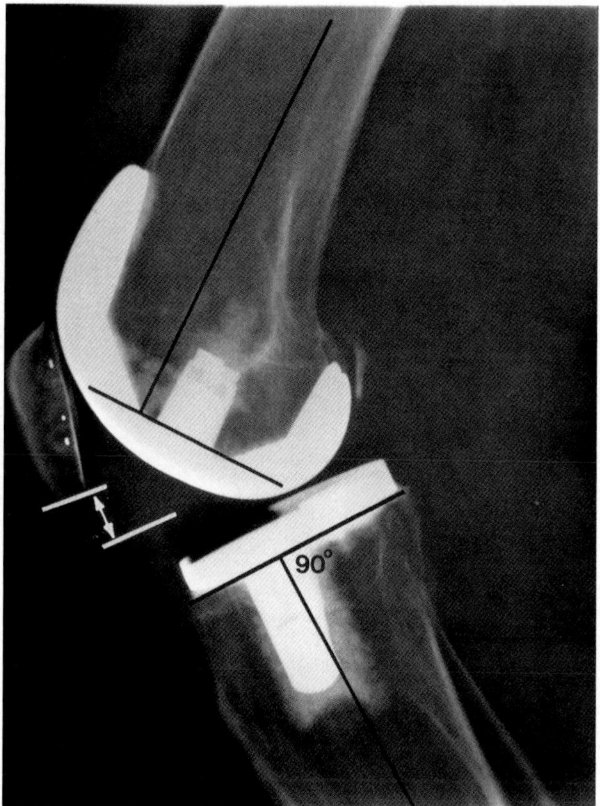


A

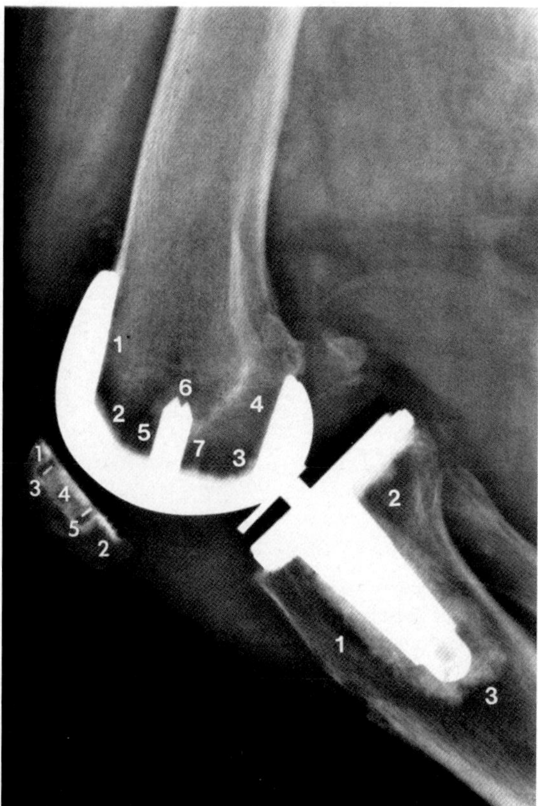


B

Fig. 6-63 A: Lateral radiograph demonstrating the normal angles of the tibial tray and femoral component with the tibial and fibular shafts. Both should be approximately 90 degrees. The patella should be approximately 9 to 10 mm above the anterior margin of the tibial tray (*white lines*). B: Lateral radiograph demonstrating the zones of the tibial and femoral components. The patellar component is numbered as well and varies with the number of fixation lugs.

component on the lateral view has three zones with 1 anterior, 2 posterior, and 3 for the stem or central zone if there is no stem (Fig. 6-63B).

## Merchant View

The patellar component is evaluated on the lateral (Fig. 6-63) and Merchant views. The patellar component should be centered over the femoral trochlea on the Merchant view and the surfaces should be parallel. Patellar tilt may indicate extensor mechanism imbalance, which can lead to failure. The interface with the native patella should be evaluated for lucent lines. Zones are also used on this view with zone 1 reserved for the medial side, 2 for the lateral side, and 3 to 5 vary depending on the number of fixation lugs (see Fig. 6-64).

## Computed Tomography

CT is not only a valuable tool for evaluating complications but is also useful for evaluating component rotation on the femur or tibia, which can lead to pain and patellar tracking disorders. Axial CT images (see Fig. 6-65) at the transepicondylar axis of the

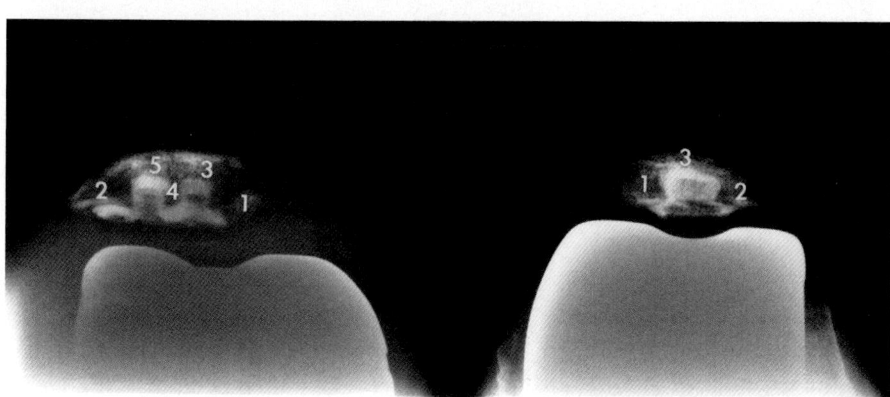


Fig. 6-64 Merchant views with one fixation lug on the right (zones *1* to *3*) and two lugs on the left with zones *1* to *5*. The right patella is centered over the trochlea. The left patella is subluxed laterally.

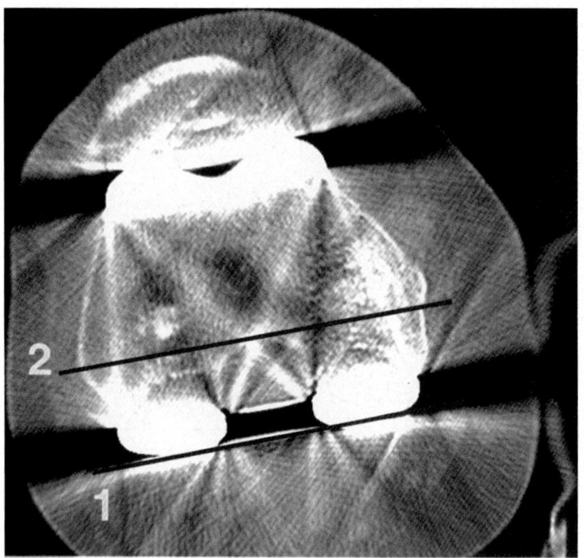


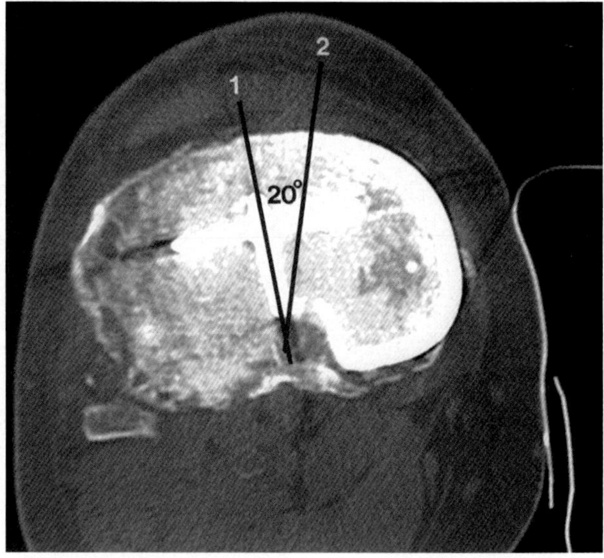


**Fig. 6-65** Computed tomographic (CT) images for component position and rotation in the axial plane. **A:** Femoral rotation is measured by a line along the posterior component margins (*1*) and a second line from the lateral condylar eminence and the medial sulcus of the medial epicondyle (*2*). The lines are parallel indicating no rotation. **B:** Axial image through the tibial component with line (*1*) through the center of the component and line (*2*) transposed from the tuberosity forming an 20 degrees, which is within normal limits (18 degrees ± 2.6).

femoral component and tibial tray–osseous interface are used to evaluate component rotation and associated patellofemoral complications. CT scans are obtained with the knee extended and axial images are obtained perpendicular to the mechanical axis (Fig. 6-53). Images are obtained at four levels: epicondyle of the femur, tibial component, tibial plateau, and tibial tuberosity. In the femur, a line is drawn along the femoral prosthesis posteriorly and a second line is drawn connecting the lateral epicondylar prominence and medial sulcus of the medial condyle (Fig. 6-65A). The tibial component is evaluated by determining the geometric center of the plateau and transposing the position of the tibial tuberosity. The angle formed indicates the degree of internal rotation (Fig. 6-65B). The normal relationship is 18 degrees ± 2.6. When the combined femoral and tibial angles exceed normal by up to 4 degrees, there is associated patellar tilt and lateral tracking. Moderate increases (3 to 8 degrees) correlated with patellar subluxation and larger degrees of internal rotation of the components (7 to 17 degrees)

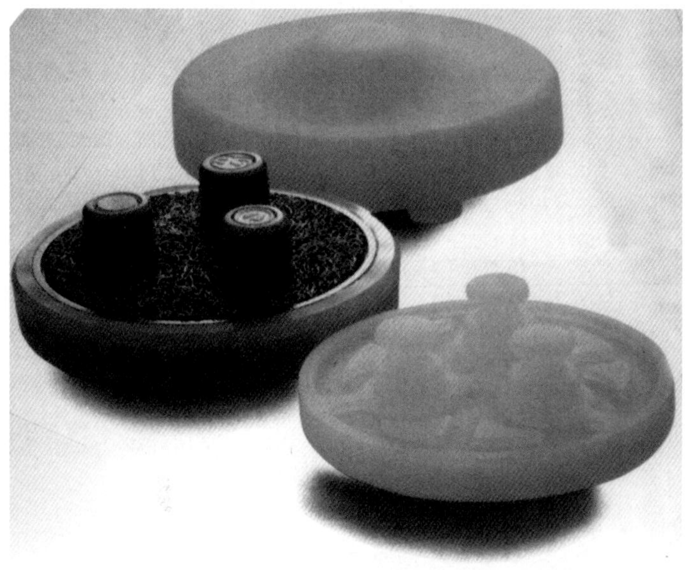


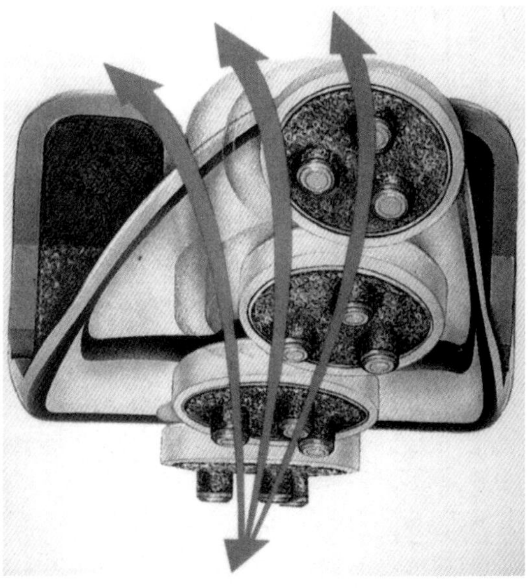


**Fig. 6-66** Patellar components. **A:** Illustration of mesh metal-backed and all polyethylene patellar components. **B:** Illustration of normal patellar tracking. (Courtesy of Zimmer, Warsaw, Indiana.)

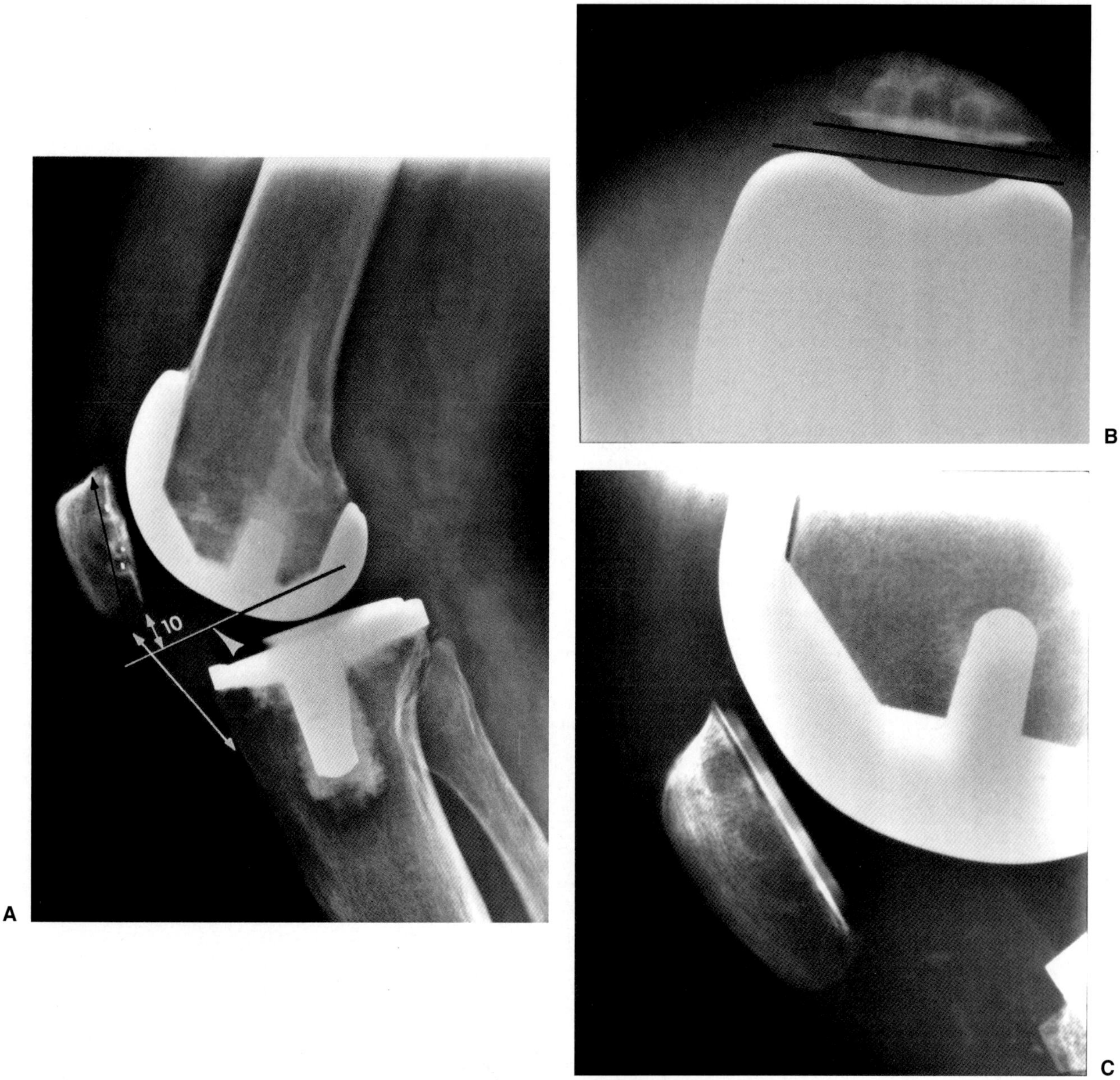

B

10

A

C

Fig. 6-67 Normal patellar position: A: Lateral radiograph demonstrating the normal position at 10 mm above the anterior tibial implant margin or patellar height (*black* and *white double arrows*) essentially the same as the patellar tendon with the knee flexed 30 degrees. B: Merchant view demonstrating the polyethylene patellar component symmetrically positioned in the trochlea of the femoral component with no significant patellar tilt (*lines*). C: Fluoroscopically positioned lateral of the patella component interface.

Fig. 6-68 Patellar tilt and abutment. Merchant views of the knee demonstrating patellar tilt and early lateral osseous changes (*arrow*) due to abutment and extensor mechanism imbalance.

correlated with early patellar dislocation and patellar component failure.

## Suggested Reading


Anouchi YS, Whiteside LA, Kaiser AD, et al. The effects of axial rotational alignment of the femoral component on knee stability and patellar tracking in total knee arthroplasty demonstrated on autopsy specimens. *Clin Orthop*. 1993;287: 170–177.

Berger RA, Rubash HE, Seel MJ, et al. Determining rotational alignment of the femoral component in total knee arthroplasty using the epicondylar axis. *Clin Orthop*. 1992;286:40–47.

Berquist TH. Imaging of joint replacements. *Radiol Clin North Am*. 2006;44:419–437.

Ewald FC. The Knee Society total knee arthroplasty roentgen evaluation and scoring system. *Clin Orthop*. 1989;248:9–12.

Math KR, Zaidi SF, Petchprapa C, et al. Imaging of total knee arthroplasty. *Semin Musculoskelet Radiol*. 2006;10:47–63.


### Imaging of Postoperative Complications

Complications following knee replacement may be related to the procedure, component selection, and patient compliance. Extensor mechanism problems are among the most common complications, followed by loosening, infection, osteolysis, and instability. Heterotopic ossification is less common compared to hip replacement and this is usually not symptomatic in the knee.

**EXTENSOR MECHANISM** Extensor mechanism problems occur in 4% to 41% of knee replacements and they are the most common cause for knee revision. Multiple problems can occur related to soft tissue support (extensor mechanism imbalance), patellar tracking, subluxation, dislocation, implant loosening, anterior knee pain, and gait disturbances. As noted earlier, the rotational alignment of the components is important for appropriate patellar tracking. Studies have demonstrated that excessive internal rotation of the components effects knee stability and patellar tracking most significantly. Problems are reduced with neutral position (Fig. 6-65) and tracking is improved when the femoral component is slightly externally rotated ($\leq$5 degrees).

Most problems can be detected on serial radiographs (see Figs. 6-66 to 6-70), (see also Fig. 6-12). Patellar tracking can be evaluated with Merchant views in different degrees of flexion and extension and with CT (Fig. 6-70) to evaluate component rotation.

**COMPONENT LOOSENING** Component loosening occurs in 2% to 5% of patients. As noted earlier, the Knee Society has described zones that can be used for component changes. Ideally, at least the baseline study following surgery should be fluoroscopically

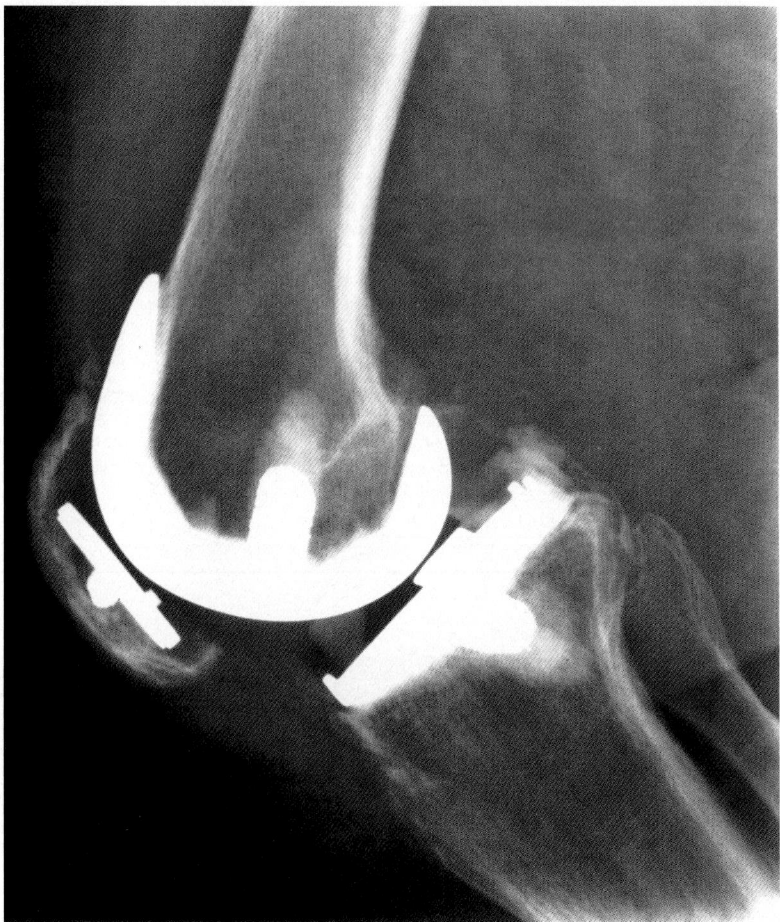

Fig. 6-69 Lateral radiograph demonstrating gross loosening and fragmentation of the metal backed patellar component.

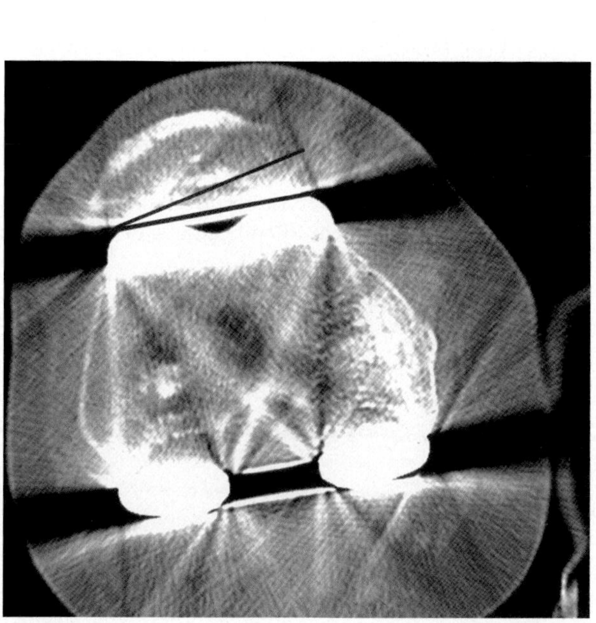

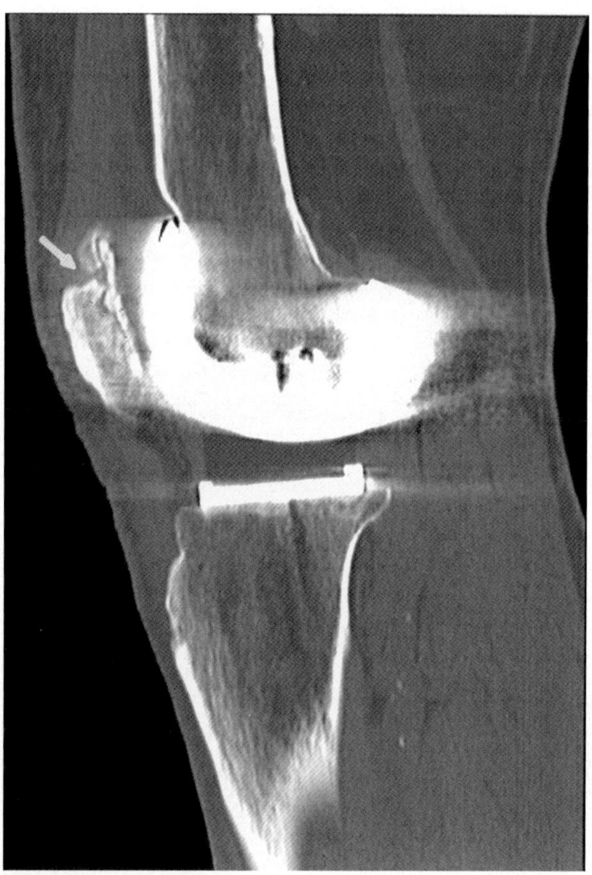

Fig. 6-70 Patellar tracking disorder. Computed tomographic (CT) images in the axial (A) and sagittal (B) planes demonstrate patellar tilt (*lines*) and subluxation with subtle loosening and fragmentation (*arrow*) of the patella on the sagittal image (B).

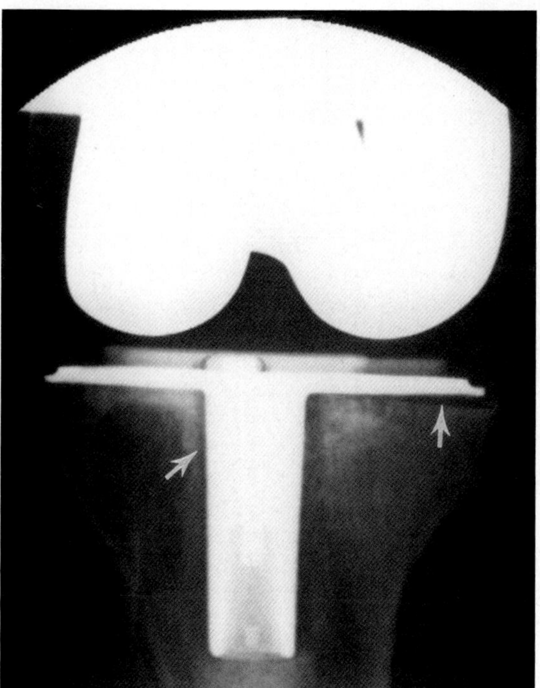

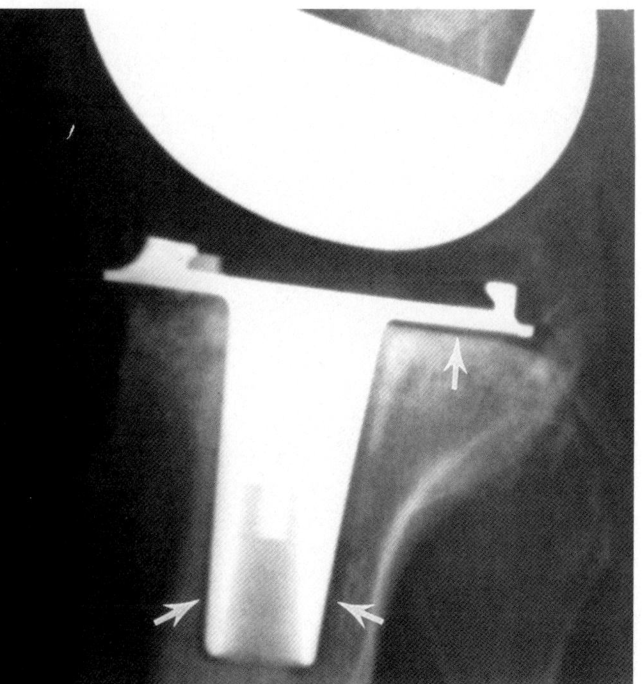

Fig. 6-71 Loose tibial component. Fluoroscopically positioned anteroposterior (AP) (A) and lateral (B) images demonstrate lucency about the tibial tray and stem (*arrows*) due to loosening.

positioned. Following this evaluation, conventional radiographs may be adequate, but fluoroscopic positioning should be considered in subtle cases. The main signs of loosening are lucent lines >2 mm at the bone–cement interface of cemented components or any lucency about uncemented components and change in component position. Keep in mind that normally slight lucency can be identified 1 to 2 years after implantation due to stress shielding. This is more common with hip implants and knee revision implants. Lucency and loosening should not be used interchangeably in radiology reports because slight lucency (≤2 mm) may be totally asymptomatic.

Serial radiographs or fluoroscopically positioned images are usually diagnostic. Progression of lucent zones or migration on serial images increases the confidence that the component is loose (see Figs. 6-71 and 6-72). Tibial components tend to loosen more commonly than the femoral component. Also, significant loosening may be associated with infection.

INFECTION Superficial or wound infections and deep infections may both occur. Superficial infections usually occur in the immediate postoperative period. Deep infection is a devastating complication. The incidence of deep infection is low (1% to 2.2%) with primary knee replacements, but higher (9% to 10%) with revision knee replacements. Infections have been classified into four categories.

**Infection classification:**

**Type I**—Positive intraoperative culture
**Type II**—Early postoperative, superficial or deep
**Type III**—Acute hematogenous
**Type IV**—Late chronic infections

Clinically, patients may present with acute-onset symptoms or a more indolent course. Laboratory studies may demonstrate leukocytosis, an elevated erythrocyte sedimentation rate, or elevated C-reactive protein. Blood cultures or joint aspiration

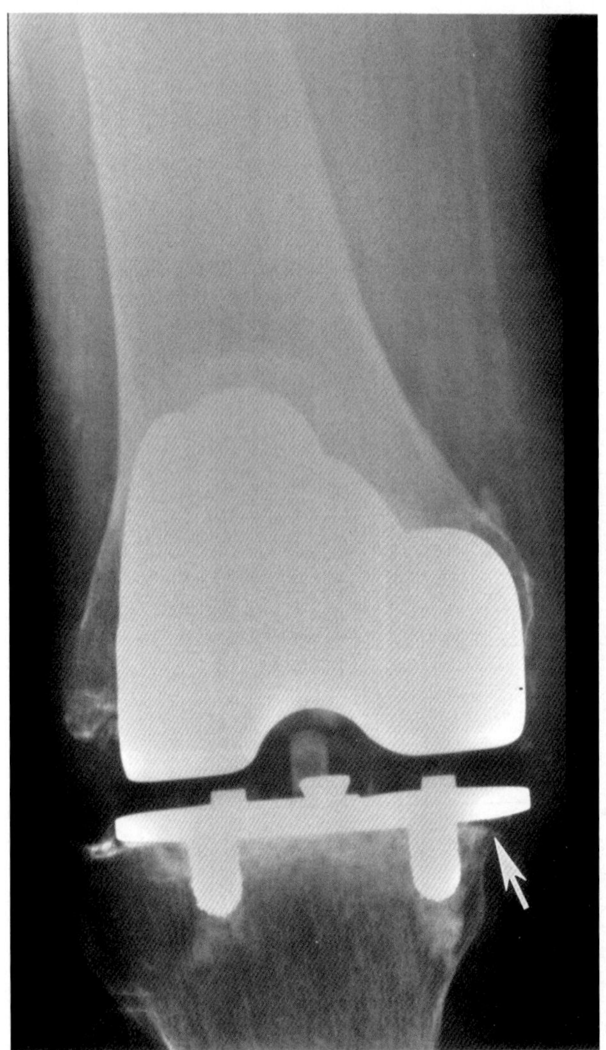


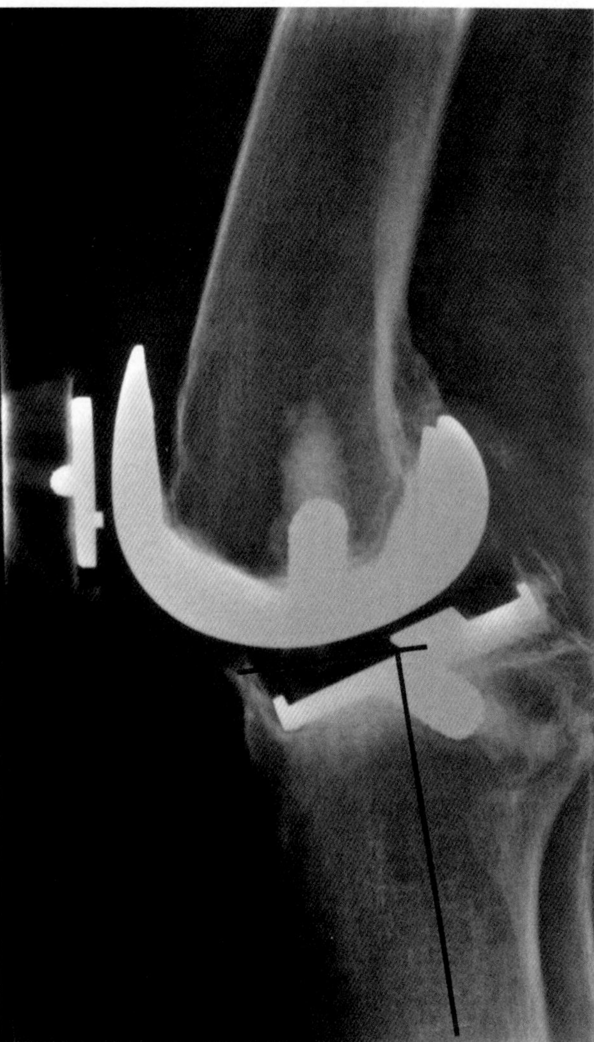


Fig. 6-72 Loosening and subsidence. Anteroposterior (AP) (A) and lateral (B) radiographs demonstrate medial displacement of the tibial tray with overhang medially (*arrow*). The anterior tray has subsided anteriorly and is not longer at 90 degrees to the tibial shaft (*lines*).

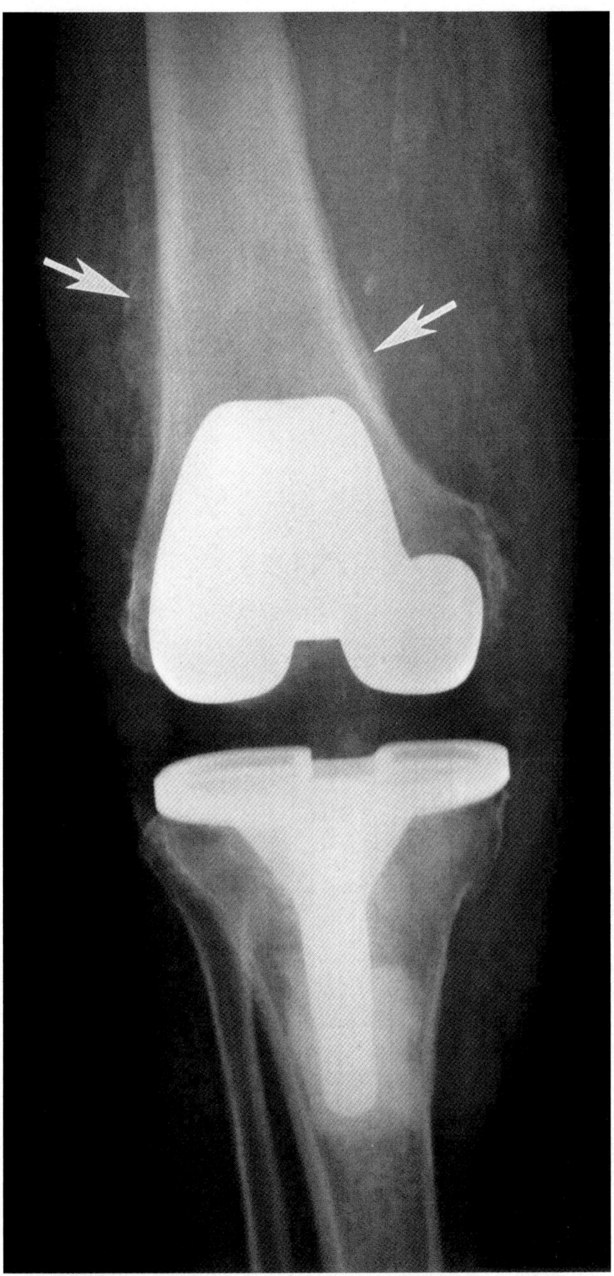

Fig. 6-73 Anteroposterior (AP) radiograph demonstrating periosteal reaction (*arrows*) in a patient with a chronic infection.

may isolate the organism. Joint aspirations are successful in 67% to 90% of cases. Infections are most commonly the result of *Staphylococcus aureus, Staphylococcus impidermidis, Pseudomonas aeruginosa, and Escherichia coli*.

Imaging of suspected infection can be complicated. Radiographic features may be subtle. Periosteal reaction, soft tissue swelling, and signs of loosening may be present (see Fig. 6-73). Conventional technetium scans can be positive for up to 1 year following surgery. After 1 year three-phase technetium scans are very sensitive (95%), but not specific. Combined radionuclide scans using Technetium Tc 99 m and indium–labeled white blood cells and/or technetium sulfur colloid are more useful for evaluating infection (see Fig. 6-74). Currently, positron emission tomographic (PET) scanning is also a useful tool for detection of periprosthetic infection.

Deep infections usually require component removal and aggressive antibiotic therapy (Fig. 6-74C and D). When the infection has cleared the knee may be revised with revision systems or an arthrodesis may be performed as an alternative.

INSTABILITY Instability occurs in up to 13% of patients following knee replacement. This is usually diagnosed with clinical examination. Fluoroscopically positioned images with varus, valgus, and AP stress may be performed. Knee dislocation is rare following total knee replacement (see Fig. 6-75).

OSTEOLYSIS AND POLYETHYLENE WEAR Osteolysis is usually the result of reaction to polyethylene wear, but may also occur as a reaction to metal particles or cement. This process typically occurs >2 years following surgery, typically at 4 to 5 years and occurs in 7% of patients. Synovial inflammation begins initially, followed by development of lytic lesions about the components. Screw in the tibial component may serve as a method of spread of the process (see Fig. 6-76). Radiographs may demonstrate the lucent lesions as well as joint asymmetry due to polyethylene wear (see Fig. 6-77). CT is the most effective method for evaluating the extent of the process and planning the management (Figs. 6-76 and 77). Smaller lesions may be grafted; however, in most cases revision surgery is performed with grafting of the lesions or augmentation wedges in the implants.

FRACTURES Fractures associated with knee replacement are uncommon, occurring in 1.2% to 3% of cases. Fractures may involve the femur, tibia, or patella and occur intraoperatively or postoperatively. Intraoperative fractures that occur during placement of the femoral or tibial components are more easily treated than postoperative fractures because there is no comminution or soft tissue injury. Postoperative stress or insufficiency fractures may occur due to increased activity compared to activity before the arthroplasty (Fig. 6-68). Complete fractures also occur, most commonly in the supracondylar region or above the femoral implant (see Fig. 6-79). Fractures may also occur in areas of osteolysis (Fig. 6-76). Patellar fractures are most common during revision of implants in osteoporotic bone. Patellar fractures following primary arthroplasty are rare (0.68% of patients with total knee replacement; Fig. 6-12). Actual implant fracture is very uncommon (see Fig. 6-80).

Detection of fractures may be accomplished with radiographs. Subtle stress or insufficiency fractures are more easily defined with CT or MRI. Management may be conservative, require internal fixation or, in some cases require revision (see Fig. 6-81).

MISCELLANEOUS COMPLICATIONS Other complications include DVT, peroneal nerve palsy (1%), dislocation of the polyethylene

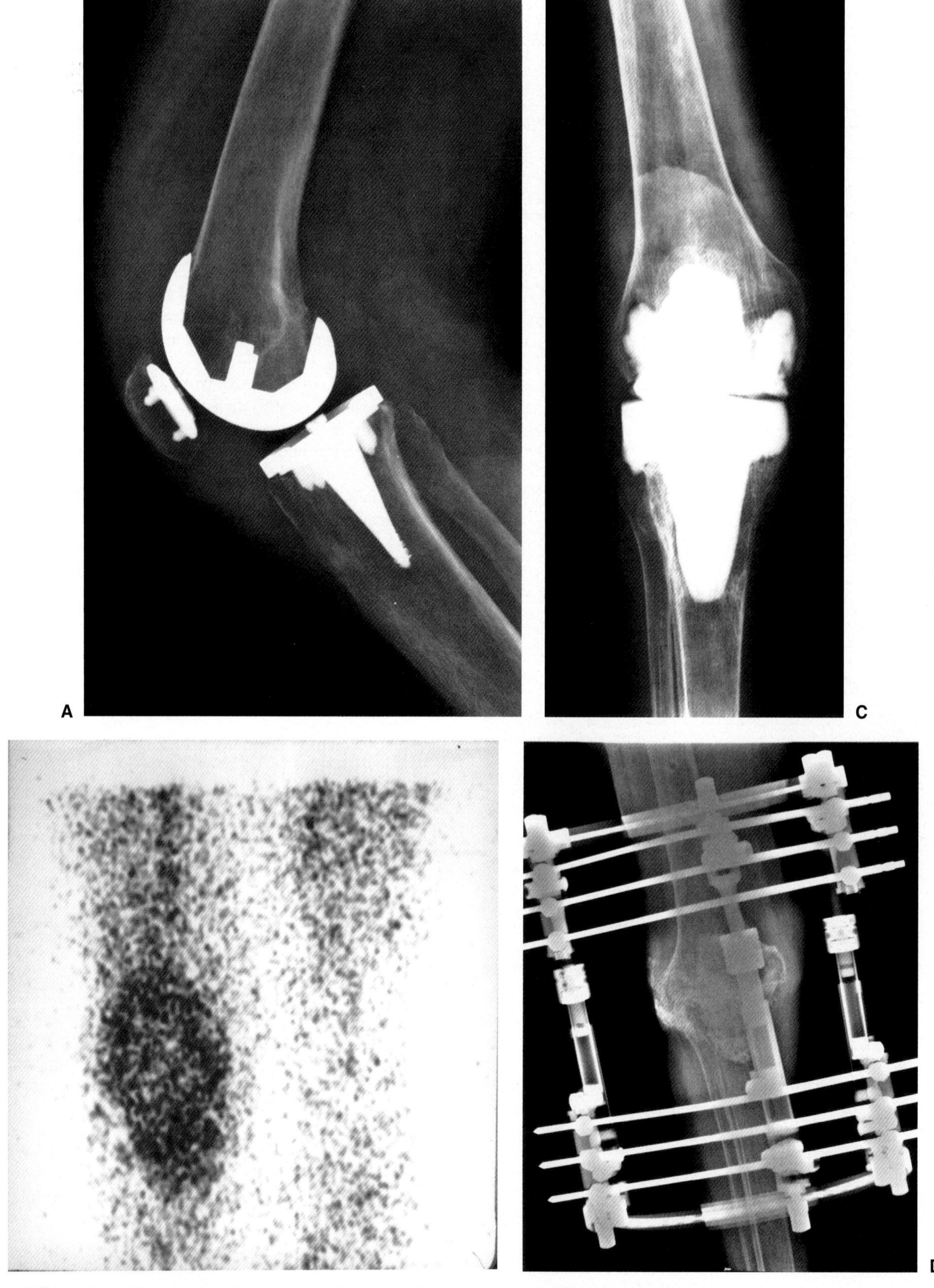

Fig. 6-74 Infected knee arthroplasty. A: Lateral radiograph demonstrates soft tissue swelling anteriorly. B: Indium labeled white blood cell scan is positive. C: Implants were removed and antibiotic impregnated methyl methacrylate spacers placed in the knee. After the infection clears the knee can be revised or in some cases an arthrodesis is performed (D) as an alternative.

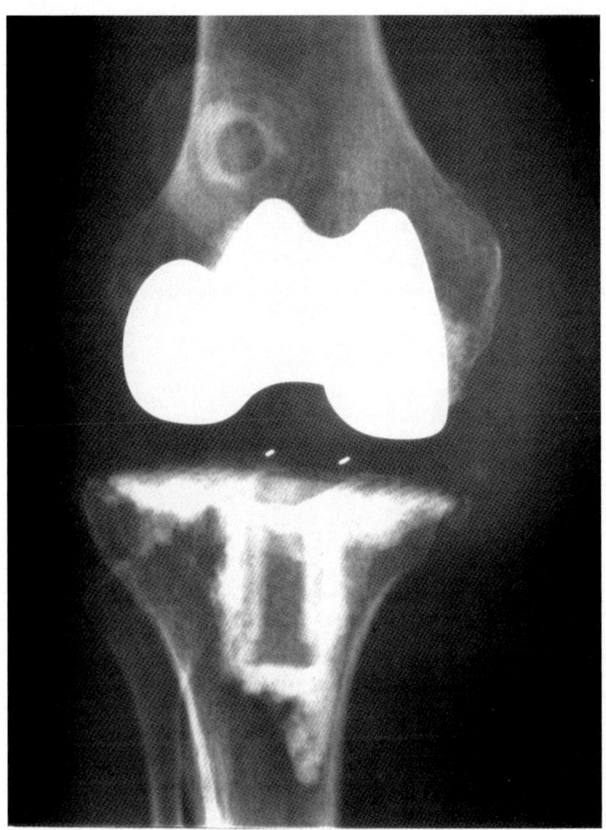

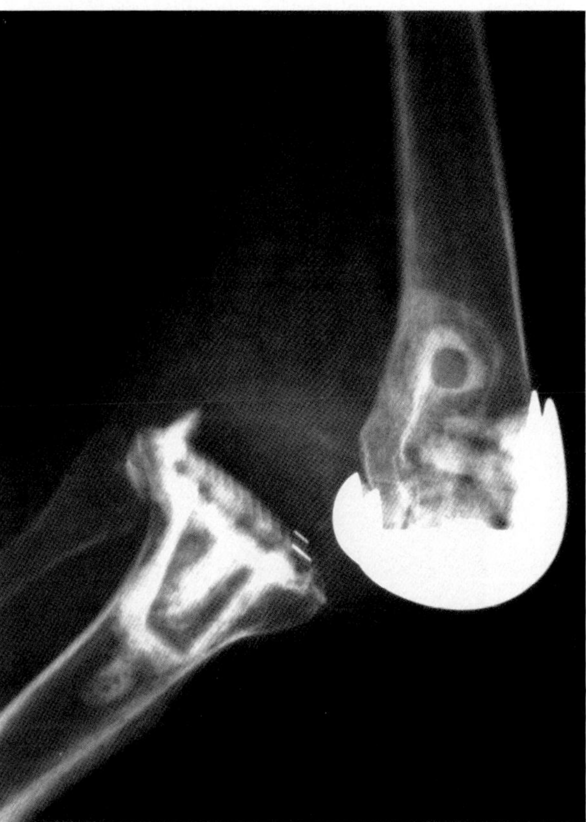

A B

Fig. 6-75 Anteroposterior (AP) (A) and lateral (B) radiographs demonstrating femorotibial and patellar dislocation.

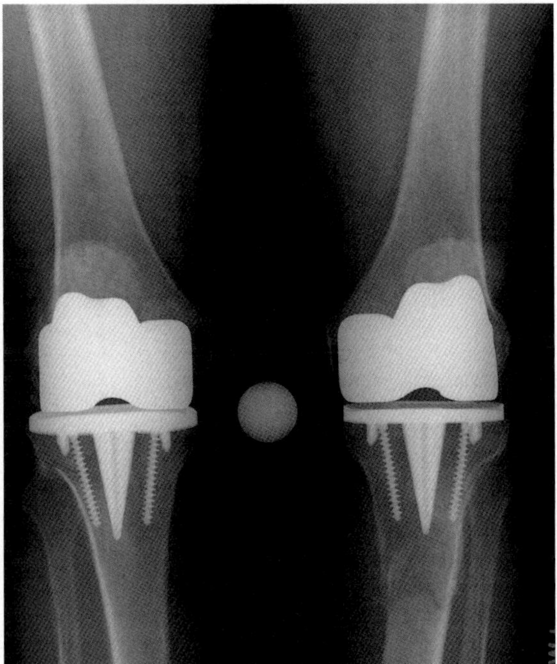

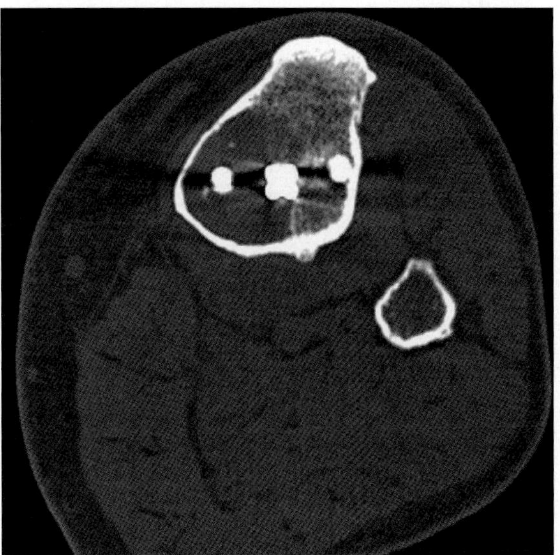

A B

Fig. 6-76 Massive osteolysis extending down from the tibial screw with pathologic fracture. A: anteroposterior (AP) radiograph demonstrates a lucent appearance in the upper tibia with a proximal shaft fracture. Axial (B), coronal (C), and sagittal (D) computed tomographic (CT) images demonstrate the aggressive osteolysis extending down from the tibial screw with a minimally displaced fracture.

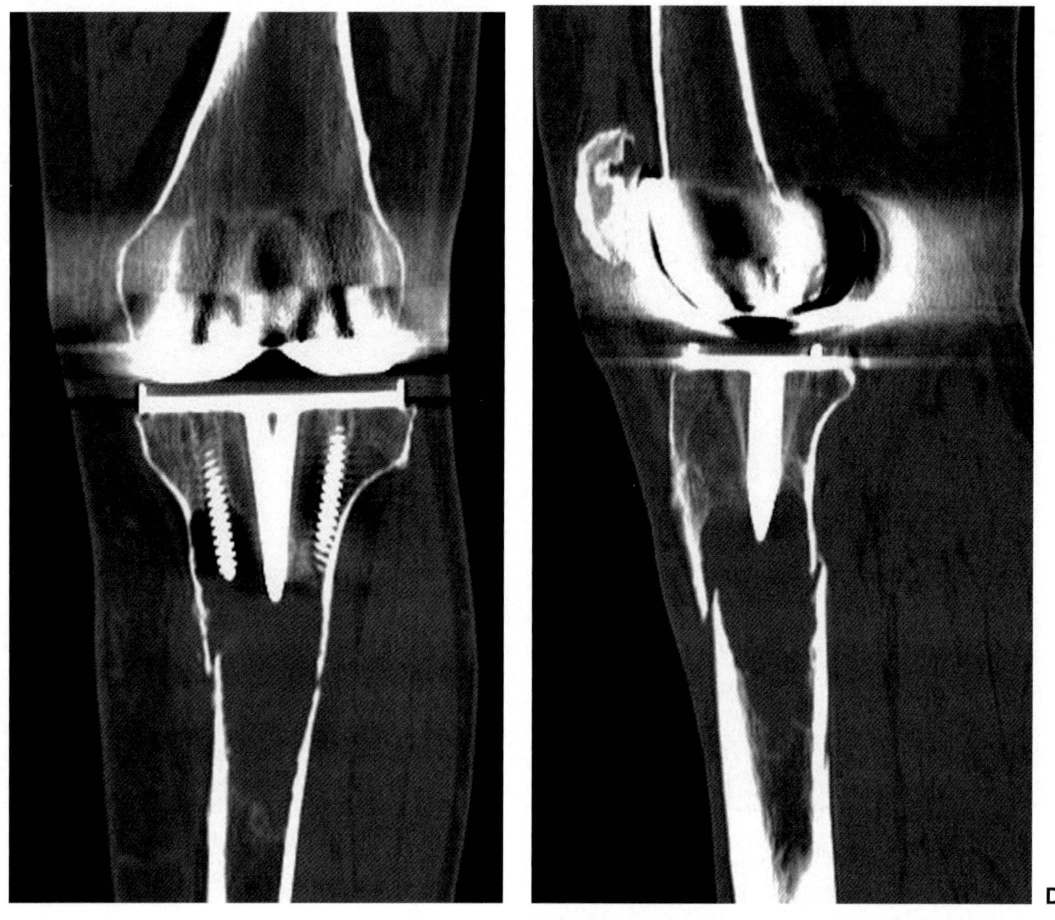

Fig. 6-76 (*Continued*)

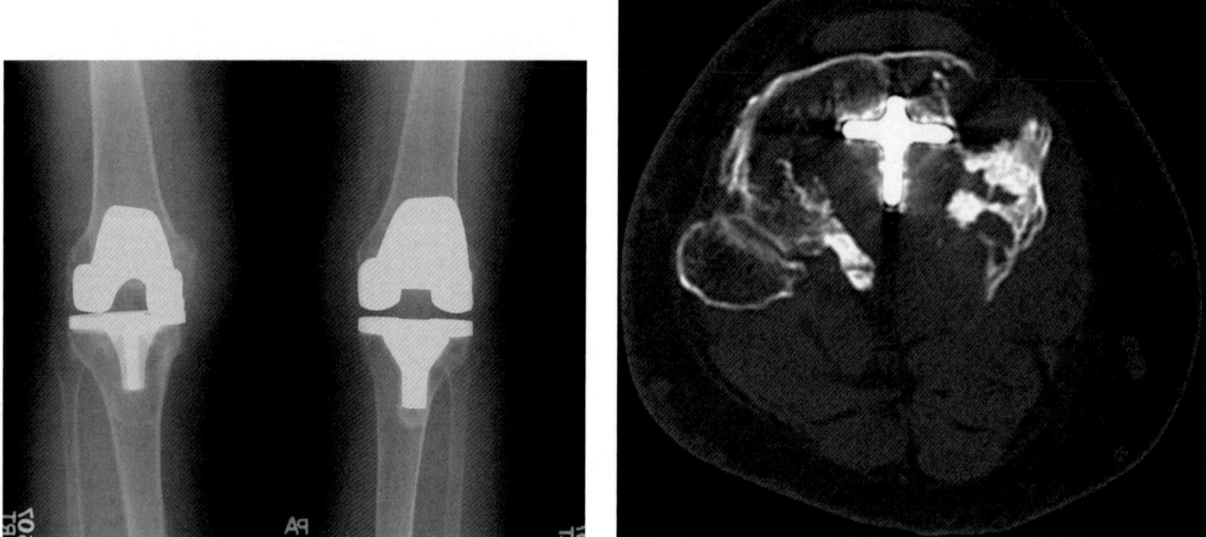

Fig. 6-77 Joint asymmetry due to polyethylene wear and associated osteolysis. **A**: Anteroposterior (AP) radiograph demonstrates bilateral knee replacements with marked narrowing medially on the right due to polyethylene wear. There is also osteolysis about the tibial component. Axial (**B**) and sagittal (**C**) computed tomographic (CT) images demonstrate extensive osteolysis with cortical breakthrough posteriorly.

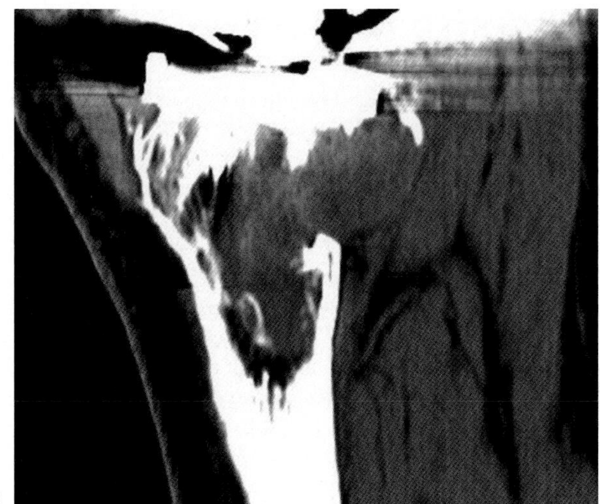

Fig. 6-77 (*Continued*)

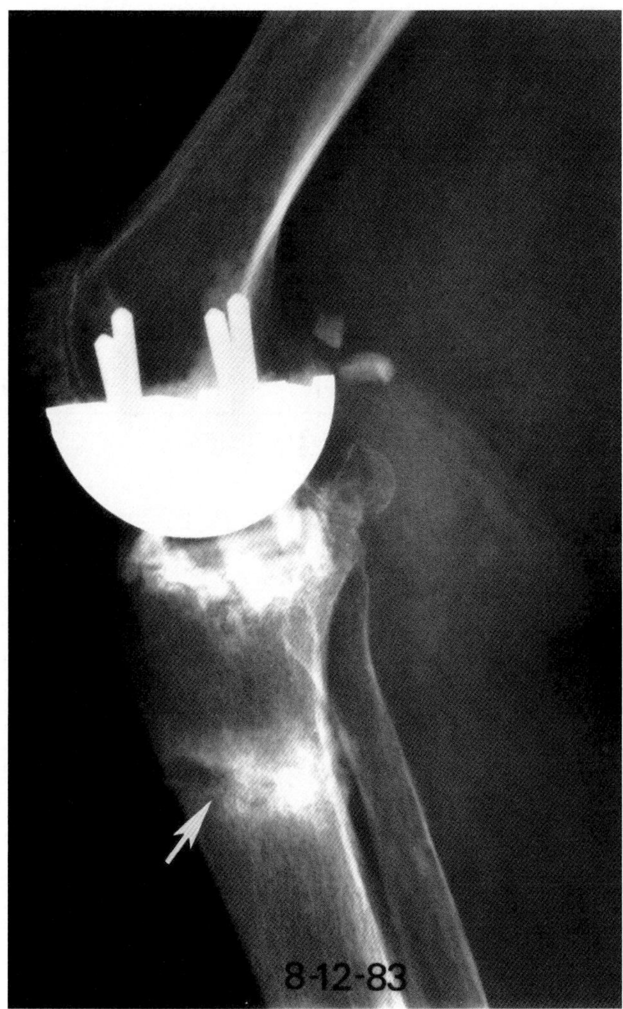


Fig. 6-78 Lateral radiograph demonstrating a stress fracture (*arrow*) following a polycentric knee replacement.

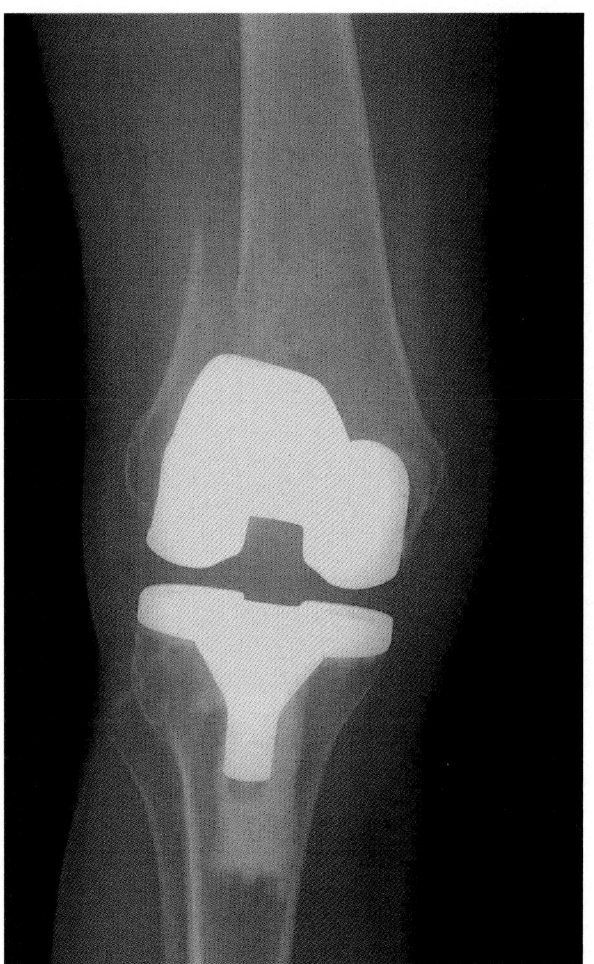

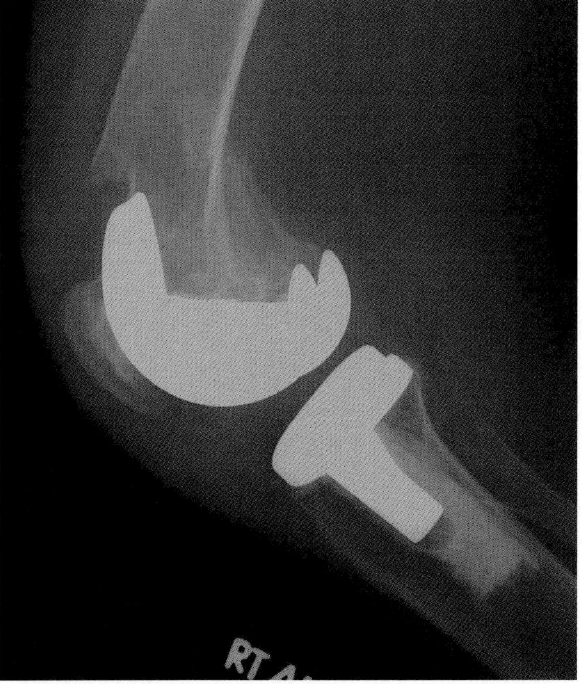

Fig. 6-79 Anteroposterior (AP) (A) and lateral (B) radiographs of a periprosthetic fracture above the femoral component with angular deformity.

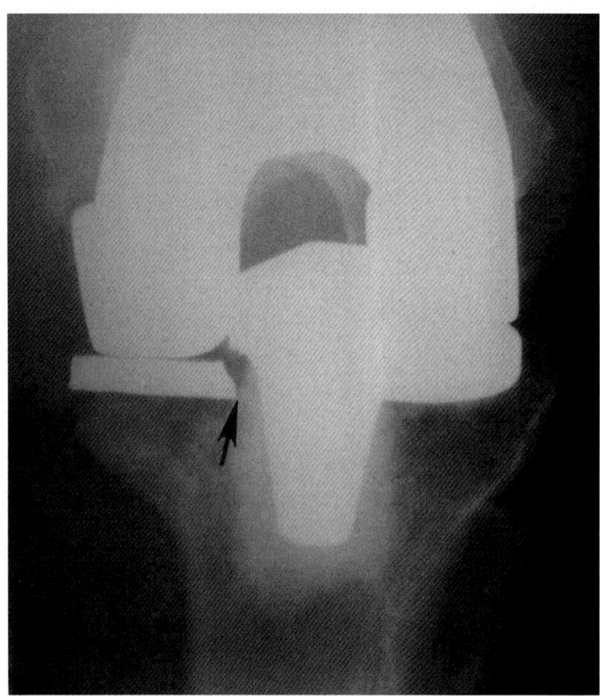

Fig. 6-80 Anteroposterior (AP) radiograph demonstrating a fracture of the tibial tray (*arrow*).

spacer, and metal synovitis. DVT is most easily evaluated with ultrasound. Nerve palsy may require MRI to define neural or perineural abnormalities. Metal synovitis is often visible on radiographs or CT. Table 6-5 summarizes complications and imaging approaches.

## Suggested Reading


Bengston S, Knutson K. The infected knee arthroplasty: a six year follow-up on 357 cases. *Acta Orthop Scand.* 1991;62: 301–311.

Berquist TH. Imaging of joint replacement procedures. *Radiol Clin North Am.* 2006;44:419–437.

Engh GA, Ammeen DJ. Periprosthetic fractures adjacent to knee implants. *J Bone Joint Surg.* 1997;79A:1100–1113.

Idusuyi OB, Morrey BF. Peroneal nerve palsy after total knee arthroplasty. *J Bone Joint Surg.* 1996;78A:177–184.

Math KR, Zaidi SF, Petchprapa C, et al. Imaging of total knee arthroplasty. *Semin Musculoskelet Radiol.* 2006;10:47–63.

Oishi CS, Grady-Benson JC, Otis SM, et al. The clinical course of deep venous thrombosis after total hip and knee arthroplasty, as determined with duplex ultrasonography. *J Bone Joint Surg.* 1994:76A:1658–1663.

Ortigera CJ, Berry DJ. Patellar fracture after total knee arthroplasty. *J Bone Joint Surg.* 2002;84A:532–540.


### Revision Knee Arthroplasty

More than 29,000 revision knee replacements were performed on the Medicare population in the United States in 2002 and the number continues to grow. Knee revisions are performed related to complications associated with primary implants described earlier and also for conversion of osteotomies (see Fig. 6-82) or unicompartmental arthroplasty to total knee replacements (see Fig. 6-83). By nature there is bone loss to be considered and revision implants are more constrained. Augmentation stems for the tibial and femoral components are used in addition to wedges for areas of bone loss (see Fig. 6-84).

**Table 6-5**

IMAGING OF KNEE ARTHROPLASTY COMPLICATIONS

| COMPLICATION (INCIDENCE) | IMAGING APPROACHES |
|---|---|
| Extensor mechanism (4%–41%) | Serial radiographs,<br>Flexion/extension Merchant images |
| Loosening (2%–5%) | Serial radiographs, CT,<br>Radionuclide scans |
| Deep infection (1%–2.2%) | Serial radiographs, joint aspiration, radionuclide scans, CT |
| Instability (13%) | Stress views |
| Osteolysis/polyethylene wear (7%) | Serial radiographs, CT |
| Fractures (1.2%–3%) | Serial radiographs, CT, MRI |
| Neurovascular (DVT, peroneal nerve) | Ultrasound, MRI |

CT, computed tomography; MRI, magnetic resonance imaging; DVT, deep venous thrombosis.

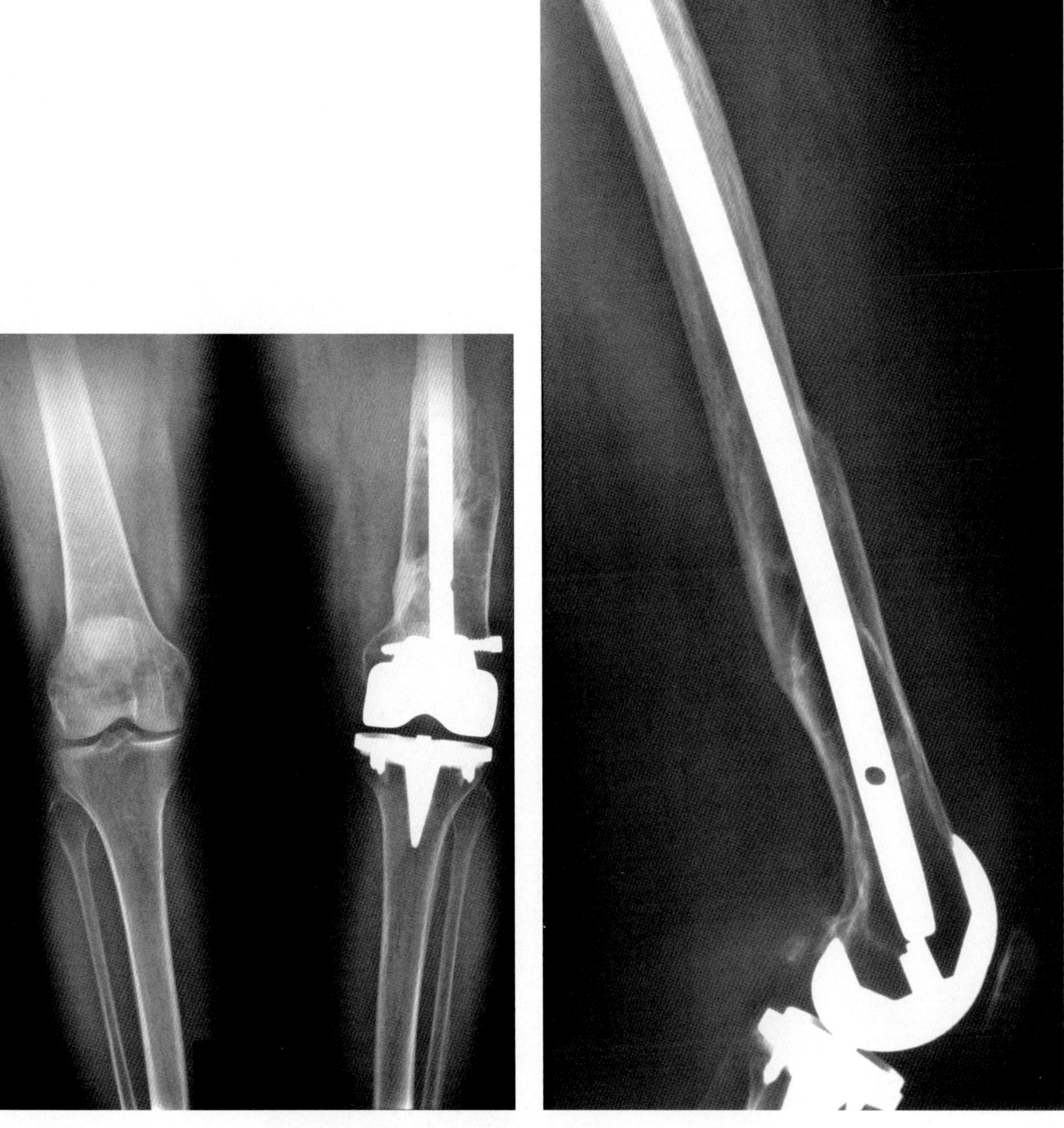

Fig. 6-81 Anteroposterior (AP) (A) and lateral (B) radiographs demonstrating a healed distal femoral fracture treated with an intramedullary nail.

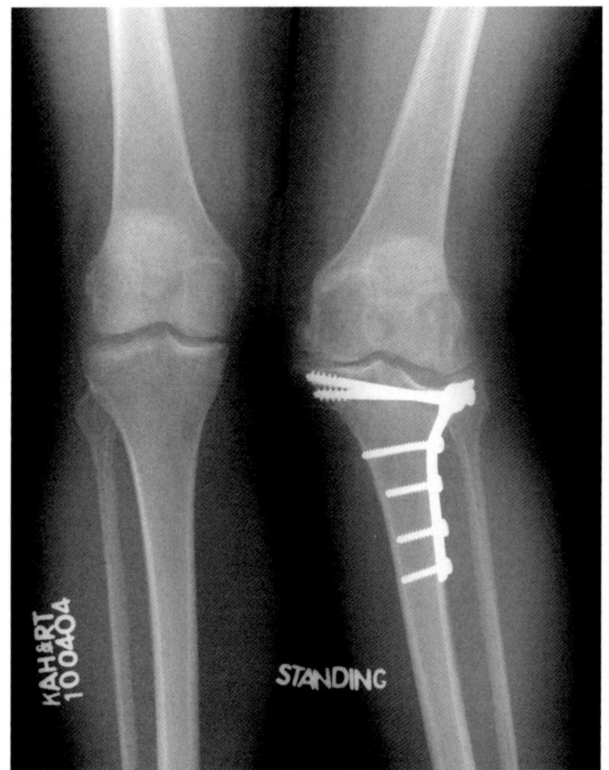


A

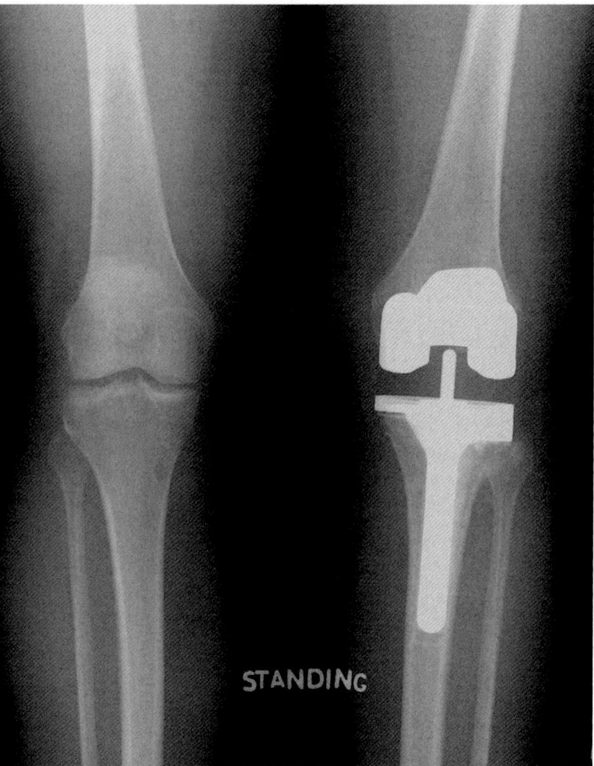


B

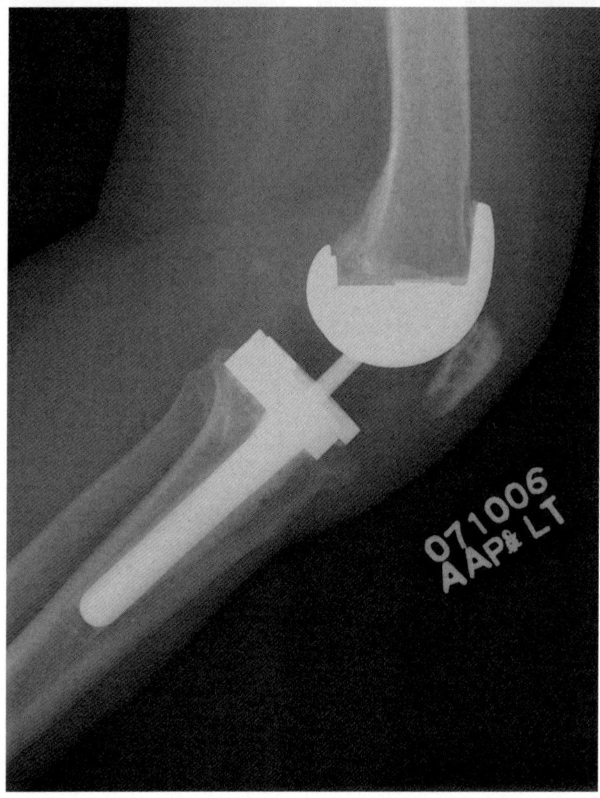


C

Fig. 6-82 Conversion of tibial osteotomy to total knee replacement using revision implants. A: Standing radiograph of the knees demonstrating a left tibial osteotomy with advanced valgus angulation and arthropathy. Anteroposterior (AP) (B) and lateral (C) radiographs following conversion to a total knee arthroplasty with revision components. There is a tibial augmentation wedge laterally and an augmentation stem. The spacer is thick to achieve joint line symmetry with the contralateral knee.

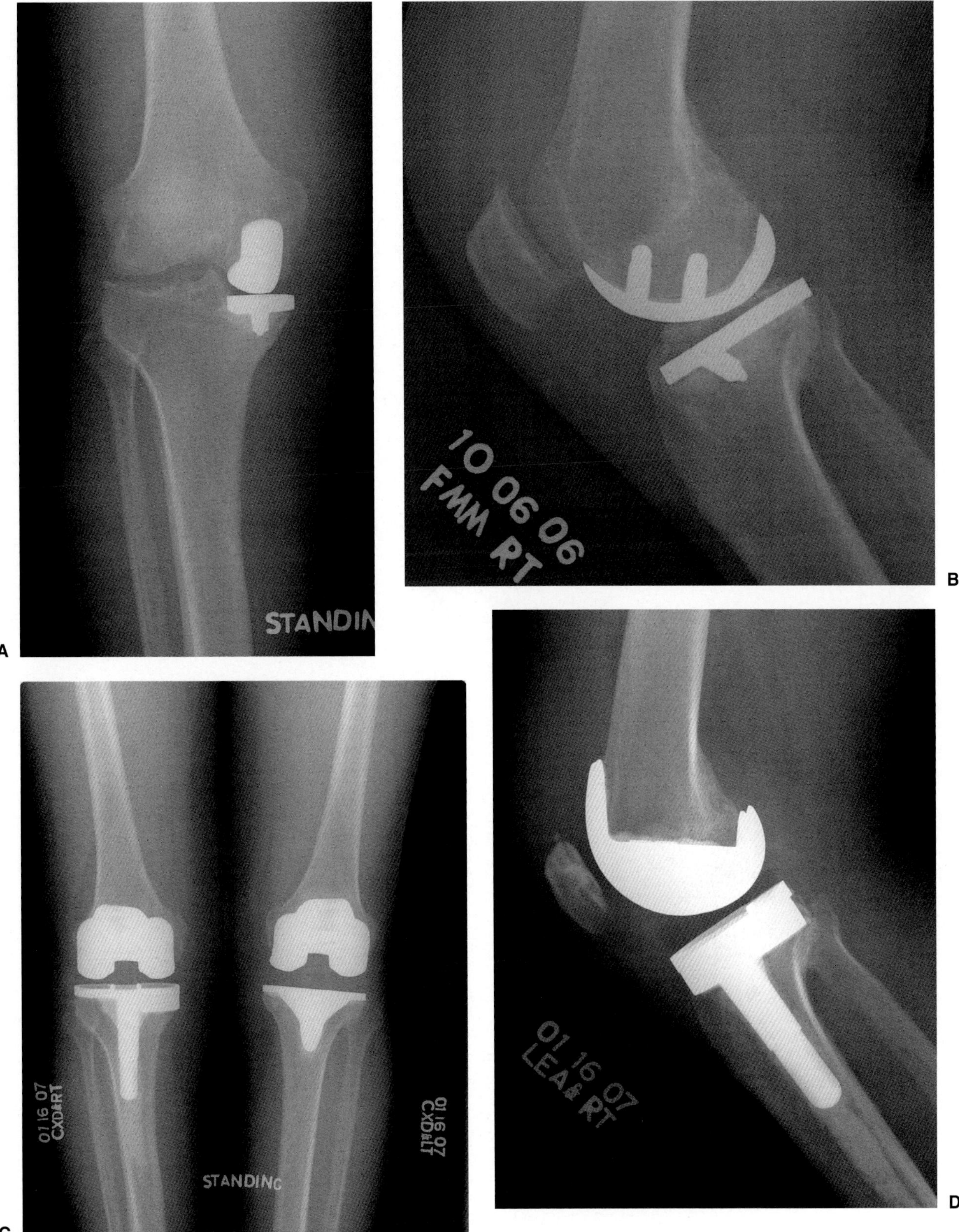


Fig. 6-83 Anteroposterior (AP) (A) and lateral (B) radiographs of the knee with a medial compartment arthroplasty on the right. There is lucency about the femoral and anterior tibial components, more evident on the lateral view (B). The knee was revised with posterior stabilized components with a medial augmentation wedge because of the bone loss from the prior implant and a long tibial stem (C and D).

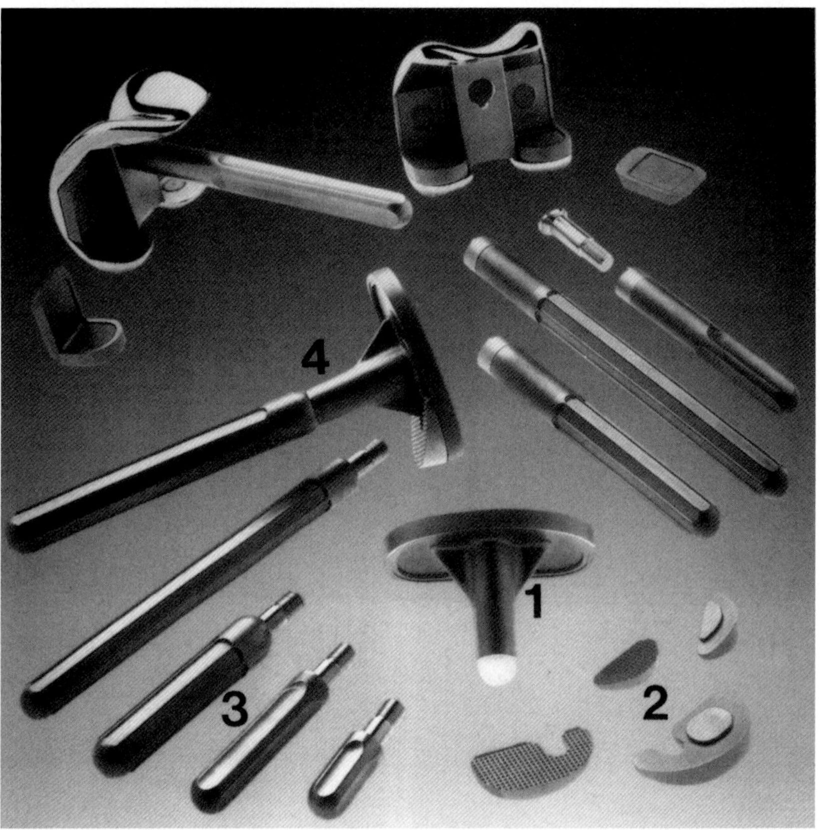


Fig. 6-84 Photograph of Johnson and Johnson modular knees with conventional tibial tray *(1)*, augmentation wedges *(2)*, augmentation stems *(3)*, and components assembled *(4)*. (Courtesy of Johnson and Johnson Orthopaedics, Raynham, MA.)

Complications following revision surgery are similar to those described with primary knee replacement (Table 6-5). However, the incidence of loosening (see Fig. 6-85) and infection is higher. The incidence of infection is 9% to 10% compared to 1% to 2.2% for primary knee replacements (see Fig. 6-86).

## Suggested Reading

Mahomed NN, Barrett J, Katz JN, et al. Epidemiology of total knee replacement in the United States medicare population. *J Bone Joint Surg*. 2005;87A:1222–1228.

Sheng P-Y, Konttinen L, Hehto M, et al. Revision total knee arthroplasty: 1990 through 2002. *J Bone Joint Surg*. 2006;88A:1425–1430.

## Miscellaneous Procedures

There are other common procedures about the knee that require instrumentation and imaging evaluation. This section will review osteotomies of the tibia and femur and knee arthrodesis.

### Osteotomy

There are multiple treatment options for younger patients with knee arthropathy. The goals in the younger population are not only to extend the natural life of the knee but also to consider the impact of the treatment selected on eventual knee replacement. Options include primary cartilage repair, ligament repair and arthroscopic debridement, osteotomy, unicompartmental arthroplasty or, if necessary, total knee replacement. Osteotomies may be performed on the distal femur or proximal tibia. Osteotomies are indicated in younger or middle-aged patients with unicompartmental disease to realign the joint and transfer the weight-bearing load to the uninvolved compartment. The treatment goal is to relieve pain and improve function. Typically, the medial compartment is involved. In this case a tibial osteotomy is performed. Distal femoral osteotomy is the procedure of choice for patients with lateral compartment disease and valgus deformity. Patellofemoral osteoarthritis is not a contraindication to osteotomy. However, patient selection is important and there are contraindications to this procedure. The ideal candidate for osteotomy is a patient in the 50s or 60s with unicompartmental disease, no patellofemoral symptoms, and normal range of motion. Patients with tricompartmental disease, severe medial compartment arthritis, systemic inflammatory arthritis, and neuropathic disease are not candidates for this procedure.

## Suggested Reading

Hanssen AD, Stuart MJ, Scott RD, et al. Surgical options for the middle-aged patient with osteoarthritis of the knee joint. *Instr Course Lect*. 2001;50:499–511.

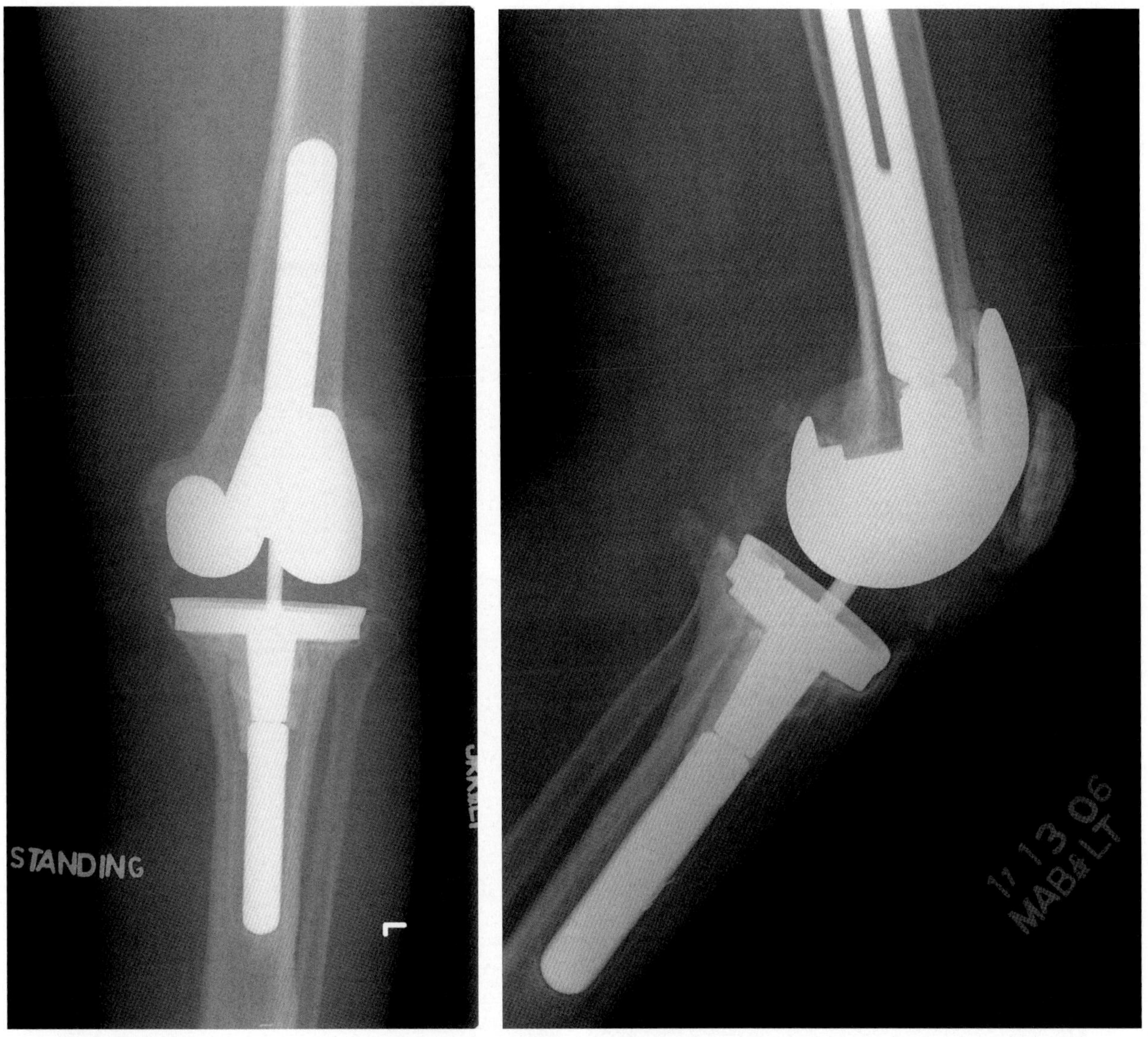


Fig. 6-85 Anteroposterior (AP) (A) and lateral (B) radiographs of a revision knee replacement. There are obvious large lucent zones about both components due to loosening.

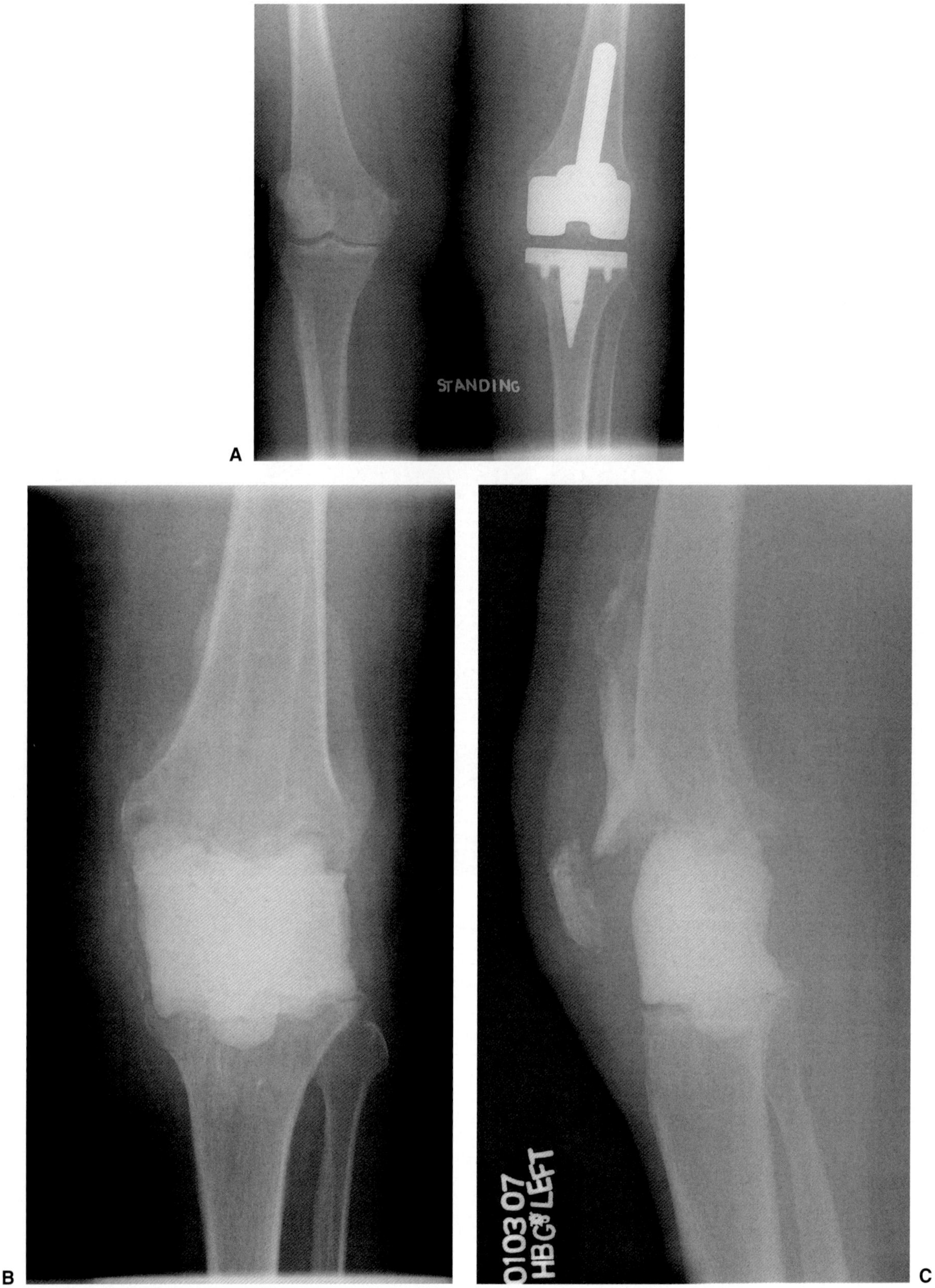

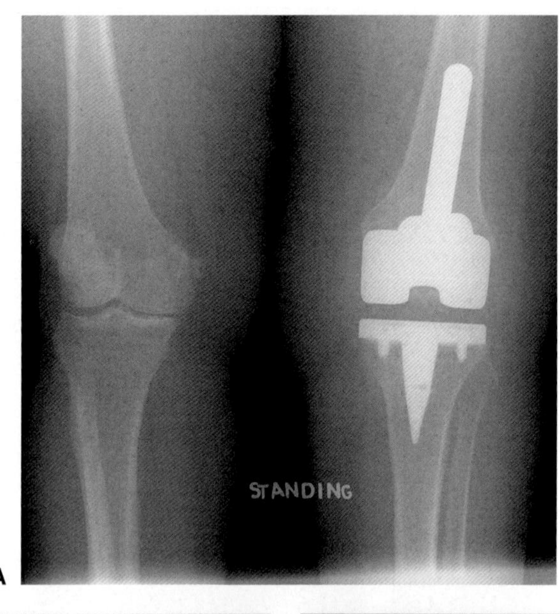


B C

Fig. 6-86 Infected revision knee arthroplasty. A: Anteroposterior (AP) radiograph demonstrates a revision implant on the left. There was no radiographic evidence of infection. The implants were removed and an antibiotic spacer (B and C) placed. AP (D) and lateral (E) radiographs 9 months after the infection cleared and a new revision knee system was placed.

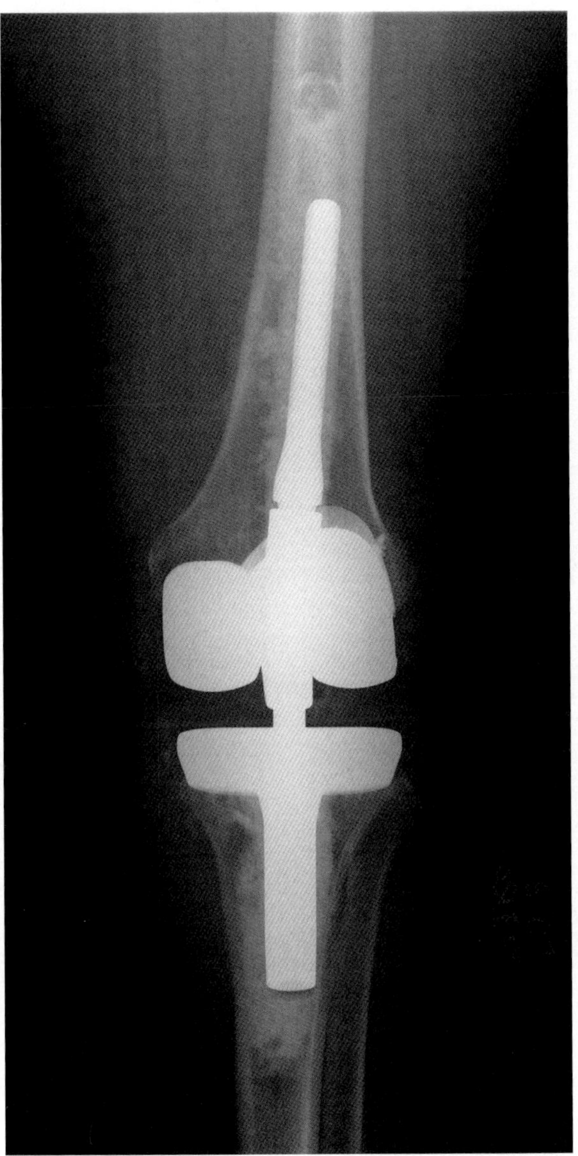
D

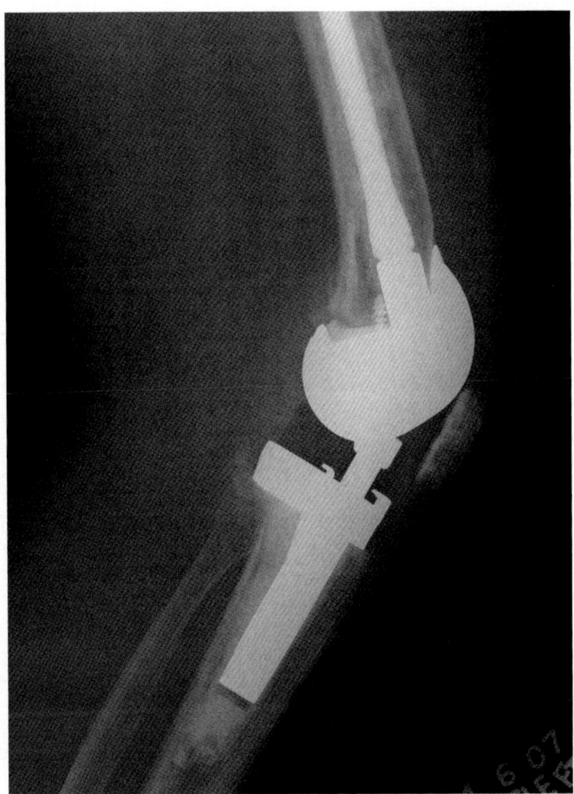
E

Fig. 6-86 *(Continued)*

## Preoperative Imaging

Preoperative images should include standing AP, lateral, and Merchant views of the knee (see Fig. 6-87). Full-length standing AP radiographs are optimal for evaluating the mechanical axis and femorotibial angle. Flexion standing PA radiographs are useful to evaluate subtle joint space abnormalities in the medial and lateral compartments. In certain cases, MRI is needed to evaluate soft tissue support and more accurately assess the articular cartilage.

# Suggested Reading

Coventry MB. Proximal tibial varus osteotomy for osteoarthritis of the lateral compartment of the knee. *J Bone Joint Surg*. 1987;69A:32–38.

Rosenberg AF, Paulos LE, Parker RD, et al. The forty-five degree posteroanterior flexion weight bearing radiograph of the knee. *J Bone Joint Surg*. 1988;70A:1479–1482.

## Distal Femoral Osteotomy

Valgus deformity with lateral compartment involvement is the ideal setting for distal femoral varus osteotomy. The osteotomy is performed on the medial side with removal of a wedge of bone. Fixation is usually accomplished using a 90-degree blade plate (see Fig. 6-88). Survival at 10 years is 64%. Osteotomies of the distal femur may also be performed for femoral deformities. This is usually performed earlier in life on patients with fracture malunion, Bount disease, and other deformities to prevent the development of osteoarthritis. In this setting, the same type of fixation or external fixation may be used.

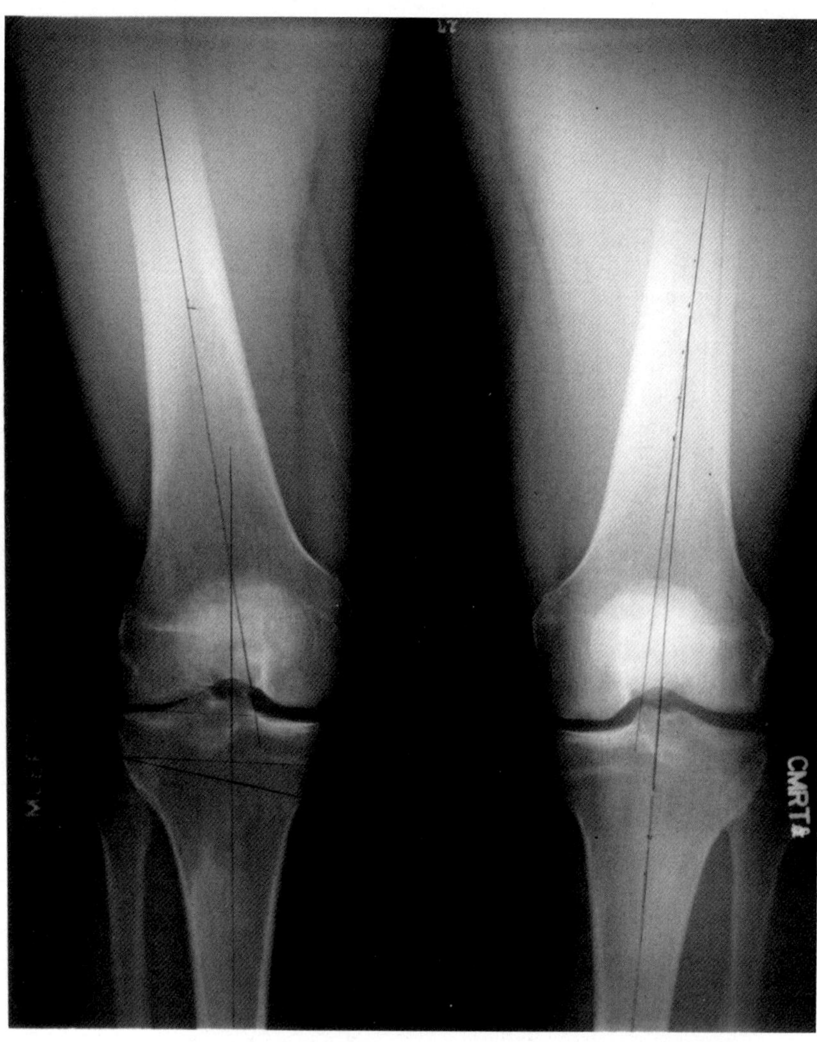

Fig. 6-87 Standing radiographs of the knee in a patient with lateral compartment osteoarthritis on the right with slight valgus deformity and lines in the upper tibia for wedge removal before osteotomy.

## Suggested Reading

Finkelstein JA, Gross AE, Davis A. Varus osteotomy of the distal part of the femur. *J Bone Joint Surg.* 1996;78A:1348–1352.

Gugenheim JJ, Brinker MR. Bone realignment with use of temporary external fixation for distal femoral valgus and varus deformities. *J Bone Joint Surg.* 2003;85A:1229–1237.

Wang J-W, HSU C-C. Distal femoral varus osteotomy for osteoarthritis of the knee. *J Bone Joint Surg.* 2006;88A:100–108.

### Upper Tibial Osteotomy

Upper tibial osteotomy was first introduced as a method for treatment of osteoarthritis of the knee in 1958. Initially the osteotomy was performed in the upper third of the tibia, below the tuberosity. However, because of excellent healing in medullary bone, proximal tibial osteotomy above the tibial tuberosity in the metaphysis replaced the initial approach. Most osteotomies involve removing or inserting a wedge of bone to realign the knee joint. Different techniques are summarized in the subsequent text.

**Upper tibial osteotomies:** (see Fig. 6-89)

**Closing wedge:** A wedge of bone is removed and the margins brought together.

**Opening wedge:** An osteotomy is performed and a wedge of bone graft is inserted (see Fig. 6-90)

**Curved osteotomies:** A curved osteotomy is performed above or below the tibial tuberosity, usually with fibular osteotomy

**Combined osteotomies:** Both lateral closing and medial opening performed on the same knee. Also, combined tibial osteotomy with tibial tuberosity osteotomy and transposition

Healing of tibial osteotomies usually occurs in 5 weeks. Various fixation techniques have been used including external fixation and internal fixation with staples (see Fig. 6-91) and different plate and screw systems (Fig. 6-90). With newer approaches, the survival rate may be as high as 92% at 10 years.

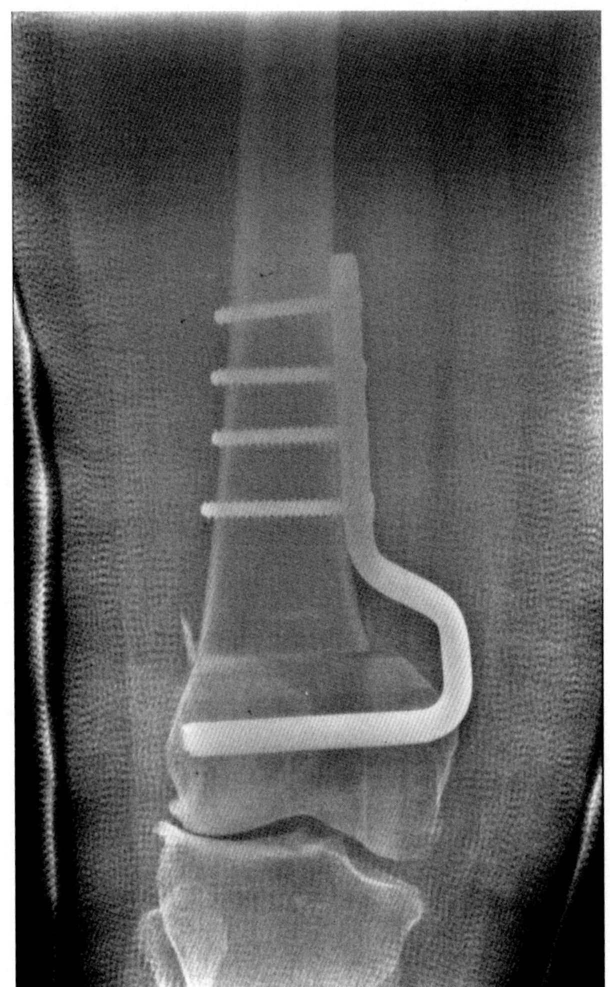


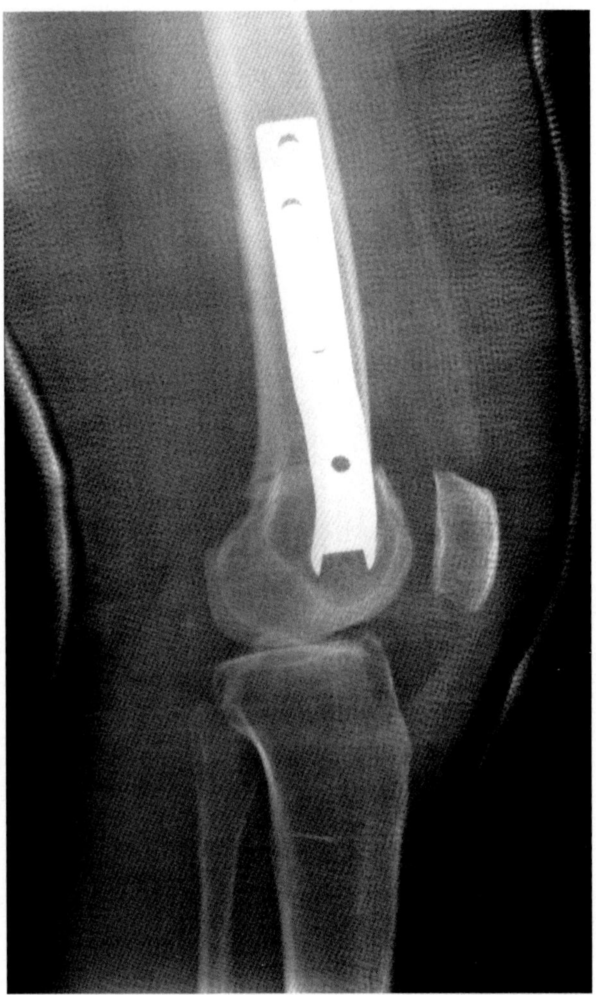


Fig. 6-88 Distal femoral osteotomy with 90-degree blade plate for fixation. Anteroposterior (AP) (A) and lateral (B) radiographs following distal femoral osteotomy with blade plate and screw fixation.

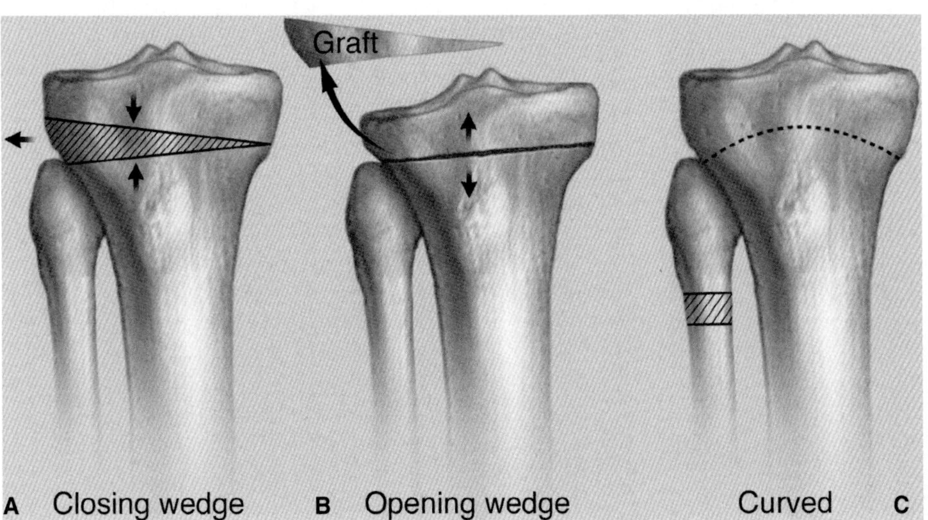


Fig. 6-89 Illustration of high tibial osteotomies. Closing wedge is performed by removing a premeasured segment and bringing the margins together (A). Opening wedge is performed by adding graft to the osteotomy site (B) and curved (C).

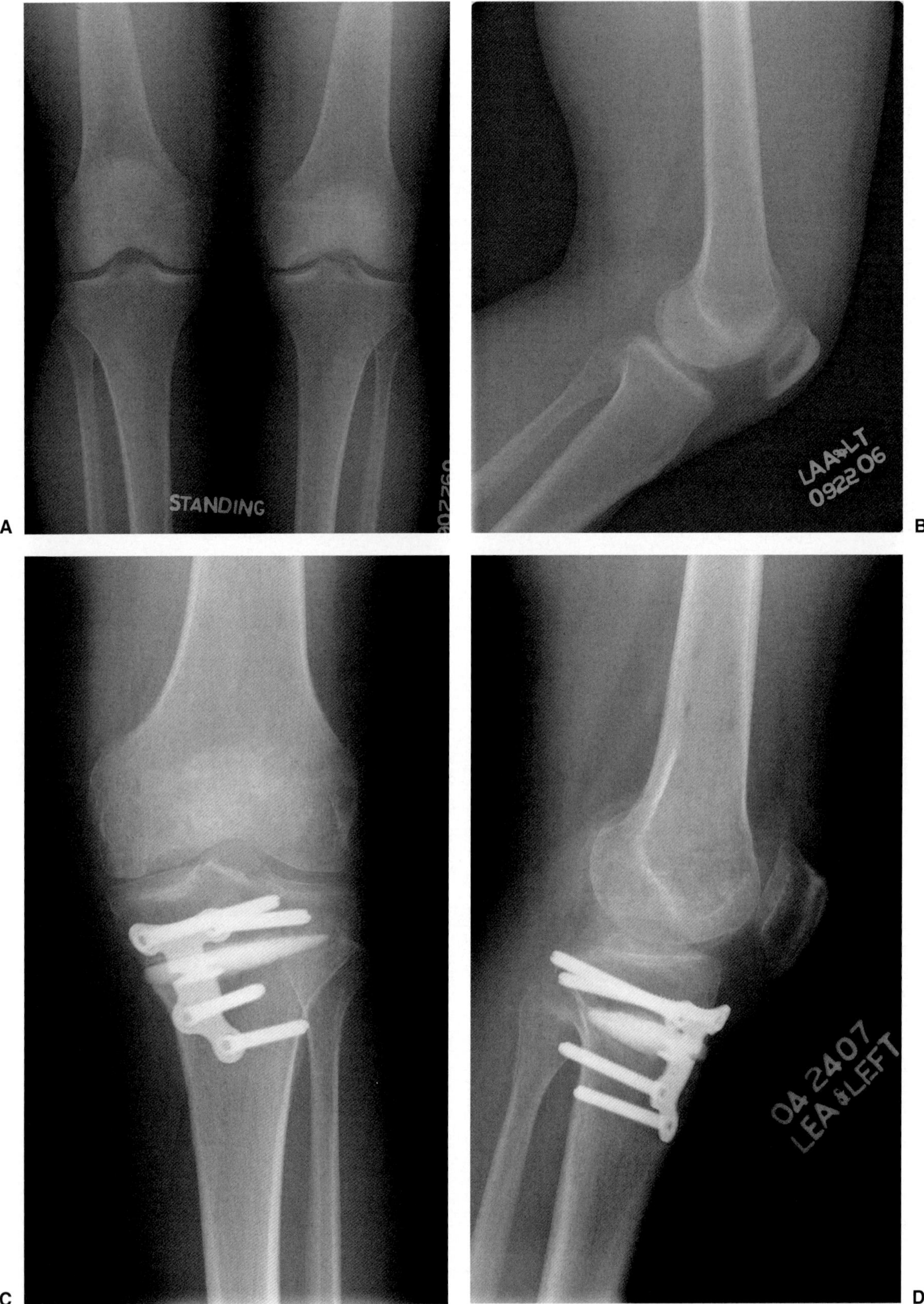


Fig. 6-90 Opening wedge osteotomy with graft in a patient with osteochondritis dissecans. Anteroposterior (AP) (A) and lateral (B) radiographs demonstrate osteochondritis dissecans involving the lateral aspect of the medial femoral condyle. AP (C) and lateral (D) radiographs following opening-wedge osteotomy with bone graft and plate and screw fixation.

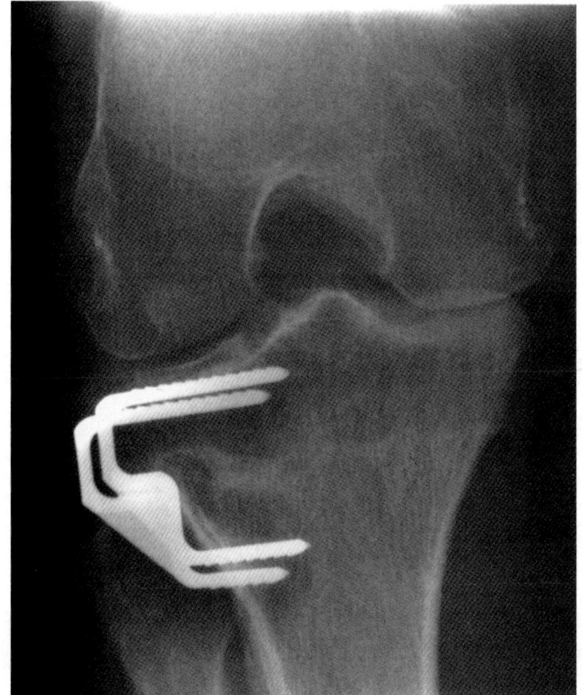


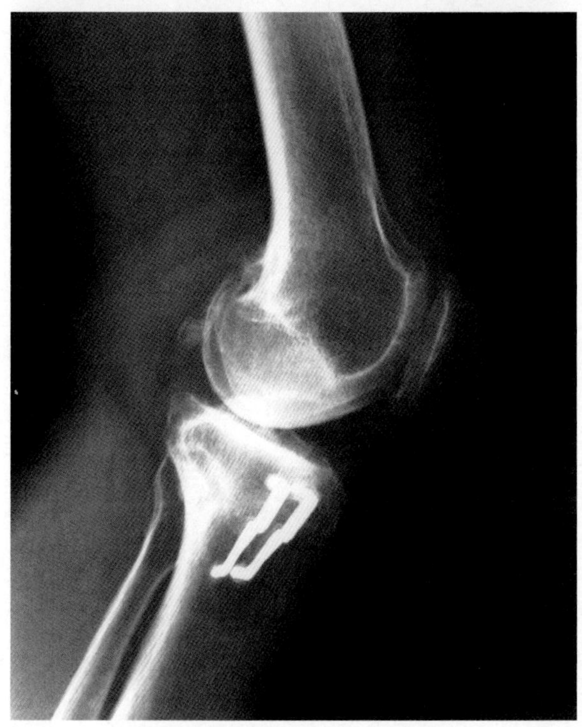


Fig. 6-91 Anteroposterior (AP) (A) and lateral (B) radiographs demonstrating a healed closed-wedge osteotomy with two barbed staples for fixation.

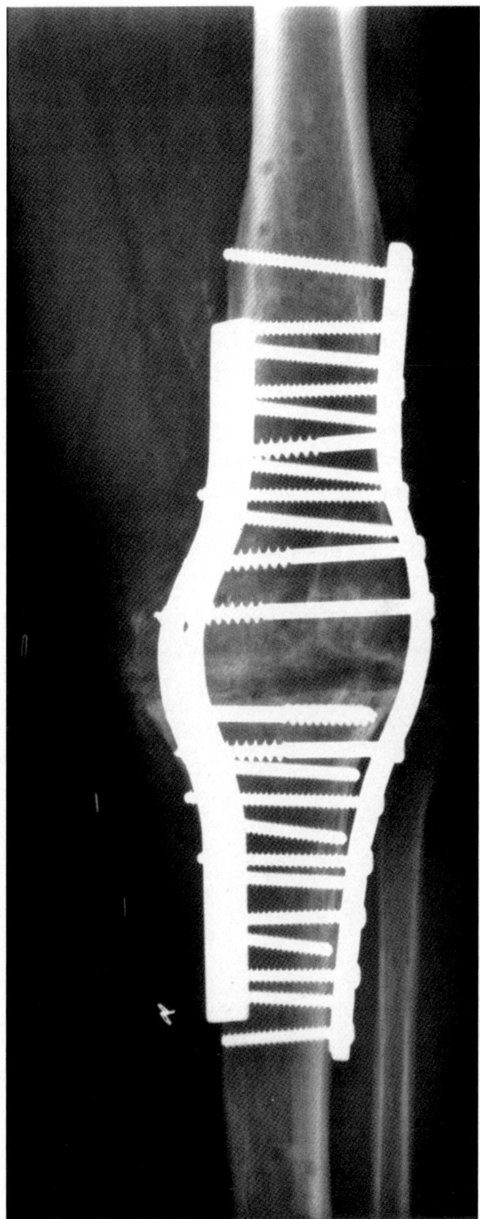

Fig. 6-92 Anteroposterior (AP) radiograph demonstrating double plate and screw arthrodesis of the knee.

## Suggested Reading


Coventry MB. Upper tibial osteotomy for osteoarthritis. *J Bone Joint Surg*. 1985;67A:1136–1140.

Jackson JP, Waugh W. The technique and complications of upper tibial osteotomy. *J Bone Joint Surg*. 1974;56B:236–245.

Nagi ON, Jumar S, Affarwal S. Combined lateral closing and medial opening-wedge high tibial osteotomy. *J Bone Joint Surg*. 2007;89A:542–549.

### Arthrodesis

Knee arthrodesis is an option to provide stability and relieve pain in patients with disability due to trauma, infected knee arthroplasty, pyarthrosis, and periarticular tumors. In the early years of this procedure, it was primarily reserved for patients with tuberculous infections or poliomyelitis. Currently, the most common indication is failed primary and revision knee arthroplasty. The primary contraindications are bilateral knee involvement and existing fusion of the hip on the involved side. Systemic conditions such as diabetes mellitus, systemic inflammatory arthropathies, vascular disease, and steroids need consideration and may impact wound healing.

Multiple fixation systems can be employed. External fixation (see Fig. 6-92) offers the advantages of limited intervention and blood loss as well as no permanent hardware. Wound access is also more accessible in patients with infection. Unilateral, ring, and hybrid external fixators can be used. Fusion rates with external fixation are lower (64% to 68%) compared to internal fixation. Compression plate and screw fixation can also be successful (see Fig. 6-93). An additional option is the use of a long intramedullary nail inserted through the piriformis fossa of the proximal femur. Fusion rates with this technique have been reported at 95%.

## SUGGESTED READING

Garberina MJ, Fitch RD, Hoffmann ED, et al. Knee arthrodesis with circular external fixation. *Clin Orthop*. 2001;382: 168–178.

MacDonald JH, Agarwal S, Lorei MP, et al. Knee arthrodesis. *J Am Acad Orthop Surg*. 2006;14:154–163.

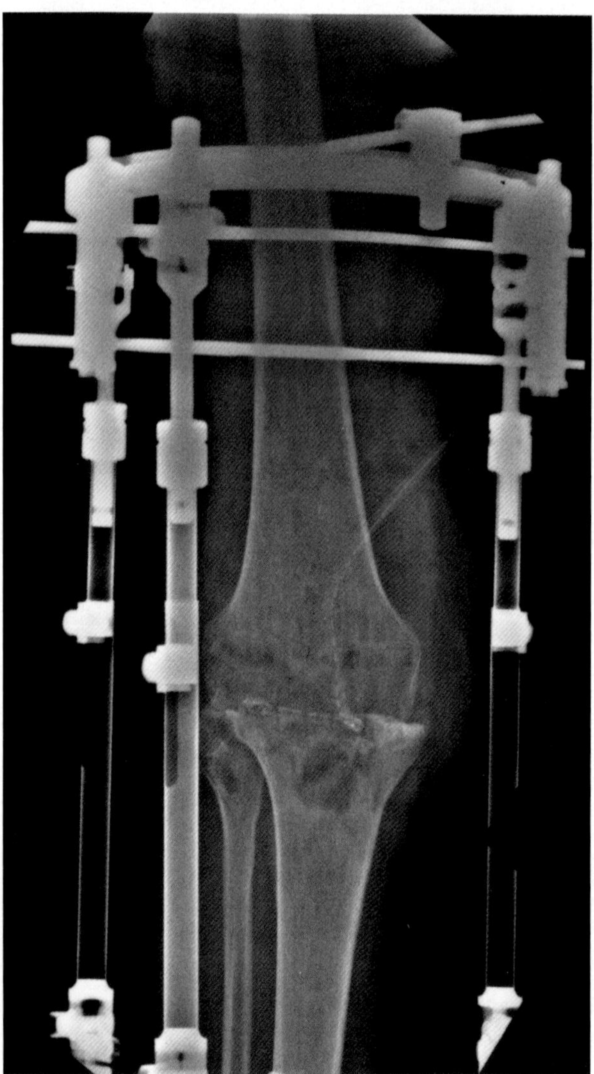
A

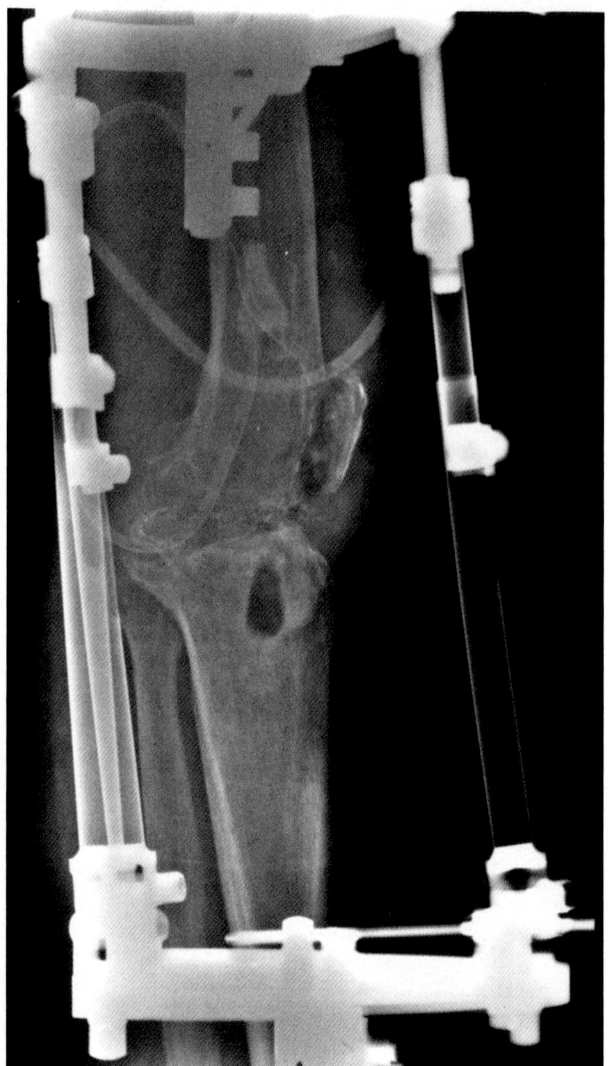
B

Fig. 6-93 Anteroposterior (AP) (A) and lateral (B) radiographs after failed knee arthroplasty treated with implant removal and arthrodesis with external fixation.

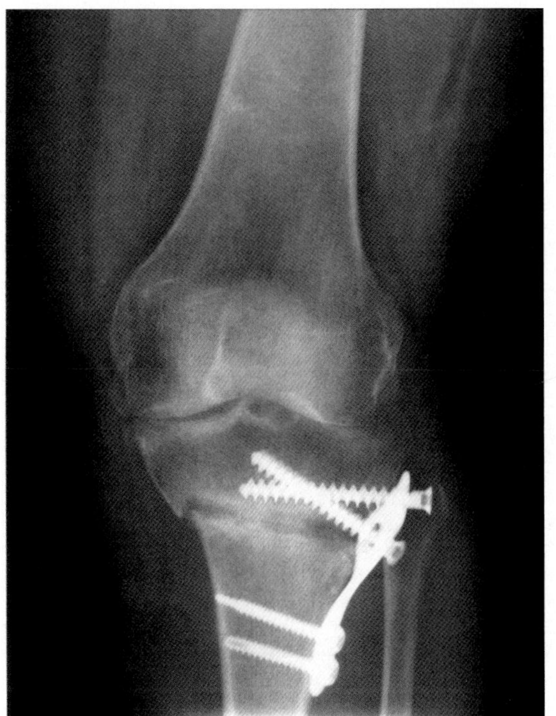


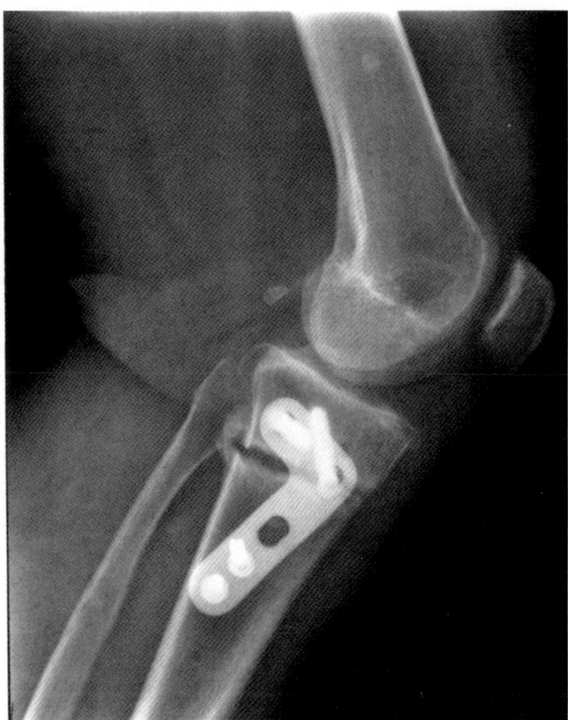


Fig. 6-94 Anteroposterior (AP) (A) and lateral (B) radiographs following upper tibial osteotomy with widening and sclerosis along the osteotomy due to nonunion.

## Complications of Osteotomy and Arthrodesis

Complications related to osteotomy and knee fusions may be related to improper patient selection (especially early failures), surgical approach, and patient compliance.

Pain following arthrodesis due to nonunion is the most common complication. Arthrodeses successfully fuse in 95% treated with intramedullary nails, in up to 100% treated with double plate and screw fixation (Fig. 6-92). However, the successful fusion using external fixation is lower (64% to 68%). Also, up to 55% of patients treated with external fixation develop pin tract infections and 32% fail to unite. Causes of nonunion include poor bone stock, poor bony contact, inadequate fixation, and persistent infection.

Complications related to osteotomy include wound infection, pin tract infection, delayed union, nonunion, failure to achieve correction, fracture into the tibial plateau, and knee stiffness. DVT, pulmonary embolus, and peroneal nerve palsy are nonmusculoskeletal complications. DVT was relatively common (up to 41%) before prophylactic use of anticoagulants. Pulmonary emboli are a significant complication but occur in <1% of patients.

Deep infection is uncommon (<1%) and superficial infections of the wound or pin tracts are more common. Pin tract infections, which can be treated locally and with antibiotics, develop in up to 55% of patients treated with external fixation. Imaging of deep infections can be accomplished with radionuclide studies or MRI.

Delayed union is most common with osteotomies performed below the tuberosity. Normally healing occurs in 5 to 6 weeks. Delayed union and nonunion may be evident on serial radiographs. Widening and sclerosis along the osteotomy are

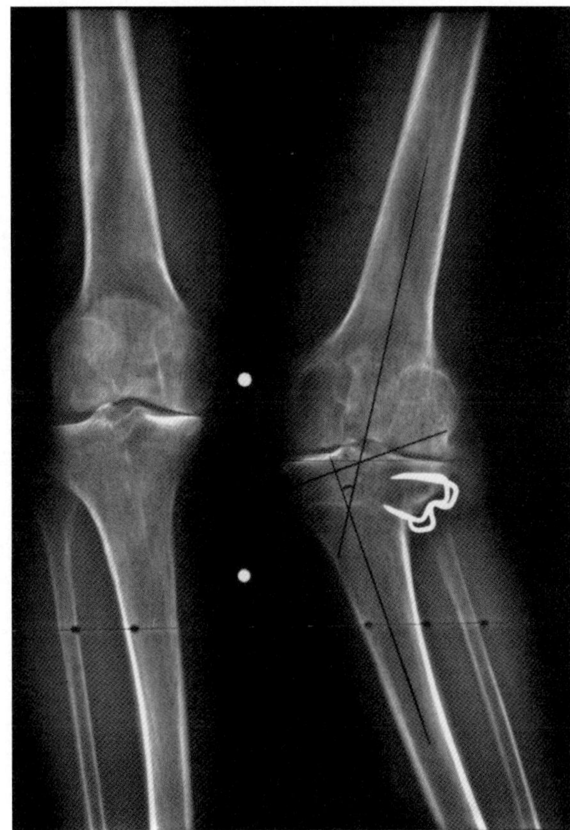

Fig. 6-95 Standing anteroposterior (AP) radiograph demonstrating loss of correction in the left knee following osteotomy with staple fixation. Note the staples have partially pulled out.

evident on radiographs (see Fig. 6-94). CT with coronal and sagittal reformatting is ideal to follow healing in patients with suspected nonunion.

Loss of correction or improper realignment is evident on radiographs. Preoperative measurements can be compared with postoperative measurements on standing images. The normal 5- to 7-degree valgus angle should be achieved if not slightly over corrected to 10 degrees (see Fig. 6-95).

Imaging of complications can be approached using the same techniques described in Table 6-5.

## Suggested Reading

Coventry MB. Upper tibia osteotomy for osteoarthritis. *J Bone Joint Surg*. 1985;67A:1136–1140.

Jackson JP, Waugh W. The technique and complications of upper tibial osteotomy. *J Bone Joint Surg*. 1974;56B: 236–245.

Finkelstein JA, Gross AE, Davis A. Varus osteotomy of the distal part of the femur. *J Bone Joint Surg*. 1996;78A:1348–1352.

MacDonald JH, Agarwal S, Lorie MP, et al. Knee arthrodesis. *J Am Acad Orthop Surg*. 2006;14:154–163.

Turner RS, Griffiths H, Heatley FW. The incidence of deep-vein thrombosis after upper tibial osteotomy. *J Bone Joint Surg*. 1993;75B:942–944.

# 7
# Tibial and Fibular Shafts

Chapter 6 included proximal tibial fractures. Chapter 8 will review distal fractures about the ankle. This chapter will focus on the shaft of the tibia and fibula with respect to fracture management and leg length discrepancy.

## Trauma

Fractures of the tibial and fibular shafts are among the most common long bone fractures in adults (average age 37), teenage males (15% of all fractures), and comprise 4% to 5% of all childhood fractures. Fibular fractures are usually associated with tibial fractures (see Fig. 7-1). Therefore, the focus will be on tibial injuries. The distal two thirds of the tibia is most often involved. Also, the lower leg is the most common site of combined osseous and soft tissue injury. The relatively exposed subcutaneous location of the tibia makes it vulnerable to direct high-velocity injury such as motor vehicle accidents or gunshot wounds. Direct trauma usually results in transverse, segmental, or comminuted fracture of the tibia with associated fibular fractures. Indirect trauma generally results in oblique or spiral fractures (see Fig. 7-2). Overuse injuries may also result in stress fractures of the tibia and fibula. Fractures should be described by precise anatomic location, pattern of the fracture line, position of the fragments, degree of comminution, and whether they are open or closed.

### Suggested Reading


Court-Brown CM, McBirnie J. The epidemiology of tibial fractures. *J Bone Joint Surg*. 1995;77B:417–421.


## Classification

Treatment of tibial shaft fractures includes closed and open approaches. Treatment choice is based on the type of fracture, whether open or closed, patient status, and surgical preference. There are multiple classification systems designed to assist with treatment and prognosis. Gustilo and Anderson's classification is specifically designed for open wounds, a common feature of tibial shaft fractures.

### Orthopaedic Trauma Association classification

**Type A:** Simple fractures
- A1—spiral fractures (Fig. 7-2)
- A2—oblique fractures
- A3—transverse fractures (see Fig. 7-3)

**Type B:** Wedge fractures (see Fig. 7-4)
- B1—spiral wedge fractures
- B2—intact bending wedge fractures
- B3—comminuted wedge fractures

**Type C:** Complex fractures (see Fig. 7-5)
- C1—spiral complex fractures
- C2—segmental complex fractures

### Gustilo and Anderson classification

**Type I:** Wound clean and $<1$ cm
**Type II:** Wound larger than 1 cm without extensive soft tissue damage
**Type IIIA:** Extensive soft tissue wound ($\geq 10$ cm), periosteum intact
**Type IIIB:** Periosteal stripping requiring flap coverage
**Type IIIC:** Above plus vascular injury requiring vessel repair (see Fig. 7-6)

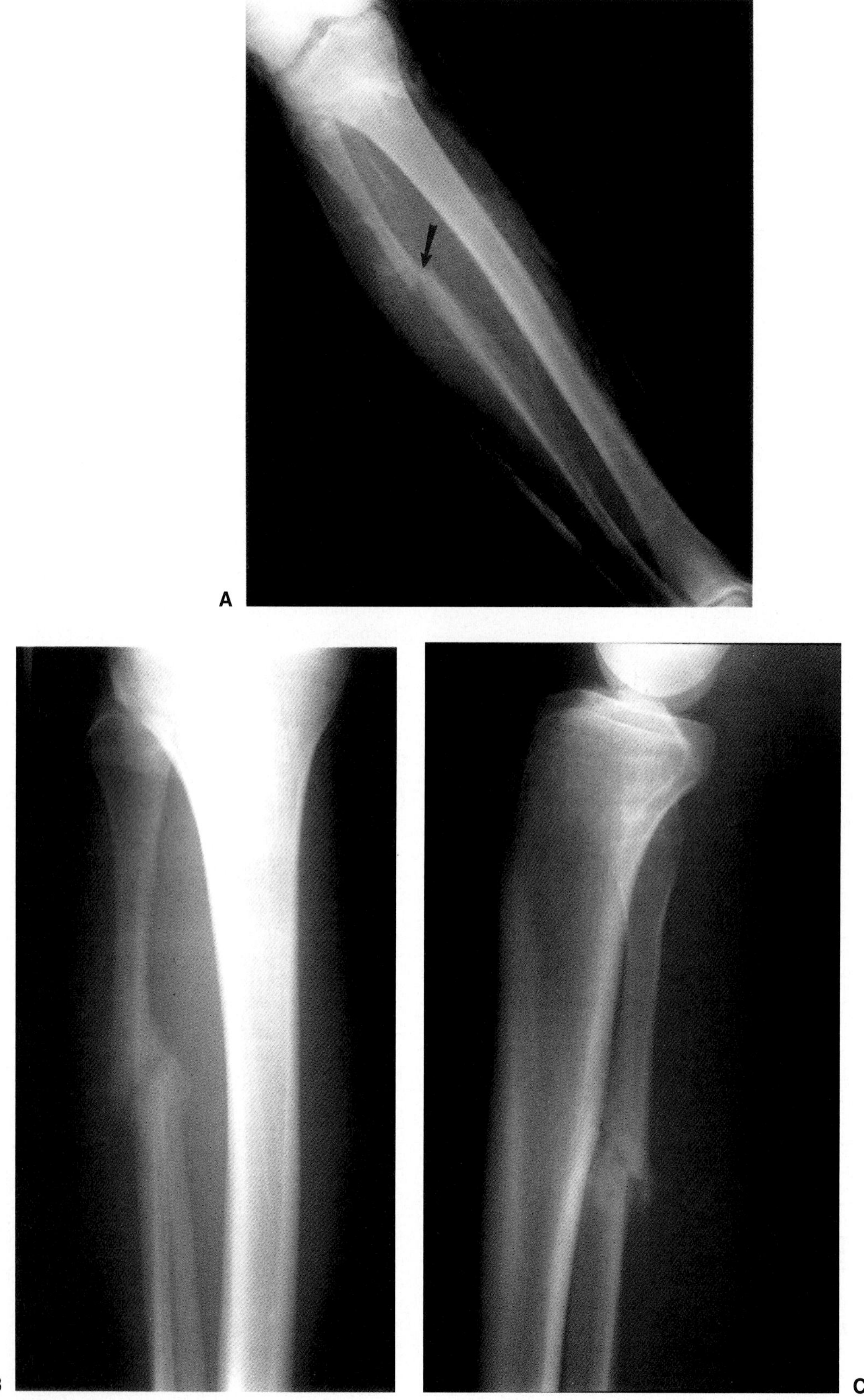


Fig. 7-1 A: Isolated fibular fracture (*arrow*) due to a direct blow. Cast immobilization. Anteroposterior (AP) (B) and lateral (C) radiographs at 6 weeks demonstrate organizing callus formation.

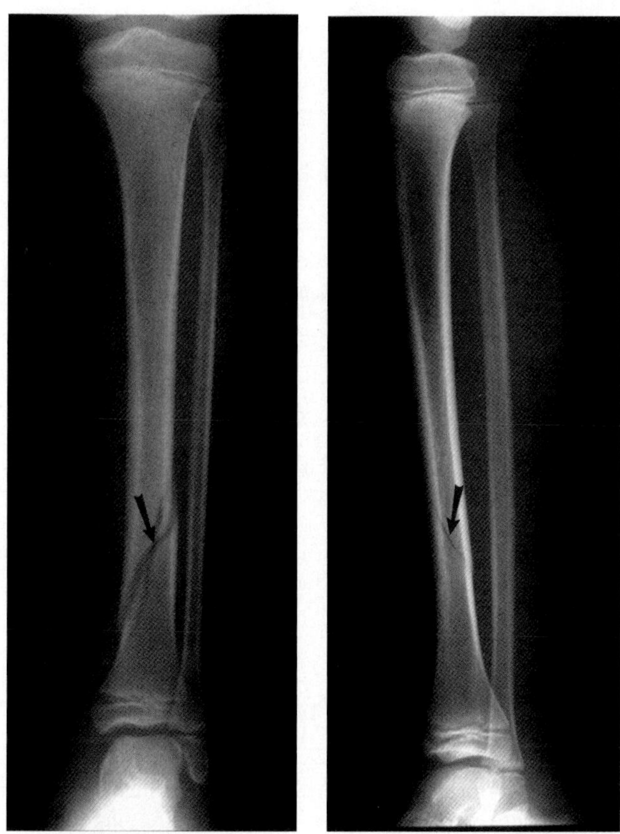


Fig. 7-2 Minimally displaced spiral fracture of the distal tibia due to a twisting injury in soccer. Anteroposterior (AP) (A) and lateral (B) radiographs demonstrate the tibial fracture (*arrow*) with no associated fibular fracture.

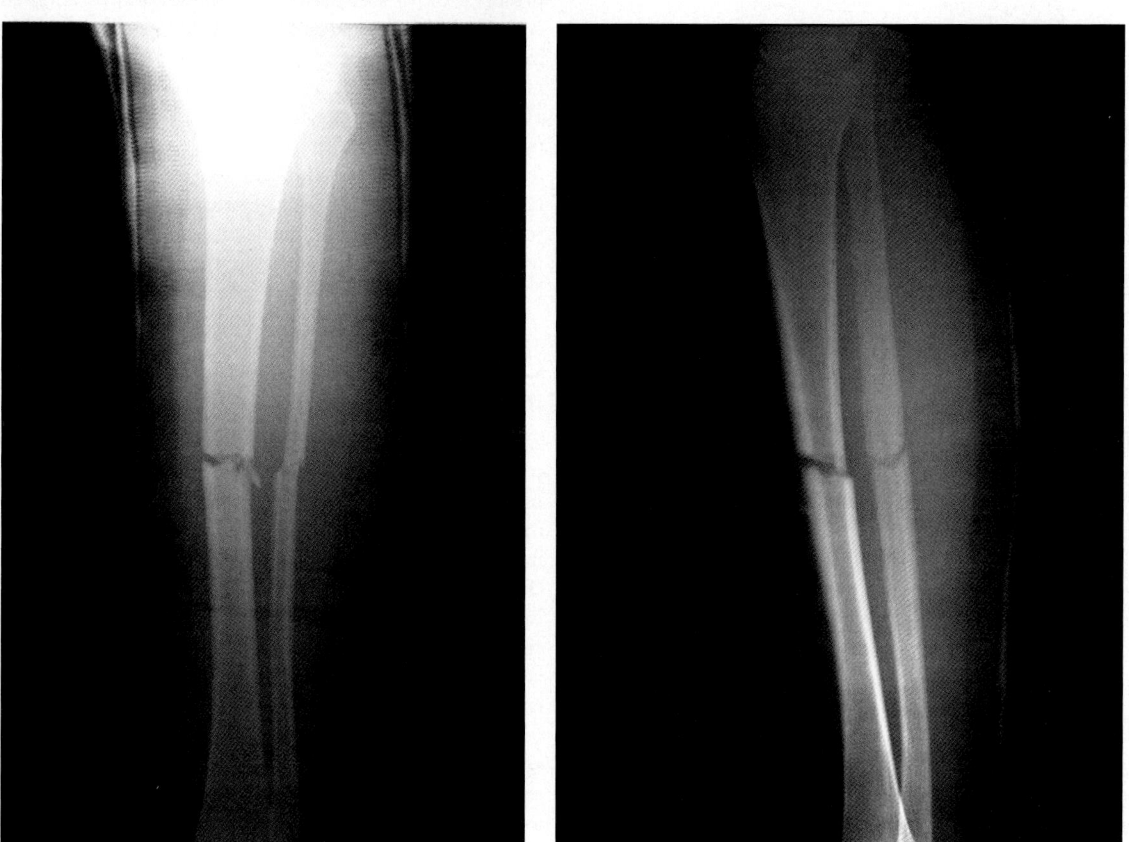


Fig. 7-3 Anteroposterior (AP) (A) and lateral (B) radiographs of minimally displaced transverse fractures of the mid tibia and fibula with cast immobilization.

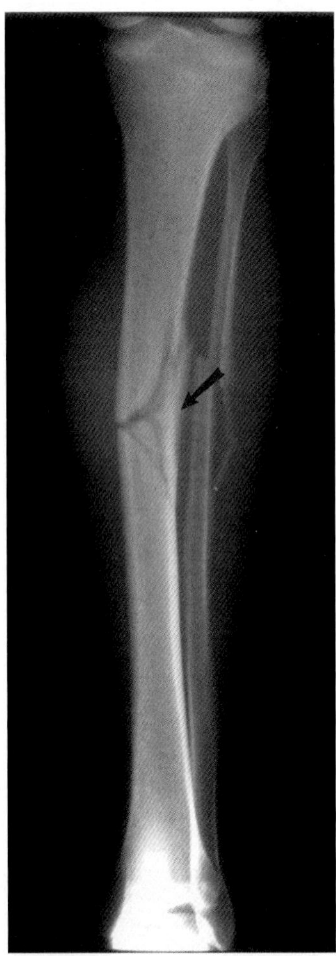

Fig. 7-4 Anteroposterior (AP) radiograph demonstrating a wedge (butterfly fragment) fracture (*arrow*) of the proximal tibia with adjacent comminuted fibular fracture.

## Suggested Reading

Gustilo RB, Anderson JT. Prevention of infection in treatment of 1025 open fractures of the long bones. *J Bone Joint Surg.* 1976;58A:453–458.

Lenehan B, Fleming P, Walsh S, et al. Tibial-shaft fractures in amateur footballers. *Br J Sports Med.* 2003;37:176–178.

Muller ME, Nazarin D, Koch P, et al. *Comprehensive classification of fracture of the long bones*. Springer-Verlag: Berlin; 1990.

Okike K, Bhattacharyya T. Trends in management of open fractures. *J Bone Joint Surg.* 2006;88A:2739–2748.

# Imaging Techniques

Imaging of tibial and fibular shaft injuries can be accomplished with anteroposterior (AP) and lateral radiographs for complete fractures (Figs. 7-1 to 7-5). Knee and ankle should be included. Subtle stress injuries or undisplaced fractures may be more easily assessed with magnetic resonance imaging (MRI). Radionuclide scans can also be useful for detection of subtle fractures. However, magnetic resonance (MR) features are typically more specific. Angiography may be required in patients with advanced soft tissue injury who may require vascular repair (Gustilo and Anderson IIIC) (Fig. 7-6).

## Suggested Reading

Bender CE, Campbell DC, Berquist TH. The tibia, fibula and calf. In: Berquist TH, ed. *Imaging of orthopaedic trauma*, 2nd ed. New York: Raven Press; 1992:433–454.

Mashru RP, Herman MJ, Pizzutillo PD. Tibia shaft fractures in children and adolescents. *J Am Acad Orthop Surg.* 2005;13: 345–352.

Tervonen O, Junila J, Ojala R. MR imaging of tibial-shaft fractures. A potential method for early visualization of delayed union. *Acta Radiol.* 1999;40:410–414.

# Treatment Options

Goals for management of tibial fractures include maintaining length, restoring normal weight-bearing alignment, and preservation of soft tissues. Alignment and rotation should be corrected to near anatomic position. The ankle and knee joints must be parallel. There should be no >5 degrees of varus or valgus angulation, 10 degrees of anterior or posterior angulation, 10 degrees of rotation, and 1 cm or less of leg length discrepancy (see Fig. 7-7). In children younger than 8 years, apposition is less critical. In older children, at least 50% apposition should be achieved (see Fig. 7-8). Treatment options include closed reduction with cast or brace immobilization, external fixation, intramedullary nailing, and open reduction with plate and screw fixation.

### Closed Reduction with Cast or Brace Immobilization

Initially, all tibial fractures should be treated with a long posterior splint with the knee in flexion and the ankle in neutral position. Compartment syndrome is a concern and should be monitored. Stable undisplaced fractures can be treated with cast immobilization in 3 to 5 days after initial swelling has decreased (Fig. 7-8). There are several cast approaches including long leg casts with slight knee flexion and patellar-tendon bearing (PTB) casts (see Fig. 7-9). In either situation, early weight bearing is important. In adolescents long leg cast immobilization for 6 weeks is followed by progressive weight bearing in a PTB cast for an additional 4 to 6 weeks. A brace can also be used after several weeks of cast immobilization to increase joint motion and facilitate weight bearing. Serial radiographs are important to assure fracture stability. Callus begins to form at approximately 6 to 8 weeks following the injury.

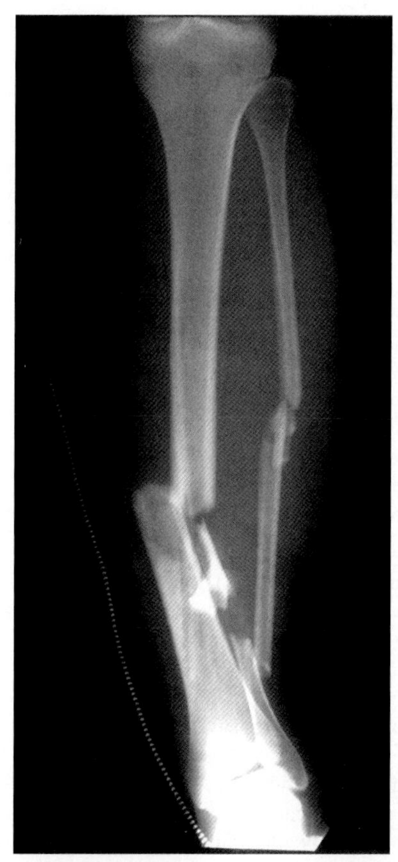

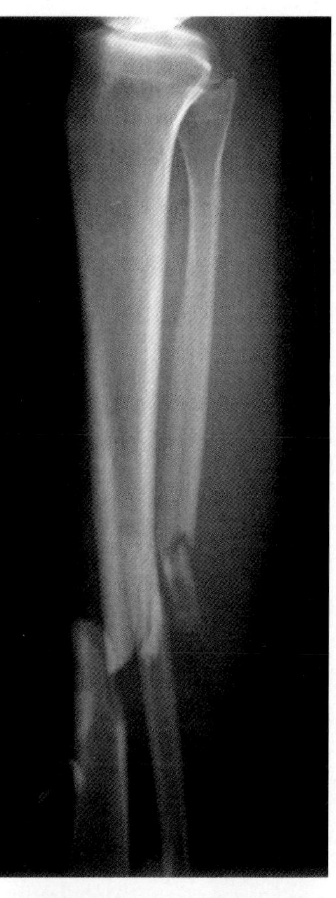

Fig. 7-5 Complex open fracture. Anteroposterior (AP) (A) and lateral (B) radiographs of a complex open fracture with displaced comminuted fractures of the tibia and a comminuted segmental fibular fracture.

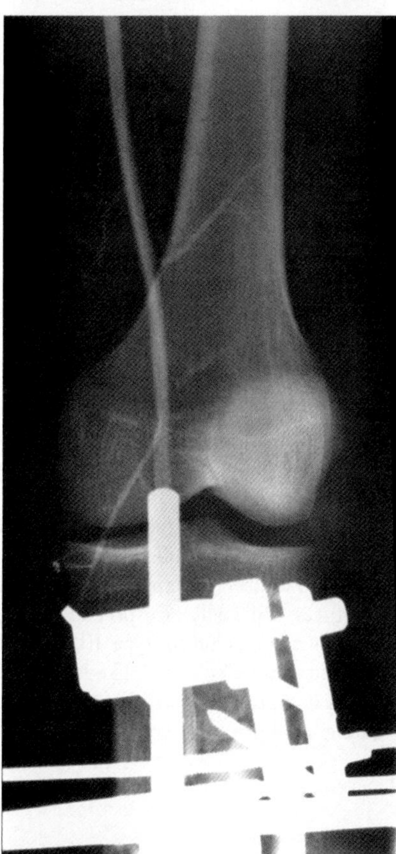

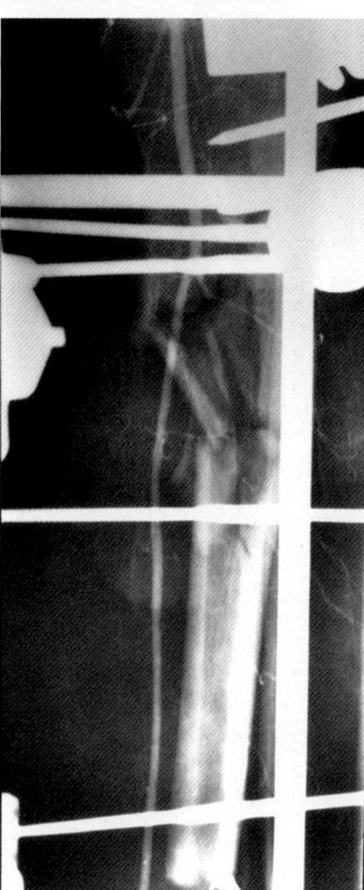

Fig. 7-6 Gustilo and Anderson type IIIC injury. Anteroposterior (AP) angiographic views of the knee (A) and leg (B) demonstrating a complex open fracture with occlusion of all but the posterior tibial artery below the trifurcation.

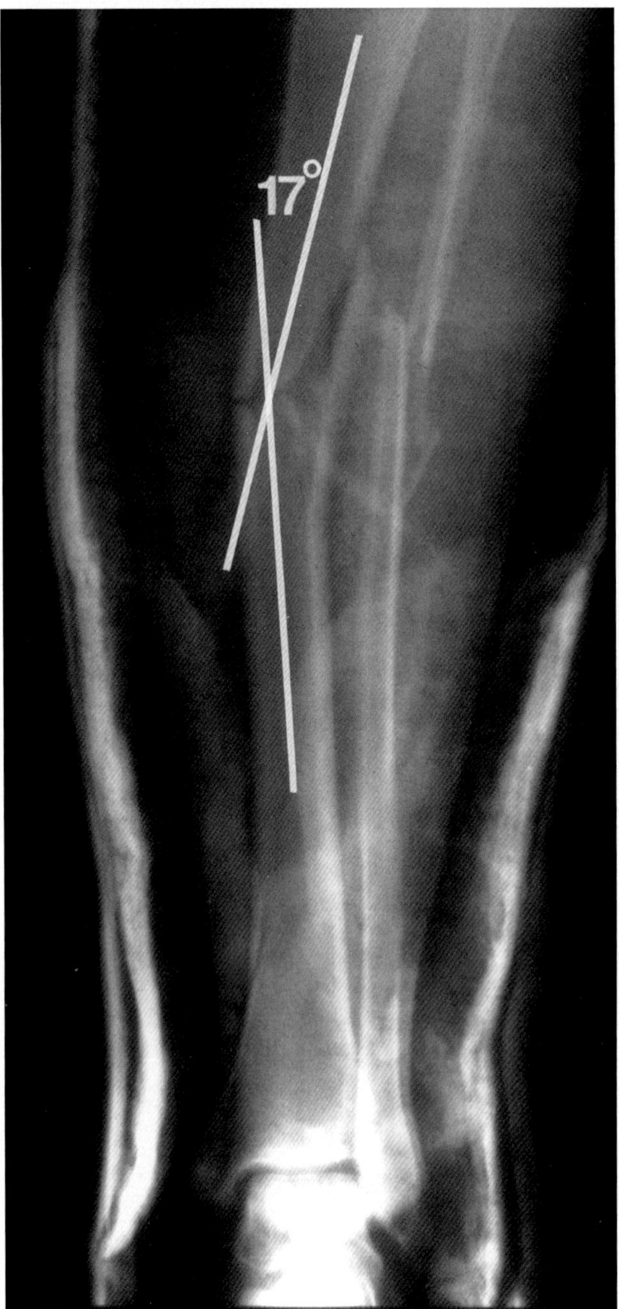


Fig. 7-7 Anteroposterior (AP) radiograph following closed reduction of comminuted mid tibial and fibular fractures. There is 17 degrees of medial angulation at the tibial fracture site and the ankle is not parallel to the knee.

## External Fixation

External fixation approaches are commonly used with tibial shaft fractures due to the relatively high frequency of open fractures with varying degrees of soft tissue injury. Fixation is easily applied and allows adjustability of fragments and access to soft tissue wounds (see Fig. 7-10). Pin or wire placement is accomplished to avoid critical anatomic structures such as neurovascular areas (see Fig. 7-11).

### Indications for external fixation

- Open fractures with soft tissue injuries (see Fig. 7-12)
- Management of fractures with bone loss
- Closed severely unstable fractures
- Closed fractures in patients with:
  - Burns
  - Head injuries
  - Neurosensory deficits
  - Compartment syndromes
- Bone lengthening procedures
- Treatment of the following:
  - Nonunion
  - Infected nonunion
  - Malunion

External fixation (see Chapter 2) is accomplished using unilateral, ring, or hybrid fixation devices. There are advantages and disadvantages to external fixation techniques.

### Advantages

- Stabilization away from fracture site
- Wound access
- Wide variety of fixation options
- Adjustable during treatment
- Minimal interference with adjacent joints
- Mobilization of patients with weight bearing

### Disadvantages

- Soft tissue injury and contractures
- Pin tract infection
- Loss of reduction

External fixation can be converted to intramedullary nail fixation (see Fig. 7-13) or uncommonly internal fixation with plate and screw fixation.

## Intramedullary Nail Fixation

Intramedullary nails (see Fig. 7-14) are commonly used in adult tibial fractures with exception of proximal third fractures where results are less than optimal. Intramedullary nails may be placed with or without reaming using open or closed techniques. In children, this technique has not been used extensively due to the potential of proximal physeal injury and growth disturbance. Flexible intramedullary nails can be used in certain situations. Intramedullary techniques are most optimal with closed fractures. The risk of infection is increased with open fractures, especially Gustilo and Anderson type II or III injuries. However, excluding type IIIB and IIIC injuries, the success of intramedullary nail fixation of both closed and open fractures is high. In closed fractures reaming is preferred with healing at 4 months compared to longer

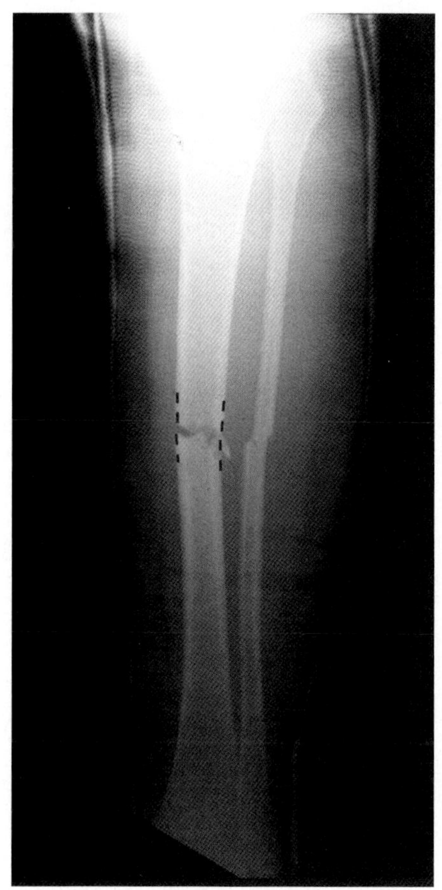

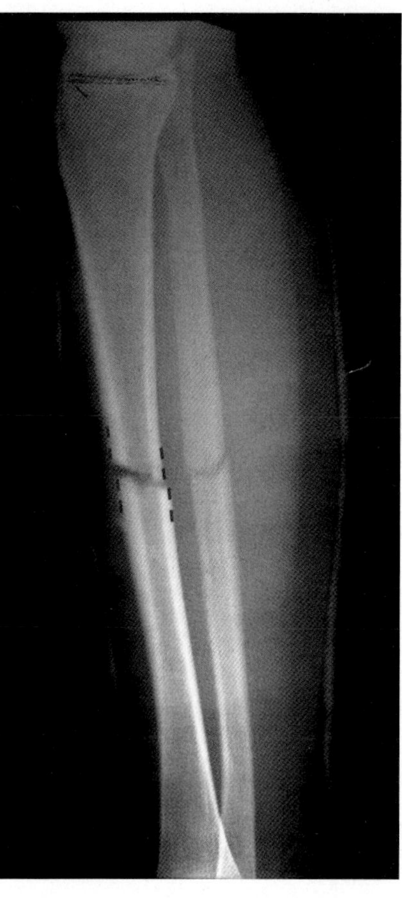

Fig. 7-8 Anteroposterior (AP) (A) and lateral (B) radiographs following closed reduction in a teenager with transverse mid shaft fractures of the tibia and fibula. There is excellent cortical apposition (*broken lines*).

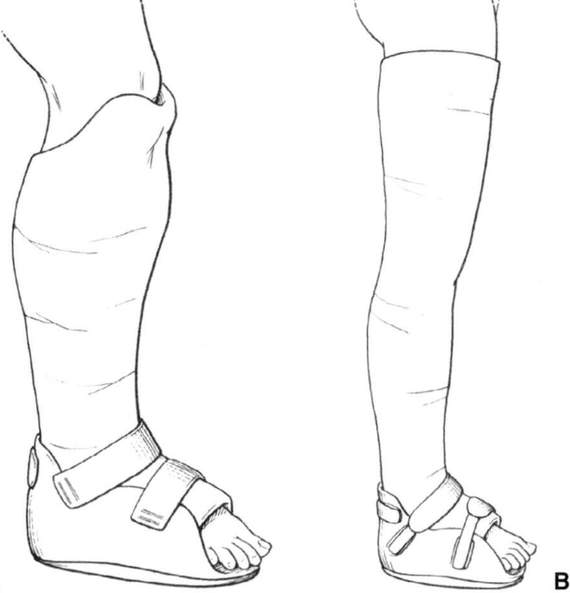

Fig. 7-9 Illustration of a patellar-tendon bearing cast (A) and long leg cast (B).

healing times for unreamed nail fixation (6.5 months) (see Fig. 7-15).

## Plate and Screw Fixation

Open reduction with internal fixation using plate and screw fixation (see Fig. 7-16) has largely been replaced by intramedullary nails. However, there are certain indications for plate and screw techniques, which are improved with the new less invasive stabilization systems and locking plates (see Fig. 7-17).

### Indications

Noncomminuted fractures
Fractures extending into the knee or ankle
Nonunion or malunion

### Advantages

Reduced mean healing time
Improved anatomic reduction

### Disadvantages

Increased risk of infection
Longer non–weight bearing to prevent implant failure
Refracture through screw tracts

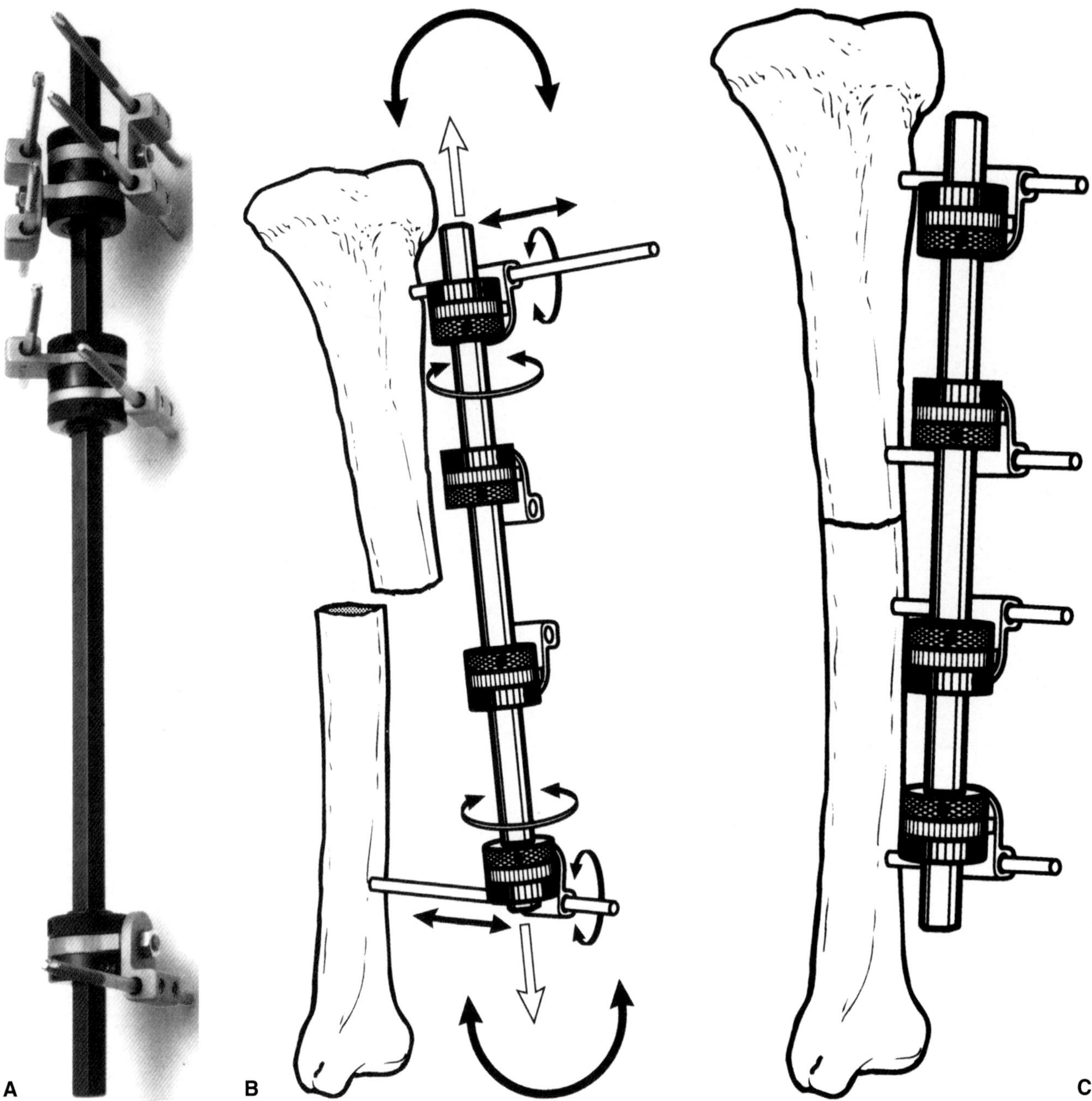


Fig. 7-10 A: Hex-Fix unilateral fixator. External fixation allows fragment position (B) to be adjusted (C) and access to open wounds. D: Ilizarov ring fixator. (Courtesy Smith and Nephew Richards, Memphis, Tennessee.)

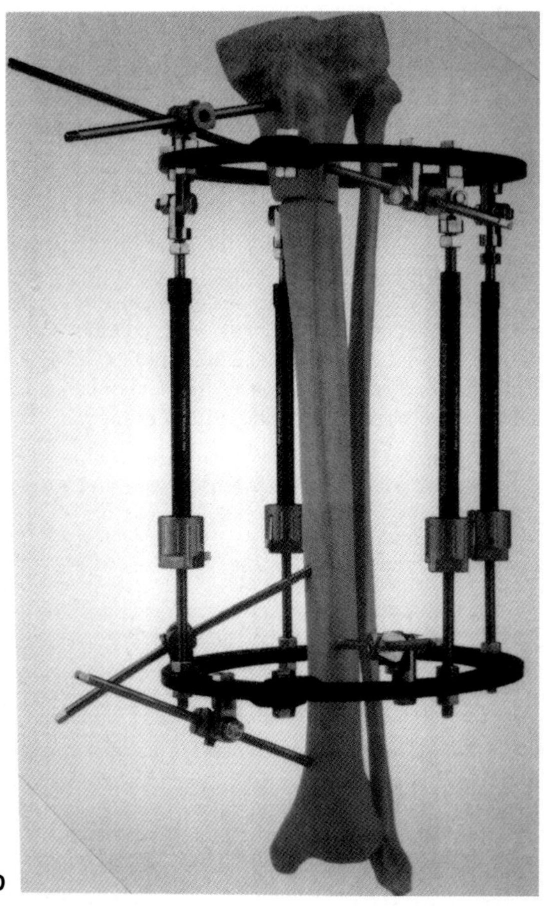


Fig. 7-10 *(Continued)*

## Suggested Reading


Behrens F. General theory and principles of external fixation. *Clin Orthop*. 1989;241:15–23.

Finkemeier CG, Schmidt AH, Kyle RF, et al. A prospective randomized study of intramedullary nails inserted with and without reaming for treatment of open and closed fractures of the tibial shaft. *J Orthop Trauma*. 2000;14:187–193.

Giannoudis PV, Papkostidis C, Roberts C. A review of management of open fractures of the tibia and femur. *J Bone Joint Surg*. 2006;88B:281–289.

Lang GJ, Cohen BE, Bosse MJ, et al. Proximal third tibial fractures. *Clin Orthop*. 1995;315:64–74.

Mashru RP, Herman MJ, Pizzutillo PD. Tibial-shaft fractures in children and adolescents. *J Am Acad Orthop Surg*. 2005;13: 345–352.

McGraw JM, Lim EV. Treatment of open tibial-shaft fractures. External fixation and secondary intramedullary nailing. *J Bone Joint Surg*. 1988;70A:900–911.

Smith WR, Ziran BH, Angel JO, et al. Locking Plates: Tips and tricks. *J Bone Joint Surg*. 2007;89A:2298–2307.

Vallamshetla VRP, De Silva U, Bache CE, et al. Flexible intramedullary nails for unstable tibial fractures in children. *J Bone Joint Surg*. 2006;88B:536–540.


## Postoperative Imaging and Complications

Complications following fractures of the tibial shaft with or without associated fibular fractures are related to the extent

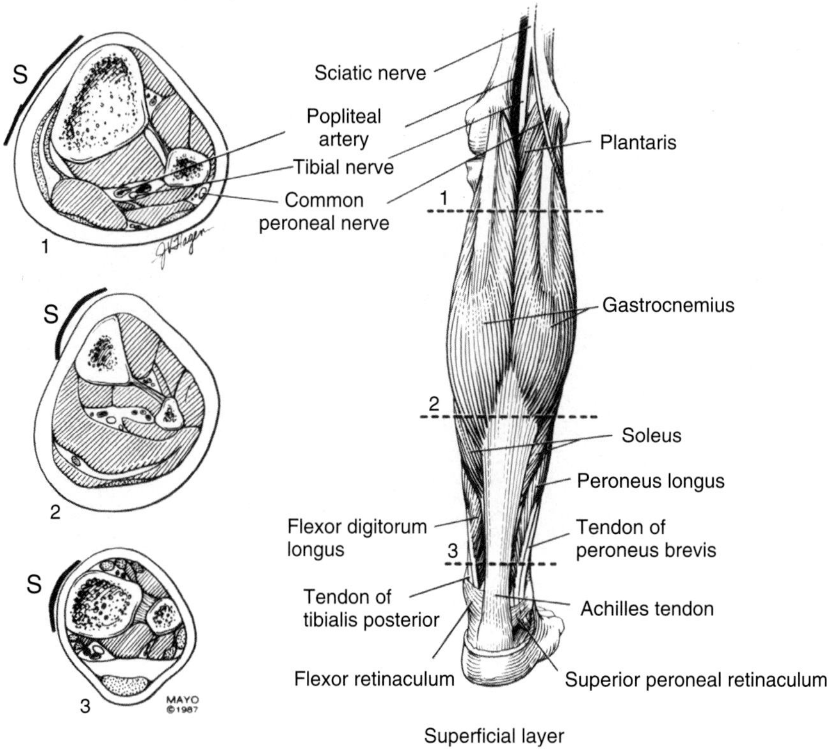

Fig. 7-11 Anatomic illustration of the leg with axial anatomy at three levels showing the regions for safe (S) pin placement at these levels.

of osseous and soft tissue injury and the treatment method or methods selected. In any case, close radiographic follow-up is required to assure stable position of the fragments (see Fig. 7-18). Other complications require additional imaging techniques depending on the suspected problem.

## Infection

Infection is one of the most difficult problems, especially with open wounds. The incidence varies significantly with the type of injury (Gustilo and Anderson type I—1.4%; type II—3.6%, and type III—22.7%). The incidence of infection also varies with treatment selection. Deep infection occurs in 16.2%, pin tract infection in 32%, and chronic osteomyelitis develops in 4.2% of patients treated with external fixation (see Fig. 7-19). Deep infections in patients treated with unreamed (7% to 33%) and reamed nails (6.4%) also vary, although the incidence of chronic osteomyelitis is only 0.7% with either method. The data is somewhat skewed because patients with the worst open wounds are more likely to be treated, at least initially with external fixation.

Imaging of infections also varies depending on the type and extent of infection. Pin tract infections may be identified on serial radiographs or if the pin is removed by fluoroscopically positioned images down the barrel of the tract demonstrating ring sequestra. Deep infections, even in the presence of fixation devices, may be studied with MRI, computed tomography (CT), or combination radionuclide studies (see Fig. 7-20). Multiple approaches have been used with radionuclide imaging including three-phase bone scans with Technetium Tc 99 m

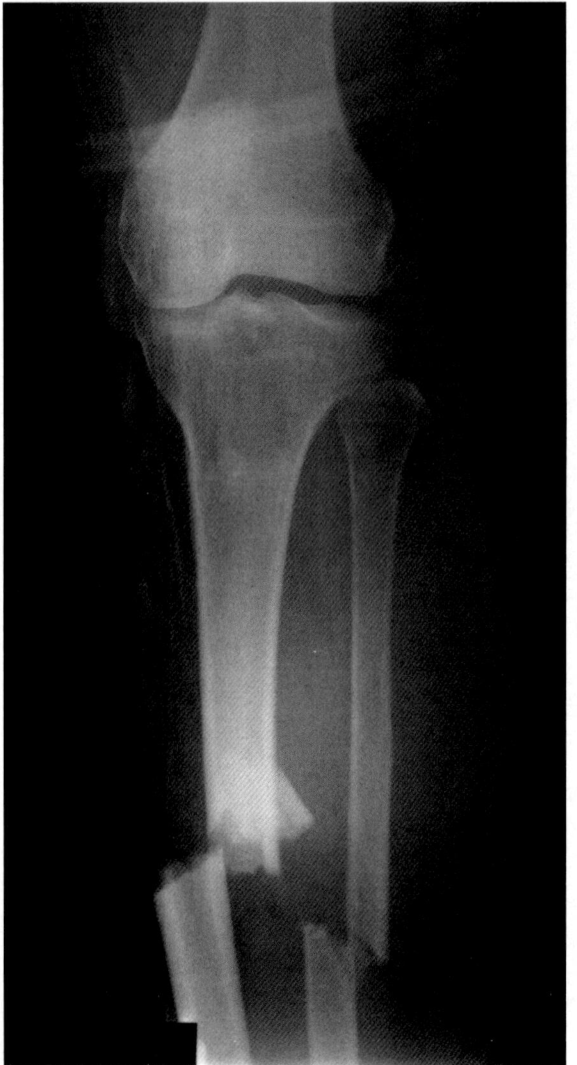

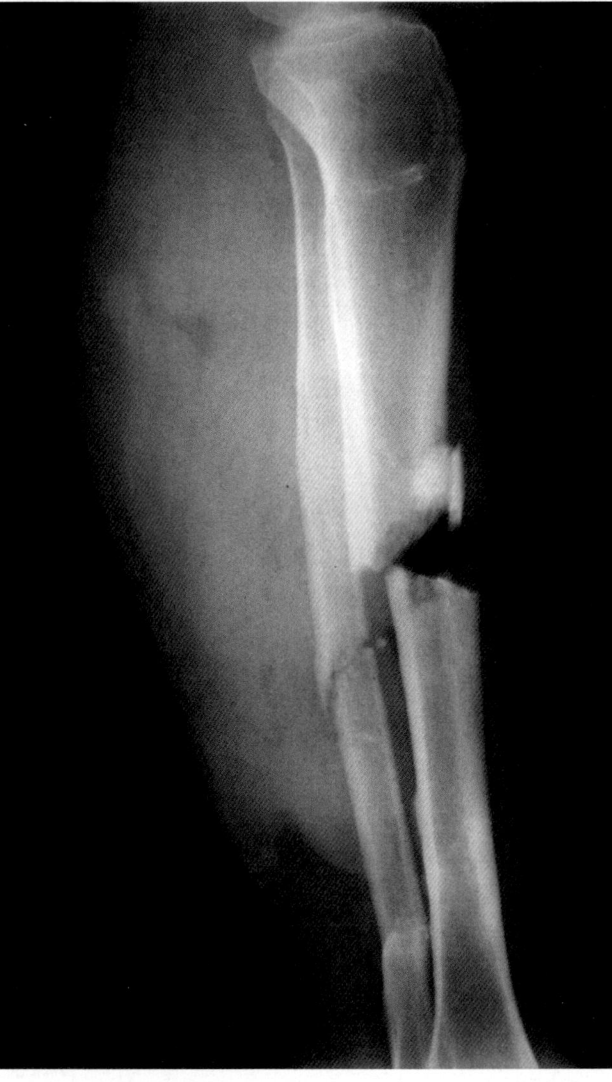

A B

Fig. 7-12 Complex fracture with open wound (Gustilo and Anderson type IIIA). Anteroposterior (AP) (A) and lateral (B) radiographs demonstrate complex mid tibial and fibular shaft fractures. Following external fixation with a ring fixator, the fragments, specifically the tibia, have been reduced (C). Radiographs 6 months (D) later show the healed fractures.

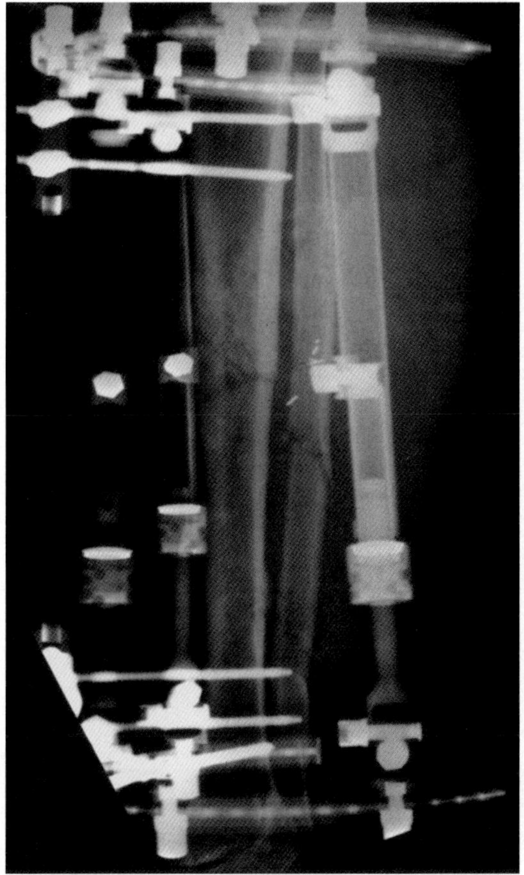

C

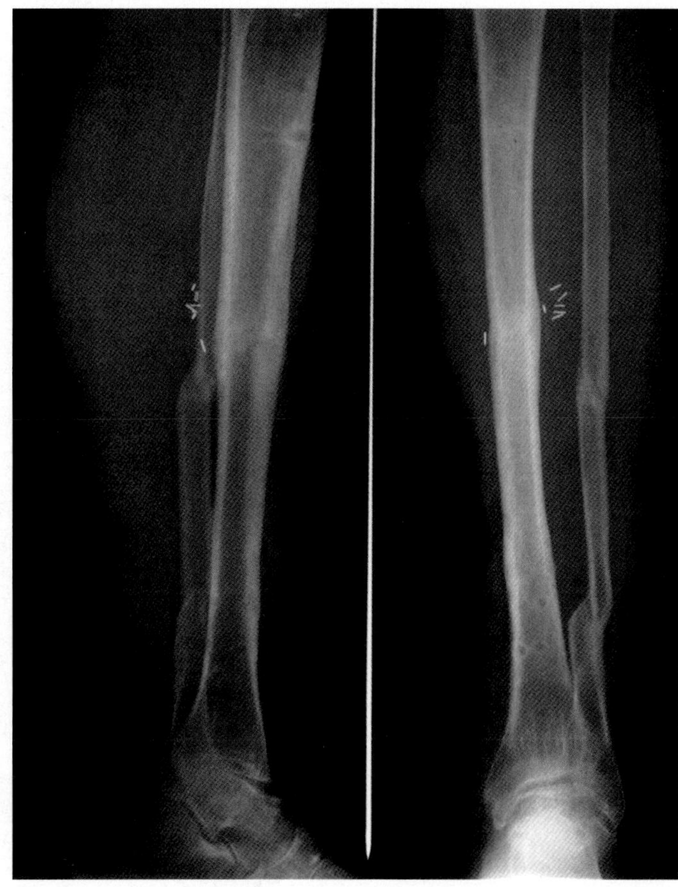

D

Fig. 7-12 *(Continued)*

methylene-diphosphonate (MDP), technetium-labeled white blood cells, antigranulocyte antibody–labeled technetium, Indium In 111–labeled white blood cells, and more recently, F-18 fluorodeoxyglucose positron emission tomography (PET) imaging. Technetium-labeled white blood cells disassociate at a rate of 5% to 7% per hour following injection. This results in significant unwanted background activity. PET studies report sensitivities of 92% and specificities in the 97% range (see Fig. 4–80). In 111–labeled white blood cells remain the gold standard in our practice. Sensitivity ranges from 84% to 96% with specificity exceeding 96%.

## Delayed Union/Nonunion

Delayed union or nonunion is not uncommon (Fig. 7-13). The former occurs in 15% of distal tibial fractures in adults. The incidence increases with more comminuted fractures. In children, delayed union occurs in only 2% of patients with closed fractures but increases to 25% with open fractures. Delayed union and nonunion also vary with treatment approaches. Problems with union result in a second procedure in 68% of patients treated with external fixation. Union rates are similar with reamed and unreamed intramedullary nails, although delayed union is reported in up to 22%. The incidence of nonunion is higher (31%) for proximal third tibial fractures treated with intramedullary nails. Loss of reduction and refracture occur in more than 20% of patients treated with external fixation.

Imaging of delayed union and nonunion can be accomplished with serial radiographs. However, CT with reformatted images is preferred in the coronal and sagittal planes to evaluate callus and healing (Fig. 7-20).

## Malunion

Poor results with alignment, rotation, leg length, and angulation also occur. Malunion with external fixation may occur in up to 20% of patients compared to 10% treated with unreamed and 6% treated with reamed intramedullary nails. The incidence is higher (84%) in proximal third tibial fractures treated with intramedullary nails and lower than any of the above-mentioned methods with plate fixation. Serial radiographs are generally adequate for evaluation of malunion.

## Implant Failure

Implant failure is uncommon, but as expected is more common with complex injuries (Fig. 7-16). Implant fracture or loosening

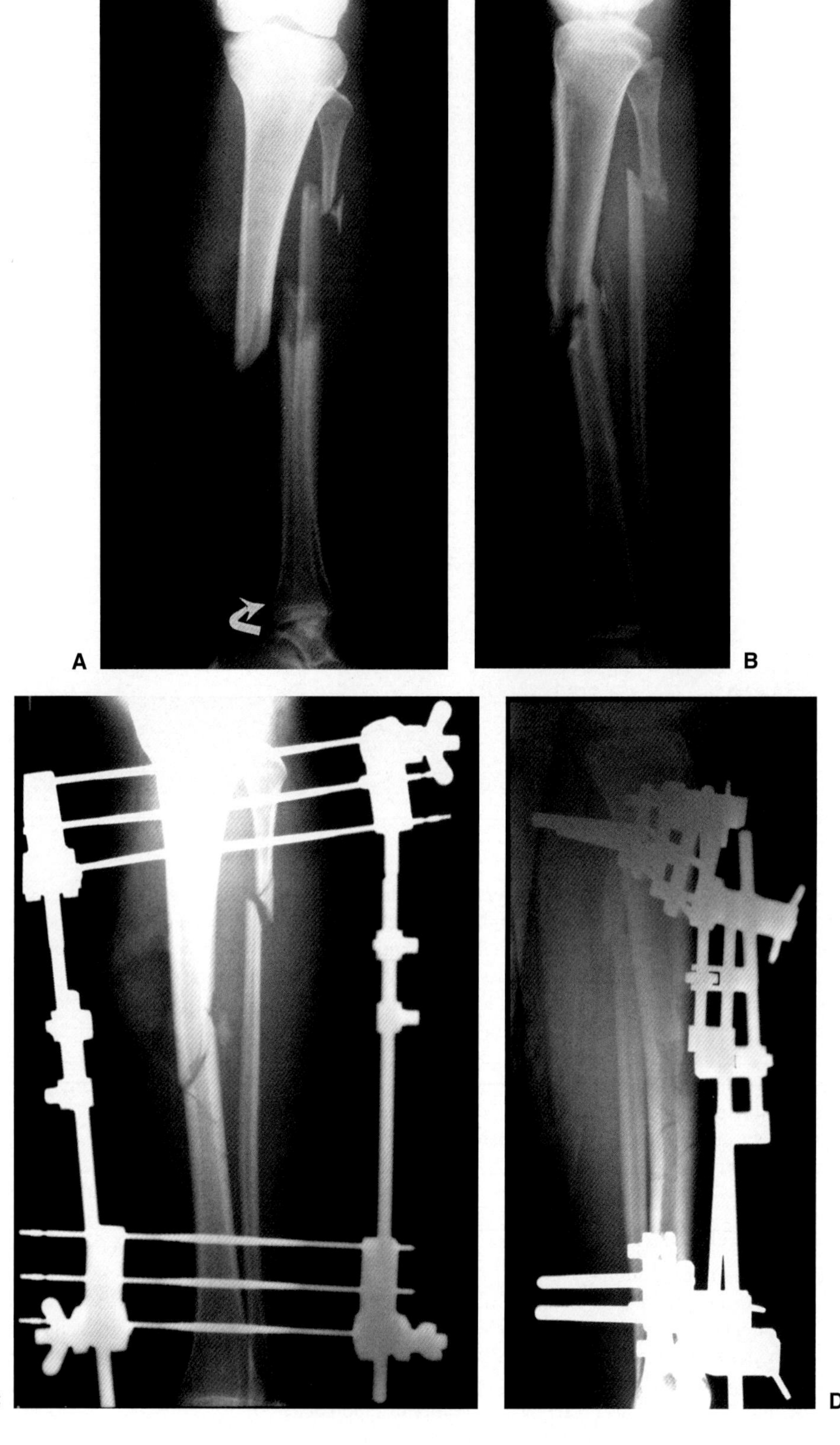


**Fig. 7-13** Anteroposterior (AP) (**A**) and lateral (**B**) radiographs of a complex fracture. Note the distal tibial fragment is externally rotated 90 degrees. AP (**C**) and lateral (**D**) radiographs following external fixation demonstrate good alignment of the tibial fracture. At 5 months (**E**), there are signs of nonunion with sclerosis of the fracture margins. Therefore, the fracture line was debrided and an intramedullary nail positioned (**F**). AP (**G**) and lateral (**H**) radiographs 2 months later demonstrate that the fracture has healed.

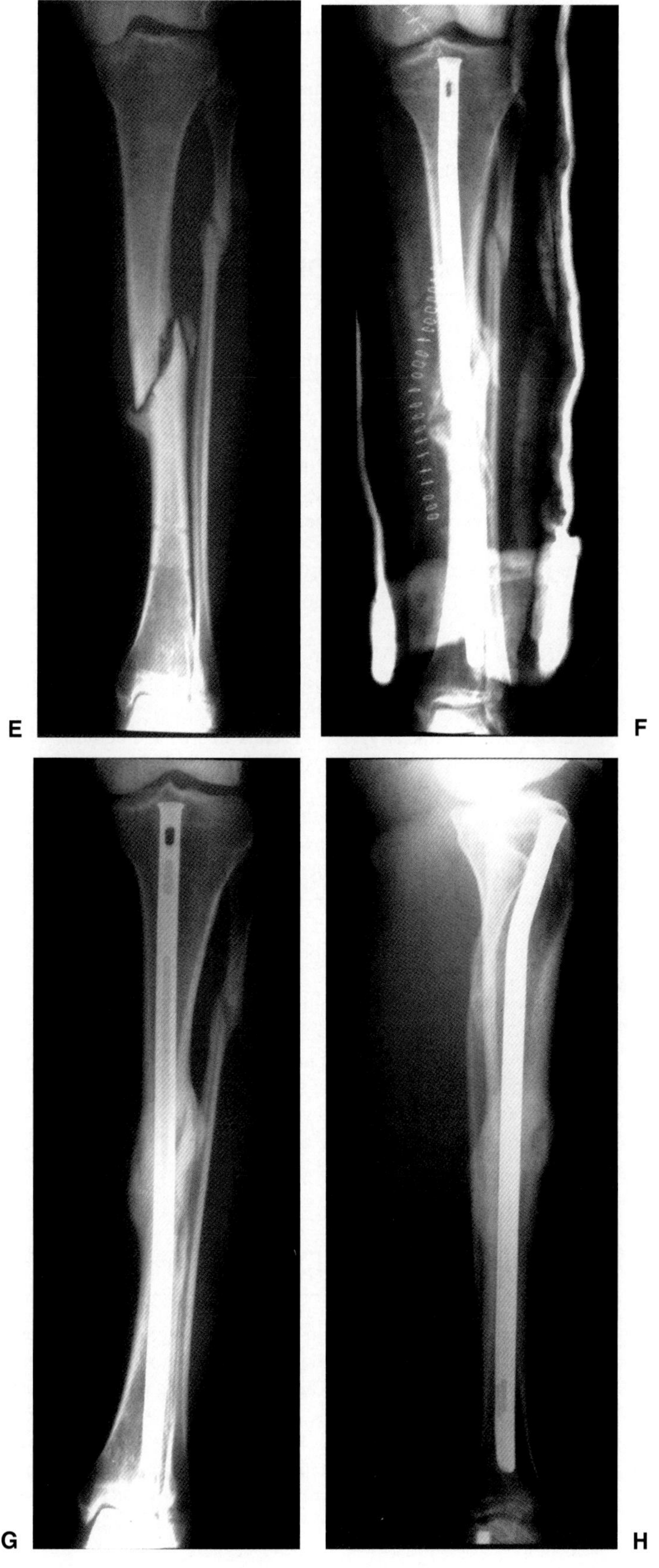


Fig. 7-13 (*Continued*)

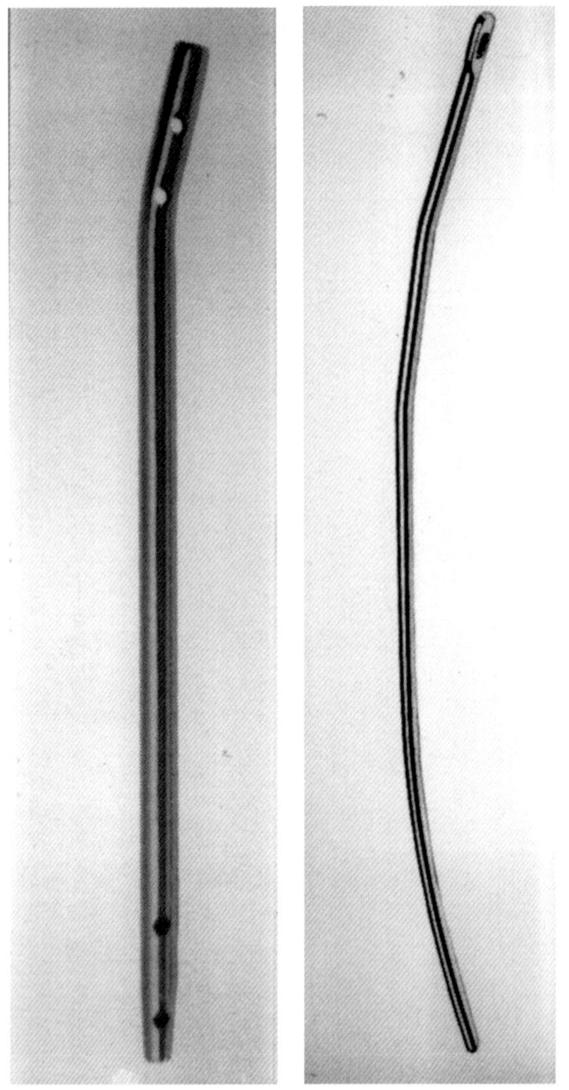


Fig. 7-14 Intramedullary nails. A: Russell Taylor nail with screw holes at both ends to allow dynamic or static fixation. B: Flexible Ender rod.

occurs in 2.7% of patients treated with external fixation, 3% of patients treated with reamed nails, and 12.4% of patients treated with unreamed nails (see Fig. 7-21). Serial radiographs are adequate for detection of implant failure.

### Compartment syndrome

Compartment syndrome can occur with open and closed fractures with an incidence ranging from 1% to 9%. The incidence is highest with more complex fractures. Soft tissue injury and arterial injury may result in bleeding or edema in the four compartments of the leg. The compartments include the anterior, lateral, superficial, and deep posterior compartments. Increased pressure (>25 to 30 mm Hg) may result in ischemia. Patients may have paresthesias, pain, and decreased pulses. Once diagnosed, patients are treated with fasciotomy to reduce the compartment pressure.

Neurovascular injuries may occur as isolated events due to the injury or treatment method in the absence of compartment syndrome. Depending on the implants, MRI or CT may be useful for imaging these complications.

## Suggested Reading

Giannoudis PV, Papakostidis C, Roberts C. A review of the management of open fractures of the tibia and fibula. *J Bone Joint Surg*. 2006;88B:281–289.

Gratz S, Rennen HHM, Boerman OC. $^{99m}$Tc-HMPAO-labeled autogenous vs. heterogenous leukocytes for imaging of infection. *J Nucl Med*. 2002;43:918–924.

Lang GJ, Cohen BE, Bosse MJ, et al. Proximal third tibial fractures. Should they be nailed. *Clin Orthop*. 1995;315: 64–74.

Mashru RP, Herman MJ, Pizzutillo PD. Tibial-shaft fractures in children and adolescents. *J Am Acad Orthop Surg*. 2005; 13:345–352.

McGraw JM, Lim EV. Treatment of open tibial-shaft fractures. External fixation with secondary intramedullary nailing. *J Bone Joint Surg*. 1988;70A:900–911.

Okike K, Bhattacharyya T. Trends in management of open fractures. A critical analysis. *J Bone Joint Surg*. 2006;88A: 2739–2748.

Termaat MF, Raijmakers PGHM, Scholten HJ, et al. The accuracy of diagnostic imaging for assessment of chronic osteomyelitis: A systematic review and meta-analysis. *J Bone Joint Surg*. 2005;87A:2464–2471.

Tornetta P, Templeman D. Compartment syndrome associated with tibial fracture. *J Bone Joint Surg*. 1996;78A:1438–1444.

Webb LX, Bosse MJ, Castillo RC, et al. Analysis of surgeon controlled variables in treatment of limb-threatening Type III open tibial diaphyseal fractures. *J Bone Joint Surg*. 2007; 89A:923–928.

Zalavras CG, Marcus RE, Levin LS, et al. Management of open fractures and subsequent complications. *J Bone Joint Surg*. 2007;89A:884–895.

# Leg Length Discrepancy

Approximately 15% of adults have some degree of leg length discrepancy. Leg length discrepancies are common problems with multiple etiologies. The need for surgical intervention depends on multiple factors. Discrepancy of 2 cm or less can be managed with shoe lifts. With this degree of discrepancy, abnormal gait results if not properly managed with orthotics. Epiphysodesis of the uninvolved extremity can be performed

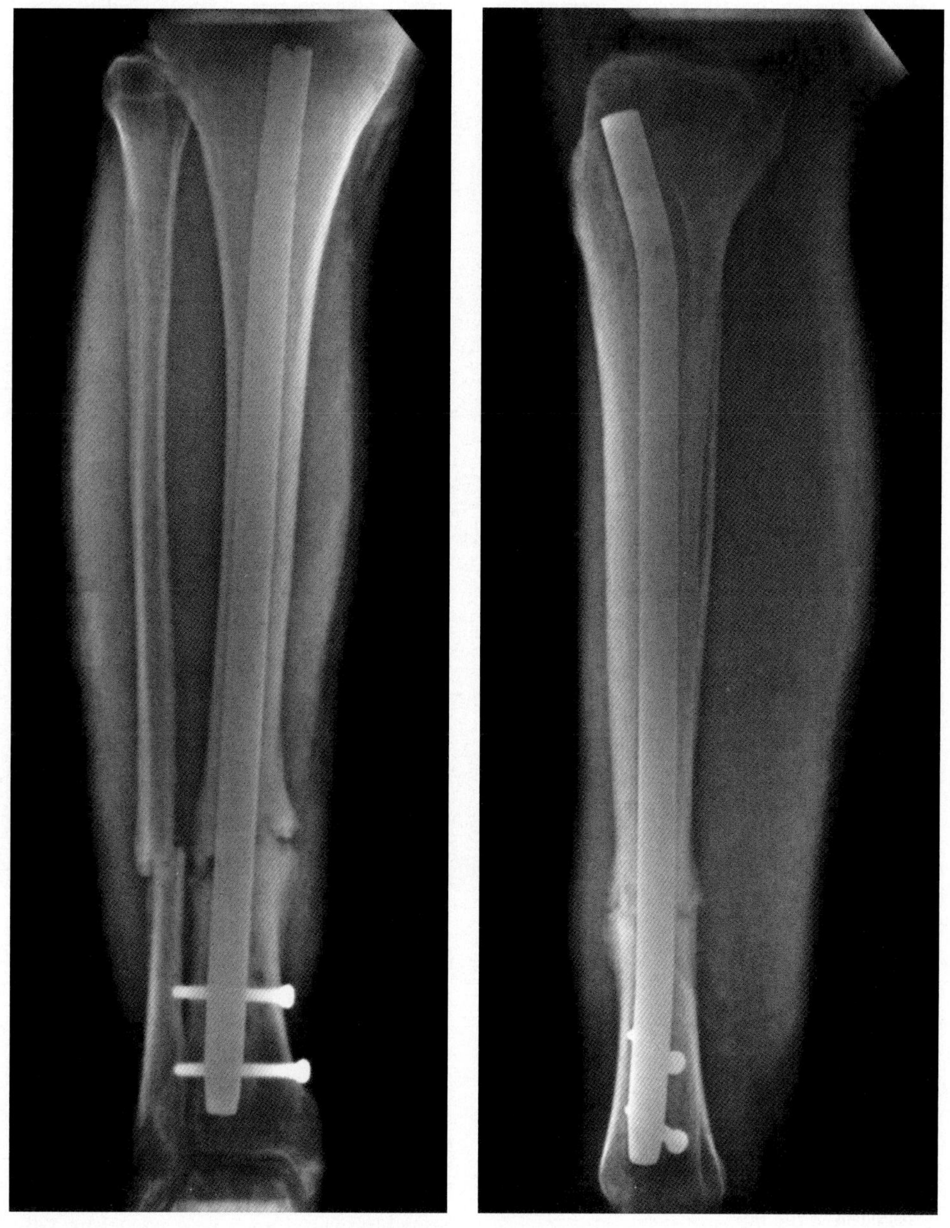


Fig. 7-15 Anteroposterior (AP) (A) and lateral (B) radiographs following intramedullary nail fixation of a distal tibial fracture. There are two distal screws with no proximal screws.

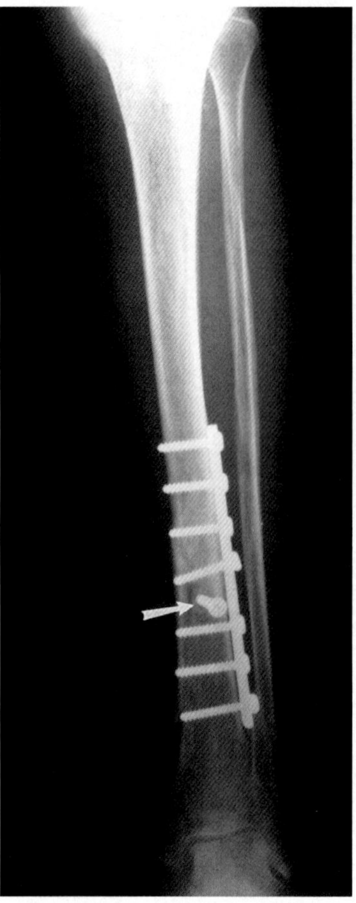


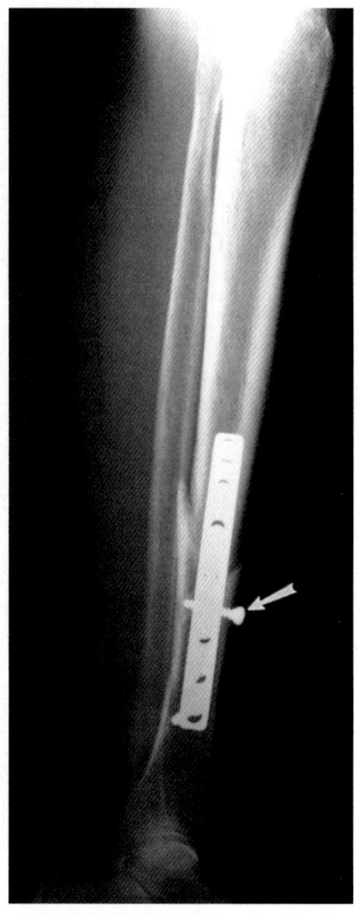


**Fig. 7-16** Comminuted wedge fracture of the distal tibia reduced with internal fixation using a dynamic compression plate and screws. There is an interfragmentary screw (*arrow*) as well that has pulled out and extends into the anterior soft tissues.

if the discrepancy is 5 cm or less. Step-cut osteotomy of the tibia may also be used for shortening. More significant length discrepancies may require lengthening procedures.

## Etiologies of Leg Length Discrepancy

**Congenital**

- Proximal focal femoral deficiency
- Developmental dysplasia of the hip
- Tibial hemimelia
- Congenital tibial bowing
- Hereditary exostoses

**Physeal abnormalities**

- Blount disease
- Ischemic physeal arrest
- Trauma
- Slipped capital femoral epiphysis

**Hyperemia**

- Post-traumatic overgrowth
- Chronic infection
- Inflammatory arthropathies
- Arteriovenous malformations

**Neuromuscular disorders**

- Poliomyelitis
- Spastic hemiplegia
- Spinal cord anomalies

## Suggested Reading

Broughton NS, Olney BW, Menelaus MB. Tibial shortening for leg length discrepancy. *J Bone Joint Surg*. 1989;71B: 242–245.

Guichet JM, Spivak JM, Trouilloud P, et al. Lower limb-length discrepancy. An epidemiologic study. *Clin Orthop*. 1991;272:235–241.

Stricker SJ, Hunt T. Evaluation of leg length discrepancy in children. *Int Pediatr*. 2004;19:134–142.

# Imaging Techniques

Radiographic, CT, and MRI techniques have all been used to define leg length discrepancy. Radiographic scanograms are

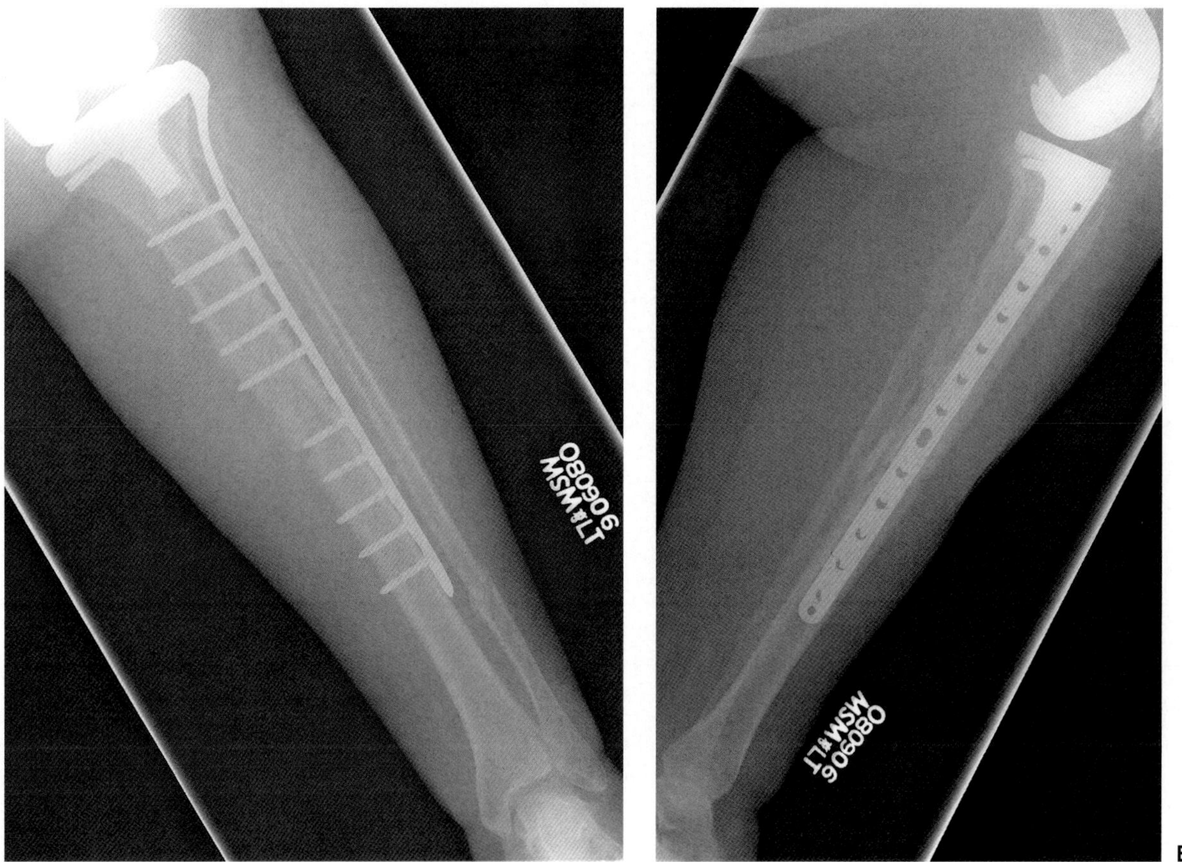

Fig. 7-17 Anteroposterior (AP) (A) and lateral (B) radiographs following locking plate fixation of a mid tibial fracture in a patient with a knee arthroplasty. There are associated fibular fractures.

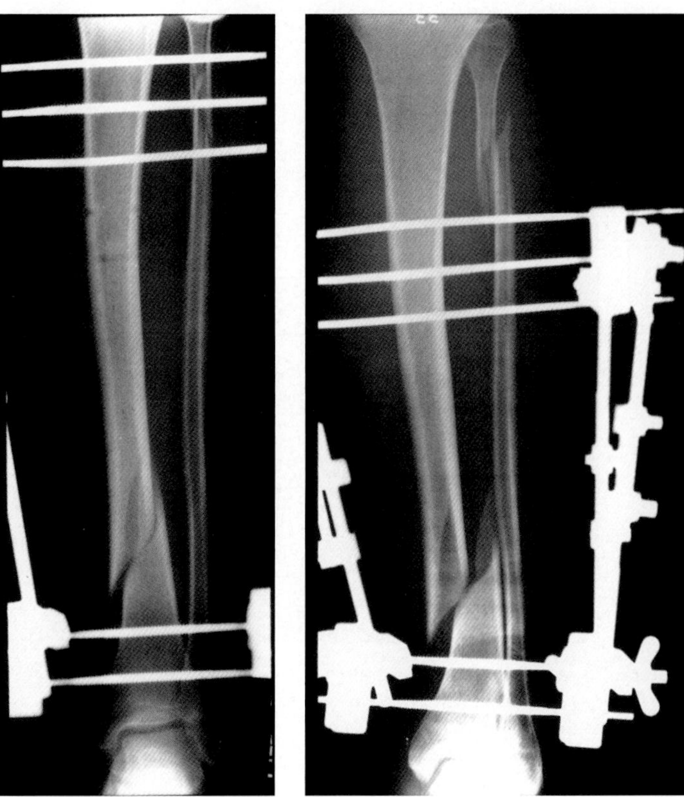

Fig. 7-18 External fixation of spiral fractures of the distal tibia and proximal fibula. A: Radiograph following positioning of the fixation device. B: Radiograph obtained the following day with loss of position and shortening.

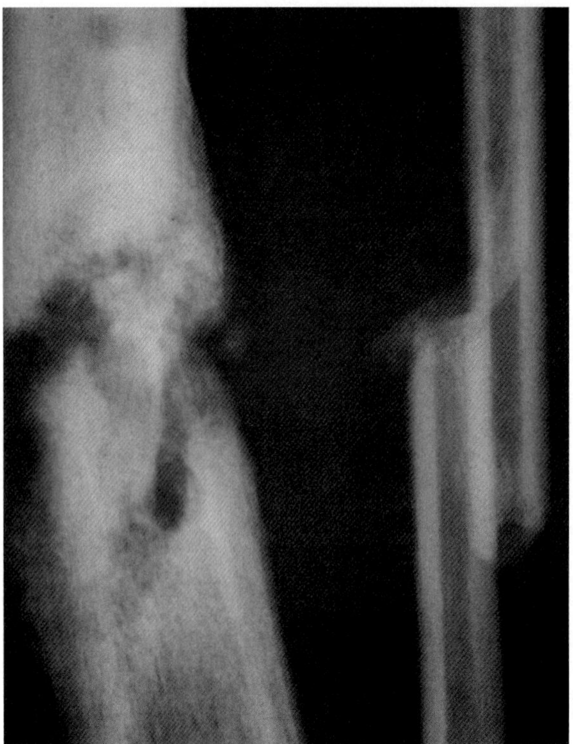

Fig. 7-19 Radiographic spot image of an infected nonunion. The external fixation device has been removed.

obtained with the patient supine and ruler between the legs. Three separate exposures are made centered over the hips, knees, and ankles to avoid magnification. This technique is most appropriate for older children who are able to maintain a fixed position during the exposures. Radiographic scanograms are also suboptimal in patients with angular deformities.

Biplanar CT scanograms are more appropriate in patients with angular deformities or joint contractures. CT studies can also be performed with lower radiation doses.

## Suggested Reading

Helms CA, McCarthy S. CT scanograms for measuring leg length discrepancy. *Radiology*. 1984;151:802.

Thaller PH, Baumgart R, Burghardt S, et al. Digital imaging in lower limb bone deformities-standards and new perspectives. *Int Congr Ser*. 2005;1281:154–158.

## Treatment Options

Treatment options vary with the underlying disorder and degree of leg length discrepancy. As noted earlier, discrepancy of 2 cm or less is treated conservatively. Discrepancy of 2 to 5 cm may be treated with limb-shortening procedures. Discrepancy of >5 cm

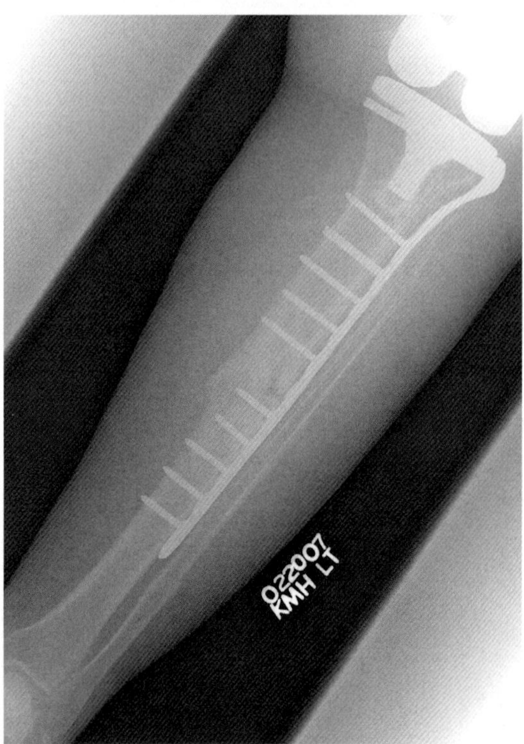


A

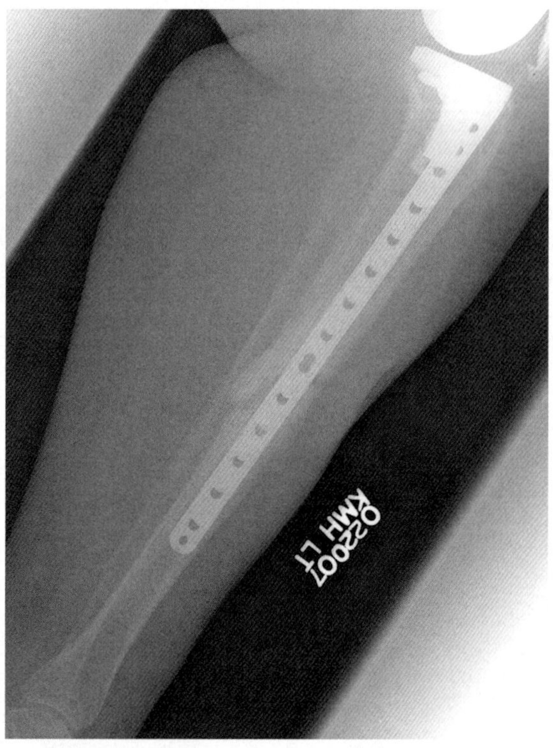


B

Fig. 7-20 Tibial nonunion. Anteroposterior (AP) (A) and lateral (B) radiographs demonstrate sclerosis along the fracture line in a patient with locking plate fixation. C: Technetium Tc 99m methylene-diphosphonate (MDP) scan demonstrates intense uptake at the fracture site. An indium In 111–labeled white cell scan was negative. Coronal (D) and sagittal (E) reformatted computed tomographic (CT) scans clearly demonstrate the hypertrophic nonunion.

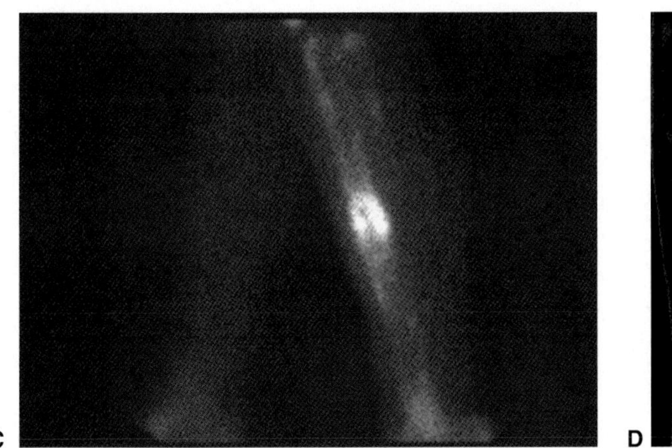

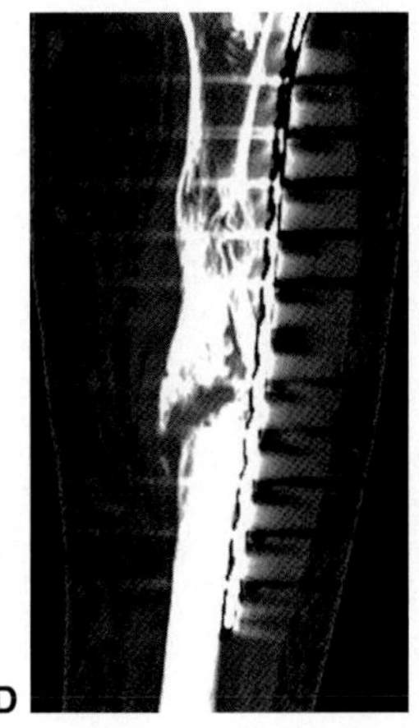

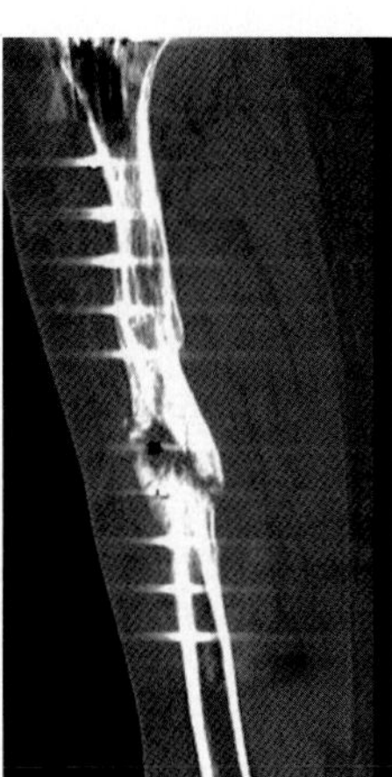

Fig. 7-20 *(Continued)*

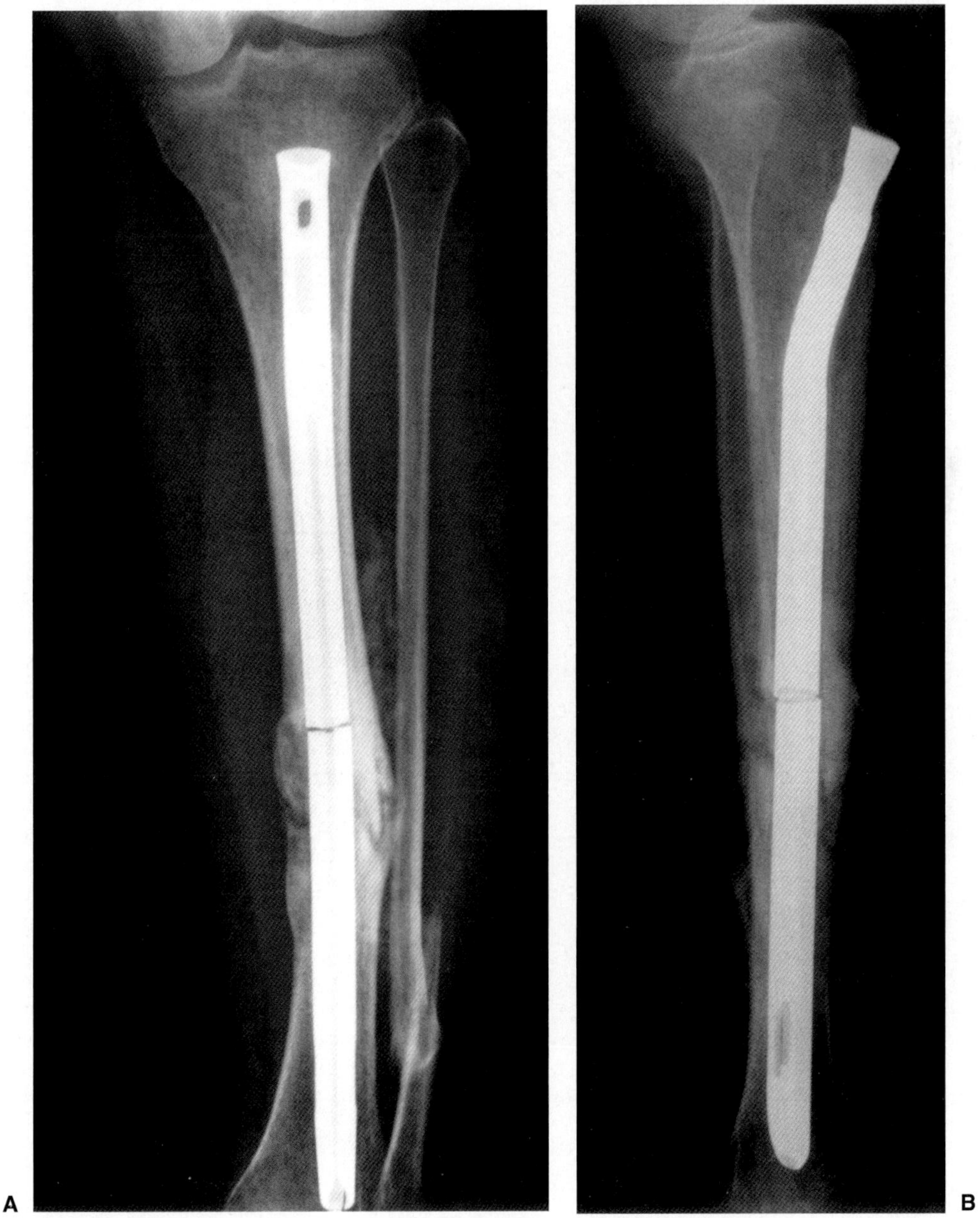

Fig. 7-21 Anteroposterior (AP) (A) and lateral (B) radiographs of a fractured intramedullary nail.

is more often treated with lengthening techniques. Leg length discrepancy >5 cm is at higher risk for complications.

## Shortening Procedures

**Epiphysodesis:** Stapling or closing of the epiphysis of the longer limb; most optimal in patients with significant growth potential

**Step-cut osteotomy:** Tibia shortened with stair step configuration osteotomy with screw fixation. Fibular osteotomy at a different level

**Progressive shortening:** Osteotomy with external fixation and reduction in length at 1 mm per day increments until desired length achieved

## Lengthening Procedures

**Wagner technique:** Stage 1—diaphyseal osteotomy with 0.5 to 1.0 cm distraction increased by 1 mm per day to the desired length with external fixator; stage 2—insertion of iliac bone graft when desired length achieved and plate and screw fixation; stage 3—plate removal and protected weight bearing

**Distraction epiphysodesis:** External fixator applied with 0.25 mm of epiphyseal distraction four times a day until endpoint reached; best used in patients just before growth plate closure

**Ilizarov technique:** Distraction osteogenesis; cortical osteotomy with controlled distraction 5 to 7 days after osteotomy at 0.25 mm every 6 hours (see Fig. 7-22).

**Callotasis:** Gradual distraction after callus is evident on radiographs, usually 10 to 15 days; distraction at 0.25 mm every 6 hours

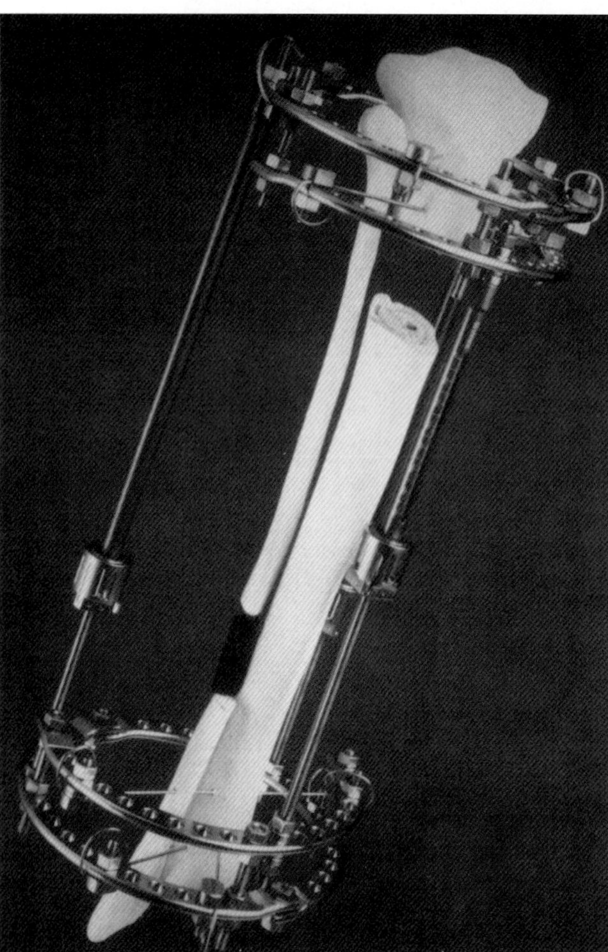

Fig. 7-22 Illustration of leg lengthening using an Ilizarov ring fixator with tibial corticotomy and distal fibular resection. (Courtesy of Smith and Nephew Richards, Memphis, Tennessee.)

# Suggested Reading

Abdlslam KM, Oleksak M, Saleh M. Tibial shortening for correction of leg length discrepancy and deformity: A new technique. *J Pediatr Orthop.* 2003;12:264–268.

Broughton NS, Olney BW, Menelaus MB. Tibial shortening for leg length discrepancy. *J Bone Joint Surg.* 1989;71B: 242–245.

Stricker SJ, Hunt T. Evaluation of leg length discrepancy in children. *Int Pediatr.* 2004;19:134–142.

Walker CW, Aronson J, Kaplan PA, et al. Radiographic evaluation of limb-lengthening procedures. *AJR Am J Roentgenol.* 1991;156:353–358.

# Imaging of Postoperative Complications

Complications and incidence following limb discrepancy procedures vary widely in the literature. However, there is agreement that major complications are reduced from the range 69% to 75% to the range 25% to 35% with increased surgical experience. Complications increase with discrepancies that require >5 cm of correction. Osseous complications include nonunion, malunion, fracture, joint deformities, pin loosening, and infection. Angular deformities are more common with unilateral fixators compared to ring or hybrid external fixation systems. Osseous infection is more common with larger threaded pins and is unusual with small wires used in ring fixators. Soft tissue complications include diminished muscle function, neurovascular injury, and compartment syndrome and infection. Serial radiographs can detect most osseous complications (see Fig. 7-23). However, CT with coronal and sagittal reformatting is preferred to evaluate healing and callus formation. Soft tissue complications may require angiography, CT, or MRI depending on the type of fixation in place. Complex wire or pin configurations may cause too much image distortion on MR images.

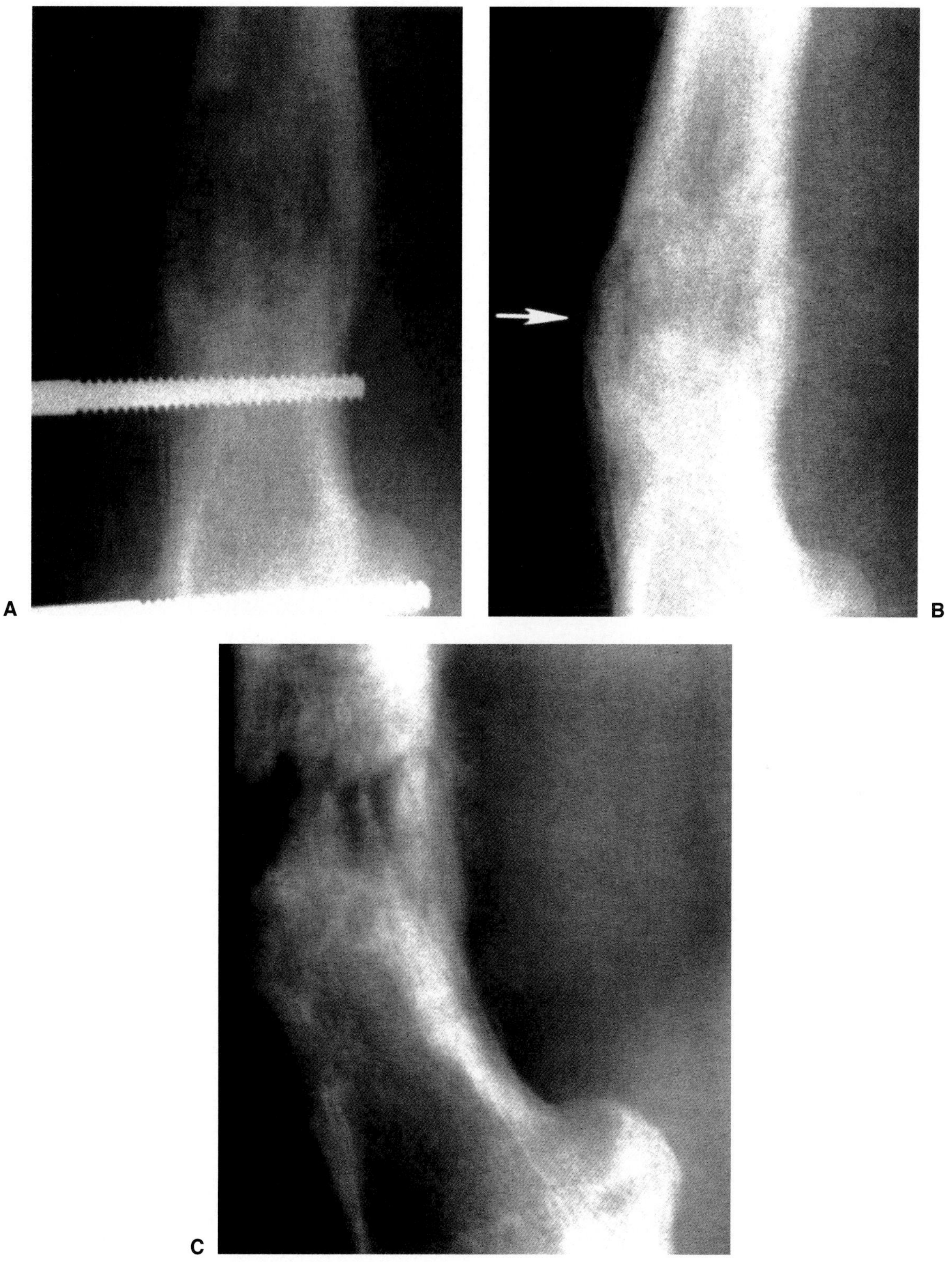


Fig. 7-23 Serial radiographs before (A) and after (B and C) removal of the external fixator. A subtle fracture (*arrow*) with varus angulation is present in B after fixator removal. This was overlooked and marked varus angulation developed (C). (From Walker CW, Aronson J, Kaplan PA, et al. Radiologic evaluation of limb-lengthening procedures. *AJR Am J Roentgenol.* 1991; 156:353–358.)

## SUGGESTED READING

Aronson J. Limb-lengthening, skeletal reconstruction and bone transport with the Ilizarov method. *J Bone Joint Surg*. 1997; 79A:1243–1259.

Paley D. Current techniques in limb lengthening. *J Pediatr Orthop*. 1988;8:73–92.

Walker CW, Aronson J, Kaplan PA, et al. Radiologic evaluation of limb-lengthening procedures. *AJR Am J Roentgenol*. 1991; 156:353–358.

# 8

# The Foot and Ankle

This chapter will focus on foot and ankle disorders requiring orthopaedic instrumentation including trauma, common orthopaedic procedures, and joint replacement. Clinical evaluation, treatment options, and complications will be reviewed. Preoperative imaging and imaging of complications will be emphasized.

## Trauma

The management of foot and ankle fractures is a common problem for orthopaedic surgeons, emergency physicians, family physicians, and radiologists. Imaging plays an important role in detection and classification of bone and soft tissue injuries so that appropriate treatment plans can be instituted.

Discussion of specific injuries is most easily accomplished by anatomic regions. Therefore, ankle, hind foot, mid foot, and forefoot injuries will be discussed separately.

## Ankle Fractures

Approximately 10% of emergency department visits are related to ankle injuries, typically presenting as sprains. The number of ankle injuries in adults (especially those older than 50 years) has been constantly increasing. The highest incidence is in women aged 75 to 84 years. Most fractures involve the lateral malleolus with isolated malleolar fractures accounting for 67% of ankle fractures. Most fractures involve the lateral malleolus with isolated fractures accounting for 67% of ankle fractures. Twenty five percent of ankle fractures are bimalleolar and about 7% trimalleolar. Approximately 2% of adult ankle fractures are open injuries. In children, ankle fractures account for 5% of all skeletal fractures and 15% of physeal injuries. Adult and pediatric ankle fractures are managed somewhat differently and will be reviewed separately.

### Adult Ankle Fractures

When evaluating ankle fractures, an accurate assessment of fracture location, appearance, and displacement is critical. Associated soft tissue or ligament injuries are also important to detect for appropriate management of the injury. When evaluating ankle injuries, it is helpful to consider the bones and ligaments as a ring-like structure. The ring is made of the medial malleolus, tibial plafond, distal tibiofibular ligaments (TFLs) and

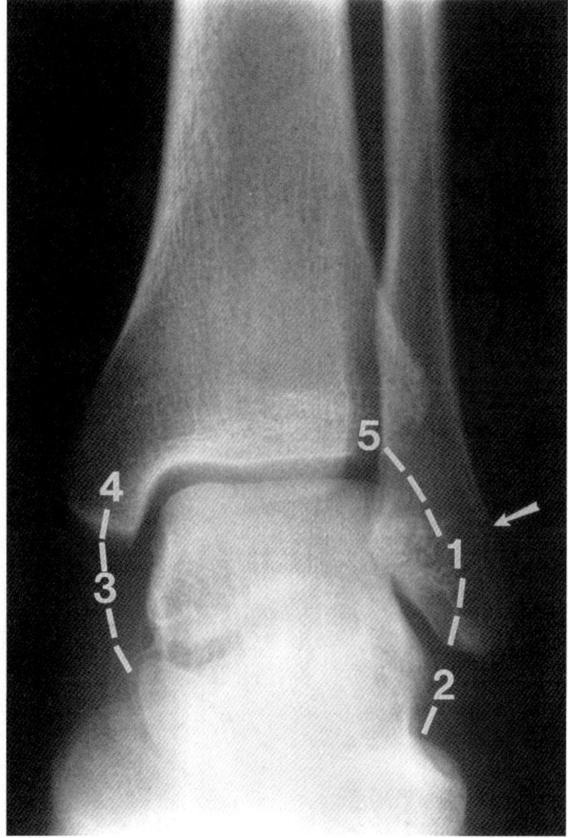


Fig. 8-1 Anteroposterior (AP) radiograph demonstrating the ring concept created by bones and ligaments of the ankle. Common breaks in the ring are (*1*) the lateral malleolus, (*2*) lateral ligaments, (*3*) medial ligaments, (*4*) medial malleolus, and (*5*) the distal tibiofibular ligaments and syndesmosis. Note the subtle fracture in the lateral malleolus (*arrow*).

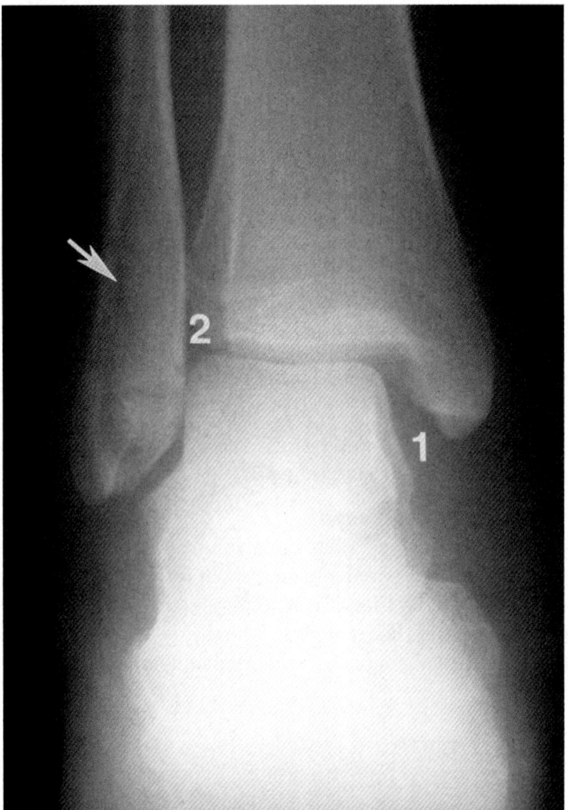


Fig. 8-2 Anteroposterior (AP) radiograph demonstrating widening of the medial ankle mortise (*1*) due to medial ligament tear, widening of the syndesmosis (*2*) due to distal tibiofibular ligament and syndesmotic tears, and a subtle (*arrow*) distal fibular fracture.

syndesmosis, the lateral malleolus, lateral ligament complex, talus, and medial ligaments. Breaks in the ring commonly occur at five sites, either alone or in combination (see Fig. 8-1). Breaks in the ring resulting in asymmetry in the position of the talus in the ankle mortise require fracture or ligament injury involving two of these locations (see Fig. 8-2).

## Classifications

Most ankle injuries are the result of inversion (supination) or eversion (pronation) forces. However, the mechanism of injury is rarely pure with rotational, abduction, or adduction forces to the foot and axial loading occurring as well (see Figs. 8-3, 8-4, 8-5, and 8-6). There are multiple classification systems, but the Lauge-Hansen, Danis-Weber, and Orthopaedic Trauma Association systems will be reviewed. Common fracture eponyms will also be listed following the classification section.

The Lauge-Hansen classification is based on the position of the foot and direction of the forces at the time of injury. This system is very accurate in predicting associated ligament injuries. Determining the mechanism of injury is based on the appearance of the fibular fracture and position of the talus. Table 8-1 describes the stages of injury and radiographic features of the Lauge-Hansen classification.

The Danis-Weber classification is based on the location of the fibular fracture. Type A fractures are below the level of the ankle joint. Type B fractures are at the level of the ankle with the distal TFLs intact. Type C fractures are above the ankle joint with disruption of the ligaments and syndesmosis (see Fig. 8-7).

The Orthopaedic Trauma Association classification expands upon the Weber, Lauge-Hansen, and AO (Arbeitsgemeinshaft

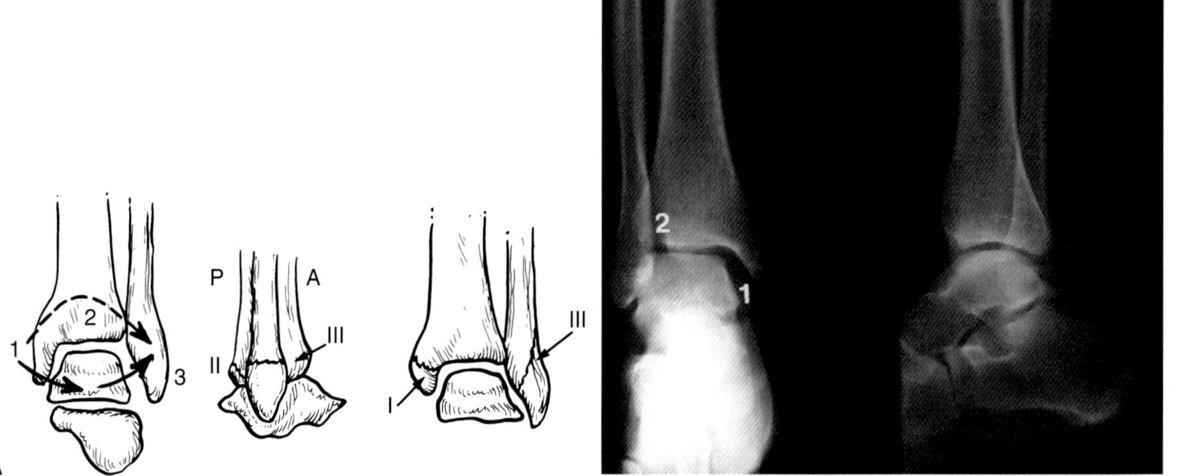


Fig. 8-3 Pronation (eversion)-abduction injury. **A:** Illustration of the three stages that occur if the force continues. Stage I—transverse fracture of the medial malleolus or deltoid ligament tear. State II: posterior tibial fracture of distal tibiofibular ligament tear. Stage III: Oblique fibular fracture beginning at the joint level and best seen on the anteroposterior (AP) radiograph. Traction forces cause the medial injury and impaction the lateral fracture. **B:** AP and lateral radiographs demonstrate widening of the ankle mortise medially (*1*) with no fibular fracture but disruption of the distal tibiofibular ligaments (stage II).

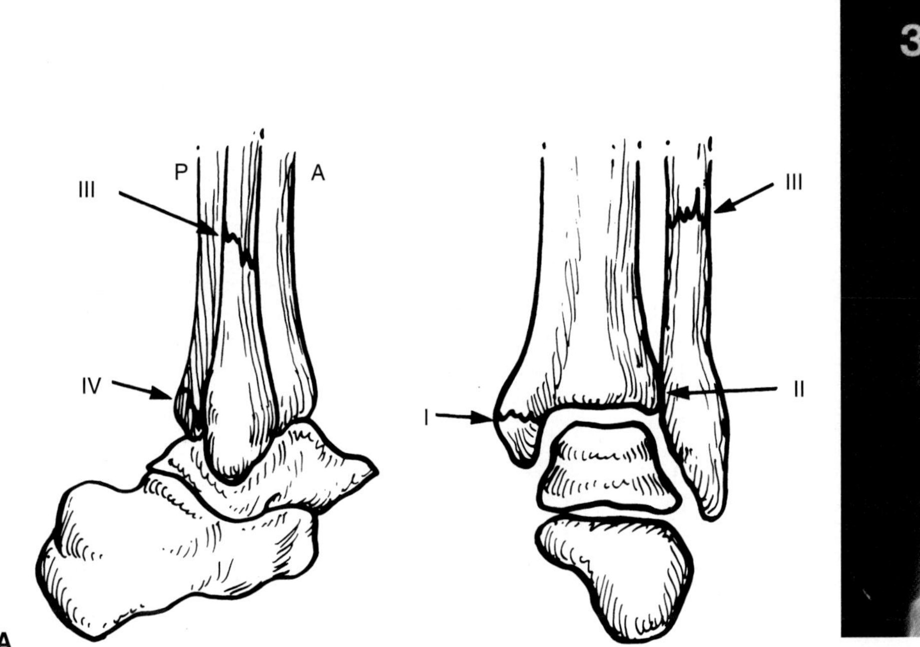


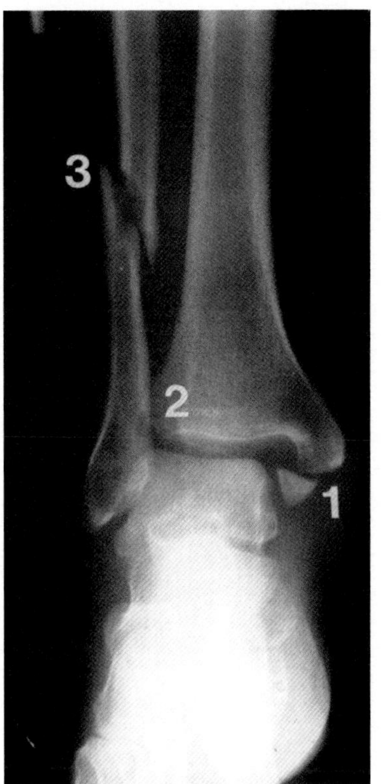


Fig. 8-4 Pronation (eversion)-lateral rotation injury. A: Illustration of the four stages of a pronation-lateral rotation injury. Stage I—deltoid ligament rupture or transverse medial malleolar fracture. Stage II: disruption of the anterior distal tibiofibular ligament and syndesmosis. Stage III: high fibular fracture typically >6 cm above the joint line. Stage IV: posterior tibial fracture or posterior distal tibiofibular ligament tear. B: Anteroposterior (AP) radiograph demonstrating a stage III pronation-lateral rotation injury with a transverse medial malleolar fracture (*1*), widening of the syndesmosis due to disruption of the anterior distal tibiofibular ligament and syndesmosis (*2*), and a high fibular fracture (*3*).

fur Osteosynthesefragen) classifications with three major groups (A to C) divided into three subgroups with multiple additional subgroups (see Figs. 8-8, 8-9, and 8-10). The features are similar to the classifications mentioned in the preceding text and when appropriate will be included in Table 8-2.

Chapter 2 contains common fracture eponyms for fractures and ligament injuries involving the ankle.

## Tibial Plafond Fractures

Tibial plafond fractures do not fit neatly into the commonly used ankle fracture classifications mentioned earlier. Most (77%) occur in patients younger than 50 years. Fractures are the result of axial loading after falls from significant heights or high-velocity motor vehicle accidents. Fractures usually extend up the tibial shaft in an oblique or spiral manner. Severe comminution with multiple articular fragments (pilon fracture) is common. In addition, 20% of plafond fractures are open.

The Orthopaedic Trauma Association classification of plafond fractures expands the AO classification with subgroups, but Table 8-3 and the illustrations (see Figs. 8-11 through 8-13) demonstrate the complexity of these injuries.

Isolated dislocations of the ankle without fractures are rare. Most occur with plantar flexion and inversion resulting in posteromedial dislocations.

## Suggested Reading

Arimoto HR, Forrester DM. Classification of ankle fractures: An algorithm. *AJR Am J Roentgenol.* 1980;135:1057–1063.

Berquist TH. *Radiology of the foot and ankle*, 2nd ed. Philadelphia: Lippincott Williams & Wilkins; 2000:171–280.

Lauge-Hansen N. Fractures of the ankle. II. Combined experimental-surgical and experimental-radiological investigations. *Arch Surg.* 1950;60:957–985.

Orthopaedic Trauma Association Committee for Coding and Classification. Fracture and dislocation compendium. *J Orthop Trauma.* 1996;10:1–155.

Ovadia DN, Beals RK. Fractures of the tibial plafond. *J Bone Joint Surg.* 1986;68A:543–551.

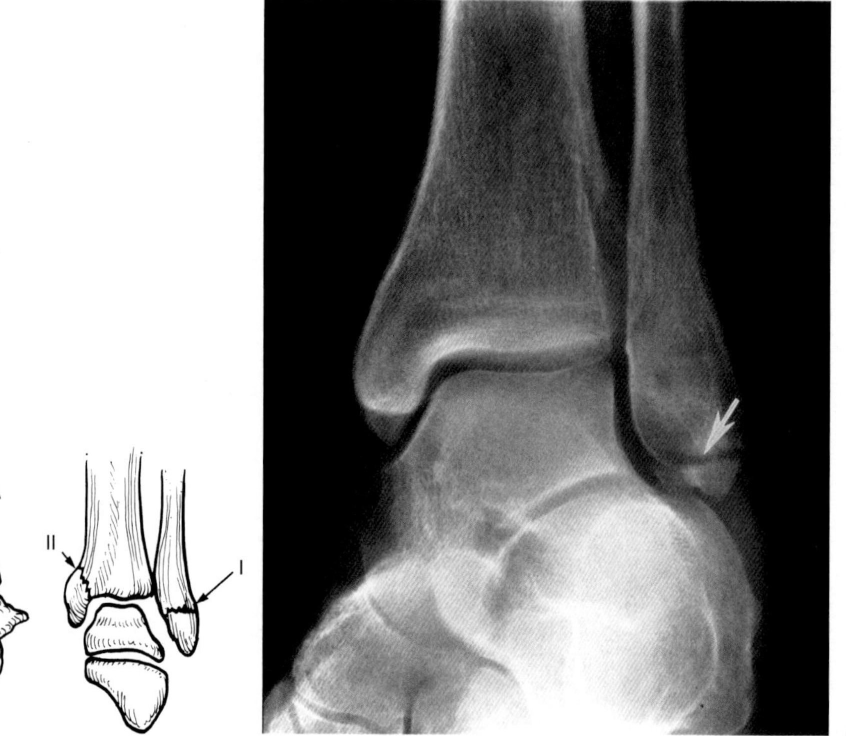

**Fig. 8-5** Supination (inversion)-adduction injury. **A:** Illustration of the two stages of injury. Stage I: lateral ligament tear or transverse fracture of the lateral malleolus below the joint line. Stage II: lateral ligament tear or transverse fracture of the lateral malleolus below the joint line with a steep oblique medial malleolar fracture. **B:** Mortise view demonstrating a transverse (traction) fracture of the distal lateral malleolus (*arrow*).

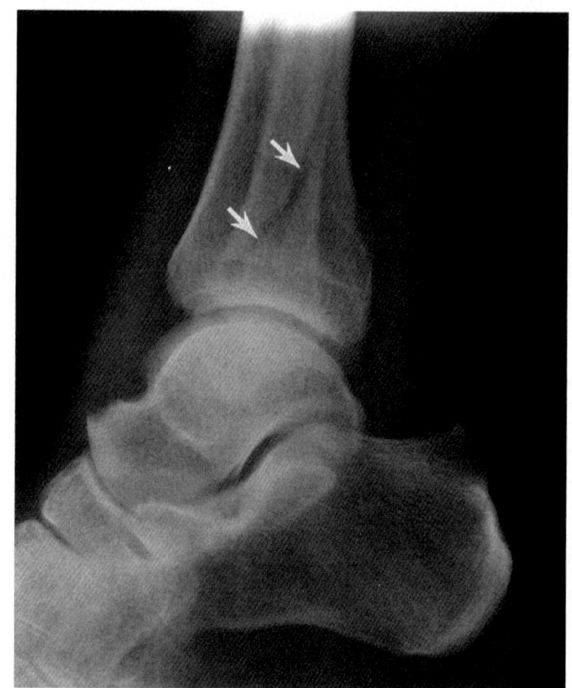

**Fig. 8-6** Supination (inversion)-lateral rotation injury. **A:** Illustration of the four stages of injury. Stage I: disruption of the anterior tibiofibular ligament. Stage II: spiral fracture of the distal fibula best seen on the lateral view. Stage III: above plus disruption of the posterior distal tibiofibular ligament. Stage IV: above plus transverse fracture of the distal medial malleolus. **B:** Lateral radiograph demonstrating an oblique fibular fracture (*arrows*) not clearly seen on the anteroposterior (AP) view.

Table 8-1

LAUGE-HANSEN CLASSIFICATION

| STAGE | RADIOGRAPHIC FEATURES |
|---|---|
| Pronation-abduction (Fig. 8-3) | |
| Stage I | Ruptured deltoid ligament or transverse medial malleolar fracture at or below the joint |
| Stage II | Posterior tibial fracture or distal tibiofibular ligament tear |
| Stage III | Oblique fibular fracture best seen on the anteroposterior (AP) radiograph |
| Pronation-lateral rotation (Fig. 8-4) | |
| Stage I | Ruptured deltoid ligament or transverse medial malleolar fracture at or below the joint |
| Stage II | Rupture of the anterior distal tibiofibular ligament and syndesmosis |
| Stage III | Fibular fracture well above (≥6 cm) the joint line |
| Stage IV | Posterior tibial margin fracture or posterior tibiofibular ligament tear |
| Supination-adduction (Fig. 8-5) | |
| Stage I | Lateral ligament tear or transverse fracture of the lateral malleolus below the joint line |
| Stage II | Stage I plus steep oblique medial malleolar fracture |
| Supination-lateral rotation (Fig. 8-6) | |
| Stage I | Disruption of the anterior tibiofibular ligament |
| Stage II | Spiral fracture of the distal fibula near the joint line and best seen on the lateral view |
| Stage III | Above plus rupture of the posterior tibiofibular ligament |
| Stage IV | Above plus transverse fracture of the medial malleolus |

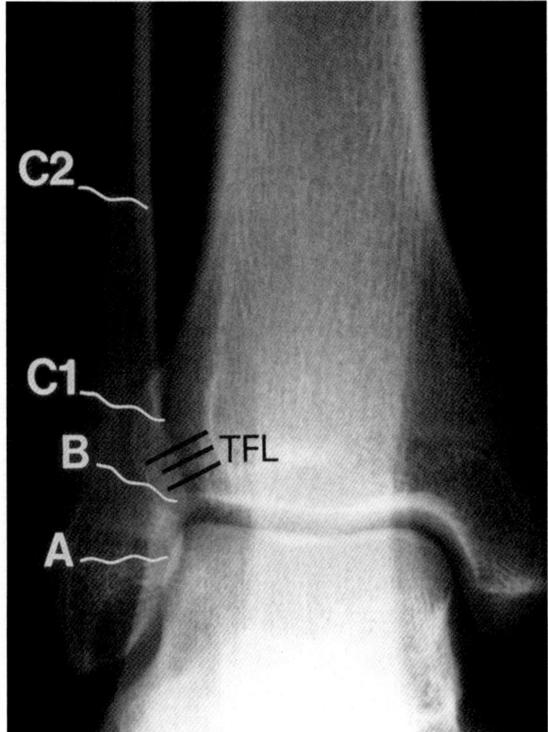


Fig. 8-7 Radiograph demonstrating the Danis-Weber classification for ankle fractures based on the location of the fibular fracture. Type A: below the level of the joint. Type B: at the level of the ankle with tibiofibular ligament (TFL) intact. Type C: above the joint with syndesmotic and distal TFL rupture (*C1*) and higher fibular fracture (*C2*).

## Pediatric Ankle Fractures

The appearance of ankle fractures in children depends on the age (growth plate development), relationship of the ligaments, and mechanism of injury. Fractures most commonly occur in boys aged 8 to 15 years. The age cutoff for pediatrics may be arbitrarily set at 18 or when the growth plates are closed. Ligament injuries are unusual in children. The mechanisms of injury are similar to those described in the adult.

Several classification systems are commonly used including the Salter-Harris (see Fig. 8-14 and Table 8-4) and the Dias-Tachdjian (see Fig. 8-15 and Table 8-5) classifications. The latter is similar to the Lauge-Hansen system with integration of the Salter-Harris classification.

Two additional pediatric injuries include the juvenile Tillaux fracture and triplane fractures. The distal tibial growth plate fuses medial to lateral placing the lateral physis at greater risk in adolescents. With external rotation forces, the distal TFL displaces the lateral epiphysis resulting in a Salter-Harris III fracture of the lateral tibia (see Fig. 8-16).

Triplane fractures are more complex physeal fractures resulting in poorer prognosis. These injuries account for 5% to 7% of ankle fractures in children. Triplane fractures have components in the sagittal, coronal, and axial planes which may result in two- (see Fig. 8-17), three-, or four-part fractures. Three-part fractures differ from two-part fractures in that an additional fracture line separates the anterolateral epiphyseal fragment from the posteromedial tibial fragment (see Fig. 8-18).

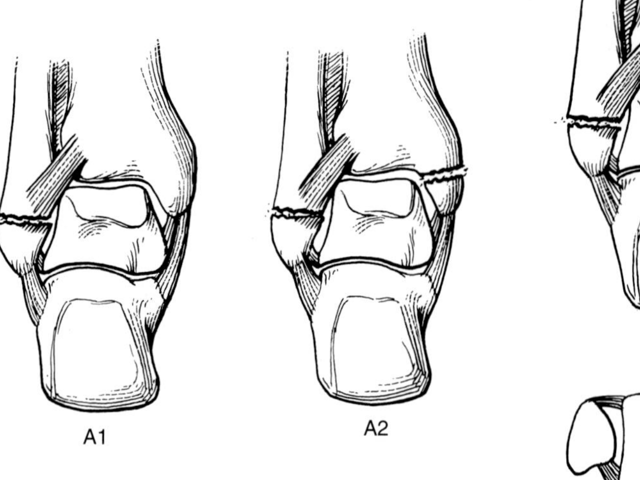


**Fig. 8-8** AO (Arbeitsgemeinshaft fur Osteosynthesefragen)/Orthopaedic Trauma classification. Type A: infrasyndesmotic fractures. Type A1: isolated malleolar fracture below the syndesmosis (see also Lauge-Hansen supination-adduction Stage I in Fig. 8-5B). Type A2: medial and lateral malleolar fractures below the syndesmosis. Type A3: medial and lateral malleolar fractures with a posteromedial tibial fragment.

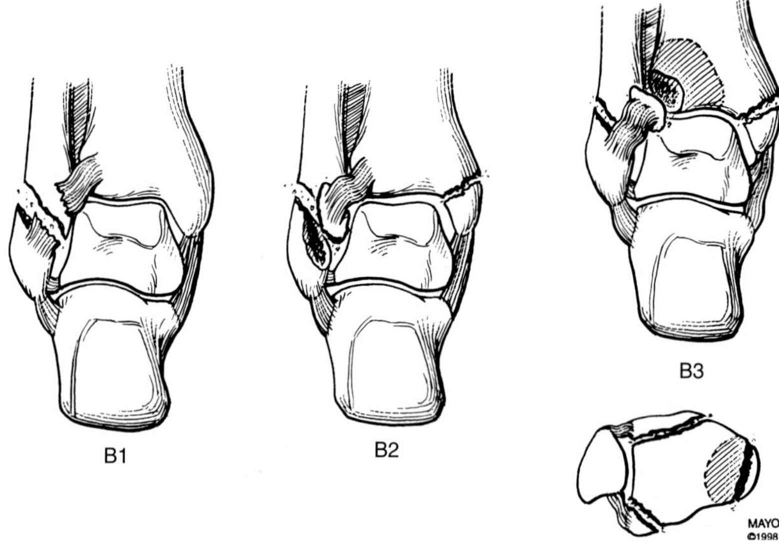


**Fig. 8-9** AO (Arbeitsgemeinshaft fur Osteosynthesefragen)/Orthopaedic Trauma classification. Type B: transsyndesmotic fractures. Type B1: isolated lateral malleolar fracture at the syndesmosis. Type B2: with associated medial malleolar fracture. Type B3: bimalleolar with avulsions of the anterior and posterior tibiofibular ligaments.

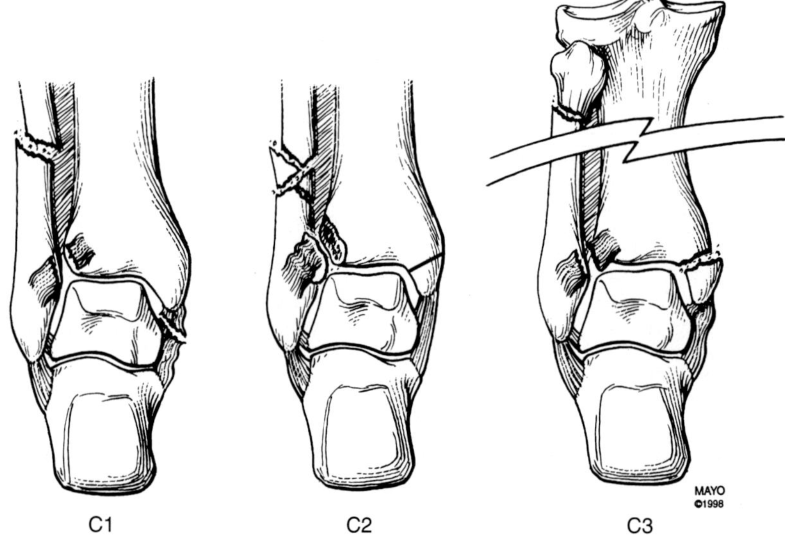


**Fig. 8-10** AO (Arbeitsgemeinshaft fur Osteosynthesefragen)/Orthopaedic Trauma Association. Type C: fibular fracture well above the syndesmosis. Type C1: fibular fracture in the distal diaphysis with associated syndesmotic and medial ligament tears (see also Lauge-Hansen pronation-lateral rotation stage III in Fig. 8-4). Type C2: similar to C1, but with complex fibular fracture. Type C3: similar secondary features with proximal fibular fracture and more extensive interosseous membrane disruption.

**Table 8-2**

ORTHOPAEDIC TRAUMA ASSOCIATION CLASSIFICATION ANKLE FRACTURES

| TYPE | RADIOGRAPHIC FEATURES |
|---|---|
| Type A (Fig. 8-8) | Below the syndesmosis |
| A1 | Isolated malleolar (Weber A, Lauge-Hansen supination-adduction stage I, or pronation-abduction stage I) |
| A2 | Bimalleolar below the syndesmosis |
| A3 | Bimalleolar with posteromedial tibial fracture |
| Type B (Fig. 8-9) | Transsyndesmotic fractures |
| B1 | Isolated fibular fracture |
| B2 | Transsyndesmotic fibular and medial malleolar fracture |
| B3 | B2 with anterior and posterior distal tibiofibular ligament avulsions |
| Type C (Fig. 8-10) | High fibular fractures (Weber C) |
| C1 | Fibular fracture well above the syndesmosis with medial malleolar or medial ligament and syndesmotic tears (Lauge-Hansen pronation-lateral rotation stage III) |
| C2 | Multifragmentary high fibular fracture with other features similar to C1 |
| C3 | Proximal fibular fracture with other features similar to C1 |

**Table 8-3**

ORTHOPAEDIC TRAUMA ASSOCIATION CLASSIFICATION TIBIAL PLAFOND FRACTURES

| TYPE | RADIOGRAPHIC FEATURES |
|---|---|
| Type A (Fig. 8-11) | Extra-articular |
| A1 | Metaphyseal, simple |
| A2 | Metaphyseal wedge |
| A3 | Metaphyseal complex |
| Type B (Fig. 8-12) | Partial articular |
| B1 | Pure split |
| B2 | Split with depression |
| B3 | Complex depression |
| Type C (Fig. 8-13) | Complex articular |
| C1 | Articular simple |
| C2 | Articular simple, complex metaphyseal |
| C3 | Articular complex |

## Suggested Reading

Cooperman DR, Spiegel PG, Laros CG. Tibial fractures involving the ankle in children: The so-called triplane epiphyseal fracture. *J Bone Joint Surg*. 1978;60A:1040–1046.

Dias LS, Tachdjian MO. Physeal injuries to the ankle in children: Classification. *Clin Orthop*. 1978;136:230–233.

Kay RM, Matthys GA. Pediatric ankle fractures: Evaluation and treatment. *J Am Acad Orthop Surg*. 2001;9:268–278.

## Imaging Evaluation

Ankle radiographs account for 10% of all radiographs requested in the emergency department. In many cases, an adequate physical examination is not performed before ordering radiographs. Following the Ottowa ankle rules, imaging should be performed if the patient has the following findings: (a) inability to bear weight; (b) point tenderness over the medial malleolus, or posterior edge or inferior tip of the lateral malleolus, or talus or calcaneus; and (c) inability to ambulate for four steps in the emergency department.

At most institutions and according to the American College of Radiology appropriateness criteria, anteroposterior (AP), lateral, and mortise radiographs should be obtained if patients meet the Ottowa ankle rules. Additional views or radiographs of the foot may be obtained as indicated.

Patients with a joint effusion frequently have a subtle, easily overlooked fracture. In fact, fractures that may mimic ankle sprains need to be considered and include the base of the fifth metatarsal, anterior calcaneal process fractures, talar dome fractures, and lateral and posterior talar process fractures. Up to 50% of talar dome and process fractures are overlooked on radiographs. When an effusion is present or there is question about a possible fracture, computed tomography (CT) with thin sections and reformatting for complete evaluation are recommended. CT may also be required to classify complex adult fractures and physeal fractures in children. Magnetic resonance imaging (MRI) is rarely warranted in the acute setting, but is useful for evaluating soft tissue structures and more subtle marrow changes if symptoms persist.

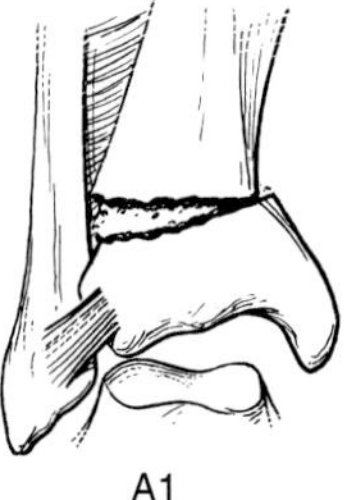


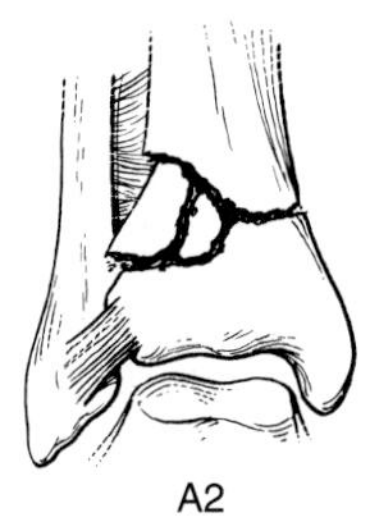


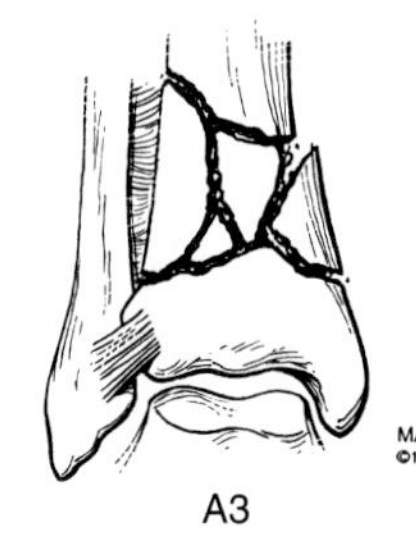


**Fig. 8-11** Orthopaedic Trauma Association classification for tibial plafond fractures. Type A: extra-articular. Type A1: simple metaphyseal. Type A2: metaphyseal wedge. Type A3: metaphyseal complex.

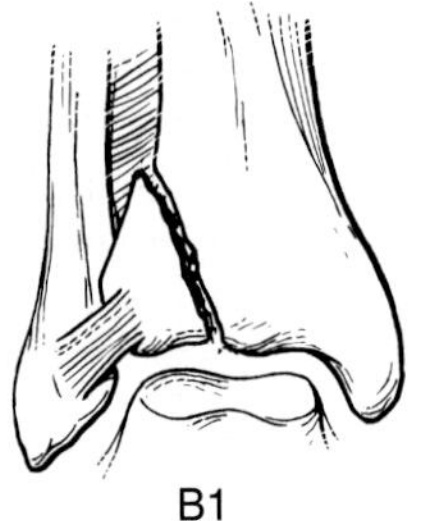


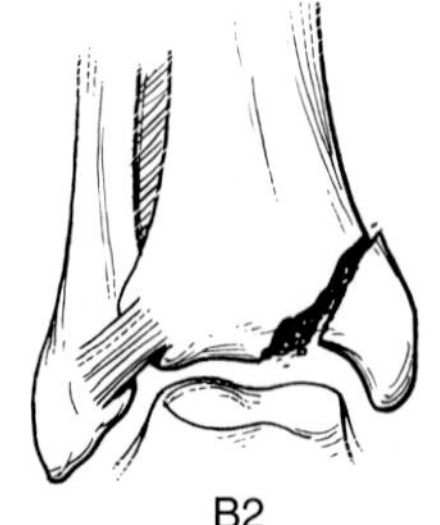


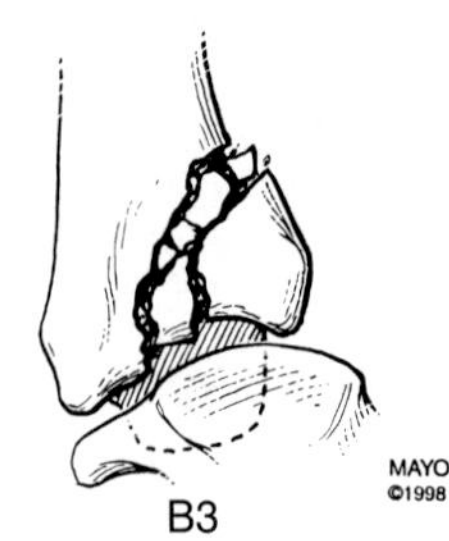


**Fig. 8-12** Orthopaedic Trauma Association classification for tibial plafond fractures. Type B: partial articular. Type B1: pure split. Type B2: split with depression. Type B3: complex depression.

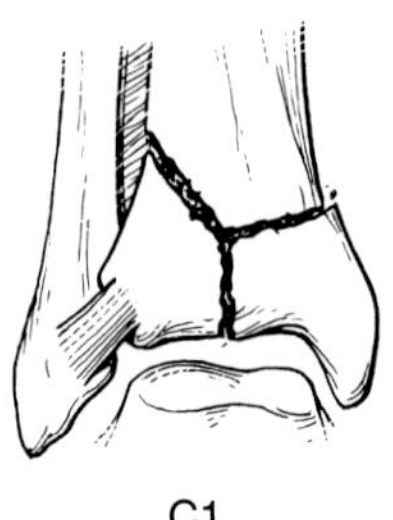


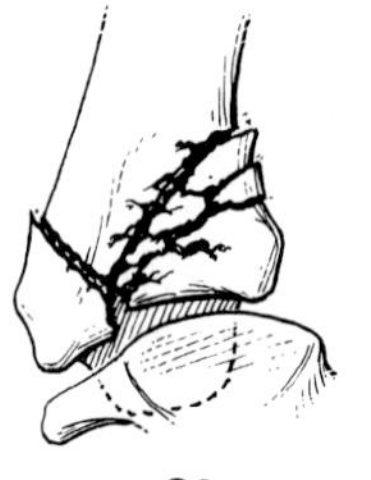


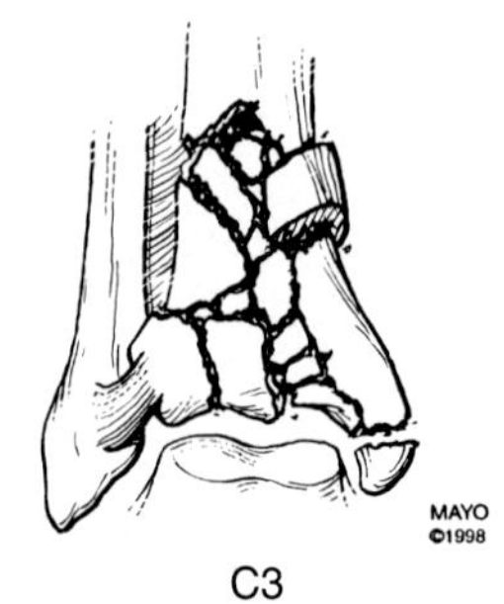


**Fig. 8-13** Orthopaedic Trauma Association classification for tibial plafond fractures. Type C: complex articular. Type C1: articular simple. Type C2: articular simple, complex metaphyseal. Type C3: complex articular.

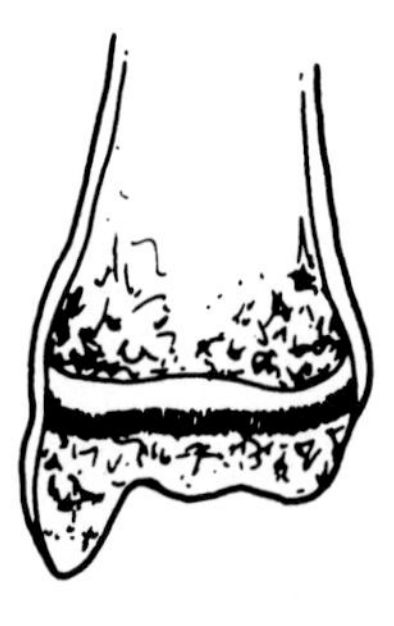


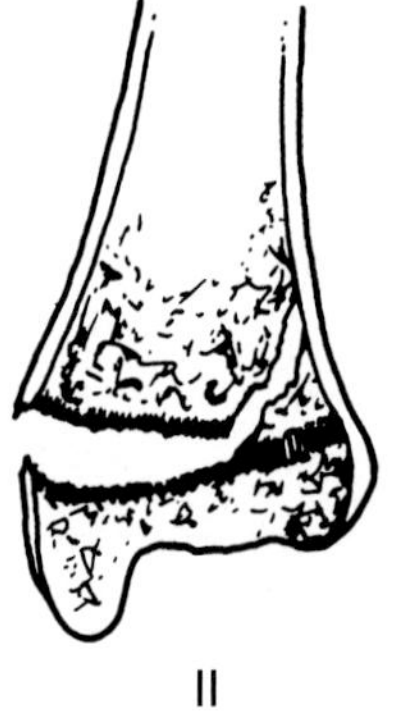


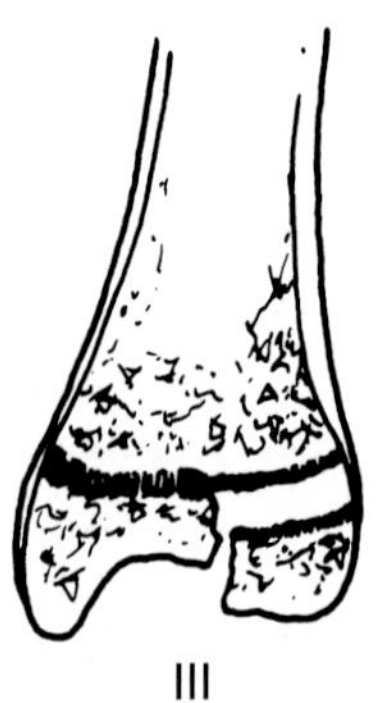


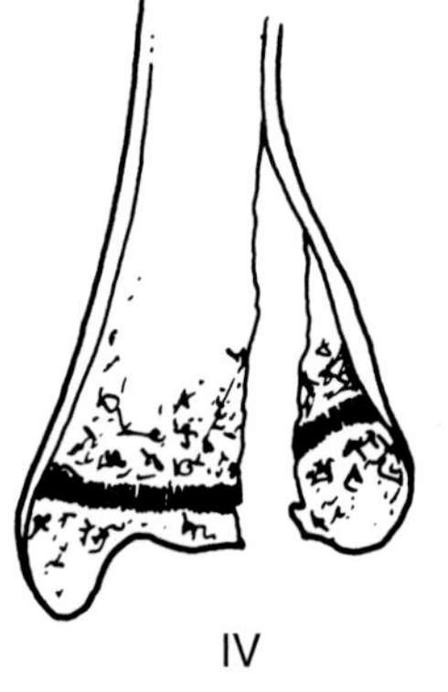


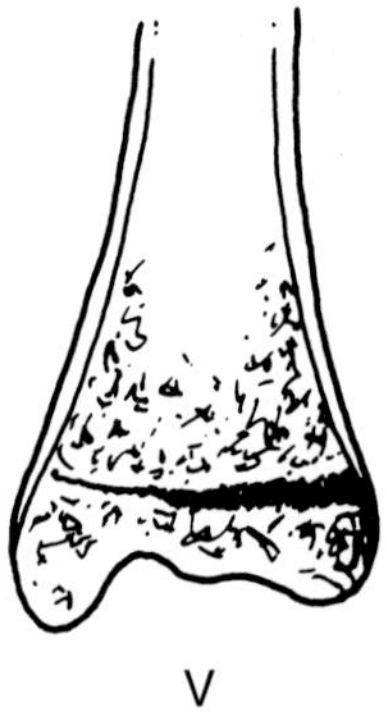


**Fig. 8-14** Illustration of the Salter-Harris classification for physeal injuries. Type I: fracture through and isolated to the growth plate. Type II: growth plate fracture extending through the metaphysic. Type III: growth plate fracture extending through the epiphysis. Type IV: fracture extending through the metaphysic, physis, and epiphysis. Type V: growth plate compression.

**Table 8-4**

SALTER-HARRIS CLASSIFICATION

| TYPE (INCIDENCE) | RADIOGRAPHIC FEATURES |
|---|---|
| Type I (15%) | Fracture isolated to growth plate |
| Type II (40%) | Fracture of the growth plate exiting through the metaphysis |
| Type III (25%) | Fracture of the growth plate extending through the epiphysis to the joint surface |
| Type IV (10%–25%) | Fracture extending through the epiphysis growth plate and metaphysic |
| Type V (1%) | Compression of growth plate |

See Figure 8-14.

## Suggested Reading

Dalinka MK, Alazraki NP, Daffner RH, et al. ACR appropriateness criteria for suspected ankle fractures. *Am Coll Radiol.* 2005:1–4.

Magid D, Michelson JD, Ney DR, et al. Adult ankle fractures: Comparison of plain films and interactive two- and three-dimensional CT scans. *AJR Am J Roentgenol.* 1990;154:1017–1023.

Stiell IG, McKnight RD, Greenberg GH, et al. Implementation of the Ottowa ankle rules. *JAMA.* 1993;269:1127–1132.

## Treatment Options for Ankle Fractures

Treatment approaches vary with the type of injury, degree of displacement, and whether there is still significant growth potential in children (≤2 years remaining). In adults, the goals of treatment are accurate anatomic reduction, parallel articular surface, and early motion to reduce stiffness or adhesive capsulitis.

Fractures of the medial or lateral malleolus without secondary fracture or ligament injury may be treated conservatively with closed reduction if displacement is <2 mm. Immobilization for 6 weeks is usually adequate. If displacement exceeds 2 mm, internal fixation is indicated. Medial malleolar fractures can be treated with one or two cannulated screws or malleolar screws, K-wire, and tension band or bioabsorbable fixation devices. Placement of malleolar screws is important to avoid abutment with the posterior tibial tendon (see Fig. 8-19). Fibular fractures can be treated with interfragmentary screws or plate and screw fixation (see Fig. 8-20).

When both malleoli are involved a similar approach is used in both structures. A syndesmotic screw may also be required to secure the distal tibiofibular relationship when the ligament is disrupted (Lauge-Hansen pronation–lateral rotation). The screw should not be too tightly placed as complications may result. Also, if the screw is too proximal the tibia may displace laterally. Posterior tibial fragments are usually fixed internally with one or more screws if they involve >25% of the articular surface.

Tibial plafond fractures (Figs. 8-11 to 8-13) are particularly difficult to manage (see Fig. 8-21). Significant separation of

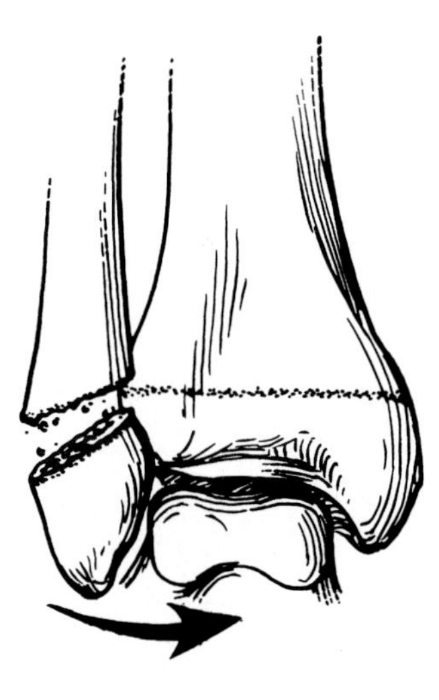


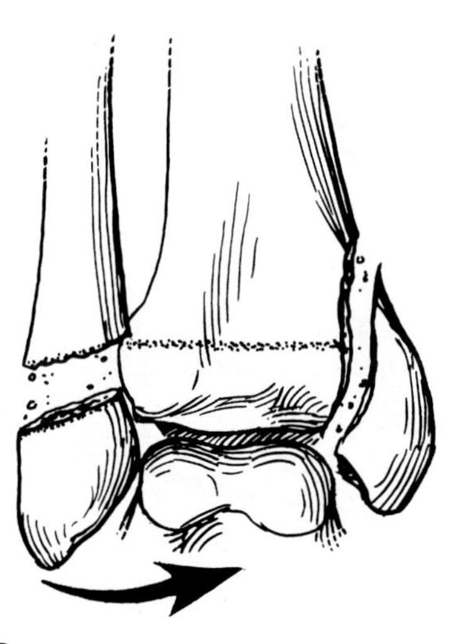


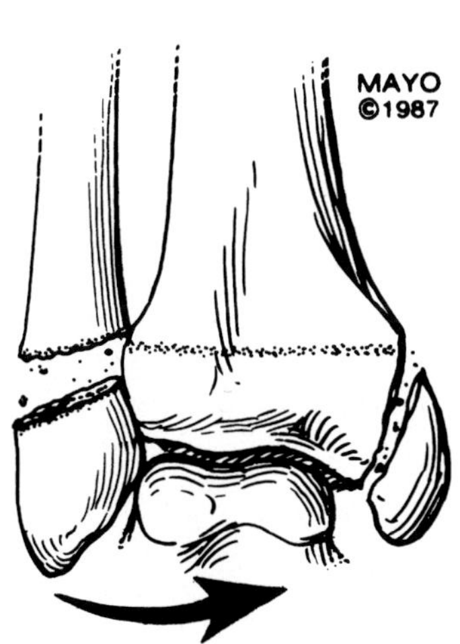


**Fig. 8-15** Illustration of the Dias-Tachdjian classification of pediatric ankle fractures combining the Lauge-Hansen and Salter-Harris classifications. **A–C:** Supination-inversion injures. Stage I: Salter-Harris I or II fibular fracture. Stage II: Salter-Harris I or II fibular fracture with steep oblique medial malleolar fracture (Type IV Salter-Harris in this case). **D:** Supination-plantar flexion injury: Salter-Harris I or II of the tibia best seen on the lateral view. **E:** Supination-external rotation injury: Stage I: Salter-Harris II or oblique fracture of the distal tibia; Stage II: Stage I plus fibular fracture well above the growth plate. **F:** Pronation–eversion-external rotation injury. Salter-Harris II of the tibia plus high fibular fracture.

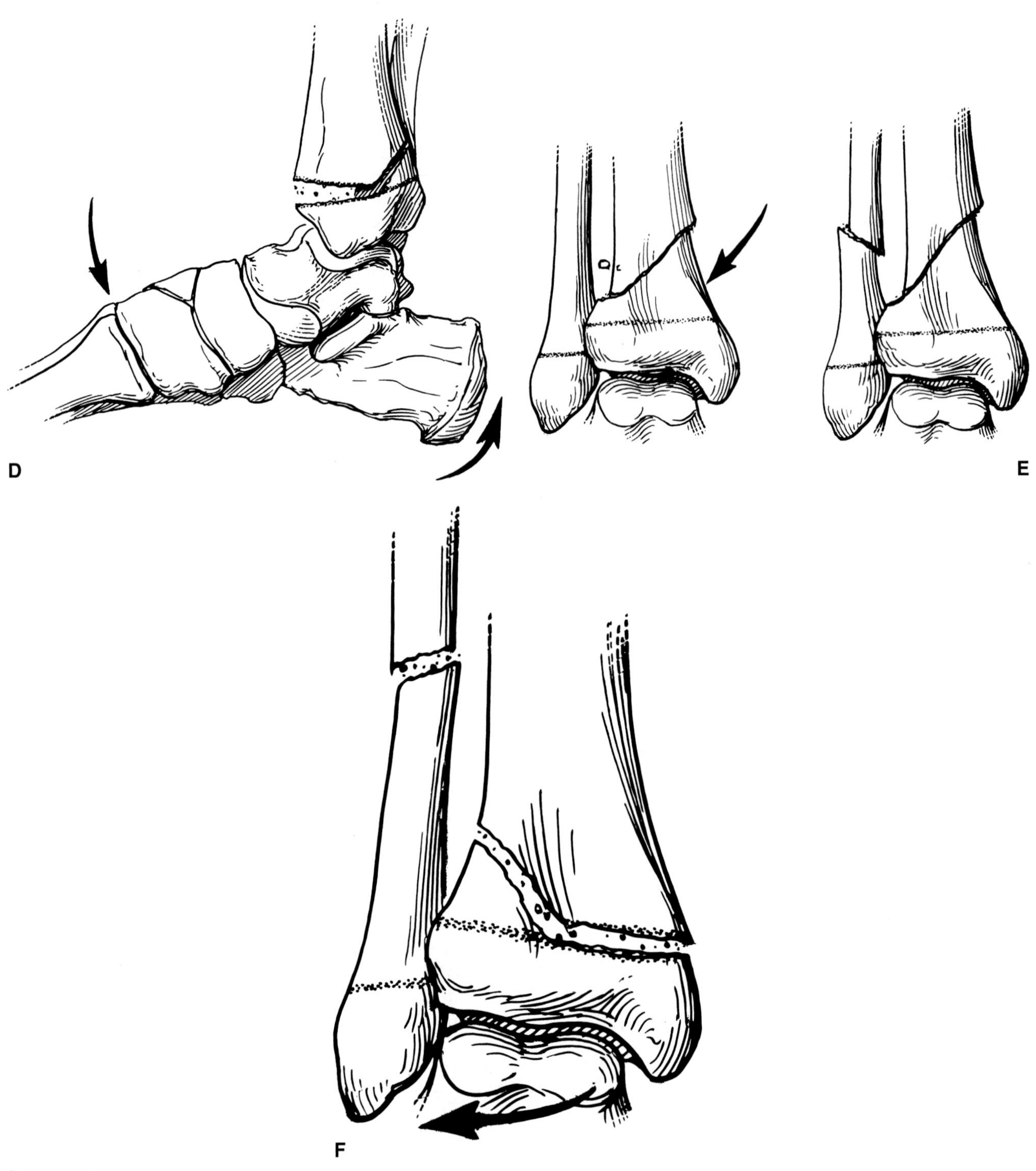


Fig. 8-15 *(Continued)*

**Table 8-5**

**DIAS-TACHDJIAN CLASSIFICATION FOR PEDIATRIC ANKLE FRACTURES**

| STAGE | RADIOGRAPHIC FEATURES |
|---|---|
| Supination-inversion (Fig. 8-15A-C) | |
| Stage I | Traction on lateral ligaments leads to Salter-Harris I or II of fibula |
| Stage II | Continued force leads to associated steep Salter-Harris III or IV of the medial Malleolus |
| Supination-plantar flexion (Fig. 8-15D) | Salter-Harris I or II of tibia best seen on the lateral view |
| Supination-external rotation (Fig. 8-15E) | |
| Stage I | Salter-Harris II or oblique distal tibial fracture |
| Stage II | Stage I plus high fibular fracture |
| Pronation-eversion—external rotation (Fig. 8-15F) | Salter-Harris II of the distal tibia with high fibular fracture |

See Figure 8-15.

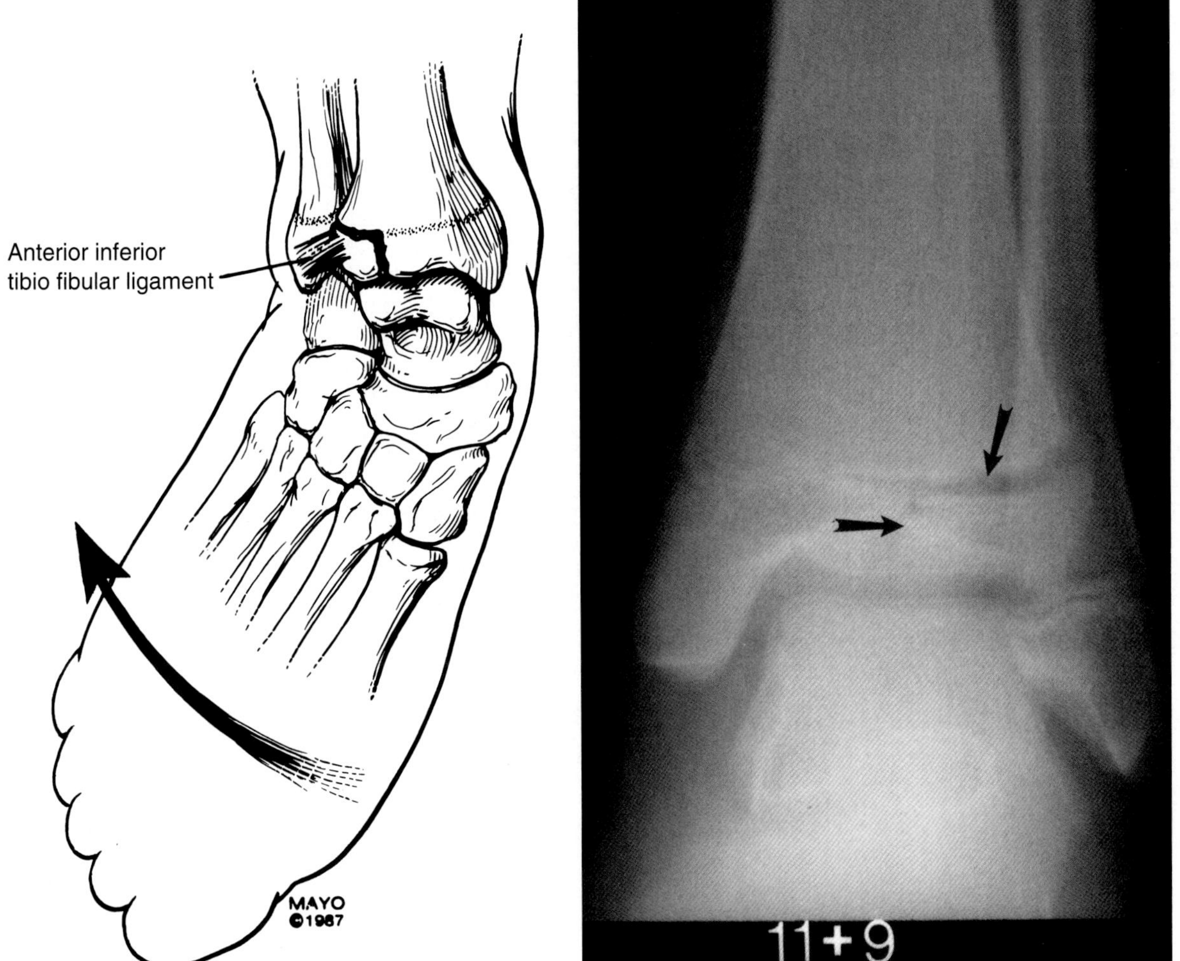


**Fig. 8-16** Juvenile Tillaux fracture. **A:** Illustration of the mechanism of injury with external rotation of the foot causing avulsion of the lateral tibial epiphysis. **B:** Anteroposterior (AP) radiograph of a juvenile Tillaux fracture (*arrows*).

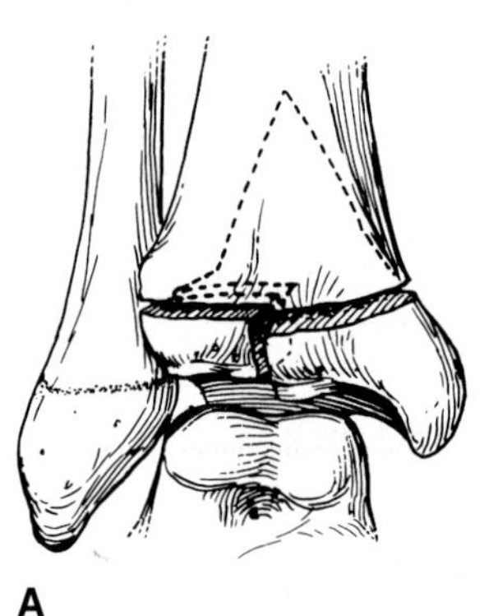

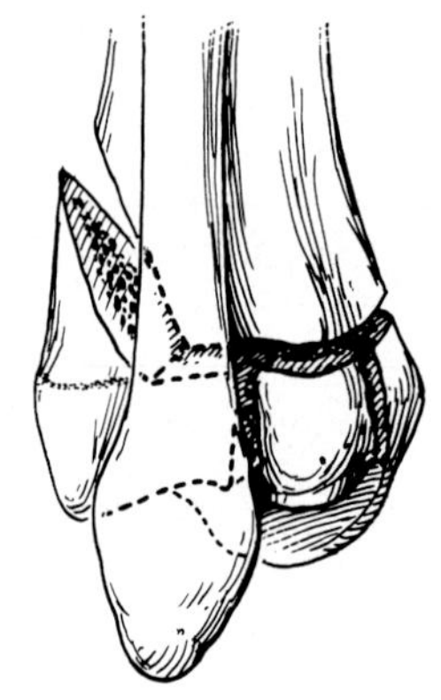
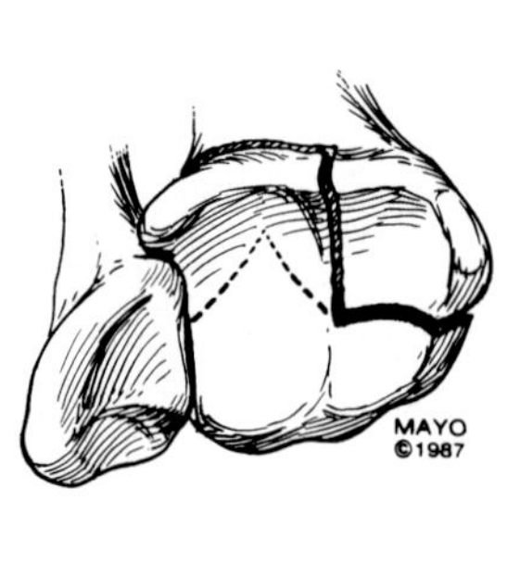

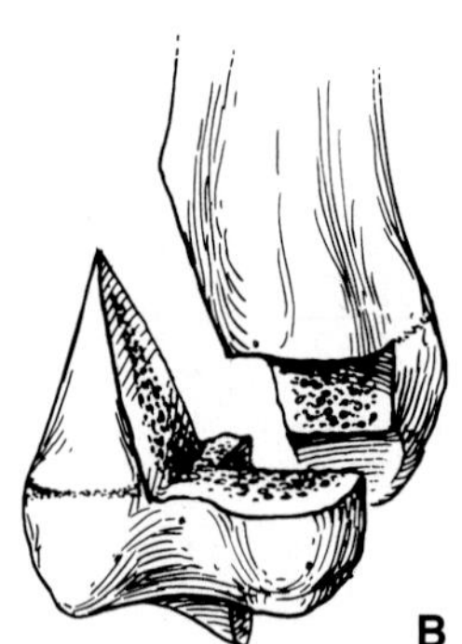


**Fig. 8-17** Two-part triplane fracture. A: Coronal and sagittal plane illustrations. B: Axial plane and separated fragments.

the fragments and loss of articular cartilage may be present. CT with reformatting in the coronal and sagittal planes or three-dimensional reconstruction may be required to plan the surgical approach. Bone grafting may be required to support the articular surface and to fill in bone voids. It is not unusual (15%) to proceed to arthrodesis in more complex injuries.

Pediatric ankle fractures are approached differently, especially if there is significant growth potential remaining. Physeal fracture should be reduced with care to avoid further damage to the growth plate. In most cases, closed techniques with a short leg cast or brace yields good results. Isolated fibular fractures heal in approximately 3 weeks. When the tibia is also involved it can be reduced and the fibula realigns.

Salter-Harris I and II tibial fractures with <2 mm displacement can be treated with cast immobilization for 4 to 6 weeks. If reduction cannot be maintained or the displacement exceeds 2 mm, cannulated screws or K-wires can be placed parallel to the physis. Similar approaches can be used for displaced (>2 mm) Salter-Harris III, triplane, and juvenile Tillaux fractures (see Fig. 8-22). Physeal compression injuries are uncommon. In this setting, excision of the damage growth plate and bone grafting may be required. Leg length discrepancy may be an issue that can be dealt with later as indicated.

## Suggested Reading


Femino JE, Gruber BF, Karunakar MA. Safe zone for placement of medial malleolar screws. *J Bone Joint Surg*. 2007;89A:133–138.

Kay RM, Matthys GA. Pediatric ankle fractures: Evaluation and treatment. *J Am Acad Orthop Surg*. 2001;9:268–278.

Ovadia DN, Beals RK. Fractures of the tibial plafond. *J Bone Joint Surg*. 1986;68A:543–551.

Tejwani NC, McLauring TM, Walsh M, et al. Are outcomes of bimalleolar fractures poorer than those of lateral malleolar fractures with medial ligamentous injury? *J Bone Joint Surg*. 2007;89A:1438–1441.


# Imaging of Ankle Fracture Complications

Complications vary in children and adults and may be related to the initial injury or treatment method selected. For example, bimalleolar fractures have a poorer prognosis than isolated malleolar fractures. In adults, the most common complication is

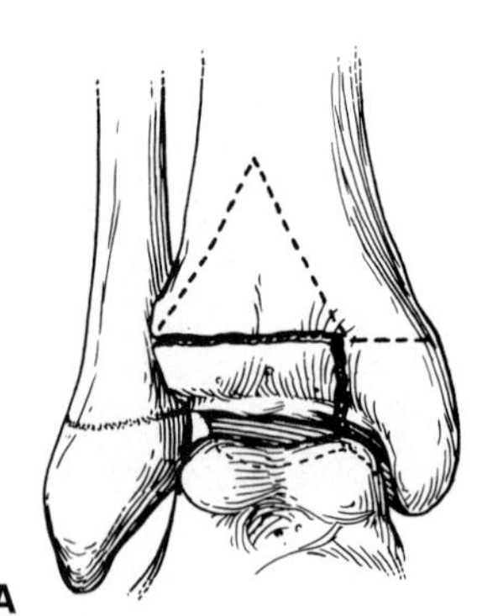

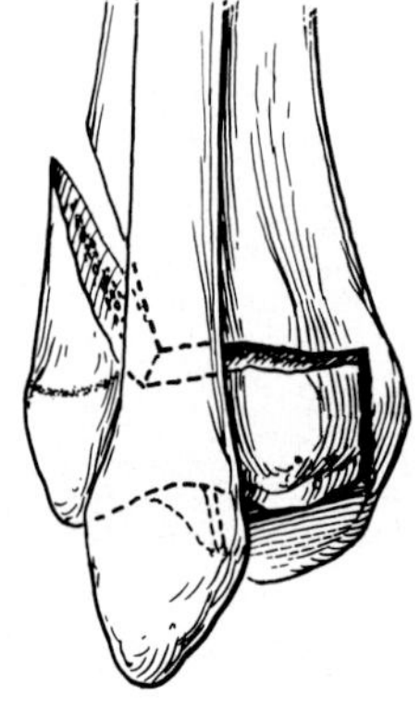
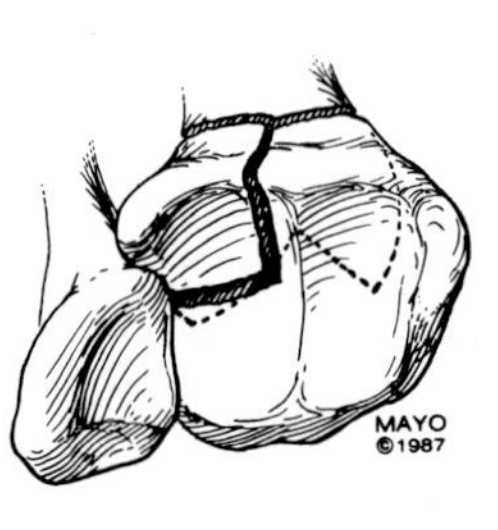

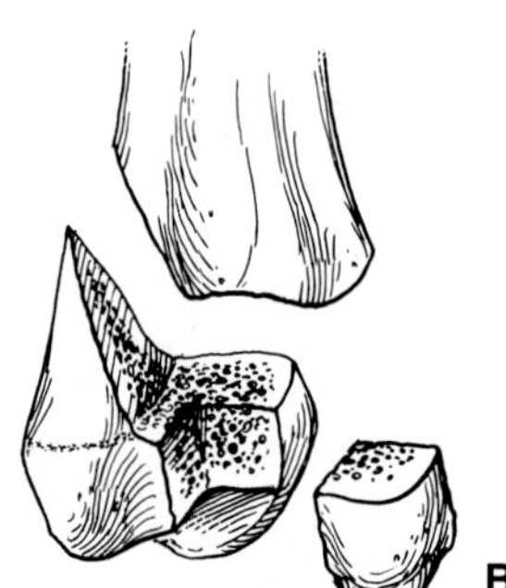


**Fig. 8-18** Three-part triplane fracture. A: Coronal and sagittal plane illustrations. B: Axial plane and separated fragments.

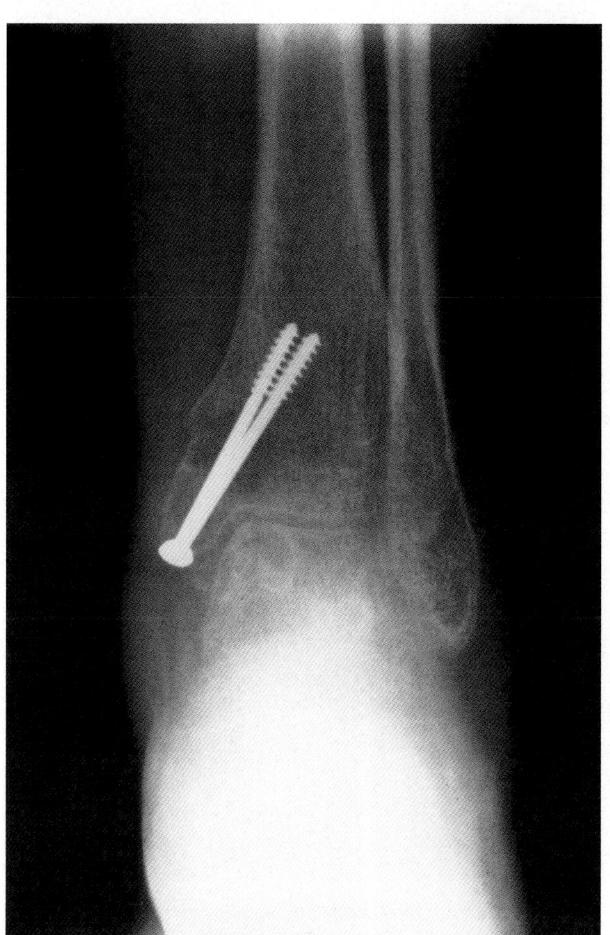

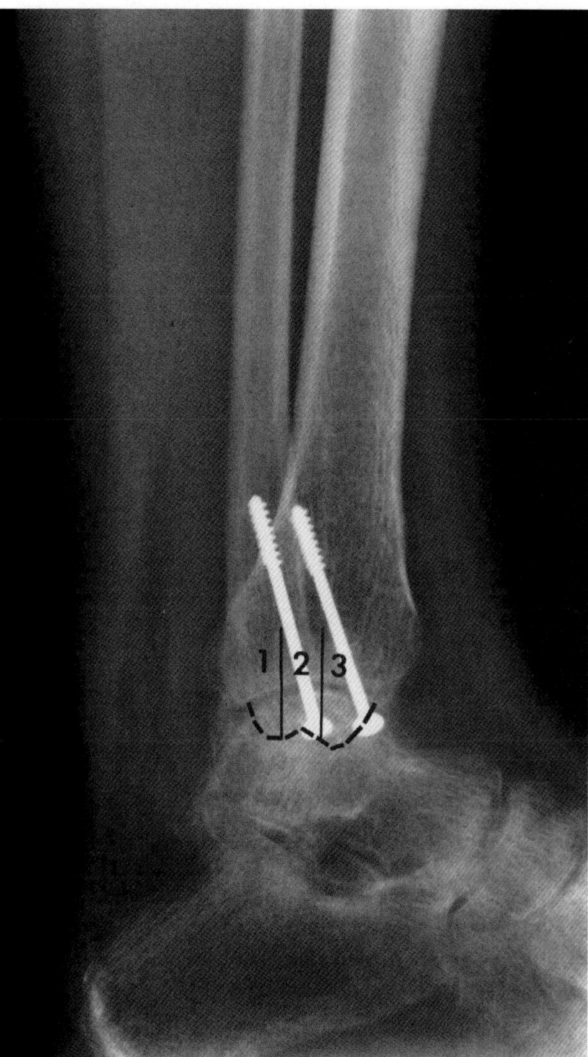


A B

Fig. 8-19 Anteroposterior (AP) (A) and lateral (B) radiographs of a healed medial maleollar fracture with two malleolar fixation screws. Broken lines indicate the malleolar margins with the three zones divided by vertical lines. Zone 1 is the safe zone. Zone 2 is within 2 mm of the posterior tibial tendon increasing the risk of tendon abutment. Screws placed in zone 3 will likely cause abutment. In this case the anterior screws are in zones 2 and 3.

posttraumatic arthrosis, which occurs in 30% to 40% of cases. The incidence is highest in complex plafond fractures, when the syndesmosis is not adequately reduced and in older patients. Serial radiographs are adequate for diagnosis, although in certain cases CT or even MRI may be required before consideration of ankle fusion (see Fig. 8-23).

Ankle pain related to internal fixation hardware occurs in up to 31% of patients. This may be related to superficial or deep soft tissue irritation or bony impingement. Up to 23% of patients with internal fixation request removal of the hardware. However, symptomatic improvement occurs in only 50% of the cases. Hardware failure with plate fracture or screw pullout may also cause pain. Overcorrection or cross-union may also occur with syndesmotic screws. This may be obvious on radiographs, but may require CT or MRI for confirmation and syndesmotic evaluation (see Fig. 8-24).

Malunion, delayed union, and nonunion are uncommon. In a larger series of 260 patients, the incidence of nonunion was <1%. Nonunion is reported to occur more frequently with medial malleolar fractures (10% to 15%) (see Fig. 8-25). The incidence is much higher with closed reduction compared to internal fixation. Evaluation of healing can be accomplished with CT or MRI in subtle cases.

Reflex sympathetic dystrophy is a syndrome of refractory pain, neurovascular changes of swelling, and vasomotor instability affecting the bone and soft tissues. The etiology is unclear. Most consider the syndrome related to posttraumatic reflex spasm leading to loss of vascular tone and aggressive osteoporosis. Osteoporosis may be patch or diffuse involving cortical and medullary bone. Radionuclide bone scans may demonstrate impressive changes early (see Fig. 8-26). Table 8-6 lists complications of adult ankle fractures and imaging approaches.

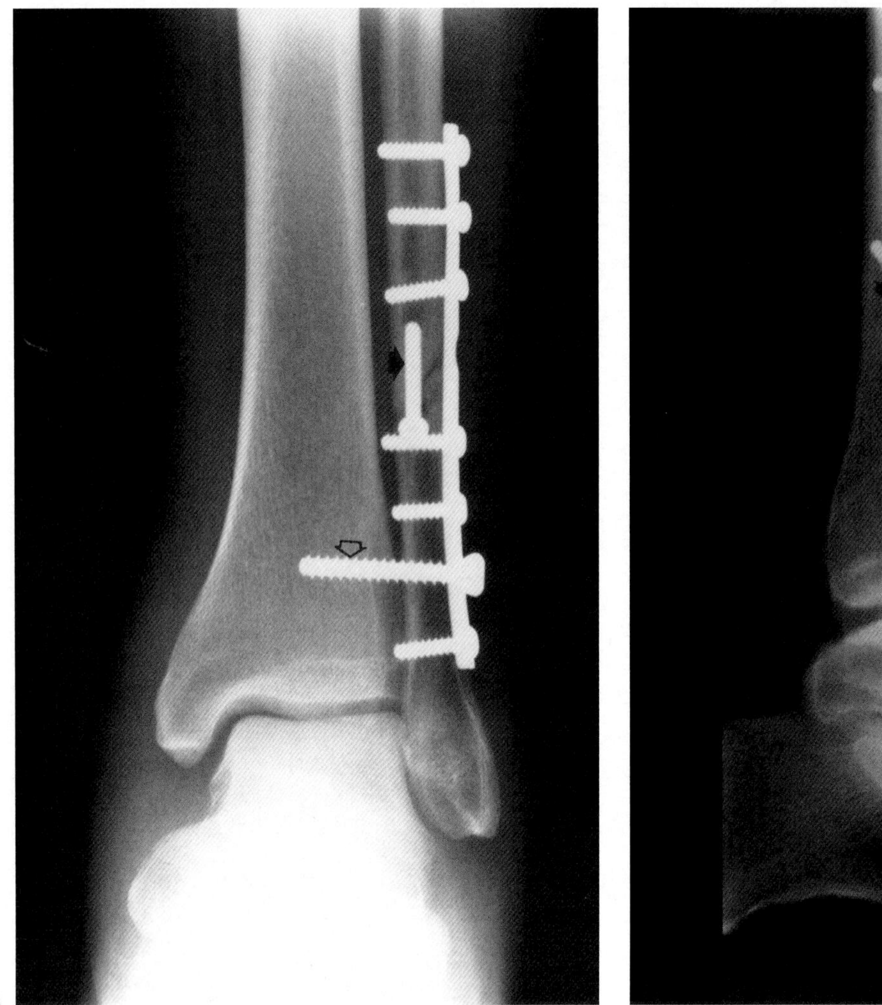


Fig. 8-20 Anteroposterior (AP) (A) and lateral (B) radiographs with one third tubular plate and cortical screw fixation of a high fibular fracture. There is also an interfragmentary screw (*arrow*) and a syndesmotic screw (*open arrow*) to reduce the ligament and interosseous membrane disruption.

Pediatric ankle fracture complications can be similar, but are more often related to the patient age and status of the growth plates. The most common problem is premature or asymmetric closure of the growth plates (see Fig. 8-27). Salter-Harris III and IV fractures of the tibia have the poorest prognosis resulting in leg length discrepancy and joint asymmetry. Leg length discrepancy >1 to 2 cm may require lengthening of the involved extremity or epiphysodesis of the contralateral tibia. In patients with asymmetric physeal closure, the bony bar may be excised if it involves <50% of the growth plate. Angular deformities >10 degrees may be treated with wedge osteotomy.

Spiegel et al. divided physeal fractures into three groups based on complication rates. Low-risk (Salter-Harris I and II fibular fractures and type I tibial fractures) injuries had a 6.7% complication rate. High-risk fractures included type III and IV tibial fractures with >2 mm displacement, juvenile Tillaux fractures, comminuted epiphyseal fractures, and type V fractures (32% complication rate). Type II tibia fractures were considered more unpredictable with a 16.7% complication rate.

Long-term osteoarthritis is also more common with Salter-Harris III and IV fractures (29%) compared to lesser injuries (12%). Serial radiographs are usually adequate to follow these

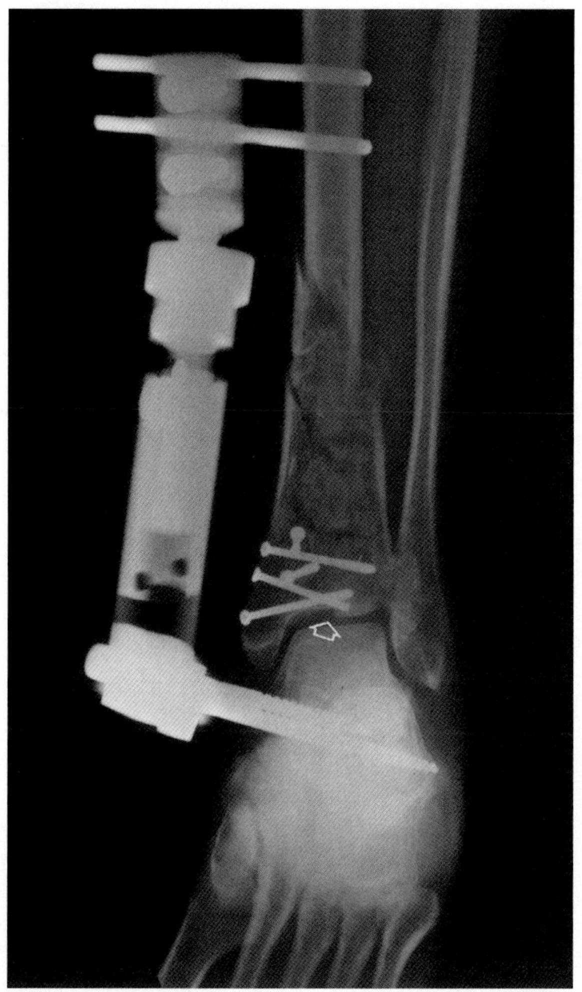
A

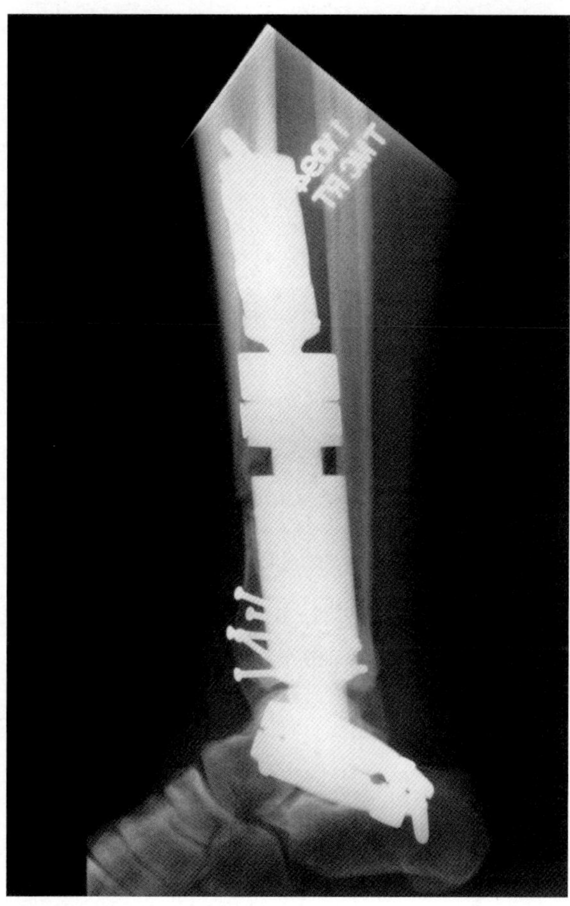
B

Fig. 8-21 Anteroposterior (AP) (A) and lateral (B) radiographs following reduction of a complex tibial fracture involving the plafond. There is slight articular deformity (*open arrow*) following screw fixation of the distal tibial fragments and external fixation to maintain tibial length.

patients. Ankle stiffness due to bone and soft tissue injury occurs in approximately 6% of patients.

Reflex sympathetic dystrophy also occurs in children and is much more common in females (up to 84% of patients).

## Suggested Reading

Brown OL, Dirschl DR, Obremskey WT. Incidence of hardware-related pain and its effect on functional outcomes after open reduction and internal fixation of ankle fractures. *J Orthop Trauma*. 2001;15:271–274.

Femino JE, Gruber BF, Karunakar MA. Safe zone for placement of medial malleolar screws. *J Bone Joint Surg*. 2007;89A:133–138.

Kay RM, Matthys GA. Pediatric ankle fractures: Evaluation and treatment. *J Am Acad Orthop Surg*. 2001;4: 268–278.

Spiegel PG, Cooperman DR, Laros GS. Epiphyseal fractures of the distal ends of the tibia and fibula. *J Bone Joint Surg*. 1978;60A:1046–1050.

Tejwani NC, McLaurin TM, Walsh M, et al. Are outcomes of bimalleolar fractures poorer than those of lateral malleolar fractures with medial ligament injury? *J Bone Joint Surg*. 2007;89A:1438–1441.

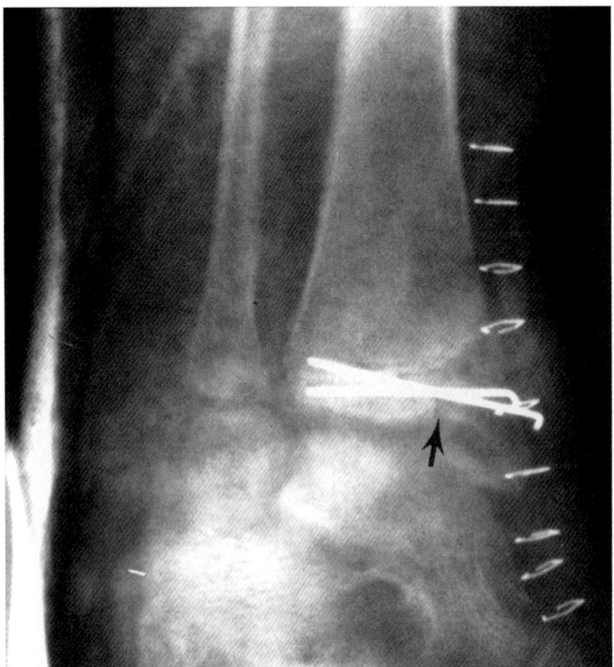

Fig. 8-22 Mortise view of the ankle with K-wire fixation of a Salter-Harris III (*arrow*) medial malleolar fracture. The wires are placed parallel to, but not through, the growth plate.

## Talar Fractures and Dislocations

Talar fractures account for <1% of all skeletal fractures. However, the talus is the second most common tarsal fracture after the calcaneus. Talar fractures are rare in children compared to adults. Less than 1% of all pediatric fractures and 2% of foot fractures involve the talus. In adults, talar neck fractures account for 30% to 50% of talar fractures, followed by talar body fractures (40%) and associated dislocations (15%). Talar head fractures account for 3% to 10% of talar fractures. Subtalar dislocations account for only 1.3% of all dislocations. Fractures of the talar dome, posterior process, and lateral talar process (snowboarder's fracture) may be subtle. In fact, up to 50% are initially overlooked on radiographs.

There are certain key features regarding the talus. First, its articulations account for 90% of the motion in the ankle and foot. Also, due to the extensive articular surface area the vascular supply is tenuous. Therefore, avascular necrosis (AVN) is not uncommon, especially following displaced talar neck fractures.

### Talar Neck Fractures

Talar neck fractures account for 30% to 50% of talar fractures and 6% of all foot and ankle injuries. Fractures are the

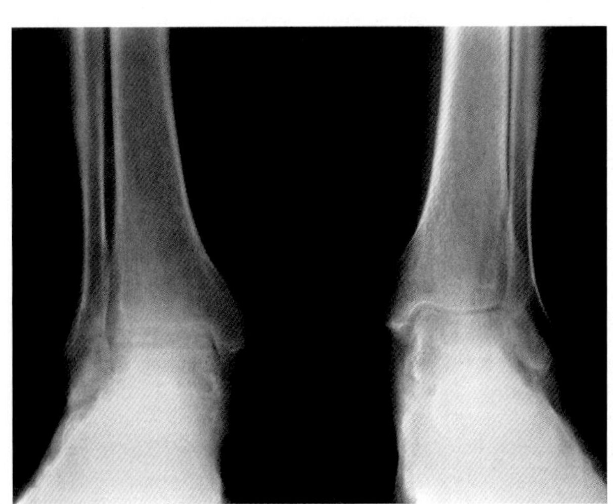

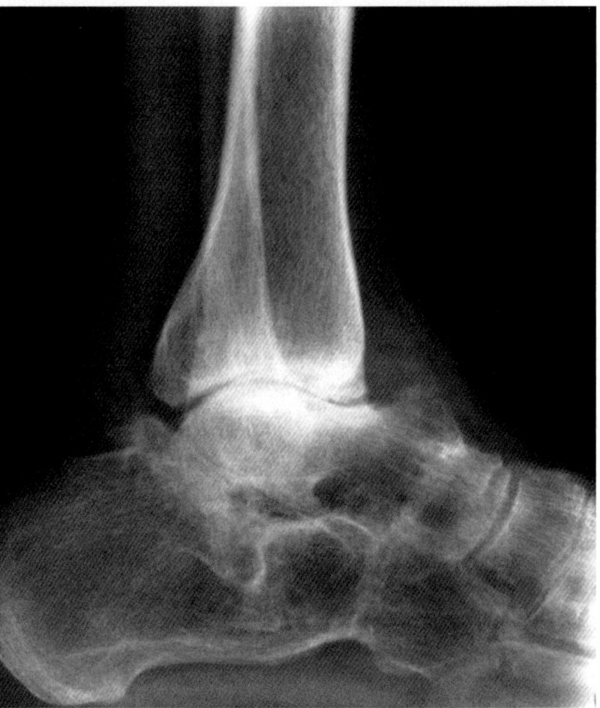

Fig. 8-23 Posttraumatic arthrosis. Anteroposterior (AP) (A) and lateral (B) radiographs demonstrate posttraumatic arthritis on the right. The patient was treated with ankle arthrodesis with screw fixation and fibular osteotomy with buttress graft (C and D).

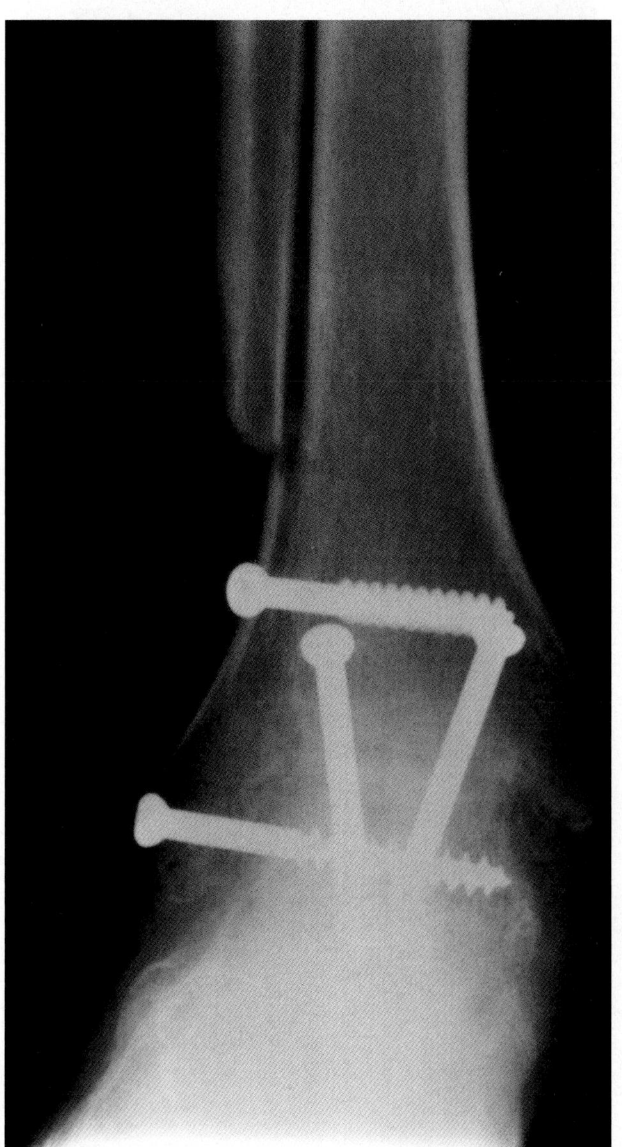


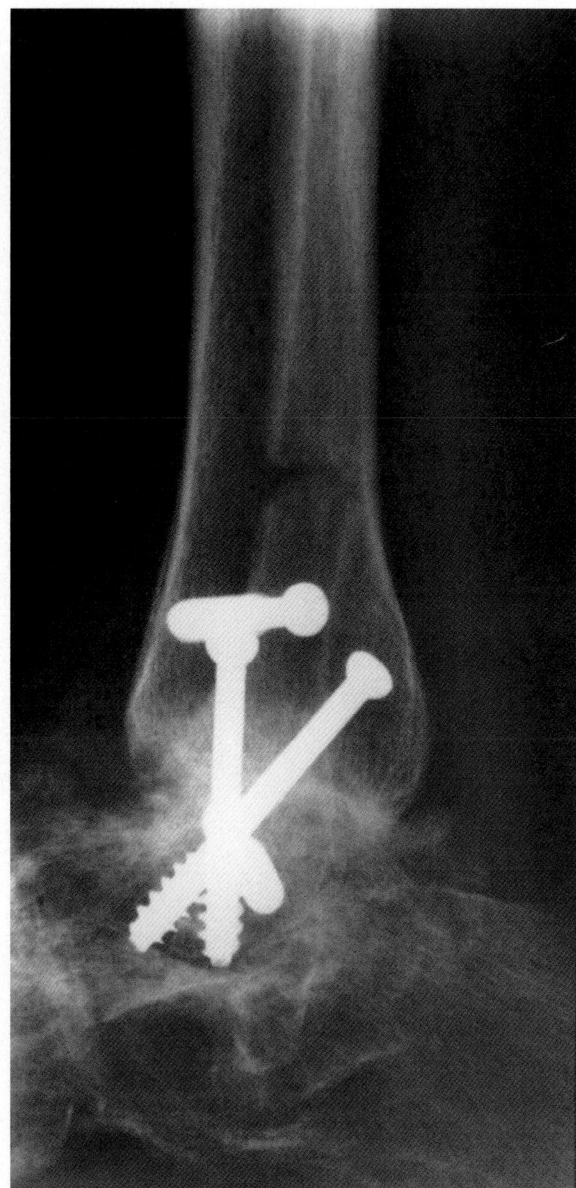


Fig. 8-23 *(Continued)*

result of abrupt dorsiflexion of the foot impacting the talus against the tibia. Injuries typically occur during motor vehicle accidents or significant falls. Supination-lateral rotation injuries may also result in talar neck fracture. Associated fractures are not uncommon. Up to 26% of patients have associated fractures of the medial malleolus and 15% have talar head fractures with associated fractures of the medial and lateral malleoli.

The Orthopaedic Trauma Association classification considers talar neck fractures as extra-articular. A common classification is the Hawkins classification (see Fig. 8-28).

## Talar Body Fractures

There is a wide range of talar body fractures including osteochondral fractures, talar process fractures, and complex crush or shearing fractures. Table 8-7 summarizes the incidence and mechanism of injury of talar body fractures.

Lateral talar process and talar dome fractures are overlooked on initial radiographs in up to 50% of patients. Talar dome fractures are more common and may involve the lateral or medial talar dome or both simultaneously. Medial lesions are deeper and not always associated with acute trauma (see Fig. 8-29). Lateral lesions are more subtle and flake-like

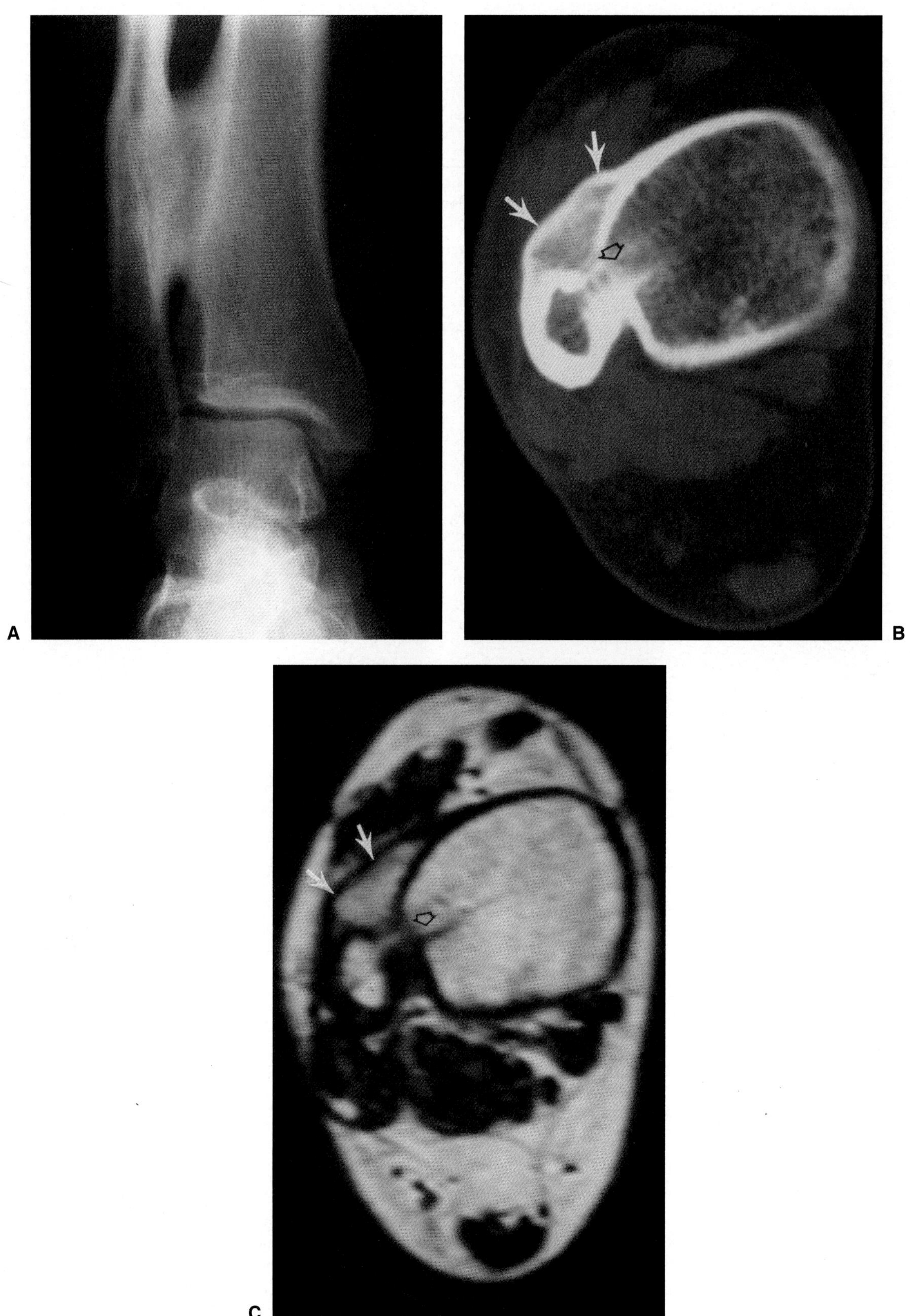


Fig. 8-24 Syndesmotic cross-union. Anteroposterior (AP) (A) radiograph demonstrates an old healed fibular fracture with cross-union of the tibia and fibula. Axial computed tomography (CT) (B) and T1-weighted magnetic resonance (MR) images show the bony union (*arrows*) and the prior syndesmotic screw tract (*open arrow*).

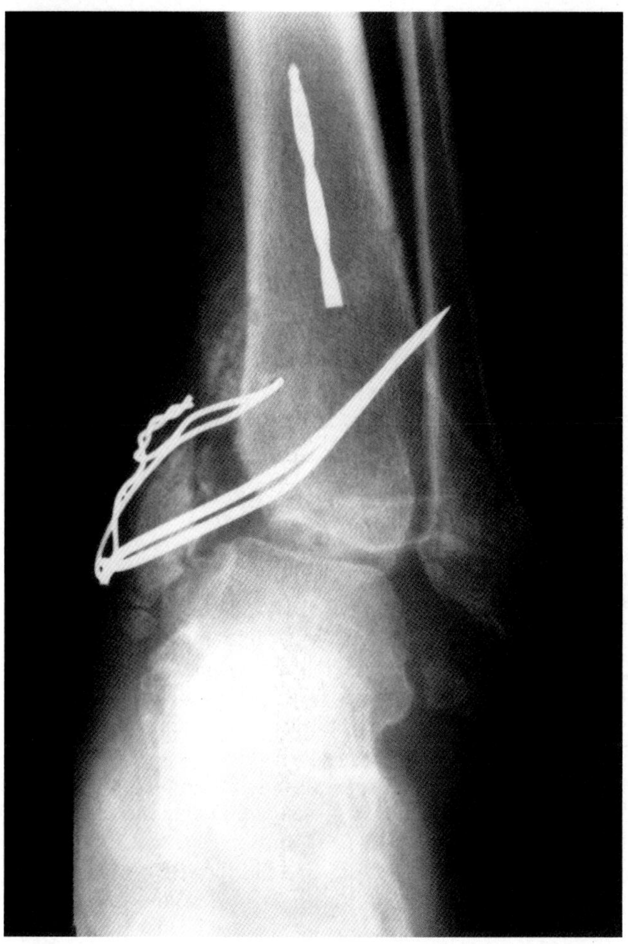

Fig. 8-25 Medial malleolar fracture treated with K-wire and tension band with nonunion and marked asymmetry of the ankle mortise.

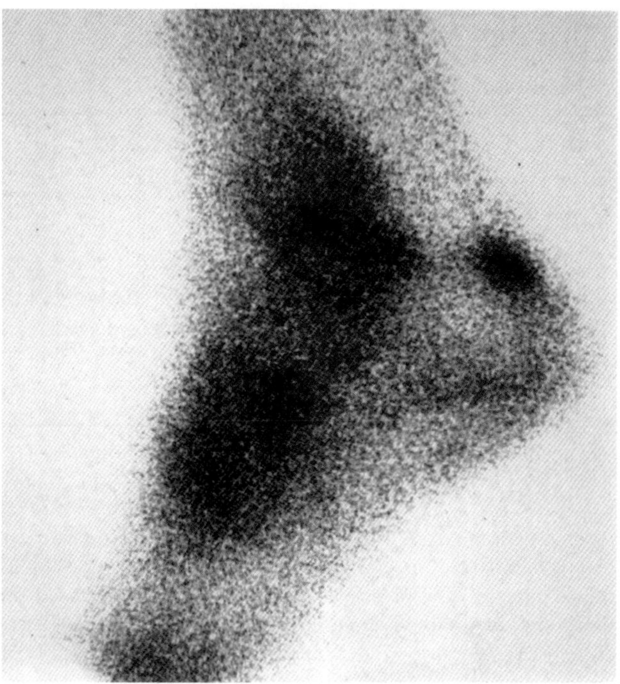

Fig. 8-26 Reflex sympathetic dystrophy. Technetium Tc 99m methylene diphosphonate (MDP) bone scan demonstrate increased tracer in the ankle and mid foot.

(see Fig. 8-30). The Berndt and Harty classification is applied to talar dome fractures. Stage I lesions are compressions of the talar dome without associated ligament ruptures and intact overlying cartilage. Stage II lesions are partially elevated fractures. Stage III lesions are complete fractures without displacement and stage IV lesions are displaced. Stage II to IV lesions can be easily overlooked due to the associated ligament injuries.

### Talar Head Fractures

Talar head fractures are uncommon, although some reports indicate that they account for 3% to 10% of talar fractures. Fractures may be easily overlooked on radiographs. Injuries result from extreme dorsiflexion of the foot or associated with subtalar dislocations when the talar head is impacted against the navicular.

## Suggested Reading

Berndt AL, Harty M. Transchondral fractures (osteochondritis dissecans) of the talus. *J Bone Joint Surg*. 1959;41A:988–1020.

Canale ST, Kelly FB. Fractures of the neck of the talus. *J Bone Joint Surg*. 1978;60A:143–156.

Fortin PT, Balazsy JE. Talus fractures: Evaluation and treatment. *J Am Acad Orthop Surg*. 2001;9:114–127.

Hawkins LG. Fractures of the neck of the talus. *J Bone Joint Surg*. 1970;52A:991–1002.

Kay RM, Tang CW. Pediatric foot fractures: Evaluation and treatment. *J Am Acad Orthop Surg*. 2001;9:308–319.

Valderrabono V, Perreu T, Ryf C, et al. "Snowboarders" talus fracture-treatment outcome of 20 cases after 3.5 years. *Am J Sports Med*. 2005;33:871–880.

### Imaging of Talar Fractures

Imaging of talar fractures begins with routine AP, lateral, and oblique views of the foot and ankle (see Fig. 8-31). Both internal and external oblique views of the ankle may be helpful for subtle fractures (see Fig. 8-32). Special subtalar oblique projections have also been described. However, if radiographs are equivalent or fractures are defined, most institutions obtain CT with coronal and sagittal reformatting or three-dimensional

**Table 8-6**

IMAGING OF ADULT FRACTURE COMPLICATIONS

| COMPLICATION | IMAGING APPROACHES |
|---|---|
| Osteoarthritis | Serial radiographs |
| Chronic instability | Stress views, MRI |
| Nonunion | Serial radiographs, MRI, CT |
| Implant failure | Serial radiographs |
| Reflex sympathetic | Radionulcide scans dystrophy |
| Adhesive capsulitis | Distension arthrography |
| Tendon rupture | MRI |

MRI, magnetic resonance imaging; CT, computed tomography.

**Table 8-7**

TALAR BODY FRACTURES

| TYPE | INCIDENCE | MECHANISM OF INJURY |
|---|---|---|
| Crush/shearing | 28%–33% | Axial compression, shearing |
| Talar dome | 1%–6% | Inversion, eversion, rotation |
| Lateral process | Uncommon | Dorsiflexion-inversion (snowboarder's fracture) |
| Posterior process | Uncommon | Avulsion, plantar flexion |

reconstructions to fully evaluate the fracture and articular involvement (see Fig. 8-33). CT is particularly important in subtle injuries. The presence of a joint effusion (best seen on the lateral view) should suggest further imaging (CT or MRI) to exclude subtle injuries to the talar dome or talar processes. MRI is useful for detection of subtle stress injuries, bone bruises, early AVN, and soft tissue injuries (see Fig. 8-34).

## Suggested Reading

Berquist TH. *Radiology of the foot and ankle*, 2nd ed. Philadelphia: Lippincott Williams & Wilkins; 2000:171–280.

DeSmet AA, Fisher DR, Burnstein MI, et al. Value of MR imaging in staging osteochondral lesions of the talus (osteochondritis dissecans): Results in 14 patients. *AJR Am J Roentgenol.* 1990;154:555–558.

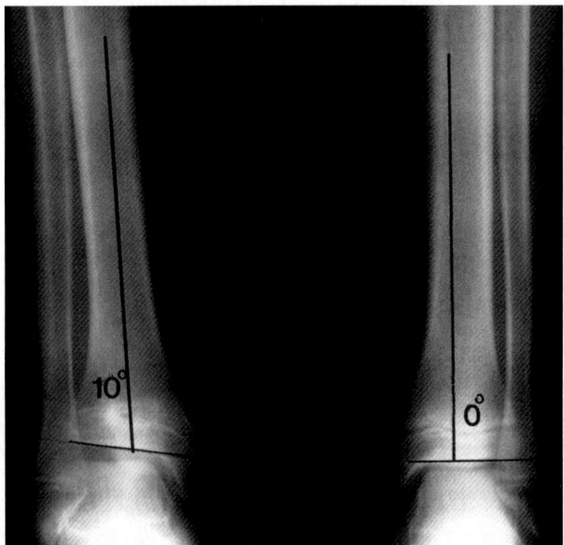


**Fig. 8-27** Standing radiographs of the legs with parallel articular surfaces on the left and 10-degree angular deformity on the right due to premature closure laterally.

### Treatment Options

Treatment options vary with the type of injury, articular involvement, open wounds, patient condition, and surgical preference. Both closed reduction and open reduction with internal fixation may be used in the appropriate settings.

Treatment of talar neck fractures varies with the extent of the lesion. Type I undisplaced fractures or minimally displaced type II injuries can be managed with cast immobilization for 6 weeks. Open reduction and internal fixation is preferred for failed closed reduction of type II and initial treatment of type III and IV lesions (Fig. 8-31). Twenty-five percent of type III fractures are open, thereby increasing the risk of infection. In this setting, internal fixation with delayed wound closer to 3 to 5 days is preferred.

Complex talar body fractures have a high complication rate with closed reduction (see Fig. 8-35). Therefore, open reduction with internal fixation is preferred to restore articular anatomy and preserve as much function as possible.

Talar dome and process fractures are frequently overlooked. Talar process fractures (lateral or posterior) can be managed with cast immobilization if there is <2 mm of displacement. Comminuted fractures may require removal of the small fragments with internal fixation or major fragments. Talar dome fractures that are undisplaced (types I to III) may be treated conservatively. If closed reduction fails, arthroscopic drilling of type II and debridement of type III lesions should be considered. Displaced fragments (type IV) usually result in chronic symptoms and should be removed (see Fig. 8-36).

Talar head fractures with minimal articular deformity or involving only a small portion of the articular surface may be managed with cast immobilization for 6 weeks. If the fragment is displaced or causes incongruency of the talonavicular joint, open reduction and internal fixation with screws or bioabsorbable pins is preferred (see Fig. 8-37).

Isolated dislocations or those associated with other injuries are managed with immobilization that is in concert with treatment of the other injuries. CT images should be obtained following reduction to fully evaluate the joint spaces and any osteochondral fragments that may not have been initially recognized.

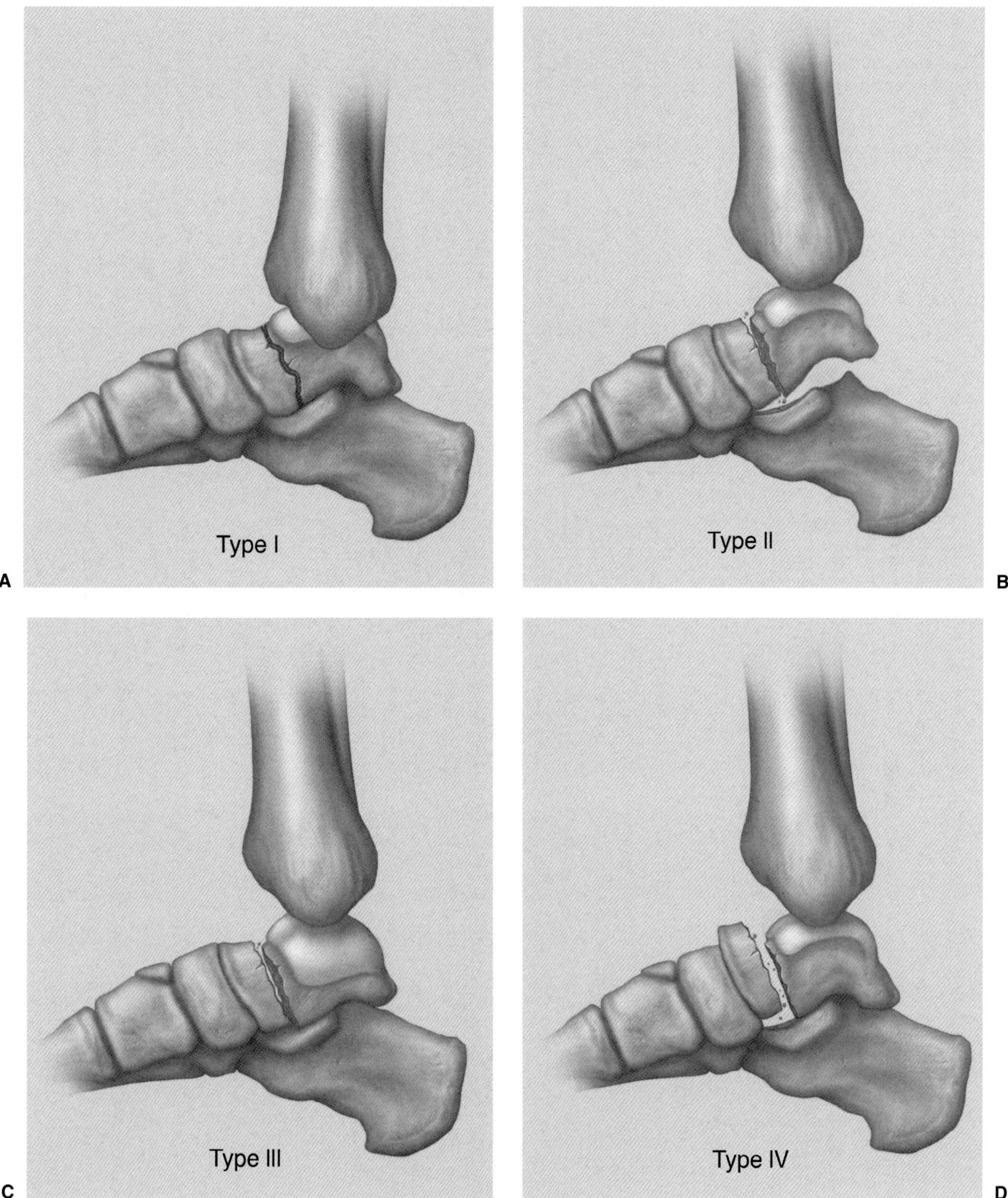


Fig. 8-28 Illustration of the Hawkins classification for talar neck fractures. A: Type I—undisplaced neck fracture. B: Type II—neck fracture with subluxation or dislocation of the subtalar joint. C: Type III—fracture of the neck with displacement of the body from both the ankle and subtalar joints. D: Type IV—fracture of the neck with dislocation with ankle or subtalar subluxation/dislocation and talonavicular subluxation/dislocation.

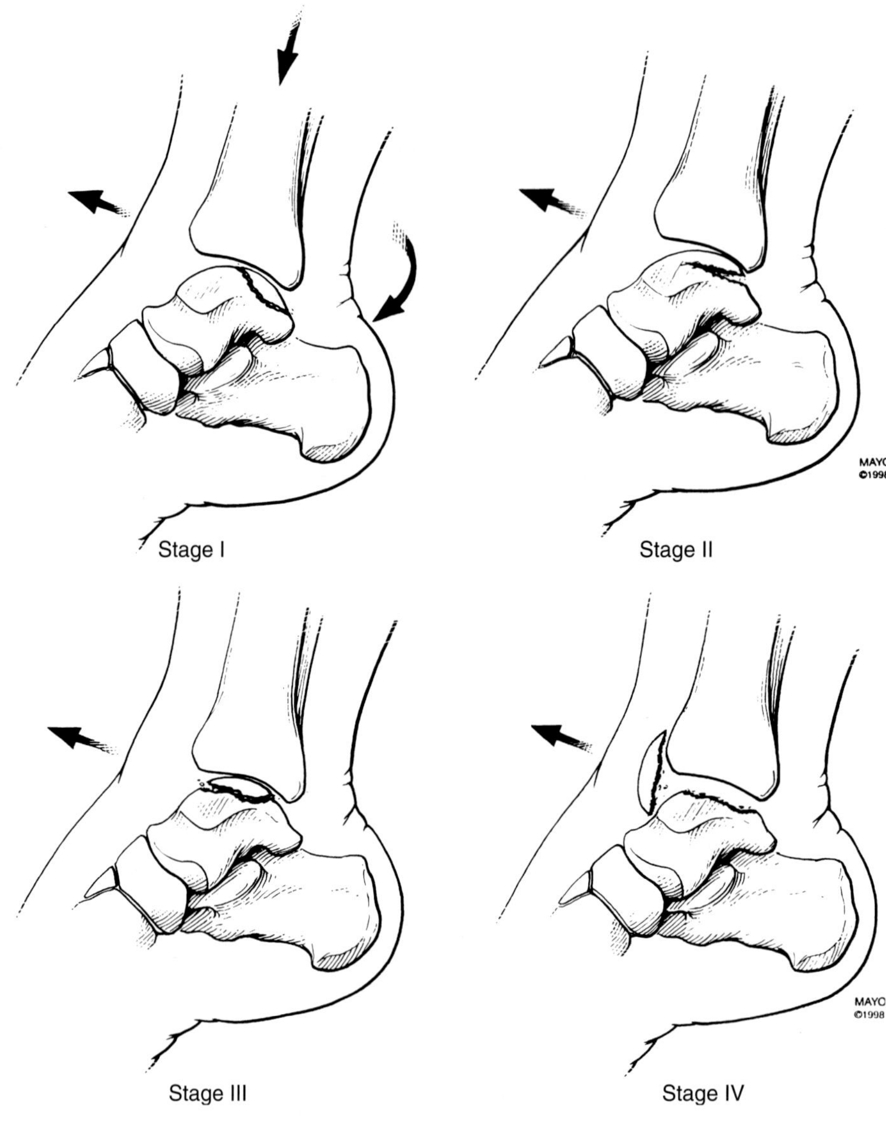


**Fig. 8-29** Illustration of the mechanism of injury of medial talar dome fractures. The injury occurs with plantar flexion, axial loading, and inversion-lateral rotation. Stage I—compression, stage II—fracture with partial elevation, stage III—complete fracture with no displacement, and stage IV—displaced fracture. (From Berquist TH. *Radiology of the foot and ankle*, 2nd ed. Philadelphia: Lippincott Williams & Wilkins; 2000.)

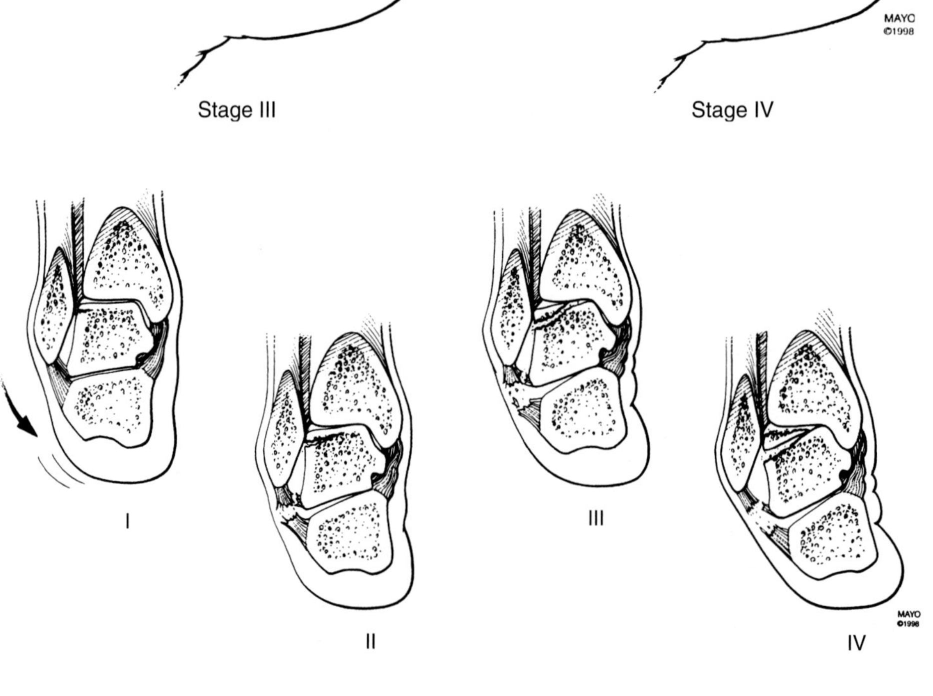


**Fig. 8-30** Illustration of the mechanism of injury and classification of lateral talar dome fractures. Inversion causes the lateral talar dome to impact on the fibula. Stage I—compression injury, stage II—partial elevation with lateral ligament tear, stage III—complete fracture without displacement and ligament tear, and stage IV—displaced fracture with ligament tear. (From Berquist TH. *Radiology of the foot and ankle*, 2nd ed. Philadelphia: Lippincott Williams & Wilkins; 2000.)

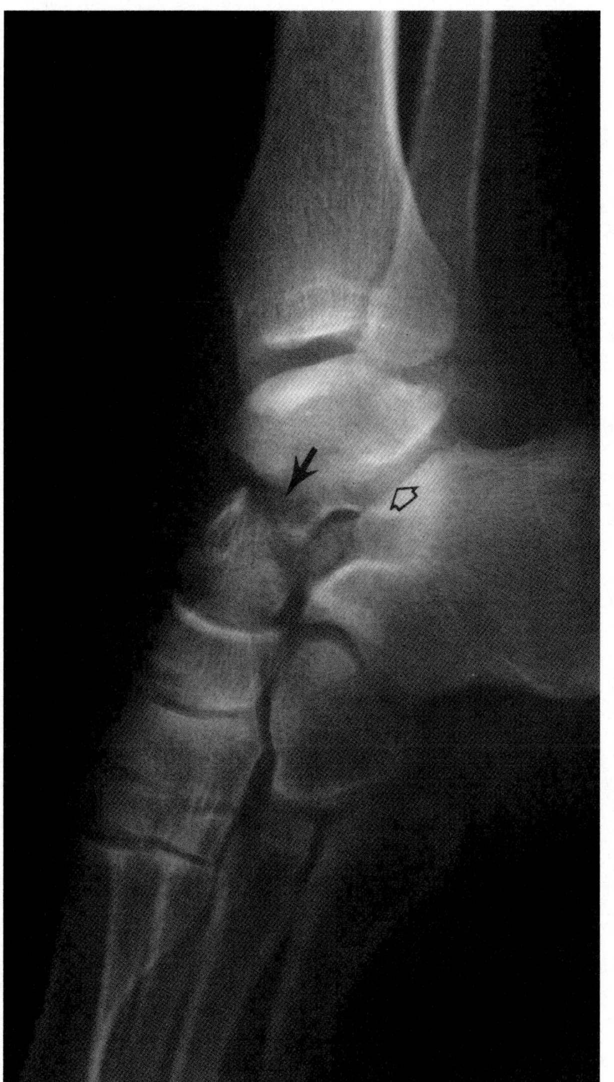


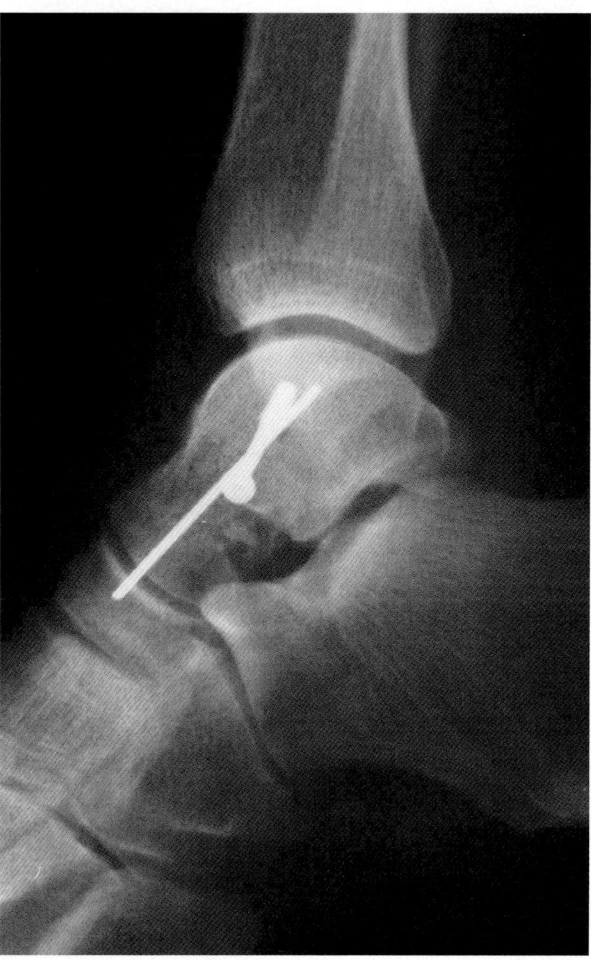


**Fig. 8-31** Hawkins type II talar neck fracture. **A:** Lateral radiograph demonstrates a displaced talar neck fracture (*arrow*) with subluxation of the subtalar joint (*open arrow*). The fracture was treated (**B**) with open reduction using a K-wire and screw for fixation.

## Suggested Reading

Canale ST, Kelly FB. Fractures of the neck of the talus. *J Bone Joint Surg*. 1978;60A:143–156.

Fortin PT, Balazsy JE. Talus fractures: Evaluation and treatment. *J Am Acad Orthop Surg*. 2001;9:114–127.

### Imaging of Complications

Complications following talar fracture/dislocations include AVN, posttraumatic arthritis, malunion or nonunion, and infection. AVN is common following displaced talar neck fractures and complex talar body fractures. The incidence of AVN is only 0% to 13% with Hawkins type I fractures, but increases to 20% to 58% with type II and 83% to 100% with type IV fractures (see Table 8-8). The incidence of AVN with complex body fractures is 40%. AVN is less common with talar process and talar dome fractures. Radiographs following fractures may demonstrate changes of AVN within 6 to 8 weeks. Normally, there is subchondral osteopenia due to hyperemia. When this is absent or bone sclerosis is evident (Hawkins sign), the area is ischemic (see Fig. 8-38). MRI is more specific and can demonstrate changes earlier (see Fig. 8-39).

Posttraumatic arthrosis involving the tibiotalar and subtalar joints is common following all types of talar fractures. Following complex talar body fractures (Fig. 8-35) the incidence ranges from 48% to 90%. Arthrosis occurs in 54% of patients with talar neck fractures and 50% with talar dome fractures. Serial radiographs are usually adequate for evaluation. However, based on the symptoms and when arthrodesis is considered, CT with coronal and sagittal reformatting is useful for treatment planning purposes.

Fracture healing may be delayed or result in malunion or nonunion. Nonunion occurs in only 4% of patients with

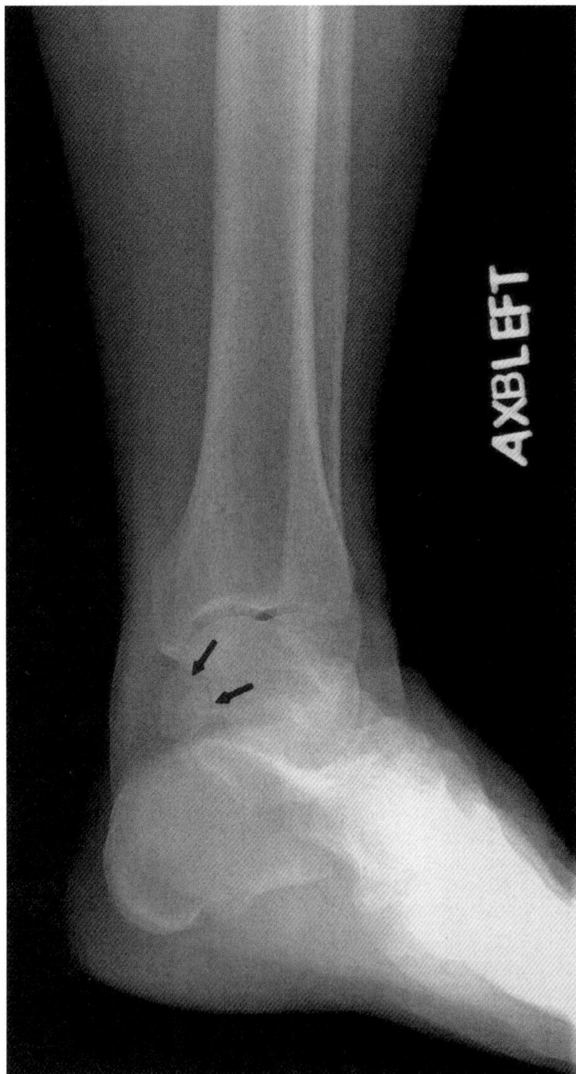


Fig. 8-32 Subtle posteromedial talar fracture (*arrows*) seen only on the external oblique view.

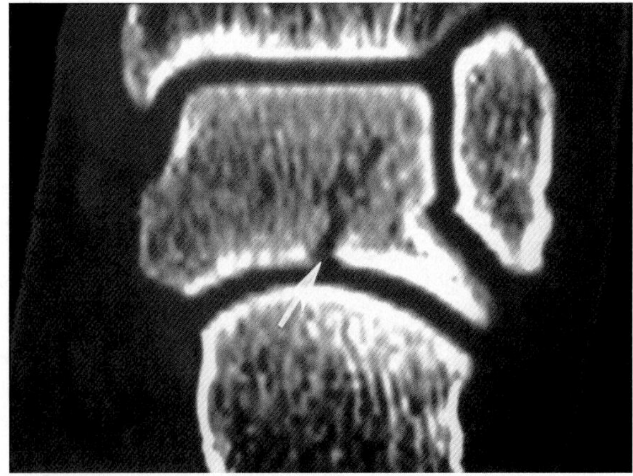

Fig. 8-33 Coronal reformatted computed tomographic (CT) image of a talar body fracture (*arrow*) with subtalar joint involvement.

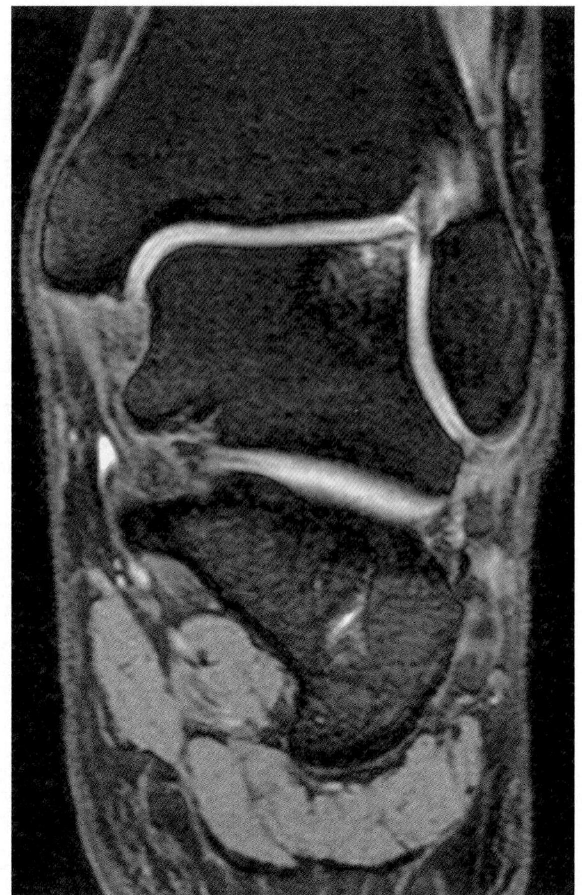


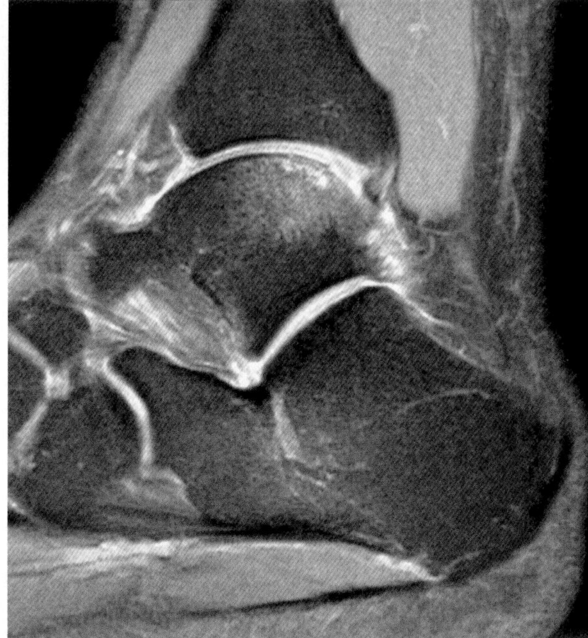


Fig. 8-34 Coronal (A) and sagittal (B) fat-suppressed fast spin-echo T2-weighted sequences demonstrating a talar dome fracture medially. At least two image planes are important to evaluate the size of the lesion and overlying articular cartilage.

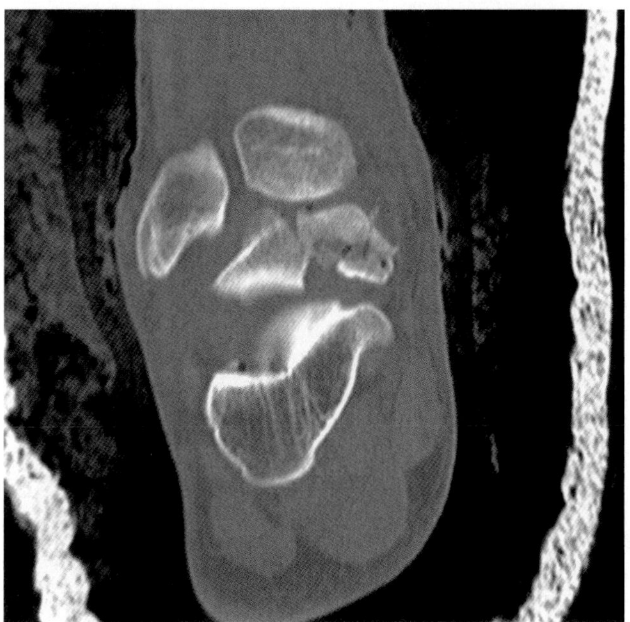

Fig. 8-35 Coronal computed tomographic (CT) image demonstrating a complex talar body fracture with extensive tibiotalar and subtalar articular deformity.

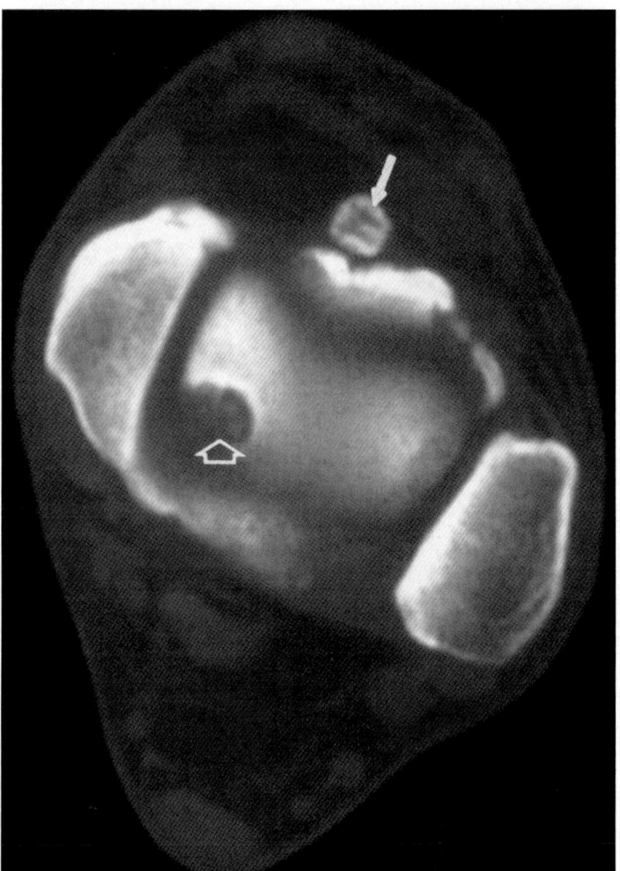

Fig. 8-36 Type IV talar dome lesion. Axial computed tomographic (CT) image demonstrates an osteochondral defect (*open arrow*) with the displaced fragment anteriorly (*arrow*).

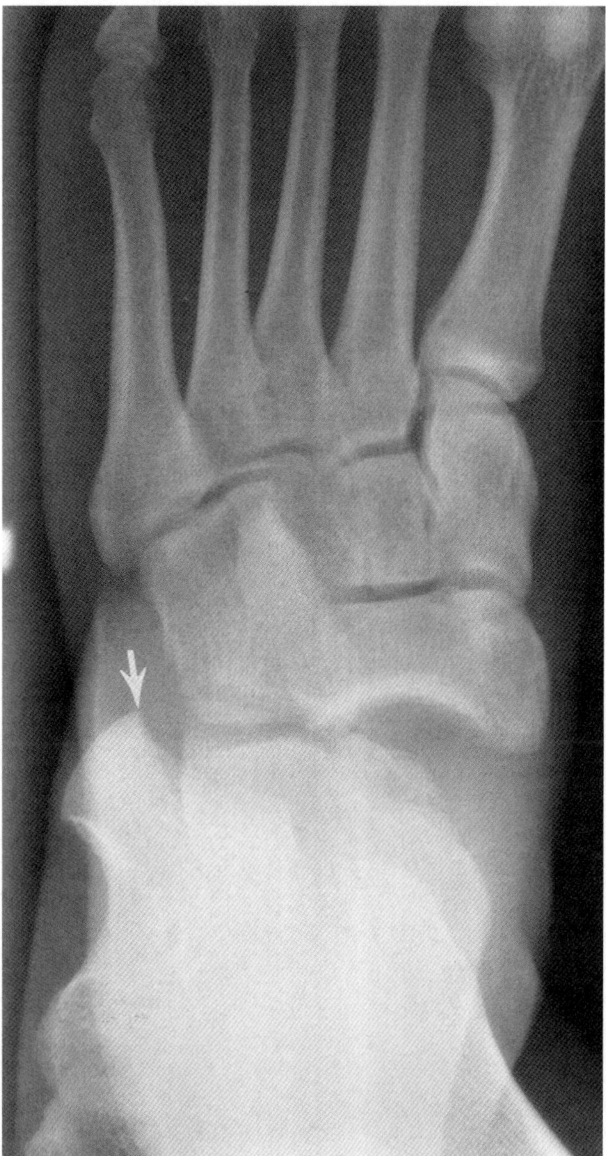

Fig. 8-37 Radiograph of a complex Hawkins IV fracture with talonavicular dislocation and a large displaced talar head fragment (*arrow*).

talar neck fractures, although delayed union is common (15%). Delayed union is considered in fractures that have not healed by 6 months. Malunion following talar neck fractures is also common (32%). CT is preferred to evaluate healing in patients with talar fractures.

Infection is a relatively common problem due to the incidence of open wounds associated with talar fracture dislocations. More than 50% of Hawkins type III and IV fractures are associated with open wounds. Infection and skin slough are the most difficult complications to manage. Implant removal and placement of antibiotic spacers may be required for treatment. MRI or combined technetium Tc 99m and labeled white blood cells or antigranulocyte antibodies are useful to define infection. Aspirations can also be used to isolate the organisms.

Table 8-8

HAWKINS CLASSIFICATION FOR TALAR NECK FRACTURES

| TYPE | INCIDENCE (%) | RADIOGRAPHIC FEATURES |
|---|---|---|
| I | 11–21 | Undisplaced neck fracture (Fig. 8-28A) |
| II | 10–24 | Displaced neck fracture with subluxation or dislocation of the subtalar joint (Fig. 8-28B) |
| III | 23–47 | Displaced neck fracture with subluxation or dislocation of both the subtalar and ankle joints (Fig. 8-28C) |
| IV | 5 | Same as type III with talonavicular dislocation or subluxation (Fig. 8-28D) |

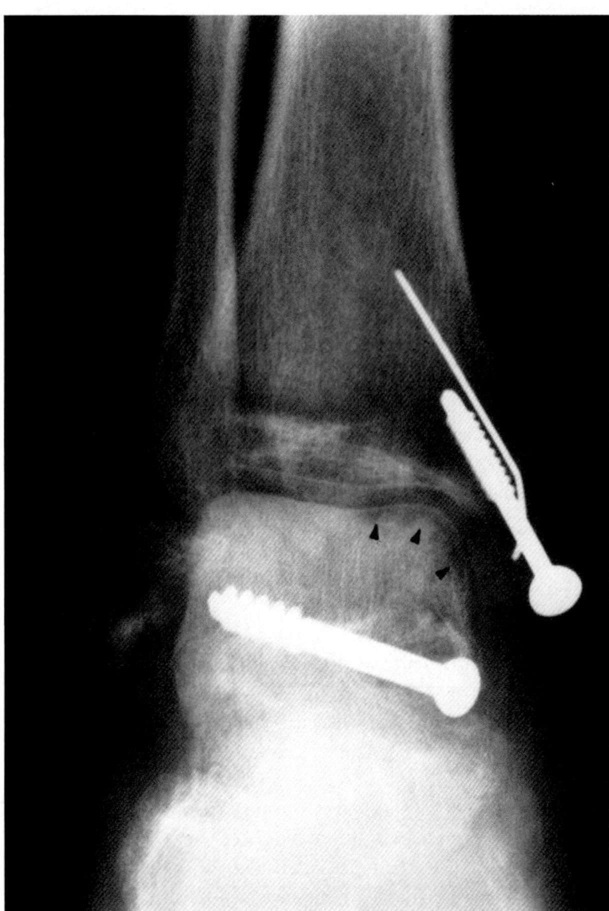

Fig. 8-38 Anteroposterior (AP) radiograph following reduction of a talar neck fracture with a single screw and internal fixation of the associated medial malleolar fracture. Note the subchondral osteopenia (*small arrowheads*) in the vascularized portion of the talus and the sclerotic appearance laterally due to avascular necrosis (AVN).

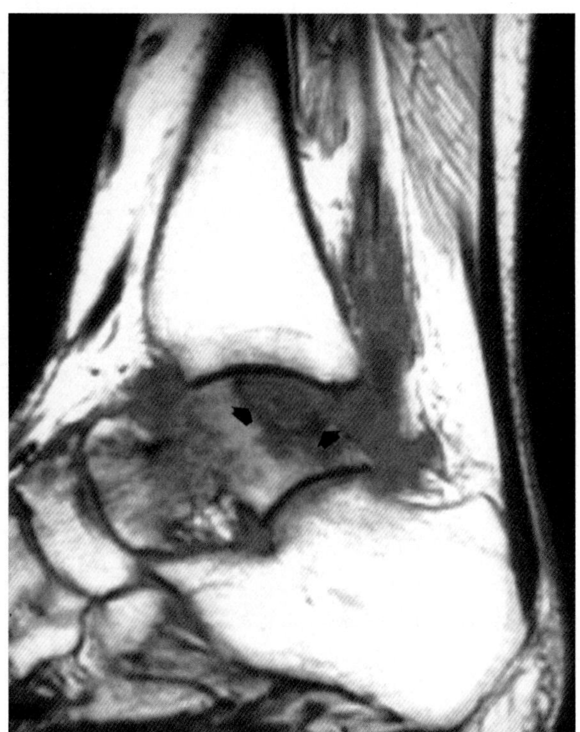


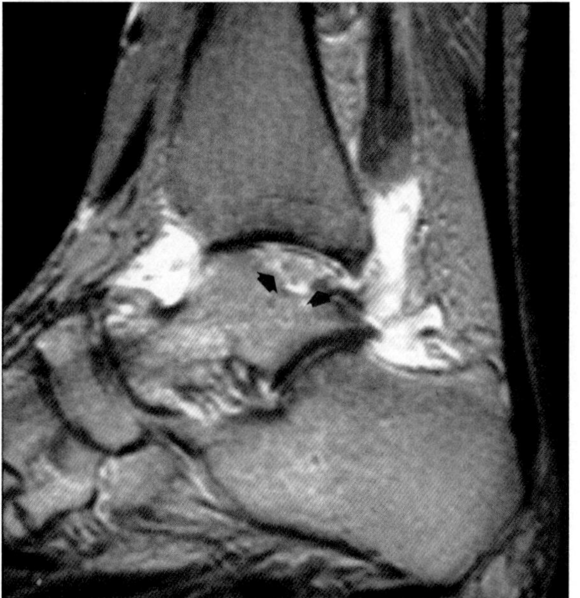


Fig. 8-39 Avascular necrosis (AVN) of the talus. **A:** Sagittal T1- and T2-weighted (**B**) images demonstrating a focal area of AVN (*arrows*).

## Suggested Reading


Berquist TH. *Radiology of the foot and ankle*, 2nd ed. Philadelphia: Lippincott Williams & Wilkins; 2000:171–280.

Canale ST, Kelly FB. Fractures of the neck of the talus. *J Bone Joint Surg*. 1978;60A:143–156.

Fortin PT, Balazsy JE. Talus fractures: Evaluation and treatment. *J Am Acad Orthop Surg*. 2001;9:114–127.

Vallier HA, Nork SE, Benirschke SK, et al. Surgical treatment of talar body fractures. *J Bone Joint Surg*. 2003;86A:1711–1724.

## Calcaneal Fractures

The calcaneus is the most commonly fractured tarsal bone, but accounts for only 2% of all skeletal fractures. All age-groups are affected with 5% occurring in children. Extra-articular fractures are more common in children compared to adults. The mechanism of injury may be a fall from a significant height which results in bilateral calcaneal fractures in 5% to 9% and associated thoracic or lumbar compression fractures in 10% of patients. Fractures also occur in motor vehicle accidents. Other associated injuries include ankle fractures (25%), compartment syndrome (10%), peroneal tendon dislocation, and flexor hallucis longus entrapment between bone fragments. Fracture patterns may be intra-articular (70% to 75%) or extra-articular (25% to 30%).

### Extra-articular Fractures (25% to 30%)

Extra-articular fractures include all fractures that do not involve the posterior facet. Injuries may be caused by twisting, avulsion, or compression forces. The posterior, anterior, or medial calcaneus may be involved. Patients with anterior calcaneal process fractures often present with symptoms similar to ankle sprain. Therefore, it is not uncommon for these fractures to be overlooked (see Fig. 8-40).

Fractures of the calcaneal body spare the facets, but may result in joint incongruency and articular deformity. Although the prognosis is better than articular fractures, there may still be considerable calcaneal deformity. Fractures of the peroneal tubercle or lateral calcaneal process are uncommon. This injury is usually related to inversion plantar flexion forces or direct trauma. Once again, patients typically present with symptoms of ankle sprain.

Calcaneal tuberosity fractures result from Achilles avulsion and are more common in younger patients and elderly osteoporotic or diabetic patients (see Fig. 8-41). Fractures of the medial calcaneal process are more likely the result of vertical shearing forces than avulsion of the plantar fascia, adductor hallucis, or flexor digitorum muscles.

### Intra-articular Fractures (70% to 75%)

Two fracture patterns occur with intra-articular fractures due to shearing or compression forces. A shear fracture line

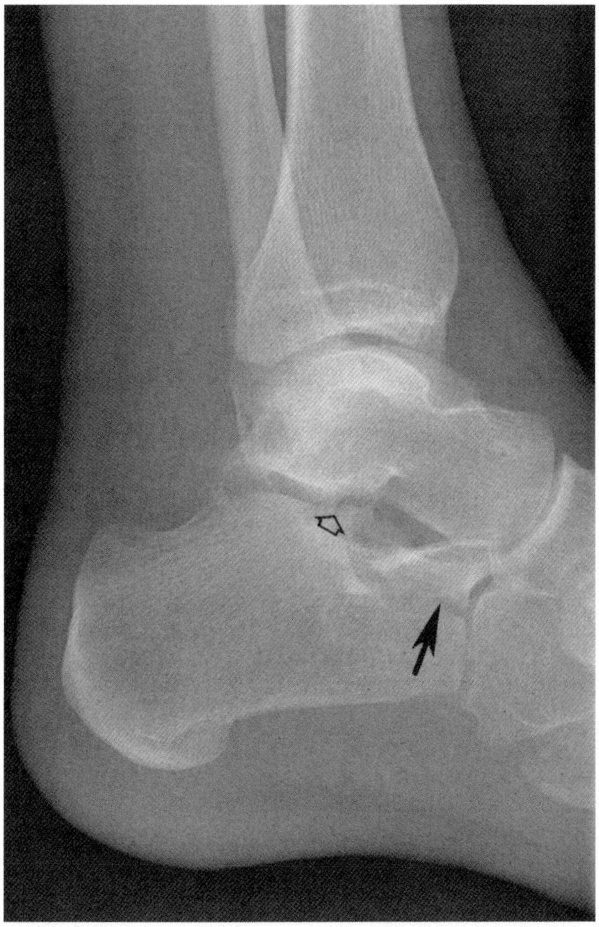

**Fig. 8-40** Lateral radiograph demonstrating an anterior calcaneal process fracture (*arrow*). There is also a subtle talar articular fracture (*open arrow*).

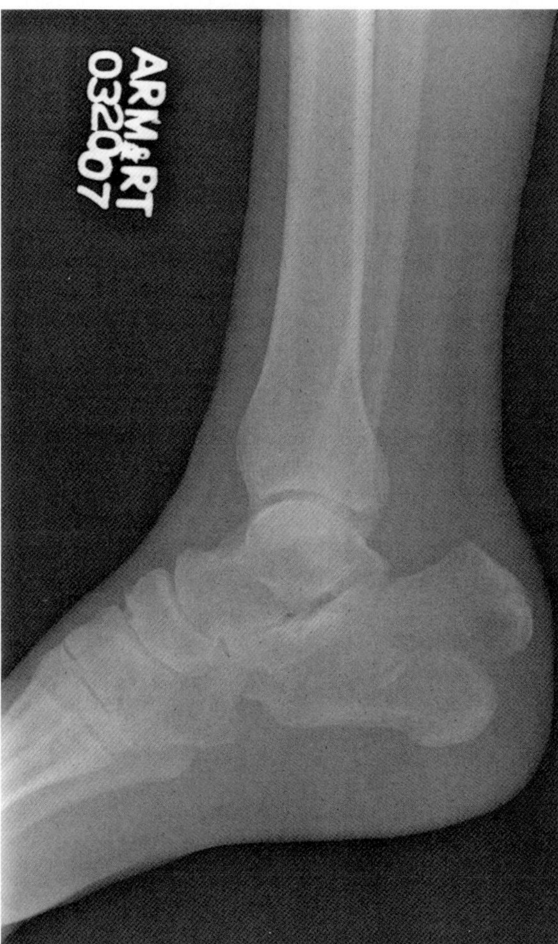

**Fig. 8-41** Lateral radiograph demonstrating a displaced tuberosity fracture.

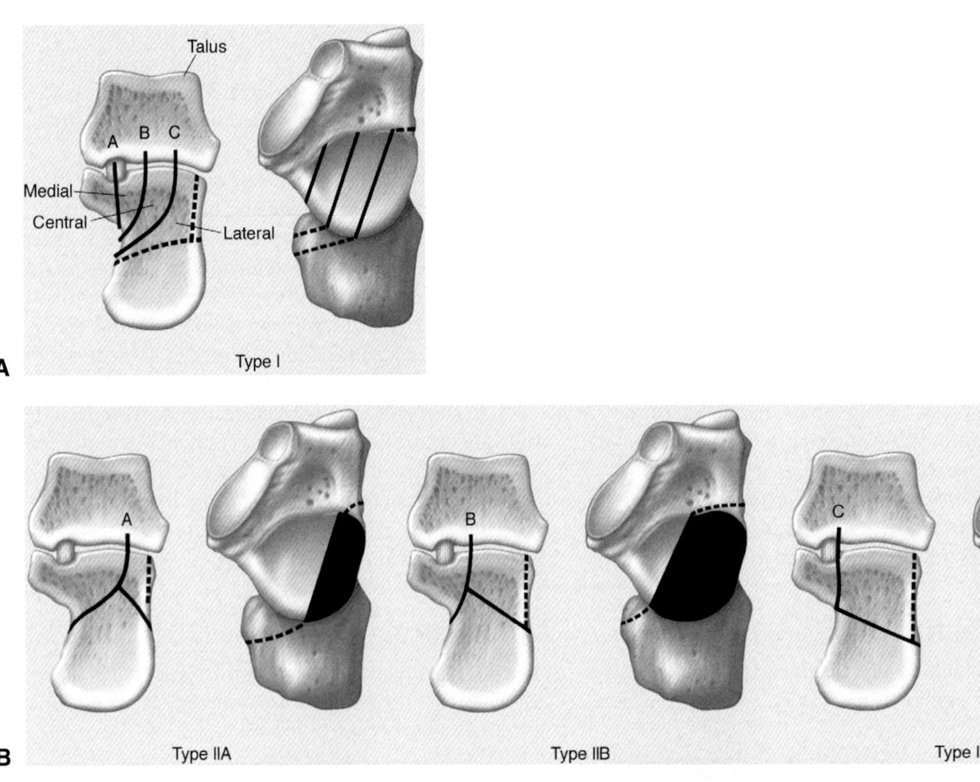


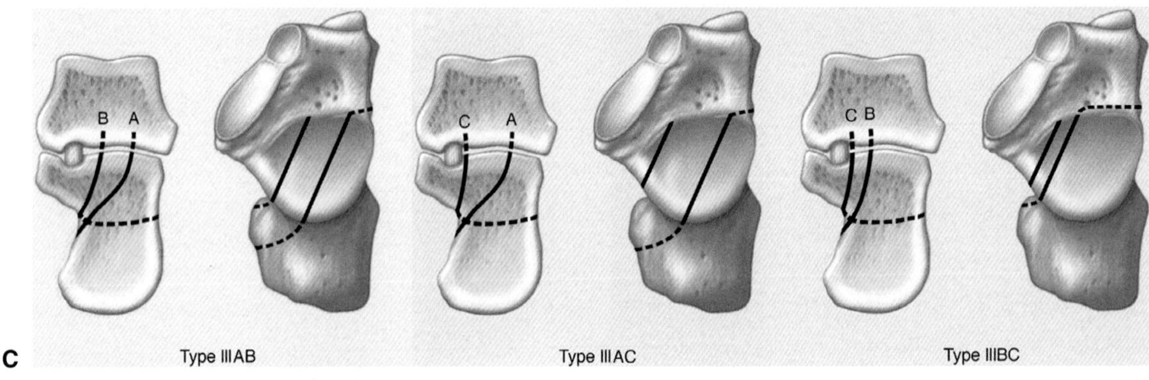


C
Type IIIAB
Type IIIAC
Type IIIBC

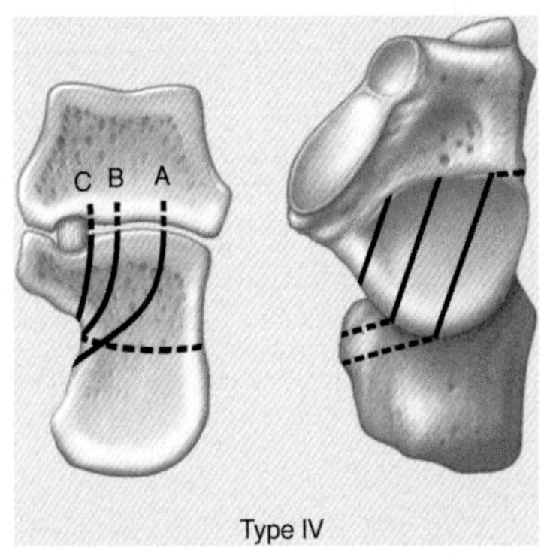


Fig. 8-42 Illustration of the Sanders computed tomography (CT) classification of calcaneal fractures involving the posterior facet. **A:** The widest undersurface of the posterior facet is divided by two lines (*A* and *B*) into three columns—medial, central, and lateral. Line *C* separates the medial column and sustentaculum. **B:** Type II—two-part fractures. IIA—fracture lateral or line *A*; Type IIB—fracture central or line *B*; Type IIC—fracture medial or line *C*. **C:** Type III—three-part posterior facet fractures with central depression. IIIAB—fracture lines lateral and central or *A* and *B*; Type IIIAC—fracture lines lateral and medial or *A* and *C*; Type IIIBC—fracture lines central and medial or *B* and *C*. **D:** Type IV—four-part or highly comminuted posterior facet fractures or lines *A*, *B*, and *C*.

occurs in the sagittal plane involving the posterior facet that may extend to the calcaneocuboid articulation. This fracture separates the calcaneus into sustentacular (anteromedial) and tuberosity (posterolateral) fragments. Compression injuries cause displacement of the anterolateral calcaneus into the angle of Gissane. This results in loss of calcaneal height, widening of the calcaneus, and articular deformity in the posterior facet.

### Fracture Classifications

Calcaneal fracture classifications have been modified over the years from the Rowe, Essex-Lopresti, Orthopaedic Trauma Association, and in recent years several classifications based upon CT findings, specifically related to the posterior facet. The Sanders classification is useful for correlating image features with prognosis and treatment approaches. With this method the coronal image with the widest undersurface of the posterior talar facet is divided by two lines (A and B) into three columns. The two lines separate the posterior calcaneal facet into three segments—medial, central, and lateral. A third line (C) separates the margin of the posterior facet from the sustentaculum resulting in four potential fragments. The lines are named A, B, and C moving from lateral to medial as the more medial the fracture the more difficult the reduction (see Fig. 8-42).

Almost all calcaneal fractures should be evaluated with CT to exclude articular involvement. Therefore, this classification has more application for imagers than some of the other fracture classifications.

## Suggested Reading

Daftary A, Haims AH, Baumgaertner MR. Fractures of the calcaneus: A review with emphasis on CT. *Radiographics* 2005; 25:1215–1226.

Fitzgibbons TC, McMullen ST, Mormino MA. Fractures and dislocation of the calcaneus. In: Bucholtz RW, Hechman JD, eds. *Rockwood and Green's fractures in adults*, 5th ed. Philadelphia: Lippincott Williams & Wilkins; 2001:2133–2179.

Kay RM, Tang CW. Pediatric foot fractures: Evaluation and treatment. *J Am Acad Orthop Surg*. 2001;9:308–319.

Sanders R, Fortin P, DiPasquale T, et al. Operative treatment of 120 displaced intra-articular calcaneal fractures: Results using a prognostic computed tomography scan classification. *Clin Orthop*. 1993;290:87–95.

### Imaging of Calcaneal Fractures

Radiographs should be obtained as the initial screening examination for suspected calcaneal fractures. Lateral and axial projections are obtained. The latter is useful to evaluate calcaneal width although the articulations may not always be identified (see Fig. 8-43). There are two key measurements that should be made routinely on the lateral radiograph. The Bohler angle (normal 25 to 40 degrees) (see Fig. 8-44) is a useful measurement for evaluating calcaneal height. The angle is formed by a line from the posterior superior calcaneal margin to the upper margin of the posterior calcaneal facet. A second line is drawn from the posterior superior margin of the facet

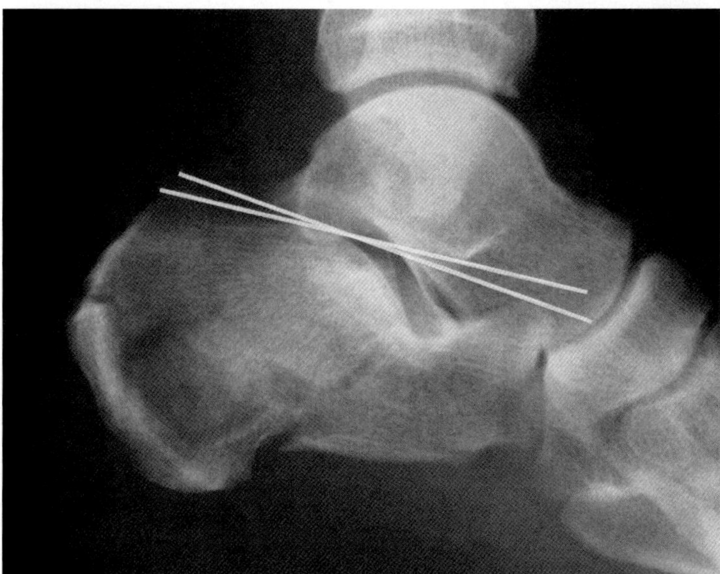


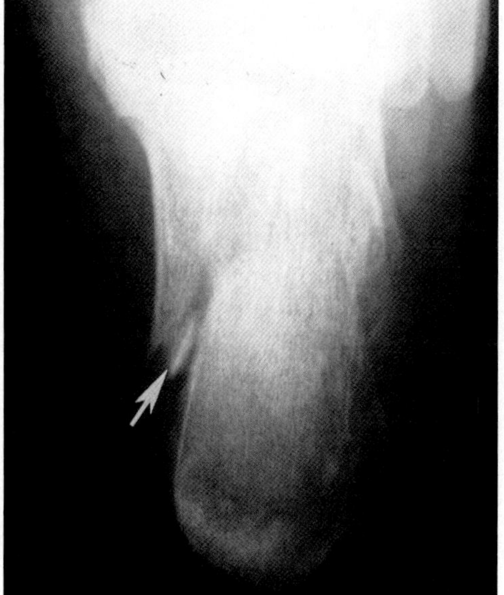


**Fig. 8-43** Lateral (A) and axial (B) views of the calcaneus in a patient with a complex fracture and marked reduction in Bohler angle (*lines*). The axial view (B) demonstrates the fracture (*arrow*) and calcaneal widening.

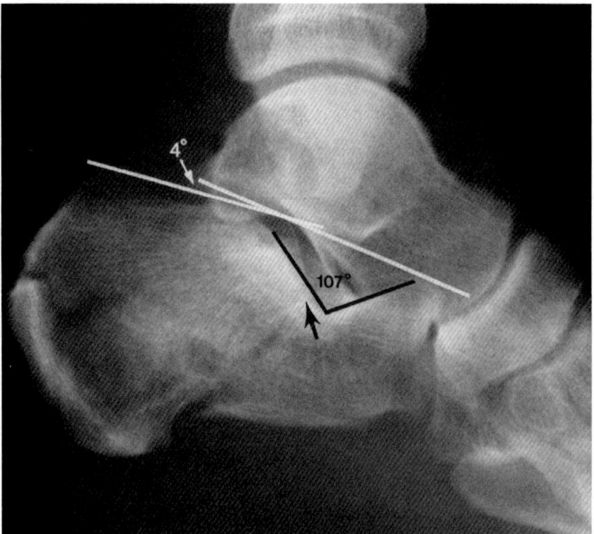


Fig. 8-44 Measurements on the lateral radiograph. Complex calcaneal fracture. The Bohler angle is formed by a line from the posterior superior calcaneal margin to the upper margin of the posterior calcaneal facet. The second line is from the margin of the facet to the superior margin of the anterior calcaneal process. The angle (*white lines*) is decreased to 4 degrees (normal 25 to 40 degrees). The crucial angle of Gissane is formed by lines along the posterior facet and anterior calcaneal process (*black lines*). The angle is increased to 107 degrees (normal ~100 degrees). The fracture (*arrow*) enters the posterior facet.

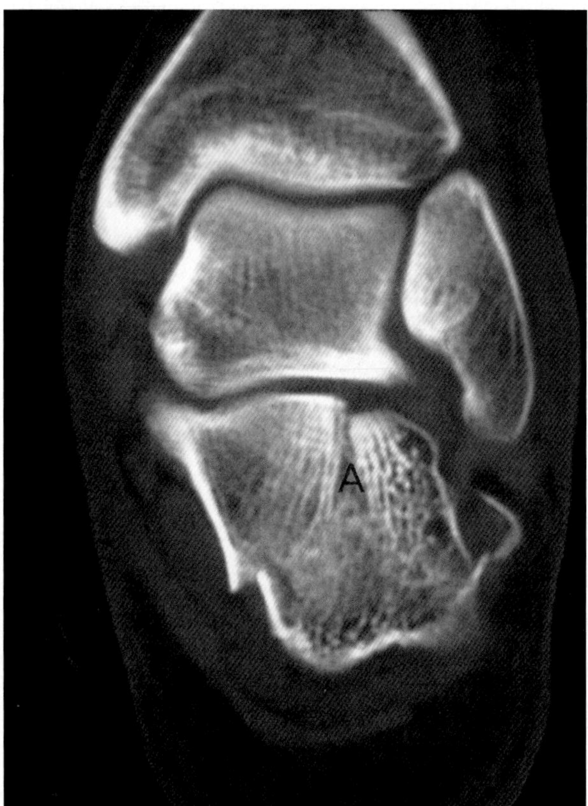


Fig. 8-45 Coronal computed tomographic (CT) image of the posterior facet demonstrating a single fracture line laterally (A) with displacement or Sanders type II fracture.

to the upper margin of the anterior calcaneal process. The crucial angle of Gissane (normal ~100 degrees) (Fig. 8-44) is formed by lines along the posterior facet and anterior calcaneal process.

CT with reformatting in the coronal and sagittal planes is essential to classify the type of injury and plan appropriate management (see Fig. 8-45). Coronal and sagittal reformatted images are aligned from the axial images along the axis of the talus to best define the posterior facet. Three-dimensional reconstructions can also be obtained although they typically do not add significant new information.

MRI is useful for subtle osseous injuries, such as stress fractures, tubercle, or process fractures (see Fig. 8-46) and to evaluate the soft tissues to exclude peroneal tendon dislocation, tendon entrapment, and compartment syndrome.

## Suggested Reading

Daftary A, Haims AH, Baumgaertner MR. Fractures of the calcaneus: A review with emphasis on CT. *Radiographics* 2005;25:1215–1226.

Ouellette H, Salamipour H, Thomas BJ, et al. Incidence and MR features of fractures of the anterior process of calcaneus in a consecutive patient population with ankle and foot symptoms. *Skeletal Radiol.* 2006;35:833–837.

Petrover D, Schweitzer ME, Laredo JD. Anterior process calcaneal fractures: A systematic evaluation of associated conditions. *Skeletal Radiol.* 2007;36:627–632.

### Treatment Options

Treatment of calcaneal fractures has varied considerably over the years in an attempt to reduce the high incidence of long-term disability. The goals of treatment are to restore calcaneal height, length and axis, reduce articular deformities, and restore function. Treatment approaches vary with the type of injury (intra-articular versus extra-articular), the degree of displacement, and other patient factors.

Extra-articular fractures do not involve the posterior facet. Although frequently obvious on radiographs, CT is still preferred to confirm the extent of injury. Anterior calcaneal process fractures can be treated with closed reduction if <25% of the articular surface is involved and there is <3 mm of displacement (Fig. 8-40). Other extra-articular fractures can also be managed conservatively unless there is displacement or widening of the calcaneus that may result in peroneal tendon dysfunction.

Treatment options for intra-articular fractures included no reduction and early motion, closed reduction and fixation, open reduction with grafting and fixation, or primary arthrodesis depending on the extent of injury. Sanders type I fractures can be treated conservatively. Patients with posterior facet fracture displacement ≥3 mm should be treated surgically (Figs. 8-43 to 8-45). Surgery is typically performed in the first 3 weeks using reconstruction plates or special calcaneal plates and screws (see Fig. 8-47). Anatomic reduction varies with the type of injury. In Sanders type II (two-part fractures of the posterior facet) fractures, 86% had anatomic reduction confirmed on CT

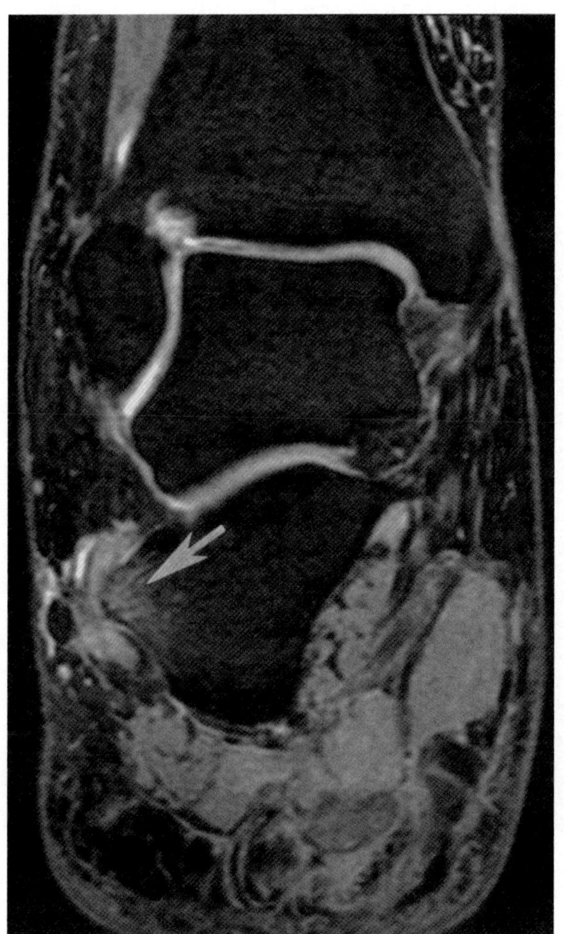


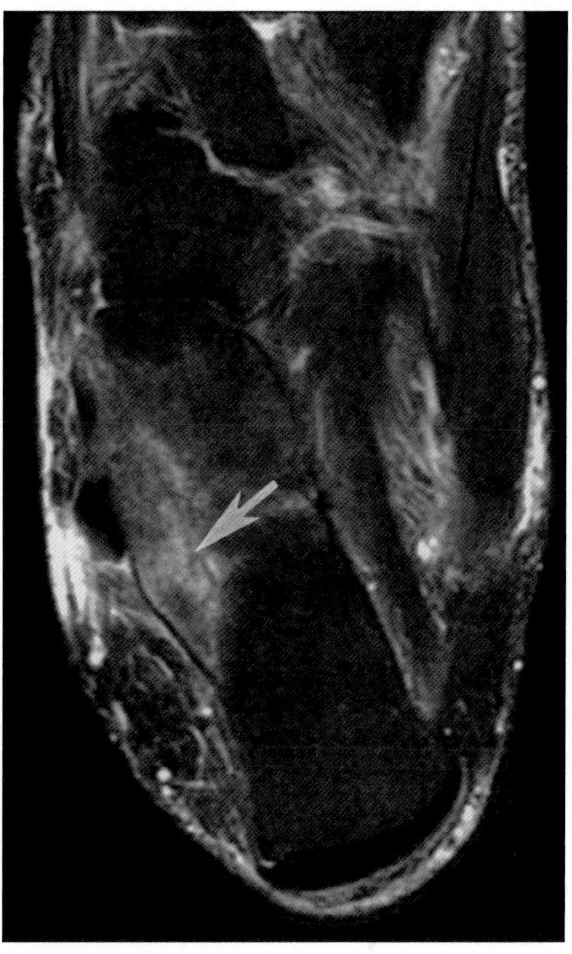


**Fig. 8-46** Coronal dual echo steady state (DESS) (A) and axial fat-suppressed T2-weighted images demonstrating increased signal intensity (*arrow*) due to an undisplaced lateral tubercle fracture adjacent to the peroneal tendons.

images. Anatomic reduction was achieved in 60% of type III and none of type IV fractures (see Table 8-9 and Fig. 8-42).

## Suggested Reading


Kay RM, Tang CW. Pediatric foot fractures: Evaluation and treatment. *J Am Acad Orthop Surg*. 2001;9:308–319.

Sanders R, Fortin P, DiPasquale T, et al. Operative treatment of 120 displaced intra-articular calcaneal fractures: Results using a prognostic computed tomography scan classification. *Clin Orthop*. 1993;290:87–95.

Zwipp H, Rammelt S, Barthel S. Calcaneal fractures: Open reduction and internal fixation. *Injury* 2004;35:SB46–SB54.


### Imaging of Complications

Complications related to calcaneal fracture may occur early or late with long-term disability. Early complications include skin necrosis, compartment syndrome, and neural injuries. Later complications may be related to the initial injury or treatment. Late complications include nonunion, malunion, subfibular impingement, peroneal and flexor tendon injuries, neurovascular injury, and complex regional pain syndrome (reflex sympathetic dystrophy).

The most common problem is prolonged pain and disability. This commonly lasts for several months and subsides in approximately 2 years. However, only approximately 32% of patients are pain-free after 2 years. Loss of motion occurs in 74% to 89% of patients and contributes to symptoms. Fibular calcaneal abutment syndrome is associated with widening of the calcaneus (see Fig. 8-48).

Soft tissue complications including tendon disorders and nerve compression syndromes may be evaluated with CT with coronal and sagittal reformatting if metal artifact degrades MR images significantly. Peroneal tendon disorders are particularly common with bone entrapment in 12%, subluxation in up to 33%, and dislocation in 14%. Overall, abnormalities in the peroneal tendons occur in >50% of patients following acute fracture of the calcaneus.

Associated fractures of the lower extremity occur in 20% to 46% of patients. Spinal compression fractures, typically lumbar, occur in 10% to 30% of patients with calcaneal fractures. The incidence of associated fractures or soft tissue injuries in

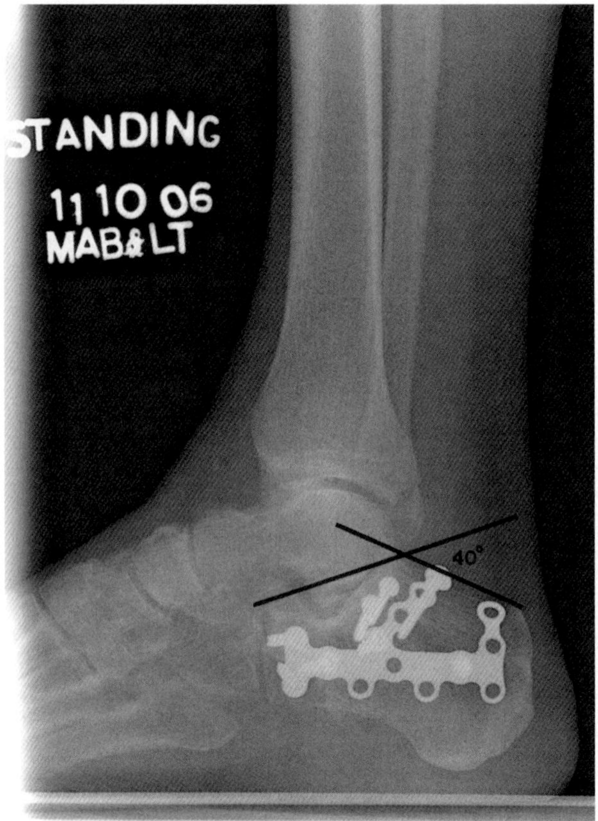


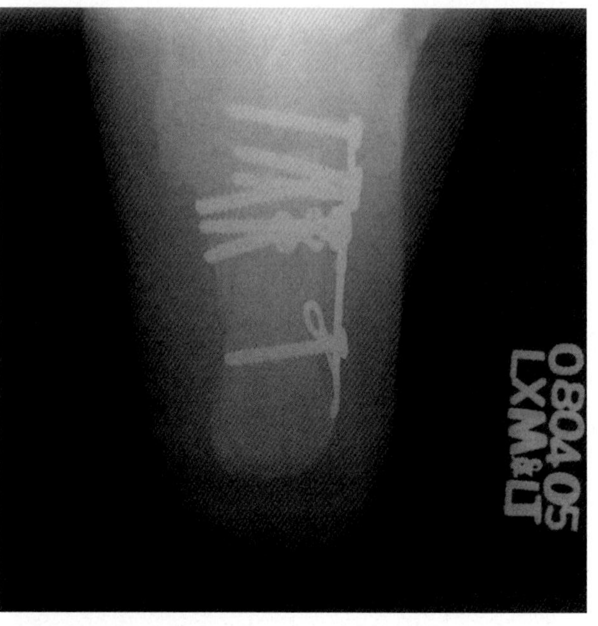


Fig. 8-47 Lateral (A) and axial (B) radiographs following calcaneal plate and screw fixation of an intra-articular fracture. The width has been restored and the Bohler angle improved to 40 degrees.

Table 8-9

SANDERS CLASSIFICATION FOR CALCANEAL FRACTURES

| TYPE | CT IMAGE FEATURES |
|---|---|
| Type I (Fig. 8-42A) | All undisplaced fractures regardless of the number of fragments |
| Type II (Fig. 8-42B) | Two-part fractures of posterior facet |
| IIA | Fracture lateral or line A |
| IIB | Fracture line central or line B |
| IIC | Fracture line medial or line C |
| Type III (Fig. 8-42C) | Three-part posterior facet fractures with central depression |
| IIIAB | Fracture lines lateral and central or A and B |
| IIIAC | Fracture lines lateral and medial or A and C |
| IIIBC | Fracture lines central and medial or B and C |
| Type IV (Fig. 8-42D) | Four part or highly comminuted posterior facet fractures |

CT, computed tomography.

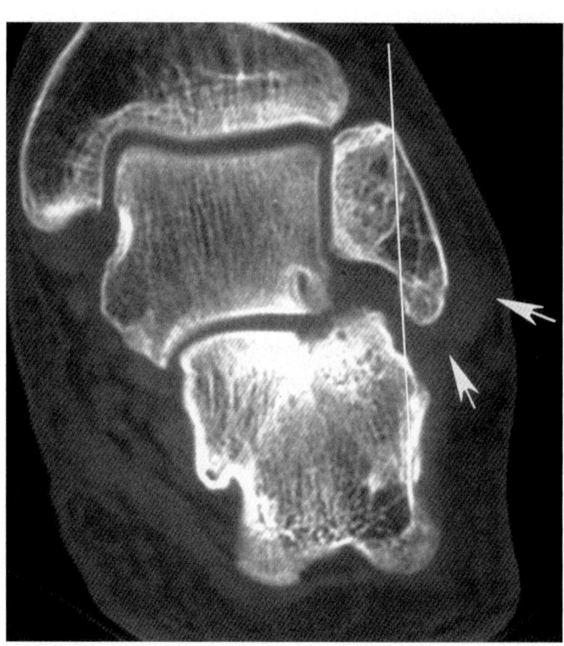

Fig. 8-48 Coronal computed tomographic (CT) image with widening of the calcaneus and the fibular line extending into the displaced calcaneus. There is also thickening (*arrows*) of the peroneal tendons due to chronic tendinopathy.

children approaches 57%. Most associated injuries occur in children older than 12 years of age.

## Suggested Reading


Berquist TH. *Radiology of the foot and ankle*, 2nd ed. Philadelphia: Lippincott Williams & Wilkins; 2000:171–280.

Sanders R, Fortin P, DiPasquale T, et al. Operative treatment of 120 displaced intra-articular calcaneal fractures: Results using a prognostic computed tomography scan classification. *Clin Orthop*. 1993;290:87–95.

Schmidt TL, Weiner DS. Calcaneal fractures in children. An evaluation of the nature of injury in 56 children. *Clin Orthop*. 1982;171:150–155.

Slatis P, Kroduoto O, Santavista S, et al. Fractures of the calcaneus. *J Trauma*. 1979;19:939–943.


# Midfoot Fracture/Dislocations

The mid foot is the anatomic region distal to Chopart's joint and proximal to Lisfranc's joint line. The osseous structures include the navicular, cuboid and medial, intermediate (middle), and lateral cuneiforms. There is no weight-bearing contact in the mid foot. The osseous structures are supported by strong plantar ligaments. The mid foot is divided into columns. The medial column consists of the talonavicular, navicular cuneiform, and first and second metatarsal articulations. The lateral column is comprised of the calcaneocuboid articulation, the cuboid, and the fifth metatarsal. The medial column is more rigidly fixed than the lateral column (see Fig. 8-49).

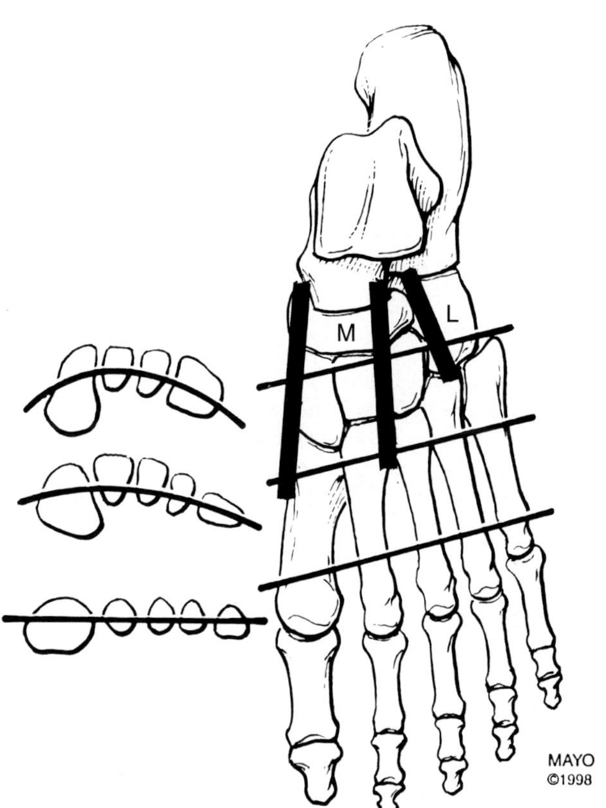


Fig. 8-49 Illustration of the medial (*M*, thick black lines) and lateral (*L*, thick black line) columns of the mid foot with the arches in the coronal plane on the right.

## Navicular Fractures

The navicular is the key structure in the medial longitudinal arch of the foot. The proximal concave facet articulates with the talus and the three distal facets with the three cuneiforms. There is a medial tuberosity for attachment of the posterior tibial tendon. Commonly there is an accessory ossicle (os tibiale externum) within the distal tendon (25%). Most of these ossicles are bilateral (90%).

Multiple navicular fracture patterns have been described. Acute fractures may involve the tuberosity, cortical avulsions, or the body of the navicular. Stress fractures also develop due to repetitive microtrauma. Dorsal avulsion fractures occur with twisting injuries or with inversion and plantar flexion. This fracture (see Fig. 8-50) is the most common navicular fracture (47%). Navicular tuberosity fractures are due to avulsion at the attachment of the deltoid ligament and posterior tibial tendon.

Navicular body fractures are uncommon (see Fig. 8-51). The mechanism of injury is axial loading or direct trauma. Fractures may be transverse in the coronal plane with a dorsal fragment involving <50% of the body. More commonly, the fracture line passes dorsolateral to plantar medial with the dorsomedial fragment the larger of the two fragments. Central comminution may also occur with associated subluxation or dislocation of the calcaneocuboid articulation.

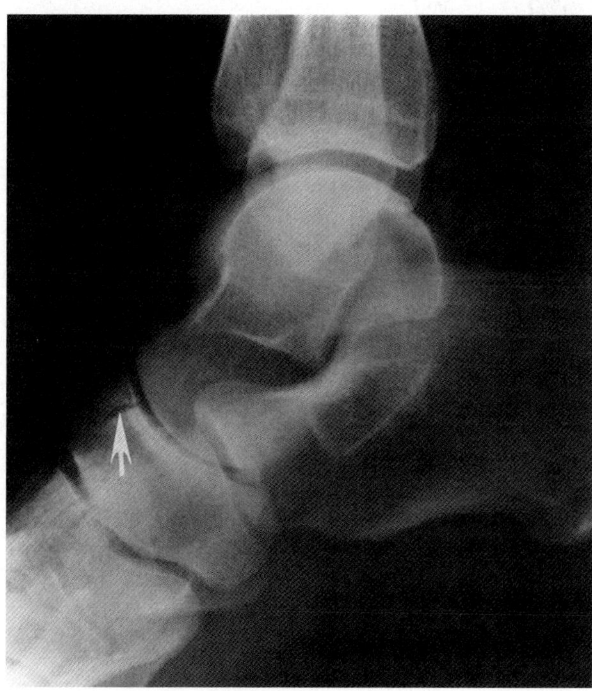

Fig. 8-50 Lateral radiograph of the mid foot demonstrating a dorsal avulsion fracture (*arrow*).

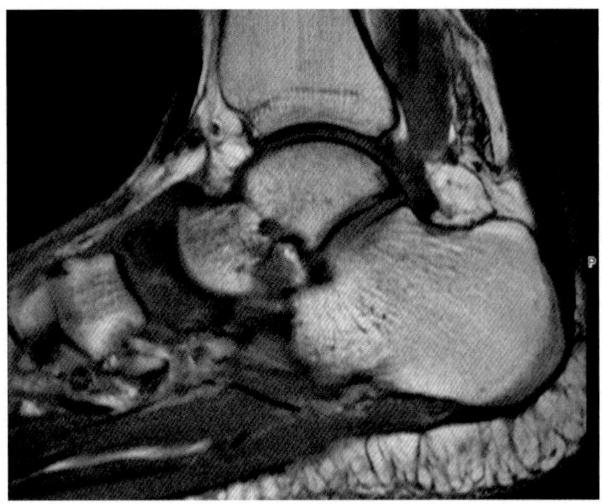
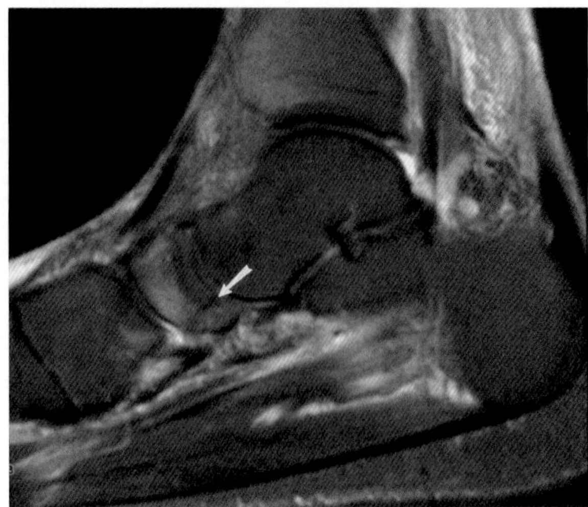

Fig. 8-51 Navicular body fracture. Sagittal T1- (A) and fat-suppressed fast spin-echo T2-weighted (B) images demonstrating a fracture (*arrow*) with marrow edema.

## Cuboid Fractures

The cuboid maintains the lateral column (Fig. 8-49). Therefore, fractures may have significant functional consequences. Isolated cuboid fractures are rare. There are usually associated injuries of the talonavicular articulation, midfoot fractures, or a Lisfranc injury. Medial or dorsal avulsions of the navicular should lead one to search carefully for an associated cuboid fracture.

Cuboid fractures are due to direct trauma to the lateral foot or a fall with an associated twisting injury. Fractures may be simple avulsions (see Fig. 8-52), coronal plane fractures, or comminuted crush injuries.

Fig. 8-52 Anteroposterior (AP) radiograph demonstrating avulsion fractures (*arrows*) at the calcaneocuboid articulation.

## Cuneiform Fractures

Cuneiform injuries are related to direct trauma or indirect axial loading. They are almost always associated with more complex tarsometatarsal fracture/dislocations (see Fig. 8-53). Isolated cuneiform fractures are rare. Again, fractures may be related to avulsion injuries, involve the articular surface or consist of comminuted fragments.

## Tarsometatarsal Fracture/Dislocations

The anatomy of the Lisfranc articulations is important. This includes the articulations and ligament supporting structures of the cuboid, cuneiforms, and five metatarsal bases (see Fig. 8-54). The lateral metatarsals (second through fifth) are connected proximally by the transverse metatarsal ligaments. The second metatarsal is situated in a mortise formed by the medial and lateral cuneiforms. Ligament support is provided by the transverse ligament laterally and the oblique ligament (OL) medially (Fig. 8-54). The OL extends from the medial cuneiform to the second metatarsal base (Fig. 8-54). Avulsion fractures can occur at the attachment. The plantar ligaments are strongest; therefore, dislocations tend to occur dorsally (see Fig. 8-55). The dorsalis pedis artery is at risk as it passes between the first and second metatarsals to form the plantar arch.

Injuries to the Lisfranc articulations may be mild or complex. Findings on radiographs are often subtle with 20% of injuries overlooked on initial radiographs (see Fig. 8-56). Mild ligament sprains may occur with athletic injuries. More significant injuries are related to high-velocity motor vehicle accidents and direct or indirect loading injuries. Direct loading dorsally from a heavy object falling on a stationary foot can result in fracture and soft tissue injury (see Fig. 8-57A). Indirect forces applied to a plantar flexed foot is more common (Fig. 8-57B) and may be associated with fractures of the cuneiforms, cuboid, and metatarsal bases. The second metatarsal is most commonly

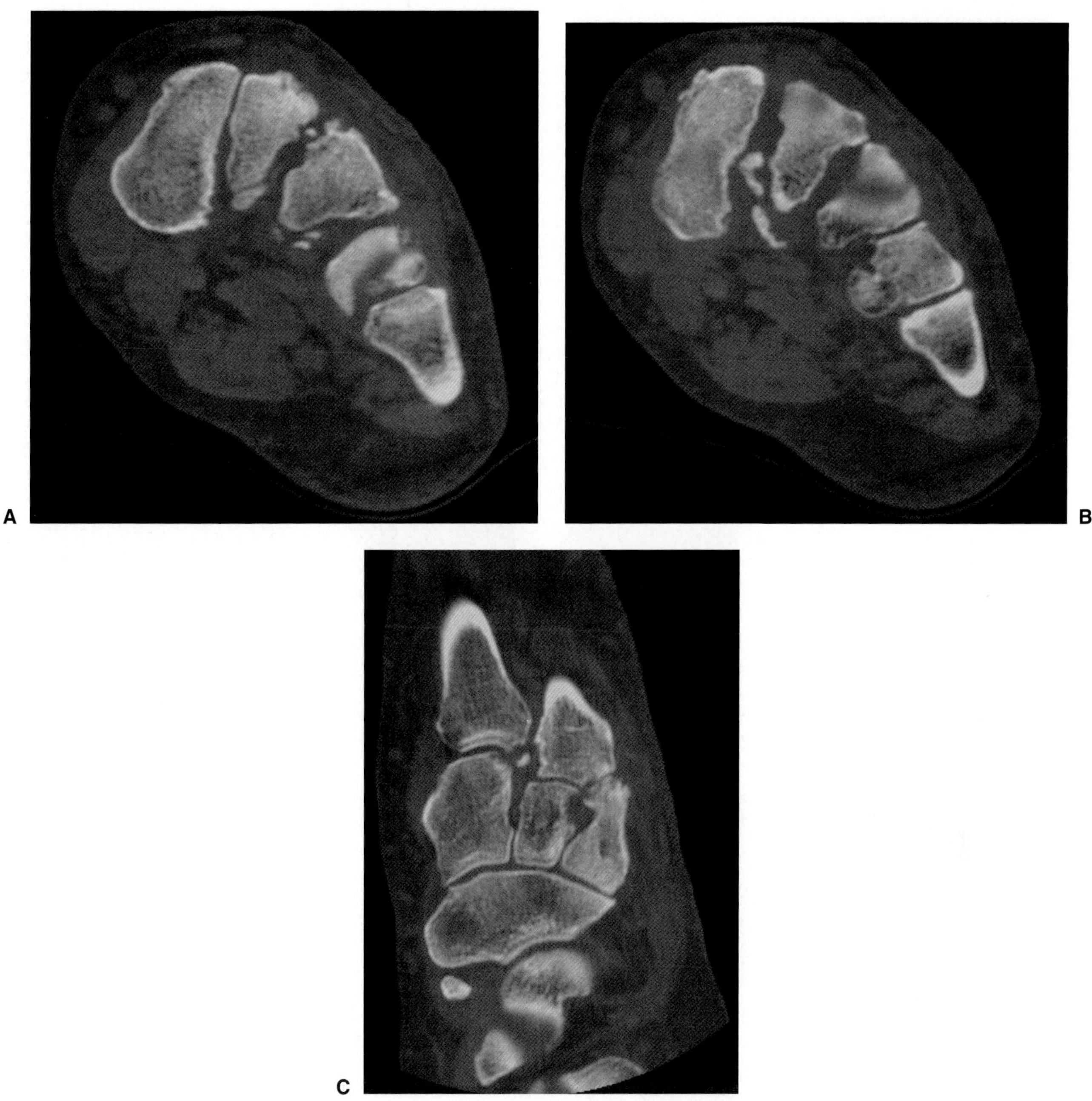


Fig. 8-53 Cuneiform fractures associated with a Lisfranc injury. Axial (A and B) and coronal (C) computed tomographic (CT) images demonstrate multiple small cuneiform avulsion fragments.

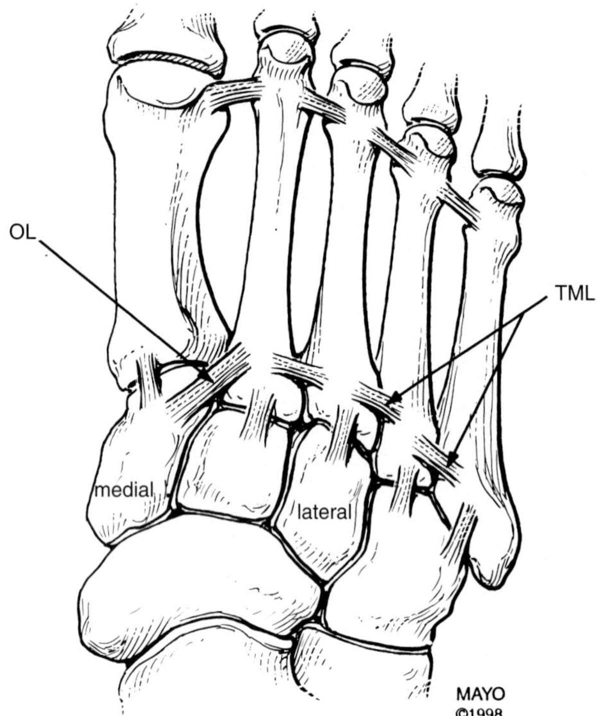


Fig. 8-54 Illustration of the supporting ligaments of the Lisfranc articulations. The transverse metatarsal ligaments (TMLs) connect the metatarsal bases. The second metatarsal lies in a mortise formed by the medial and lateral cuneiforms. The oblique ligament (OL) extends from the medial cuneiform to the second metatarsal base.

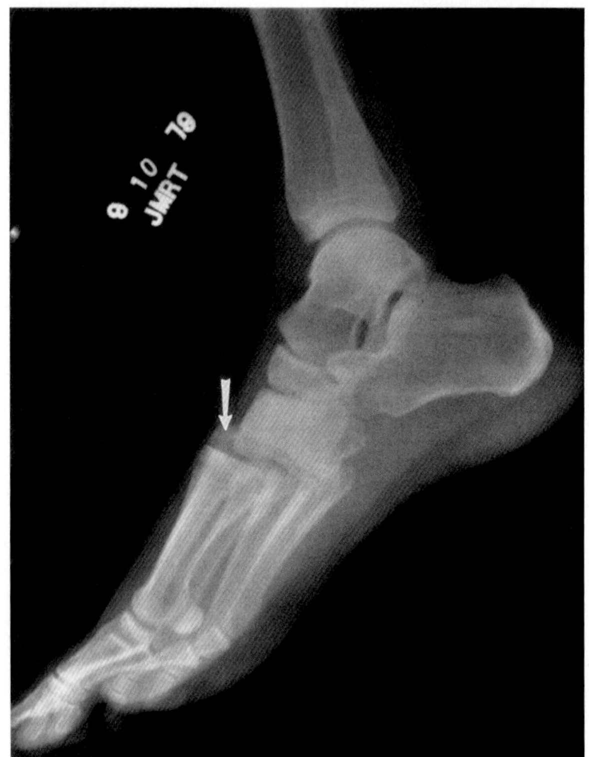


Fig. 8-55 Lateral radiograph demonstrating dorsal subluxation (*arrow*) of the tarsometatarsal joints.

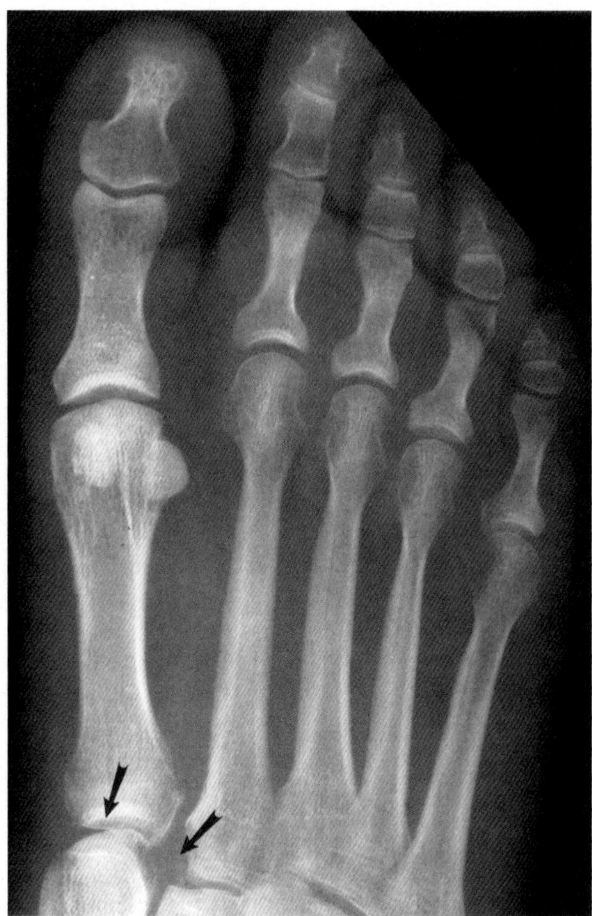

Fig. 8-56 Anteroposterior (AP) radiograph following Lisfranc injury. The only findings are slight widening of the 1 to 2 metatarsal bases (*arrow*) and first tarsometatarsal joint (*arrow*).

involved due to its position in the mortise between the medial and lateral cuneiforms. Several patterns have been described, but none are useful for treatment planning due to their complexity. The homolateral pattern (total incongruency) occurs when all five metatarsals are displaced (see Fig. 8-58). Displacement is almost always lateral, but medial displacement can also occur. The divergent pattern occurs when the first metatarsal fractures at the base and the shaft displaced medially accompanied by lateral displacement of the second through fifth metatarsals. Associated cuneiform and navicular fractures are common with this displacement pattern (see Fig. 8-59).

## Suggested Reading

Hardcastle PH, Seschauer R, Kutcha-Lissberg E, et al. Injuries of the tarsometatarsal joint. Incidence, classification and treatment. *J Bone Joint Surg*. 1982;64B:349–356.

Karasick D. Fractures and dislocations of the foot. *Semin Roentgenol*. 1994;29:152–175.

Richter M, Thermann H, Huefner T, et al. Aetiology, treatment and outcome of Lisfranc joint dislocations and fracture dislocation. *J Foot Ankle Surg*. 2002;8:21–32.

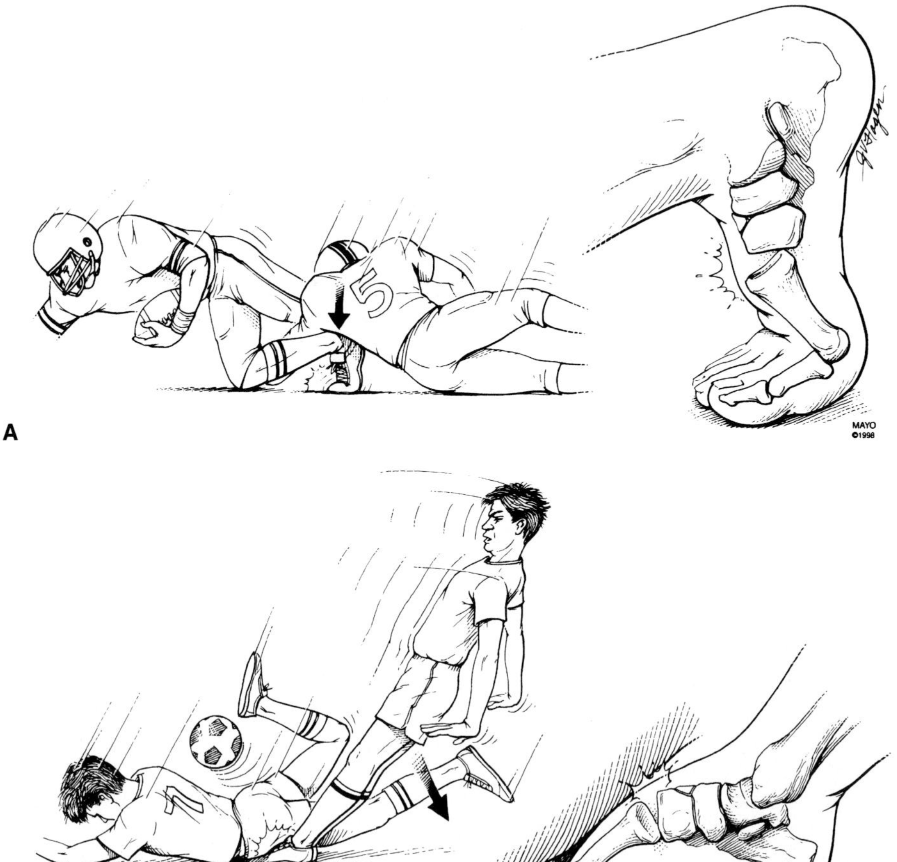


Fig. 8-57 Illustrations of the mechanism of injury of Lisfranc fracture/dislocations. A: Axial loading of the foot due to a heavy object or weight applied to the foot. B: Indirect force due to a fixed plantar flexed foot.

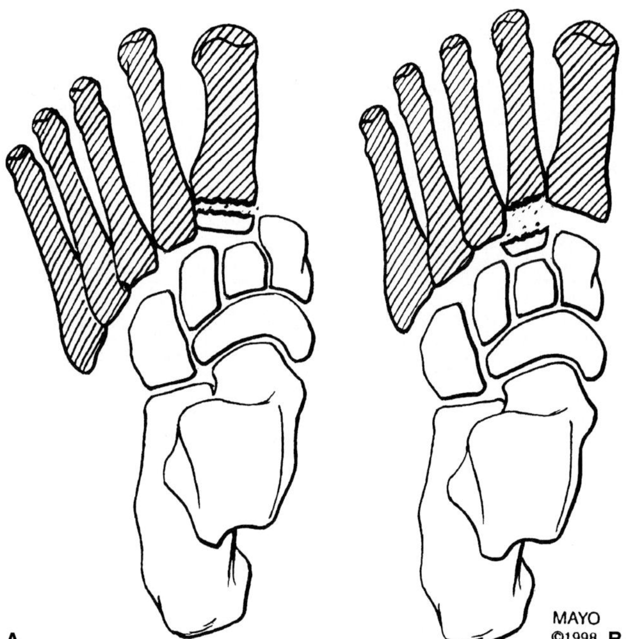


Fig. 8-58 Illustration of homolateral (all five metatarsals displaced) Lisfranc pattern with lateral (A) and dorsal (B) displacement.

## Imaging of Midfoot Fracture/Dislocations

Radiographs in the AP, lateral, and oblique projections are usually adequate for displaced fractures and dislocations of the mid foot (Figs. 8-50, 8-52, 8-55, and 8-56). However, subtle Lisfranc injuries are easily overlooked. The only finding may be slight widening of the first–second metatarsal bases (Fig. 8-56) or subtle dorsal metatarsal displacement on the lateral view (Fig. 8-55). When symptoms dictate or radiographs are equivocal, CT with multiplanar reformatting should be obtained (Fig. 8-53). More subtle osseous or ligament injuries may only be detectable on MR images.

# Suggested Reading

Karasick D. Fractures and dislocations of the foot. *Semin Roentgenol.* 1994;29:152–175.

Sartoris DJ. Diagnosis of foot trauma. The essentials. *J Foot Ankle Surg.* 1993;32:539–550.

## Treatment Options

Isolated fractures of the navicular, cuboid, and cuneiforms are uncommon. Undisplaced fractures of the navicular and cuboid

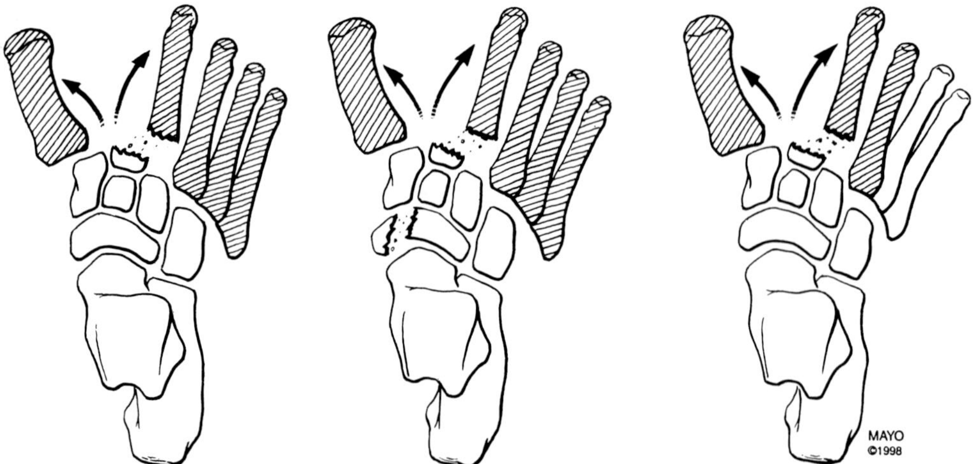


Fig. 8-59 Illustration of the divergent pattern with medial displacement of the first metatarsal and lateral displacement of the lesser metatarsal with or without associated navicular and cuneiform fractures.

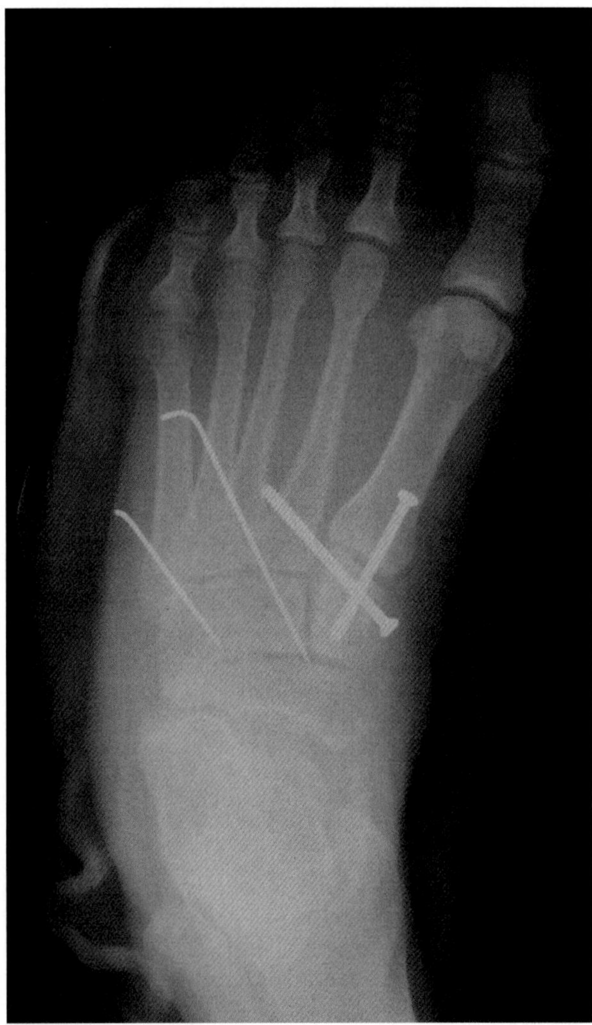

Fig. 8-60 Anteroposterior (AP) radiograph following internal fixation of a Lisfranc fracture/dislocation with cannulated screws for fixation of the first and second metatarsal bases and K-wires for the lesser metatarsals.

can be treated with closed reduction and cast immobilization. Open reduction with screw fixation is reserved for displaced fractures (≥2 mm) or when conservative treatment fails. Navicular fractures can be particularly difficult to manage, especially in athletes. Screw fixation is more often required and only approximately half the number of patients return to full activity. Cuneiform fractures, except small avulsions, are treated with internal fixation due to their importance in structural stability.

Lisfranc injuries may be subtle and easily overlooked or more complex. In either setting, CT is important to completely evaluate the injury before treatment planning. Injuries with no evidence of instability on weight bearing can be managed with cast immobilization with partial weight bearing for 6 weeks. When injuries are reduced with closed reduction, but not considered stable, percutaneous K-wires or screws can be used to maintain position. Open reduction and internal or combined internal and external fixation are used in more complex injuries (see Fig. 8-60). Fusion of the fourth and fifth metatarsal bases is avoided when possible.

## Suggested Reading

Early JS. Fractures and dislocations of the mid foot and forefoot. In: Bucholtz RW, Heckman JD, eds. *Rockwood and Green's fractures in adults*, 5th ed. Philadelphia: Lippincott Williams & Wilkins; 2001:2181–2245.

Kay RM, Tang CW. Pediatric foot fractures: Evaluation and treatment. *J Am Acad Orthop Surg*. 2001;9:308–319.

Richter M, Thermann H, Huefner T, et al. Aetiology, treatment and outcome of Lisfranc joint dislocations and fracture dislocation. *J Foot Ankle Surg*. 2002;8:21–32.

### Imaging of Complications

Imaging of Lisfranc fracture/dislocations can be difficult with 20% overlooked initially on radiographs. Also, 8% to 9% of injuries are bilateral. The most common complication is persistent pain (20% to 30%) and arthrosis. Less commonly, vascular injury and AVN of the second metatarsal base may also occur. Postoperative infection is uncommon.

Imaging can be accomplished with serial radiographs and CT when indicated. MRI is useful for suspected AVN.

## Suggested Reading

Kay RM, Tang CW. Pediatric foot fractures: Evaluation and treatment. *J Am Acad Orthop Surg*. 2001;9:308–319.

Richter M, Thermann H, Huefner T, et al. Aetiology, treatment and outcome of Lisfranc joint dislocations and fracture dislocation. *J Foot Ankle Surg*. 2002;8:21–32.

Vuori JP, Aro HT. Lisfranc joint injuries: Trauma mechanisms and associated injuries. *J Trauma*. 1993;35:40–45.

# Forefoot Fractures and Dislocations

Fractures of the metatarsals and phalanges are common. Dislocations may occur as an isolated event or with associated fractures. Sesamoid injuries are also common, especially in long-distance runners.

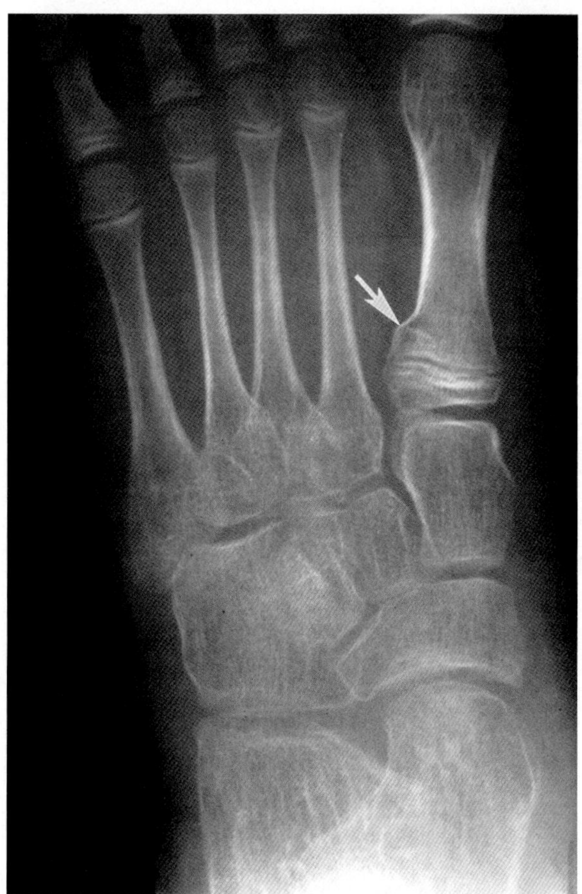

Fig. 8-61 Anteroposterior (AP) radiograph demonstrating a torus fracture (*arrow*) of the first metatarsal.

## Metatarsal Fractures

The first metatarsal is shorter and wider than the lesser metatarsals. The anatomic position and ligaments at the metatarsal bases were reviewed in the last section and impact the fracture patterns. Metatarsal fractures may be extra- or intra-articular. Fractures may occur in isolation or as part of a more complex injury pattern. Fractures of the second through fifth metatarsals are more common than the first metatarsal in adults. In children, metatarsal fractures account for 60% of pediatric foot fractures and 22% if foot fractures involve the fifth metatarsal base. Fractures of the first metatarsal are more common than in adults with first metatarsal fractures (see Fig. 8-61) accounting for 73% of tarsal and metatarsal fractures in children younger than 5 years, but only 12% of foot fractures in older children. In children, up to 20% of first metatarsal fractures were initially overlooked (Fig. 8-61).

Fractures of the fifth metatarsal are common and occur with different mechanisms of injury. The fifth metatarsal is divided into three zones (see Fig. 8-62). Zone 1 fractures are avulsion injuries due to the attachment of the lateral band of the plantar aponeurosis and to a lesser degree, the peroneus brevis insertion (see Fig. 8-63). Zone 2 fractures are Jones fractures caused by adduction of the forefoot (see Fig. 8-64). Zone 3 fractures are usually stress fractures commonly seen in athletes with repetitive microtrauma. Distal shaft fractures have been termed *Dancer's* fractures.

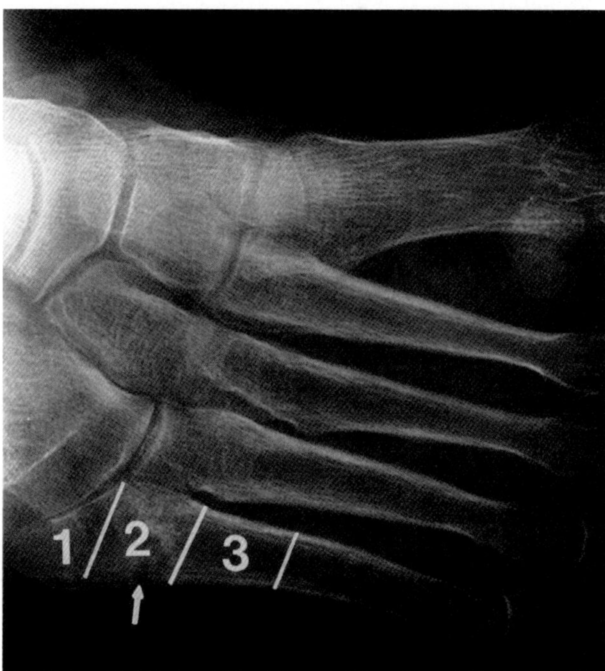


Fig. 8-62 Radiograph demonstrating the zones of the fifth metatarsal base. Zone 1 injuries tend to be avulsion fractures, zone 2 fractures or Jones fractures are due to adduction of the forefoot, and zone 3 fractures are more commonly stress fractures in athletes. In this case there is a Jones fracture (*arrow*).

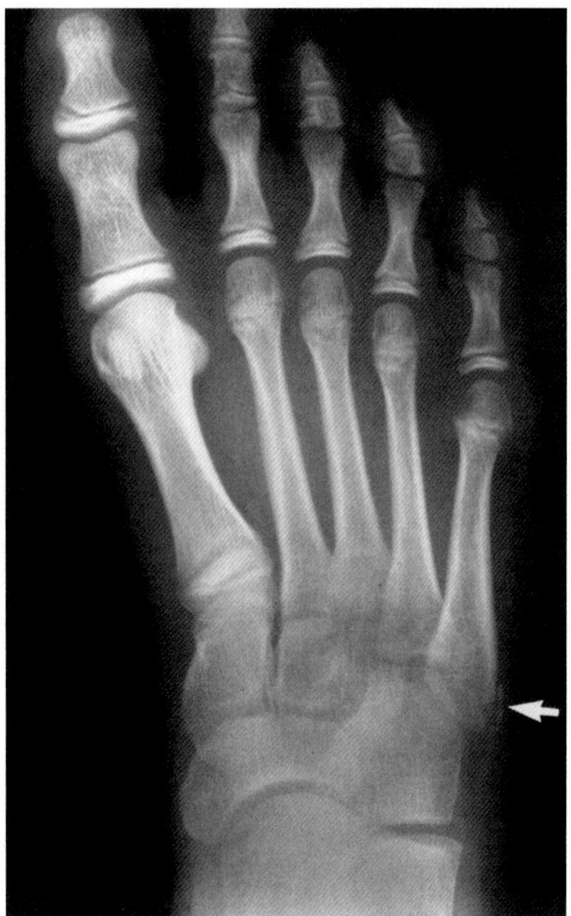


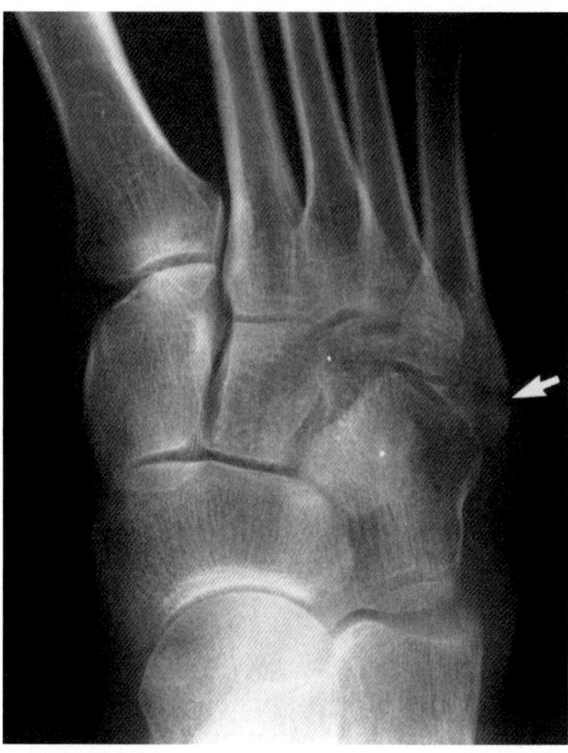


Fig. 8-63 A: Anteroposterior (AP) radiograph of the normal fifth metatarsal apophysis (*arrow*) that aligns parallel to the shaft. B: Zone 1 fracture (*arrow*) is perpendicular to the shaft.

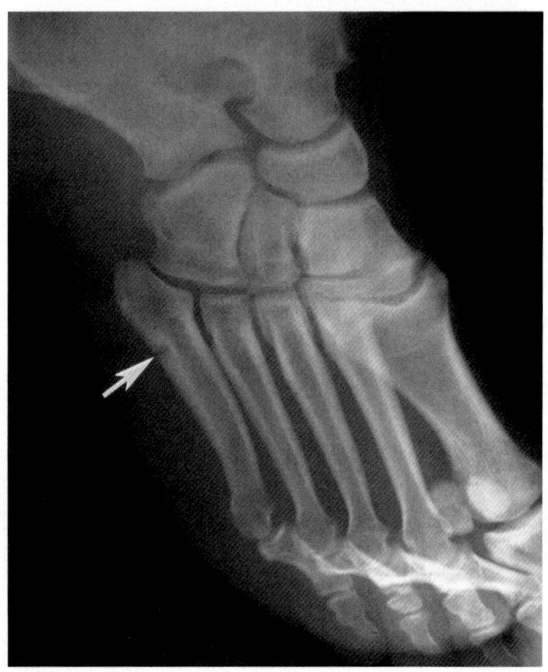

Fig. 8-64 Oblique radiograph demonstrating and incomplete Jones fracture (*arrow*).

## Phalangeal Fractures

Phalangeal fractures are the most common forefoot fractures in adults and account for 18% of pediatric foot fractures (see Fig. 8-65). The proximal phalanx of the fifth digit is most often involved (see Fig. 8-66). A direct blow from a heavy object or jamming the toe creates the fractures. Fracture may involve the articular surface and be comminuted.

## Metatarsophalangeal and Interphalangeal Dislocations

Dislocations of the metatarsophalangeal or interphalangeal joints may be isolated or related to more complex injuries. Metatarsophalangeal dislocations are usually due to hyperextension injuries with the proximal phalanx forced dorsal to the metatarsal. This results in disruption of the plantar capsule. The first metatarsophalangeal joint is most commonly involved (see Fig. 8-67). Interposition of the plantar plate or sesamoid may prevent reduction. This results in persistent widening of the joint space on radiographs.

Phalangeal dislocations most commonly involve the proximal interphalangeal joint (see Fig. 8-68). The mechanism of injury is similar to metatarsophalangeal dislocations.

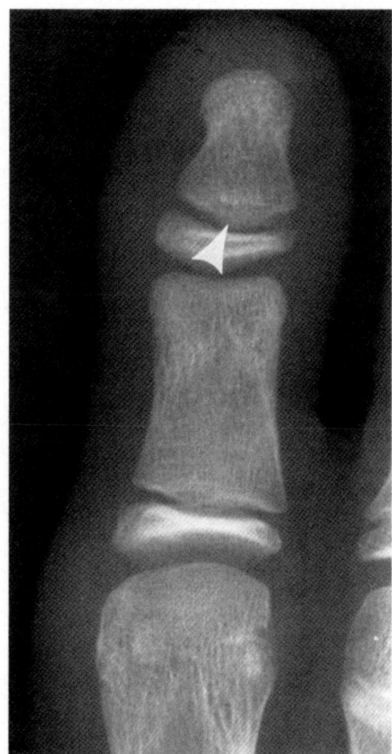

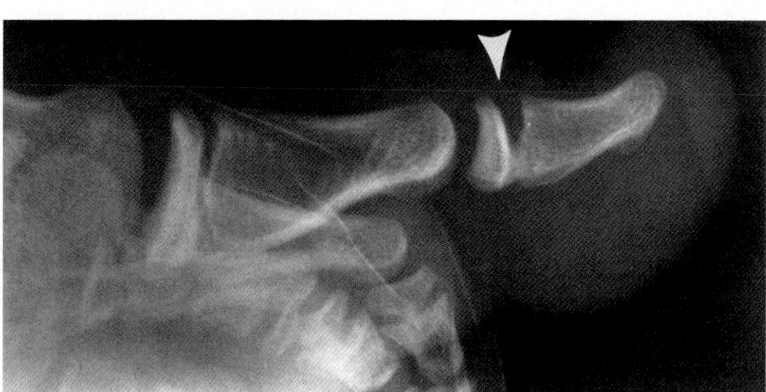

A B

Fig. 8-65 Anteroposterior (AP) (A) and lateral (B) radiographs of a Salter-Harris type I fracture of the physis of the phalanx of the great toe.

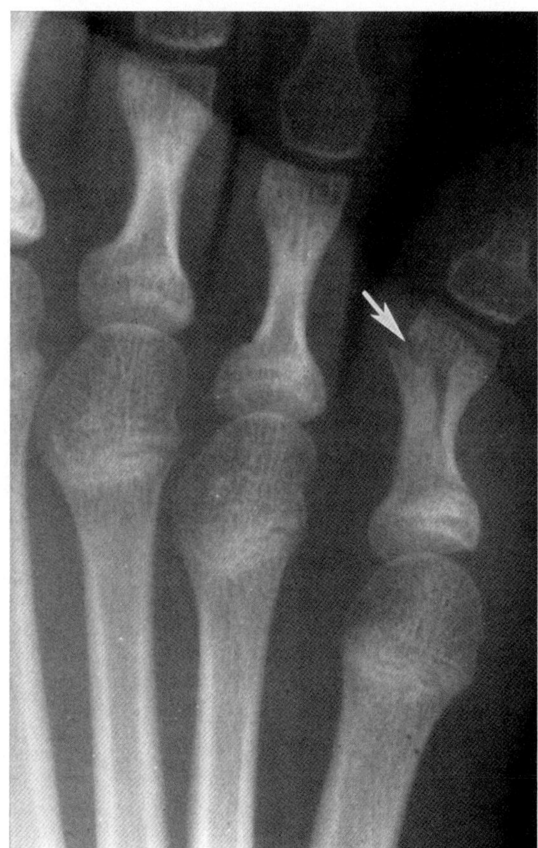

Fig. 8-66 Anteroposterior (AP) radiograph of a displaced fracture of the fifth proximal phalanx.

## SUGGESTED READING


Brunet J, Tubin S. Traumatic dislocation of the lesser toes. *Foot Ankle* 1997;18:406–411.

Dameron TB. Fractures and anatomic variations of the proximal portion of the fifth metatarsal. *J Bone Joint Surg.* 1975;57A:788–792.

Ekrol I, Court-Brown CM. Fractures of the base of the fifth metatarsal. *Foot.* 2004;14:96–98.

Karasick D. Fractures and dislocations of the foot. *Semin Roentgenol.* 1994;29:152–175.

Kay RM, Tang CW. Pediatric foot fractures: Evaluation and treatment. *J Am Acad Orthop Surg.* 2001;9:308–319.

Theodorou DJ, Theodorou SJ, Kakitubata Y, et al. Fractures of the fifth metatarsal base: Anatomic imaging evidence of pathogenesis of avulsion of the plantar aponeurosis and short peroneal muscle tendon. *Radiology* 2003;226:857–865.


### Imaging of Forefoot Fracture/Dislocations

Detection of most forefoot fractures and dislocations is easily accomplished with AP, lateral, and oblique radiographs in most situations (Figs. 8-61 to 8-68). Fractures of the second through fourth metatarsal bases may be difficult to detect due to bone overlap (see Fig. 8-69). In this setting, CT with reformatting or MRI may be necessary to define the fracture and associated injuries. MRI is also useful for stress injuries or stress reaction (see Fig. 8-70) and to evaluate associated soft tissue injuries. Bone scans can also be used to evaluate subtle fractures.

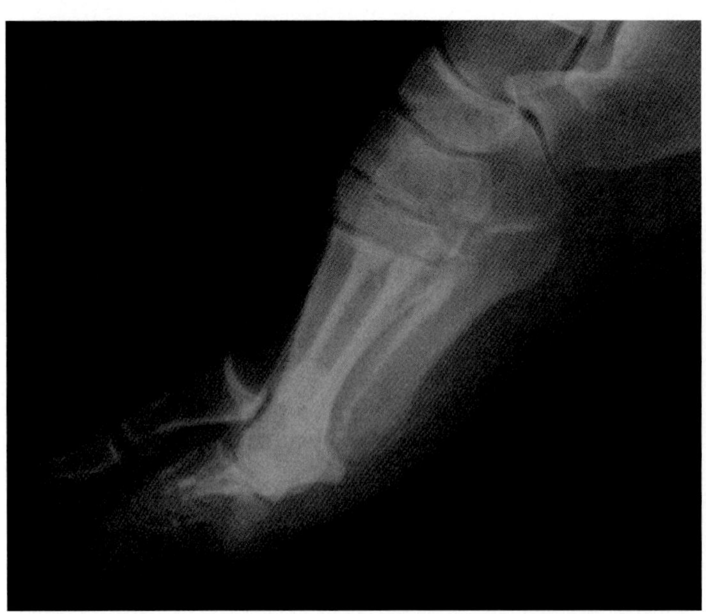


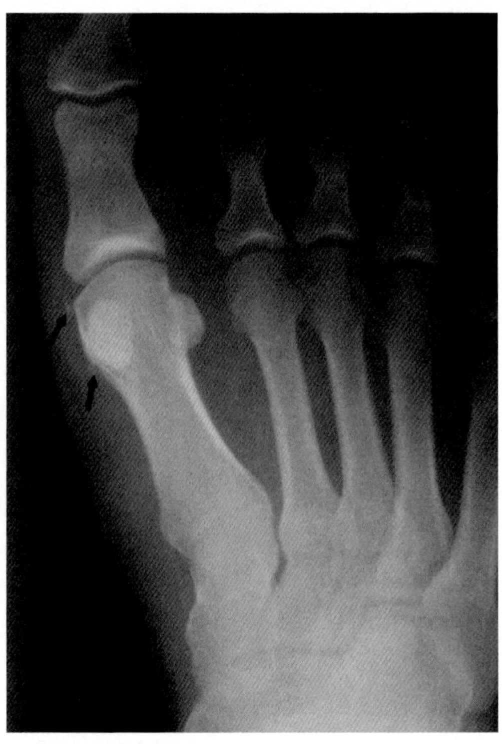


Fig. 8-67 Dislocation of the first metatarsophalangeal joint. A: Lateral radiograph demonstrating dislocation of the first metatarsophalangeal joint. B: Anteroposterior (AP) radiograph following reduction demonstrates small osteochondral fragments medially (*arrows*).

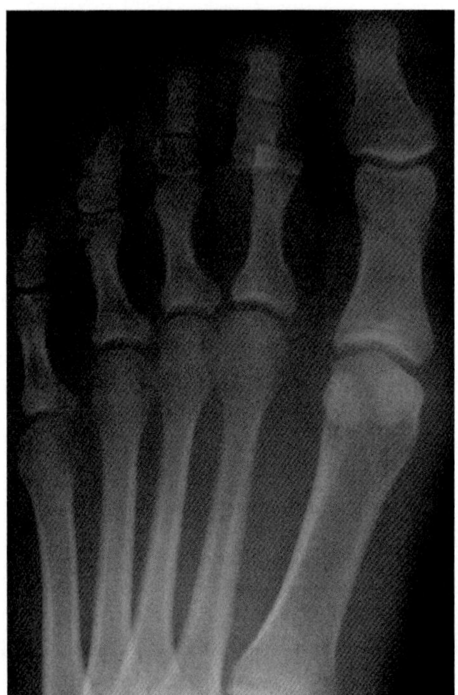


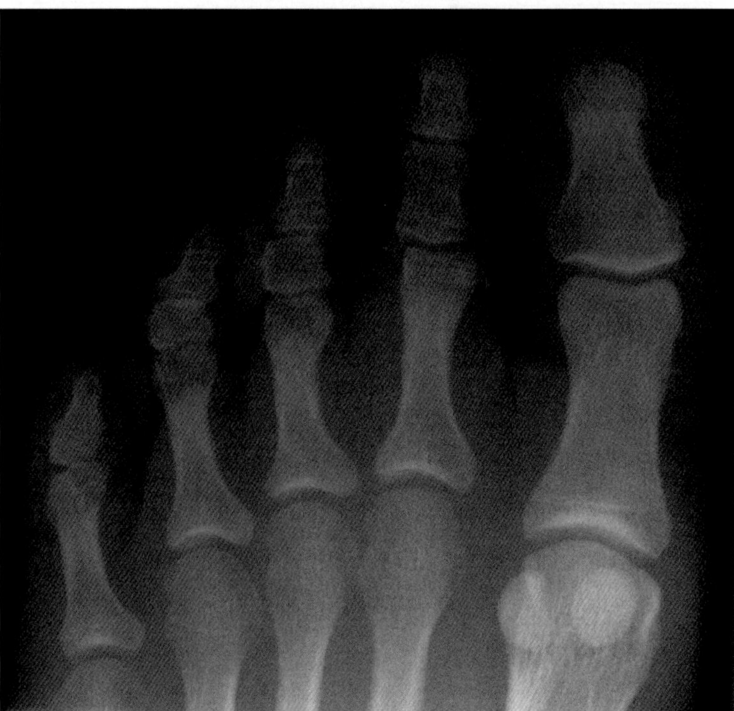


Fig. 8-68 A: Anteroposterior (AP) radiograph demonstrating a dorsal dislocation of the second proximal interphalangeal joint (*arrow*). B: Following reduction there is an osteochondral fragment laterally (*arrow*).

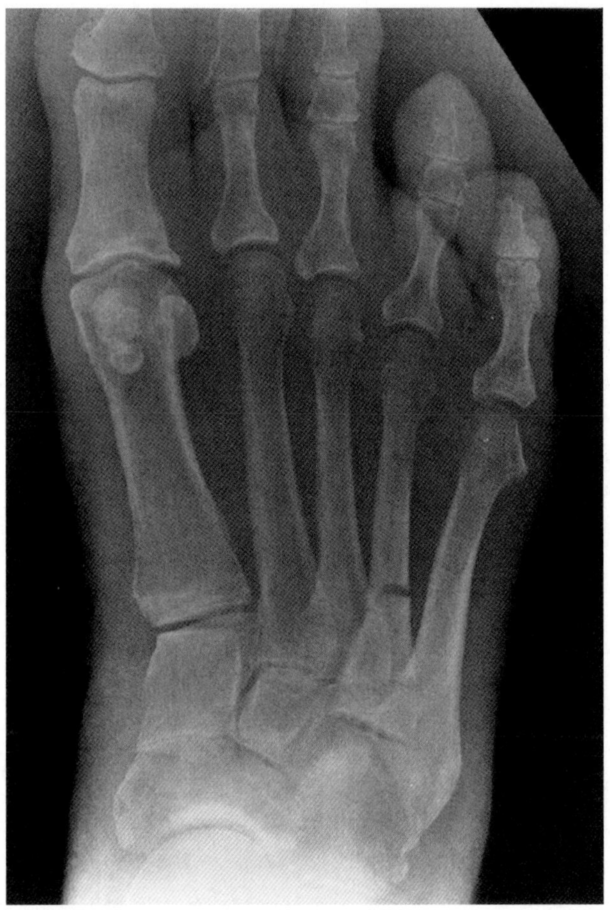

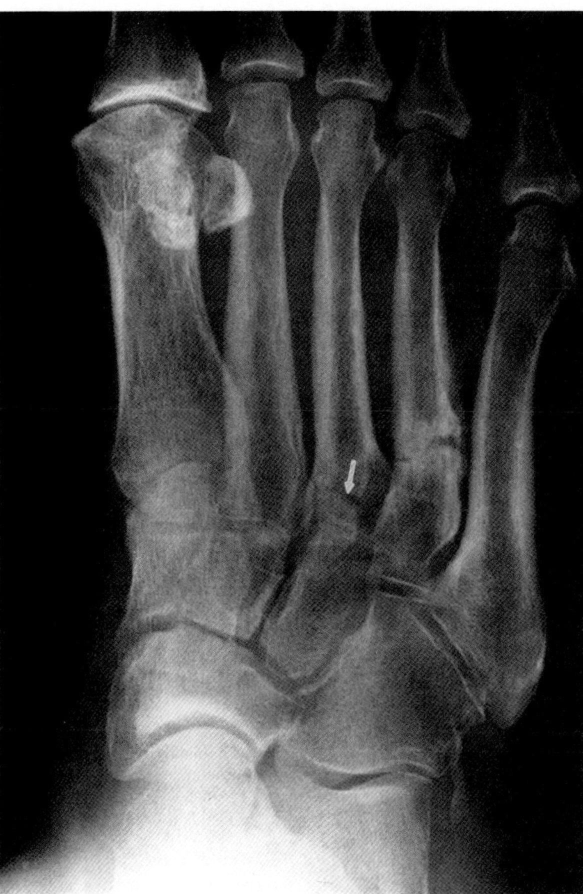

Fig. 8-69 A: Anteroposterior (AP) radiograph demonstrates a fracture of the proximal fourth metatarsal (*arrow*). Note the overlap of the metatarsal bases. B: Follow-up radiograph demonstrates a fracture (*arrow*) of the third metatarsal base that was overlooked on the initial radiograph.

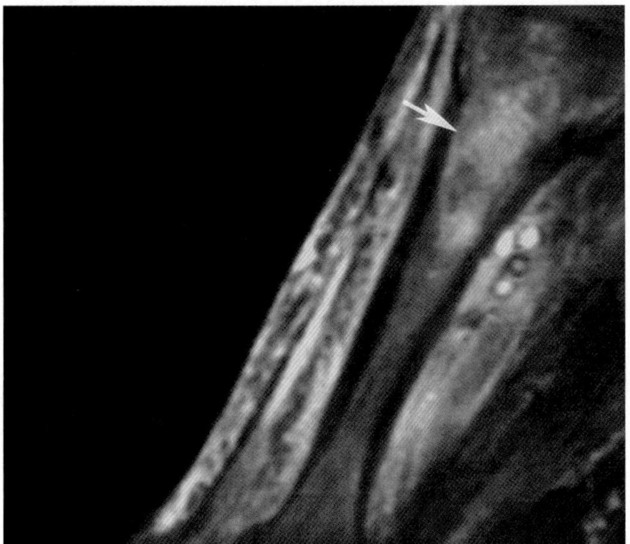

Fig. 8-70 Fat-suppressed fast spin-echo T2-weighted magnetic resonance (MR) image demonstrates increased signal intensity in the proximal metatarsal (*arrow*) due to stress reaction in an athlete.

## Suggested Reading

Karasick D. Fractures and dislocations of the foot. *Semin Roentgenol.* 1994;29:152–175.

Major NM. Role of MRI in Prevention of Metatarsal Stress Fractures in Collegiate Basketball Players. *Am J Roentgenol.* 2006;186:255–258.

Morris G, Nix K, Goldman FD. Fracture of the second metatarsal base: An overlooked cause of chronic mid foot pain. *J Am Podiatr Med Assoc.* 2003;93:6–10.

### Treatment Options

Most minimally displaced metatarsal and phalangeal fractures can be treated with closed reduction. Metatarsal fractures require cast immobilization (see Fig. 8-71), whereas most phalangeal fractures are treated with buddy taping to the adjacent uninvolved digit. Displaced fractures cannot be reduced with closed techniques and open fractures require internal fixation (see Fig. 8-72).

Management of fractures of the first and fifth metatarsals can be more difficult. Isolated first metatarsal fractures are uncommon. If there is displacement or evidence of instability, internal

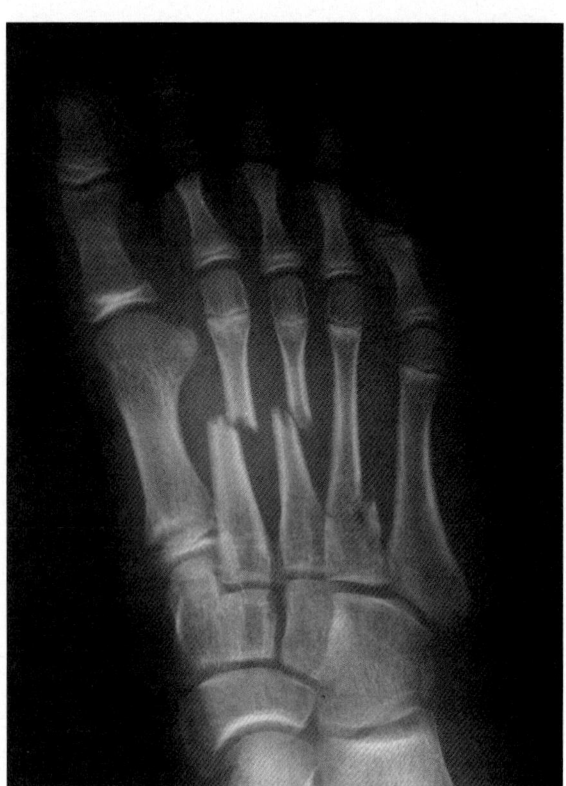

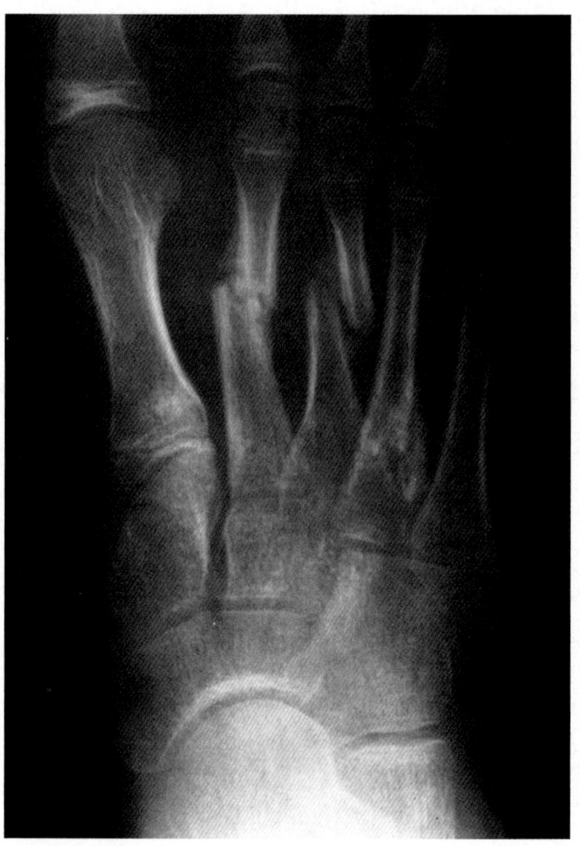

Fig. 8-71 Anteroposterior (AP) radiographs demonstrating fractures of the second through fourth metatarsals following injury (A) and with callus formation and healing 6 weeks later (B).

fixation with plate and screw fixation is usually performed. Fifth metatarsal fracture treatment is more controversial. Zone 1 (avulsion) fractures and fractures of the distal shaft can be treated with cast immobilization. Fractures in zone 2 and stress fractures in zone 3 are approached more aggressively. Although cast immobilization may result in healing, screw fixation is often used to avoid nonunion (see Fig. 8-73).

Dislocations are reduced and treated conservatively unless there are large osteochondral fragments that require pinning.

## Suggested Reading

Ekrol I, Court-Brown CM. Fractures of the base of the fifth metatarsal. *Foot* 2004;14:96–98.

Kay RM, Tang CW. Pediatric foot fractures: Evaluation and treatment. *J Am Acad Orthop Surg*. 2001;9:308–319.

Reese KA, Litsky A, Kaeding C, et al. Cannulated screw fixation of Jone's fractures–a clinical and biomechanical study. *Am J Sports Med*. 2004;32:1736–1742.

### Imaging of Complications

Complications related to forefoot fracture dislocations are similar to those described in previous sections. Nonunion, malunion, and delayed union occur with greater frequency in some locations. Fractures in zones 2 and 3 of the fifth metatarsal are particularly prone to delayed union or nonunion (see Fig. 8-74).

In children, growth arrest due to physeal fractures occurs in the metatarsals and phalanges. Metatarsal shaft fractures may result in overgrowth. Pain and stiffness are not uncommon following phalangeal fractures.

Compartment syndrome can develop in complex fractures (Fig. 8-72) with high-velocity trauma. The diagnosis can usually be made clinically. MRI is useful for anatomic definition of the involved compartments and neurovascular structures.

## Suggested Reading

Anderson LD. Injuries to the forefoot. *Clin Orthop*. 1977; 122:18–27.

Kay RM, Tang CW. Pediatric foot fractures: Evaluation and treatment. *J Am Acad Orthop Surg*. 2001;9:308–319.

Silas SI, Herzenberg JE, Myerson MS, et al. Compartment syndrome in the foot in children. *J Bone Joint Surg*. 1995; 77A:356–361.

# Joint Reconstruction Procedures

Joint replacement procedures in the foot and ankle are most commonly performed on the ankle and metatarsophalangeal

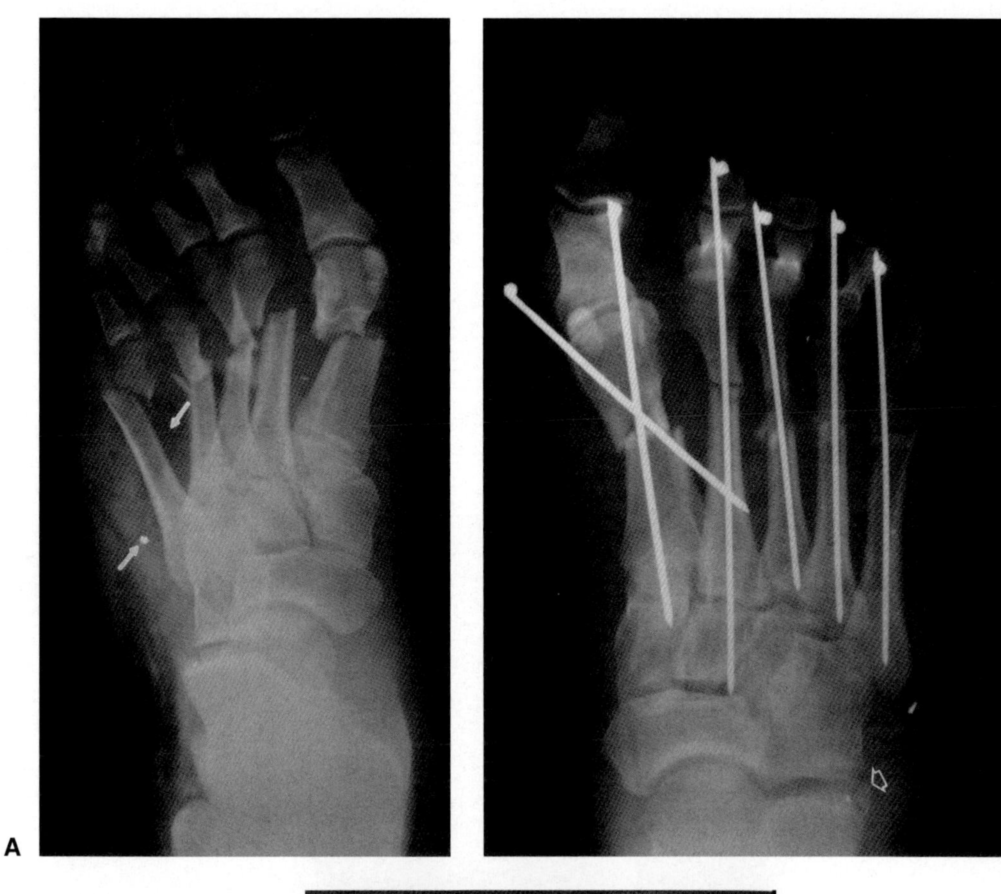


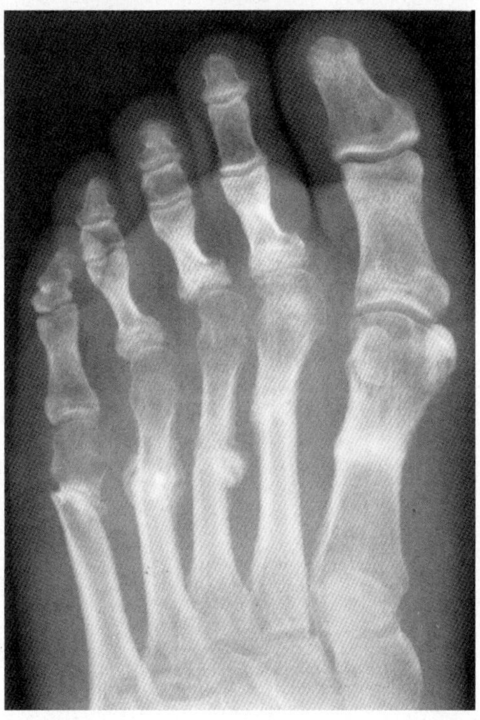


Fig. 8-72 Complex open fractures of the metatarsals. A: Anteroposterior (AP) radiograph demonstrates displaced fractures of the distal first through fifth metatarsals with air and foreign bodies in the soft tissues (*arrows*). B: Fractures were fixed with large caliber K-wires. There is also a fracture subluxation of the calcaneocuboid articulation (*open arrow*) which was not apparent on the initial image. C: Radiograph after K-wire removal and fracture healing.

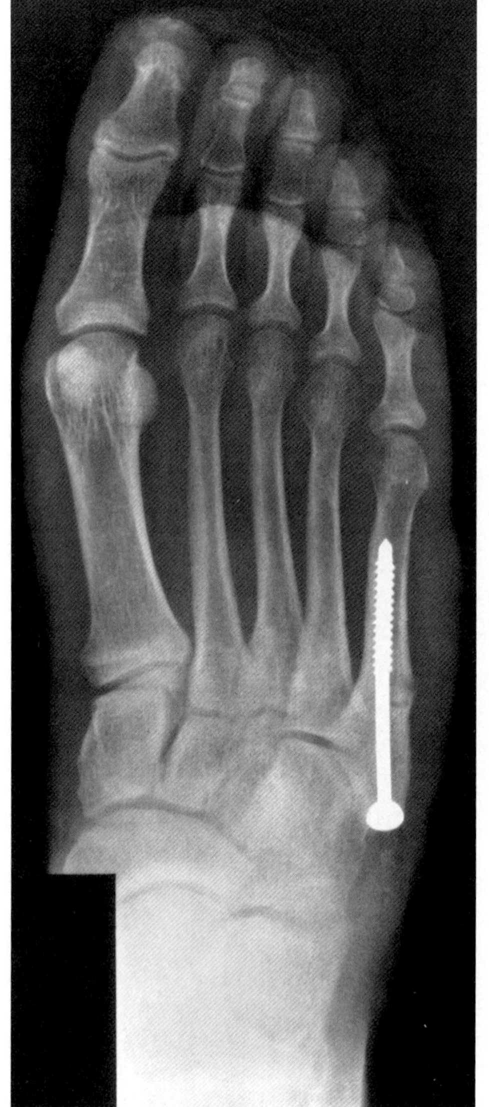


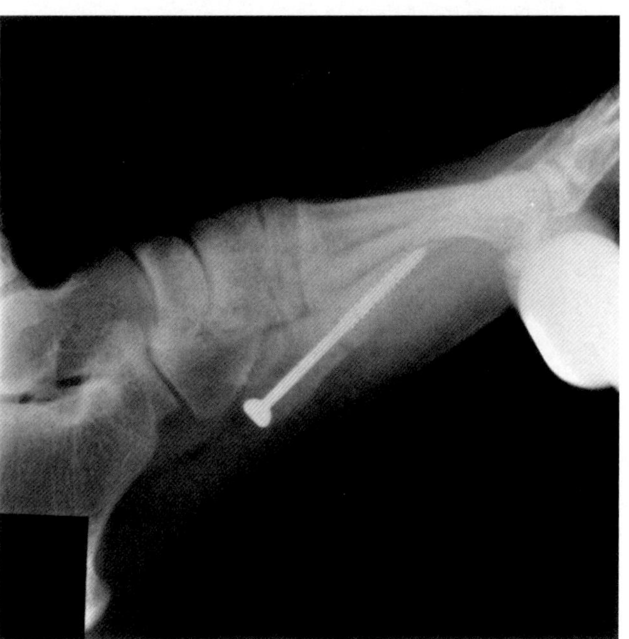


Fig. 8-73 Anteroposterior (AP) (A) and lateral (B) radiographs of a zone 3 fracture treated with screw fixation.

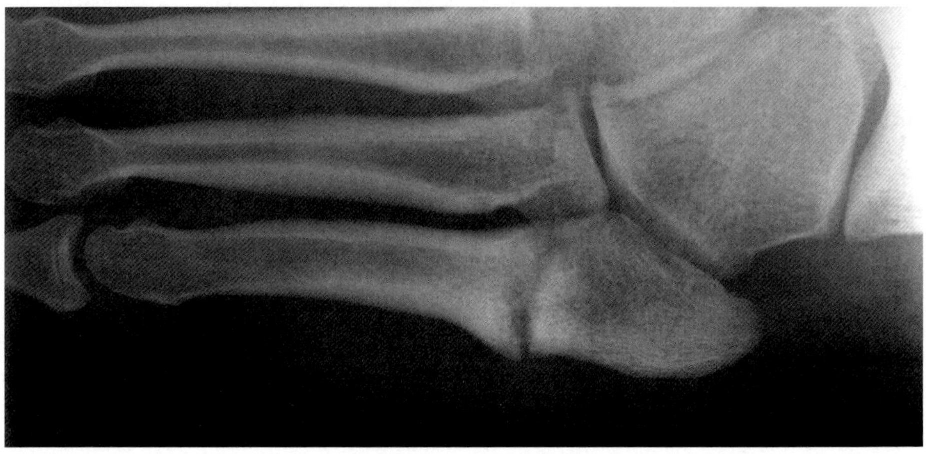

Fig. 8-74 Radiograph demonstrating widening of the fracture line with hypertrophic sclerotic margins due to nonunion.

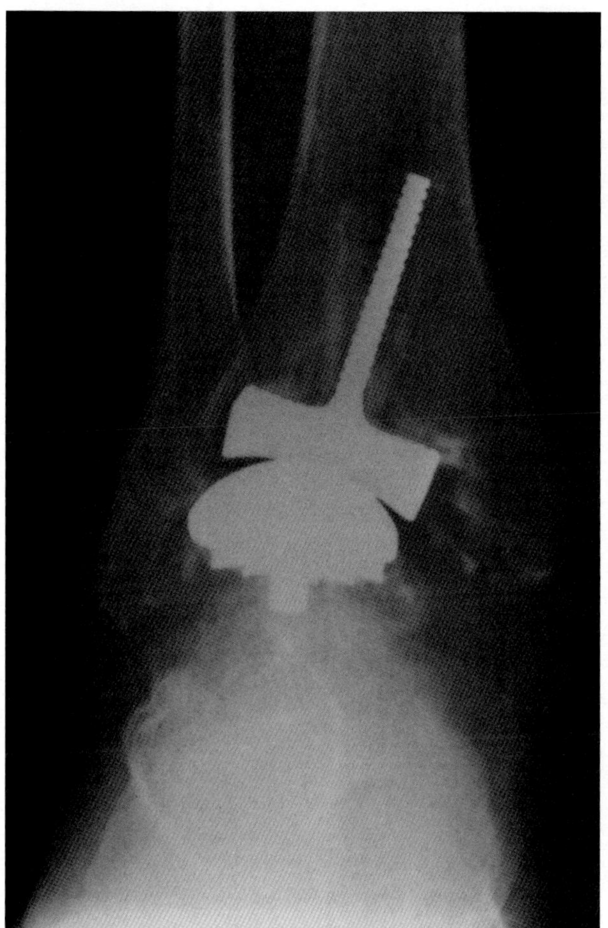


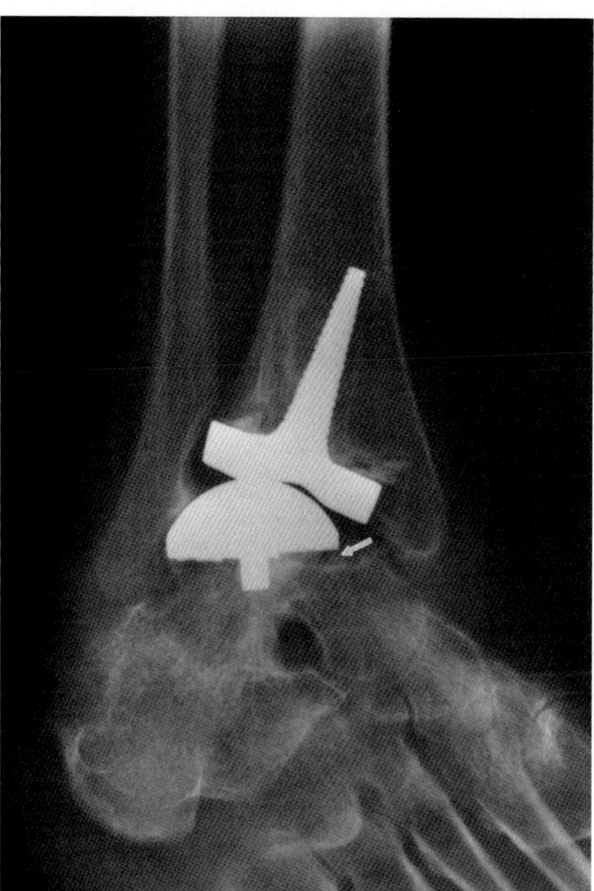


Fig. 8-75 First generation total ankle replacement. Anteroposterior (AP) (A) and oblique (B) radiographs demonstrate loosening with toggling of the tibial stem and migration (*arrow*) of the talar component.

joints. Indications, preoperative imaging, component or procedure selection, and postoperative imaging and complications will be reviewed.

## Ankle Arthroplasty

Early first-generation ankle replacements had high failure rates compared to the alternative of ankle arthrodesis. Osteolysis, loosening, impingement, infection, and soft tissue breakdown caused disappointing results (see Fig. 8-75). Improvements in hip and knee components translated to less constrained ankle implants with less bone resection and improved fixation. There is also now a better understanding of the importance of soft tissue support with ankle arthroplasty.

Indications for ankle joint replacement continue to be refined as patient selection is critical to successful outcomes. Ankle arthroplasty can be performed for osteoarthritis, rheumatoid arthritis, and posttraumatic arthropathy. The last accounts for 80% of patients considered for ankle replacement. Older patients with low demand and multiarticular involvement are the best candidates. Younger patients with posttraumatic arthritis tend to have a poorer prognosis. Contraindications for total ankle replacement include infection, peripheral vascular disease, inadequate soft tissue support, and neuropathic arthropathy.

As with the hip and knee, clinical scoring systems have been developed for the foot and ankle by the American Orthopaedic Foot and Ankle Society. The system for the foot and ankle (ankle-hindfoot scale) grades the ankle, subtalar, talonavicular, and calcaneocuboid joints. The system can be used for multiple procedures in addition to ankle arthroplasty. There are a maximum of 100 points in categories of pain (40 points), function (50 points), and alignment (10 points). There are multiple subcategories with decreasing points as pain increases and function decreases. Table 8-10 summarizes the ankle-hindfoot scale.

# Suggested Reading

Easley ME, Vertullo CJ, Urban WC, et al. Total ankle arthroplasty. *J Am Acad Orthop Surg.* 2002;10:157–167.

Kitaoka HB, Alexander IJ, Adelaar RS, et al. Clinical rating systems for the ankle-hindfoot, mid-foot, hallux and lesser toes. *Foot Ankle Int.* 1994;15:349–353.

Kitaoka HB, Patzer GL. Clinical results of the Mayo total ankle arthroplasty. *J Bone Joint Surg*. 1996;78A:1658–1664.

### Preoperative Imaging

Radiographs of the ankle (AP, lateral, mortise views) and foot (AP and lateral standing, oblique views) are required to assess the articular anatomy and evaluate the extent of arthropathy in the ankle, subtalar joint, and the joints of the mid and forefoot (see Fig. 8-76). In certain cases, CT with reformatting is important to evaluate bone stock, subchondral cysts, and more accurately assess the extent of ankle and hindfoot arthropathy (see Fig. 8-77). In addition, diagnostic injections are performed to assess the extent of pain relief in a given joint before considering the surgical approach. Injections are especially useful if arthroplasty needs to be combined with arthrodesis of the subtalar or other tarsal articulations.

Table 8-10

ANKLE-HINDFOOT SCORING SYSTEM AMERICAN ORTHOPAEDIC FOOT AND ANKLE SOCIETY

| CATEGORY | POINTS |
|---|---|
| Pain (40 points) | |
| No pain | 40 |
| Mild, occasional | 30 |
| Moderate, daily | 20 |
| Severe, constant | 0 |
| Function (50 points) | |
| Activity limitations | |
| No limitations | 10 |
| Severe limitations, walker or crutches | 0 |
| Maximum walking distance | |
| Greater than six blocks | 5 |
| Less than one block | 0 |
| Walking surfaces | |
| No surface issues | 5 |
| Severe difficulty uneven terrain, stairs, ladders | 0 |
| Gait abnormality | |
| None | 8 |
| Obvious | 4 |
| Marked | 0 |
| Sagittal motion | |
| Normal or mild reduction | 8 |
| Moderate restriction | 4 |
| Marked restriction | 0 |
| Hindfoot motion | |
| Normal | 6 |
| Moderate restriction | 3 |
| Marked restriction | 0 |
| Ankle-hindfoot stability | |
| Stable | 8 |
| Unstable | 0 |
| Alignment | 10 |

MRI is useful for evaluation of soft tissue support, AVN, and articular cartilage.

## SUGGESTED READING

Berquist TH. Diagnostic and therapeutic injections as an aid to musculoskeletal diagnosis. *Semin Interv Radiol.* 1993;10: 326–343.

Lucas PE, Hurwitz SR, Kaplan PA, et al. Fluoroscopically guided injections in the foot and ankle: Localization of the source of pain to guide treatment-prospective study. *Radiology* 1997;204:411–415.

Mitchell MJ, Bielecki D, Bergman AG, et al. Localization of specific joint causing hindfoot pain: Value of injecting local anesthetic into individual joints during arthrography. *AJR Am J Roentgenol.* 1995;164:1473–1476.

### Treatment Options

Ankle arthroplasty is an alternative to arthrodesis. There are multiple implants that can be used for ankle replacement. Currently, there are four commonly used systems in the United States and in the author's practice. These include the Agility, INBONE, Scandinavian Total Ankle Replacement (STAR), and Salto Talaris ankle replacements.

The Agility (DePuy, a Johnson and Johnson Company, Warsaw, Indiana) ankle consists of a tibial component, a cobalt-chromium talar component, and an ultra–high molecular weight polyethylene (UHMWPe) insert (see Fig. 8-78). This system is semiconstrained with different component sizes that provide a choice of 11 different combinations. The system is U.S. Food and Drug Administration (FDA) approved.

The INBONE ankle system (INBONE Technologies, Boulder, Colorado) consists of a titanium tibial stem with tibial tray and talar stem with titanium plasma spray coating, a highly polished cobalt-chromium talar dome, and a polyethylene (UHMWPe) insert (see Fig. 8-79). Again, multiple sizes are available. This total ankle system is also FDA approved.

The STAR (Link Orthopaedics, Rockaway, New Jersey) is a mobile-bearing system that requires less bone removal and allows more normal motion. The system comprises cobalt-chromium alloy tibial and talar components with titanium plasma spray coating on the bone interfaces and a polyethylene (UHMWPe) insert (see Fig. 8-80). There are five choices for each of the three components. The FDA panel recommended clearance in April 2007. This ankle system is used without cement.

The Salto Talaris Anatomic Ankle (Tornier, Stafford, Texas) has cobalt-chromium alloy tibial and talar components with titanium plasma spray on the bone interface surfaces and a polyethylene (UHMWPe) insert (see Fig. 8-81). There are three tibial and four talar sizes. This implant was FDA approved in 2006.

A talar prosthesis has also been used for treatment of crush injuries and AVN of the talus. This technique is not commonly employed in the United States.

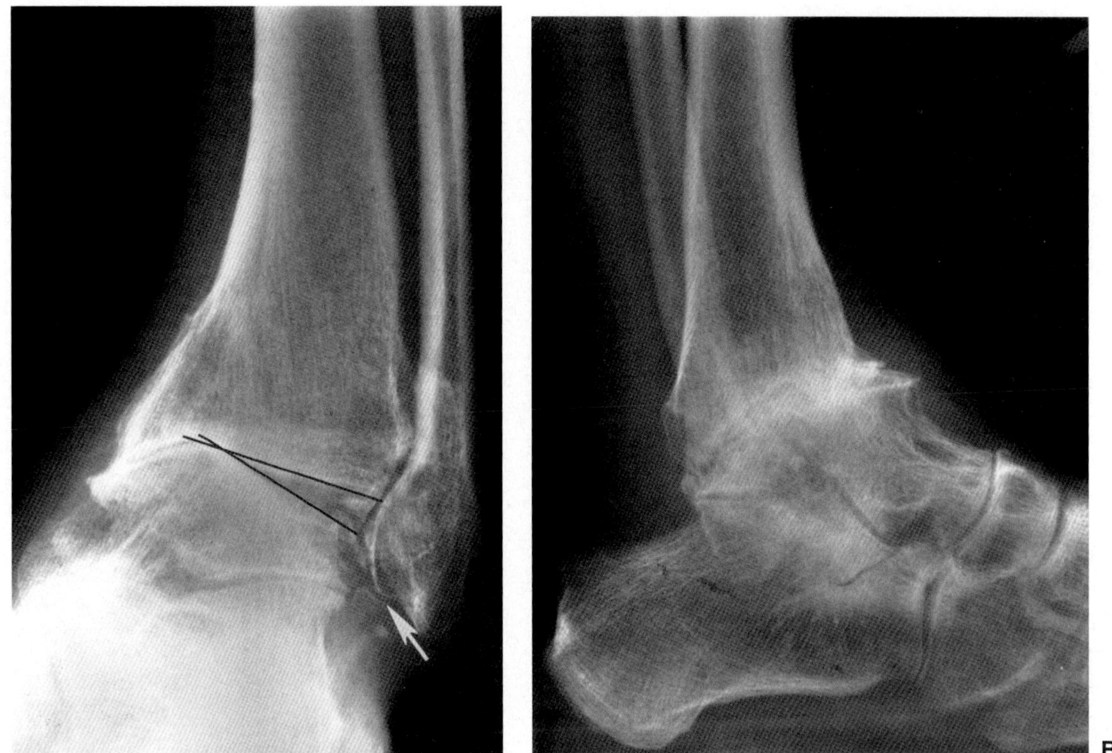


Fig. 8-76 Anteroposterior (AP) (A) and lateral (B) radiographs demonstrate marked posttraumatic arthropathy with asymmetry (lines) of the tibiotalar articulation and calcaneofibular abutment (*arrow*). The subtalar joint is also narrowed.

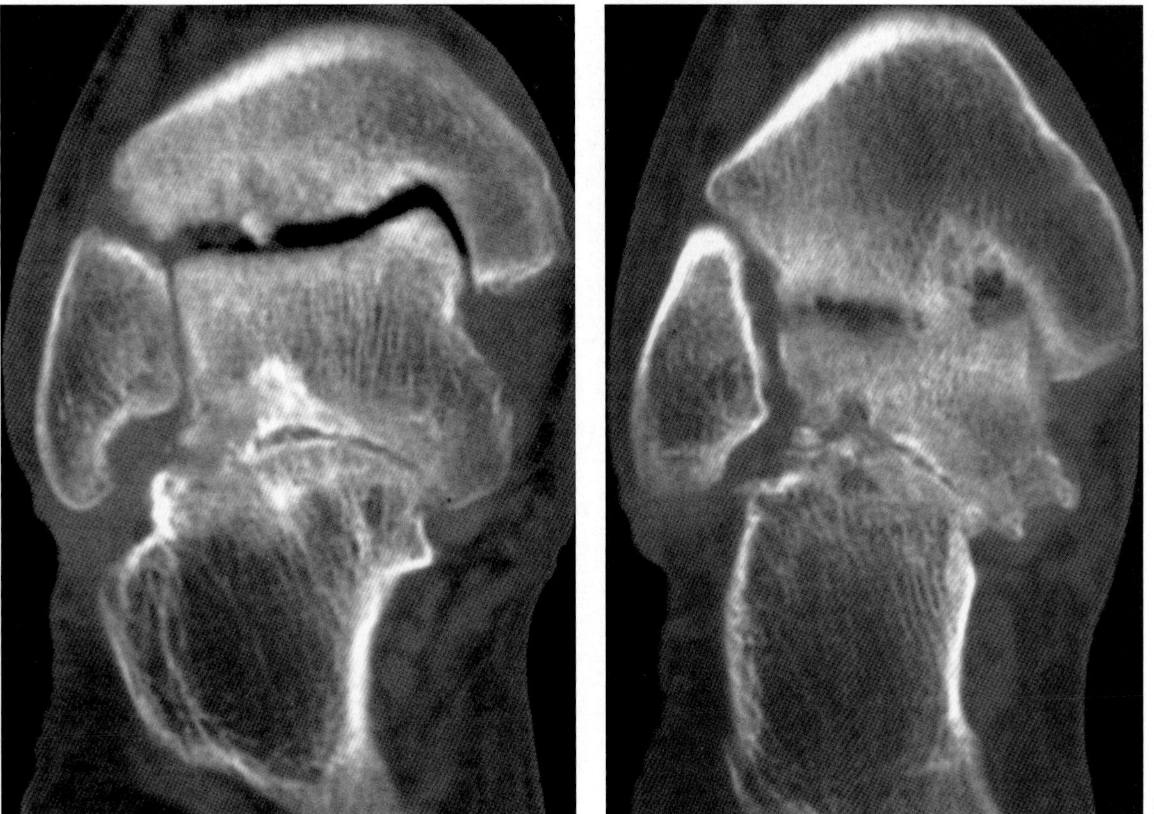


Fig. 8-77 Coronal computed tomographic (CT) images (A and B) demonstrate extensive tibiotalar and subtalar arthrosis.

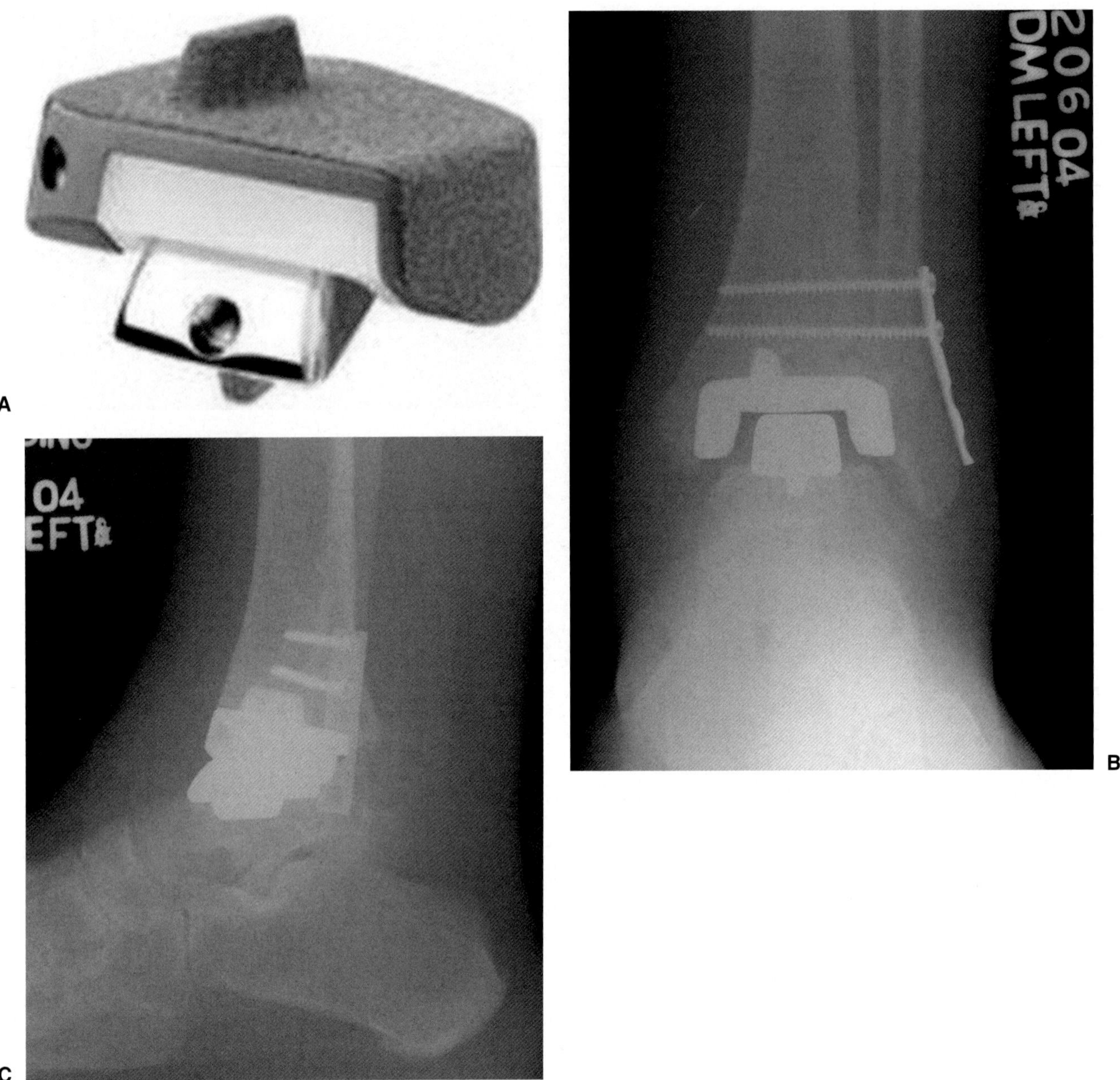


Fig. 8-78 A: Photograph of the components of the Agility ankle replacement (Courtesy DePuy, a Johnson and Johnson Company, Warsaw, Indiana). Anteroposterior (AP) (B) and lateral (C) radiographs of an Agility arthroplasty with fibular side plate and syndesmotic screws.

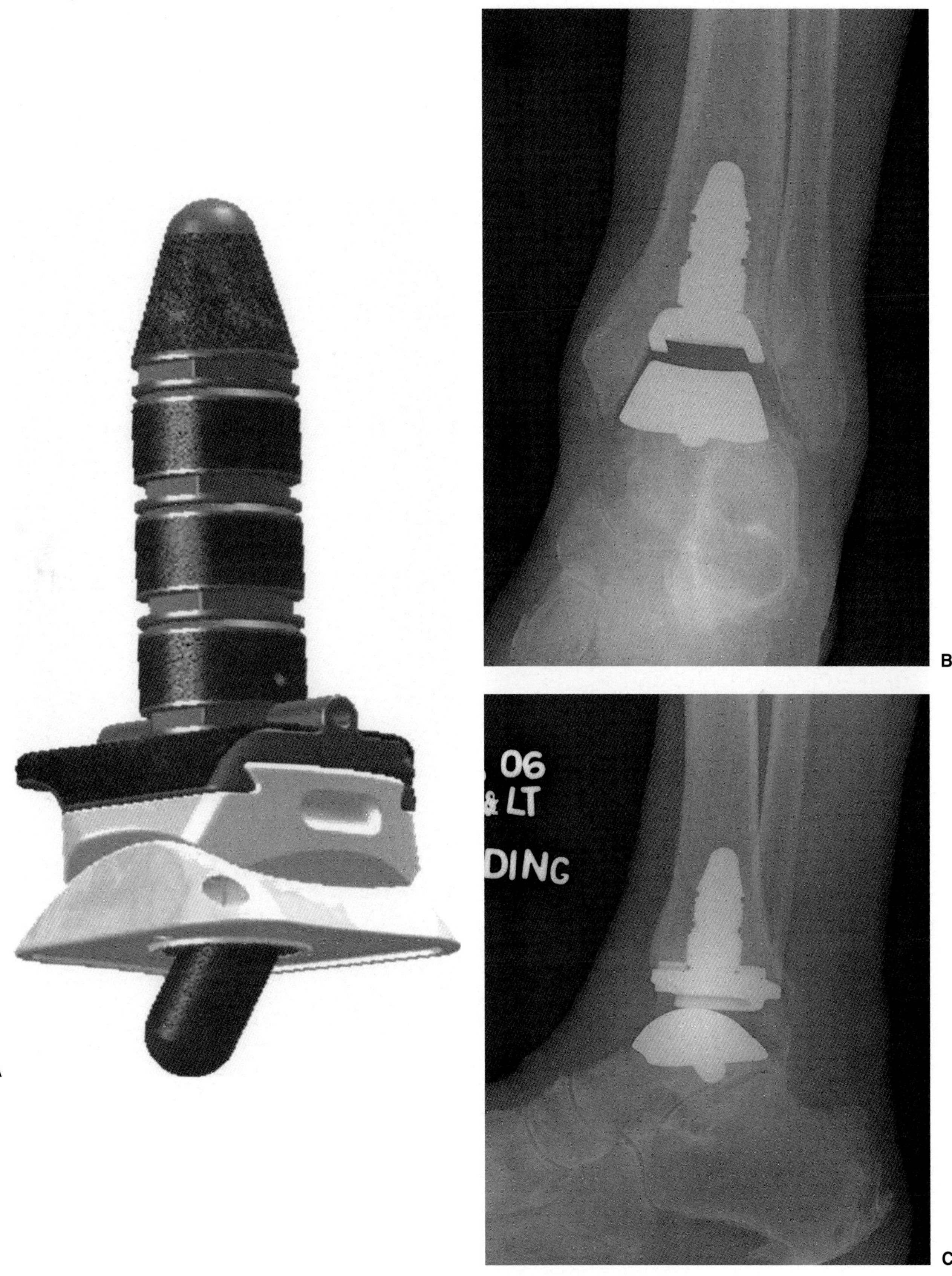


Fig. 8-79 A: Photograph of an INBONE ankle replacement (Courtesy of INBONE Technologies, Boulder, Colorado). Anteroposterior (AP) (B) and lateral (C) on the INBONE ankle replacement.

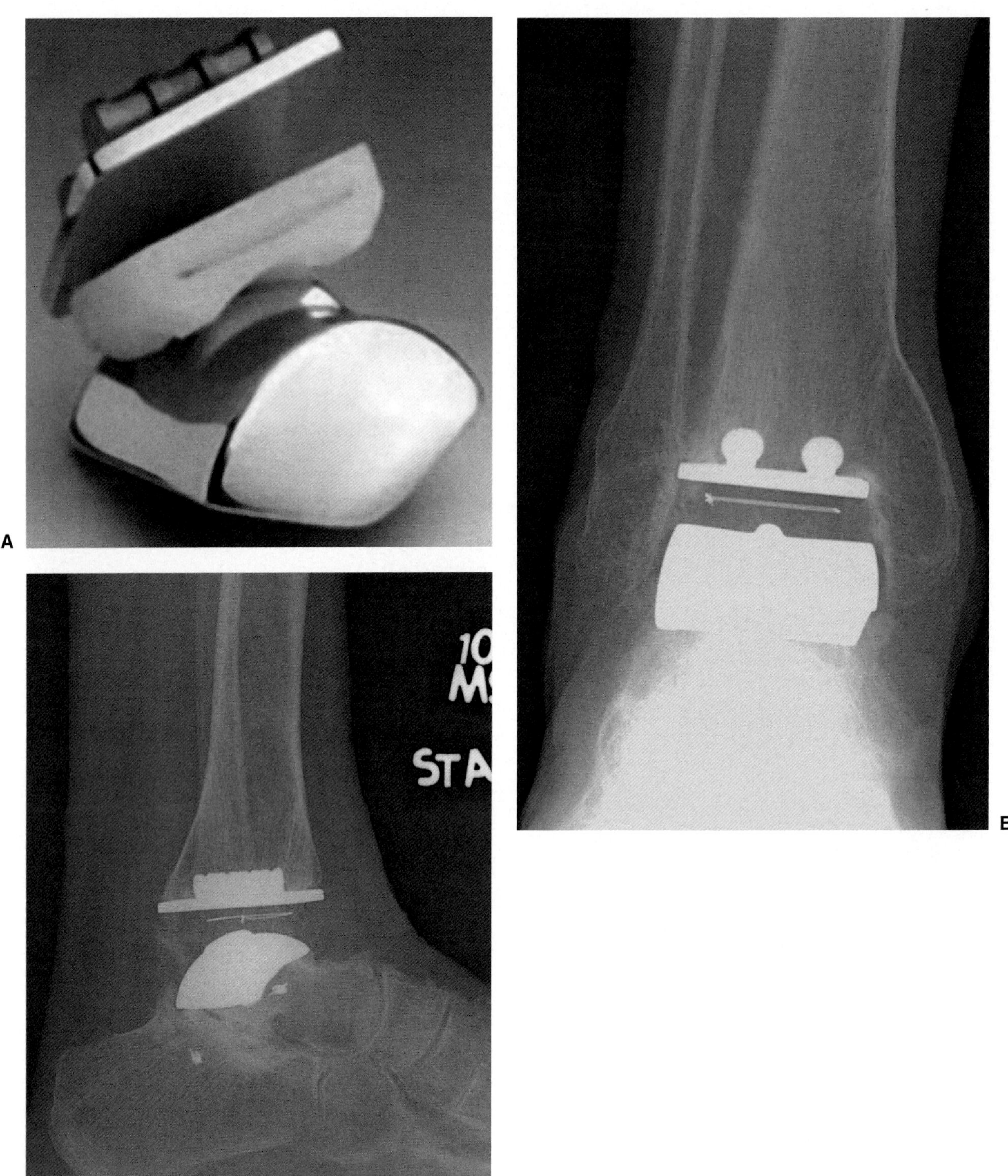


Fig. 8-80 A: Photograph of the Scandinavian Total Ankle Replacement (STAR) (Courtesy of Link Orthopaedics, Rockaway, New Jersey). Anteroposterior (AP) (B) and lateral (C) radiographs of the STAR ankle replacement. There are soft tissue anchors in the talus and calcaneus due to ligament repair.

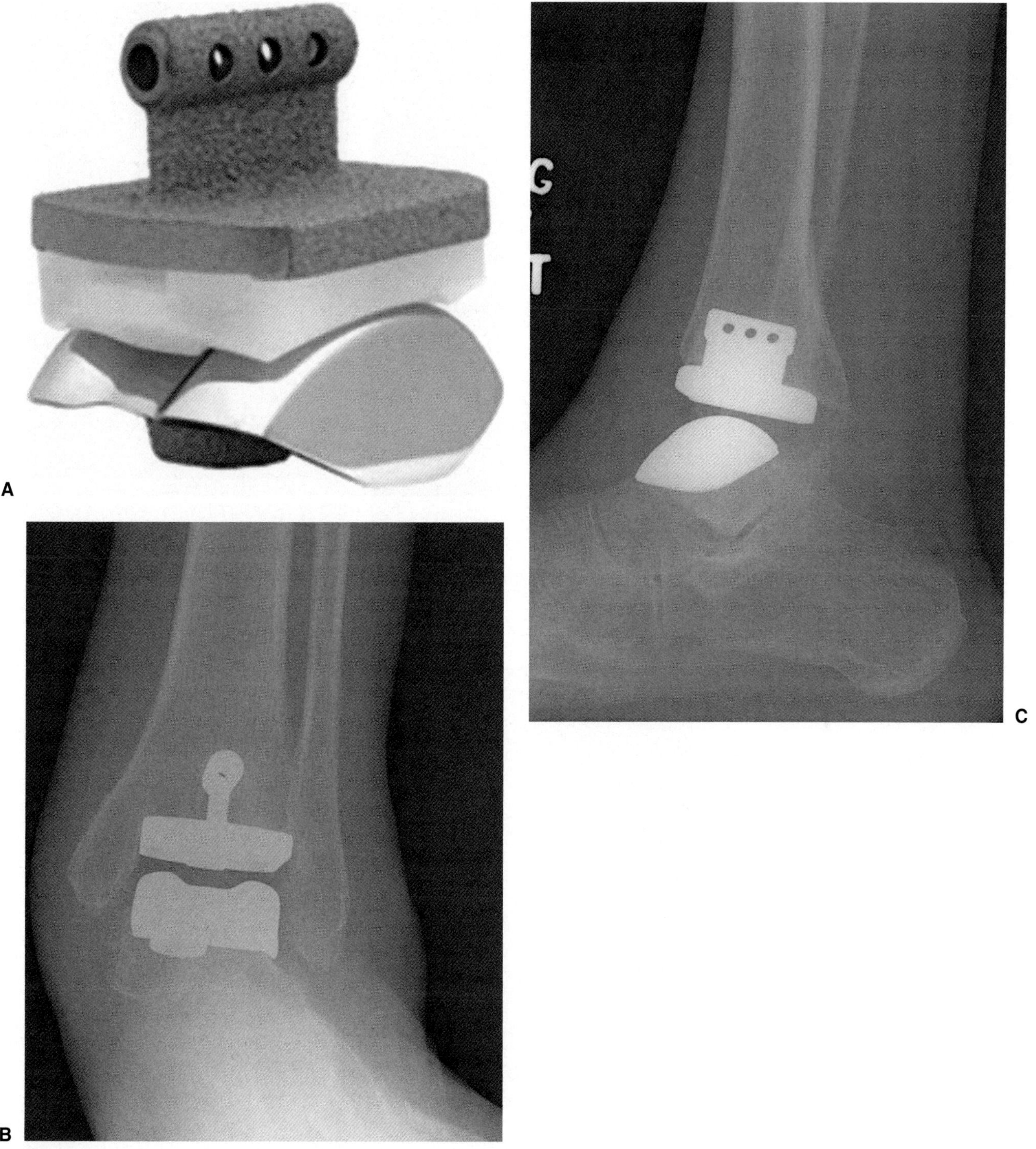


Fig. 8-81 A: Photograph of a Salto Talaris Anatomic Ankle (Courtesy of Tornier, Stafford, Texas). Anteroposterior (AP) (B) and lateral (C) radiographs of a Salto Talaris arthroplasty.

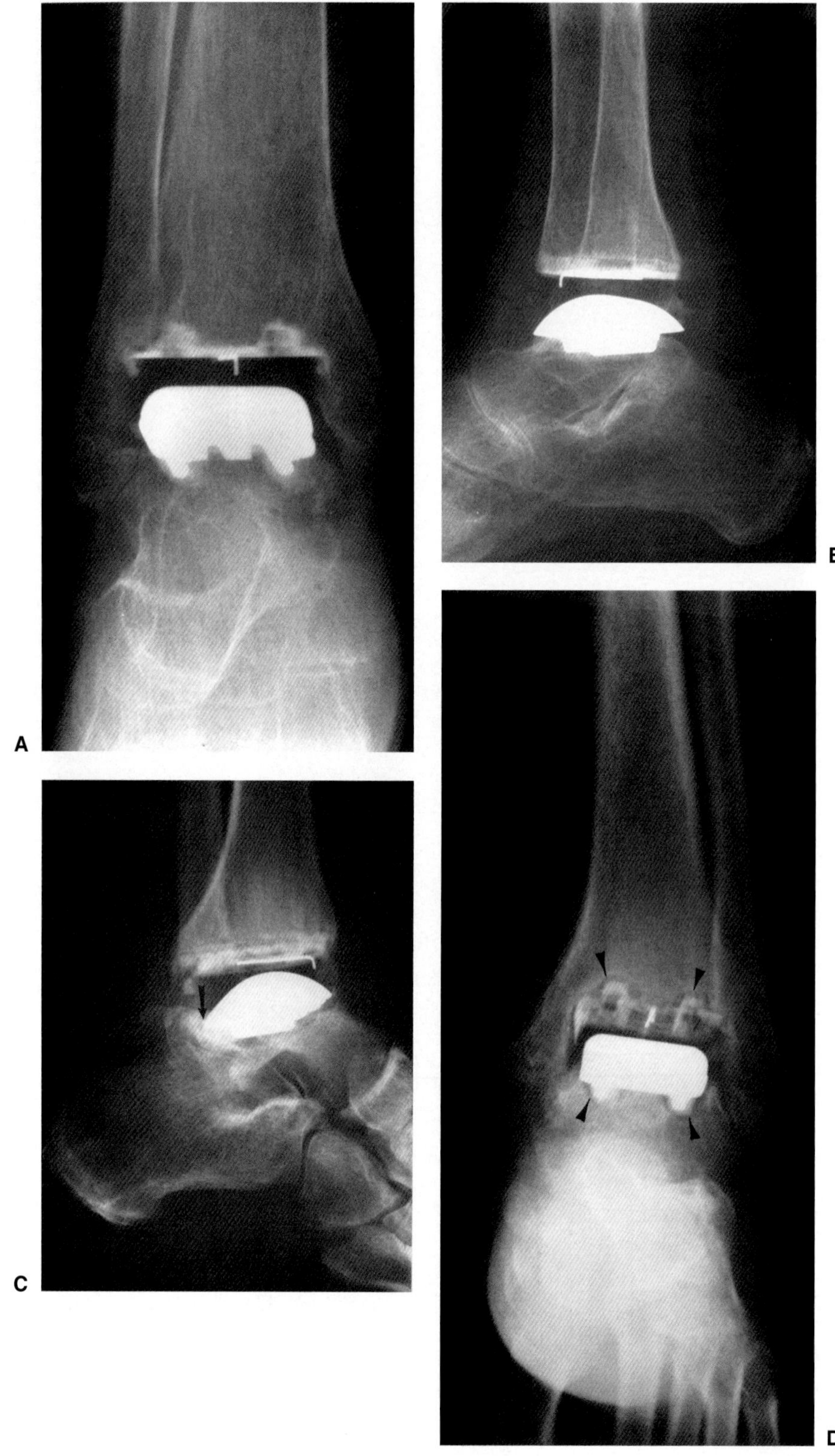


**Fig. 8-82** Component loosening. Normal Mayo ankle replacement seen on anteroposterior (AP) (**A**) and lateral (**B**) radiographs. Lateral radiograph (**C**) demonstrating posterior subsidence of the talar component. **D:** AP radiograph in a different patient demonstrating obvious lucent lines about the tibial and talar (*arrowheads*) components due to loosening.

## Suggested Reading


Bonnin M, Judet T, Colombier JA, et al. Midterm results of the Salto total ankle prosthesis. *Clin Orthop*. 2004;424:6–18.

Easley MA, Vertullo CJ, Urban WC, et al. Total ankle arthroplasty. *J Am Acad Orthop Surg*. 2002;10:157–167.

Harnoongroj T, Vanadurongwan V. The Talar prosthesis. *J Bone Joint Surg*. 1997;79A:1313–1322.

Murnaghan JM, Warnock DS, Henderson SA. Total ankle replacement. Early experience with the STAR prosthesis. *Ulster Med J*. 2005;74:9–13.


# Postoperative Imaging and Complications

Complications related to ankle replacement may occur during the procedure, in the early postoperative period, or late. Complications at the time of surgery occur in up to 29% of patients. Fractures of the medial malleolus occurred in 56% of patients with intraoperative complications, fractures of the anterior distal tibia in 15%, and 19% had fractures of the lateral malleolus. Screw fixation was required in 33% of cases with the remainder treated with cast immobilization.

Early postoperative complications include delayed wound healing (7% to 8%), early deep infection (3%), and early spontaneous fractures of the distal tibia in osteopenic patients (4%). For early complications, radiographs are usually adequate if imaging is required.

Imaging of late complications can be more complex. Serial radiographs remain most useful for detection of heterotopic ossification, fractures, impingement, and loosening. More complex imaging is required for deep infection. In this setting, combined radionuclide scans (Tc 99m methylene diphosphonate [MDP] and labeled white blood cells) may be useful due to artifact from implants on MR images. CT is most useful to assess bone stock and evaluate osteolysis before revision surgery or arthrodesis.

Component loosening varies with the type of implant used. Therefore, the incidence varies from 6% to 26%. Features are similar to those described with hip and knee replacements with progressive lucent lines (>2 mm), component migration, and subsidence. Subsidence most often involves the talar component. Changes in component position >5 degrees indicate radiographic failure. Serial radiographs are adequate for following component position and changes and loosening in most cases (see Figs. 8-82 and 8-83).

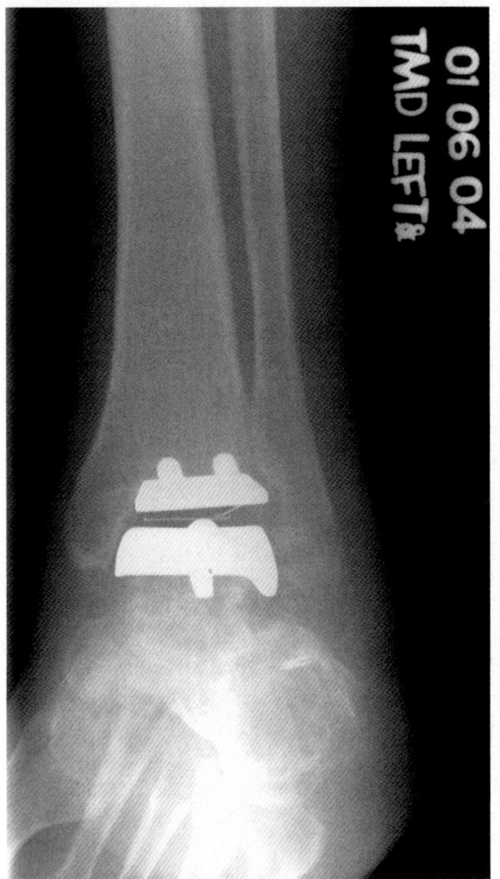


A

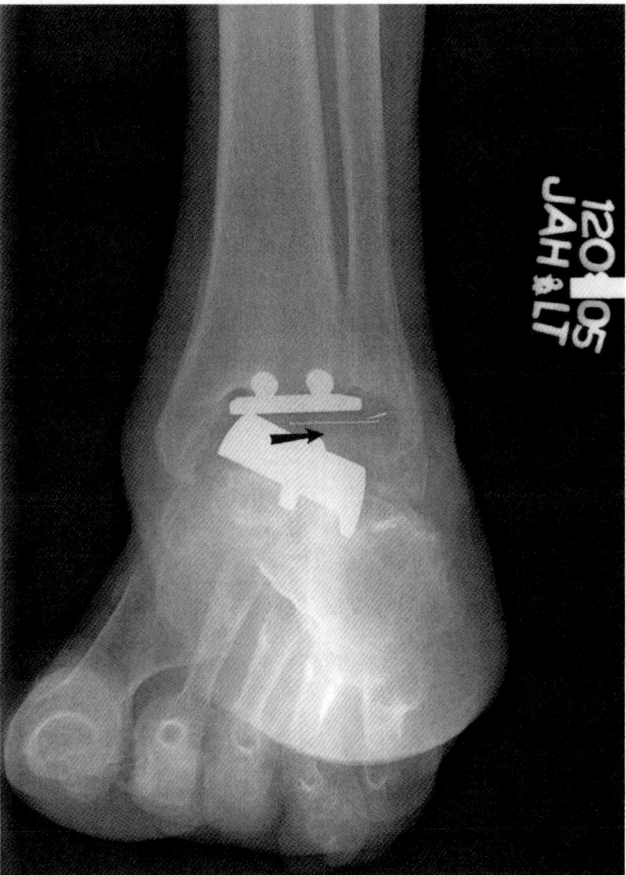

B

Fig. 8-83 Scandinavian Total Ankle Replacement (STAR) ankle prosthesis. Anteroposterior (AP) radiographs postoperatively (A) and 14 months later (B) demonstrate subsidence with tilt of the talar component, loosening of the tibial component, and lateral displacement (*arrow*) of the polyethylene insert.

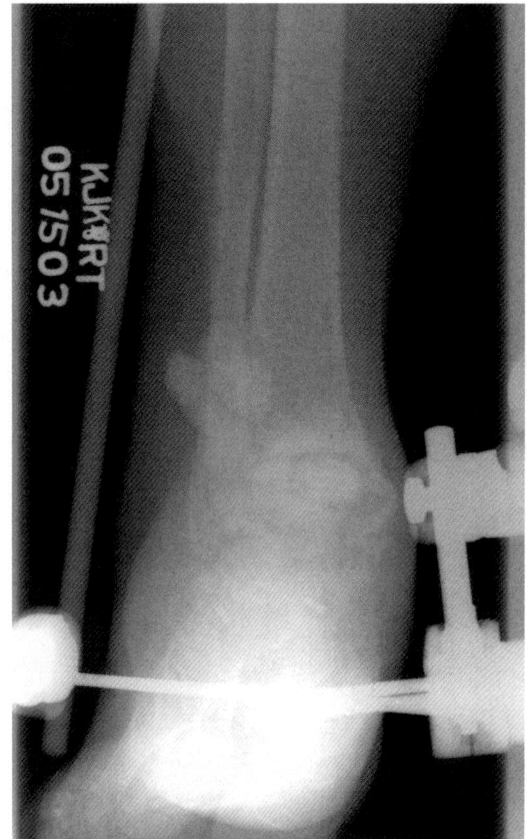

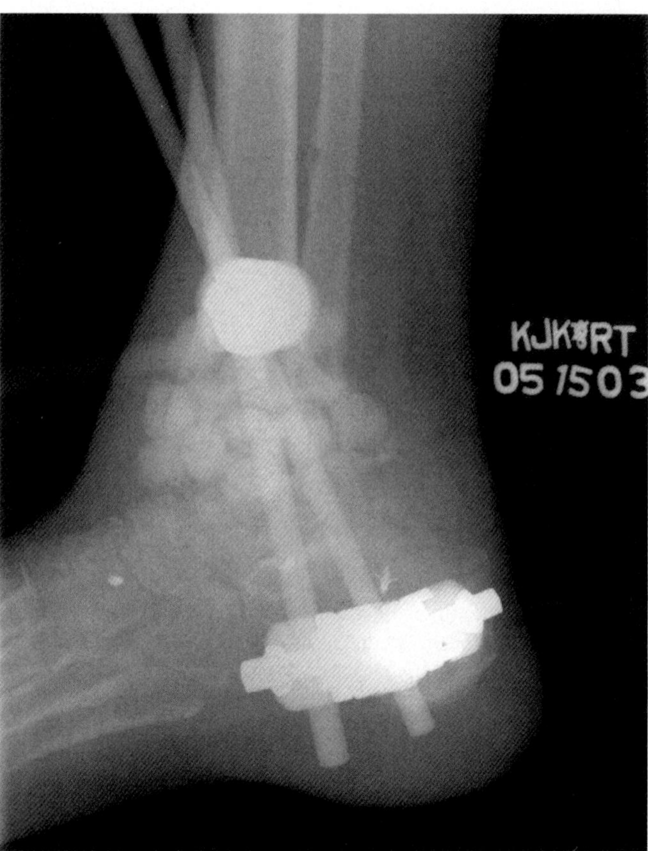

**Fig. 8-84** Deep infection. Anteroposterior (AP) **(A)** and lateral **(B)** radiographs following component removal and insertion of antibiotic-impregnated methacrylate beads. Stability achieved with an external fixator.

Both superficial and deep infections (2% to 3.7%) occur. Serial radiographs may demonstrate signs of loosening and periosteal reaction. Radiographic findings are often subtle requiring additional imaging studies and joint aspiration to confirm the infection. Tc 99m MDP combined with labeled white blood cell scans using $^{111}$Indium ($^{111}$In) or Tc are useful to confirm infection. Patients with deep infection usually require component removal (see Fig. 8-84).

Distal tibial fractures and malleolar fractures are not uncommon during and following the procedures. Stress or insufficiency fractures also occur in osteoporotic patients. Serial radiographs are adequate for detection in most cases.

Malleolar impingement is also a cause of postoperative ankle pain. This may occur as an isolated event or in association with implant subsidence or migration or excessive bone resection during implant placement. Fibular calcaneal impingement occurs most frequently, but tibiotalar involvement is not uncommon. Again, serial radiographs are adequate for diagnosis along with clinical features (see Fig. 8-85). Similarly, heterotopic ossification in the periarticular soft tissues is a common problem (up to 63%) frequently requiring debridement to correct symptoms of impingement and reduced range of motion.

Osteolysis also occurs with ankle replacement related to particle disease similar to the hip and knee. This may be associated with loosening and infection (see Fig. 8-86). The incidence is not as well documented compared to the hip and knee.

Instability may occur with or without implant failure. Although serial radiographs may indicate joint space asymmetry, fluoroscopically positioned stress views are more reliable for demonstrating instability. Anesthetic injection may be required in patients with significant pain in order to perform an accurate study.

Osteoarthritis in the subtalar and talonavicular joints frequently develops following ankle replacement procedures. This may reduce the long-term functional outcome of the procedure. In certain cases, arthrodesis of these joints is later performed or in the case of the subtalar joint may be performed with the arthroplasty. If arthrodesis is a consideration, it may be useful to perform diagnostic anesthetic injections to confirm the source of pain before fusion.

Table 8-11 summarizes complications and imaging approaches for ankle arthroplasty.

Arthroplasty failures have been decreased with improved newer generation systems. Newer implants report 5-year survival rates in the range of 74% to 95% and 14-year survival rates in the 72% to 75% range. Despite the improvements, failure rates have been reported in the range of 16% to 28%. Up to 28% of patients require resurgery, which may include debridement of heterotopic ossification (35%), correction of

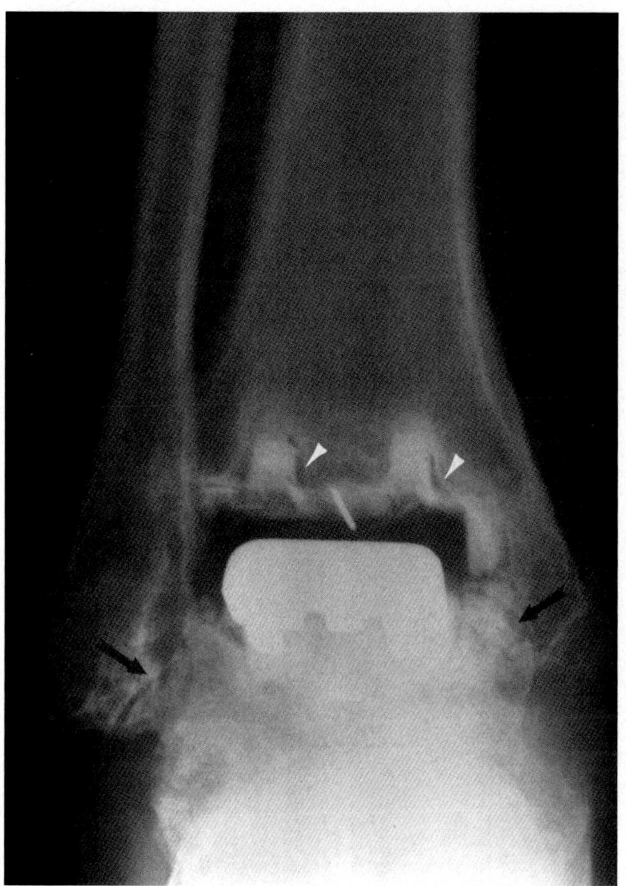

Fig. 8-85 Impingement. Anteroposterior (AP) radiograph demonstrating malleolar impingement (*black arrows*) and incomplete lucency (*arrowheads*) about the tibial component.

component alignment (24%), and component replacement (18%). It is not unusual to proceed to arthrodesis (Fig. 8-86) for failed ankle arthroplasty (14% of original implants).

## Suggested Reading


Doets HC, Brand R, Nelissen RGGH. Total ankle arthroplasty in inflammatory joint diseases with use of two mobile-bearing designs. *J Bone Joint Surg*. 2006;88A:1272–1284.

Easley ME, Vertullo CJ, Urban WC, et al. Total ankle arthroplasty. *J Am Acad Orthop Surg*. 2002;10:157–167.

Lacomte AR, Singh SK, Fitzgerald F, et al. Small joint arthroplasty. *Semin Musculoskelet Radiol*. 2006;10:64–78.

Lucas PE, Hurwitz SR, Kaplan PA, et al. Fluoroscopically guided injections into the foot and ankle: Localization of the source of pain as a guide to treatment-prospective study. *Radiology* 1997;204:411–415.

Murnaghan JM, Warnock DS, Henderson SA. Total ankle replacement. Early experiences with the STAR prosthesis. *Ulster Med J*. 2005;74:9–13.

Spirt AA, Assal M, Hansen ST. Complications and failure after total ankle arthroplasty. *J Bone Joint Surg*. 2004;86A: 1172–1178.


## Metatarsophalangeal Arthroplasty

Joint replacement arthroplasty in the foot is most commonly performed on the first metatarsophalangeal joint. This procedure was developed as an alternative to resection arthroplasty, arthrodesis, and cheilectomy. Resection arthroplasty is performed by resection of the first metatarsal head (Mayo procedure) or proximal phalanx (Keller procedure). Cheilectomy (resection of the dorsal osteophytes) is used for treatment of hallux rigidus. The other procedures noted earlier were most commonly performed for hallux rigidus, osteoarthritis, and hallux valgus.

Joint replacement arthroplasty indications include hallux valgus, hallux rigidus, degenerative joint disease, rheumatoid arthritis, and failed surgical procedures. Most procedures are performed on the great toe. However, the lesser toes may also be managed in this manner in patients with Freiberg infraction, rheumatoid arthritis, subluxations, and bunionette deformities.

The goals of treatment are to improve function and relieve pain. As with other joint replacement procedures, the orthopaedic surgeon or pediatrist uses a clinical scoring system as part of the decision-making process and preoperative evaluation. There are scales for the great toe and lesser toes based on the degree of pain (40 points), function (45 points), and alignment (15 points) for a total of 100 points. The factors are similar to those listed in Table 8-10. Functional factors include footwear requirements, motion, and stability. Alignment measures the degree of deformity of the articulations.

## Suggested Reading


Craccihiolo A III, Kitaoka HB, Leventen EO. Silicone implant arthroplasty of second metatarsophalangeal joint disorders with and without hallux valgus deformities. *Foot Ankle*. 1988;9:10–18.

Grace DL. The surgical management of the rheumatoid foot. *Br J Hosp Med*. 1996;56:473–480.

Kitaoka HB, Alexander IJ, Adellaar RS, et al. Clinical rating system for the ankle-hindfoot, mid-foot, hallux and lesser toes. *Foot Ankle Int*. 1994;15:349–353.

Papagelopoulos PJ, Kitaoka HB, Ilstrup DM. Survivorship analysis of implant arthroplasty for the first metatarsophalangeal joint. *Clin Orthop*. 1994;302:164–172.


### Preoperative Imaging

Preoperative radiographs should include standing AP and lateral images along with oblique views. There are numerous features that should be assessed on preoperative radiographs. On the lateral radiograph, one should evaluate joint alignment, the talar-first metatarsal angle, the first metatarsophalangeal relationship, and digital deformities. Dorsal osteophytes seen with hallux rigidus are also easily appreciated on the lateral view (see Fig. 8-87).

Standing AP images should be evaluated to determine the extent of articular disease, erosions, subluxation, and angulation. Specific measurements include the metatarsophalangeal

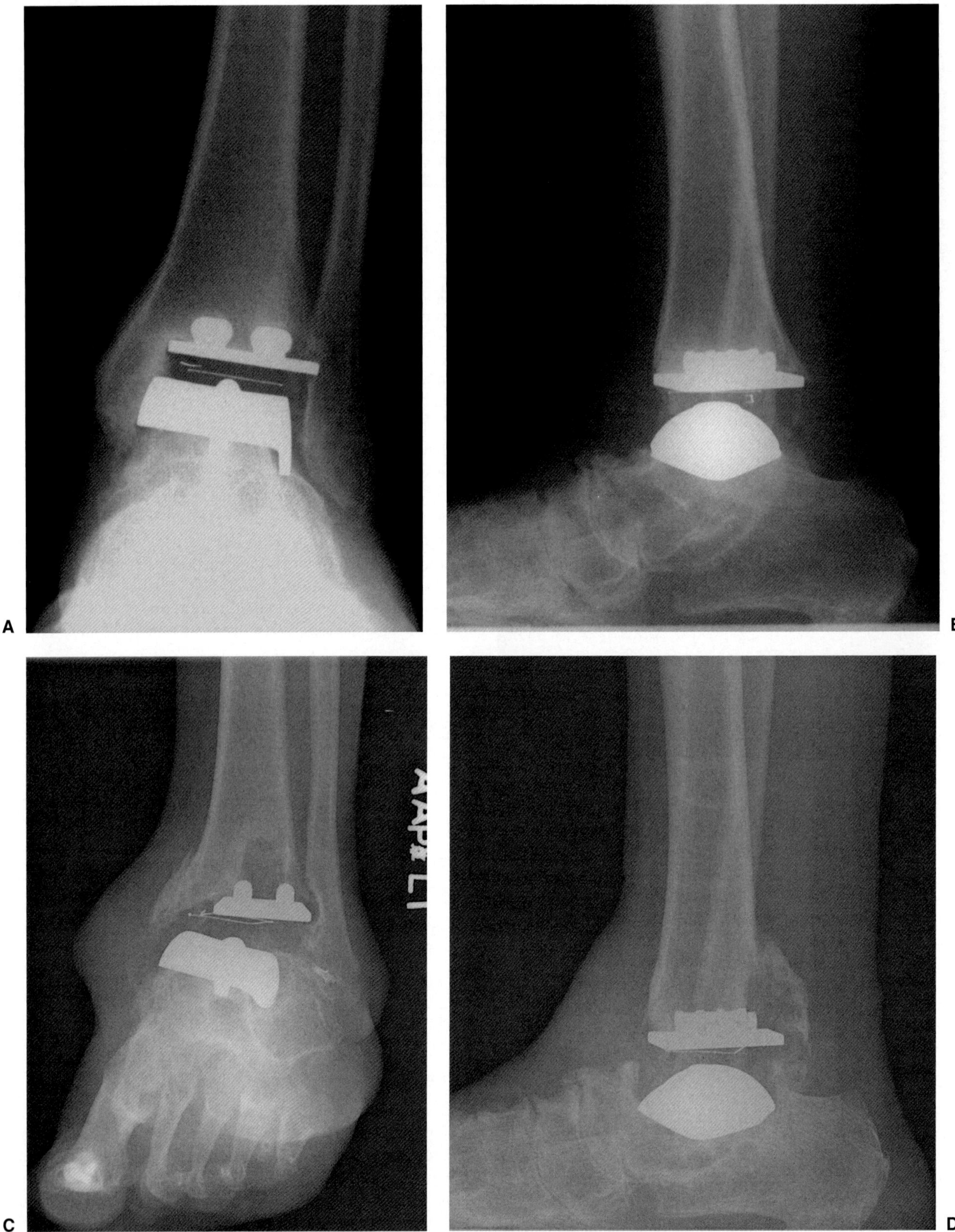


Fig. 8-86 Osteolysis. AP (A) and lateral (B) radiographs following Scandinavian Total Ankle Replacement (STAR) ankle arthroplasty. Follow-up radiographs (C and D) 4 years later demonstrate a medial malleolar fracture, subsidence of the talar component, shift of the tibial component with subluxation of the insert, and extensive tibial osteolysis. AP (E) and lateral (F) radiographs following component removal and arthrodesis with a retrograde intramedullary nail and bone graft.

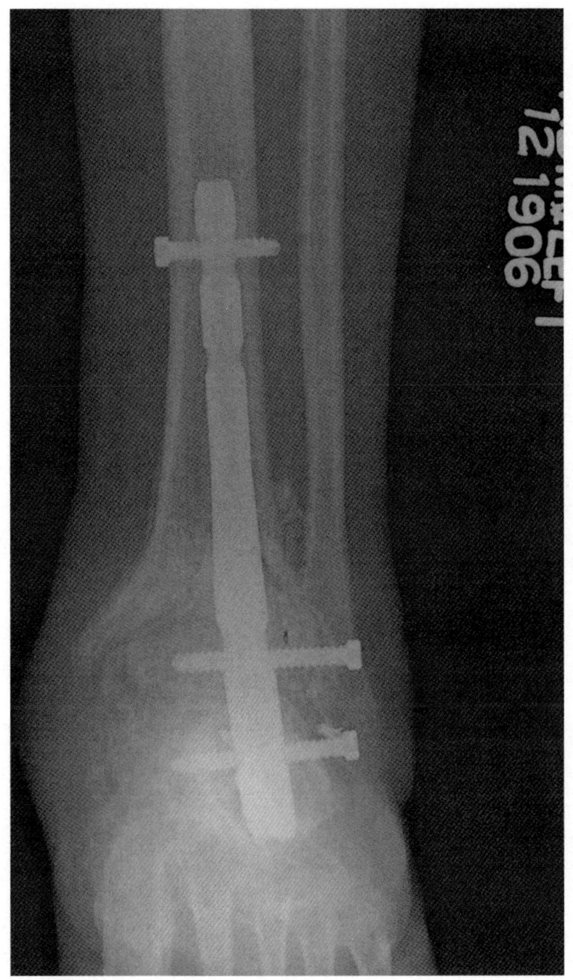


E

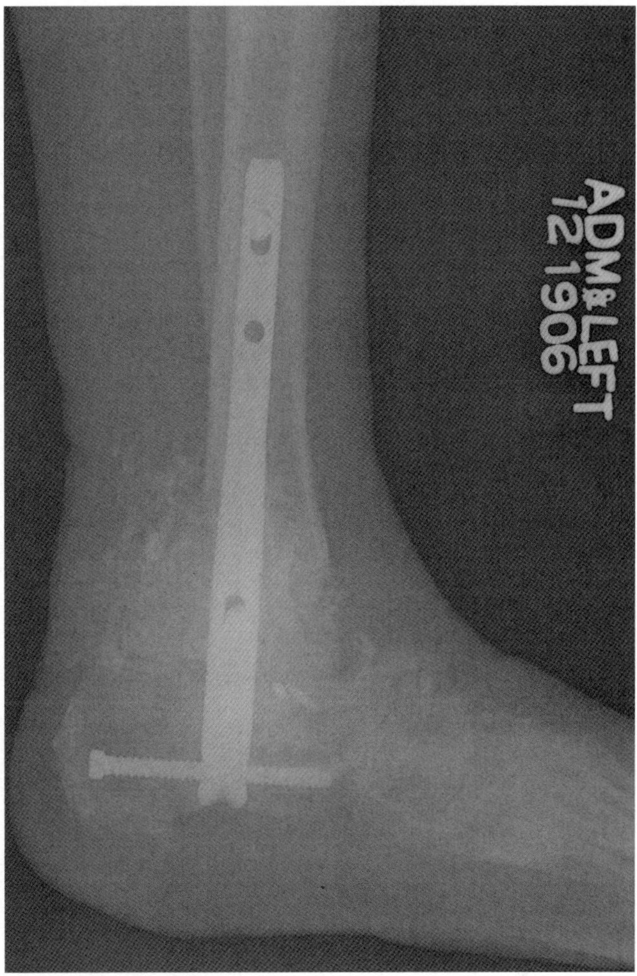


F

Fig. 8-86 *(Continued)*

**Table 8-11**

**ANKLE ARTHROPLASTY IMAGING OF COMPLICATIONS**

| COMPLICATION (INCIDENCE) | IMAGING APPROACHES |
|---|---|
| Component loosening (6%–26%) | Serial radiographs, CT |
| Deep infection (2%–3.7%) | Serial radiographs, radionuclide scans |
| Fractures (15%–20%) | Serial radiographs |
| Impingement/heterotopic ossification | Serial radiographs, CT |
| Osteolysis | Serial radiographs, CT |
| Instability | Stress views |
| Adjacent arthrosis | Radiographs, CT, diagnostic injections |

CT, computed tomography.

angles, first-second metatarsal angle, phalangeal angles, joint congruency, and the position of the sesamoids (see Fig. 8-88). When the lateral sesamoid is covered by the metatarsal it is considered in position. When it is shifted 10% to 50% it is considered subluxed and if >50% of the sesamoid is uncovered it is considered dislocated (Fig. 8-88B).

Additional imaging may be required in selected cases. CT is useful to evaluate bone loss and articular surfaces. MRI is best for evaluation of AVN, subtle articular cartilage changes, and soft tissue abnormalities. Joint aspiration or diagnostic injections are usually not required in the forefoot.

## Suggested Reading

Berquist TH. *Radiology of the foot and ankle*. Philadelphia: Lippincott Williams & Wilkins; 2000:479–526.

Lucas PE, Hurwitz SR, Kaplan PA, et al. Fluoroscopically guided injections into the foot and ankle: Localization of the source of pain as a guide to treatment-prospective study. *Radiology* 1997;204:411–415.

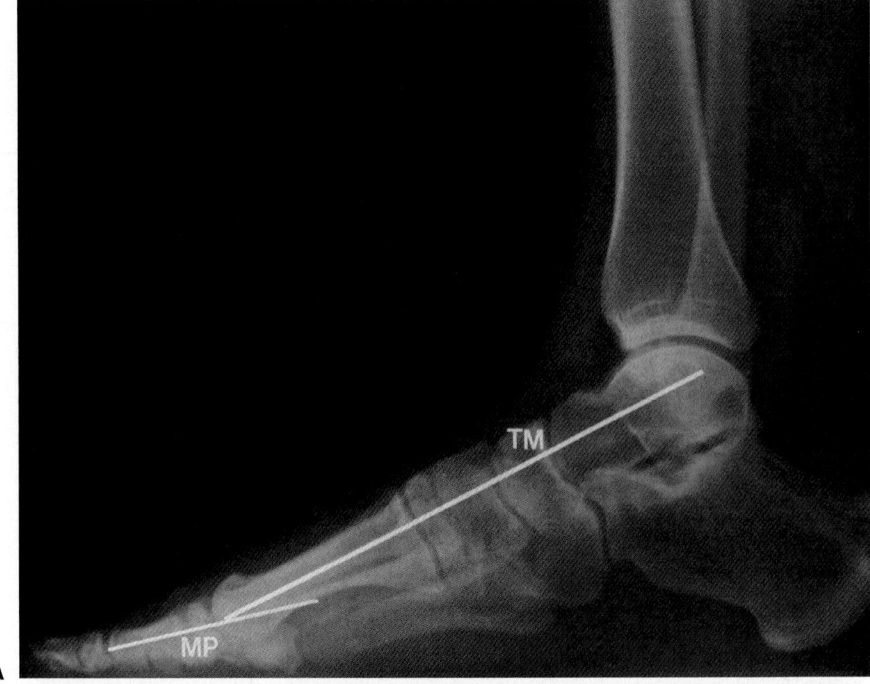


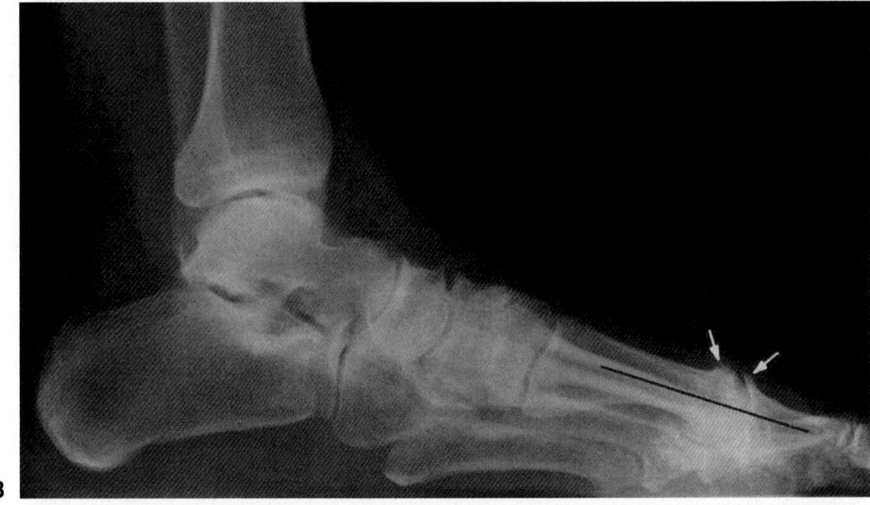


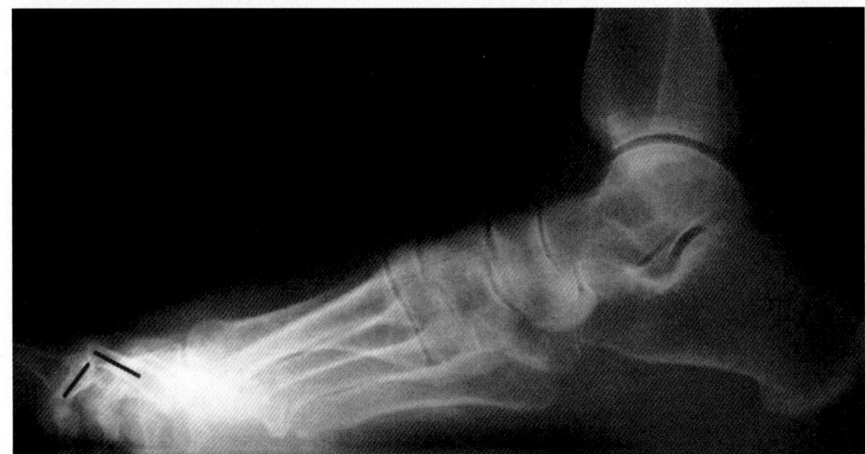


**Fig. 8-87** Lateral radiographic evaluation. **A:** The first metatarsal and talus (TM, talar-first metatarsal angle) are aligned. The first metatarsal phalangeal (MTP) relationship is defined. **B:** The alignment and prominent dorsal osteophytes (*arrows*) are clearly seen on the lateral image. **C:** There is dorsal swelling and hammer toe (*black lines*) deformities of the lesser toes.

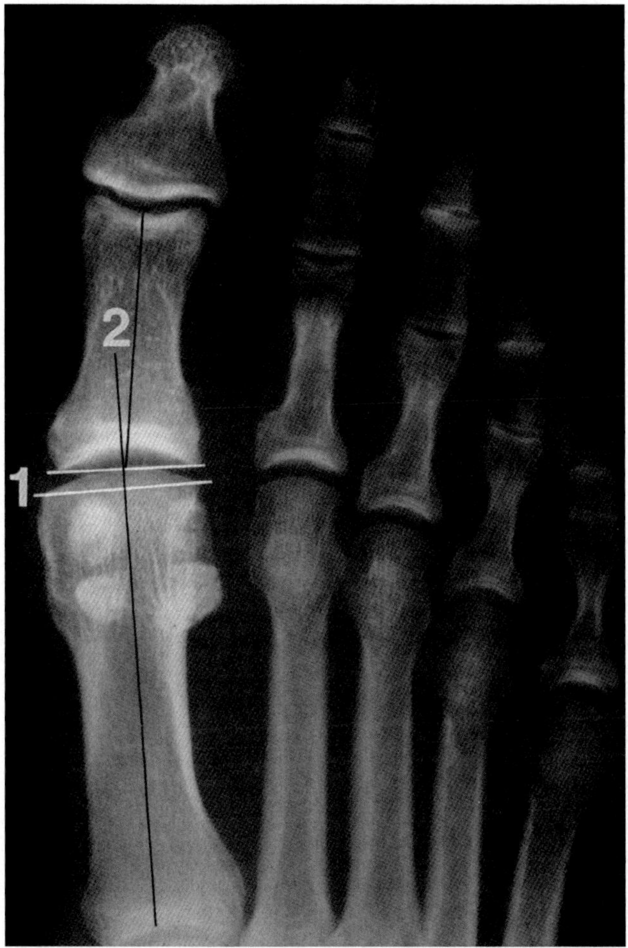


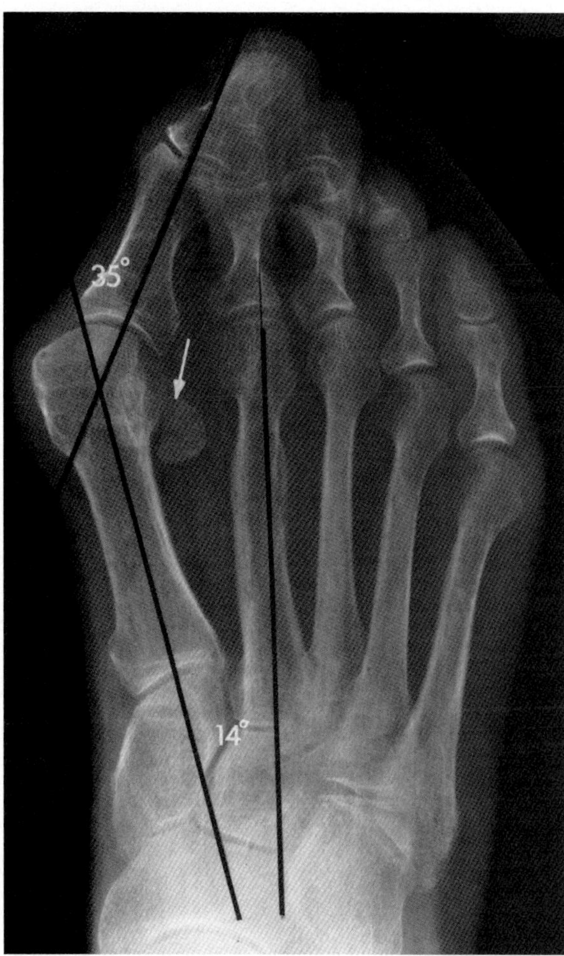


**Fig. 8-88** Standing anteroposterior (AP) evaluation. **A:** Coned image of the forefoot demonstrating early osteoarthritis of the first metatarsal phalangeal (MTP) joint (*1—white lines*) with slight incongruency. The metatarsophalangeal angle (*2—black lines*) is <10 degrees. **B:** Standing AP radiograph in a patient with hallux valgus (35 degrees), the lateral sesamoid is completely uncovered (*arrow*-dislocated) and a first-second metatarsal angle of 14 degrees (range 4 to 23 degrees).

## Treatment Options

There are multiple component types similar to arthroplasty techniques discussed in prior chapters and sections. Single- or double-stemmed silicone implants have been designed by several manufactures (see Figs. 8-89 and 8-90). Some designs include metal grommets to protect the adjacent bone (see Fig. 8-91). Metal and polyethylene as well as ceramic components are also available (see Fig. 8-92).

## Suggested Reading

Granberry WM, Noble PC, Bishop JO, et al. Use of hinged silicone prosthesis for replacement arthroplasty of the first metatarsophalangeal joint. *J Bone Joint Surg.* 1991;73A: 1453–1459.

Swanson AB, de Groot Swanson G, Mayhew DE, et al. Flexible hinge results of implant arthroplasty of the great toe. *Rheumatology* 1987;11:136–152.

## Postoperative Imaging and Complications

Baseline postoperative radiographs should be obtained using the same projections listed earlier. In some cases, fluoroscopic positioning may be indicated to optimally align the component–bone interfaces. Radiographs should be evaluated to assess component position, joint congruency, lucent zones, and osteophyte formation (see Fig. 8-93).

Lucent zones are evaluated similar to other joint replacement procedures with progression of zones >2 mm considered indications of loosening. Changes of osteolysis or silicone synovitis may also be evident on radiographs. Osteophyte formation at the cut metatarsal and phalangeal implant junctions is graded based on the extent of joint involvement. Formation of small osteophytes without joint encroachment is considered minimal; moderate osteophytes cause <50% encroachment into the joint and severe osteophytes >50% (see Fig. 8-94).

Loosening occurs over time in up to 56% of implants (Fig. 8-92). Lucency has been reported more commonly about the distal stem (35%) compared to 9% for the metatarsal stem. Lucent zones about the entire implant indicate probable

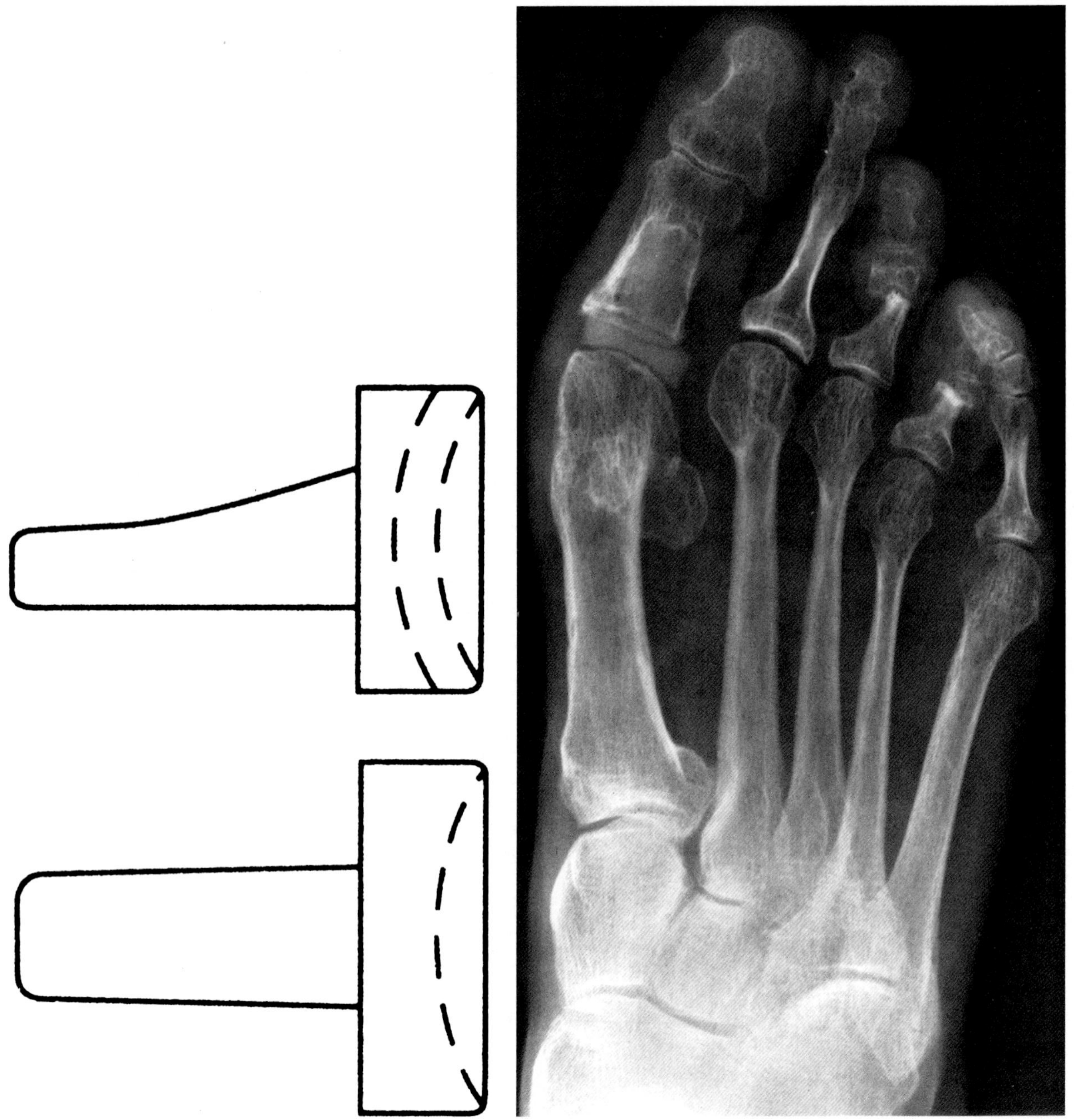


Fig. 8-89 Single-stem silicone implant. A: Illustration of single-stemmed silicone implants seen from the front and side. (Courtesy Sutter, San Diego, California.) B: Standing anteroposterior (AP) radiograph of a single-stemmed silicone implant. There are also prior resection arthroplasties of the third and fourth proximal interphalangeal joints with fusion of the second digit.

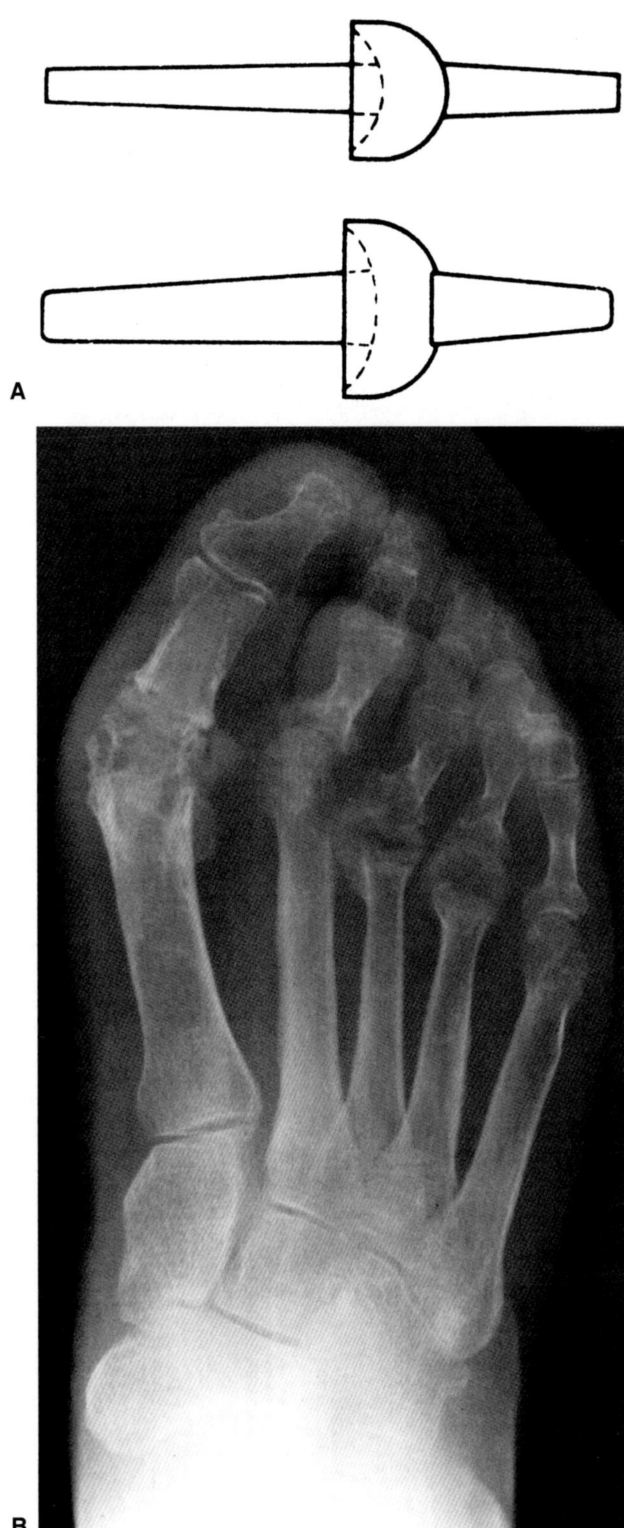

Fig. 8-90 Lesser toe double-stemmed implants. A: Illustration of lesser toe double-stemmed implants. (Courtesy of Sutter, San Diego, California.) B: Standing radiograph demonstrating lesser toe silicone implants of the third and fourth metatarsal phalangeal (MTP) joints. There is also a single-stemmed first MTP implant.

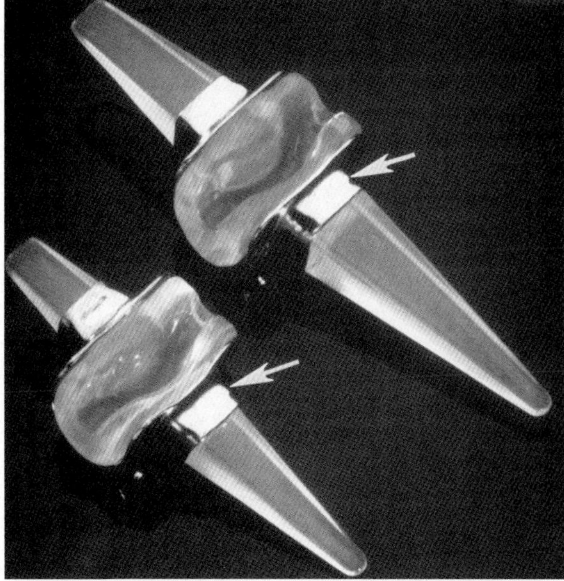

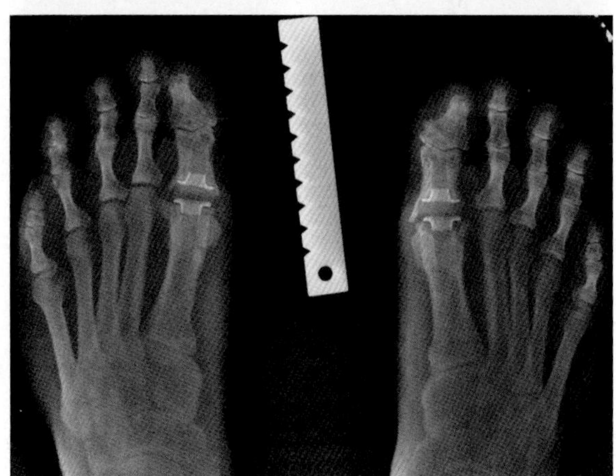

Fig. 8-91 Double-stemmed implant with grommets. A: Photograph of the Swanson double-stemmed silicone implants with metal grommets for the bone interfaces. (Courtesy of Wright Medical Technologies, Arlington, Tennesse and Dr. A.B. Swanson.) B: Radiograph of bilateral double-stemmed great toe implants with metal grommets. There is marginal osteophyte formation.

loosening (see Fig. 8-95) while component migration is the most accurate feature.

Deep infection occurs in up to 5% of cases. Serial radiographs may demonstrate osteolysis or periosteal reaction. Silicone implants can be evaluated with MRI as there are no artifacts with these implants, and minimal artifact when grommets are in place. Combination radionuclide scans described earlier are an alternative. Joint aspiration is also useful to isolate the organisms.

Implant wear, deformity, or fracture occurs in up to 25% of patients, but is not always symptomatic (see Fig. 8-96). Serial radiographs or CT are useful for evaluation of these changes as well as classification of new joint deformity and osteophyte formation (Fig. 8-94).

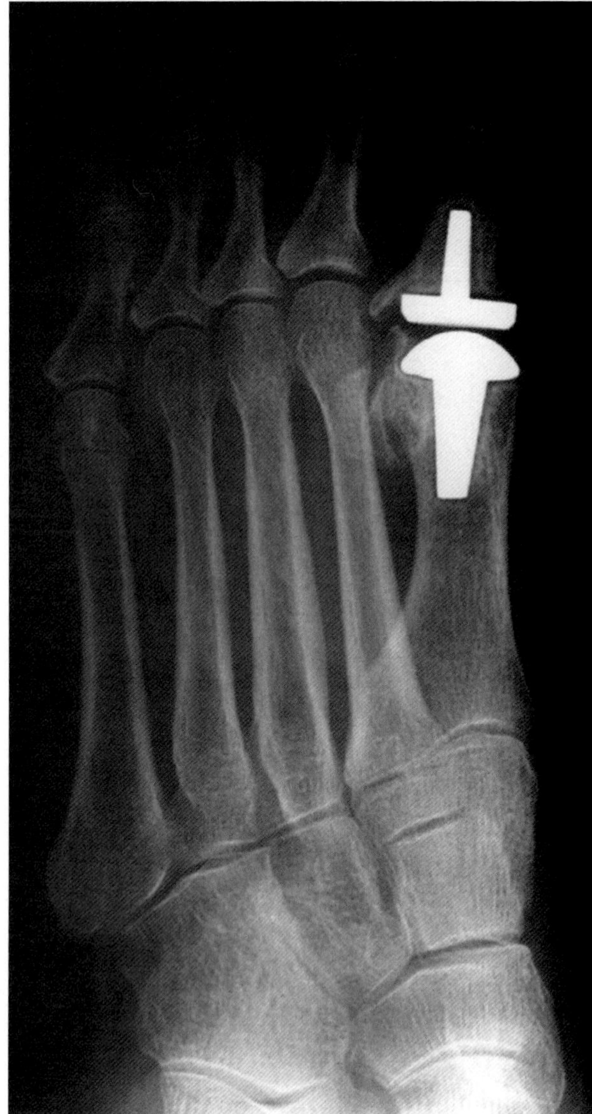

Fig. 8-92 Radiograph of a metal on metal implant with lucency about the implants due to loosening.

Stress fractures occur in 2.2% of cases and may be evident on serial radiographs. Early changes and stress reaction are more easily appreciated with MRI.

Silicone synovitis may be obvious on radiographs (see Fig. 8-97). However, MRI with postcontrast fat-suppressed T1-weighted images is preferred to evaluate the extent of the process.

Certain conditions such as painful callus formation (69%) do not require imaging. Transfer metatarsalgia results in plantar forefoot pain in the lesser toes and occurs in 11% of cases.

Overall survival of implants improves with age. Ten-year survival treatment results were 82% for patients younger than age 57 as compared to 90% for patients older than 57 years. The overall survival at 15 years is also approximately 82%. Up to 16% of patients require resurgery. Table 8-12 summarizes complications of metatarsophalangeal arthroplasty with imaging approaches. Not all complications warrant imaging.

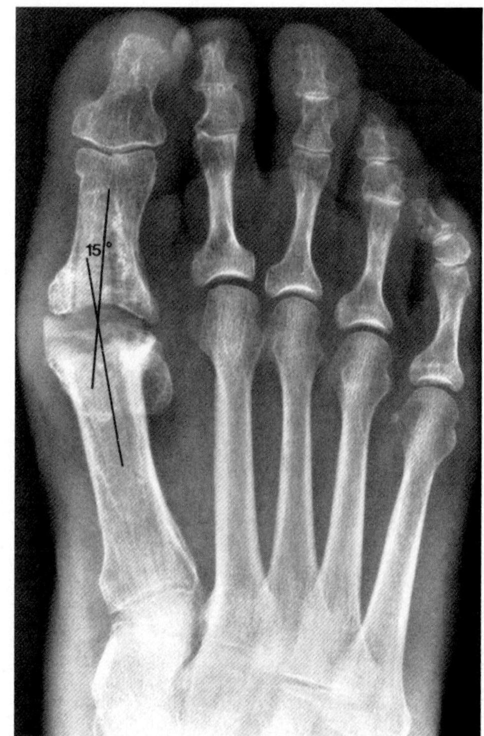


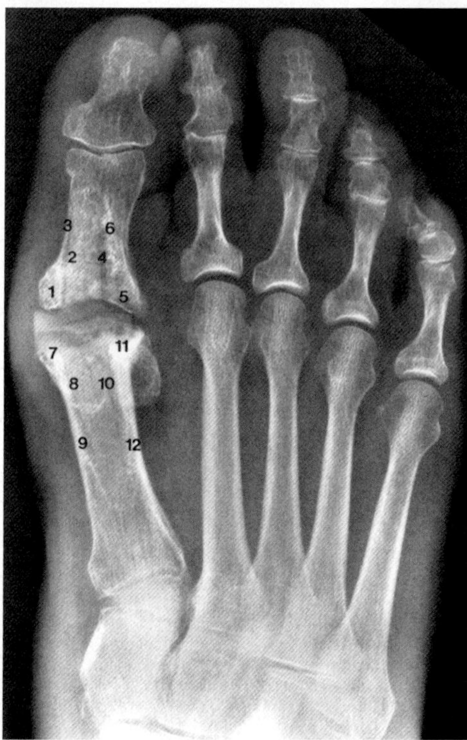


Fig. 8-93 Baseline postoperative assessment of metatarsophalangeal arthroplasty. A: Standing anteroposterior (AP) radiograph following placement of a double-stemmed silicone implant without grommets. The metatarsophalangeal angle is 15 degrees. There is slight joint incongruency. B: Same patient as A with zones marked used to describe any areas of lucency and osteophyte formation. C: Standing lateral radiograph demonstrates the metatarsophalangeal relationship (16 degrees) and a dorsal osteophyte (*open arrow*).

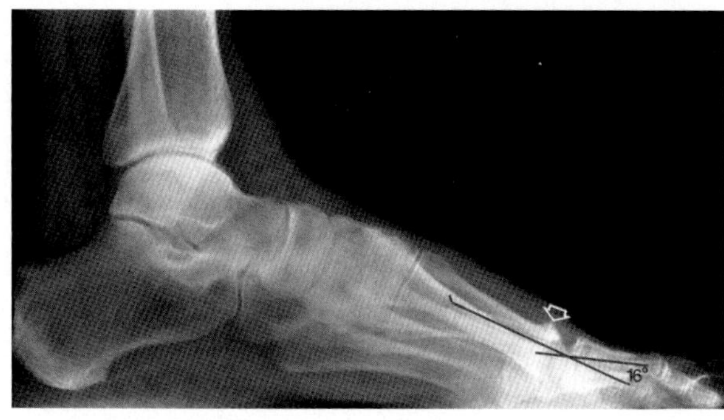


C

Fig. 8-93 *(Continued)*

## SUGGESTED READING


Cracchiolo A III, Weltmer JB Jr, Lian G, et al. Arthroplasty of the first metatarsophalangeal joint with double-stemmed silicone implant. Results in patients who have degenerative joint disease failure of previous surgeries or rheumatoid arthritis. *J Bone Joint Surg.* 1192;74A:552–563.

Granberry WM, Noble PC, Bishop JO, et al. Use of hinged silicone prosthesis for replacement arthroplasty of the first metatarsophalangeal joint. *J Bone Joint Surg.* 1991;73A: 1453–1459.

Lecomte AR, Singh SK, Fitzgerald B, et al. Small joint arthroplasty. *Semin Musculoskelet Radiol.* 2006;10:64–78.

Papagelopoulos PJ, Kitaoka HB, Ilstrup DM. Survivorship analysis of implant arthroplasty of the first metatarsophalangeal joint. *Clin Orthop.* 1994;302:164–172.


# Arthrodesis

Arthrodesis (fusion) may be performed on any articulation in the foot and ankle. The goals are to improve function and reduce or alleviate pain. Indications are similar for the ankle, hind foot, mid foot, and forefoot, although approaches and complications differ. Therefore, the procedures and imaging approaches by anatomic region will be discussed in the subsequent text.

## Ankle Arthrodesis

Indications for ankle arthrodesis in adults include osteoarthritis, rheumatoid arthritis, posttraumatic arthritis, infection, selected cases of acute injury, failed arthroplasty, and neoplasms. In children, ankle arthrodesis is most often performed for paralytic disorders, congenital anomalies, previous sepsis, or severe injury.

Preoperative decisions are based on clinical and imaging features. The same ankle-hindfoot clinical scoring system described for arthroplasty and devised by the American Orthopaedic Foot and Ankle Society (AOFAS) (Table 8-10) is used for pre- and postoperative clinical evaluation. Surgical approaches vary with patient status, patient compliance, and surgical preference. More than 30 procedures have been described for performing ankle arthrodesis including arthroscopic, internal, and external fixation techniques.

## SUGGESTED READING


Coester LM, Saltzman CL, Leupold J, et al. Long-term results following ankle arthrodesis for posttraumatic arthritis. *J Bone Joint Surg.* 2001;83A:219–228.

Cracchiolo A. Surgical arthrodesis techniques for foot and ankle pathology. *Instr Course Lect.* 1990;268:10–14.

Kitaoka HB, Patzer GL. Arthrodesis for treatment of arthrosis of the ankle and osteonecrosis of the talus. *J Bone Joint Surg.* 1998;80A:370–379.

Winson IG, Robinson DE, Allen PE. Arthroscopic ankle arthrodesis. *J Bone Joint Surg.* 2005;87B:343–347.


### Preoperative Imaging

Preoperative radiographs remain the primary screening examination for evaluating bone changes, articular deformity,

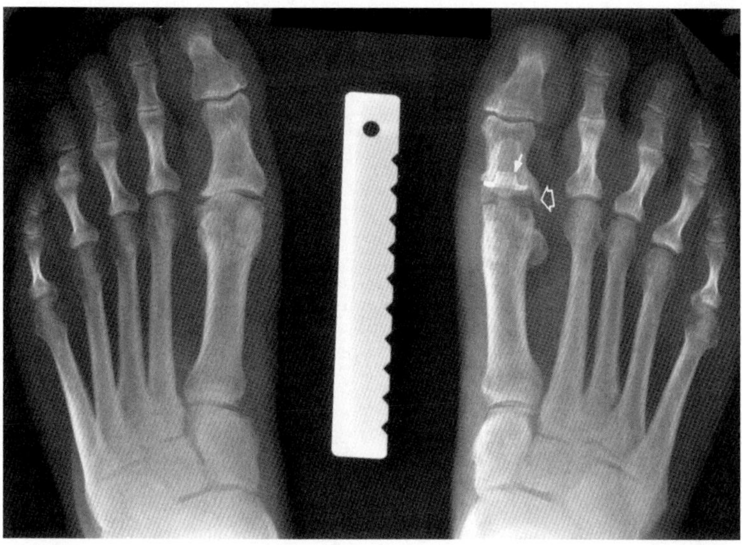

Fig. 8-94 Standing anteroposterior (AP) radiograph following placement of a double-stemmed Swanson implant on the right with a distal grommet (*small white arrow*). There is a severe osteophyte extending >50% into the joint region laterally (*open arrow*).

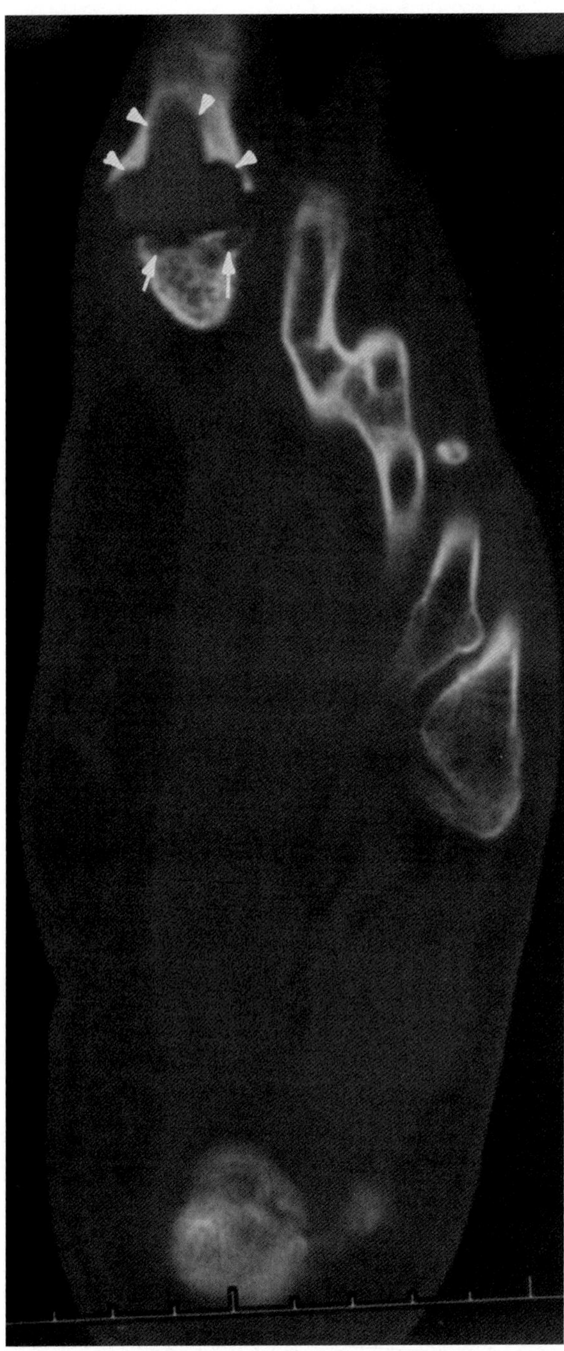

**Fig. 8-95** Coronal computed tomographic (CT) image demonstrates lucency (*arrowheads*) about the entire phalangeal portion of the component with cystic changes in the metatarsal (*small arrows*).

and alignment. Standing AP, lateral, and mortise views of the ankle are used to assess changes before surgical treatment. Osteoarthritis is categorized using all three views as grade 1 (joint space narrowing without osteophyte formation or bone sclerosis), grade 2 (joint space narrowing with moderate osteophyte formation and bone sclerosis), and grade 3 (narrowing with severe sclerosis and osteophyte formation). Change should be assessed on all three views. Several orthopaedically significant measurements should be made on the standing AP images including talocrural angle, talar tilt angle, Shenton's line, and the syndesmotic width (SW) (see Fig. 8-98). The standing lateral view can be used to assess tibiotalar position, the tibiotalar and subtalar joints, and tarsal alignment. The talar-first metatarsal angle, talocalcaneal (TC) angle, talar height, calcaneal pitch, and tibiocalcaneal angles can also be measured on the lateral view (see Fig. 8-99).

In certain cases, CT may be required to fully assess bone loss and articular deformity and MRI for assessment of AVN of the talus, articular cartilage, and soft tissue abnormalities. Diagnostic injections can be used if the sites of symptomatic articular involvement are not clear.

## SUGGESTED READING


Berquist TH. *Radiology of the foot and ankle.* Philadelphia:Lippincott Williams & Wilkins; 2000:479–526.

Cracchiolo A. Surgical arthrodesis techniques for foot and ankle pathology. *Instr Course Lect.* 1990;268:10–14.

Mazur JM, Schwartz E, Simon SR. Ankle arthrodesis: Long-term follow-up with gait analysis. *J Bone Joint Surg.* 1979; 61A:964–975.


### Treatment Options

As noted earlier, there are numerous treatment approaches to ankle arthrodesis including arthroscopic, multiple internal fixation approaches (see Fig. 8-100), and external fixation. External fixation is useful following failed arthroplasty, failed arthrodesis, and in patients with osteopenia (see Fig. 8-101). Combined ankle and subtalar fusion is not uncommon. In this setting, use of a retrograde intramedullary nail may be the preferred approach (see Fig. 8-102). This technique is most commonly performed following failed surgery or in patients with severe hindfoot deformity.

## SUGGESTED READING


Coester LM, Saltzman CL, Leupold J, et al. Long-term results following ankle arthrodesis for posttraumatic arthritis. *J Bone Joint Surg.* 2001;83A:219–228.

Felix NA, Kitaoka HB. Ankle arthrodesis in patients with rheumatoid arthritis. *Clin Orthop.* 1998;349:58–64.

Hammett R, Hepple S, Forster B, et al. Tibiotalocalcaneal (hindfoot) arthrodesis by retrograde intramedullary nailing using a curved locking nail. The results of 52 procedures. *Foot Ankle* 2005;26:810–815.

Kitaoka HB, Patzer GL. Arthrodesis for the treatment of arthrosis of the ankle and osteonecrosis of the talus. *J Bone Joint Surg.*1998;80A:370–379.

Winson IG, Robinson DE, Allen PE. Arthroscopic ankle arthrodesis. *J Bone Joint Surg.* 2005;87B:343–347.


### Postoperative Imaging and Complications

Following arthrodesis of the ankle, the patient data, imaging, and clinical scores are compared to assist in evaluating the

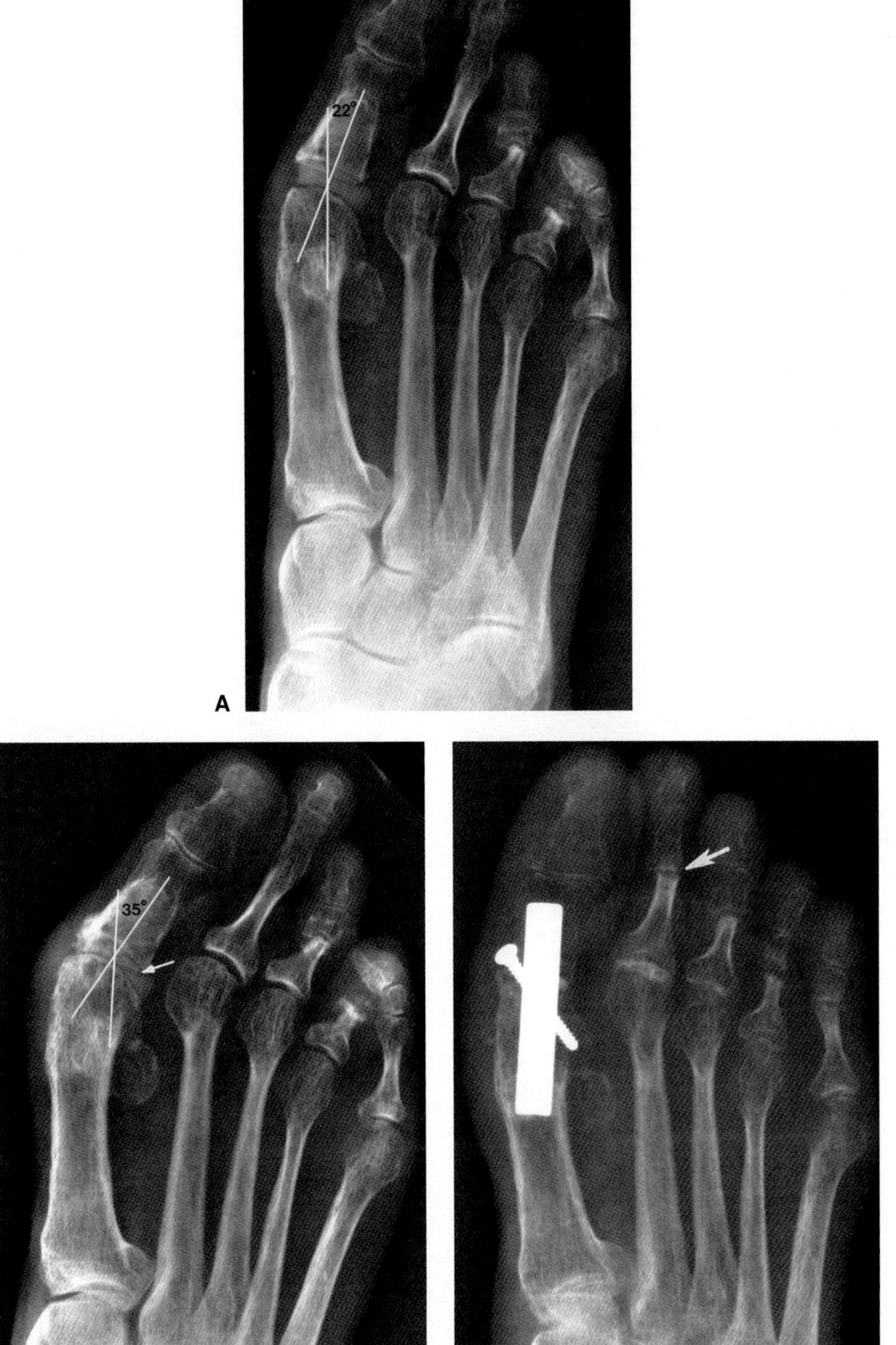


Fig. 8-96 Single-stem silicone implant with resection arthroplasty of the third and fourth interphalangeal joints and prior fusion of the second digit. A: Standing anteroposterior (AP) radiograph demonstrates the implant with metatarsophalangeal angle of 22 degrees. B: Five years later, the angle has increased to 35 degrees and the implant has fractured (*arrow*). C: The implant was removed and the joint fused with plate and screw fixation. A new resection arthroplasty (*arrow*) was also performed on the fused second digit.

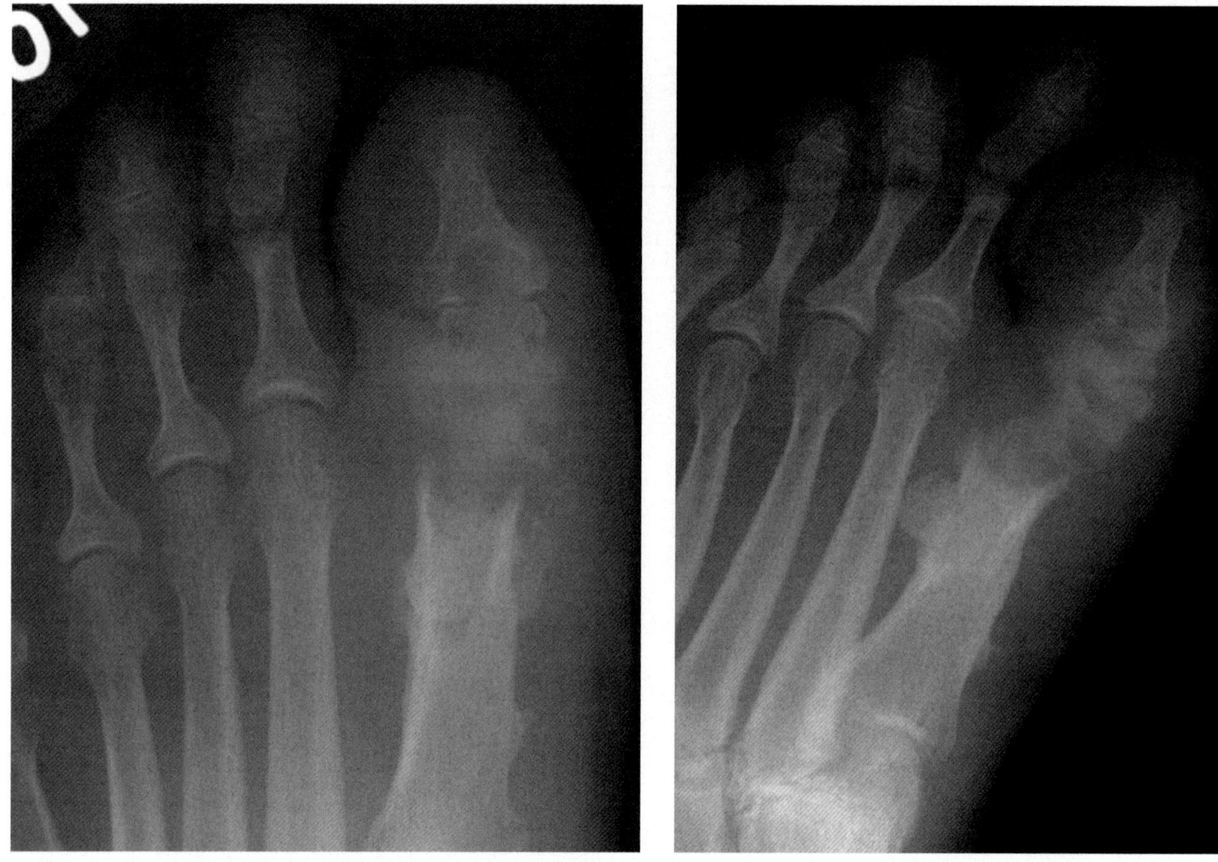

Fig. 8-97 Silicone synovitis. Anteroposterior (AP) (A) and oblique (B) radiographs demonstrate a double-stemmed silicone implant with aggressive bone destruction and soft tissue swelling due to silicone synovitis.

Table 8-12

METATARSOPHALANGEAL ARTHROPLASTY COMPLICATIONS

| COMPLICATION (INCIDENCE) | IMAGING APPROACHES |
|---|---|
| Loosening (up to 56%) | Serial radiographs, CT |
| Deep infection (5%) | Serial radiographs, MRI, radionuclide scans |
| Implant wear, fracture (25%) | Serial radiographs |
| Osteophyte intrusion | Serial radiographs, CT |
| Recurrent deformity | Serial radiographs |
| Stress fractures (2.2%) | Serial radiographs, MRI |
| Synovitis | MRI |
| Decreased motion | Stress radiographs |
| Painful plantar calluses (69%) | No imaging required |
| Transfer metatarsalgia | No imaging required |

CT, computed tomography; MRI, magnetic resonance imaging.

results. The patient's improvement in pain, activity, footwear tolerance, and ability to function without walking aids are documented. Radiographic measurements are compared to preoperative images. On the lateral radiograph, the foot should be in neutral position, although up to 5 degrees of plantar flexion is acceptable. Foot motion can be measured clinically or radiographically. Radiographs are usually obtained at 2, 6, and 12 months following surgery. Additional studies may be indicated for suspected complications.

Success rates vary with procedure and patient compliance. However, large series report pain relief and union in 80% to 100% of patients with 35% reporting excellent results, 37% good results, and 28% fair or poor results. Solid fusion usually occurs by 3 months with delay to 6 months with revision procedures.

Complications vary with the type of procedure and patient status. Patients with rheumatoid arthritis, previous surgical failures, and diabetic patients have higher complication rates. Nonunion occurs in 7% to 22% of cases. Nonunion following arthroscopic arthrodesis is reported at 7%, but increases to 22% in patients with rheumatoid arthritis. The incidence of nonunion is also higher with external fixation (21%) (see Fig. 8-103) compared to internal fixation (5% to 7%). Serial radiographs

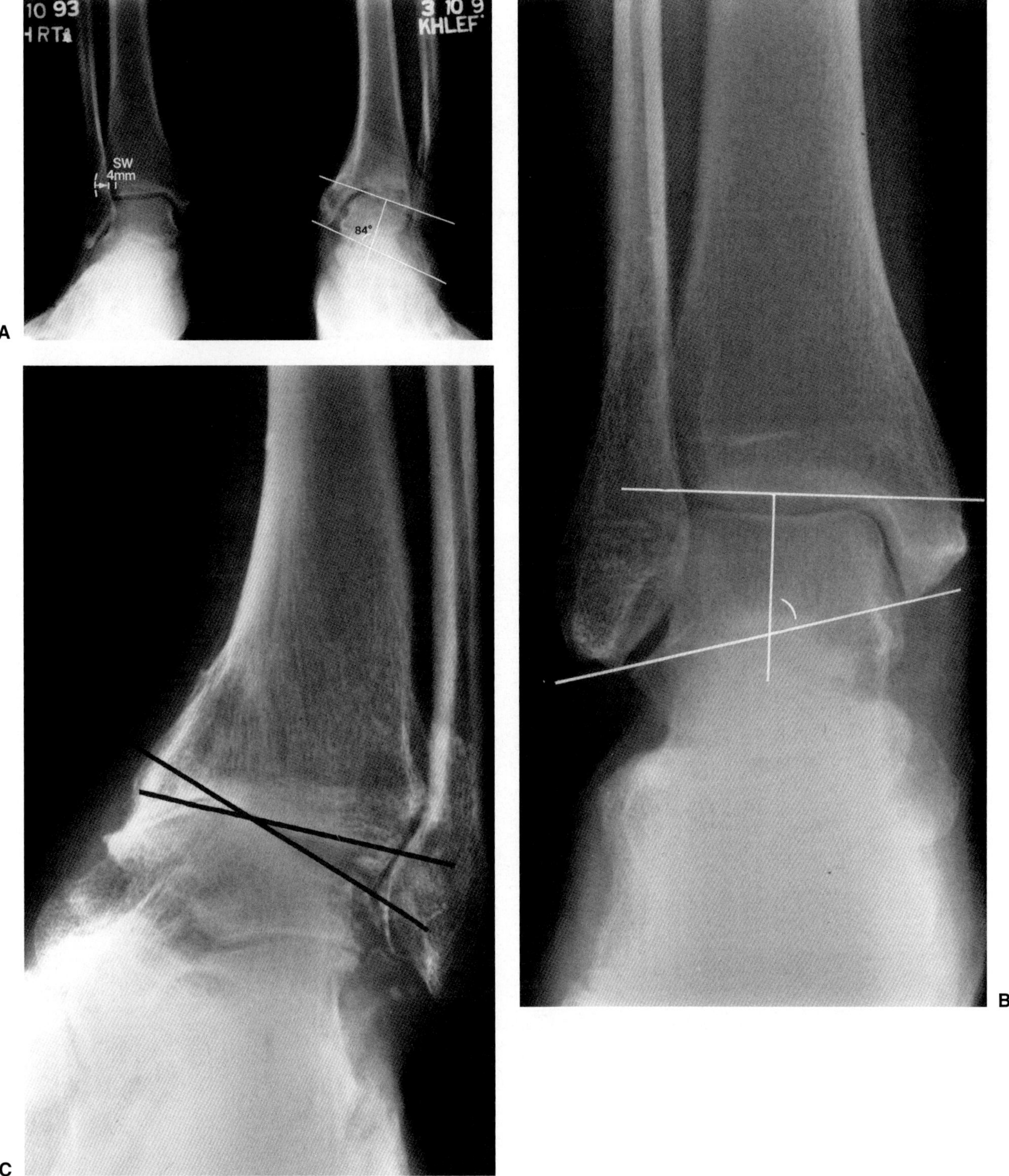


Fig. 8-98 Preoperative evaluation of the standing anteroposterior (AP) images. A: Normal right ankle and posttraumatic arthrosis on the left. The syndesmotic width (SW) is measured 1 cm proximal to the tibial articular surface (normal <5 mm). The overlap of the tibia (*broken line*) measured to the fibular margin should not exceed 1 cm. The talocrural angle is measured by a line along the tibial articular surface and a line perpendicular to this line and a line along the malleolar tips. The angle is normally 83 degrees ± 4 degrees with a difference of 2 degrees compared with the opposite ankle. B: Lines measuring the talocrural angle in a normal ankle. C: Lines along the tibial and talar surfaces demonstrating the degree of talar tilt.

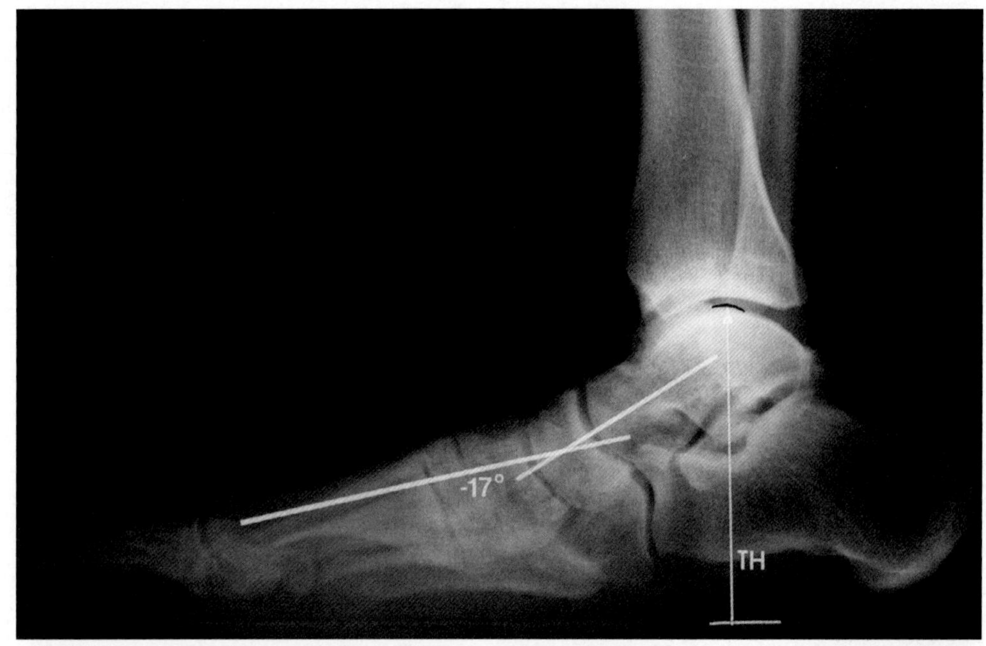


A

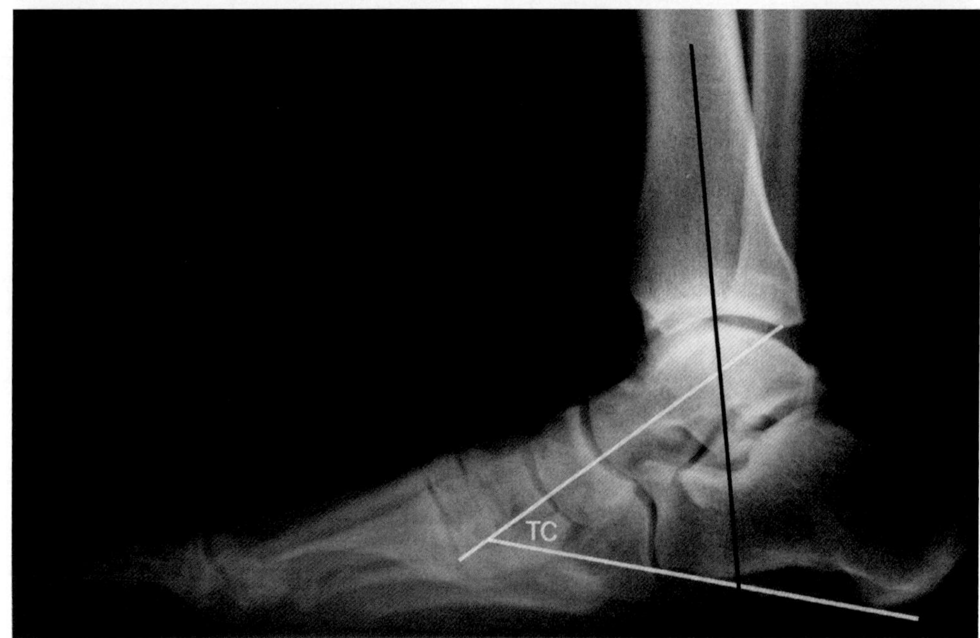


B

**Fig. 8-99** Preoperative evaluation of the standing lateral image. **A:** Standing lateral view demonstrating the measurement for talar height (TH—talar dome to the level of the foot support; normal 7.3 to 9.5 cm) and the talar-first metatarsal angle (white lines along the talar axis and first metatarsal; in this case the angle is −17 degrees). Normal is neutral or 0 degree, mild deformity is ≤15 degrees and severe is ≥15 degrees. **B:** Standing lateral view demonstrating the talocalcaneal (TC) angle which is measured by lines along the plantar calcaneus and through the talar neck. The tibiotalar and tibiocalcaneal angles can be measured by using the former lines and a line (*black line*) along the tibial axis that intersects the talar and calcaneal lines.

(see Fig. 8-104) and, in some cases, CT are useful to follow the healing process.

Infections may be superficial or deep. Superficial wound infections occur in 4% to 18% of patients. Deep infection varies with the type of procedure and patient status. Infection is reported in up to 33% of patients with rheumatoid arthritis and rates are also higher in diabetics and patients with open fractures. Nonunion and infection commonly occur together. Therefore, when nonunion is suspected (Figs. 8-103 and 8-104), additional studies (MRI or radionuclide scans) of aspiration of the pseudarthrosis should be considered. Infection can result in below-the-knee amputations in up to 5% of patients treated with ankle arthrodesis.

Serial radiographs provide the necessary information regarding implant failure, screw protrusion, stress fractures (4%), and arthrosis development in other joints. Screw removal may be necessary in up to 17% of patients. Over time, most develop osteoarthritic changes in the other joint of the ipsilateral foot. Changes may also be expected in the knee and hip on the involved side. These changes can be graded on serial radiographs.

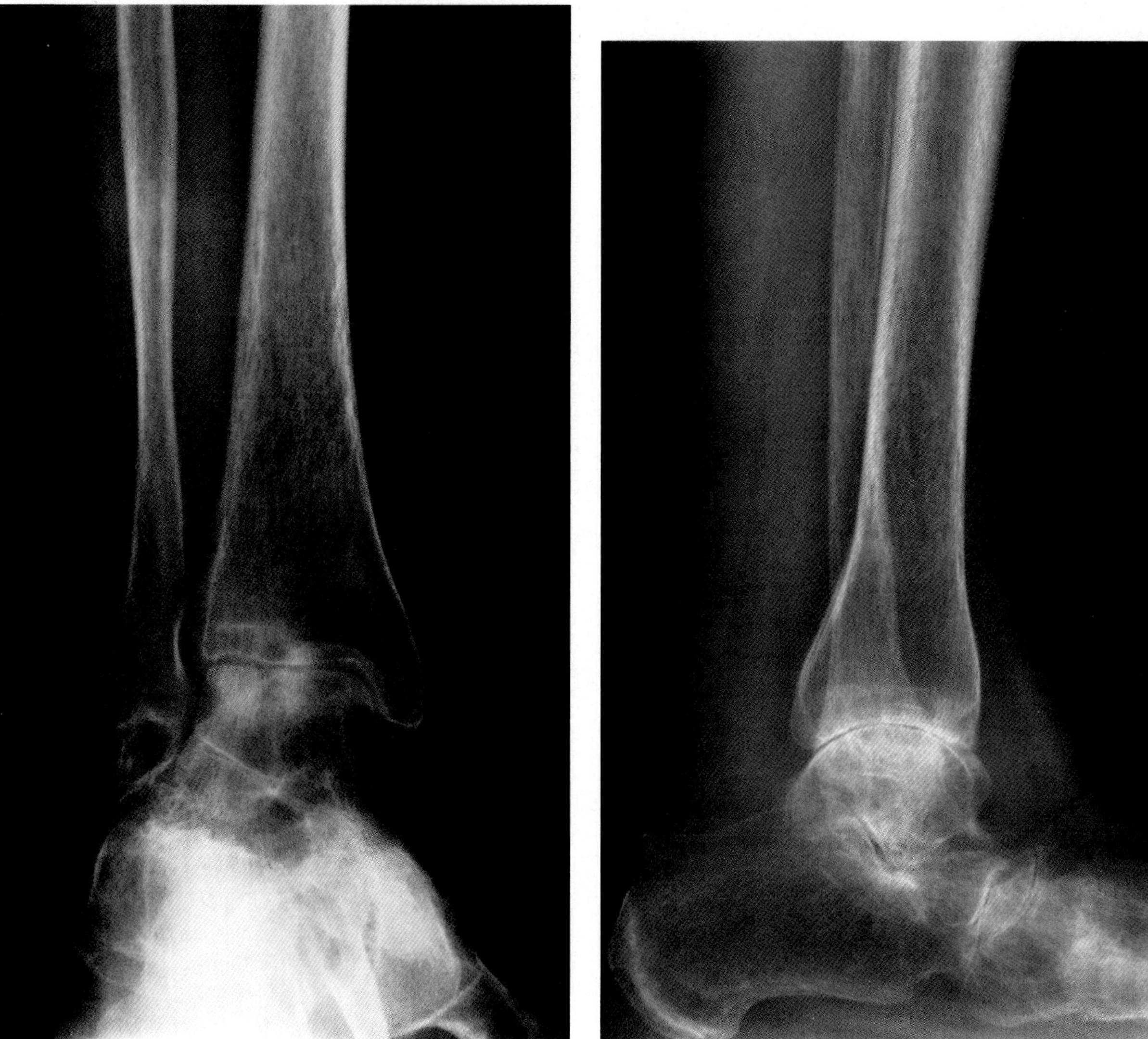


**Fig. 8-100** Ankle arthrodesis with bone graft and screw fixation. Mortise (A) and lateral (B) radiographs in a patient with posttraumatic arthrosis and sclerosis in the talus due to avascular necrosis. Anteroposterior (AP) (C) and lateral (D) radiographs following fusion using iliac bone graft and four screws with washers. The fibula was fused to the talus to enhance support.

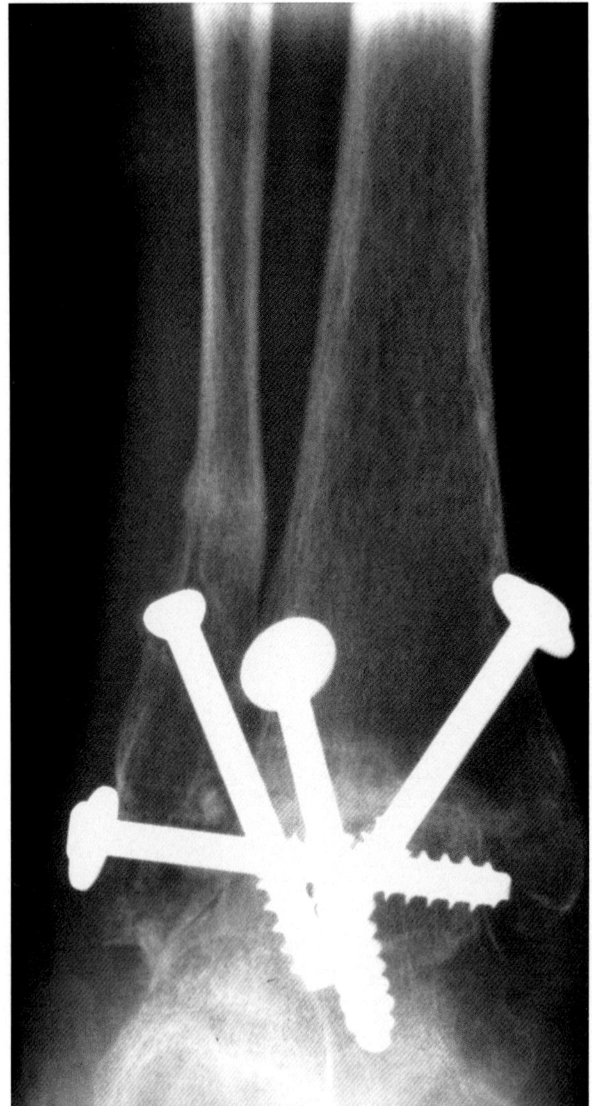

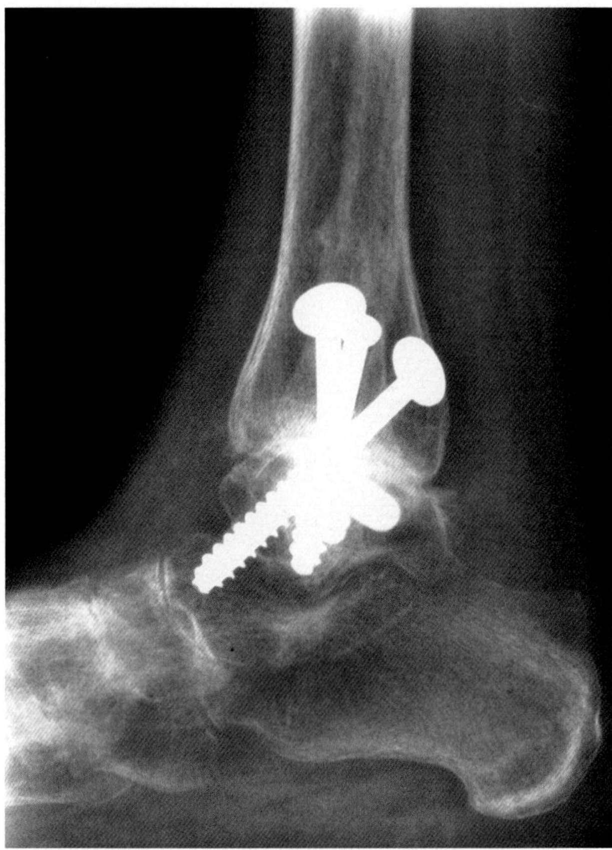

C D

Fig. 8-100 *(Continued)*

## Suggested Reading


Coester LM, Saltzman CL, Leupold J, et al. Long-term results following ankle arthrodesis for posttraumatic arthritis. *J Bone Joint Surg*. 2001;83A:219–228.

Felix NA, Kitaoka HB. Ankle arthrodesis in patients with rheumatoid arthritis. *Clin Orthop*. 1998;349:58–64.

Frey C, Halikies NM, Vu-Rose T, et al. A review of ankle arthrodesis. Predisposing factors to nonunion. *Foot Ankle Int*. 1994;15:581–584.

Haddad SL, Coetzee JC, Estok R, et al. Intermediate and long-term outcomes of total ankle arthroplasty and ankle arthrodesis. *J Bone Joint Surg*. 2007;89A:1899–1895.

Winson IG, Robinson DE, Allen PE. Arthroscopic ankle arthrodesis. *J Bone Joint Surg*. 2005;87B:343–347.


# Hind-, Mid-, and Forefoot Arthrodeses

Arthrodesis of the hind-, mid-, and forefoot are proven salvage techniques for patients with arthopathies and pain who do not respond to conservative measures. As a rule, the fewest joints possible should be fused to preserve function. Subtalar or TC arthrodesis is less technically demanding and there is less likelihood of complications compared to triple arthrodesis (TC, talonavicular, and calcaneocuboid joints fused). Triple arthrodesis was initially performed on children with polio or congenital foot deformities. Presently, selected fusion of one or more joints is common among children and adults. Arthrodesis of the first metatarsophalangeal joint is commonly performed

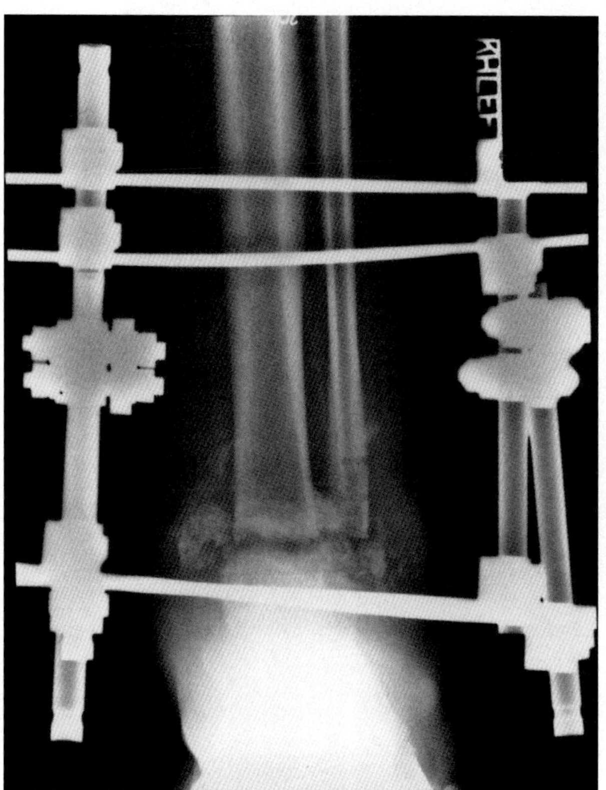


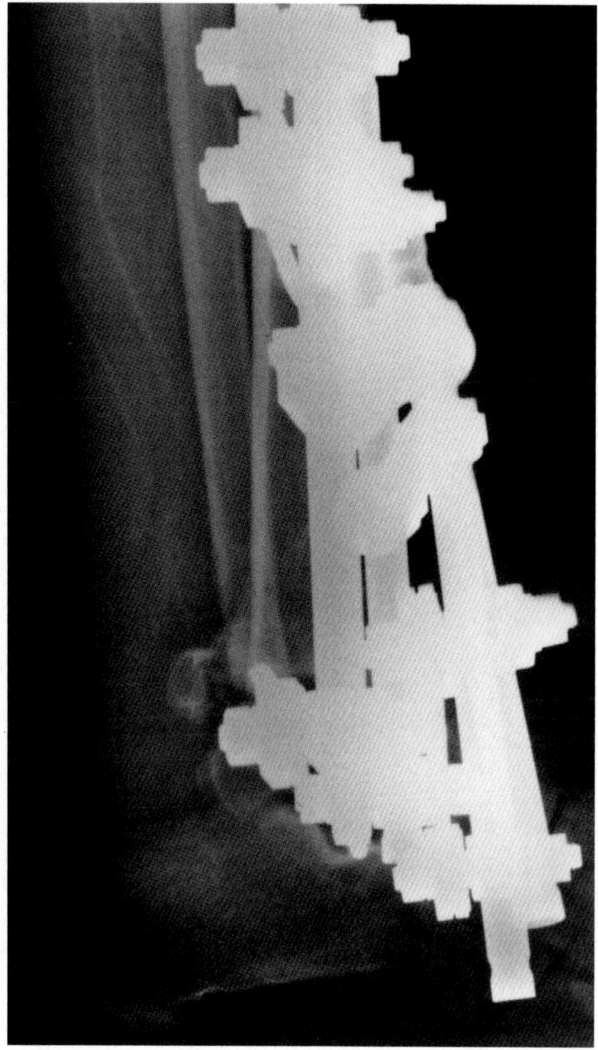


Fig. 8-101 Anteroposterior (AP) (A) and lateral (B) radiographs following failed fusion using external fixation.

for advanced arthritis. Results compete with and exceed those for arthroplasty. Indications for arthrodesis of the foot are similar to the ankle and are listed in the subsequent text:

## Indications for Arthrodesis of the Foot

Osteoarthritis
Rheumatoid arthritis
Posttraumatic arthritis
Congenital deformities
Neuropathic arthropathy
Posterior tibial tendon dysfunction

Patients are evaluated clinically using the scoring systems developed by the American Orthopaedic Foot and Ankle Society. The system for the ankle and hind foot was summarized in Table 8-10. There are similar systems for the mid- and forefoot. Pain, function, footwear requirements, alignment, and walking on different surfaces are included as before with a point total of 100 for the hind foot, mid foot, hallux metatarsophalangeal and interphalangeal joints, and the same joints in the lesser toes (2 to 5). These scoring systems are used for decision making preoperatively and for postoperative evaluation of success.

## Suggested Reading


Cracchiolo A. Surgical arthrodesis techniques for foot and ankle pathology. *Instr Course Lect.* 1990;39:49–63.

Dahm DL, Kitaoka HB. Subtalar arthrodesis with internal compression for posttraumatic arthritis. *J Bone Joint Surg.* 1998;80B:134–138.

Hammett R, Hepple S, Forster B, et al. Tibiotalocalcaneal (Hindfoot) arthrodesis by retrograde intramedullary nailing

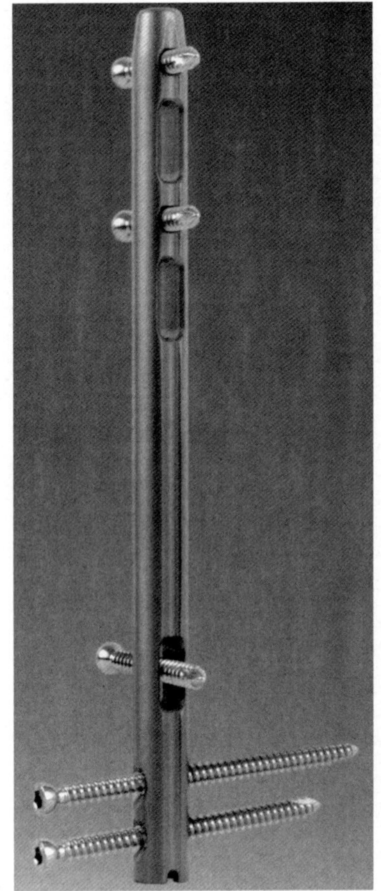

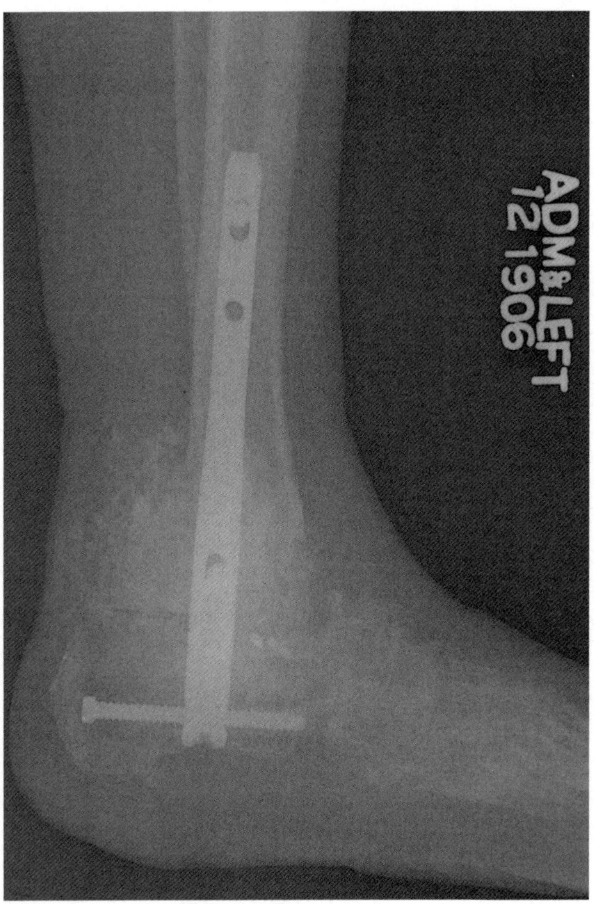


**Fig. 8-102** A: Photograph of a retrograde arthrosis nail. (Courtesy of Integra Plainsboro, New Jersey.) B: Lateral radiograph following retrograde intramedullary fusion of the ankle and subtalar joint for failed ankle arthroplasty.

using a curved locking nail. The results in 52 procedures. *Foot Ankle Int*. 2005;26:810–815.

Kitaoka HB, Alexander IJ, Adelaar RS, et al. Clinical rating systems for the ankle-hindfoot, mid-foot, hallux and lesser toes. *Foot Ankle Int*. 1994;15:349–353.

Kitaoka HB, Kura H, Luo Z-P, et al. Calcaneocuboid distraction arthrodesis for posterior tibial tendon dysfunction and flatfoot: A cadaveric study. *Clin Orthop*. 2000;381:241–247.

Kitaoka HB, Patzer GL. Arthrodesis versus resection arthroplasty for failed hallux valgus operations. *Clin Orthop*. 1998; 347:208–214.

## Preoperative Imaging

Preoperative evaluation is similar to that described for ankle arthrodesis and arthroplasty (Fig. 8-99). Standing AP, lateral, and mortise radiographs are evaluated with a number of angles and measurements used in preoperative decision making. The degree of joint space narrowing, incongruency, and osteophyte formation should be assessed. On the standing lateral radiograph, the talar height (Fig. 8-99), calcaneal inclination angle, tibiocalcaneal angle, and talar-first metatarsal angle are evaluated (see Fig. 8-105). The talar height and foot length (distance from the posterior calcaneus to the first metatarsal head) are used to calculate the height-to-length ratio. In certain cases, additional views or full-length standing radiographs from the hip to ankle are obtained when there are associated femorotibial angles and the mechanical axis in order to fuse the ankle and hind foot in the appropriate position.

CT with coronal and sagittal reformatting is frequently obtained to assess articular involvement (see Fig. 8-106). CT along with diagnostic injections can provide optimal information so that the minimum number of joints can be fused.

## Suggested Reading

Amis JA. Talus-calcaneus-cuboid (triple) arthrodesis. In: Johnson KA, ed. *The foot and ankle*. New York: Raven Press; 1994:369–400.

Berquist TH. Diagnostic and therapeutic injections as an aid to musculoskeletal diagnosis. *Semin Interv Radiol*. 1993;10: 326–343.

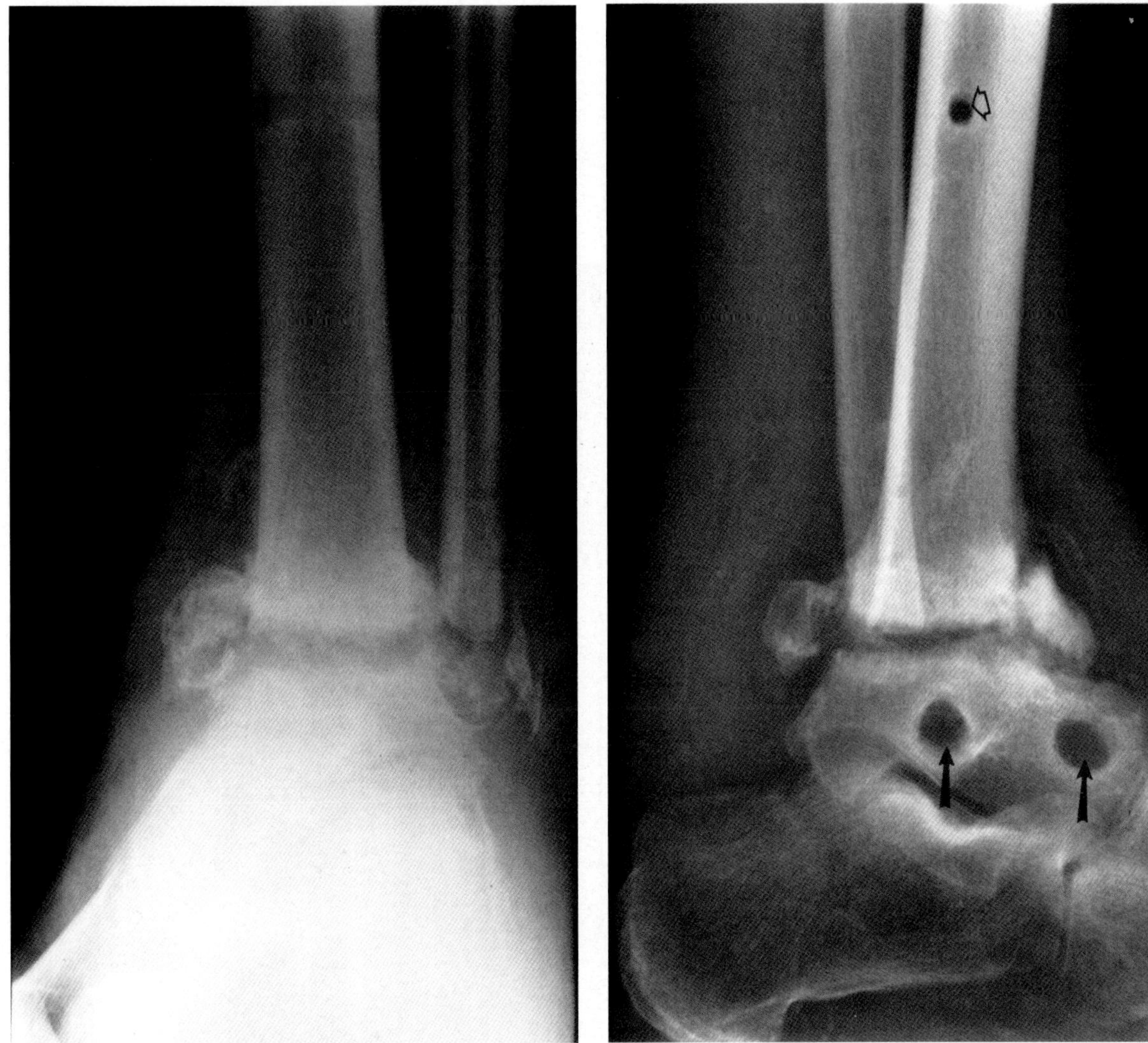

Fig. 8-103 Failed fusion using external fixation. Anteroposterior (AP) (A) and lateral (B) radiographs demonstrate failed ankle fusion with anterior tibial fragmentation. Note the size of the talar pin tracts (*arrows*) compared to the tibial tract (*open arrow*) due to motion around the talar pins. The fixation device has been removed.

## Treatment Options

Surgical approaches for hind-, mid-, and forefoot arthrodesis vary with the extent of articular involvement. Certain surgeons prefer percutaneous pinning. However, in most cases the articular surfaces are curetted to remove articular cartilage and the joints fused with or without bone graft using screws, plates, plate and screw techniques, or staples. Patients are kept non–weight bearing for 6 to 8 weeks and followed up with radiographs (see Figs. 8-107 to 8-111).

# Suggested Reading

Dahm DL, Kitaoka HB. Subtalar arthrodesis with internal compression for posttraumatic arthritis. *J Bone Joint Surg.* 1998;80B:134–138.

Kitaoka HB, Patzer GL. Subtalar arthrodesis for posterior tibial tendon dysfunction and pes planus. *Clin Orthop.* 1997; 345:187–194.

Raikin SM, Ahmad J, Pour AE, et al. Comparison of arthrodesis and metallic hemiarthroplasty of the hallux metatarsophalangeal joint. *J Bone Joint Surg.* 2007;89A:1979–1985.

Sangeorzan BJ, Smith D, Vieth R, et al. Triple arthrodesis using internal in treatment of adult foot disorders. *Clin Orthop.* 1993;294:299–307.

## Postoperative Imaging and Complications

Postoperatively, clinical scores and radiographic data are used to monitor the patients. Clinical improvement is based on pain relief, function, and flexibility with foot wear. Radiographic measurements are reevaluated and compared with preoperative image features.

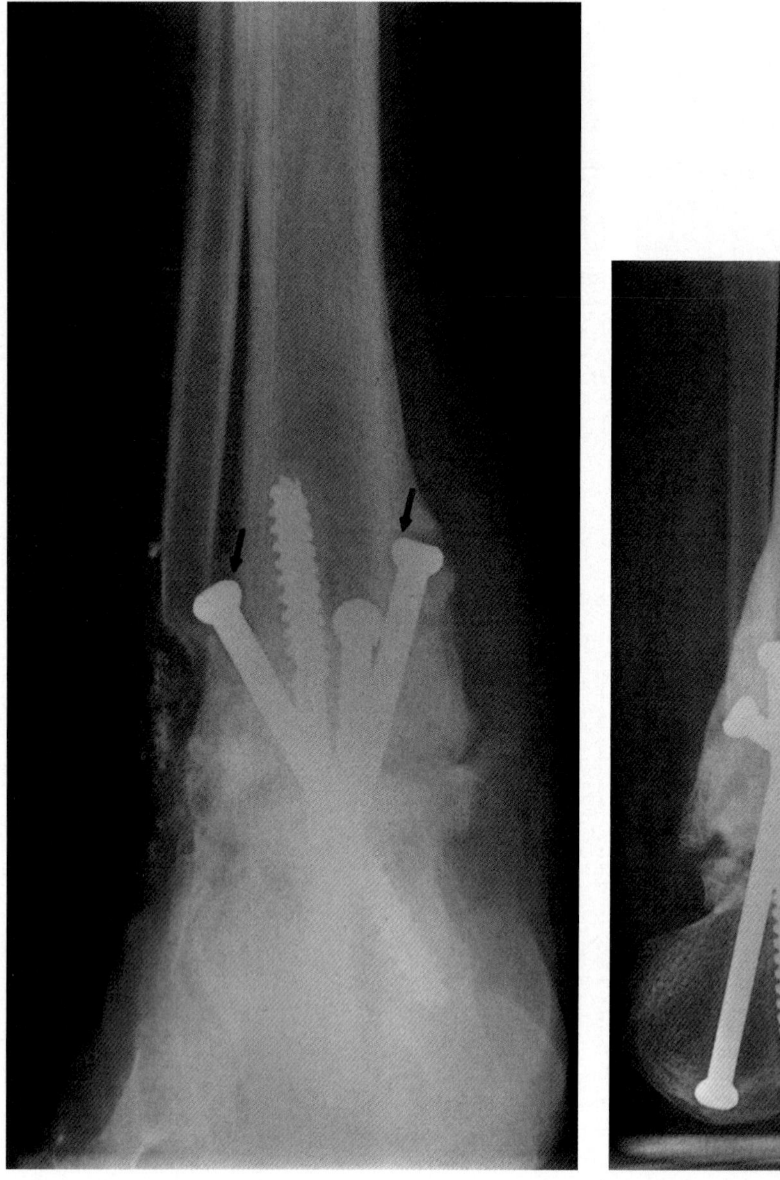


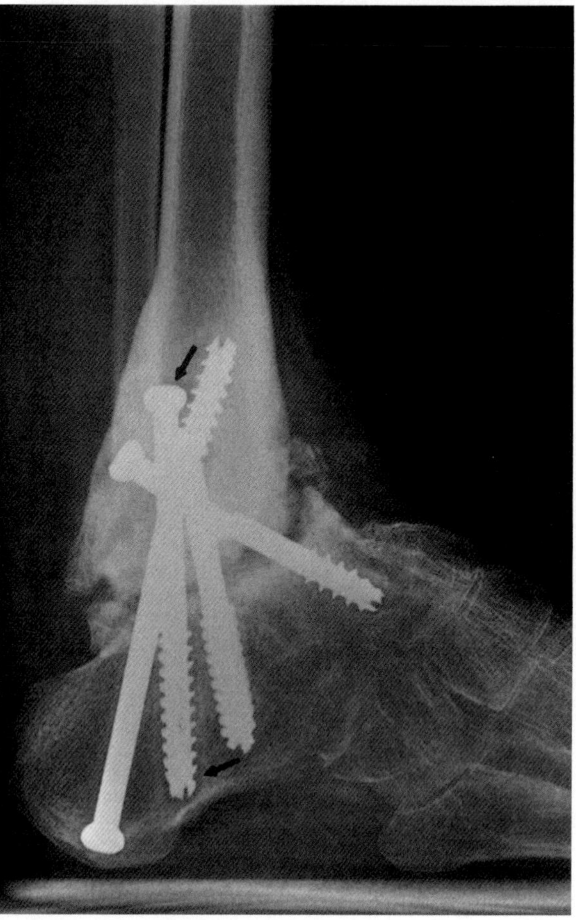


Fig. 8-104 Loosening of the screws with nonunion. Anteroposterior (AP) (A) and lateral (B) radiographs demonstrate sclerosis along the tibiotalar fusion site with lucency (*arrows*) about the screws due to motion and nonunion.

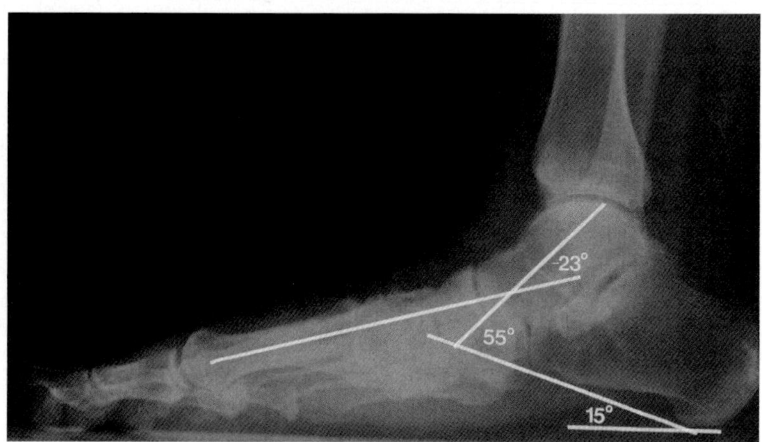


Fig. 8-105 Standing lateral images of the foot with preoperative measurements in a patient with posterior tibial tendon dysfunction. The talar-first metatarsal angle should be neutral or 0 degree. This angle is formed by lines along the metatarsal shaft and talus and in this case is −23 degrees. The talocalcaneal angle formed by lines through the axis of the talus and along the plantar surface of the calcaneus is 55 degrees (normal 25 to 50 degrees). Calcaneal inclination formed by a horizontal line on the standing device and a line along the plantar surface of the calcaneus is 15 degrees (normal 20 to 25 degrees).

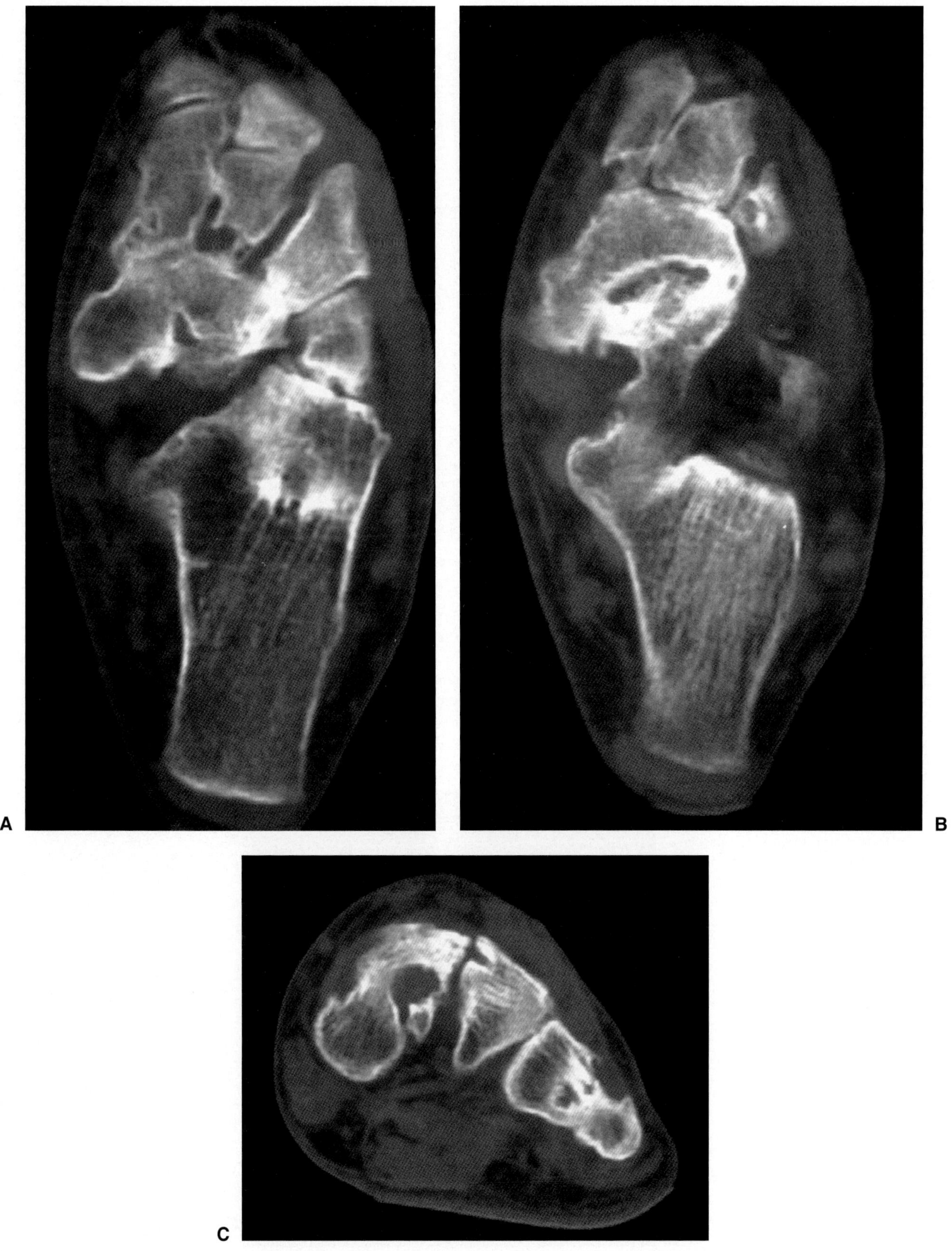


Fig. 8-106 Axial (A and B) and coronal (C) computed tomographic (CT) images demonstrating defuse talonavicular and intertarsal bone degeneration with cystic changes.

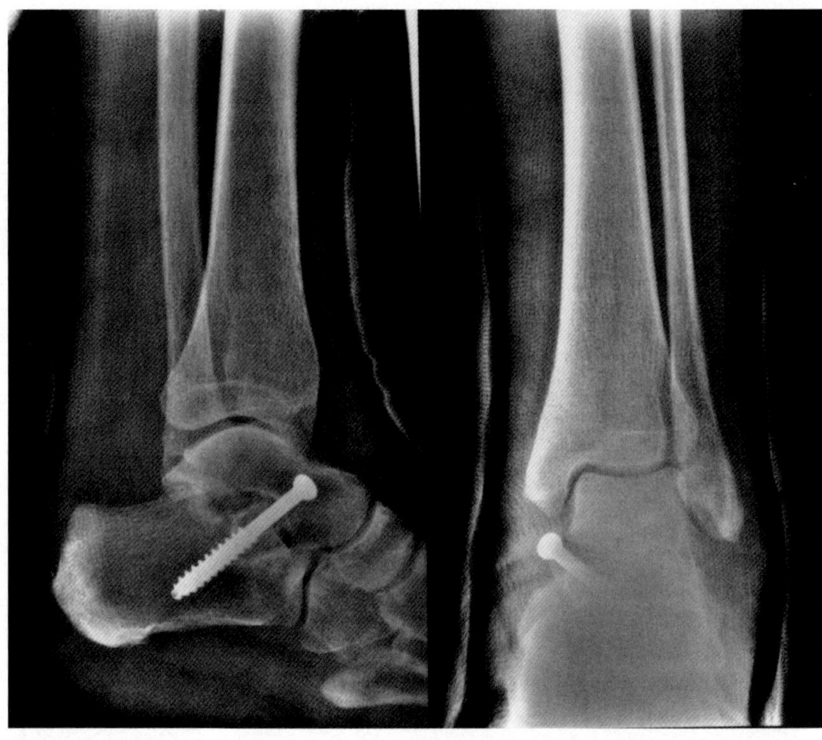

**Fig. 8-107** Subtalar arthrodesis with screw fixation. Lateral and anteroposterior (AP) radiographs following fusion with cast immobilization.

Complications following hind-, mid-, and forefoot arthrodesis vary by location and the number of articulations fused. With hindfoot arthrodesis wound infections are reported in 11%, nonunion in 4% to 17% and talofibular impingement in 5%. In patients treated with triple arthrodesis, the incidence of nonunion is highest in the talonavicular joint (37%). Progressive arthropathy in adjacent nonfused joints is not uncommon. Other complications include nerve injury, deep infection, reflex sympathetic dystrophy (complex region pain syndrome), AVN (usually the talus), and joint stiffness with gait abnormalities.

Imaging of impingement, adjacent articulation arthropathy, and reflex sympathetic dystrophy can be accomplished with serial radiographs. CT is preferred to evaluate potential nonunion, although MRI may also be useful (see Fig. 8-112). AVN and nerve injury may be most easily evaluated with MRI.

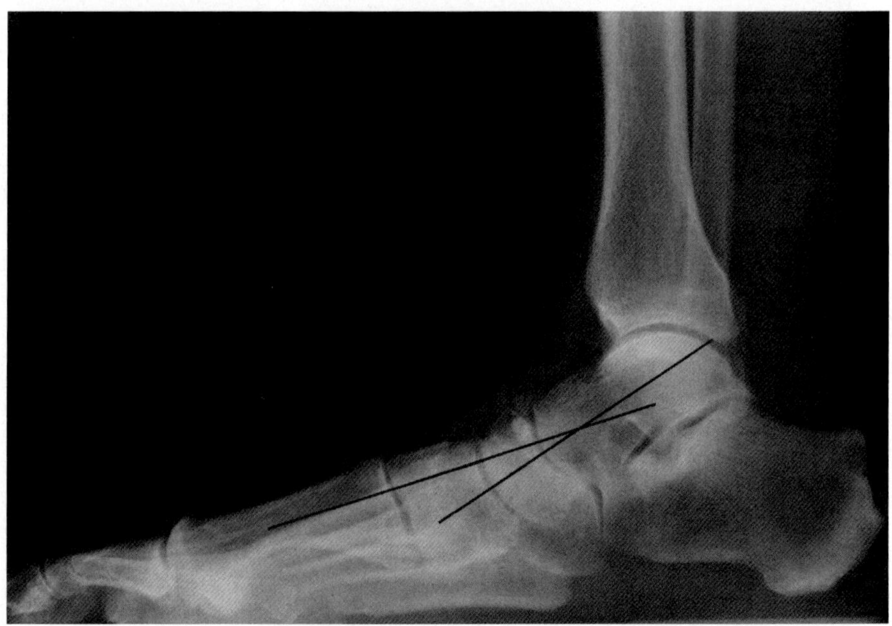


**Fig. 8-108** Isolated talonavicular fusion. **A:** Preoperative lateral view demonstrating a negative talar-first metatarsal angle. **B:** Postoperative non–weight-bearing image demonstrates improved alignment with two fixation screws and bone graft extending dorsally.

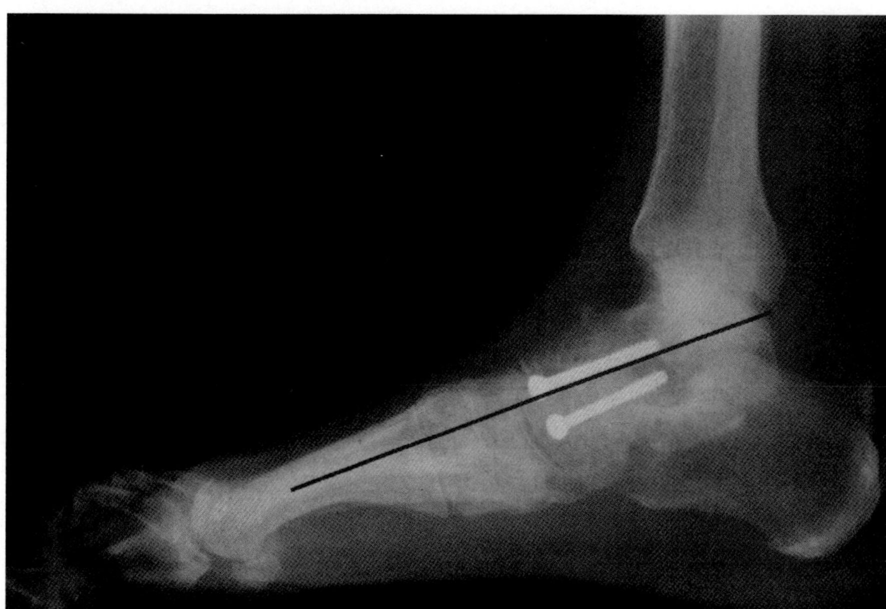

B

Fig. 8-108 (*Continued*)

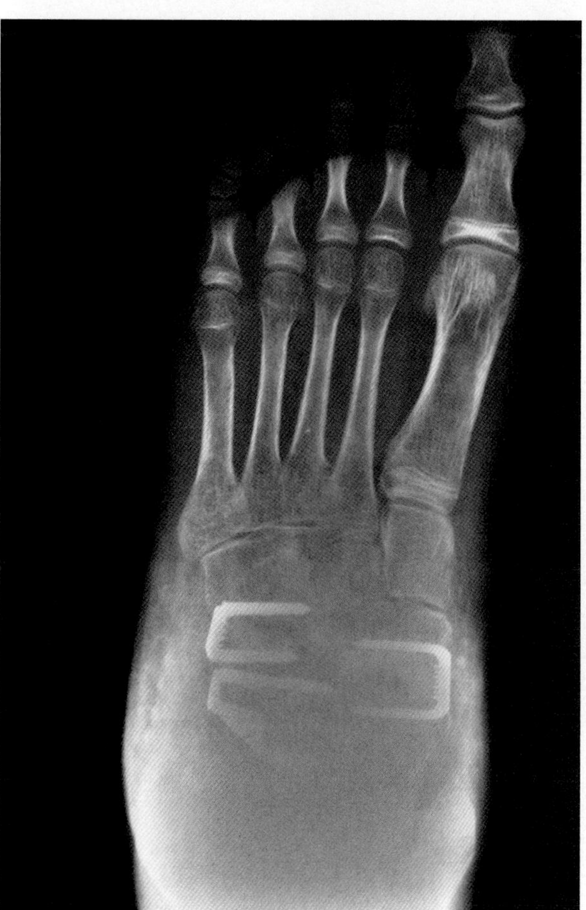

A

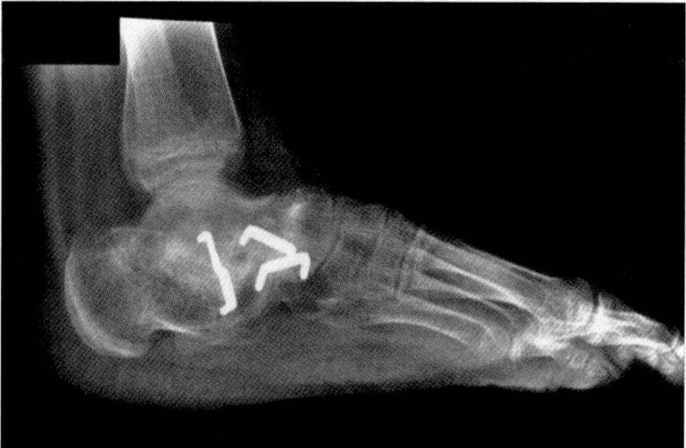

B

Fig. 8-109 Standing anteroposterior (AP) (A) and lateral (B) radiographs following triple arthrodesis (talocalcaneal, talonavicular, and calcaneocuboid articulations) with staple fixation for congenital hindfoot deformity.

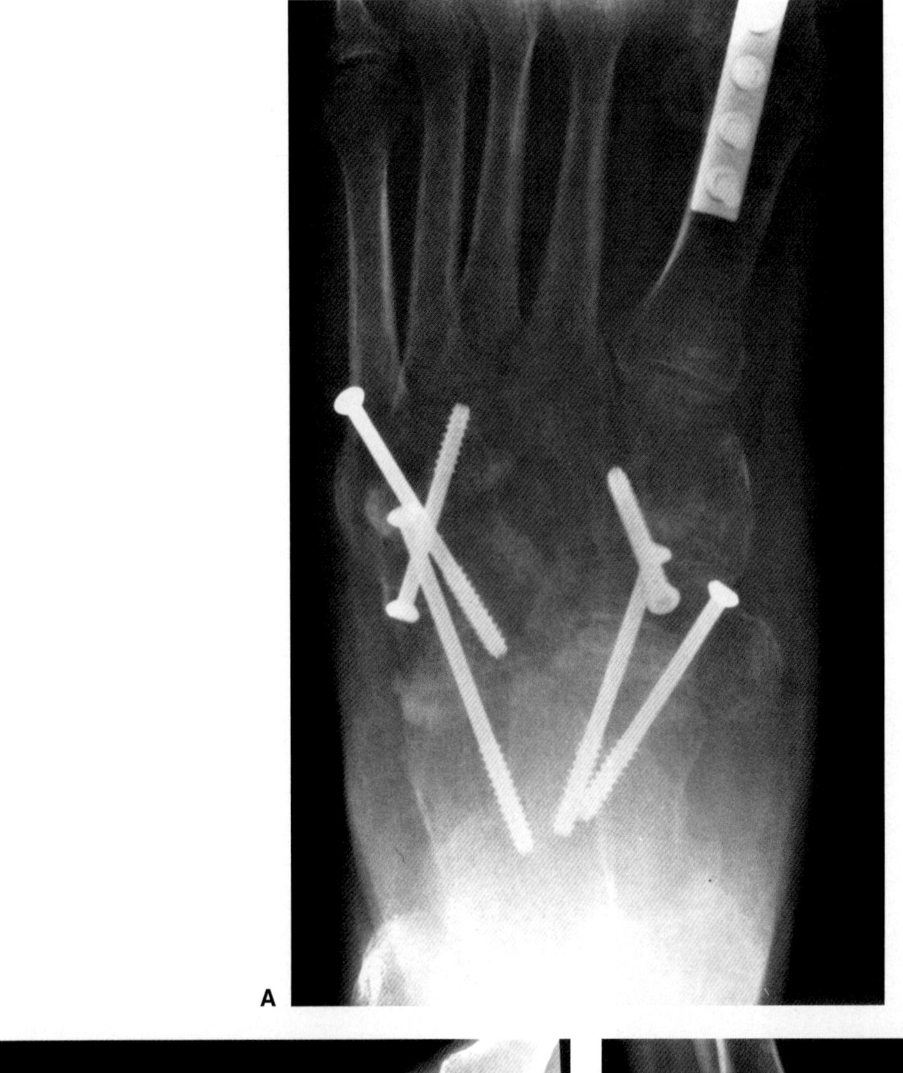

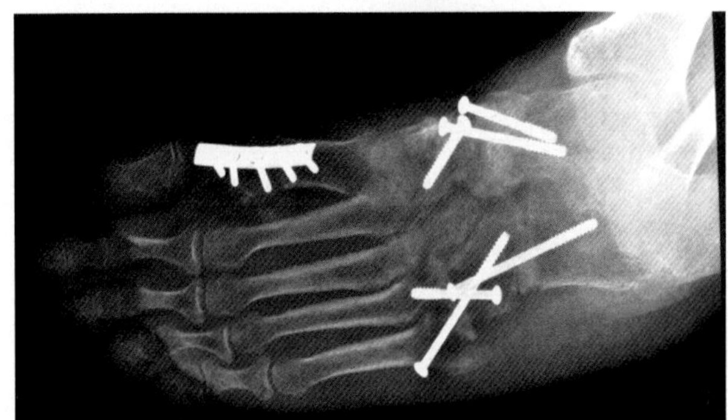

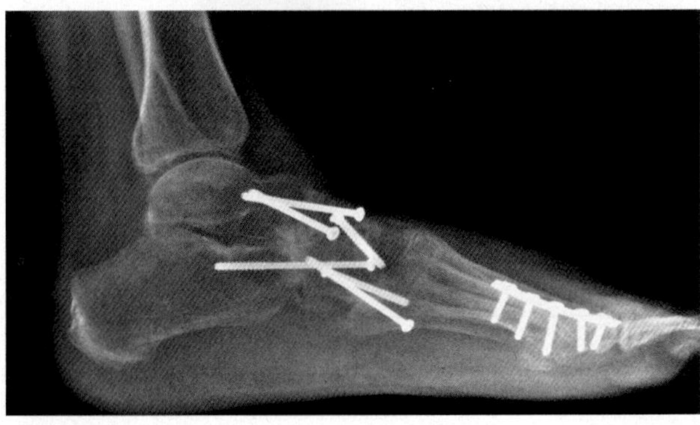

Fig. 8-110 Arthrodeses of the first tarsometatarsal joint with plate and screw fixation and screw and bone graft fusion of the calcaneocuboid and cuboid fourth and fifth metatarsal bases. There are also fusions of the talonavicular and navicular and cuneiform articulations seen on anteroposterior (AP) (A), oblique (B), and lateral (C) radiographs.

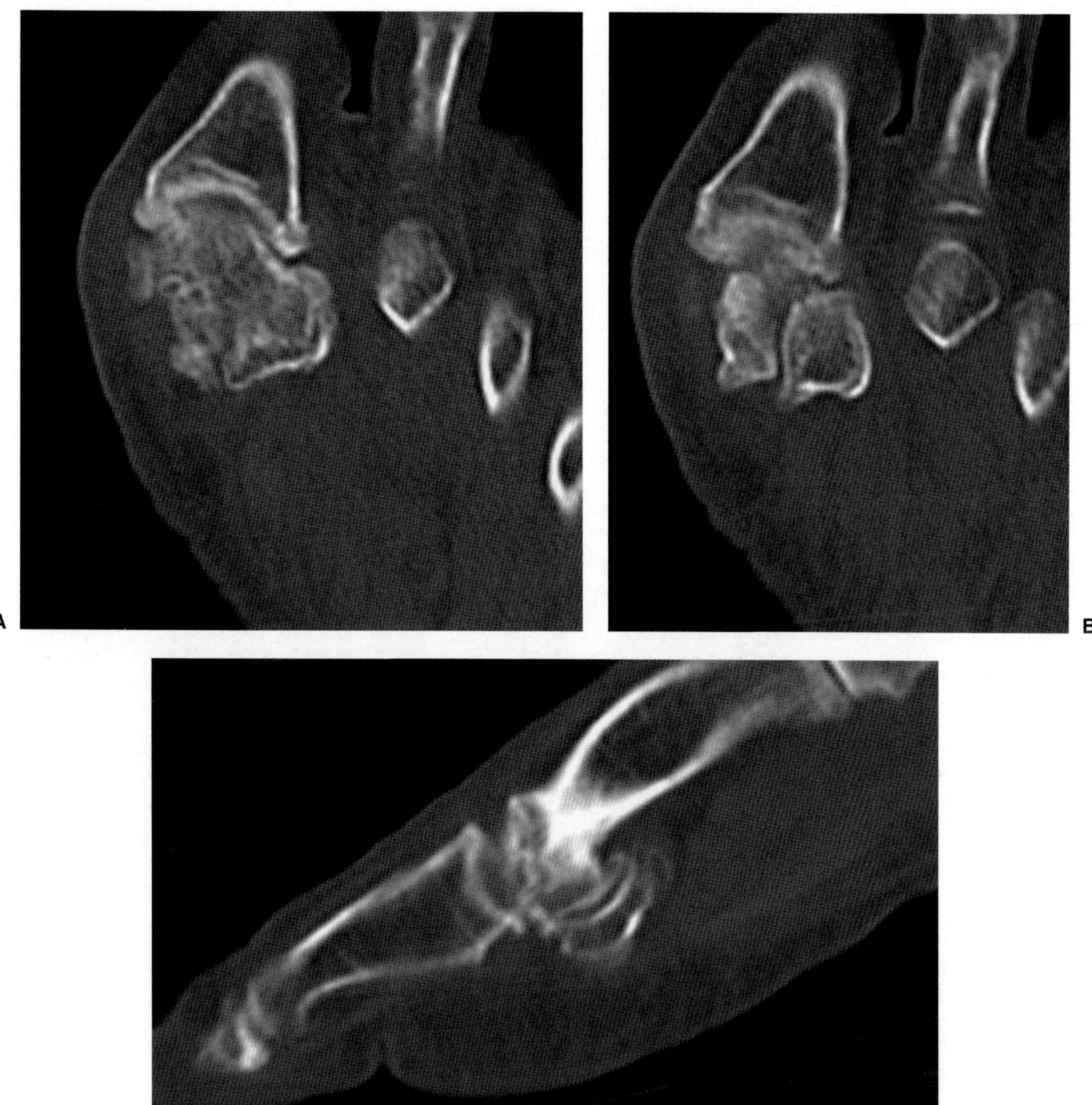


Fig. 8-111 Arthordesis first metatarsophalangeal joint. Coronal (A and B) and sagittal (C) computed tomographic (CT) images demonstrating advanced osteochondral joint deformity and rotation of the sesamoids. D: Illustration of Acumed locking mid- and forefoot plates. The locking screws do not protrude above the plate reducing soft tissue irritation. (Courtesy of Acumed, Hillsboro, Oregon.) Anteroposterior (AP) (E) and lateral (F) radiographs following arthrodesis with contoured plate and screw fixation.

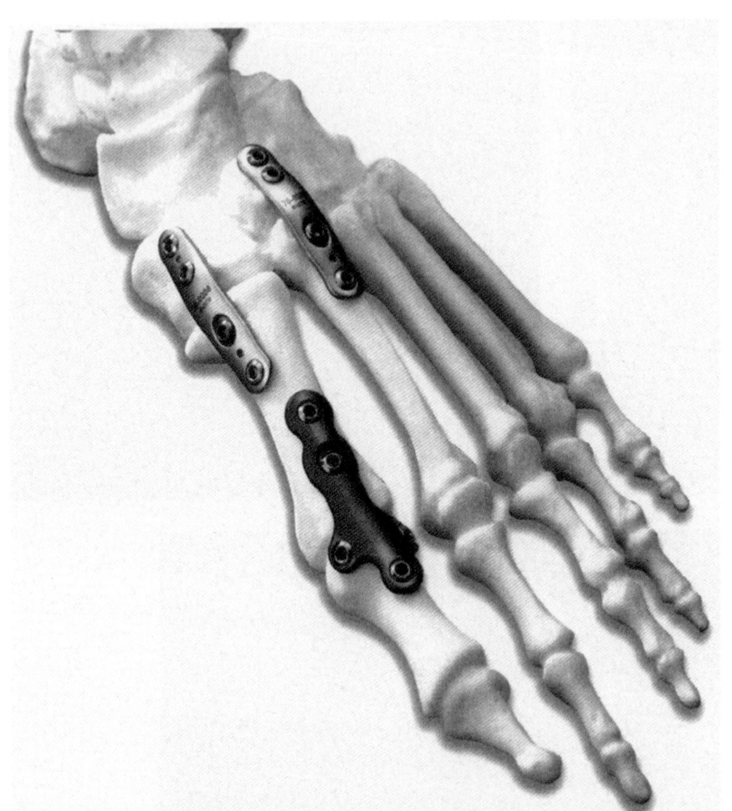
D

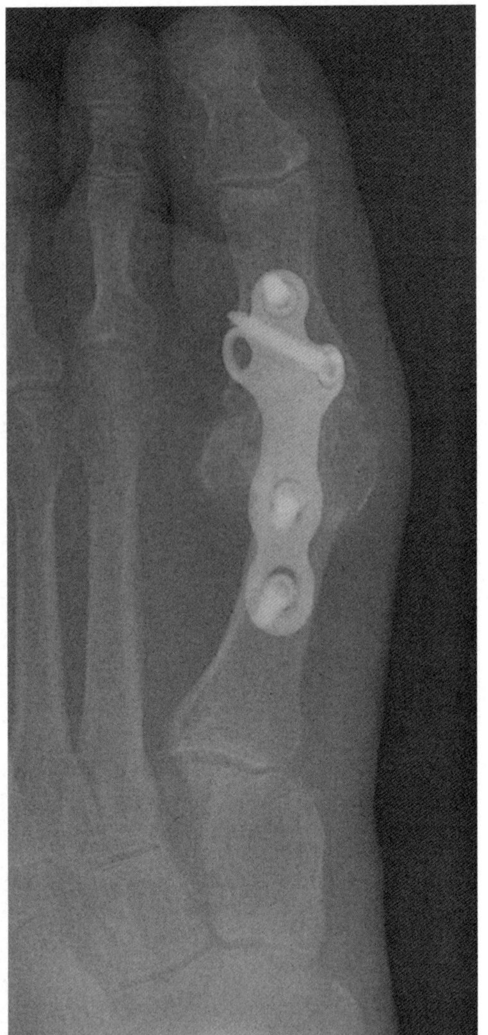
E

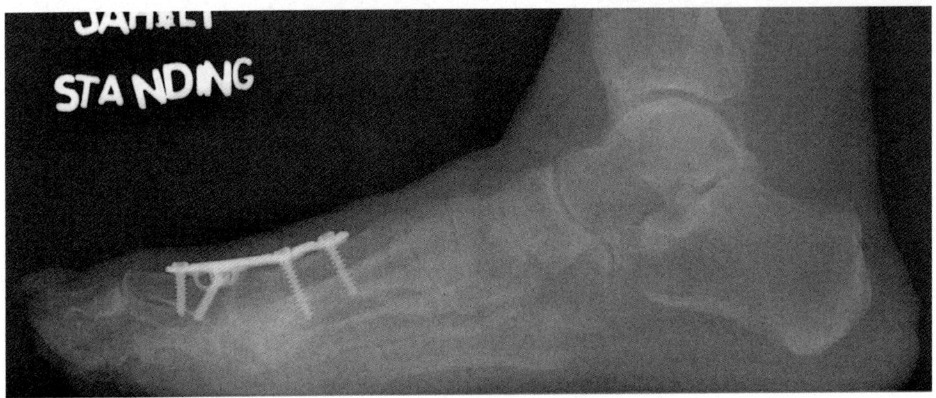

F

Fig. 8-111 *(Continued)*

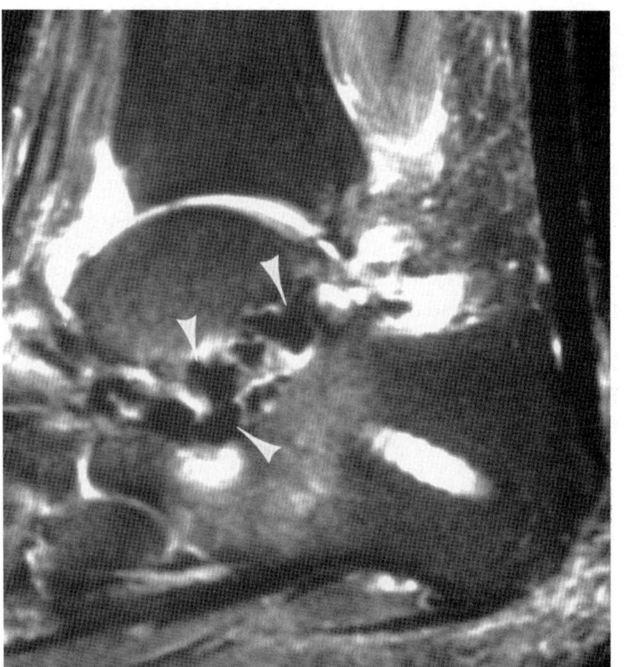

Fig. 8-112 Nonunion. Sagittal T2-weighted magnetic resonance (MR) image demonstrates a subtalar fusion with single screw fixation and bone graft. There is high signal intensity about the bone graft indicating nonfused graft material (*arrowheads*).

Radionuclide scans are useful for deep infection and reflex sympathetic dystrophy.

## Suggested Reading

Dahm DL, Kitaoka HB. Subtalar arthrodesis with internal compression for posttraumatic arthritis. *J Bone Joint Surg.* 1998;80B:134–138.

Graves SCC, Mann RA, Graves KO. Triple arthrodesis in older adults. *J Bone Joint Surg.* 1993;75A:355–362.

Raikin SM, Ahmad J, Pour AE, et al. Comparison of arthrodesis and metallic hemiarthroplasty of the hallux metatarsophalangeal joint. *J Bone Joint Surg.* 2007;89A:1979–1985.

# Hallux Valgus (bunion)/Hallux Rigidus

Hallux valgus (bunion) deformity is a common condition that typically increases with age. The condition affects approximately 3% of people aged 15 to 30 years, 9% aged 31 to 60 years, and 16% of the population older than 60 years. Females outnumber males 2–4 : 1.

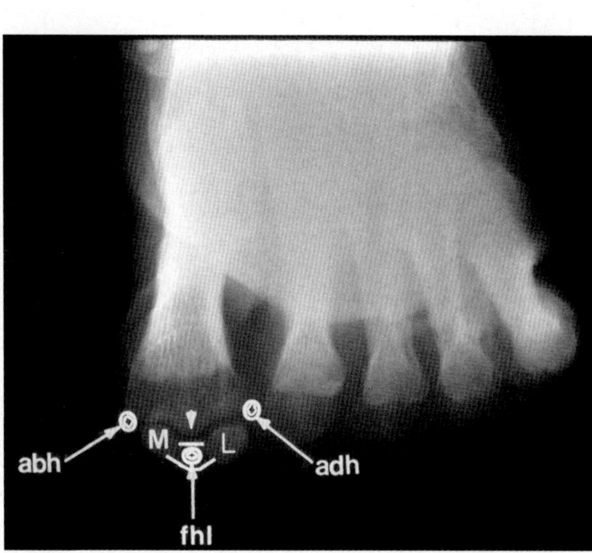



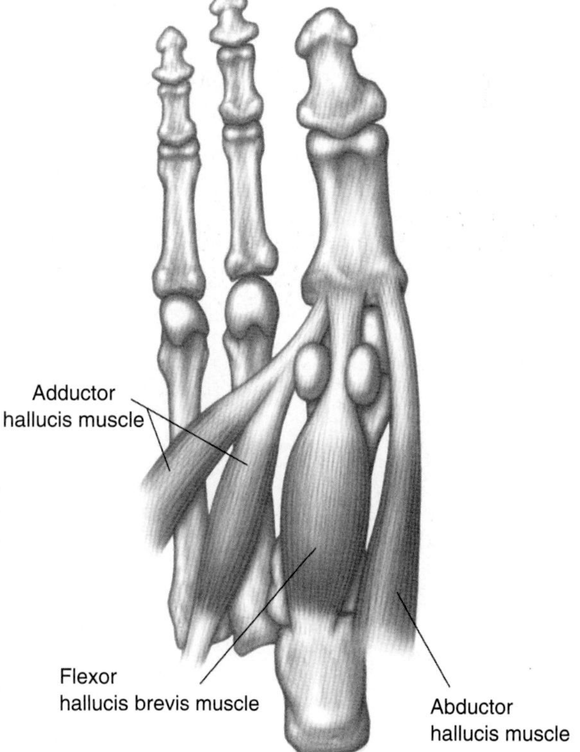



Fig. 8-113 A: Sesamoid view of the foot demonstrating the medial (*M*) and lateral (*L*) sesamoids separated by the crista (*small arrowhead*). abh—abductor hallucis tendon, fhl—flexor hallucis longus tendon, and adh—adductor hallucis tendon. Coronal (B) and axial (C) illustrations of the muscular and sesamoid anatomy.

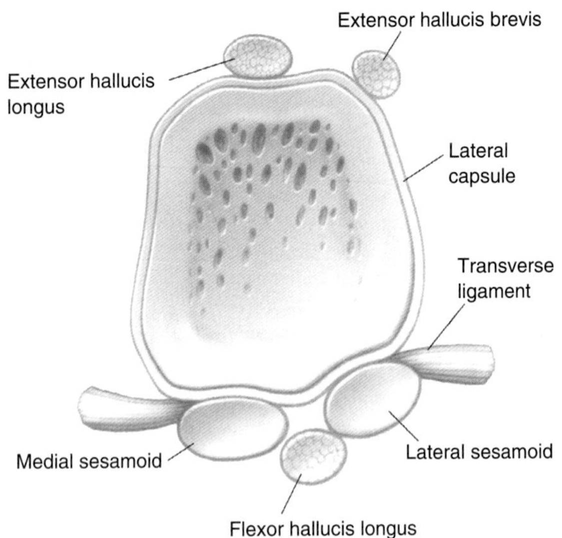


Fig. 8-113 (*Continued*)

The etiology is often attributed to footwear with restriction of the forefoot and high heels. There is also a strong familial tendency (68%). The condition advances more rapidly in the presence of pes planus. The condition is also associated with arthropathies (rheumatoid arthritis, connective tissue diseases) as well as congenital and neuromuscular disorders. Patients present with complaints of footwear restriction (80%), pain over the metatarsal head prominence (70%), cosmetic complaints (60%), and pain under the first or second metatarsal heads (40%).

A brief review of the anatomy is important for understanding the clinical and imaging aspects of the deformity. Four muscle groups are involved in the function of the first metatarsophalangeal joint and sesamoids. The extensor hallucis longus and extensor hallucis brevis extend dorsally over the articulation. The abductor hallucis is medial and the adductor hallucis muscle lateral to the great toe. The sesamoids lie on the plantar aspect of the metatarsal head separated by a notch or crista (see Fig. 8-113). The flexor hallucis longus and flexor hallucis brevis pass along the plantar aspect centrally along with the medial and lateral slips of the flexor hallucis brevis, which

20°

Fig. 8-114 Standing anteroposterior (AP) radiograph demonstrating a hullux valgus angle of 20 degrees (moderate) with 50% of the lateral sesamoid uncovered (*arrow*).

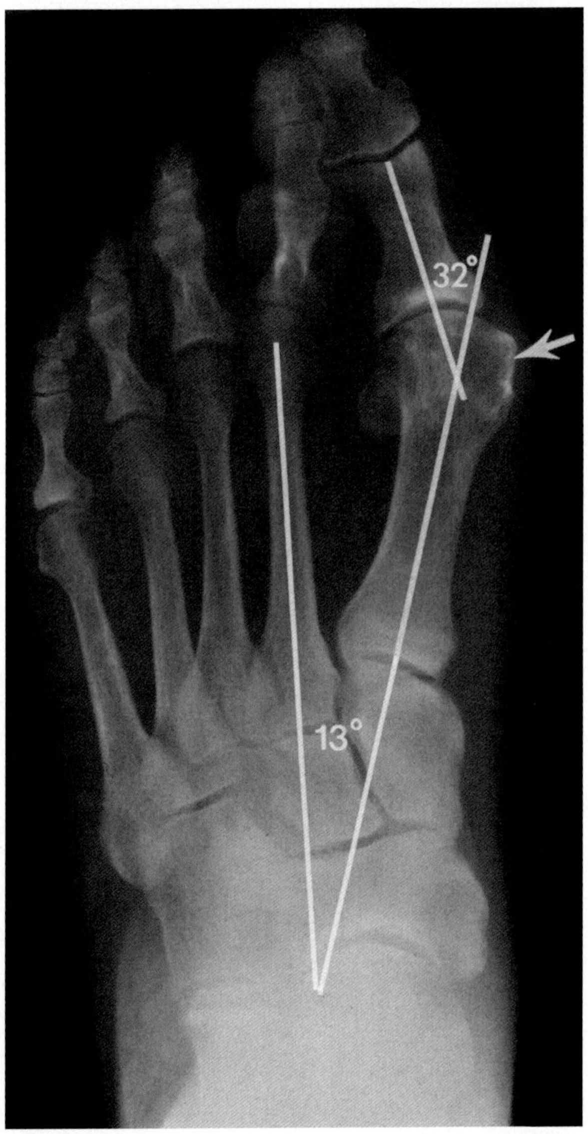


Fig. 8-115 Standing anteroposterior (AP) radiograph demonstrating moderate hallux valgus (32 degrees) with near cross-toe deformity (first and second digits touching, but not overlapped) and an intermetatarsal angle increased to 13 degrees (normal <9 degrees).

insert on the medial and lateral sesamoids. The sesamoids are attached to the base of the proximal phalanx by the plantar plate.

Pretreatment evaluation includes clinical evaluation and radiographic features. A clinical scoring system for the hallux metatarsophalangeal–interphalangeal joints has been developed by the American Orthopaedic Foot and Ankle Society, which is similar to those described in prior sections. The 100-point system includes pain (40 points), function (45 points—activity, footwear requirements, motion, callus, etc.), and alignment (15 points). Clinical data can be compared to posttreatment data to evaluate response to treatment.

## SUGGESTED READING

Johnson KA. *The foot and ankle.* New York: Raven Press; 1994.

Kitaoka HB, Alexander IJ, Adelaar RS, et al. Clinical rating systems for the ankle-hindfoot, mid-foot, hallux and lesser toes. *Foot Ankle Int.* 1994;15:349–353.

Robinson AHN, Limbers JP. Modern concepts in the treatment of hallux valgus. *J Bone Joint Surg.* 2005;87B:1038–1045.

### Preoperative Imaging

There are numerous radiographic features that are evaluated before planning conservative or surgical therapy. Standing AP, lateral and, on occasion, sesamoid views are required to plan treatment approaches. Most changes can be assessed on the standing AP and lateral views including abnormal angles, rotation, or uncovering of the lateral sesamoid and touching or cross-toe deformities in patients with severe hallux valgus. Oblique views are helpful to assess the extent or arthrosis and osteophyte formation. Measurements are listed in the subsequent text.

### Standing Anteroposterior Radiographs

**Hallux valgus angle (HVA):** Formed by lines down the shafts of the first metatarsal and proximal phalanx (see Fig. 8-114). Normal <15 degrees

- Mild hallux valgus—up to 19 degrees, intermetatarsal angle (IMA) ≤13 degrees
- Moderate hallux valgus—20 to 40 degrees, IMA 14 to 20 degrees
- Severe hallux valgus—>40 degrees, IMA >20 degrees

**Intermetatarsal (1–2) angle (IMA):** Formed by lines along the first and second metatarsal shafts (see Fig. 8-115). Normal <9 degrees

**Distal metatarsal articular angle (DMAA):** Formed by a line down the metatarsal and a second line across the articular surface. A third line perpendicular to the metatarsal line forms the angle. Normal <10 degrees (see Fig. 8-116)

**Interphalangeal angle:** Angle formed by lines through the proximal and distal phalanges. Normal ≤10 degrees (see Fig. 8-117)

**Sesamoid position:** The sesamoids normally lie medial and lateral to the crista and under the metatarsal head (see Fig. 8-118A).

- Mild hallux valgus—sesamoid covered or <50% uncovered or subluxed
- Moderate hallux valgus—sesamoid 50% to 75% uncovered
- Severe hallux valgus—sesamoid completely uncovered (Fig. 8-118B)

### Standing Lateral Radiographs

**Talar-first metatarsal angle:** Formed by lines through the talus and first metatarsal shaft. Normal 0 ± 5 degrees (see Fig. 8-119).

**Medial longitudinal arch angle:** Formed by a line along the first metatarsal and the weight-bearing device. Normal ≥20 degrees (Fig. 8-119).

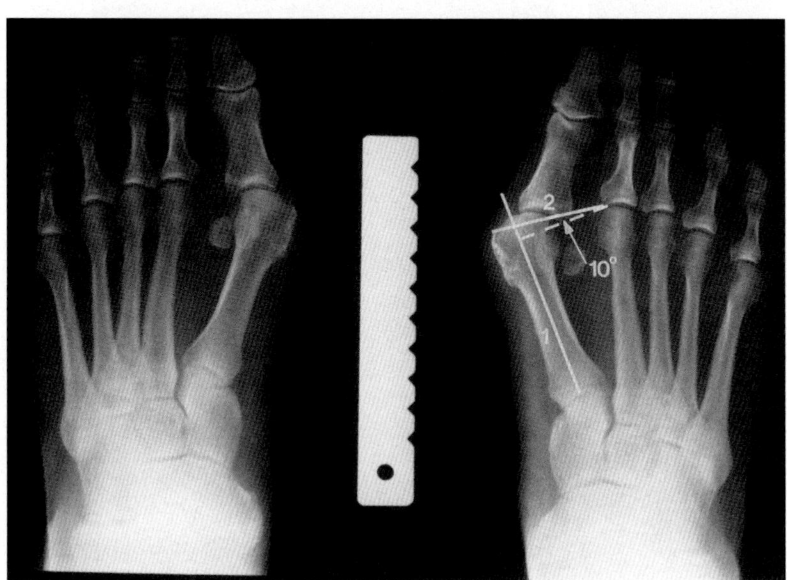


Fig. 8-116 Distal metatarsal articular angle (DMAA). A line is drawn down the first metatarsal shaft (*1*) and second line along the articular margins (*2*). A perpendicular line forms the metatarsal shaft axis (*1*) to the articular line (*2*). Broken line forms the angle, in this case 10 degrees (normal <10 degrees).

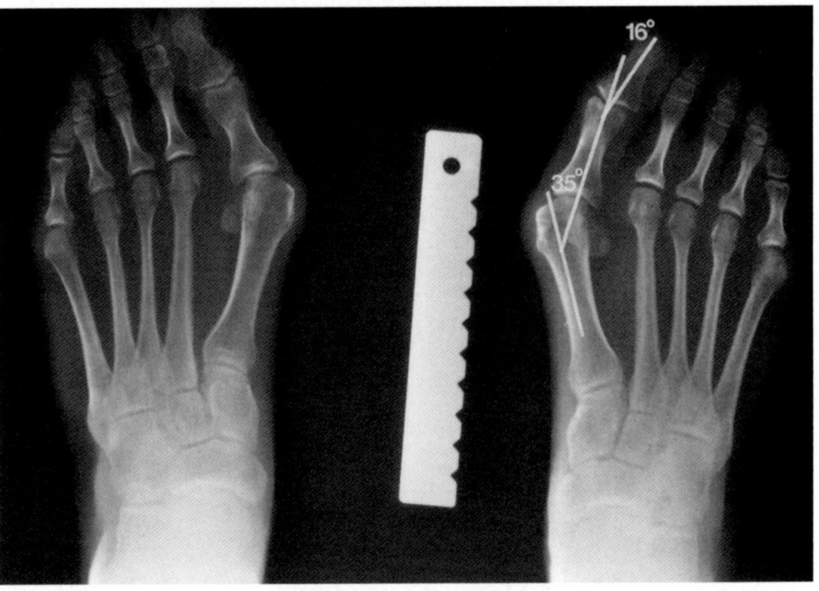


Fig. 8-117 Interphalangeal angle. Standing anteroposterior (AP) radiograph of the feet demonstrates moderate hallux valgus (35 degrees) and an interphalangeal angle of 16 degrees (normal ≤10 degrees).

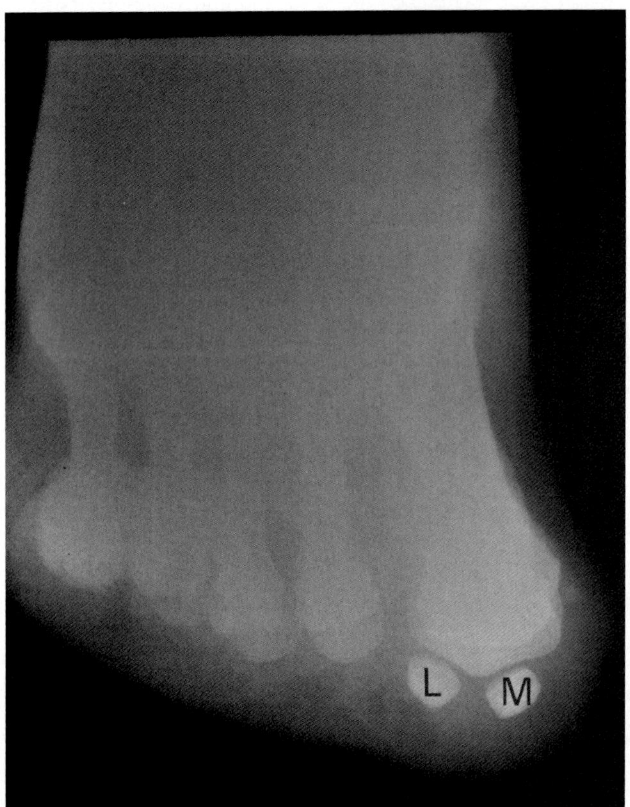


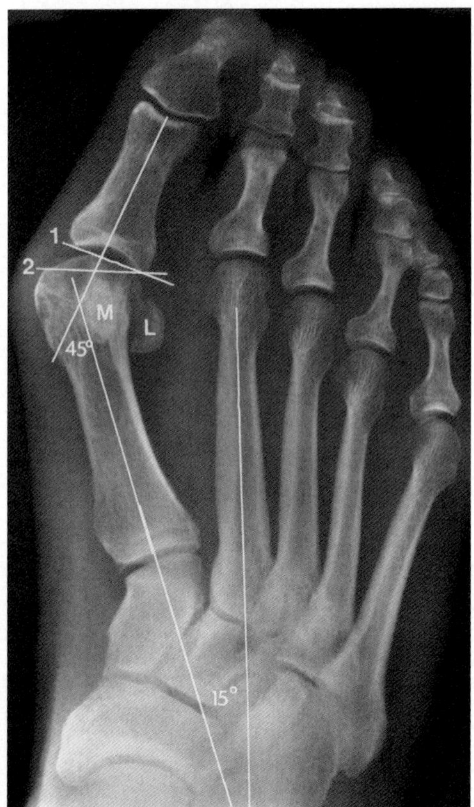


Fig. 8-118 Sesamoid position. **A:** Sesamoid view demonstrating the normal position of the medial (*M*) and lateral (*L*) sesamoids fully covered by the metatarsal head. **B:** Standing radiograph demonstrating severe hallux valgus with an intermetatarsal angle of 15 degrees, hallux valgus angle of 45 degrees (severe ≥40 degrees), and joint incongruency (lines *1* and *2*).

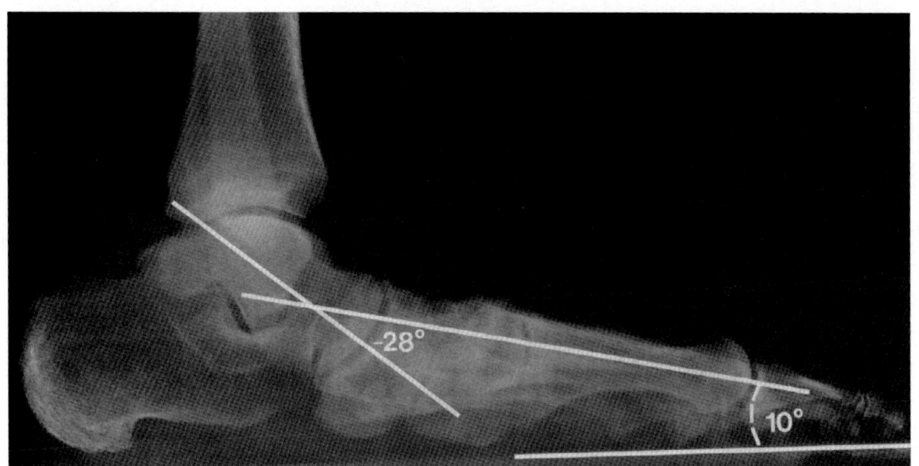


Fig. 8-119 Standing lateral radiograph demonstrates a negative talar-first metatarsal angle −28 degrees (normal 0 ± 5 degrees) and a medial longitudinal arch angle of 10 degrees (normal ≥20 degrees).

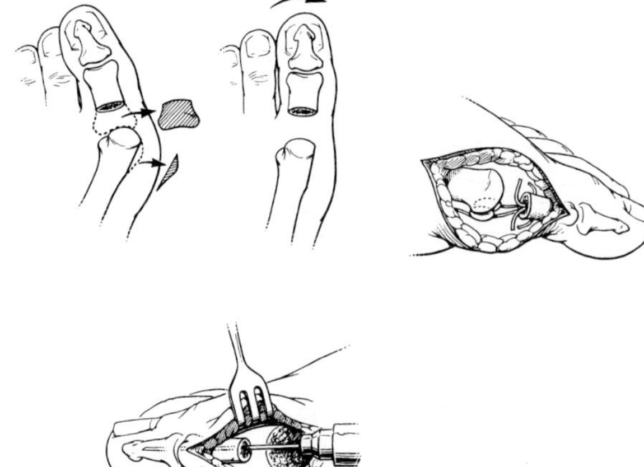


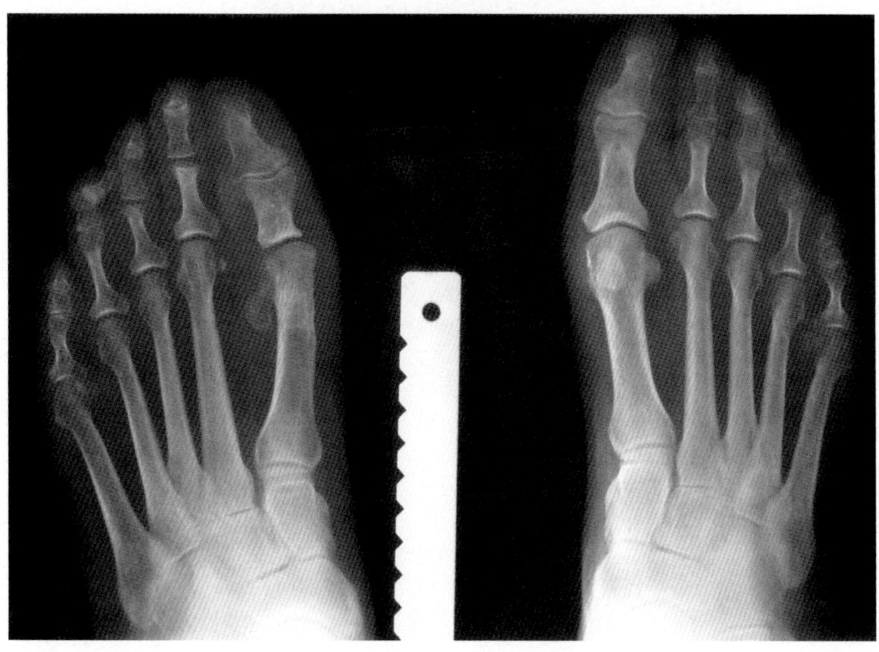


Fig. 8-120 Keller procedure. A: Illustration of the Keller procedure with resection of a portion of the proximal phalanx. B: Standing anteroposterior (AP) radiograph following resection of the proximal third of the proximal phalanx and resection of the metatarsal prominence on the left.

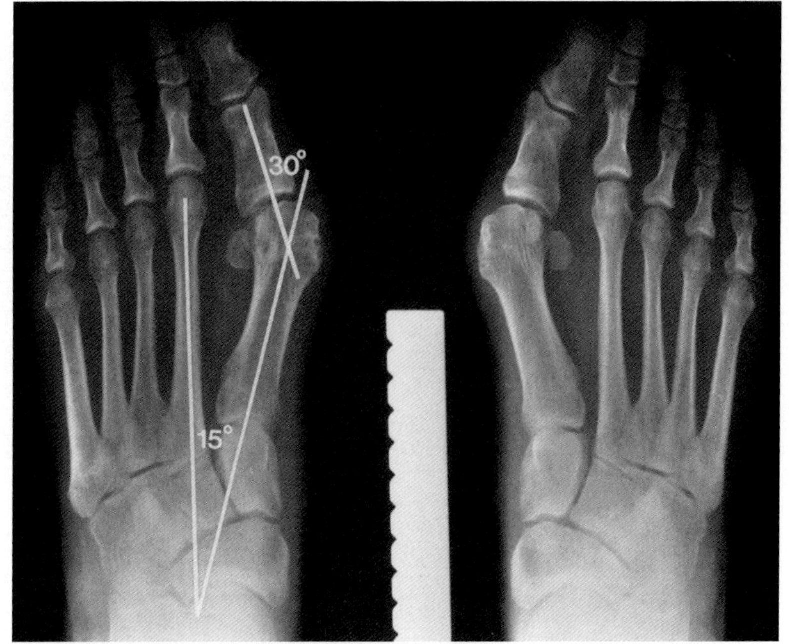


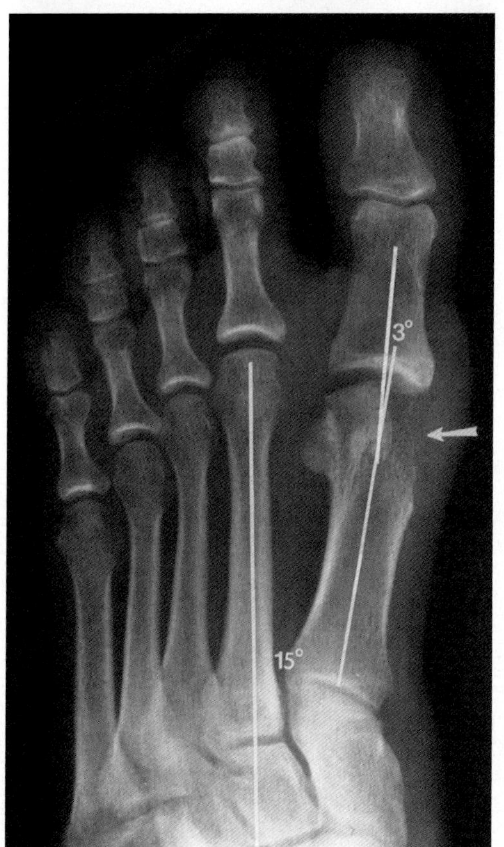


Fig. 8-121 A: Preoperative radiograph demonstrates a 30-degree hallux valgus angle and 15-degree intermetatarsal angle. B: Following soft tissue repair and resection of the median eminence (*arrow*) the hallux valgus angle is reduced to 3 degrees.

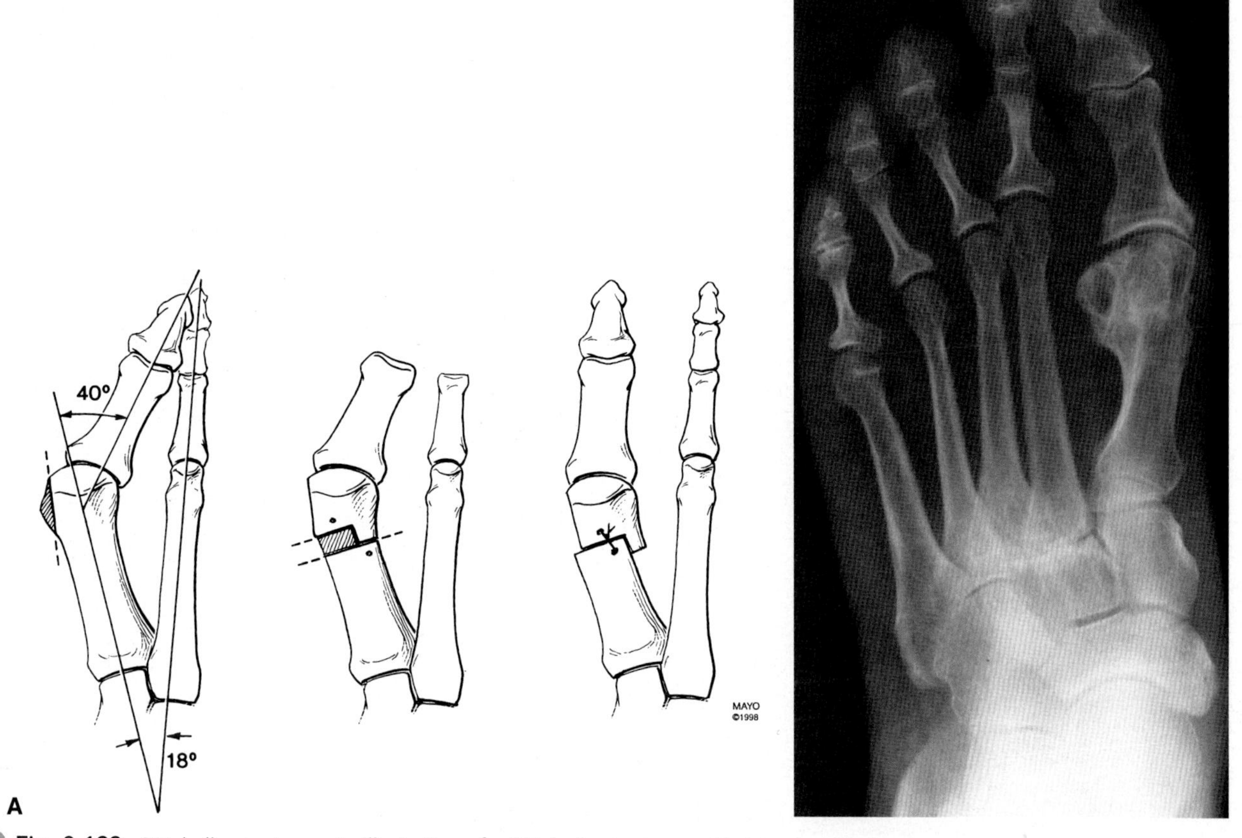


Fig. 8-122 Mitchell osteotomy. A: Illustration of a Mitchell osteotomy with lateral cortical step secured with suture and drill holes in the proximal and distal fragments. The medial eminence has been resected. B: Radiograph demonstrating a healed osteotomy.

## Suggested Reading

Eustace S, O'Bryne J, Stack J, et al. Radiographic features enable assessment of first metatarsal rotation: The role of pronation in hallux valgus. *Skeletal Radiol.* 1993;22:153–156.

Robinson AHN, Limbers JP. Modern concepts in the treatment of hallux valgus. *J Bone Joint Surg.* 2005;87B:1038–1045.

Tanoka Y, Takabura Y, Kumai T, et al. Radiographic analysis of hallux valgus. A two-dimensional coordinate system. *J Bone Joint Surg.* 1995;77A:1924–1936.

### Treatment Options

Conservative therapy with changes in footwear and orthotics is the first course of action, especially in adolescents. Patient compliance is a common problem with conservative approaches. Surgical intervention is considered when conservative therapy fails or deformity progresses. The goals of surgical intervention are to relieve pain and restore anatomic alignment along with correction of other related deformities. There are more than 130 procedures described for correction of hallux valgus and bunion deformities. Common procedures are described in the subsequent text.

**Keller procedure:** Approximately one third of the proximal phalanx is resected relaxing the lateral structures and allowing the deformity to correct. It has high recurrence rate and is best for moderate hallux valgus (≤30 degrees) (see Fig. 8-120).

**Distal soft tissue repair:** The adductor hallucis and lateral capsule are released and medial eminence of the metatarsal head resected (see Fig. 8-121)

**First metatarsal osteotomies:** Osteotomies may be performed proximally, distally, or in other diaphyseal locations.

**Distal osteotomies**

**Wilson procedure:** Oblique (distal medial to proximal lateral) osteotomy allowing lateral and proximal displacement of the metatarsal head.

**Mitchell osteotomy:** Double cut through the first metatarsal neck with lateral cortical step (see Fig. 8-122)

**Distal Chevron osteotomy:** V-shaped osteotomy through the neck with lateral displacement of the distal fragment (see Fig. 8-123)

**Diaphyseal osteotomies**

**Ludloff osteotomy:** Oblique osteotomy beginning dorsally just distal to the proximal articulation and extending distally to the plantar cortex (see Fig. 8-124)

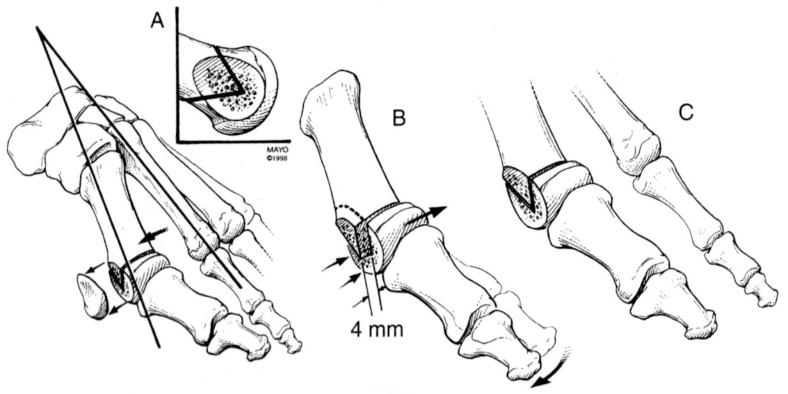

**Fig. 8-123** Distal Chevron osteotomy. **A:** Illustration of distal Chevron V-shaped osteotomy with resection of the medial eminence (*A*), lateral displacement of the distal fragment with more medial resection (*B*), and final position (*C*). Standing anteroposterior (AP) (**B**) and lateral (**C**) radiographs demonstrate the medial eminence resection (*broken line* in **B**) and the osteotomy (*small white arrows* in *C*) which is best seen on the lateral radiograph.

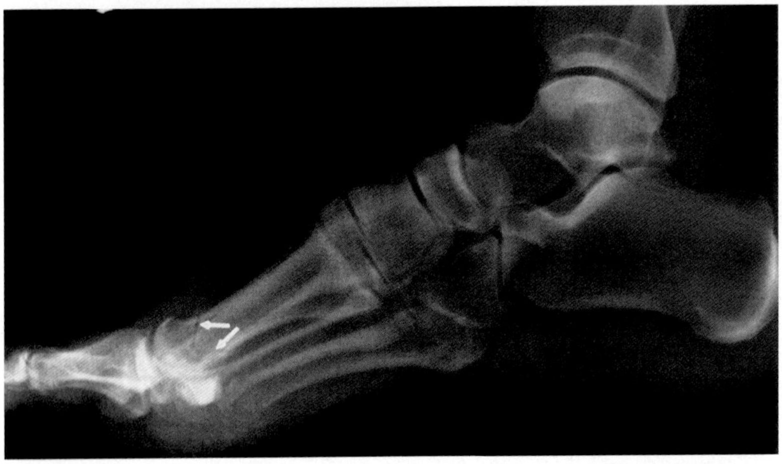

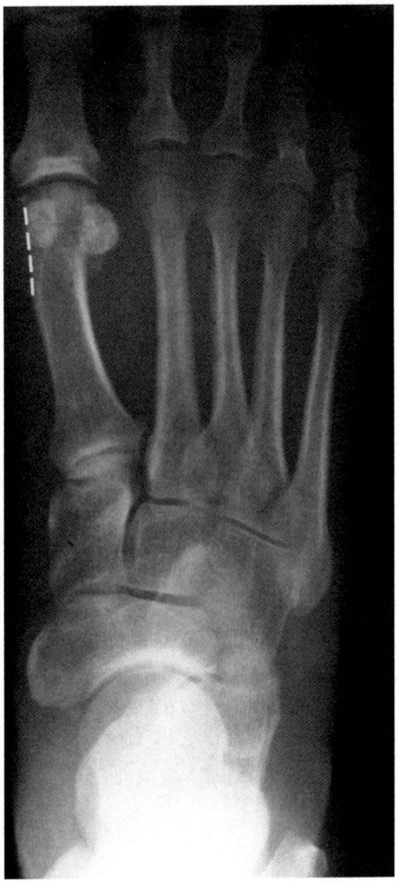

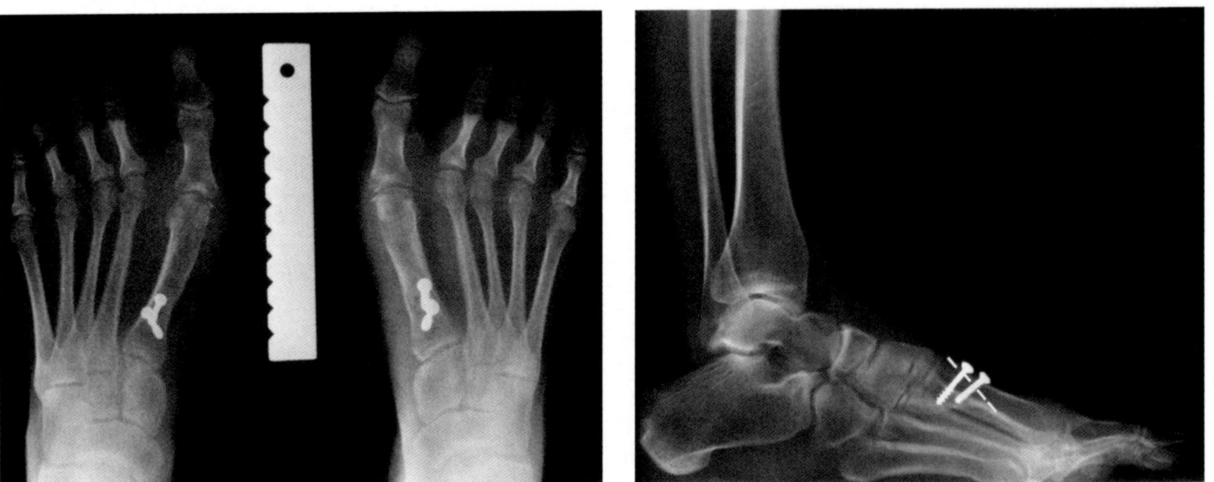


**Fig. 8-124** Ludloff osteotomy. Standing anteroposterior (AP) (**A**) and lateral (**B**) radiographs following an oblique proximal metatarsal osteotomy (*broken line* in **B**) and resection of the medial eminences bilaterally. The osteotomy is fixed with two screws.

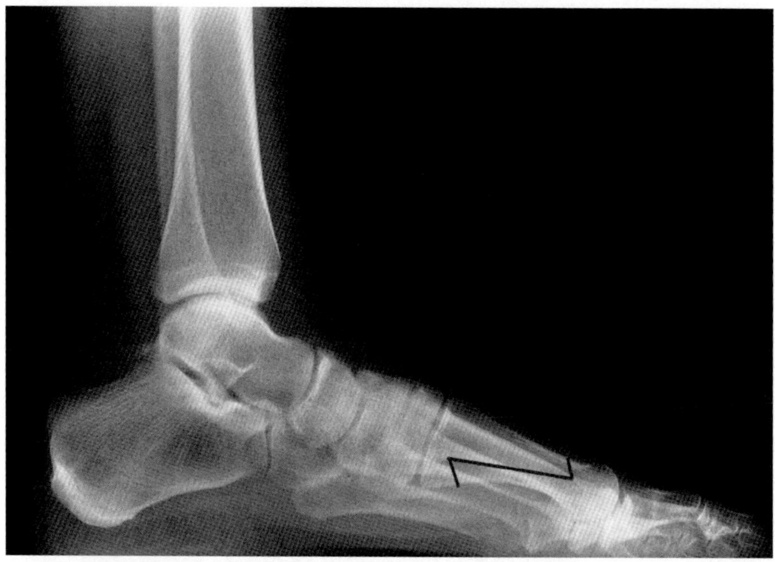

Fig. 8-125 Scarf osteotomy. Lateral radiograph demonstrating the cutting plane of the Z-shaped osteotomy. The head and plantar section are shifted laterally and held with two screws.

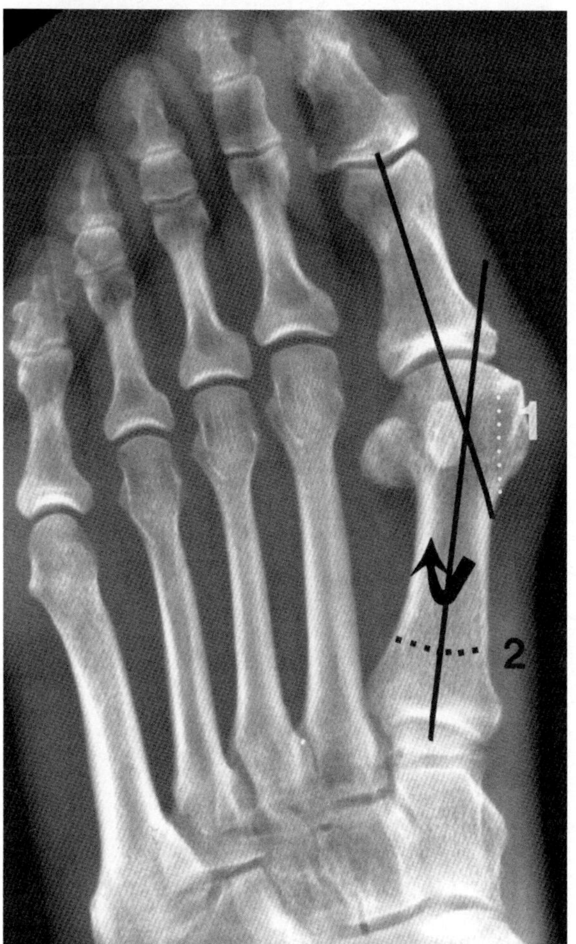


Fig. 8-126 Crescentric osteotomy. Standing anteroposterior (AP) radiograph demonstrating resection of the medial eminence (*1*) and a crescentric proximal osteotomy (*2*) concave distally. The distal fragment is rotated laterally (*curved arrow*).

**Scarf osteotomy:** Z-shaped osteotomy extending through the length of the diaphysis best seen on the lateral radiograph (see Fig. 8-125)

**Proximal osteotomies**

**Wedge osteotomy:** Opening or closing wedge. Opening causes elongation of the metatarsal and requires bone graft. Closing wedge leads to shortening.

**Crescentric osteotomy:** Distal 1 cm to the tarsometatarsal joint with concavity directed distally. Metatarsal shaft is rotated laterally and fixed with screws or K-wires (see Fig. 8-126)

**Proximal Chevron osteotomy:** V-shaped proximal osteotomy similar to the distal configuration (Fig. 8-123)

**First metatarsophalangeal arthrodesis:** Used in patients with advanced arthritis and rheumatoid arthritis (see Fig. 8-127)

**First tarsometatarsal arthrodesis:** Used in combination. Distal soft tissue repair in patients with an unstable first tarsometatarsal articulation

**Akin procedure:** Medial eminence resection and closing wedge proximal phalanx osteotomy (see Fig. 8-128)

## SUGGESTED READING

Akin OF. The treatment of hallux valgus. A new procedure and its results. *Med Sentinel.* 1925;33:678–679.

Kitaoka HB, Franco MG, Weaver AL, et al. Simple bunionectomy with medial capsulorrhaphy. *Foot Ankle* 1991;12: 86–91.

Mann RA, Coughlin MJ. Adult hallux valgus. In: Coughlin MJ, Mann RA, eds. *Surgery of the foot and ankle*, 7th ed. Vol. 1. St. Louis: Mosby; 1999:150–269.

Robinson AHN, Limers JP. Modern concepts in the treatment of hallux valgus. *J Bone Joint Surg.* 2005;87B:1038–1045.

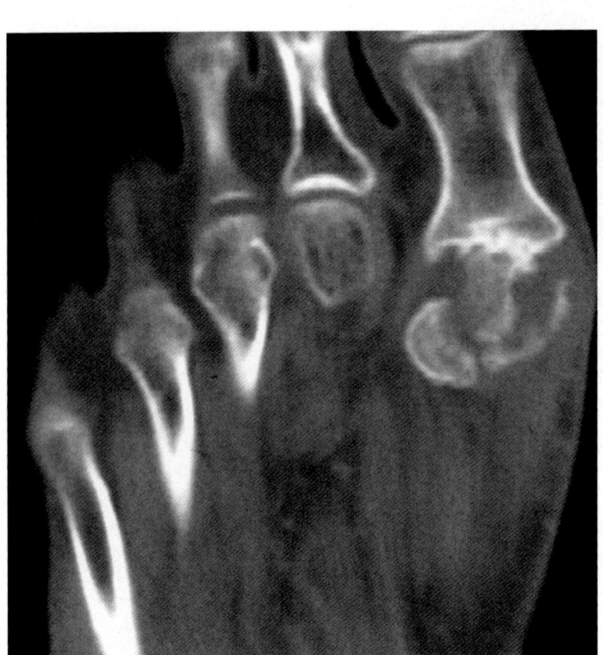
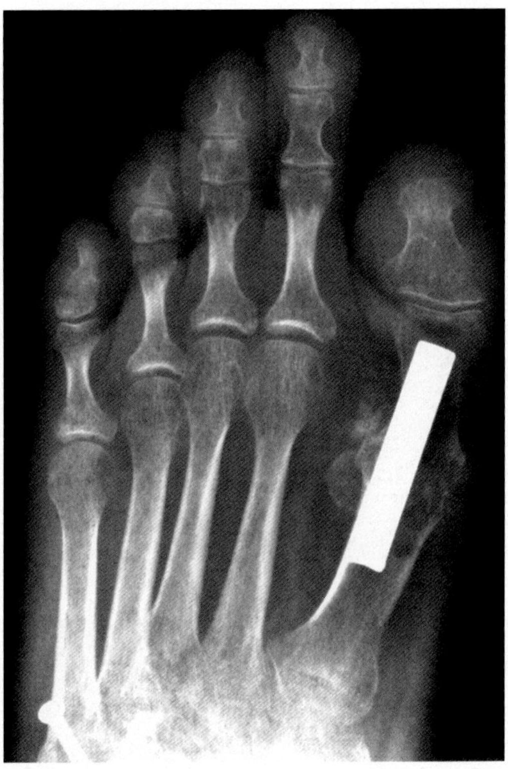

Fig. 8-127 First metatarsophalangeal arthrodesis. A: Computed tomographic (CT) image demonstrating advanced arthropathy in the first metatarsophalangeal joint. B: Anteroposterior (AP) radiograph following arthrodesis with plate and screw fixation. Note the significant shortening of the great toe.

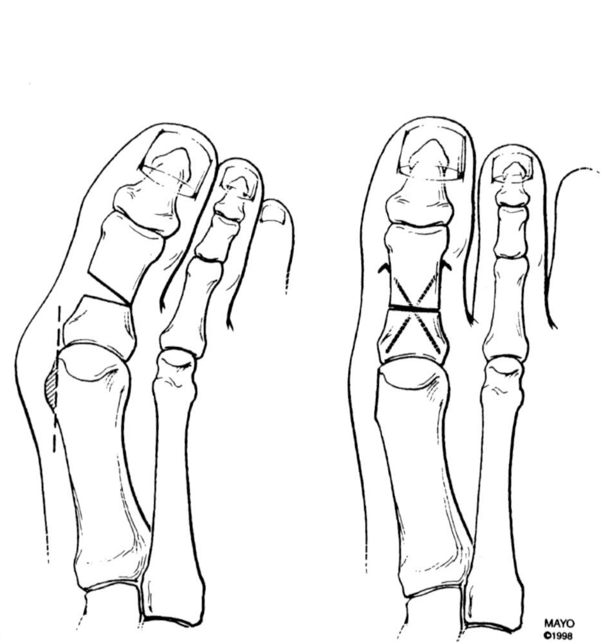

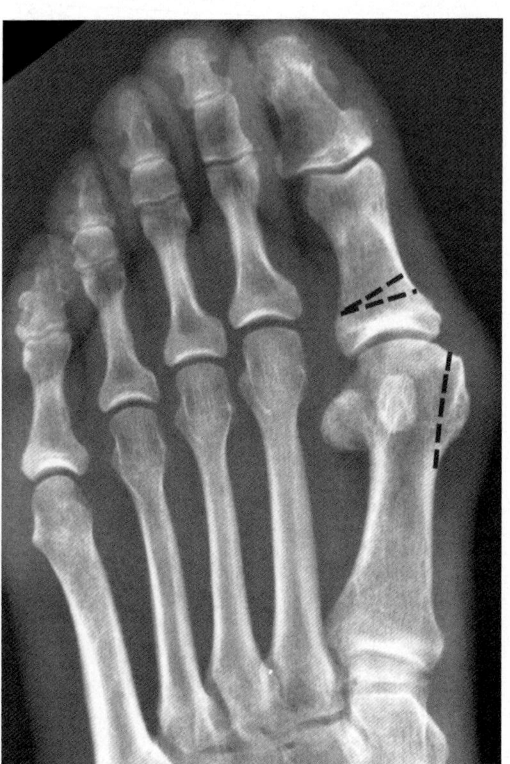

Fig. 8-128 Akin procedure. A: Illustration of the Akin procedure with resection of the medial eminence (*1*) and closing wedge medial osteotomy of the proximal phalanx (*2*) with K-wire fixation. B: Standing anteroposterior (AP) radiograph demonstrating these cuts (*broken lines*).

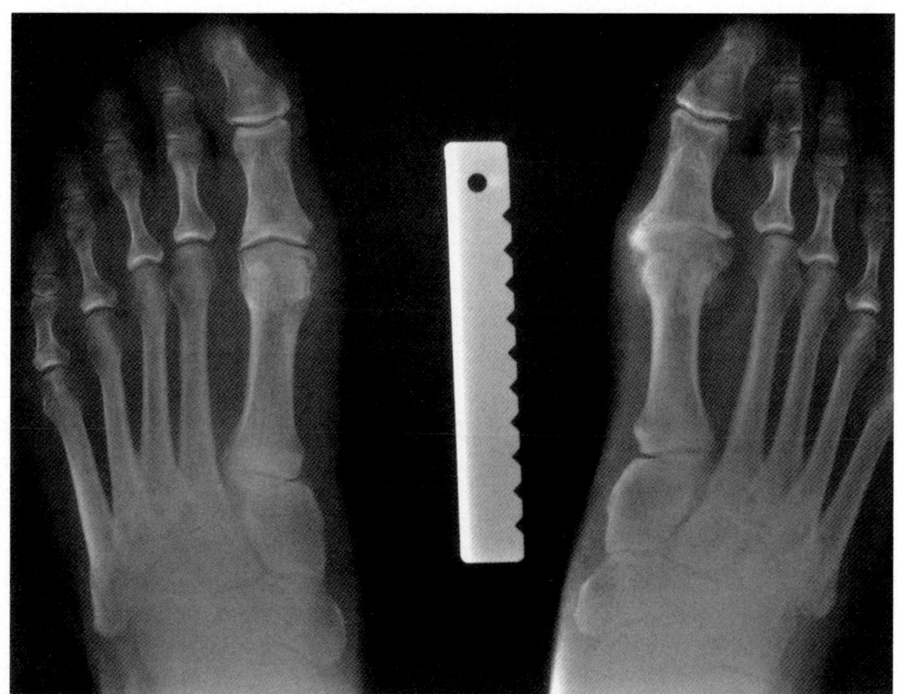

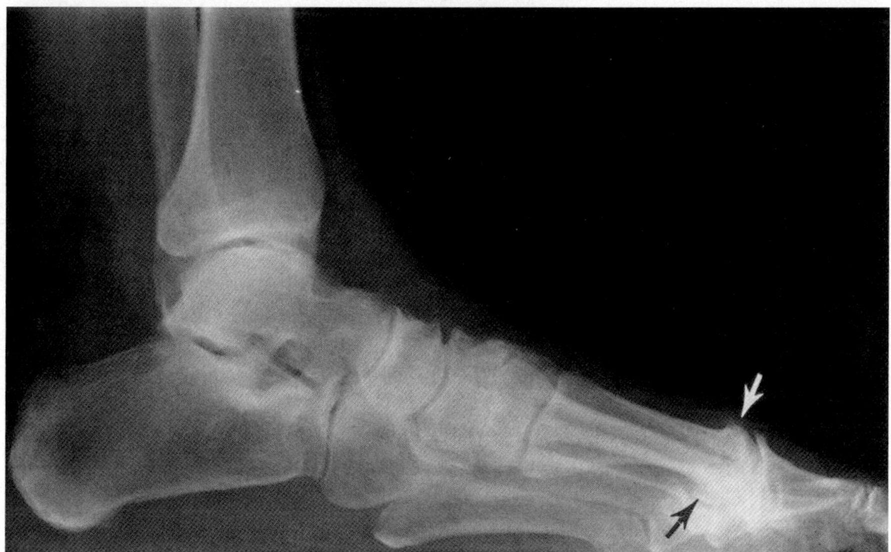

Fig. 8-129 Hallux rigidus. Standing anteroposterior (AP) (A) and lateral (B) radiographs demonstrate marked joint space narrowing and marginal osteophytes (best seen on the lateral view, *arrows*) and no hallux valgus deformity. The left foot demonstrates earlier changes.

## Hallux Rigidus

Hallux rigidus is a painful disorder of the first metatarsophalangeal joint with bone proliferation, joint space narrowing, and osteophyte formation (see Fig. 8-129). This is the second most common painful disorder of the great toe following hallux valgus. Symptoms are usually unilateral and may be related to prior trauma. Hallux rigidus is seen in adolescents and adults. The condition is progressive and can easily be graded on AP and lateral radiographs. Clinical evaluation includes range of motion, pain, and function as established by the American Orthopaedic Foot and Ankle Society similar to the grading scale used in previous sections with a total of 100 points. Clinical and radiographic features are used to grade the extent of involvement. Grade 0 changes have 40 to 60 degrees of dorsiflexion of the first metatarsophalangeal joint with normal radiographs and stiffness, but no pain. Grade I changes show loss of range of motion to 30 to 40 degrees of dorsiflexion with mild osteophyte formation (dorsal osteophyte on the lateral view is the main finding) and a normal or minimally narrowed joint space. Patients have mild or intermittent pain. Grade II hallux rigidus demonstrates progressive loss in dorsiflexion (10 to 30 degrees), moderate osteophytes with joint space narrowing, and subchondral sclerosis. The sesamoids are usually not involved. Pain is moderate to severe with consistent joint stiffness. Grade III hallux rigidus shows minimal motion and more severe changes with complete loss of joint space (Fig. 8-129).

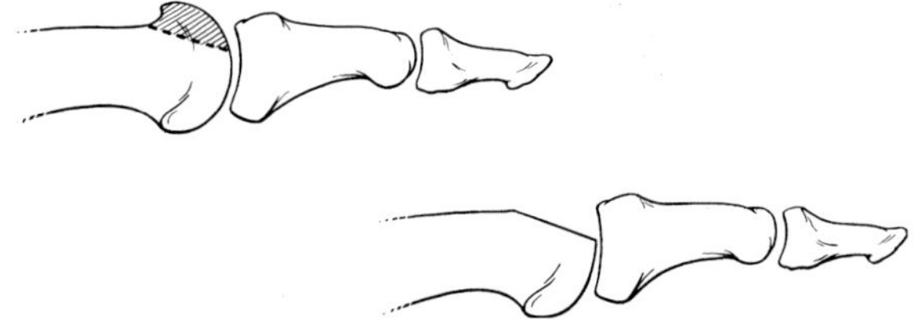

Fig. 8-130 Cheilectomy. Illustration demonstrating resection of the dorsal 20% to 30% of the metatarsal head.

Imaging is similar to that for hallux valgus and surgical treatment options are more limited. Cheilectomy, arthrodesis, resection arthroplasty with soft tissue interposition, first metatarsal osteotomy, and the Keller procedure described earlier have been employed. Joint replacement arthroplasty has been advocated, but the results have not been consistent. Cheilectomy removes 20% to 30% of the dorsal metatarsal head (see Fig. 8-130). This procedure is particularly useful when there is impingement in addition to pain in patients with grade I–II hallux rigidus. This procedure can be combined with metatarsal or phalangeal osteotomy as well as interposition arthroplasty. Patients with grade III or more advanced hallux rigidus should be treated with arthrodesis.

## Suggested Reading

Coughlin MJ, Shurnas PS. Hallux rigidus. *J Bone Joint Surg.* 2003;85A:2072–2088.

Johnson KA. *The foot and ankle.* New York: Raven Press; 1994.

Kitaoka HB, Alexander IJ, Adelaar RS, et al. Clinical rating systems for the ankle-hindfoot, mid-foot, hallux and lesser toes. *Foot Ankle Int.* 1994;15:349–353.

Mann RA, Clanton TO. Hallux rigidus: Treatment by cheilectomy. *J Bone Joint Surg.* 1988;70A:400–406.

### Imaging of Complications of Hallux Valgus and Rigidus Repairs

Postoperative evaluation of hallux valgus and rigidus repairs includes comparison with preoperative images and clinical scores. Most complications can be detected with serial standing radiographs. Complications vary with the type of procedure and patient factors including compliance. The most frequent complications include loss of reduction, recurrent deformity, malunion, nonunion, delayed union, transfer metatarsalgia, AVN of the first metatarsal head, hardware failure, and infection.

Recurrence of hallux valgus occurs in 2% to 3.5% of patients. Progressive joint deformity and recurrence of dorsal osteophytes can occur in up to 30% of patients with hallux rigidus. Hallux varus is reported in up to 11% of patients treated with distal soft tissue repair and resection of the medial eminence (see Fig. 8-131).

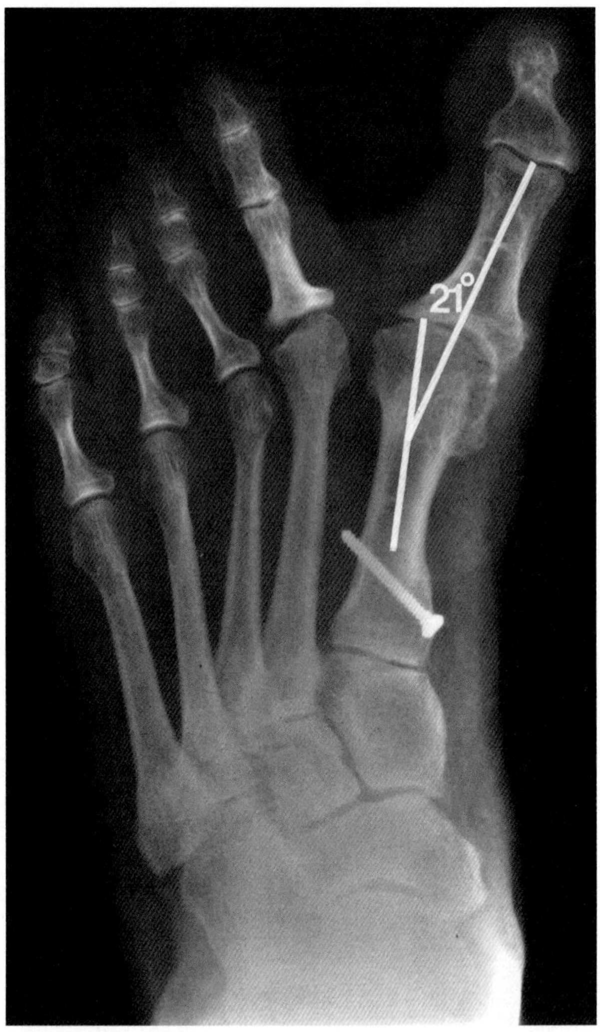


Fig. 8-131 Standing anteroposterior (AP) radiograph following proximal first metatarsal osteotomy and distal soft tissue repair with 21-degree hallux varus.

Transfer metatarsalgia is pain under the lesser metatarsal heads. This is a clinical diagnosis commonly seen following Keller procedures (20% to 40%) and Wilson and Mitchell osteotomies resulting in metatarsal shortening (10% to 30%). Symptoms are particularly common when shortening is ≥5 mm.

Malunion is much more common than nonunion (see Fig. 8-132). Dorsal malunion occurs in 38% of patients with proximal first metatarsal wedge osteotomies and 17% of patients with crescentric proximal osteotomies. Fusion rates for arthrodesis are >94%.

AVN of the first metatarsal head occurs with distal osteotomies in up to 20% of patients. This may be evident by sclerotic changes or fragmentation of the metatarsal head on serial radiographs. MRI is the technique of choice for early detection of this complication. Image features are similar to osteonecrosis in the hip with geographic signal abnormalities evident on T1- and T2-weighted sequences.

Superficial or pin tract infections occur in up to 6% of patients. This usually requires implant removal. Lucency about the implant and periosteal reaction may be evident on radiographs. More subtle changes are difficult to detect and may require MRI for early detection. Implants may also be removed due to hardware failure or pain over the implant.

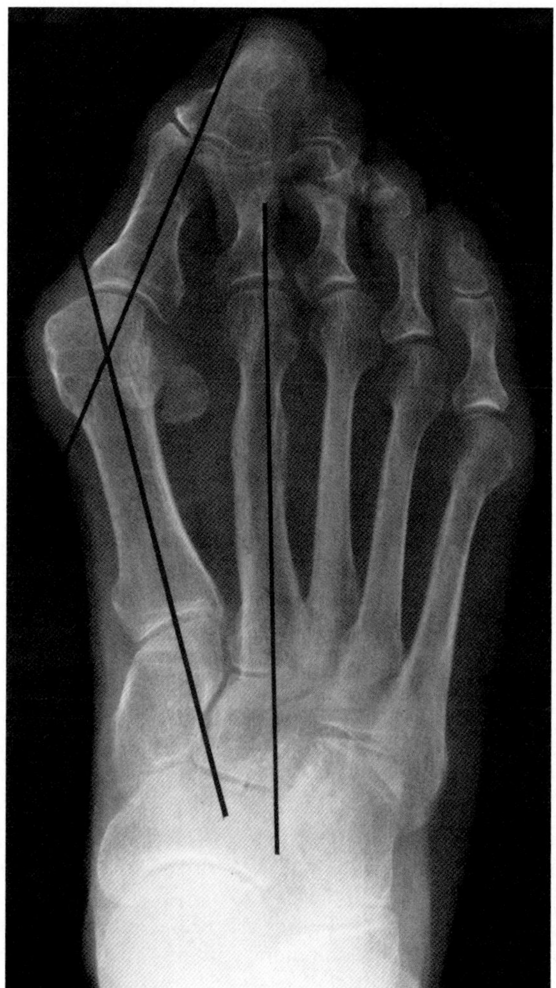


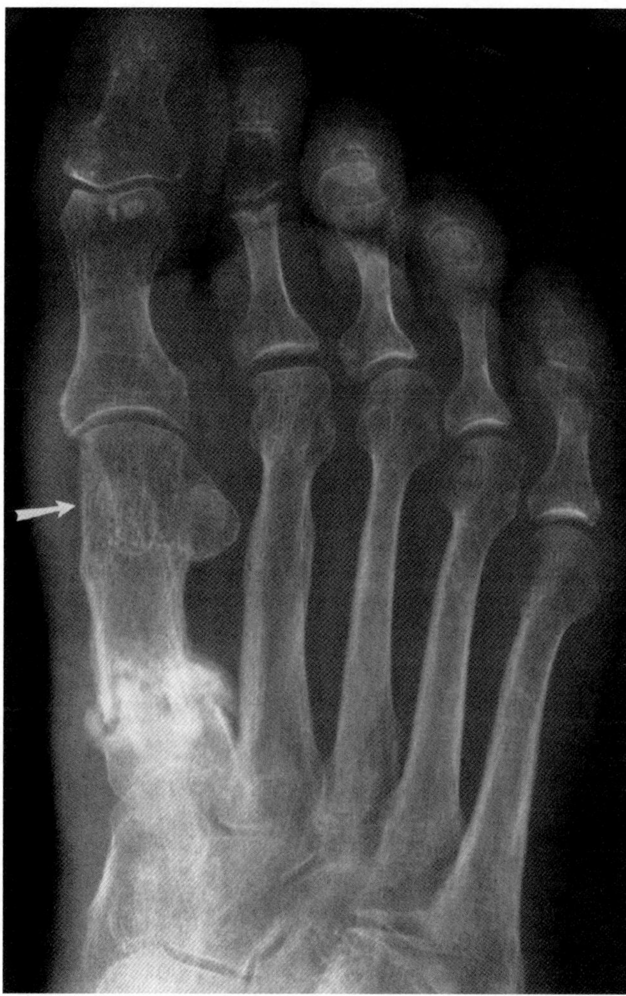


Fig. 8-132 A: Standing anteroposterior (AP) preoperative radiograph demonstrating severe hallux valgus with cross-toe deformity. B: Four months following proximal osteotomy and eminence resection (*arrow*), there is sclerosis at the osteotomy site with abundant nonbridging callus due to delayed union or nonunion.

Deep infections are uncommon (1% to 2%). MRI is most useful in this setting unless there is extensive hardware as in the case of plate and screw arthrodesis. CT may also be effective and may identify appropriate biopsy sites for culture.

## Suggested Reading


Berquist TH. *Radiology of the foot and ankle*, 2nd ed. Philadelphia: Lippincott Williams & Wilkins; 2000:479–526.

Coughlin MJ, Shurnas PS. Hallux rigidus. *J Bone Joint Surg.* 2003;85A:2072–2088.

Mann RA, Rudicel S, Graves SC. Repair of hallux valgus with a distal soft tissue procedure and proximal metatarsal osteotomy. A long-term follow-up. *J Bone Joint Surg.* 1992;74A: 124–129.

Robinson AHN, Limbers JP. Modern concepts in the treatment of hallux valgus. *J Bone Joint Surg.* 2005;87B:1038–1045.


## Lesser Toe Deformities

Digital deformities of the second through fifth toes and metatarsophalangeal joints are usually easily classified clinically. Imaging is not required except for surgical planning or to exclude associated disorders or complete evaluation of foot articulations. Deformities may be congenital (polydactyly, syndactyly, and congenital bands) or acquired. Claw and hammer toe deformities increase with age and occur in 2% to 20% of the general population. Claw toe deformity is most common in females than males (ratio 4–5:1) in the seventh and eighth decades. Common deformities are summarized in the subsequent text.

**Curly toe deformities:** This is common in children and may be referred to as *overlapping toes*. The toe is flexed at the proximal interphalangeal joint with lateral rotation and varus deformity. This condition is secondary to shortening of the flexor digitorum brevis and longus muscles.

**Overlapping fifth toe:** This condition is typically bilateral. Patients present with pain and adduction of the fifth toe over the fourth toe. The metatarsophalangeal joint is dorsiflexed. The condition is familial.

**Hammer toe:** This is a sagittal plane deformity with hyperflexion of the proximal interphalangeal joint. The metatarsophalangeal joint may be neutral, but eventually becomes dorsiflexed. The condition is usually bilateral and most commonly involves the second digit. The second metatarsal is usually elongated. (see Fig. 8-133)

**Claw toe:** This condition results in dorsiflexion of the metatarsophalangeal joint with flexion deformity of the interphalangeal joints. The condition usually involves all four lesser toes bilaterally and may be associated with pes cavus deformity. Other causes include neuropathic foot disorders, diabetes, rheumatoid arthritis, trauma, and posterior compartment syndrome (Fig. 8-133).

**Mallet toe:** This condition results in flexion deformity of the distal interphalangeal joint. Etiology is thought to be related to shortening of the flexor digitorum longus. The deformity usually involves the second digit and is also associated with elongation of the second metatarsal (Fig. 8-133).

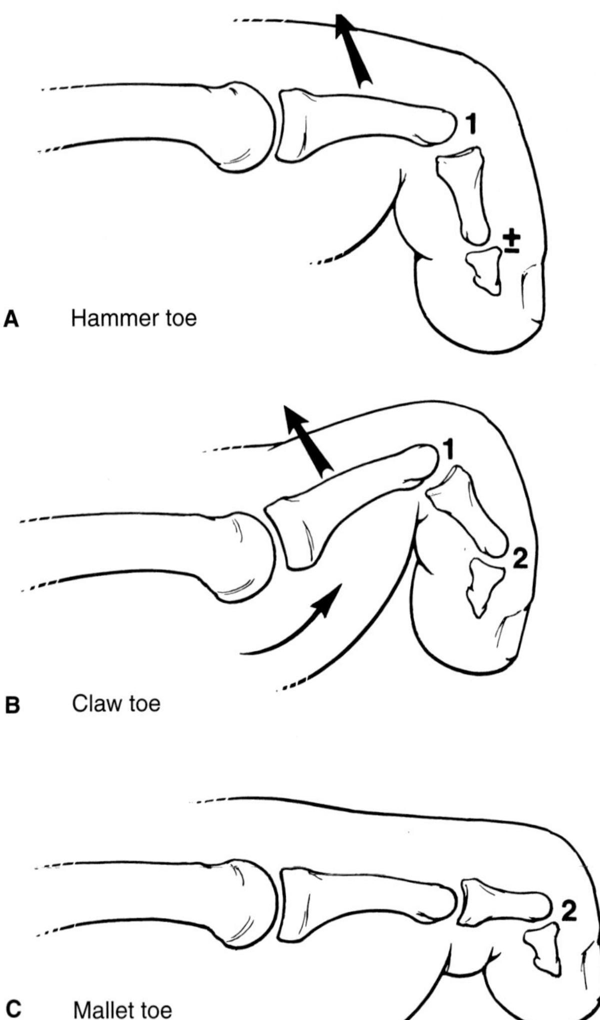


Fig. 8-133 Illustrations of common lesser toe deformities. A: Hammer toe—the proximal interphalangeal joint if flexed (*1*). The distal interphalangeal joint may be neutral or flexed (±). Metatarsophalangeal dorsiflexion (*arrow*) occurs over time. B: Claw toe—the metatarsophalangeal joint is hyperextended (*arrow*). The proximal interphalangeal joint is flexed (*1*) and the distal articulation (*2*) may also be flexed. C: Mallet toe—there is flexion deformity of the distal interphalangeal joint (*2*). The second toe is most commonly involved. The remaining articulations are neutral.

Preoperative assessment includes clinical evaluation using the American Orthopaedic Foot and Ankle Society scale for the lesser toes. This includes a 100-point system for pain (40 points), function (45 points), and alignment (15 points). Vascular evaluations are also performed to evaluate potential healing issues following surgical intervention. Electromyograms (EMGs) may also be required to assess neuropathic changes. Imaging with the standing AP, lateral, and conventional oblique radiographs may be sufficient to evaluate associated fracture deformities, inflammatory arthropathy, and position of the articulations. Rarely, contrast-enhanced MR images are required to evaluate active synovitis or AVN of the metatarsal heads.

## SUGGESTED READING

Coughlin MJ, Mann RA. Lesser toe deformities. In: Mann RA, ed. *Surgery of the foot and ankle*, 7th ed. St. Louis: Mosby; 1999:320–391.

Kitaoka HB, Alexander IJ, Adelaar RS, et al. Clinical rating systems for the ankle-hindfoot, mid-foot, hallux and lesser toes. *Foot Ankle Int*. 1994;15:349–353.

Thompson GH. Bunions and deformities of the toes in children and adolescents. *J Bone Joint Surg*. 1995;77A:1924–1936.

### Treatment Options

Conservative therapy includes changes in footwear and avoiding high-heeled or pointed styles. Metatarsal bars or pads can be added to relieve metatarsal pressure. When conservative therapy is ineffective, soft tissue repair with or without resection arthroplasty is usually indicated. K-wires are used to provide stability in the postoperative period (see Fig. 8-134). The most common complication following these procedures is pain due to recurrent deformity.

## SUGGESTED READING

Coughlin MJ, Mann RA. Lesser toe deformities. In: Mann RA, ed. *Surgery of the foot and ankle*, 7th ed. St. Louis: Mosby; 1999:320–391.

Taylor RG. The treatment of claw toes by multiple transfers of flexor into extensor tendons. *J Bone Joint Surg*. 1951;33B:539–542.

Thompson GH. Bunions and deformities of the toes in children and adolescents. *J Bone Joint Surg*. 1995;77A:1924–1936.

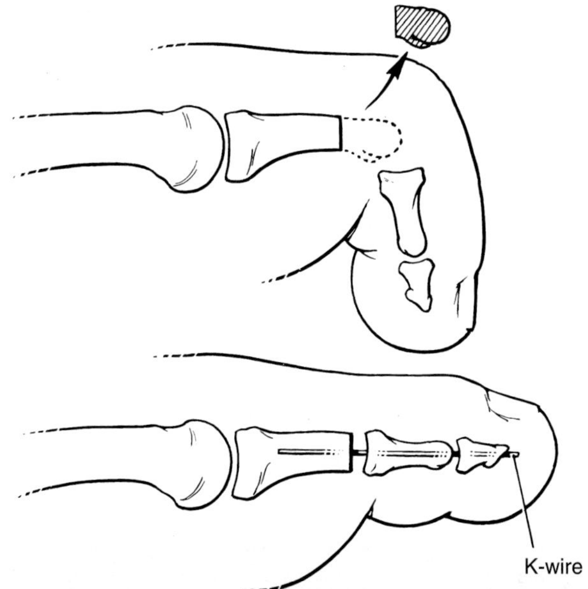


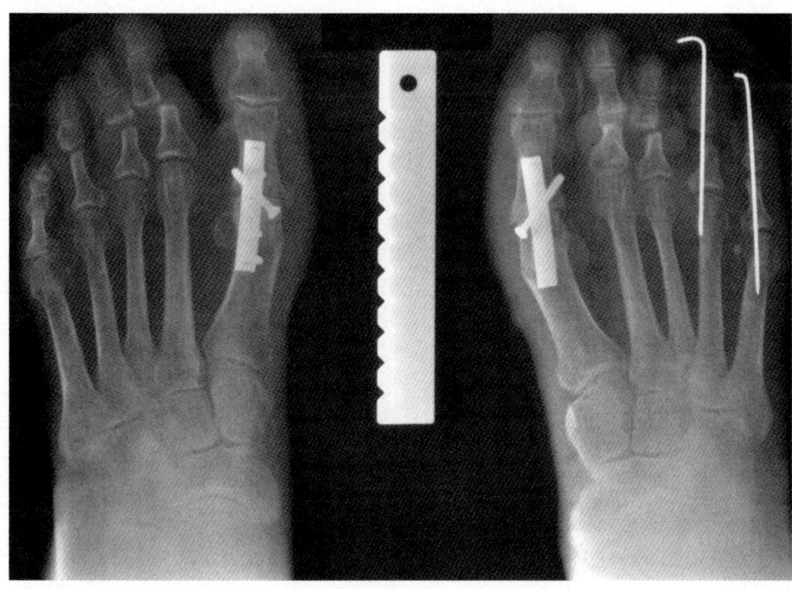


**Fig. 8-134** A: Illustration of resection arthroplasty and soft tissue repair with K-wire stabilization. B: Radiographs in a patient with failed bunion repairs and arthrodeses of the first metatarsal phalangeal (MTP) joints with plate and screw fixation. Soft tissue repairs and resection arthroplasties have been performed on the left second through fourth and right second through fifth digits with K-wire fixation of the right fourth and fifth articulations.

## Bunionette Deformities

Bunionette deformities are similar to the more common bunion deformity with hallux valgus, but they involve the lateral foot. The deformity was initially termed *tailor's bunion*. It was described in tailors who worked sitting cross-legged, thereby applying constant pressure to the fifth metatarsal head. In patients with bunionette deformity, there is a painful prominence on the fifth metatarsal head, which may be associated with overlying callus and bursal inflammation. There may also be lateral bowing of the fifth metatarsal. With more severe deformity, there is increase in the 4 to 5 metatarsal angle (see Fig. 8-135). These changes have resulted in three types of symptomatic bunionettes. Type 1 bunionette deformities present with a large metatarsal head, type 2 with lateral deviation of the fifth metatarsal, and type 3 with an increased 4 to 5 metatarsal angle (normal 8 degrees, range 3 to 10 degrees). Patients may have both bunion and bunionette deformities resulting in a splayed foot.

## Suggested Reading

Cohen BE, Nicholson CW. Bunionette deformity. *J Am Acad Orthop Surg*. 2007;15:300–307.

Karasick D. Preoperative assessment of symptomatic bunionette deformity: Radiologic findings. *AJR Am J Roentgenol.* 1995;164:147–149.

### Preoperative Imaging

Radiographic evaluation should include standing AP, lateral, and conventional oblique projections. The most critical is the standing AP radiograph as most critical measurements are obtained with this image.

**IMA:** Measured with lines along the axis of the fourth and fifth metatarsals (normal 8 degrees, range 3 to 10 degree) (Fig. 8-135A)

**Metatarsophalangeal angle:** Measured by lines along the axis of the fifth metatarsal and proximal phalanx (normal ≤10 degrees). Most symptomatic bunionettes are ≥16 degrees.

**Lateral deviation angle:** Measures lateral bowing of the distal fifth metatarsal. The angle is formed by a line along the axis of the metatarsal and a line along the proximal medial cortex (normal ≤3 degrees, most symptomatic bunionettes ≥8 degrees) (Fig. 8-135B)

**Metatarsal head width:** Measured by the greatest width perpendicular to the long axis (normal ≤13 mm).

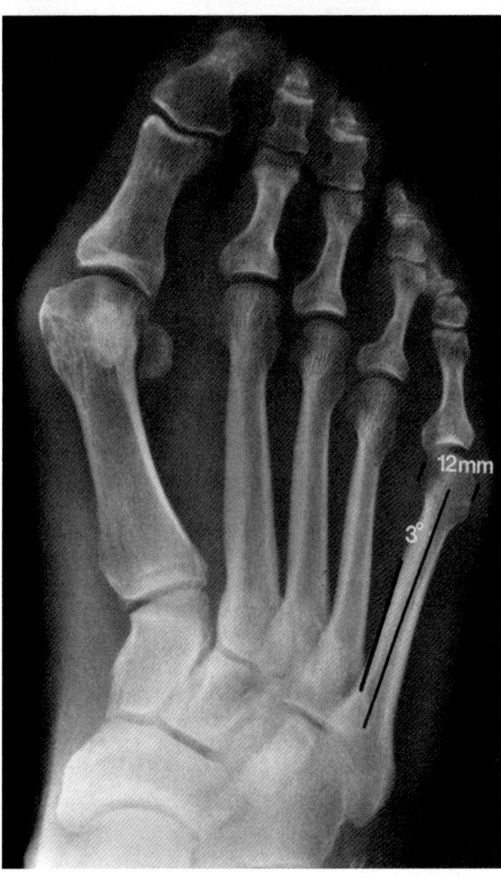


Fig. 8-135 Preoperative measurements for bunionette deformity. A: Standing anteroposterior (AP) radiographs of the feet in a patient with hallux valgus and bunion deformities. The 4 to 5 intermetatarsal angle (normal 8 degrees, range 3 to 10 degrees) measures 8 degrees. The metatarsophalangeal angle (normal ≤10 degrees) on the left measures 16 degrees. B: Standing anteroposterior (AP) radiograph demonstrating the lateral deviation angle measured by lines along the axis of the metatarsal and the proximal medial cortex (normal ≤3 degrees, most symptomatic bunionettes ≥8 degrees). In this case, the angle is normal measuring 3 degrees. The metatarsal head width measured at the widest region perpendicular to the long axis (*black line*) is 12 mm (normal ≤13 mm).

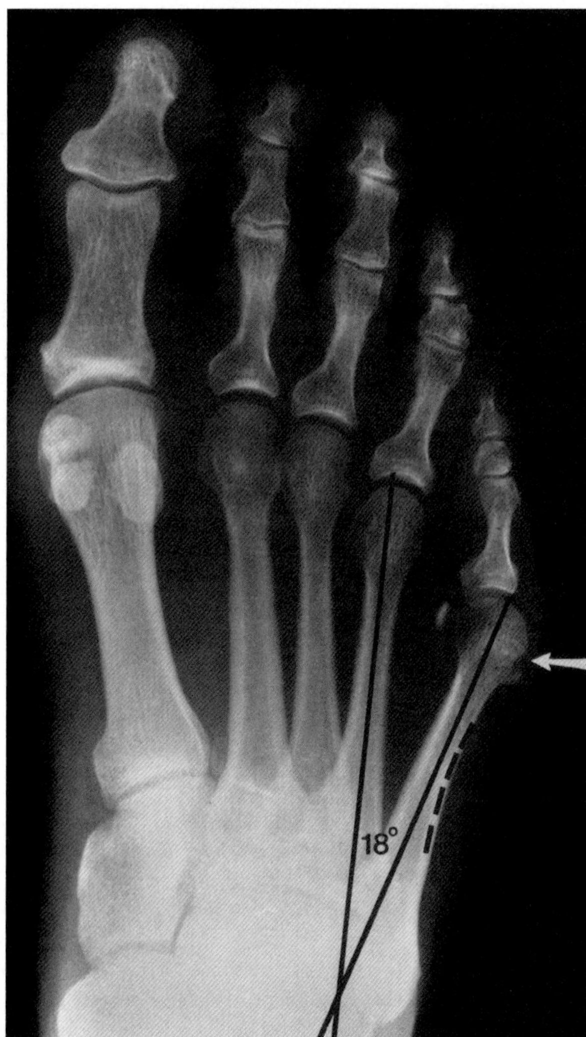


Fig. 8-136 Type 3 bunionette. Standing anteroposterior (AP) radiograph demonstrates prominence of the metatarsal head with a chronic erosion (*arrow*), lateral deviation (*broken line*) of the distal metatarsal, and an intermetatarsal angle increased to 18 degrees.

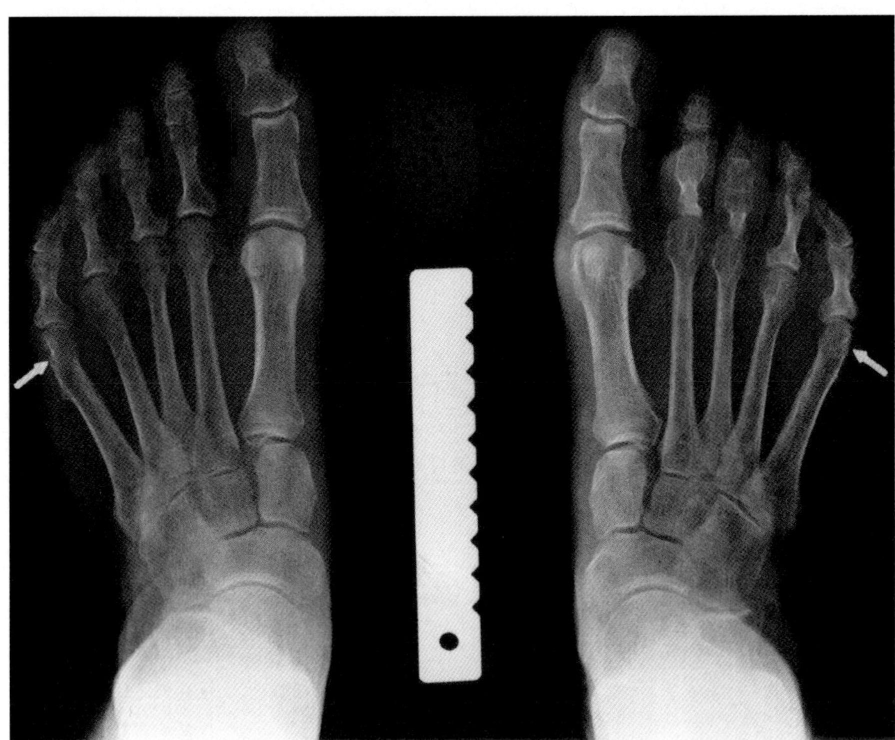

Fig. 8-137 Eminence resection and soft tissue repair. Standing anteroposterior (AP) radiographs following resection of the metatarsal head prominence (*arrows*) and reduction in the metatarsophalangeal angles.

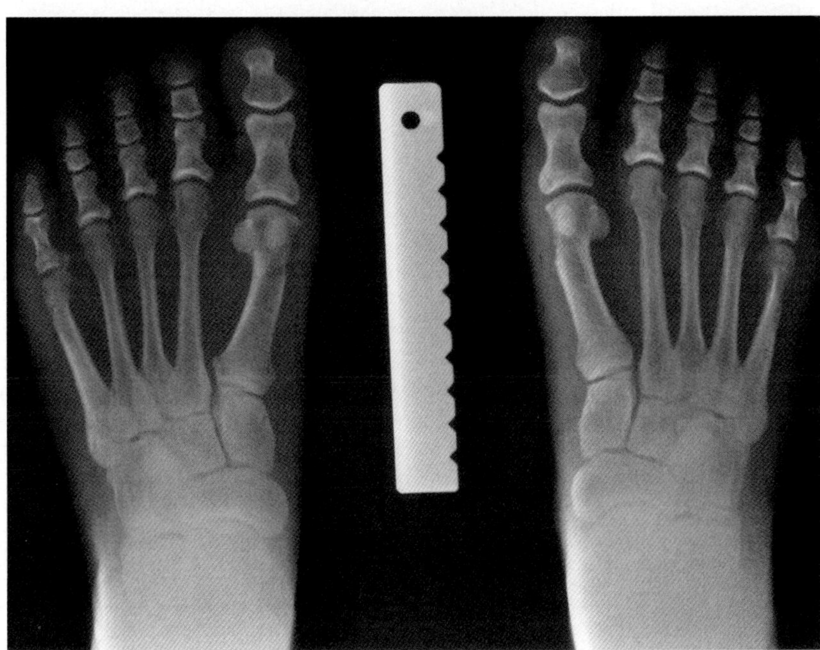

A

Fig. 8-138 Bilateral distal osteotomies for hallux valgus and bunionette repairs. Standing anteroposterior (AP) radiographs of the feet (A) demonstrate resection of the first and fifth eminences. The oblique radiographs (B and C) demonstrate the distal osteotomies of the first and fifth metatarsals.

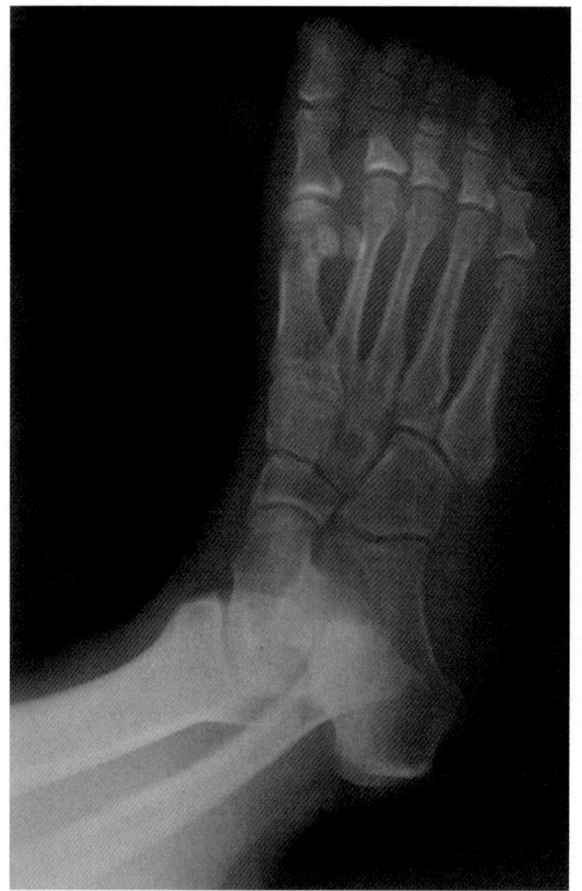

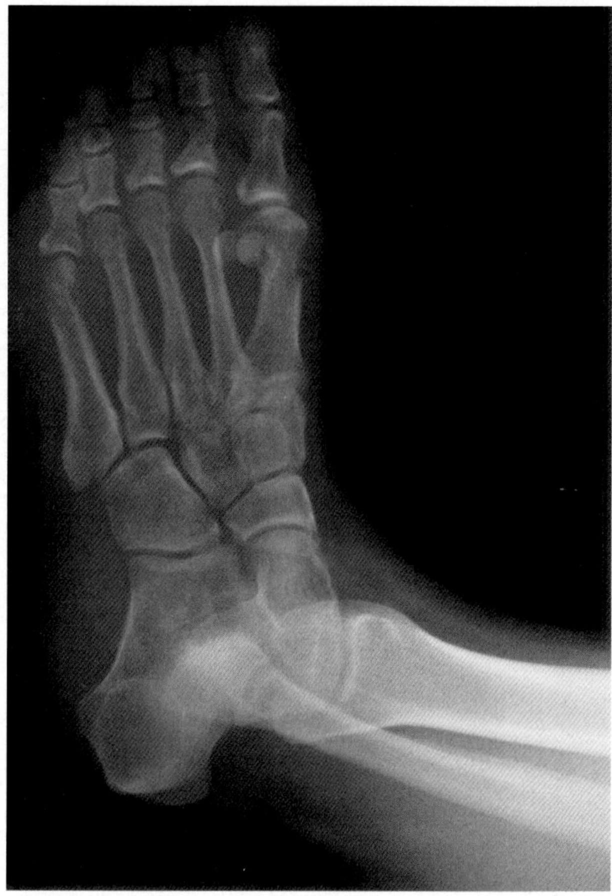

B C

Fig. 8-138 (*Continued*)

Increased width may also be due to rotation with a pronated foot (Fig. 8-135B)

## Suggested Reading


Fallot LM, Bucholz J. Analysis of tailor's bunion by radiographic and anatomic display. *J Am Podiatr Med Assoc.* 1980;70: 597–603.

Karasick D. Preoperative assessment of symptomatic bunionette deformity: Radiologic findings. *AJR Am J Roentgenol.* 1995; 164:147–149.

Kitaoka HB, Holiday A. Lateral condylar resection for bunionette deformities. *Clin Orthop.* 1991;278:183–192.


### Treatment Options

Conservative therapy includes wider shoes and padding to relieve pain. Pointed toe shoes should be avoided. Conservative therapy is ineffective in up to 20% of patients. Surgical intervention can reduce deformity, provide more stable alignment, and relieve pain. Multiple approaches can be used similar to hallux valgus repairs, including condylar or eminence resection, metatarsal head resection, and proximal, diaphyseal, or distal fifth metatarsal osteotomies. Surgical approaches are based on the type of deformity (see Fig. 8-136). Patients with a prominent metatarsal head or condyle (type 1) can be treated with resection of the eminence and soft tissue repair to improve alignment (see Fig. 8-137). In this setting the IMA is normal.

When the IMA is increased (Fig. 8-136) or the lateral deviation angle is increased, an osteotomy is the preferred approach (see Fig. 8-138). Osteotomies can be secured with K-wires or screws. Complications are similar to those described with hallux valgus repair.

## Suggested Reading


Berquist TH. *Radiology of the foot and ankle*, 2nd ed. Philadelphia: Lippincott Williams & Wilkins; 2000:479–526.

Cohen BE, Nicholson CW. Bunionette deformity. *J Am Acad Orthop Surg.* 2007;15:300–307.

Karasick D. Preoperative assessment of symptomatic bunionette deformity: Radiologic findings. *AJR Am J Roentgenol.* 1995; 164:147–149.

Kitaoka HB, Holiday A. Lateral condylar resection for bunionette deformities. *Clin Orthop.* 1991;278:183–192.

# 9 The Shoulder

This chapter will focus on imaging of shoulder trauma, arthroplasty, arthrodesis, and miscellaneous shoulder procedures requiring use of orthopaedic fixation devices and prostheses.

## Trauma

Shoulder fractures and dislocations of the glenohumeral and acromioclavicular joints are common. Conservative management may be effective in certain situations. However, operative intervention is commonly required. Clinical presentations, classifications when appropriate, treatment options, and imaging of postoperative complications will be reviewed in each section.

### Proximal Humeral Fractures

Proximal humeral fractures account for 5% of all fractures. These injuries occur most commonly in elderly osteoporotic patients and are typically associated with minor trauma, such as a fall. Morbidity is similar to hip fractures in this population. In younger patients, the mechanism of injury is more often high-velocity trauma (motor vehicle accidents, etc.).

Multiple classifications have been used for proximal humeral fractures. Fracture lines tend to follow the physeal lines that divide the humerus into four parts: (a) the head, (b) the greater tuberosity, (c) the lesser tuberosity, and (d) the shaft (see Fig. 9-1). The Neer classification was proposed in 1970. This system includes the four segments of the humerus and addresses vascular isolation of the head and the degree of displacement. As defined by Neer, fragments are considered displaced if there is >1 cm of separation or >45 degrees of angulation of a fragment with respect to the others (see Fig. 9-2). Most fractures are undisplaced (80% to 85%) using the Neer classification.

#### Neer classification

**One-part fracture:** No fragments displaced (80%)

**Two-part fracture:** One fragment displaced (13%) (Fig. 9-2)

**Three-part fracture:** Displacement of the surgical neck and either the greater or lesser tuberosity (3%)

**Four-part fracture:** Displaced fractures of the greater tuberosities and surgical neck (4%) (see Fig. 9-3)

Other classifications include the AO (Arbeitgemeinshaft fur osteosynthesefragen) classification that includes three categories based on the vascular isolation of the articular (head) fragment and the likelihood of avascular necrosis. Type A has no vascular isolation and a low incidence of avascular necrosis (extracapsular with two to four fragments). Type B fractures have partial isolation of the articular fragment and type C fractures have an isolated articular fragment with a high incidence of avascular necrosis (Fig. 9-3). There are subcategories

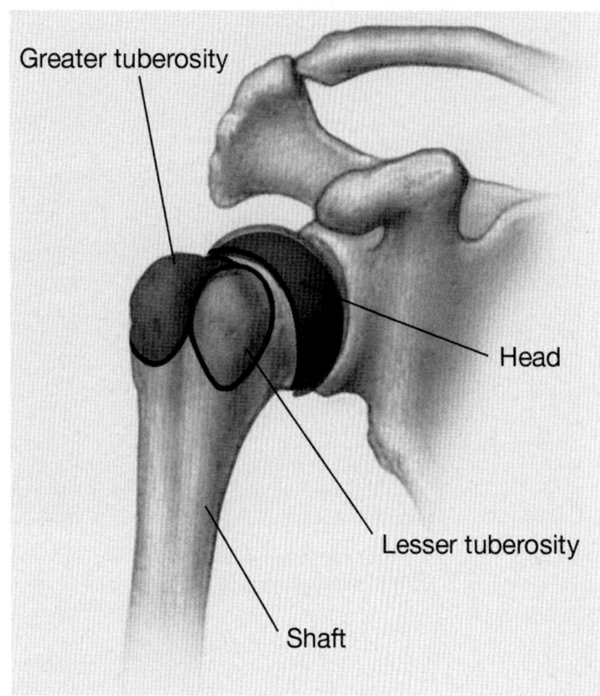


Fig. 9-1 Illustration of the proximal humerus demonstrating the four segments involved in proximal fractures.

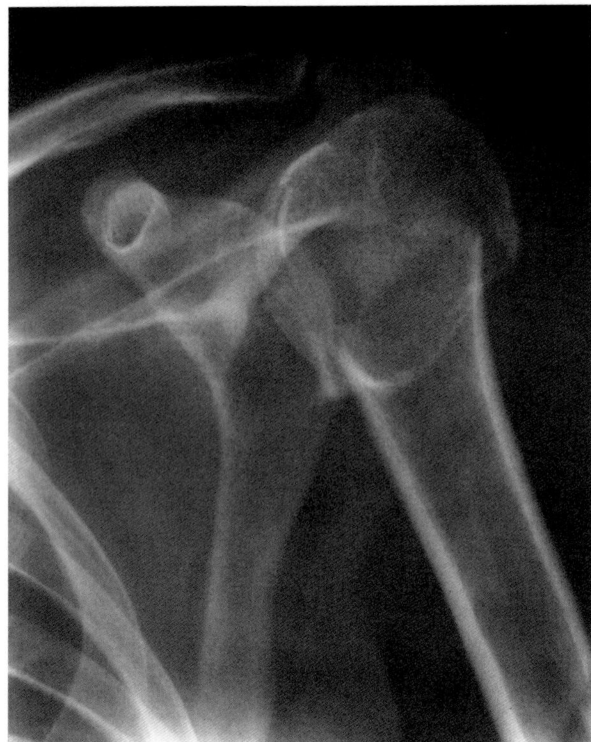


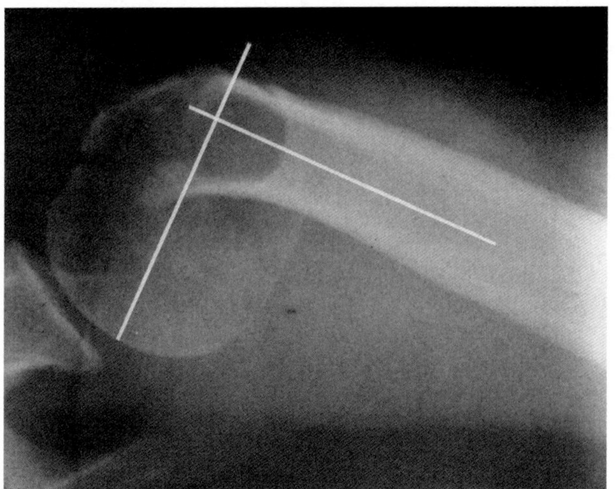


Fig. 9-2 Two-part fracture. Anteroposterior (AP) (A) and axillary (B) radiographs demonstrate a fracture of the humeral neck and tuberosity. The head is angulated over 45 degrees making this a two-part fracture.

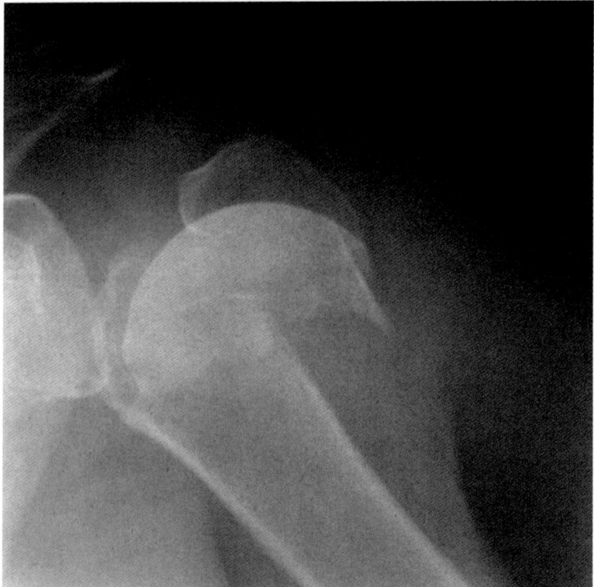


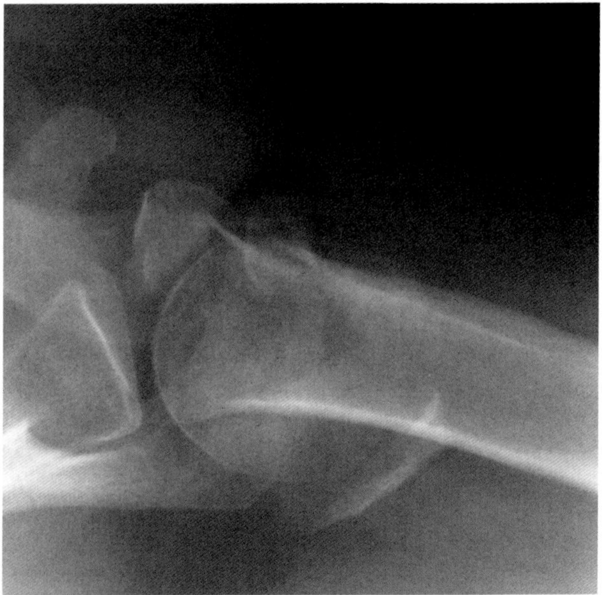


Fig. 9-3 Four-part fracture. Anteroposterior (AP) (A) and axillary (B) radiographs demonstrating displacement of >1 cm of all fragments (head, tuberosities, and shaft).

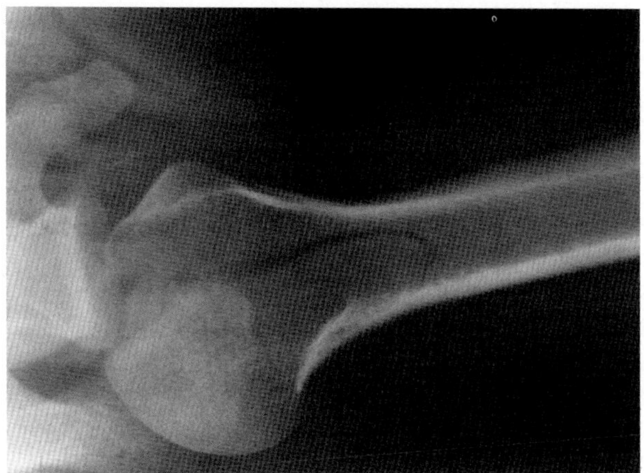

Fig. 9-4 Orthopaedic Trauma Association B3.1. Axillary radiograph demonstrates a vertical cleft fracture with the greater tuberosity intact.

with all three types due to increasing complexity. The Orthopaedic Trauma Association classification is even more complex and includes the degree of displacement of each fragment, angulation, impaction, and associated dislocations (see Fig. 9-4). Imagers should become familiar with the system used by the surgeons with whom they interact. Agreement on which classification is best is difficult due to frequent interobserver disagreement. Some use three-dimensional reconstructions of computed tomographic (CT) images to classify proximal humeral fractures.

## Suggested Reading

Edelson G, Kelly I, Vigder F, et al. A three-dimensional classification for fractures of the proximal humerus. *J Bone Joint Surg*. 2004;86B:413–425.

Neer CS II. Displaced proximal humeral fractures: Classification and evaluation. *J Bone Joint Surg*. 1970;52A:1077–1089.

Orthopaedic Trauma Association Committee on Coding and Classification. *J Orthop Trauma*. 1996;10:1–155.

### Preoperative Imaging

Imaging of patients with suspected proximal humeral fractures should include anteroposterior (AP), scapular Y, and axillary projections. The last may be difficult for some patients. Therefore, a transthoracic radiograph provides a lateral view and is excellent for evaluation of humeral head rotation (see Fig. 9-5). CT with coronal and sagittal reformatting or three-dimensional reconstruction is optimal for evaluating fragment displacement and angulation (see Fig. 9-6). Three-dimensional reconstructions may also improve the consistency for classification.

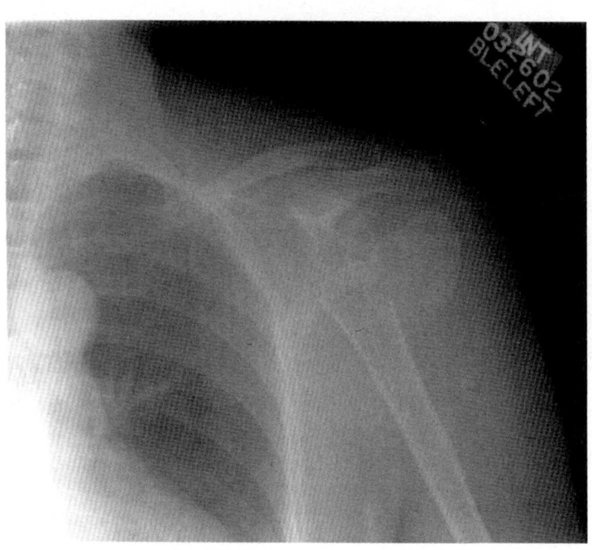


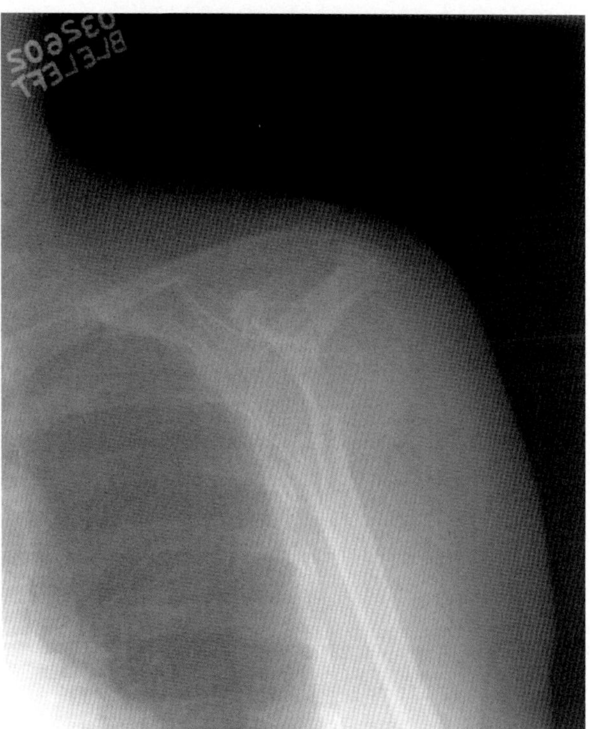


Fig. 9-5 Radiographs of a proximal humeral fracture (three part). Anteroposterior (AP) (A), scapular Y or Neer view (B), and transthoracic (C) projection of a comminuted proximal humeral fracture with displacement of the head and tuberosity. The transthoracic view provides an image at 90 degrees to the AP view and demonstrates the position of the humeral head in relation to the shaft. There is 65 degrees of posterior rotation of the humeral head in addition to the displacement.

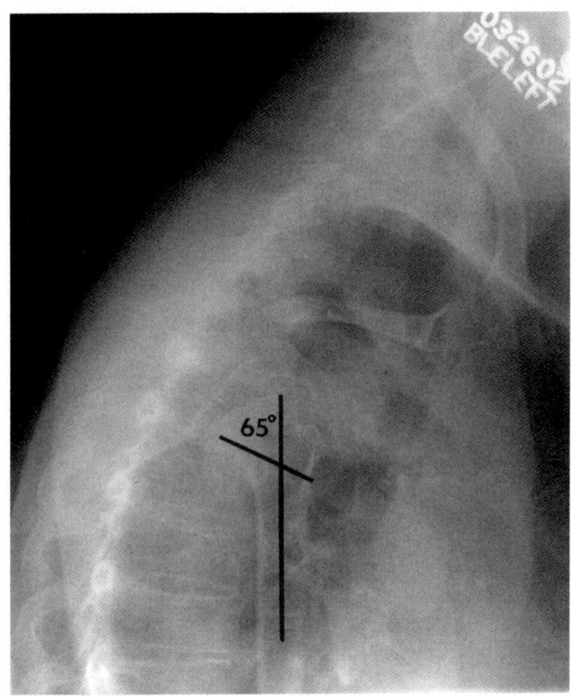


C

Fig. 9-5 *(Continued)*

## SUGGESTED READING

Burstein AH, Adler LM, Blank JE, et al. Evaluation of the Neer system of classification of proximal humeral fractures with computerized tomography scans and plain radiographs. *J Bone Joint Surg.* 1996;78A:1371–1375.

### Treatment Options

Treatment of proximal humeral fractures is based on the fracture classification, patient age, comorbidities, activity, and bone quality. Treatment options include closed reduction, open reduction and internal fixation, and arthroplasty. Hemiarthroplasty is usually performed unless there is significant glenoid articular disease.

One- and two-part fractures (Fig. 9-6) may be treated conservatively with closed reduction. Greater tuberosity fractures displaced 5 mm or more should be internally fixed to avoid loss of function and axillary nerve injury. Lesser tuberosity fractures tend to displace medially, but can usually be treated with closed reduction.

Three- and four-part fractures (Fig. 9-5) are more complex. In elderly patients with significant comorbidities, fractures may be treated with closed reduction. Significant loss of motion is

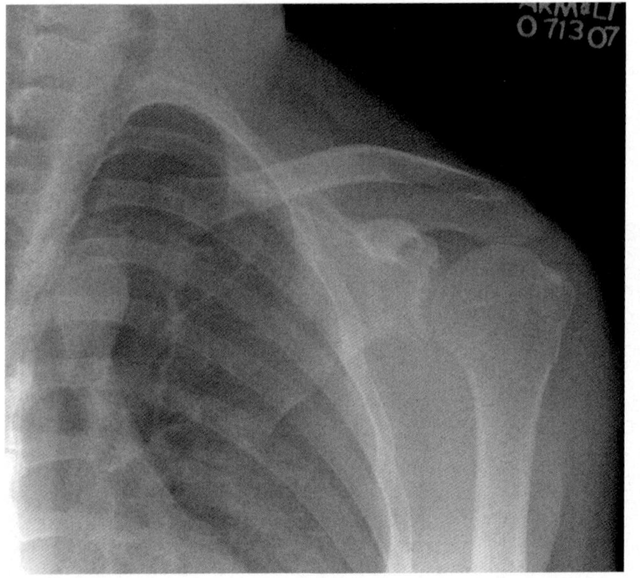

A

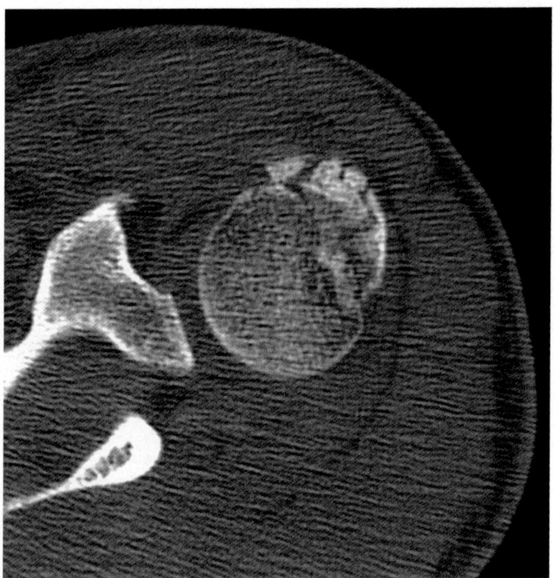

B

Fig. 9-6 Radiographic and computed tomographic (CT) images of a one-part fracture. Radiograph (A) and axial (B), coronal (C), sagittal (D), and three-dimensional (E and F) reformatted images demonstrating a minimally displaced comminuted fracture involving the greater tuberosity with sparing of the biceps groove.

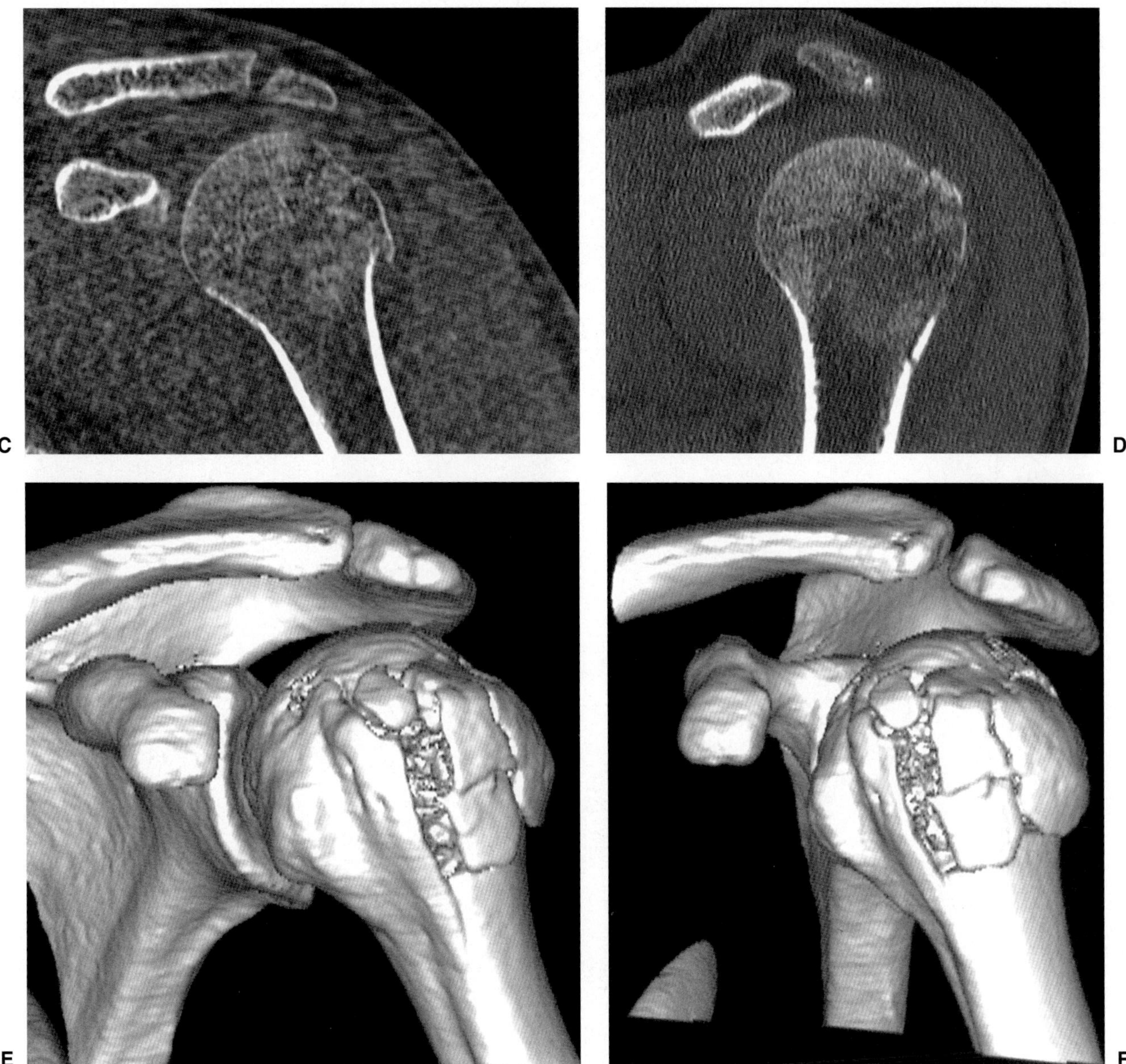


Fig. 9-6 (*Continued*)

common. Valgus-impacted head fragments are at less risk for avascular necrosis so results may be satisfactory with closed reduction. Open reduction may be accomplished with plate and screw fixation (see Fig. 9-7), intramedullary nails (see Fig. 9-8), or tension band constructs (see Fig. 9-9). Hemiarthroplasty is also an option. This approach is commonly performed on elderly patients with osteoporotic bone because internal fixation is more complex in this setting (see Fig. 9-10).

## Suggested Reading

Jacob RP, Miniaci A, Anson PS, et al. Four-part valgus impacted fractures of the proximal humerus. *J Bone Joint Surg.* 1991;73B:295–298.

Naranja RJ, Iannoti JP. Displaced three and four-part proximal humeral fractures: Evaluation and management. *J Am Acad Orthop Surg.* 2000;8:373–382.

Neer CS II. Displaced proximal humeral fractures: Part II. Treatment of three and four-part displacement. *J Bone Joint Surg*. 1970;52A:1090–1103.

## Imaging of Postoperative Complications

Complications following repair of proximal humeral fractures may be related to the initial injury or surgical approaches. Proximal humeral fractures are associated with neurovascular injuries in 21% to 36% of cases. The axillary nerve is most frequently injured and this may result in permanent motor dysfunction. Nerve injury is most common following anterior fracture dislocations. Most vascular injuries (84%) occur in elderly patients and more than half are associated with brachial plexus injuries. Diagnosis may be accomplished clinically (loss of sensation over the lateral deltoid with axillary nerve injury) or magnetic resonance imaging (MRI). Vascular injuries can be clarified with angiography because magnetic resonance (MR) angiography can be difficult following acute trauma. The rotator cuff and biceps are typically involved. Interposition

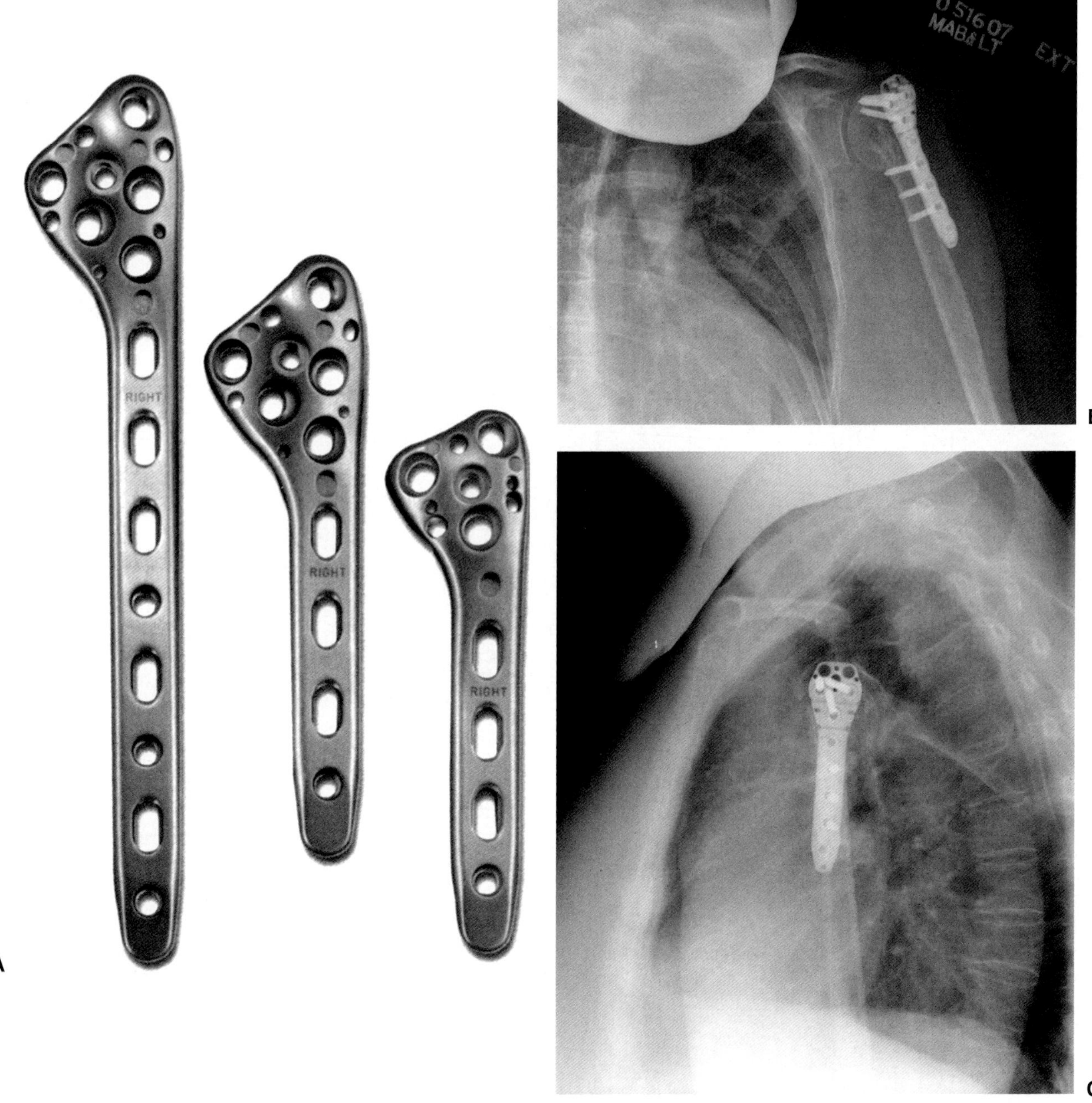


**Fig. 9-7** Internal fixation with locking plate and screws. **A:** Proximal humeral locking plates. (Courtesy of Acumed, Hillsboro, Oregon.) Anteroposterior (AP) **(B)** and transthoracic **(C)** views following plate and screw fixation of a three-part fracture.

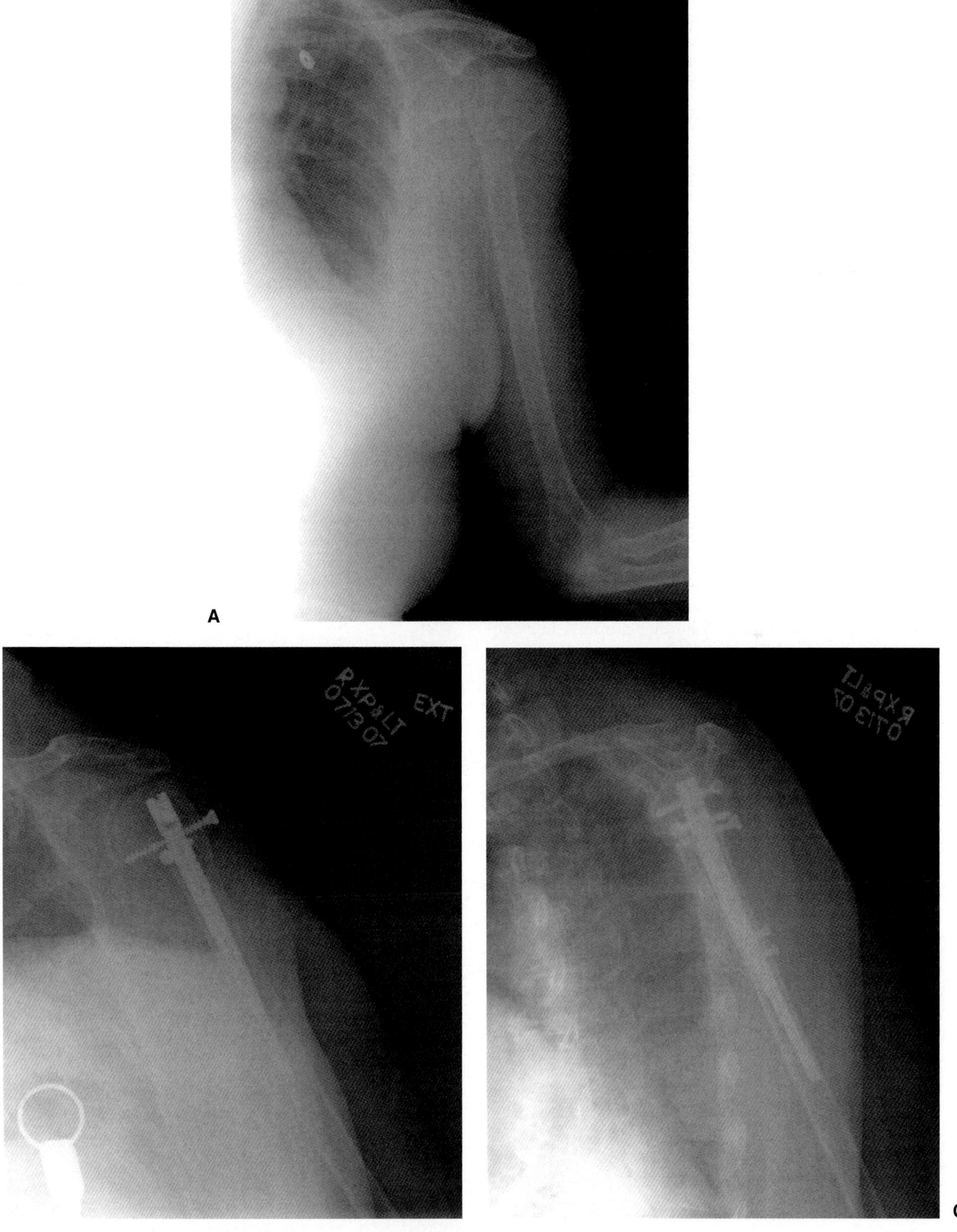


Fig. 9-8 Intramedullary nail fixation. A: Radiograph demonstrating a two-part proximal humeral fracture with undisplaced tuberosity fragments. Anteroposterior (AP) (B) and scapular Y (C) views following intramedullary nail and screw fixation of the proximal fragments with distal locking screws.

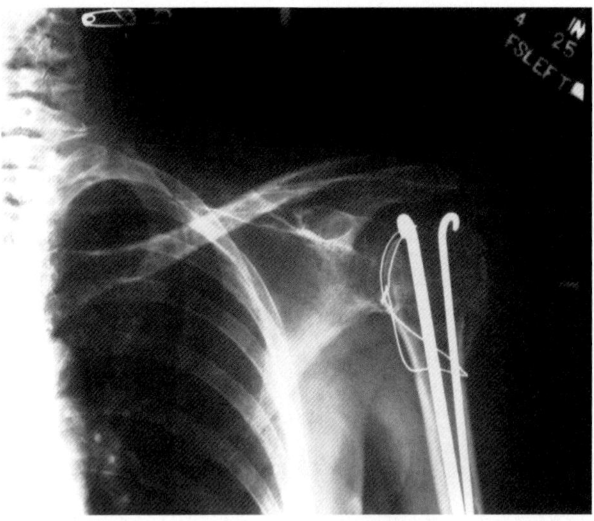


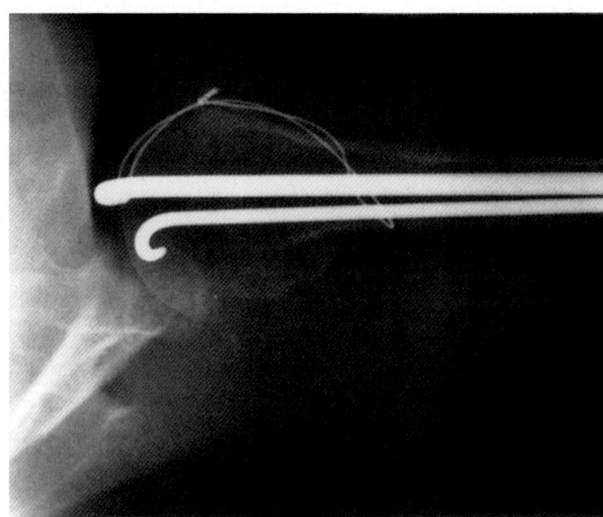

Fig. 9-9 Comminuted minimally displaced proximal humeral fracture. Anteroposterior (AP) (A) and axillary (B) radiographs demonstrate internal fixation with Rush rods and tension band wire. The Rush rods extend into the subacromial space, which may result in impingement.

of the biceps tendon between tuberosity fragments will prevent healing. Rotator cuff disruptions and tendon interposition can be evaluated with CT, MRI, or conventional arthrograms (see Fig. 9-11).

Arthrosis and loss of range of motion occur with both closed and open treatment approaches (see Fig. 9-12). Adhesive capsulitis is also fairly common following proximal humeral fractures. This may be difficult to detect unless conventional arthrography is performed and the actual capsular volume measured. Mild to moderate (5 to 10 mL) capsulitis may respond to distention arthrography.

Avascular necrosis occurs in up to 14% of three-part fractures treated with closed reduction and the incidence is higher with four-part fractures. Imaging may be hindered with internal fixation devices. However, aggressive approaches in treatment approaches for three- and four-part fractures (internal fixation or hemiarthroplasty) reduce the need to image patients following treatment. Patients treated with closed reduction or minimal internal fixation hardware can be evaluated with MRI.

Implant failure, malunion, and nonunion may be evident on serial radiographs (see Fig. 9-13). Evaluation of nonunion is most easily accomplished with CT with reformatting in the coronal and sagittal planes in the presence of orthopaedic hardware. In patients treated with closed reduction, MRI may also be helpful. The fracture margins will have low signal

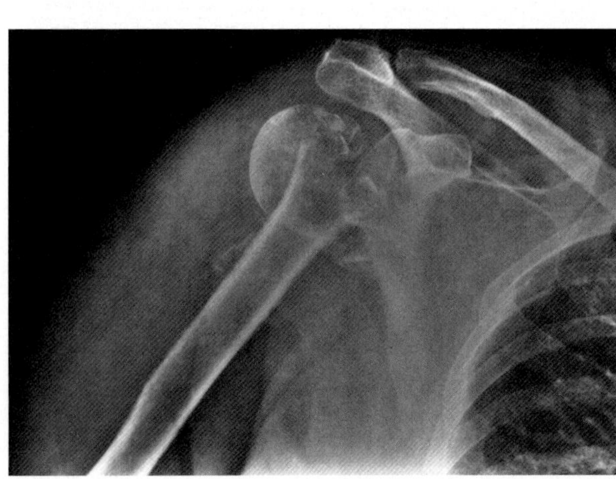

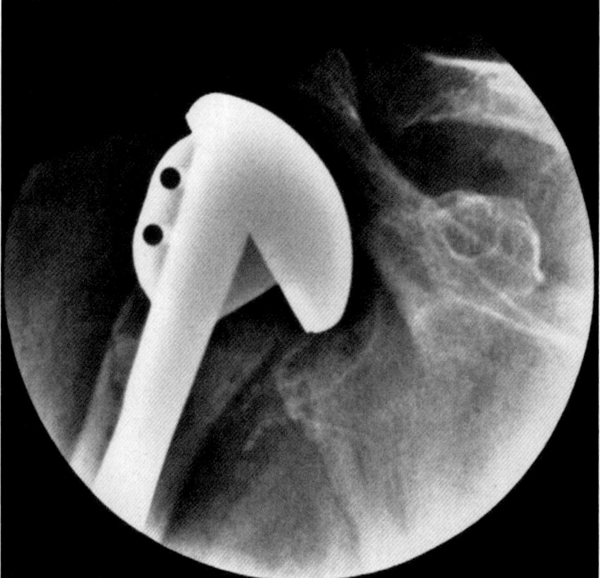

Fig. 9-10 Anteroposterior (AP) radiograph (A) demonstrating a four-part fracture in an elderly woman. B: Operative image following hemiarthroplasty.

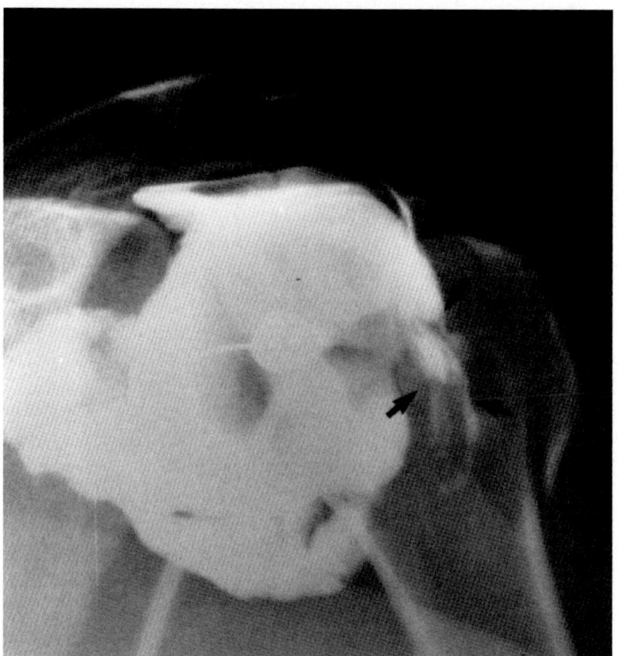

Fig. 9-11 Conventional arthrogram demonstrating entrapment of the biceps tendon (*arrows*) between the tuberosity fragments.

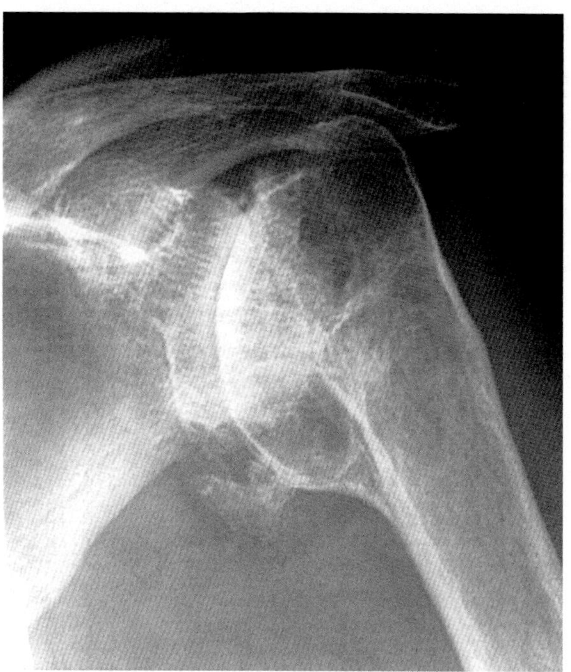

Fig. 9-12 Old three-part fracture treated with closed reduction in an 85-year old woman. There is complete loss of joint space with reduced humeroacromial space and no motion in the glenohumeral joint.

intensity with high signal intensity between the fragments on T2-weighted sequences.

## Clavicle Fractures

Clavicle fractures are common in neonates, children, and adults. Clavicle fractures account for 5% to 10% of adult fractures and 35% to 45% of shoulder-related fractures. The mechanism of injury may be direct trauma (fall on the shoulder) or a fall on the outstretched hand. Allman divided clavicular fractures by location into group I—middle third, group II—distal, and group III—proximal. Most fractures (72% to 80%) involve the

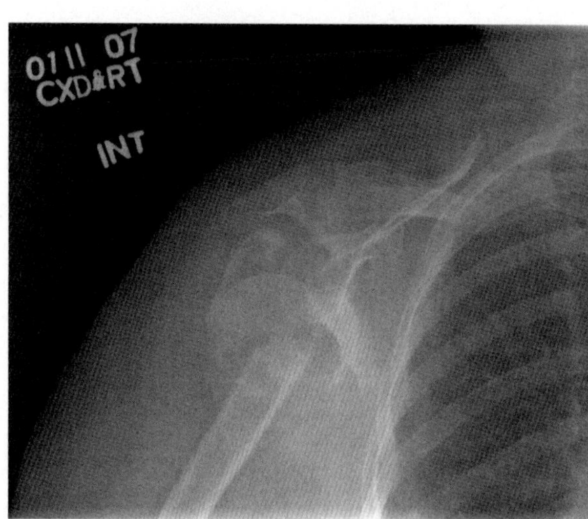


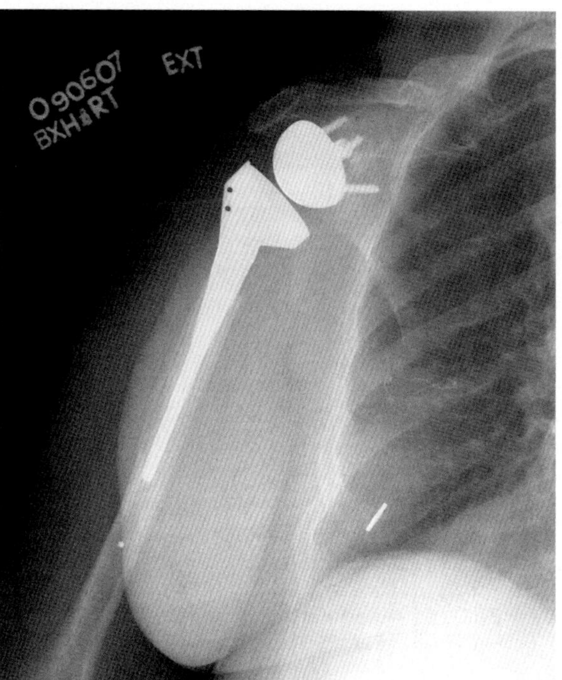


A B

Fig. 9-13 Nonunion. A: Radiograph demonstrating nonunion of a four-part fracture. B: The patient was treated with a reverse shoulder arthroplasty.

mid clavicle, whereas 20% to 30% of fractures involve the distal clavicle. Proximal or medial clavicular fractures are uncommon (2% to 5%). The Neer modification further subdivides groups II and III based on ligament and articular involvement and the degree of comminution. The Orthopaedic Trauma Association classification is more complex and is based on location, fracture line orientation, comminution, and articular involvement. The Allman classification with the Neer modification is commonly used (see Fig. 9-14).

### NEER MODIFICATION OF THE ALLMAN CLASSIFICATION (FIG. 9-14)

| | |
|---|---|
| Group I | Fractures of the middle third (Fig. 9-14A) |
| Group II | Fractures of the distal third (Fig. 9-14B) |
| Type I | Minimally displaced interligamentous (Fig. 9-14C) |
| Type II | Fragment proximal to ligaments displaced (Fig. 9-14D) |
| Type IIA | Both distal ligaments attached |
| Type IIB | One or both torn (conoid, trapezoid) |
| Type III | Fractures involve articular surface (Fig. 9-14E) |
| Type IV | Ligaments intact to periosteum |
| Type V | Comminuted |
| Group III | Fracture of the proximal third |
| Type I | Minimal displacement (Fig. 9-14F) |
| Type II | Displaced (Fig. 9-14G) |
| Type III | Articular (Fig. 9-14H) |
| Type IV | Epiphyseal separation (immature skeleton) |
| Type V | Comminuted |

## SUGGESTED READING

Allman FL Jr. Fractures and ligamentous injuries of the clavicle and its articulations. *J Bone Joint Surg*. 1967;49A:774–784.

Neer CS II. Fractures of the distal third of the clavicle. *Clin Orthop*. 1968;58:43–50.

Webber MC, Haines JF. The treatment of lateral clavicle fractures. *Injury* 2000;31:175–179.

### Pretreatment Imaging

Imaging of patients with suspected clavicular injuries should include AP and angled AP (15 degrees normally or 40 degrees cephalad for subtle injuries) projections to include the entire clavicle and acromioclavicular and sternoclavicular articulations (see Fig. 9-15). The mid and distal aspects of the clavicle are easily evaluated on these views. The medial clavicle and its articulation are more difficult to visualize due to bony overlap. Although there are several techniques that can be used to better visualize the medial clavicle, CT is most often performed to better define this region (see Fig. 9-16).

Stress views can be performed on patients with suspected ligament injury and acromioclavicular separation. However, this approach is usually reserved for stable injuries to avoid further displacement of the clavicle fracture.

## SUGGESTED READING

Cofield RH, Berquist TH. The shoulder. In: Berquist TH. *Imaging of orthopaedic trauma*, 2nd ed. New York: Raven Press; 1992:579–657.

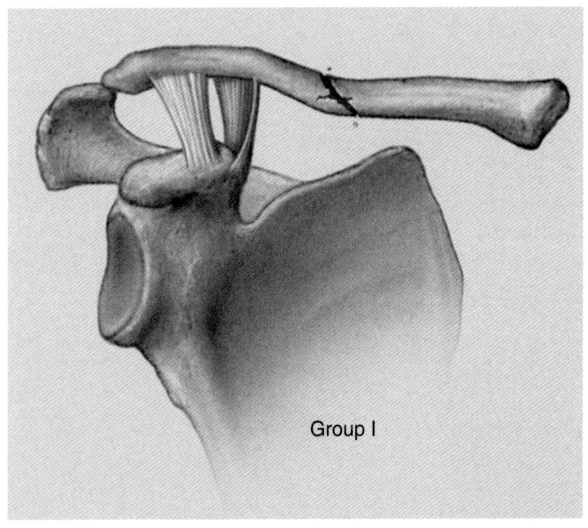


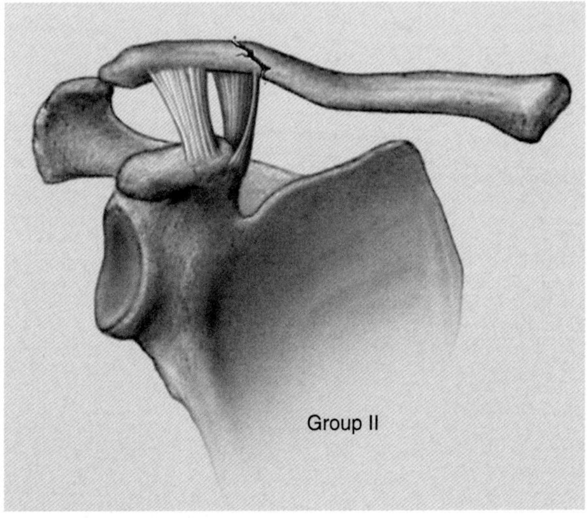


**Fig. 9-14** Neer modification of the Allman clavicle fracture classification. **A:** Group I—fractures of the middle third of the clavicle. **B:** Group II—fractures of the distal third of the clavicle. **C:** Group II, type I—fracture of the distal clavicle between the ligaments. **D:** Group II, type II—fracture of the distal clavicle proximal to the ligaments with elevated medial fragment. **E:** Group II, type III—comminuted fracture of the distal articular surface. **F:** Group III, type I—minimally displaced fracture of the medial clavicle. **G:** Group III, type II—displaced fracture of the medial clavicle with elevation of the distal fragment. **H:** Group III, type III—comminuted medial articular fracture.

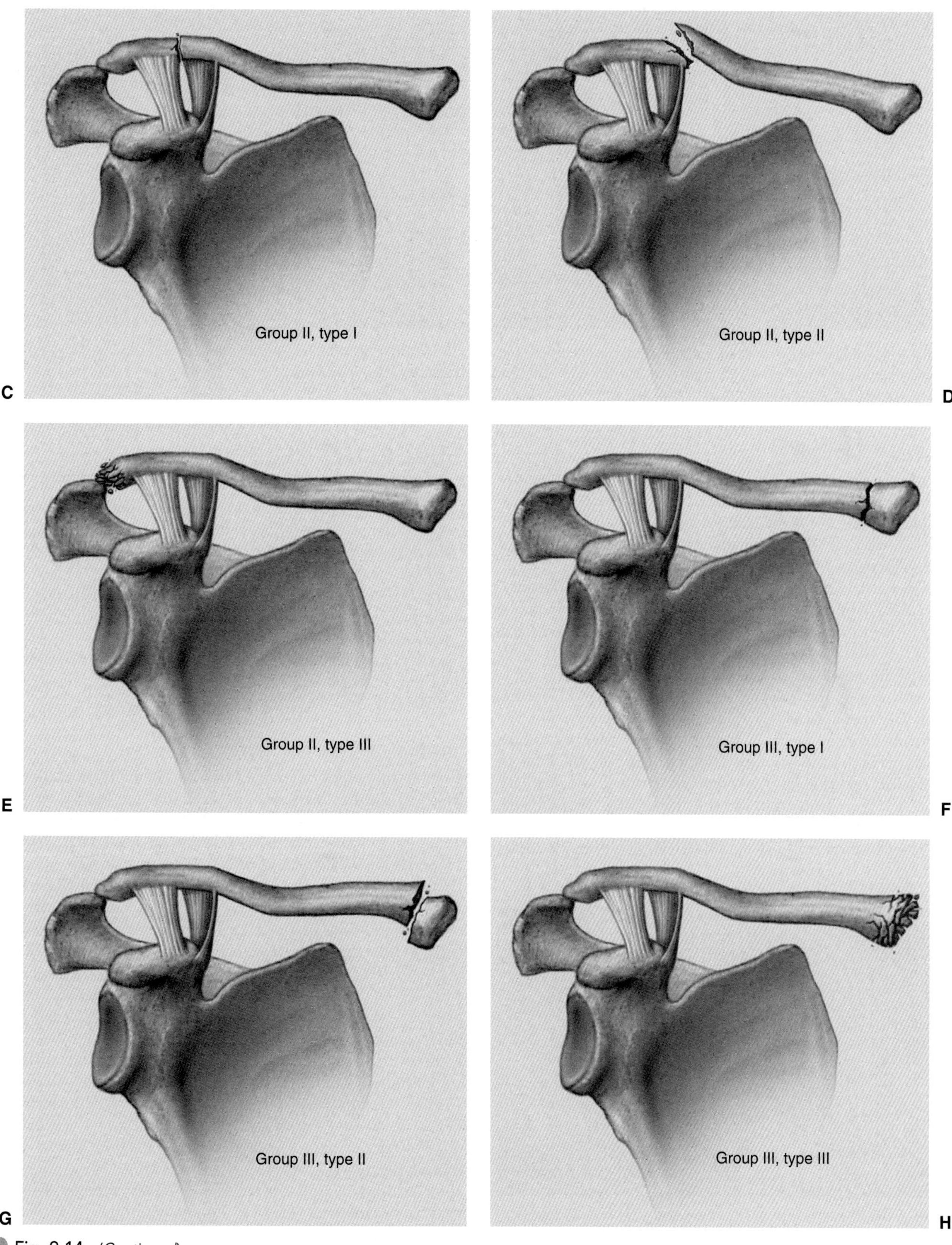


Fig. 9-14 (*Continued*)

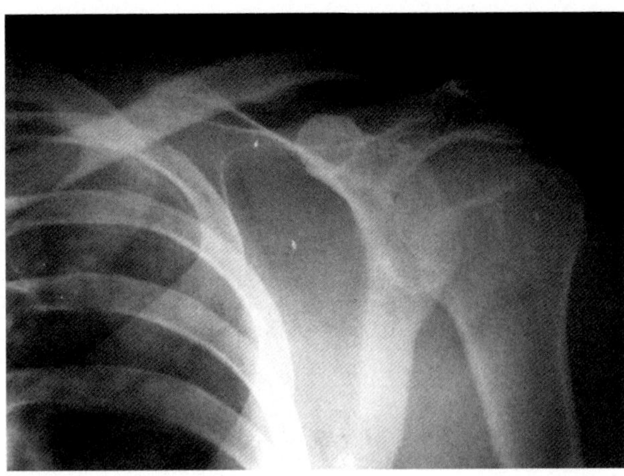

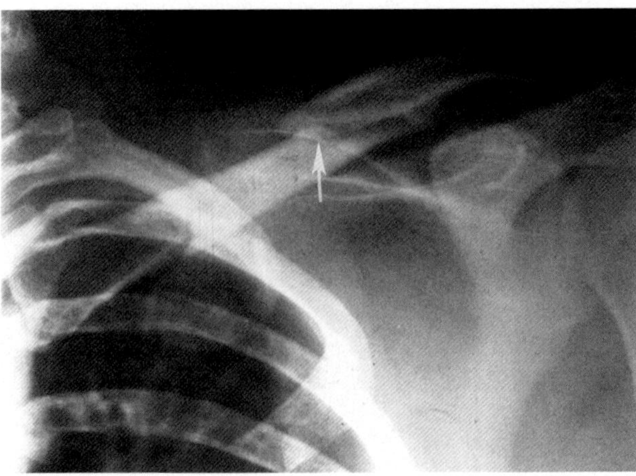

**Fig. 9-15** Minimally displaced fracture of the mid clavicle (group I). The anteroposterior (AP) (**A**) radiograph does not clearly demonstrate the fracture. The fracture is clearly identified (*arrow*) on the angled (15 degrees cephalad) view (**B**).

### Treatment Options

Conservative treatment is most often employed for treatment of clavicle fractures, specifically medial and mid-clavicle fractures. A sling or figure-of-eight brace is typically used for approximately 6 weeks with early shoulder, elbow, and hand range of motion exercises when tolerated by the patient.

Operative intervention is considered for cosmetic deformity, shortening of mid clavicle fractures >2 cm, and distal fractures. The incidence of nonunion is highest with shortening and displaced distal clavicular fractures (see Fig. 9-17). Treatment of distal third fractures has been controversial. Group II type II fractures are at the level of the coracoclavicular ligaments. Type IIA fractures are proximal to the ligaments and the ligaments remain intact. Type IIB injuries have significant displacement of the fracture fragments due to the loss of downward restraint of the coracoclavicular ligaments (see Fig. 9-18). Excellent surgical results have been reported with intramedullary pin or wire fixation and ligament repair. Plate and screw fixation is also an option (see Figs. 9-19 and 9-20).

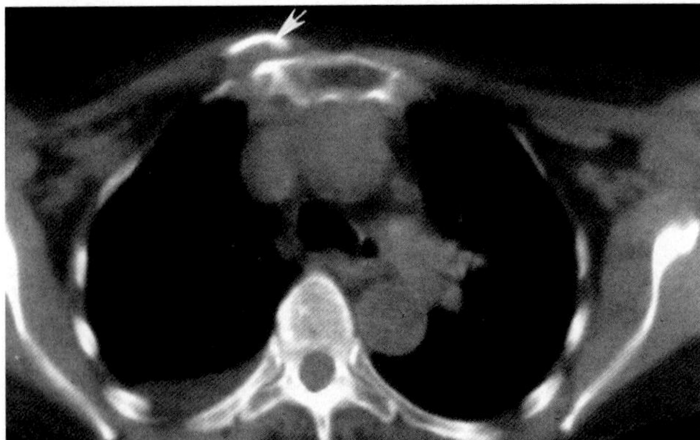

**Fig. 9-16** Axial computed tomographic (CT) image demonstrating a medial fracture dislocation (*arrow*) (group III, type III).

## Suggested Reading

Canadian Orthopaedic Trauma Society. Nonoperative treatment compared with plate fixation of displaced midshaft clavicle fractures. A multicenter, randomized clinical trial. *J Bone Joint Surg*. 2007;89A:1–10.

Chen CH, Chen WJ, Shih CH. Surgical treatment of distal clavicle fracture with coracoclavicular ligament disruption. *J Trauma*. 2002;52:72–78.

Neer CS II. Fracture of the distal clavicle with detachment of the coracoclavicular ligaments in adults. *J Trauma*. 1963; 3:99–110.

### Imaging of Complications

Complications may be related to the type of injury or treatment. In the past, the incidence of malunion and nonunion was considered to be insignificant. However, in recent years nonunion in displaced midshaft fractures has been reported to be 15% with unsatisfactory patient outcomes in up to 32% of cases. Distal third fractures are less frequent compared to midshaft fractures, but they account for half of nonunions. Imaging of nonunion can be accomplished with serial radiographs (Fig. 9-19). However, if callus and healing potential need to be better defined it is best to evaluate the fracture with CT with reformatted images in the appropriate image planes. The incidence of nonunion in displaced midshaft and distal clavicle fractures can be reduced significantly (2.2%) with operative intervention. Surgical treatment is not without complications. Migration of wires and pins has been described. Hardware removal for pain and irritation may also be necessary in up to 8% of patients. Other complications related to operative intervention include wound infection (4.8%) and transient brachial plexus neuropathy (13%). Other reported complications regardless of treatment include complex regional pain syndrome and thoracic outlet syndrome. The latter may require conventional or MR angiography for diagnosis.

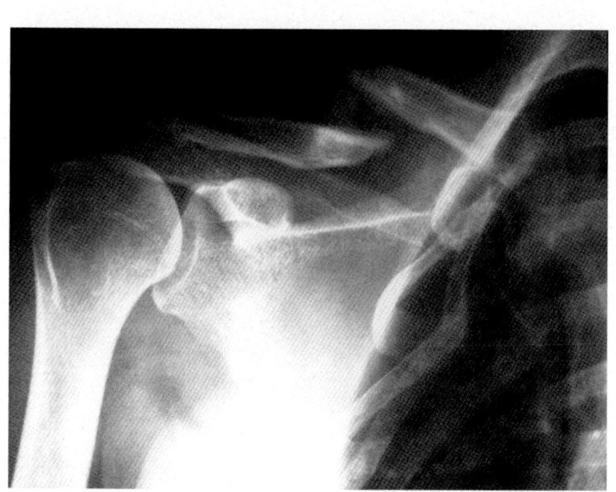

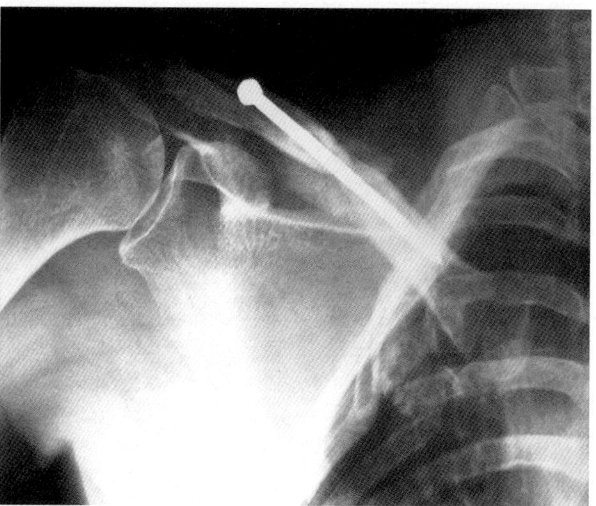

Fig. 9-17 A: Group I mid clavicle fracture with >2 cm of shortening and nonunion. B: Radiograph following reduction with an intramedullary pin.

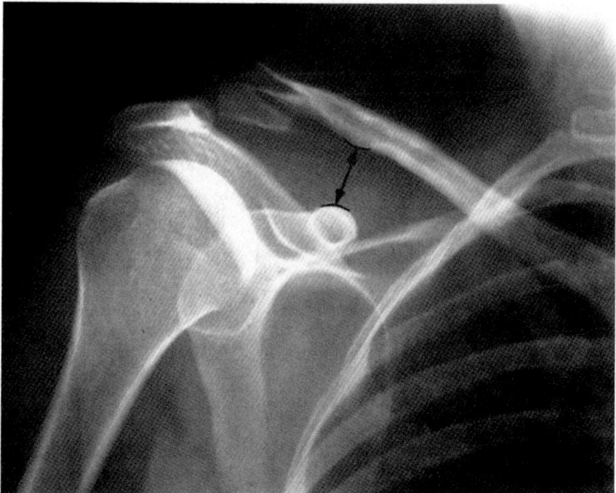

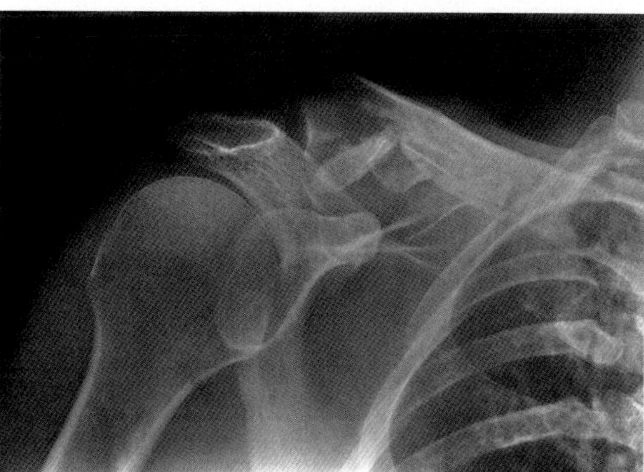

Fig. 9-18 A: Group II, type IIB fracture of the distal clavicle with upward displacement and increase in the coracoclavicular space (*curved lines, double arrow*) due to associated rupture of both the conoid and trapezoid ligaments. B: Comminuted fracture at the level of the ligaments with avulsed fragments inferiorly and elevation of the major medial fragment (group II, type V).

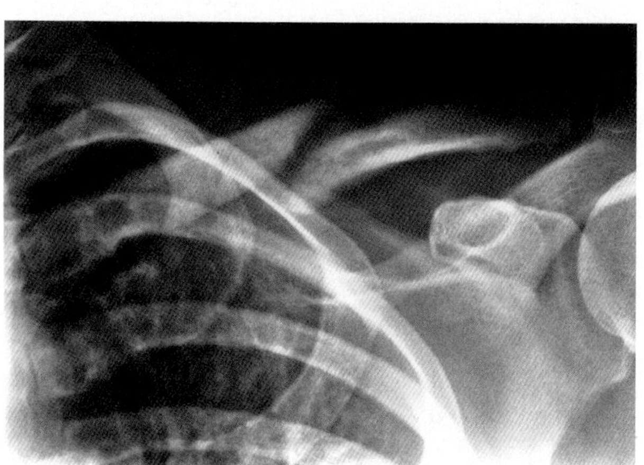

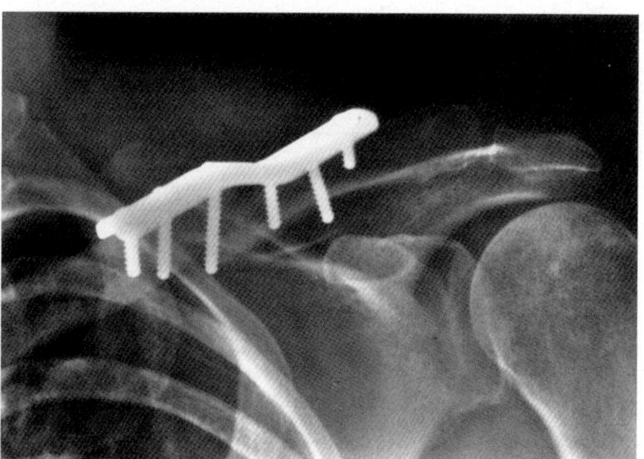

Fig. 9-19 A: Nonunion of a mid clavicle fracture treated with plate and screw fixation (B).

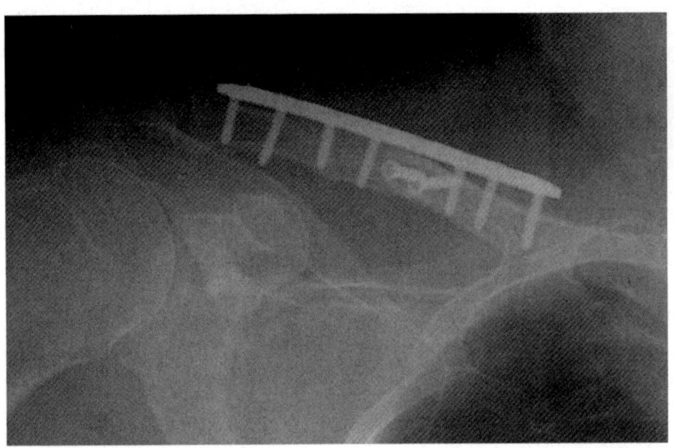

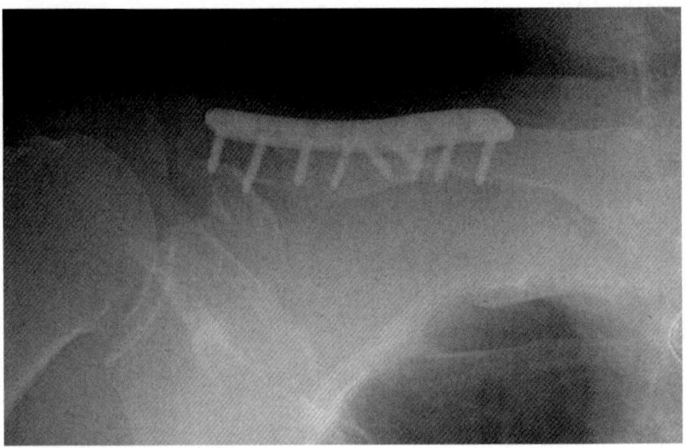

Fig. 9-20 Anteroposterior (AP) (A) and angled AP (B) radiographs following locking plate and screw fixation of a mid clavicle fracture. There are also several interfragmentary screws.

Instability or residual symptoms in the acromioclavicular joint can be evaluated with stress views once the fracture is considered healed clinically.

## Suggested Reading

Canadian Orthopaedic Trauma Society. Nonoperative treatment compared with plate fixation of displaced midshaft clavicle fractures. A multicenter, randomized clinical trial. *J Bone Joint Surg*. 2007;89A:1–10.

Connolly JF, Dehne R. Nonunion of the clavicle and thoracic outlet syndrome. *J Trauma*. 1989;29:1127–1132.

### Scapular Fractures

Scapular fractures are uncommon, accounting for only 1% of all fractures and 3% to 5% of all shoulder injuries. There is a high incidence of associated injuries due to the high velocity mechanism of injury required for complex scapular fractures. Scapular neck and body fractures are most common (see Table 9-1).

Multiple classification systems have been applied to scapular fractures. Anatomic description is important and most systems are designed to specify complexity and articular involvement. The Orthopaedic Trauma Association classification separates fractures into extra-articular, articular, and complex (see Table 9-2 and Figs. 9-21 to 9-29).

**Table 9-1**

SCAPULAR FRACTURES

| LOCATION/ INCIDENCE (%) | MECHANISM OF INJURY |
|---|---|
| Body/spine (40–75) | Direct blow |
| Acromion (8–16) | Downward blow, superior shoulder dislocations |
| Glenoid (10–25) | Fall on the flexed elbow, direct lateral blow, shoulder dislocations |
| Coracoid (3–13) | Direct blow, muscle avulsions |

**Table 9-2**

ORTHOPAEDIC TRAUMA ASSOCIATION CLASSIFICATION SCAPULAR FRACTURES

| CLASSIFICATION | IMAGE FEATURES |
|---|---|
| Type A1 (Fig. 9-21) | Scapula, extra-articular processes |
| Type A1.1 | Simple acromion |
| Type A1.2 | Acromion, comminuted |
| Type A1.3 | Coracoid |
| Type B1 (Fig. 9-21) | Articular impacted |
| Type B1.1 | Anterior rim of glenoid |
| Type B1.2 | Posterior rim of glenoid |
| Type B1.3 | Inferior rim of glenoid |
| Type A2 | Extra-articular body |
| Type A2.1 (Fig. 9-22) | Simple scapular wing |
| Type A2.2 (Fig. 9-23) | Multifragmentary |
| Type A2.3 (Fig. 9-24) | Glenoid neck |
| Type B2 | Intra-articular, nonimpacted |
| Type B2.1 (Fig. 9-22) | Anterior rim displaced |
| Type B2.2 | Posterior rim displaced |
| Type B2.3 | Anterior/posterior, glenoid neck |
| Type A3 | Extra-articular complex |
| Type A3.1 (Fig. 9-25) | Glenoid neck and body |
| Type A3.2 (Fig. 9-26) | Glenoid neck, simple clavicle |
| Type A3.3 (Fig. 9-27) | Glenoid neck, body, complex clavicle |
| Type B3 | Intra-articular complex |
| Type B3.1 (Fig. 9-25) | Multiple articular fragments |
| Type B3.2 (Fig. 9-28) | Multiple articular, neck or body |
| Type B3.3 (Fig. 9-29) | Multiple articular, clavicle |

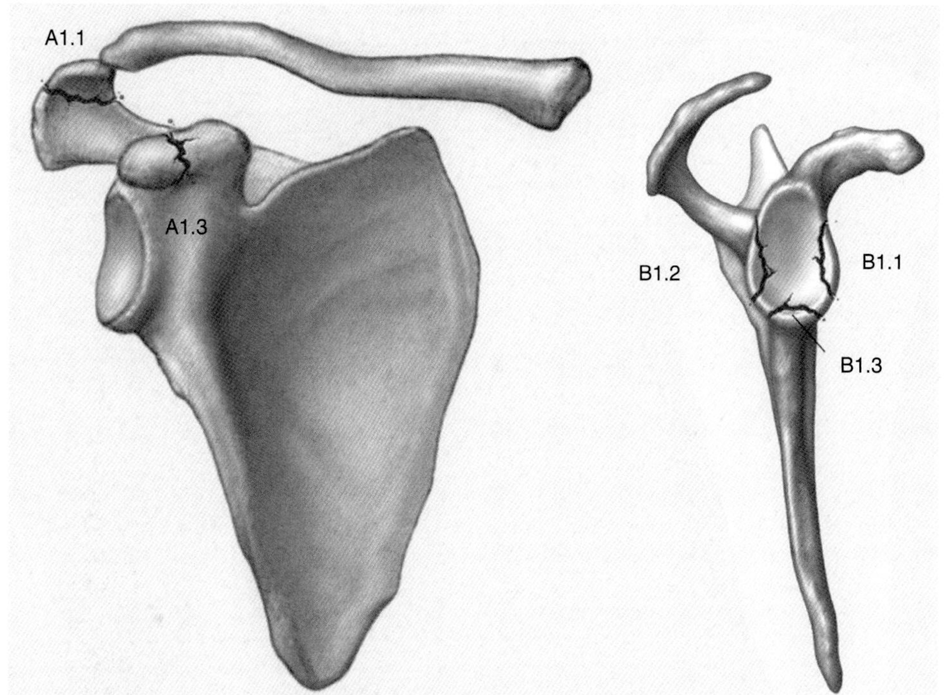


Fig. 9-21 Orthopaedic Trauma Association extra-articular processes. A: Illustration of simple fractures of the acromion (type A1.1) and coracoid (type A1.3) and (B) impacted articular fractures of the glenoid anterior rim (B1.1), posterior rim (B1.2), and inferior glenoid (B1.3).

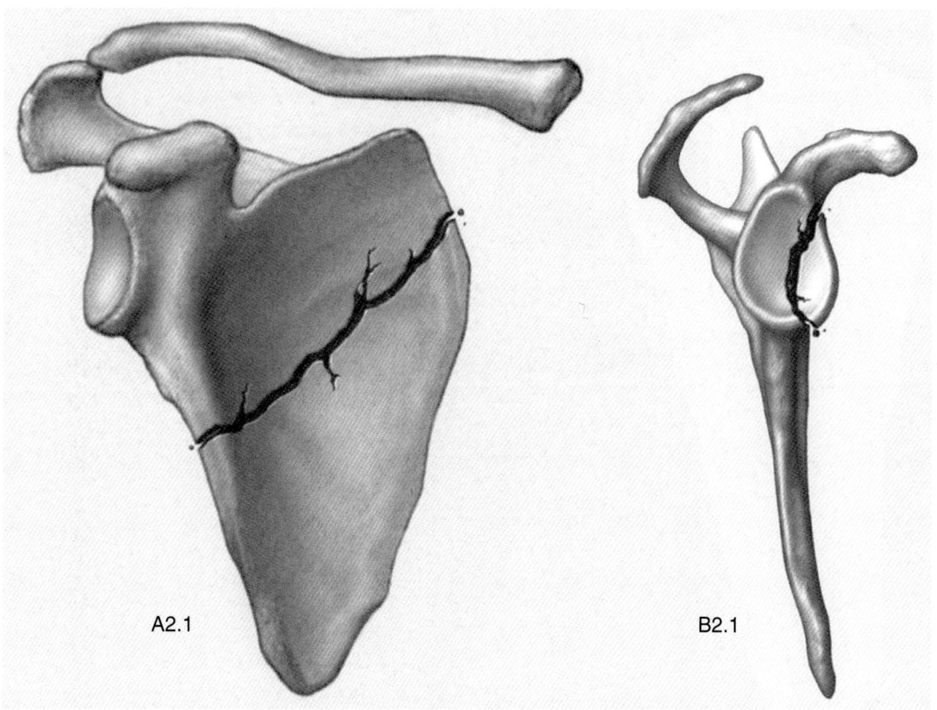


Fig. 9-22 Orthopaedic Trauma Association scapular fractures. A: Illustrations of simple scapular wing (type A2.1) and (B) displaced anterior glenoid fracture (type B2.1).

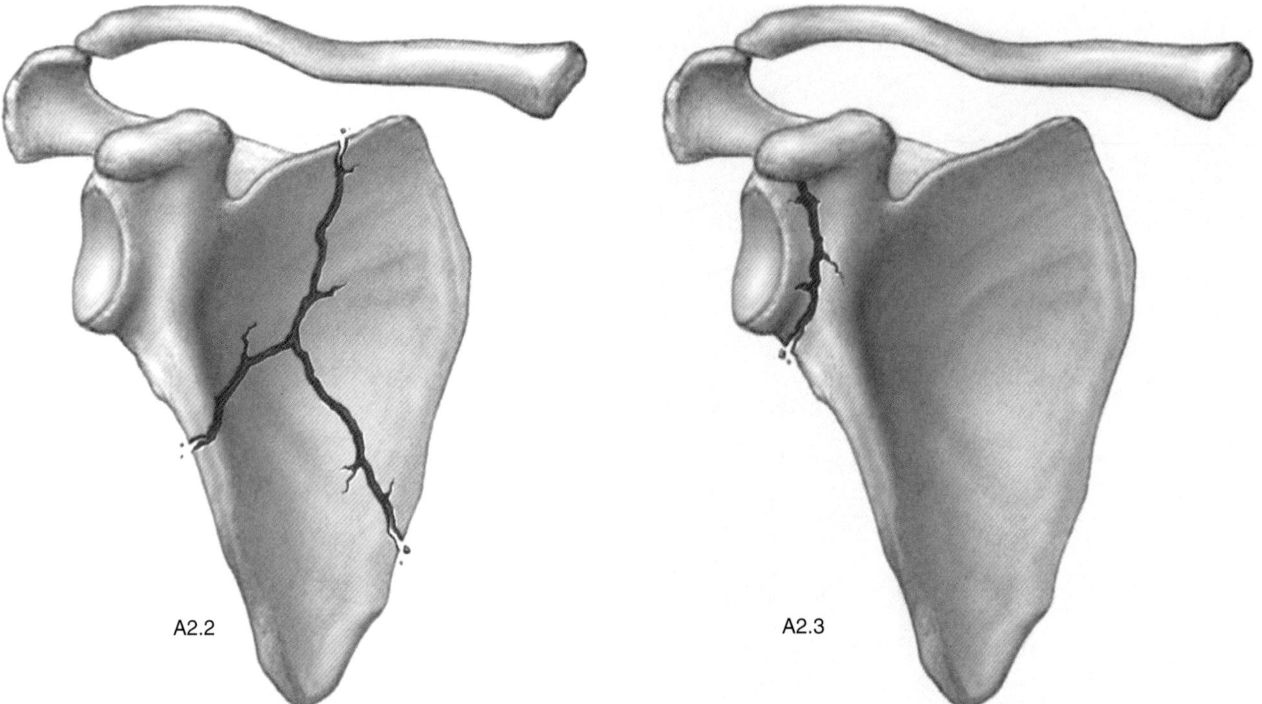


**Fig. 9-23** Orthopaedic Trauma Association complex extra-articular. Illustration of a type A2.2 fracture of the scapular body.

**Fig. 9-24** Orthopaedic Trauma Association extra-articular glenoid neck. Illustration of a glenoid neck fracture type A2.3.

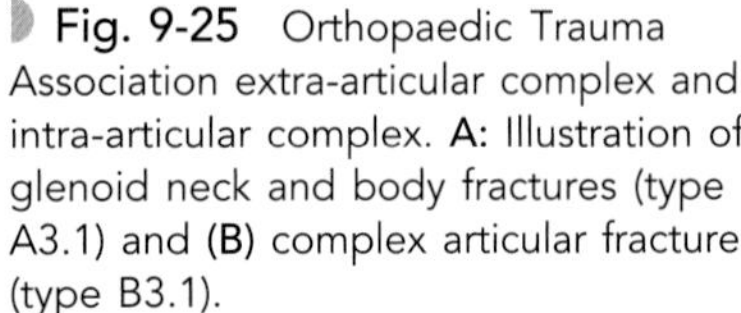

**Fig. 9-25** Orthopaedic Trauma Association extra-articular complex and intra-articular complex. **A:** Illustration of glenoid neck and body fractures (type A3.1) and **(B)** complex articular fracture (type B3.1).

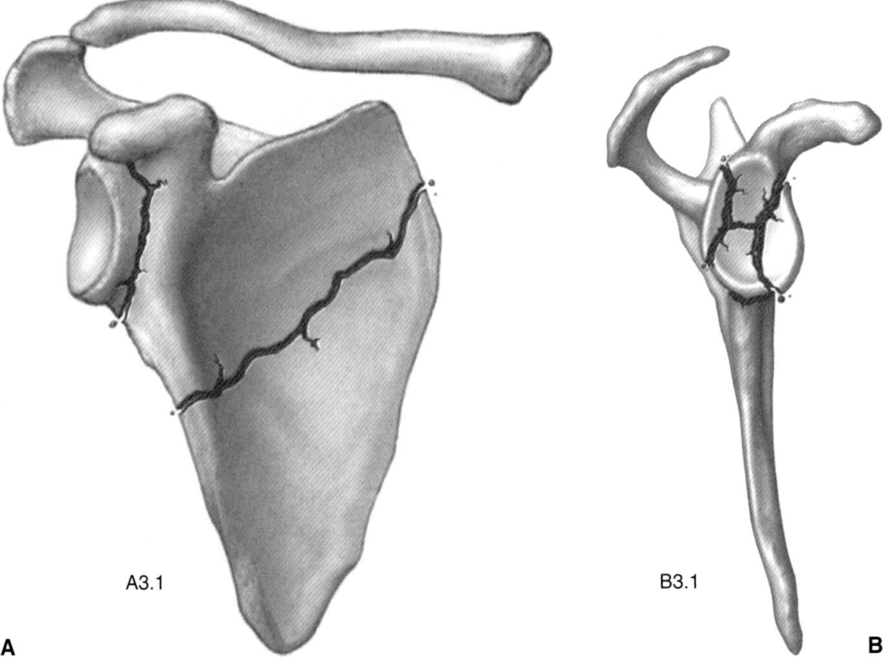

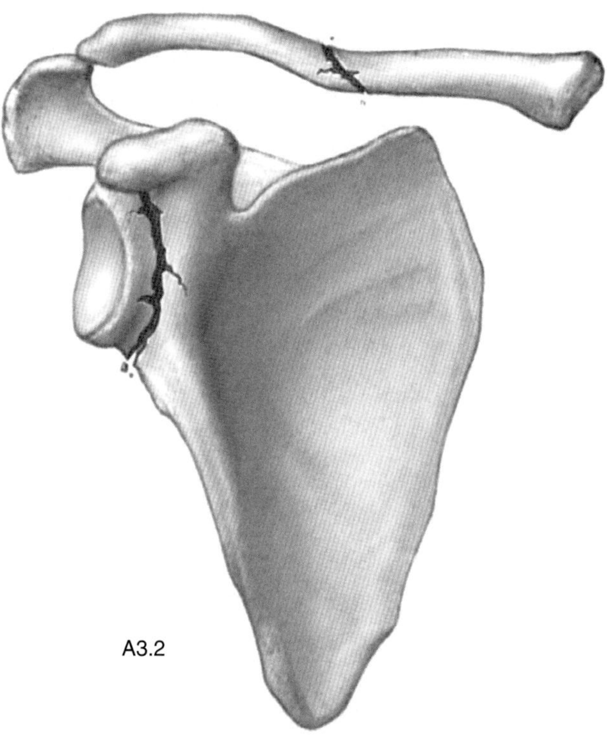


Fig. 9-26 Orthopaedic Trauma Association glenoid neck and simple clavicle. Illustration of a glenoid neck and associated simple clavicle fracture (type A3.2).

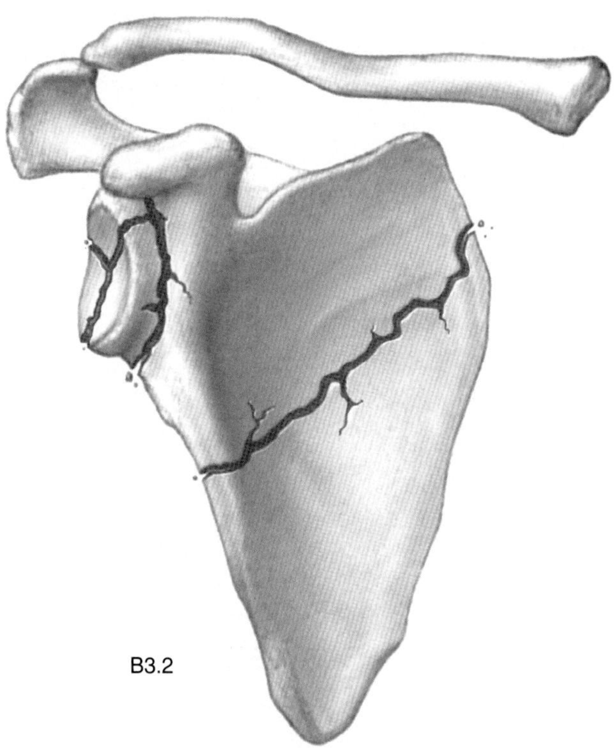


Fig. 9-28 Orthopaedic Trauma Association complex articular, glenoid neck, and body. Illustration of complex articular, glenoid neck, and body fractures (type B3.2).

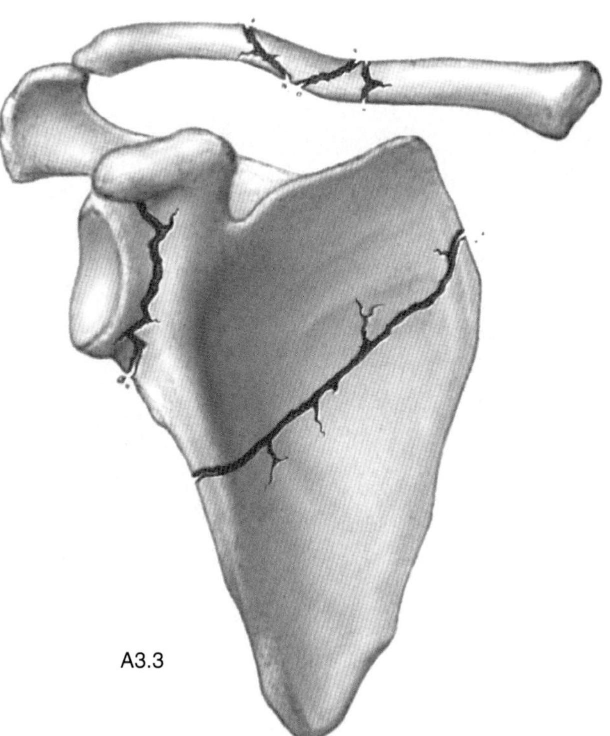


Fig. 9-27 Orthopaedic Trauma Association glenoid neck, body, and complex clavicle. Illustration of a glenoid neck, body, and complex clavicle fracture (type A3.3).

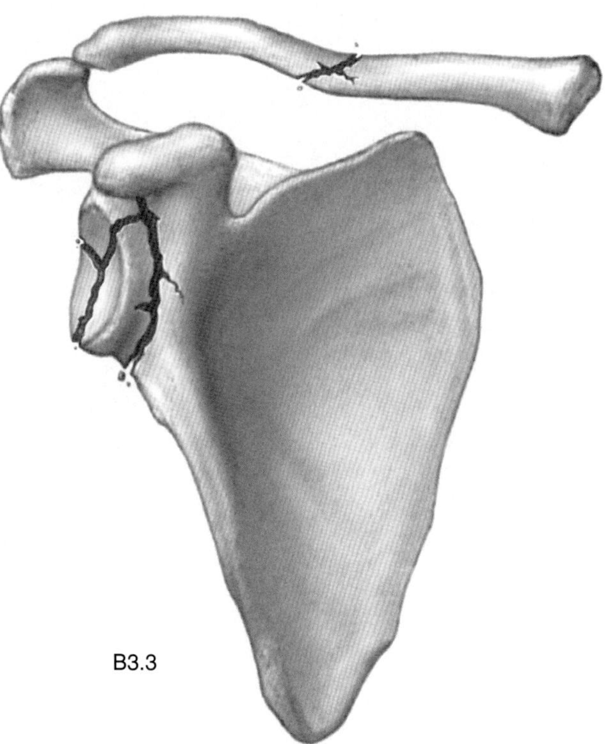


Fig. 9-29 Orthopaedic Trauma Association complex articular and clavicle. Illustration of a complex articular fracture with associated clavicle fracture (type B3.3).

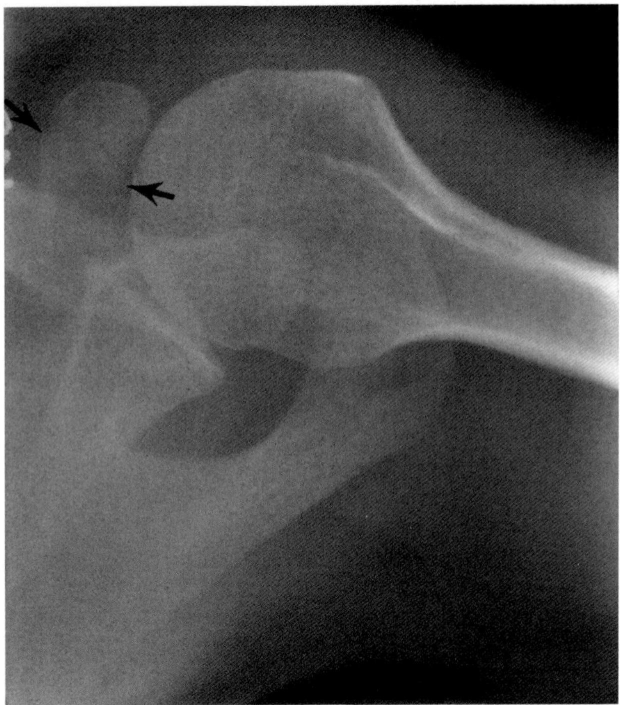

Fig. 9-30 Axillary view demonstrating an undisplaced coracoid fracture (*arrows*).

## Suggested Reading

Hardegger FH, Simpson LA, Weber BG. The operative treatment of scapular fractures. *J Bone Joint Surg*. 1984;66B: 725–731.

Orthopaedic Trauma Association Committee on coding and classification. *J Orthop Trauma*. 1996;10:1–155.

### Pretreatment Imaging

AP, lateral or scapular Y and axillary views should be obtained. The latter two projections may provide the only clear images of the coracoid and acromion (see Fig. 9-30). The most difficult problem is defining the complexity of the injury to the body and neck of the scapula and, more importantly, the articular involvement. This is difficult to assess on radiographs. When there is a question about the extent of injury, CT with reformatting or three-dimensional reconstruction should be obtained (see Fig. 9-31).

## Suggested Reading

Cofield RH, Berquist TH. The shoulder. In: Berquist TH. *Imaging of orthopaedic trauma*, 2nd ed. New York: Raven Press; 1992:579–657.

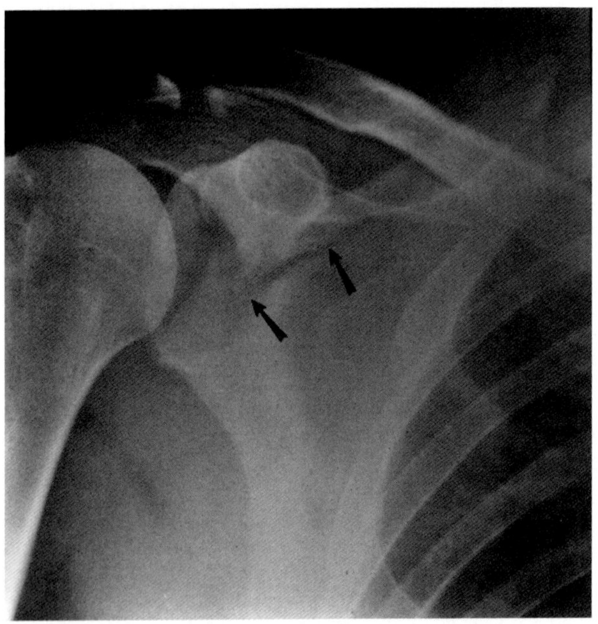



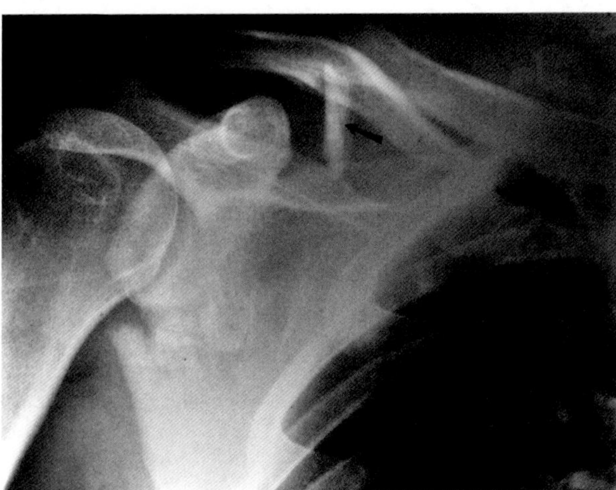



Fig. 9-31 Scapular fractures. A: Anteroposterior (AP) radiograph demonstrating a fracture that appears to involve the glenoid articular surface (*arrows*). B: Impacted glenoid neck fracture with a superiorly displaced body fragment (*arrow*). No obvious articular involvement. Computed tomography (CT) images in the axial (C) and sagittal (D and E) planes demonstrating a complex body fracture (*arrows*) with a small inferior glenoid fragment (*arrow* in E).

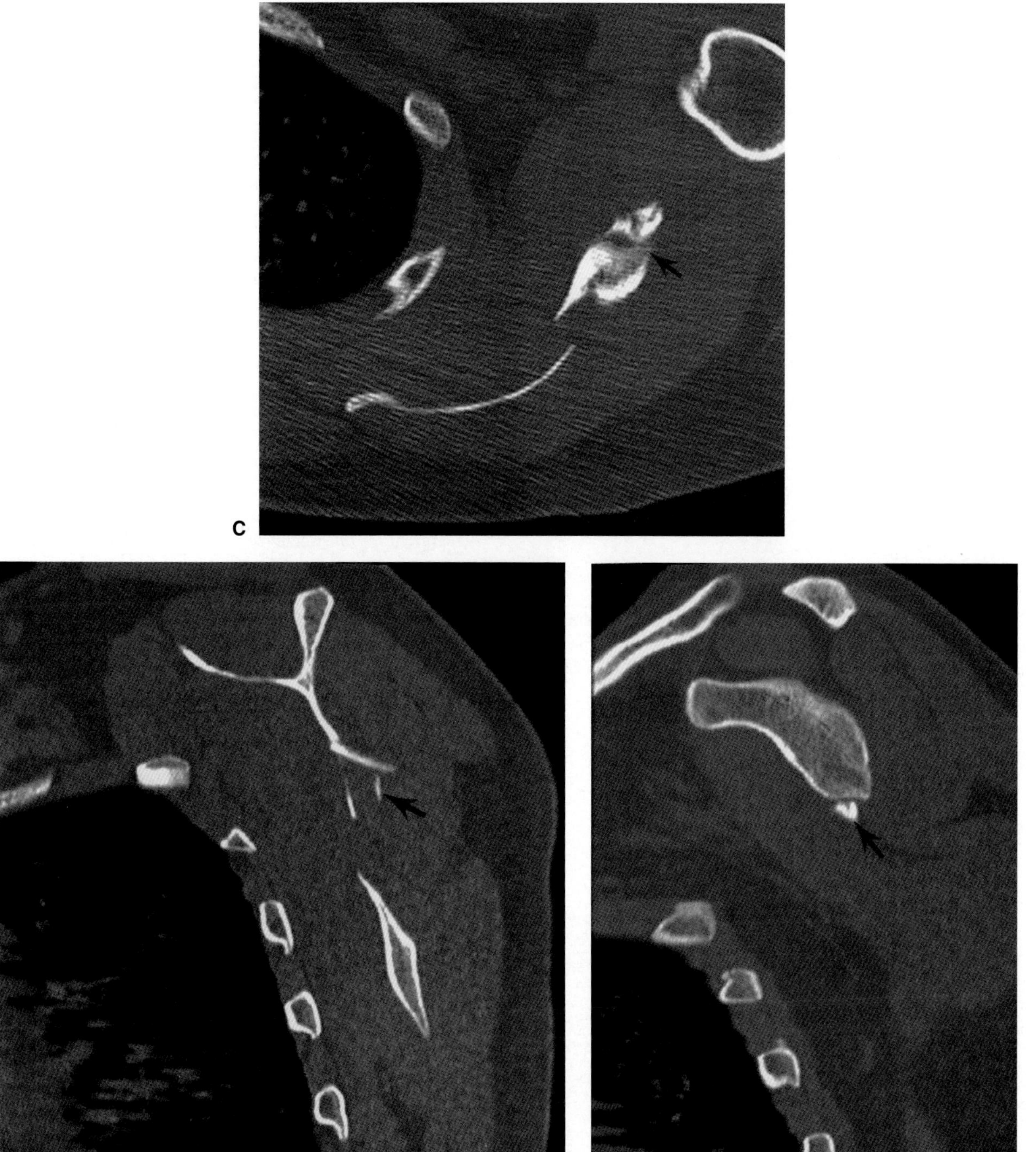


Fig. 9-31 *(Continued)*

### Treatment Options

Most scapular fractures can be treated with closed reduction. This is due to the extensive muscle support about the scapula that reduces displacement. Most fractures treated with closed reduction (90%) heal within 6 to 8 weeks. Shoulder motion should be initiated as soon as possible.

Glenoid articular fractures can be internally fixed with screws, K-wires, or reconstruction plates and screws. Similar fixation devices can be used for glenoid neck, scapular spine, and coracoid fractures.

## Suggested Reading

Hardegger FH, Simpson LA, Weber BG. The operative treatment of scapular fractures. *J Bone Joint Surg*. 1984;66B: 725–731.

Kavanagh BF, Bradway JK, Cofield RH. Open reduction and internal fixation of displaced intraarticular fractures of the glenoid fossa. *J Bone Joint Surg*. 1993;75A:479–484.

### Imaging of Complications

Complications directly related to the injury or treatment include neurovascular injury, infection, malunion, and nonunion. If not properly reduced, glenoid articular fractures can result in recurrent dislocations and instability. Instability can be diagnosed clinically. Imaging evaluation is best accomplished with MR arthrography. Capsulitis and arthrosis may also occur. Distention arthrography may be useful for releasing adhesions in patients with capsulitis.

The most significant complications are not related to the scapula. Patients frequently have complications of the upper extremity, shoulder, lung, and chest wall. Pulmonary contusions and hemothorax occur in 15% to 55% of patients. Cerebral contusions occur in up to 40% and neural deficits in 5%. Splenic laceration is not uncommon resulting in splenectomy in 8% of patients. Most of these complications can be effectively classified with CT or MRI.

## Suggested Reading

Goss TP. Fractures of the glenoid cavity. *J Bone Joint Surg*. 1992;74A:299–305.

Goss TP. Scapular fractures and dislocations: Diagnosis and treatment. *J Am Acad Orthop Surg*. 1996;52:106–115.

## Dislocations

Glenohumeral dislocations are the most common and account for 50% of all dislocations. Dislocations may also occur in the

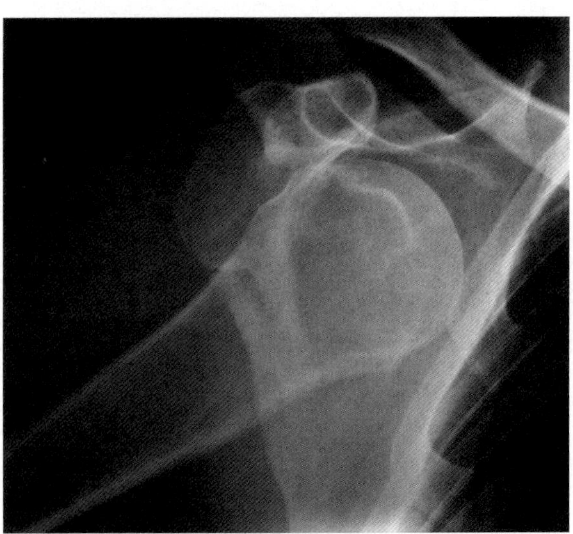


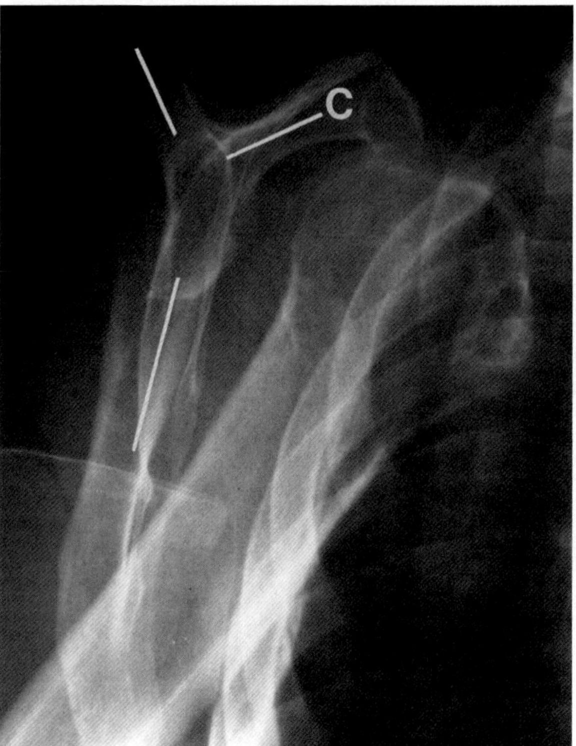


Fig. 9-32 Anterior dislocation. Anteroposterior (AP) (A) and scapular Y (B) radiographs demonstrating the typical subcoracoid position of the humeral head. On the scapular Y image (B), the humeral head should be over the glenoid at the junction of the Y formed by the scapular wing, coracoid, and spine and acromion (*lines*). In this case, it is obviously anteriorly dislocated. *C*, coracoid.

acromioclavicular joint and account for 12% of all dislocations. Sternoclavicular joint dislocations are uncommon, accounting for only 3% of all shoulder dislocations.

### Glenohumeral Dislocations

Glenohumeral dislocations are almost always anterior (96% to 98%), with posterior dislocations accounting for 2% to 4% dislocations; inferior and superior dislocations are rare. Most anterior dislocations are due to a fall with the arm abducted and externally rotated. As the humeral head is displaced anteriorly, injury to the subscapularis, anterior capsule, and glenohumeral ligaments occurs to varying degrees. There are three glenohumeral ligaments (superior, middle, and inferior) which, along with the capsule and labrum, provide anterior stability. With anterior dislocations, the inferior glenohumeral ligament, which is the primary stabilizer, is injured along with the labral complex. This results in the Bankart lesion which may also include an osseous fragment. This lesion is evident in 50% of patients. A posterolateral impaction in the humeral head (Hill-Sach lesion) occurs in 67% to 76% of patients. Greater tuberosity fractures occur in 15% of patients. When this occurs, the biceps tendon may become trapped between the humeral head and tuberosity fragment.

Posterior dislocations occur from falls with the arm internally rotated and adducted, with electroconvulsive therapy, and following direct anterior trauma. The posterior capsule, glenoid rim, and anteromedial humeral head (reverse Hill-Sachs) may also be involved. Seventy-five percent of injuries will have a reverse Hill-Sachs lesion and up to 25% of patients have associated lesser tuberosity fractures.

## Suggested Reading

Robinson M, Aderinto J. Recurrent posterior shoulder instability. *J Bone Joint Surg*. 2005;87A:883–892.

Turkel SJ, Pinto MW, Marshall JL, et al. Stabilizing mechanisms preventing anterior dislocation of the glenohumeral joint. *J Bone Joint Surg*. 1981;63A:1208–1217.

### Pretreatment Imaging

Most of the anterior and posterior shoulder dislocations are obvious on radiographs (see Fig. 9-32). Posterior dislocations may be more subtle on the AP view. The joint may appear widened, the humeral head may be fixed in internal rotation (internal and external rotation views), there may be an overlap of the glenoid and humeral head, and there may be a "trough sign" due to anteromedial impaction of the humeral head (Fig. 9-30). Use of AP, scapular Y, and axillary views will clearly demonstrate the direction of the dislocation and associated fractures in most cases (see Figs. 9-32 and 9-33). Following reduction,

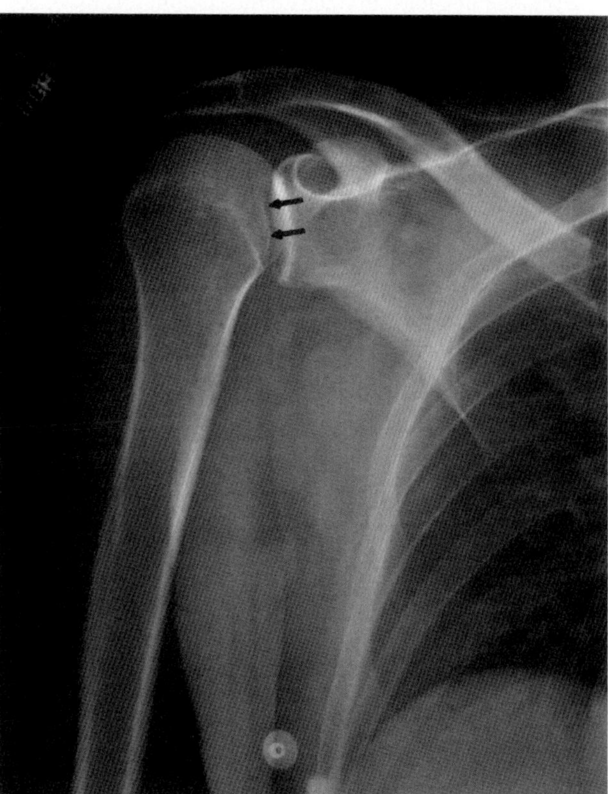


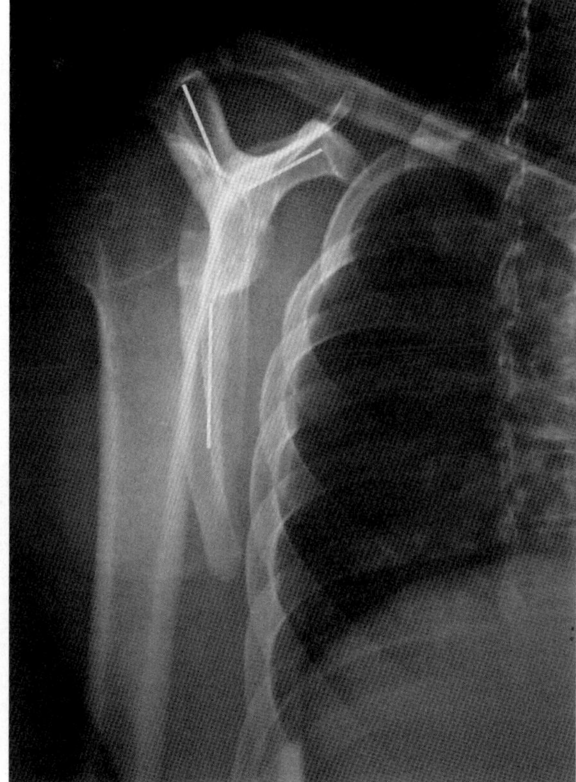


Fig. 9-33 Posterior dislocation. The anteroposterior (AP) radiograph (A) demonstrates the "trough sign" with an impaction fracture (*arrows*) of the anteromedial humeral head. The scapular Y image (B) clearly demonstrates the posterior displacement of the humeral head (lines indicate the glenoid at the junction of the limbs of the Y).

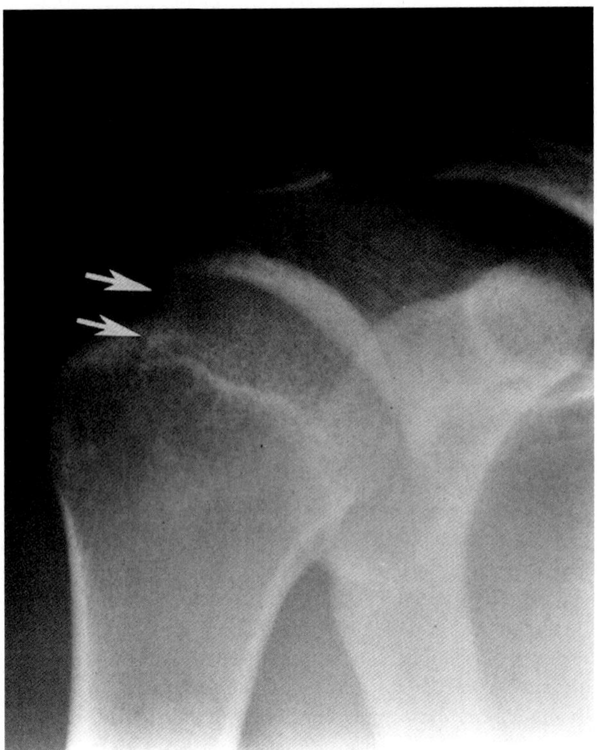

Fig. 9-34 Anteroposterior (AP) radiograph demonstrating a defect in the humeral head (*arrows*) due to a Hill-Sachs lesion after reduction of an anterior dislocation.

repeat radiographs should be obtained to assess reduction and evaluate for any subtle associated fractures. The Hill-Sachs lesion may be evident on the internal rotation image, axillary or Stryker notch view (see Fig. 9-34). CT or MRI may be required following reduction to fully evaluate the extent of injury and position of the humeral head in relation to the glenoid (see Fig. 9-35).

## Suggested Reading

Cisternino SJ, Rogers LF, Stuffleban BC, et al. The trough line: A radiographic sign of posterior dislocation. *AJR Am J Roentgenol.* 1978;130:951–954.

Cofield RH, Berquist TH. The shoulder. In: Berquist TH. *Imaging of orthopaedic trauma*, 2nd ed. New York: Raven Press; 1992:579–657.

Steinbach LS. Magnetic resonance imaging of glenohumeral joint instability. *Semin Musculoskelet Radiol.* 2005;9: 44–55.

### Treatment Options

Treatment of dislocations in the acute setting is closed manipulation and reduction. The main issue is the high incidence of recurrent dislocations. Recurrence is most common following anterior dislocations (85% to 95%) with the incidence most common if initial dislocation occurs before 22 years of age. Patients with dislocation who are older than 40 years of age have a much lower incidence or recurrence (15%).

Clinical evaluation may demonstrate the degree and directions of instability in these patients. MR arthrography is the technique of choice to evaluate the labrum, soft tissue support (capsular-ligamentous anatomy), and articular deformity (see Figs. 9-36 and 9-37).

In the past, open repair was the gold standard. Currently, arthroscopic repairs are more commonly performed with excellent results and less stiffness and morbidity resulting in improved function. This is especially important in growing athletes. There are numerous arthroscopic and open approaches

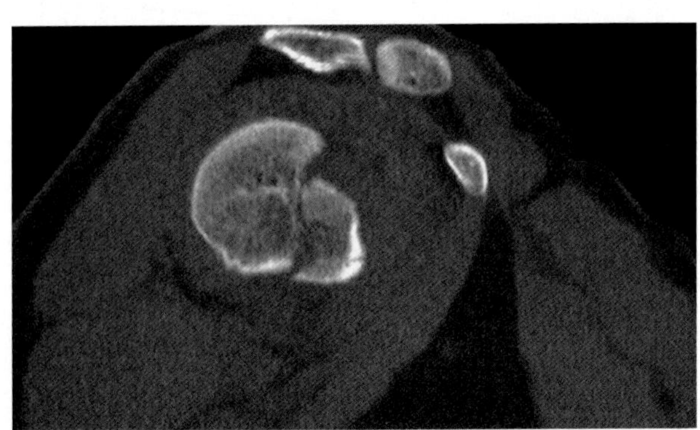



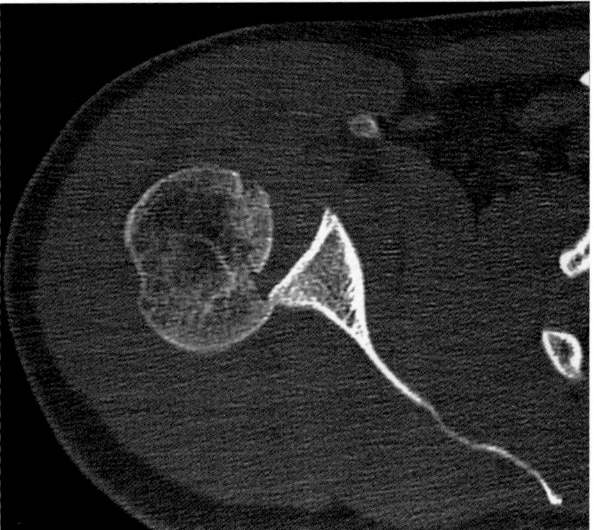



Fig. 9-35 Incomplete reduction of a posterior dislocation. Sagittal (A) and Axial (B) computed tomographic (CT) images demonstrating a humeral head fracture (reverse Hill-Sachs) with residual posterior subluxation of the humeral head.

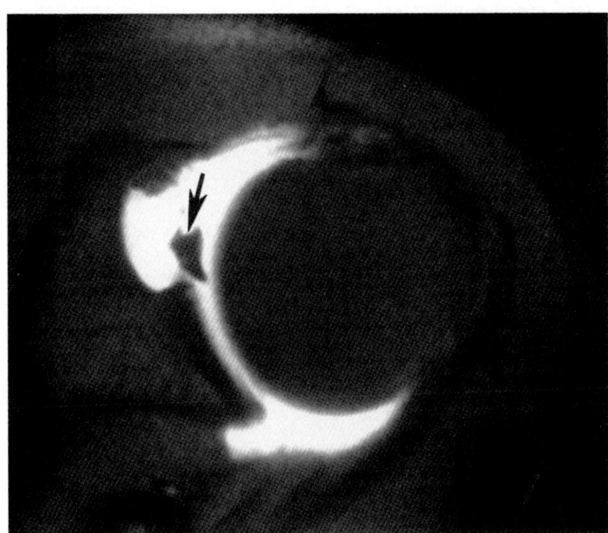

Fig. 9-36 Prior anterior dislocation. Axial magnetic resonance (MR) arthrogram demonstrating a torn anterior labrum (*arrow*).

### Table 9-3

SHOULDER INSTABILITY EPONYMS

| EPONYM | DESCRIPTION |
|---|---|
| ALPSA | Anterior ligamentous periosteal sleeve avulsion, Bankart variant |
| AMBRI | Atraumatic multidirectional bilateral instability |
| Bankart | Anterior inferior labroligamentous complex injury following anterior dislocation |
| GLAD | Glenolabral articular disruption, tear of the inferior labrum plus articular cartilage |
| HAGL | Humeral avulsion of the glenohumeral ligament |
| BHAGL | Bony avulsion or equivalent of the HAGL |
| Hill-Sachs | Posterolateral impaction of the humeral head associated with anterior dislocations |
| Hill-Sachs reverse | Anteromedial humeral head impaction associated with posterior dislocations |
| IGHLC | Inferior glenohumeral labroligamentous complex |
| Perthes lesion | Labroligamentous avulsion with intact periosteum, labrum may return to its normal position |
| SLAP | Superior labrum anterior to posterior, category of superior labral tear |
| TUBS | Traumatic, unidirectional, Bankart, surgery |

to shoulder repairs. The approach depends on the type and extent of injury. Numerous eponyms have been developed to describe injuries and instability in the shoulder (see Table 9-3).

Regardless of the operative approach, the soft tissues are sutured and labroligamentous structures repaired using metal or bioabsorbable soft tissue anchors (see Table 9-4). Osteotomies with bone transfer or rotation of the humerus have also been described.

### Table 9-4

OPERATIVE PROCEDURES FOR SHOULDER INSTABILITY

| PROCEDURE | DESCRIPTION |
|---|---|
| Bankart repair | Anterior capsule and labrum reattached to the glenoid with soft tissue anchors, 2% redislocation rate (see Fig. 9-38) |
| Bristow-Helfet | The coracoid and short head of the biceps are transferred to the inferior glenoid through a subscapularis split (see Fig. 9-39) |
| Bristow-Latarjet | Bone block from the coracoid tib is transferred to the anterior glenoid neck (see Fig. 9-40) |
| Boytchev repair | Coracoid and conjoined tendons moved deep to subscapularis and reattached to the coracoid base |
| Capsular shift | Horizontal L-shaped incision in anterior capsule with overlapped segments sutured (see Fig. 9-41) |
| Eden-Hybbinette | Coracoid extended with iliac bone graft, subscapularis is shortened |
| Gallie | Autogenous fascia used to repair capsule ligaments |
| Magnuson-Stack | Subscapularis tendon transferred to greater tuberosity, recurrence 2% |
| McLaughlin | For large anterior humeral head defects, subscapularis transferred from lesser tuberosity to the humeral head defect (see Fig. 9-42) |
| Nicola repair | Long head of the biceps transferred across anterior humerus for support |
| Putti-Platt procedure | The anterior capsule and tendons are shortened, the lateral tendon remnant is attached to the glenoid and the subscapularis is attached to the lesser tuberosity (see Fig. 9-43) |
| Saha repair | Latissimus dorsi transferred to greater tuberosity to reinforce the subscapularis |
| Weber osteotomy | Rotational humeral osteotomy with subscapularis shortening, used in younger patients |

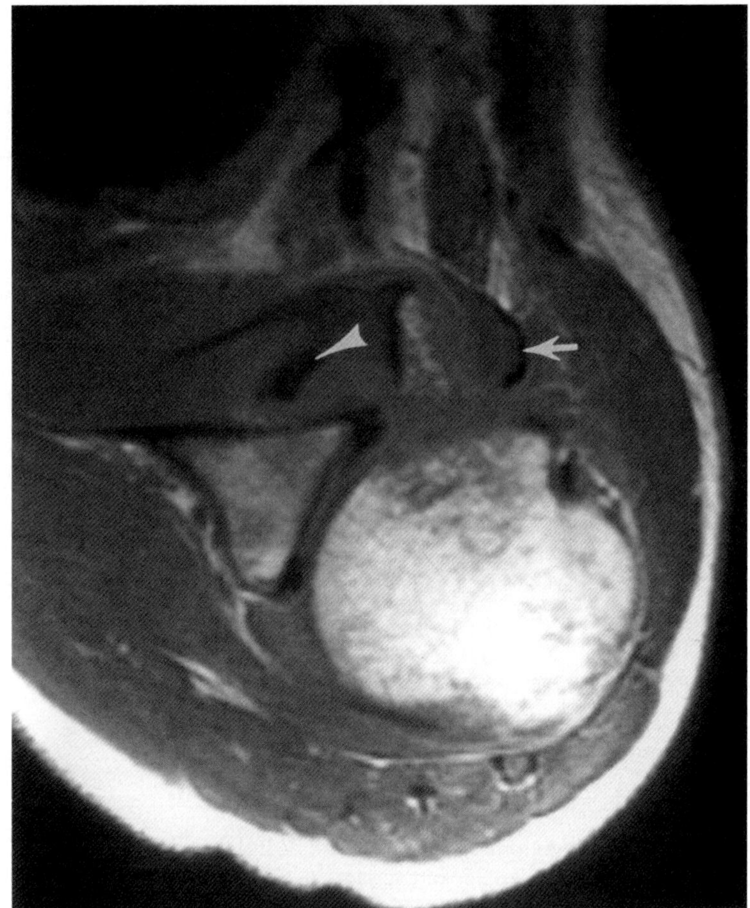


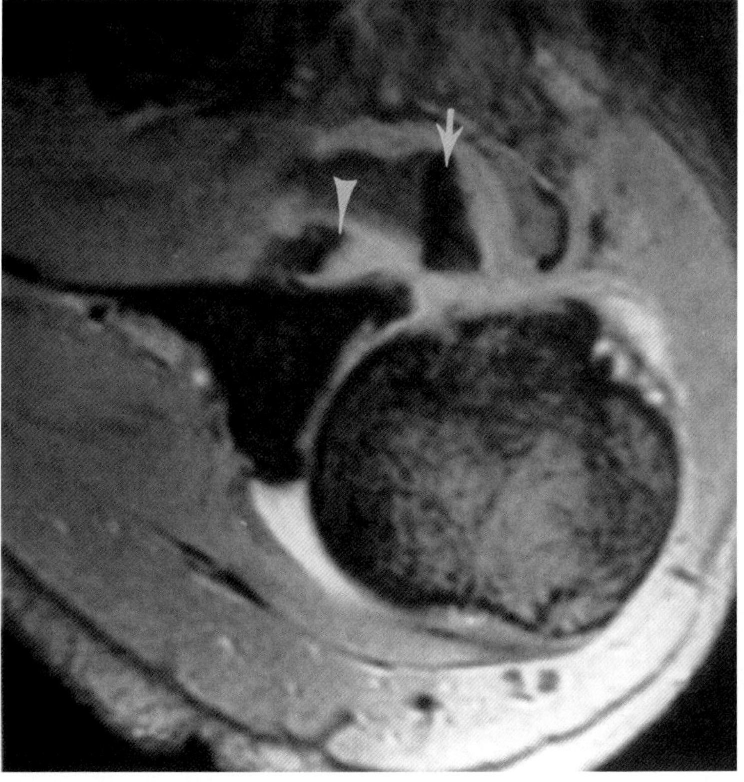


**Fig. 9-37** Prior dislocation with avulsion of the lesser tuberosity and middle glenohumeral ligament tear. Axil T1- (**A**) and T2-weighted (**B**) images demonstrate the avulsed tuberosity fragment (*arrow*) and the ligament tear (*arrowhead*).

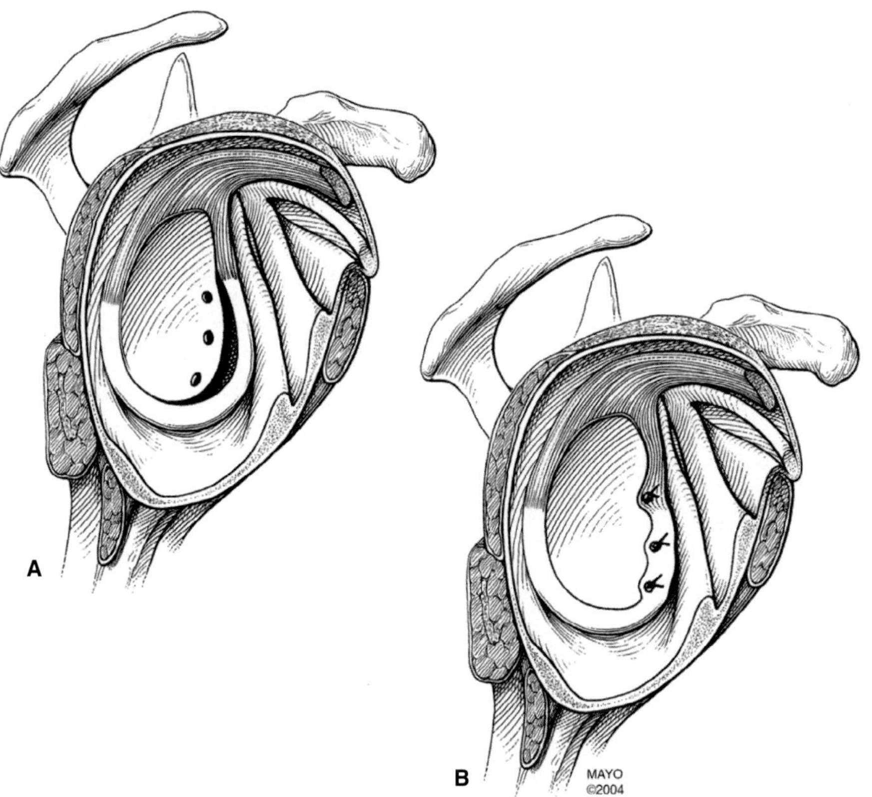


Fig. 9-38 Illustration of Bankart repair with holes at 3, 4, and 5 o'clock position (A) and suture anchors (B) to reattach the labrum. (From Berquist TH. *MRI of the musculoskeletal system*, 5th ed. Philadelphia: Lippincott Williams and Wilkins; 2006.)

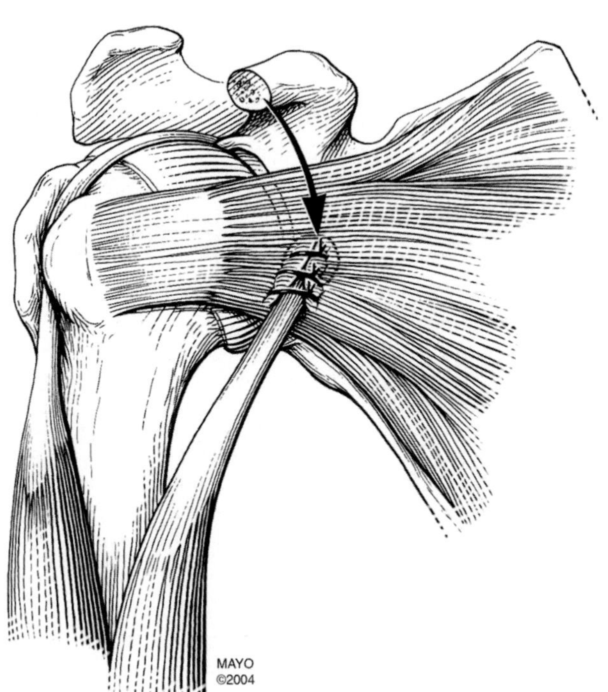


Fig. 9-39 Illustration of a Bristow-Helfet procedure. The coracoid and short head of the biceps are transferred to the anterior inferior glenoid through a subscapularis split. (From Berquist TH. *MRI of the musculoskeletal system,* 5th ed. Philadelphia: Lippincott Williams and Wilkins; 2006.)

## Suggested Reading

Berquist TH. *MRI of the musculoskeletal system*, 5th ed. Philadelphia: Lippincott Williams & Wilkins; 2006:557–656.

Budodd JE, Wolfe EM. Arthroscopic treatment of glenohumeral instability. *J Hand Surg*. 2006;31:1387–1396.

Cofield RH, Berquist TH. The shoulder. In: Berquist TH. *Imaging of orthopaedic trauma*, 2nd ed. New York: Raven Press; 1992:579–657.

Karnezis IA, Sarangi PP, Cole BJ, et al. Arthroscopic repair versus open surgery for shoulder instability. *J Bone Joint Surg*. 2001;83A:952–953.

### Imaging of Postoperative Complications

Complications related to shoulder instability may be related to the procedure or the extent of initial injury or soft tissue abnormality before repair. The most common complication is recurrent subluxations or dislocations. This may be related to the underlying disorder (unidirectional or multidirectional instability), poor patient selection, or failure to address all aspects of the pathology during the repair.

Open repair was the gold standard but reported recurrence rates from 2% to 17%. With new arthroscopic techniques, the incidence of recurrence is on the order of 2% to 5%. Diagnosis can be made clinically. However, imaging is important to evaluate the anatomy, labroligamentous structures, and degree of laxity. This can be accomplished with conventional

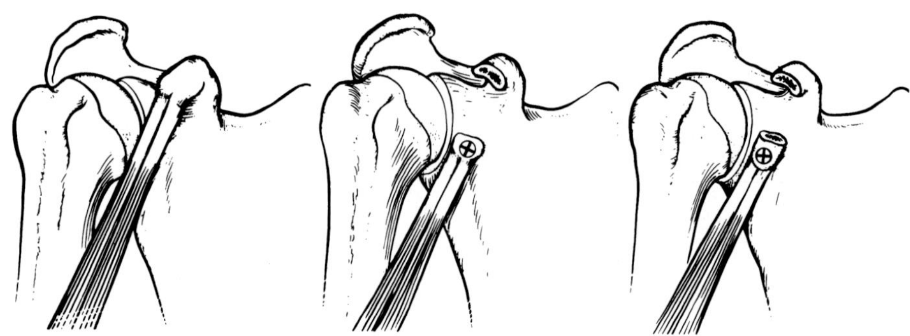

Fig. 9-40 Illustration of the Bristow-Latarjet procedure. The coracoid tip and conjoined tendon are transferred to the anterior glenoid neck.

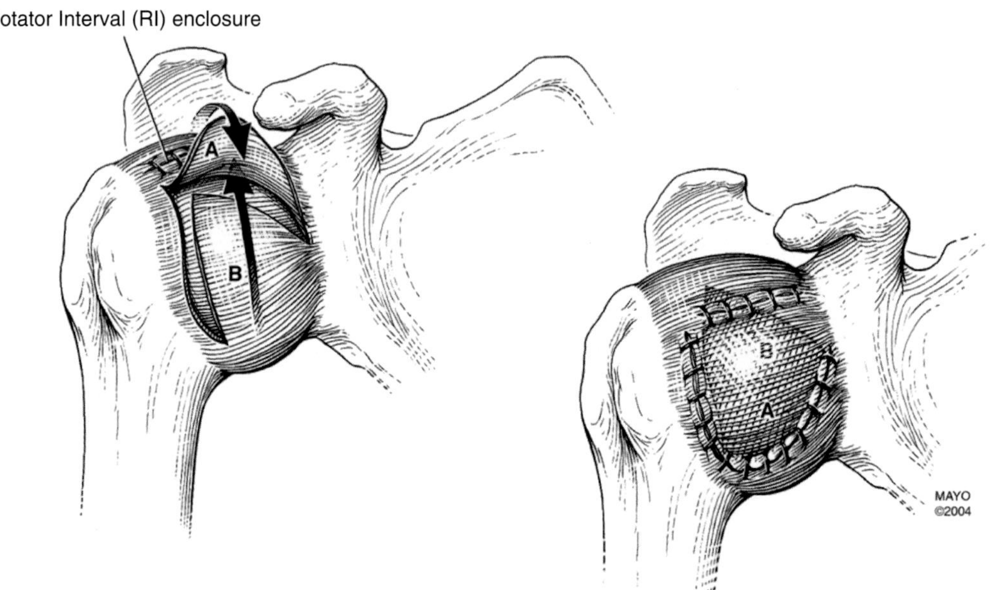


Fig. 9-41 Illustration of a capsular shift repair. (*A*) A horizontal L-shaped incision is made in the anterior capsule. (*B*) The overlapping capsule is sutured at the margins. (From Berquist TH. *MRI of the musculoskeletal system,* 5th ed. Philadelphia: Lippincott Williams and Wilkins; 2006.)

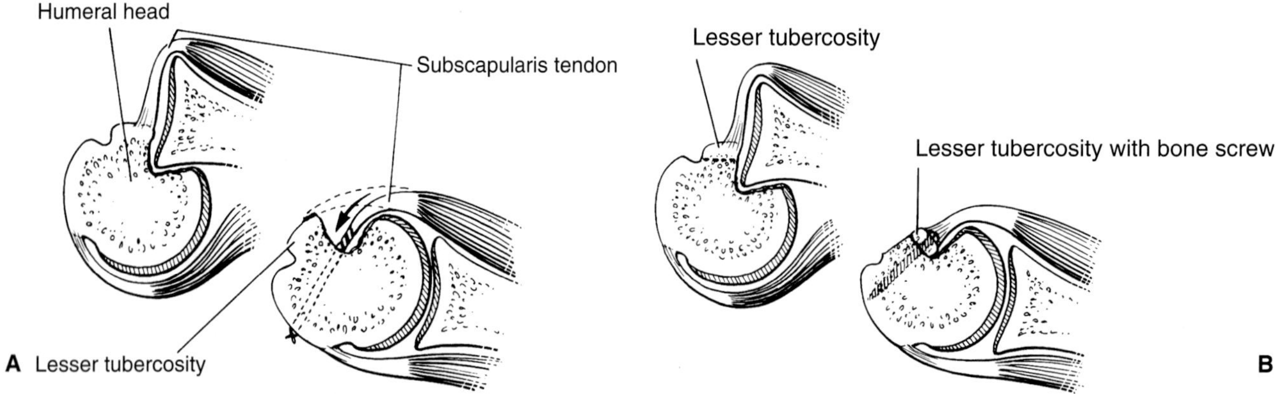


Fig. 9-42 A: Illustration of the McLaughlin procedure where the subscapularis tendon is transferred to a large anteromedial head defect. B: Neer modified this procedure by including the lesser tuberosity with the tendon.

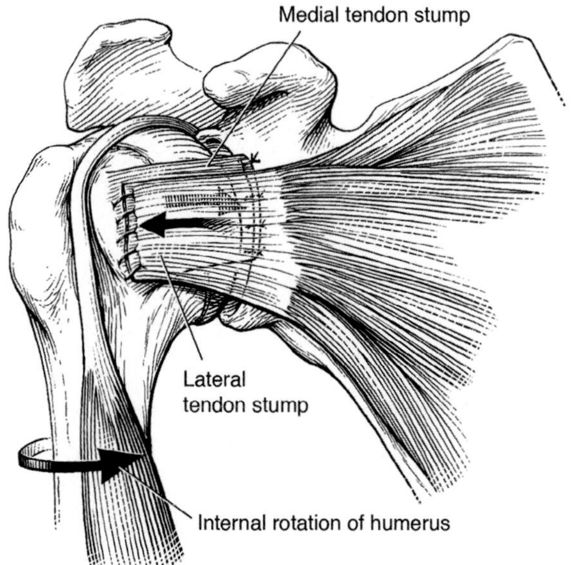


Fig. 9-43 Putti-Platt repair. Illustration demonstrating shortening of the anterior capsule and tendons. The lateral remnant is attached to the glenoid (*medially directed arrow*) and the subscapularis (*laterally directed arrow*) is attached to the lesser tuberosity. (From Berquist TH. *MRI of the musculoskeletal system,* 5th ed. Philadelphia: Lippincott Williams and Wilkins; 2006.)

arthrography and stress tests (see Fig. 9-44) or MR arthrography (see Fig. 9-45).

Stiffness and decreased range of motion may also occur. Conservative treatment with range of motion therapy and anti-inflammatory medications or steroid injections may solve the problem. When conservative treatment fails, arthroscopic intervention or distention arthrography may be required to break up adhesions and remove scar tissue.

Hardware failure or stress fractures from placing anchors too close together can also be a problem. Radiographs can detect anchor pullout when metal anchors are used (Fig. 9-44B and C). With bioabsorbable anchors, MRI or MR arthrography is preferred to evaluate anchor or suture complications (see Fig. 9-46). MR arthrography is also the optimal technique to evaluate retears in the labrum or rotator cuff.

Arthrosis is obviously a potential problem. This occurs in up to 23% of patients. Chondrolysis may also occur related to thermal injury or bupivacaine pumps. This can be evaluated with MR arthrography, but most patients require arthroscopic evaluation.

Infection and neurovascular injury may also occur. Infection can be evaluated with MRI, joint aspiration, and radionuclide scans. MRI is most effective for evaluation of neural structures. Conventional or MR angiography can be used to evaluate vascular anatomy and pathology.

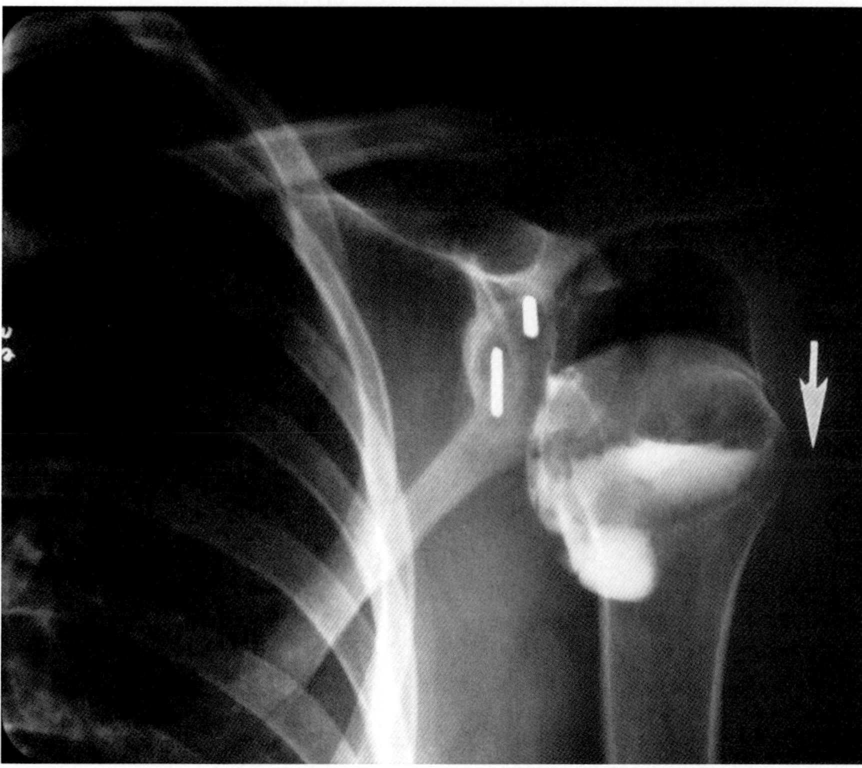


Fig. 9-44 Failed repairs for instability. A: Stress double-contrast arthrogram following anterior capsular repair demonstrating inferior instability (*arrow*). B and C: Anteroposterior (AP) (B) and axillary (C) radiographs demonstrating anterior labral repair with three Mitek soft tissue anchors. The inferior anchor has pulled out (*arrow*).

Fig. 9-44 *(Continued)*

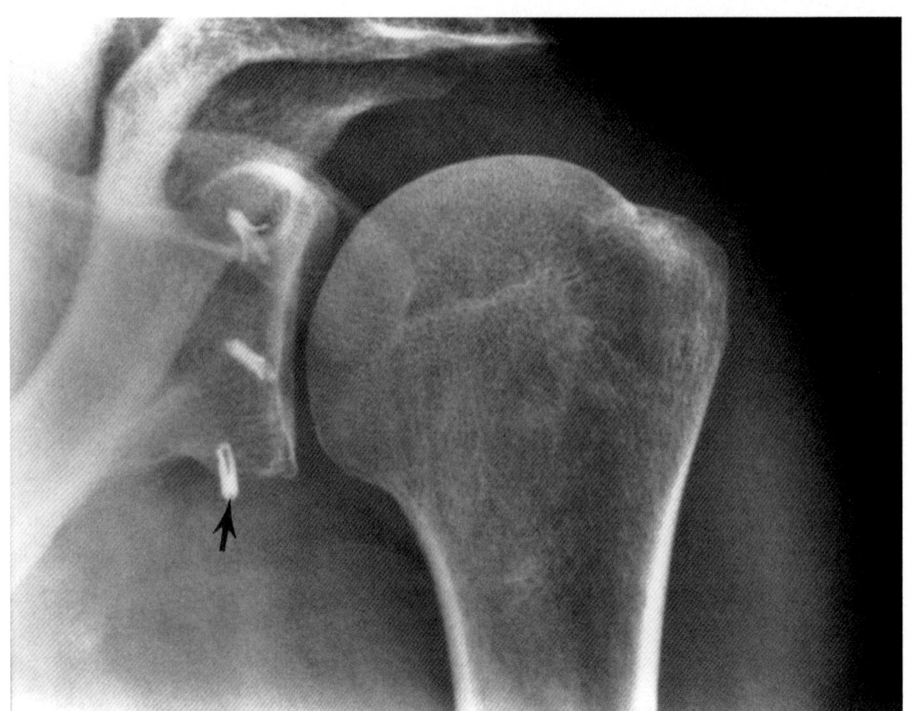


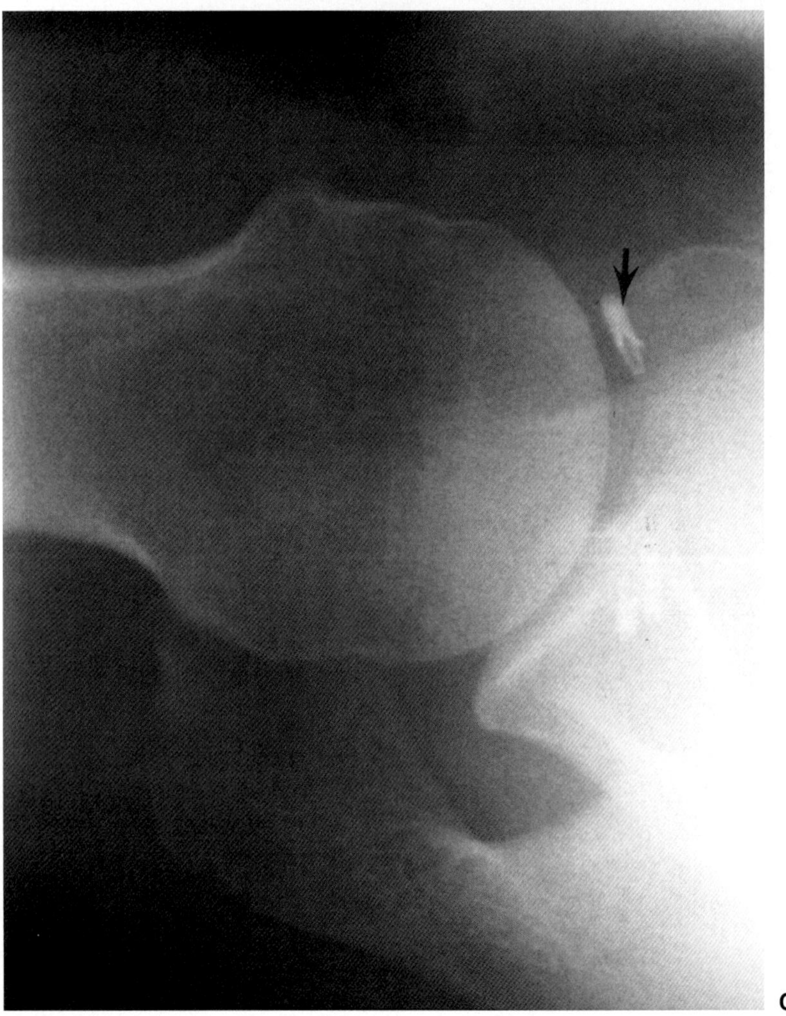

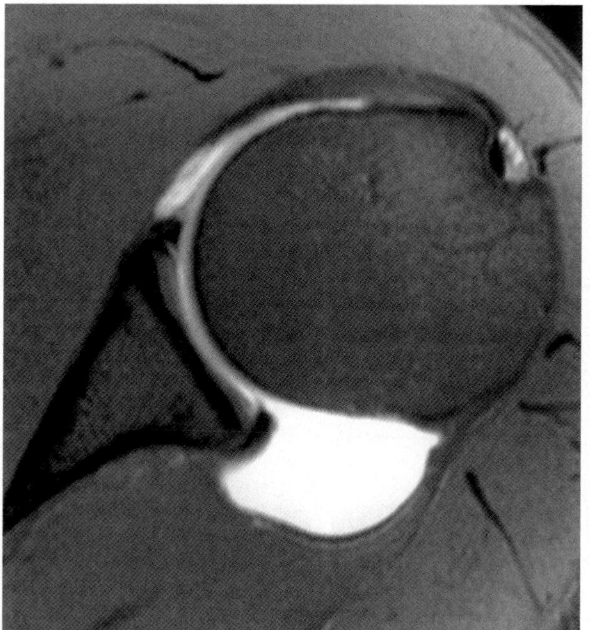


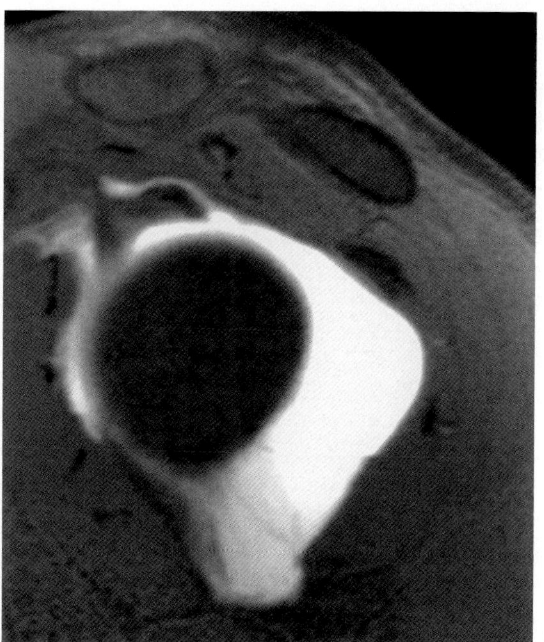


Fig. 9-45 Magnetic resonance (MR) arthrogram in a patient with recurrent posterior subluxation following dislocation and instability. Axial (A) and sagittal (B) images demonstrate an enlarged posterior capsule.

## Suggested Reading


Boileau P, Villalba M, Hery JY, et al. Risk factors for recurrence of shoulder instability after arthroscopic Bankart repair. *J Bone Joint Surg*. 2006;88A:1755–1763.

Budoff JE, Wolf EM. Arthroscopic treatment of glenohumeral instability. *J Hand Surg*. 2006;31:1387–1396.

Chu CR, Izzo NJ, Pappas NE, et al. *In vitro* exposure to 0.5% bupivacaine is cytotoxic to bovine articular chondrocytes. *Arthroscopy* 2006;22:693–699.

Levine WN, Clark AM, D'Alessandro DF, et al. Chondrolysis following arthroscopic thermal capsulorrhaphy to treat shoulder instability. *J Bone Joint Surg*. 2005;87A:616–621.

Rhee YG, Lee DH, Chun IH, et al. Glenohumeral arthropathy after arthroscopic anterior shoulder stabilization. *Arthroscopy* 2004;20:402–406.

Robinson CM, Aderinto J. Recurrent posterior shoulder instability. *J Bone Joint Surg*. 2005;87A:883–892.


# Acromioclavicular Dislocations

Dislocations of the acromioclavicular joint account for approximately 12% of all dislocations. The mechanism of injury is commonly a fall with force directed at the point of the shoulder. Less commonly, indirect force from superior displacement of the humeral head creates the dislocation.

Injuries are classified on the basis of the extent of ligament injury and displacement. The original classification proposed by Allman included three types. Type I injuries involved a few fibers, type II injuries were ruptures of the acromioclavicular ligaments and capsule, and type III injuries included coracoclavicular ligament tears. Rockwood added three additional categories (see Table 9-5 and Fig. 9-47).

## Suggested Reading


Allman FL. Fractures and ligamentous injuries of the clavicle and its articulations. *J Bone Joint Surg*. 1967;49A:774–784.

Rockwood CA, Green DP, Bucholz RW. *Rockwood and Green's fractures in adults*, 3rd ed. Philadelphia: J.B. Lippincott; 1991.


Table 9-5

ALLMAN/ROCKWOOD CLASSIFICATION FOR ACROMIOCLAVICULAR INJURIES

| CATEGORY | DESCRIPTION |
|---|---|
| Type I | Sprain of acromioclavicular (AC) ligaments |
| Type II | Disruption of AC ligaments with coracoclavicular ligaments intact |
| Type III | Disruption of the AC and coracoclavicular ligaments |
| Type IV | Disruption of both ligament complexes and posterior clavicle displacement |
| Type V | Disruption of both ligament complexes and superior clavicle displacement |
| Type VI | Disruption of both ligament complexes and anterior entrapment of the clavicle inferiorly |

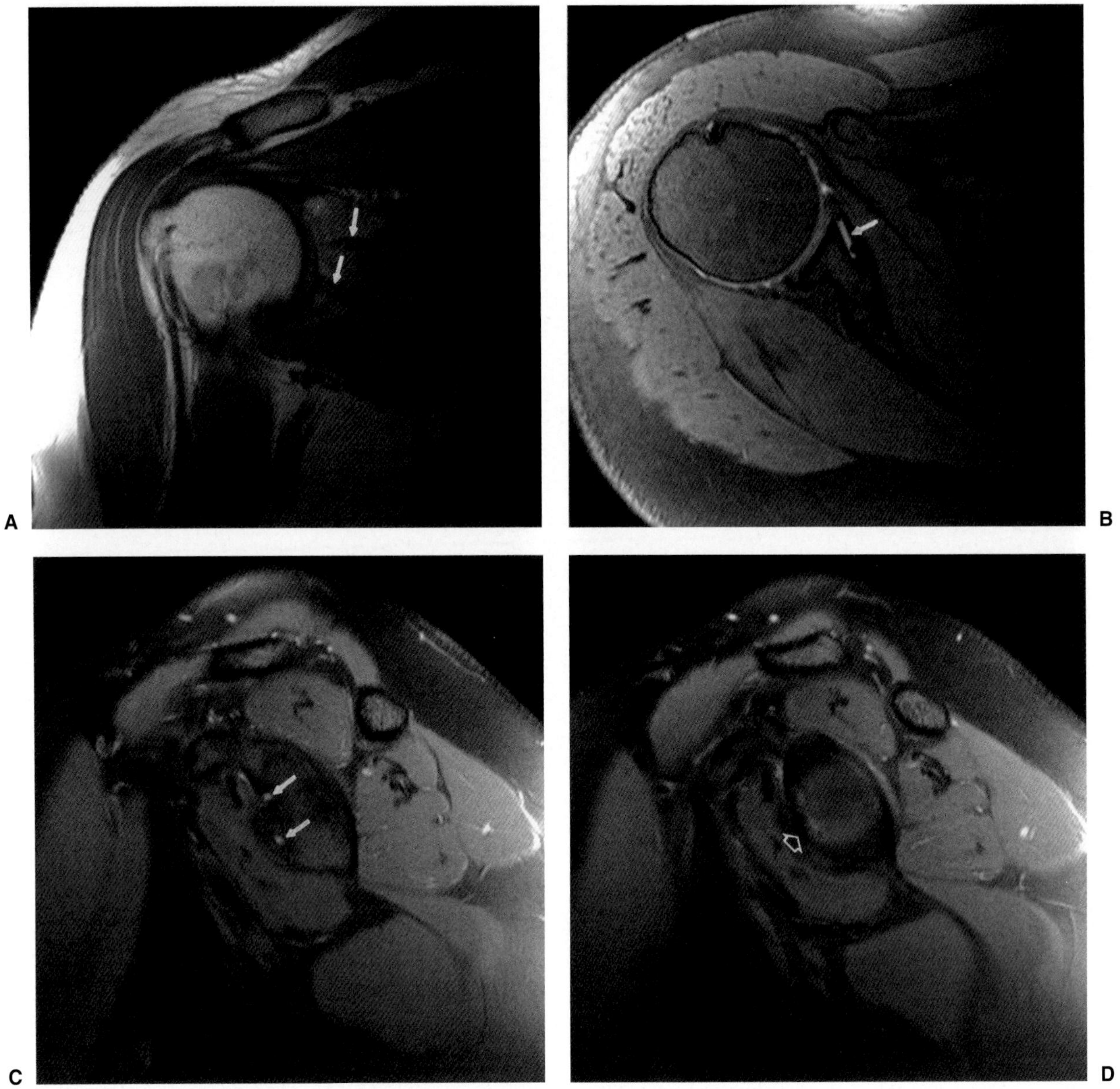

A B C D

**Fig. 9-46** Anterior repair using bioabsorbable soft tissue anchors. Coronal T1-weighted (**A**), axial dual echo steady state (DESS) (**B**), and sagittal (**C** and **D**) T2-weighted images demonstrate the soft tissue anchors (*small arrows*) and slight residual anterior labral deformity (*open arrow*). There is no artifact for the bioabsorbable anchors.

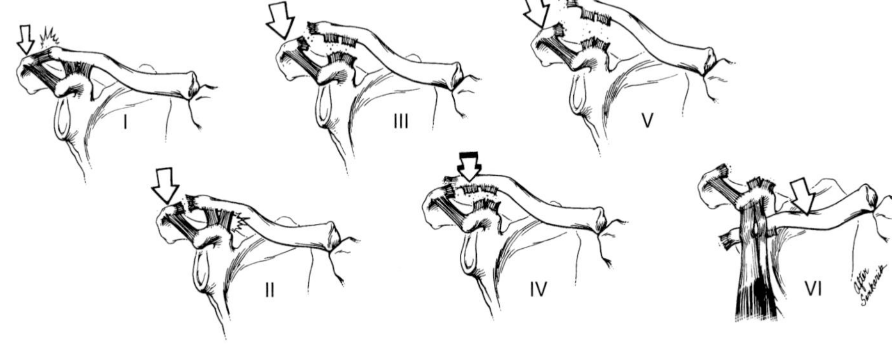


**Fig. 9-47** Acromioclavicular ligament injury classification. Type I—sprain of the acromioclavicular ligaments with intact coracoclavicular ligaments, type II—disruption of the acromioclavicular ligaments with intact coracoclavicular ligaments, type III—disruption of both ligament complexes, type IV—disruption of both ligament complexes and posterior clavicle displacement, type V—disruption of both ligament complexes and superior clavicle displacement, and type VI—disruption of both ligament complexes and anterior entrapment of the clavicle.

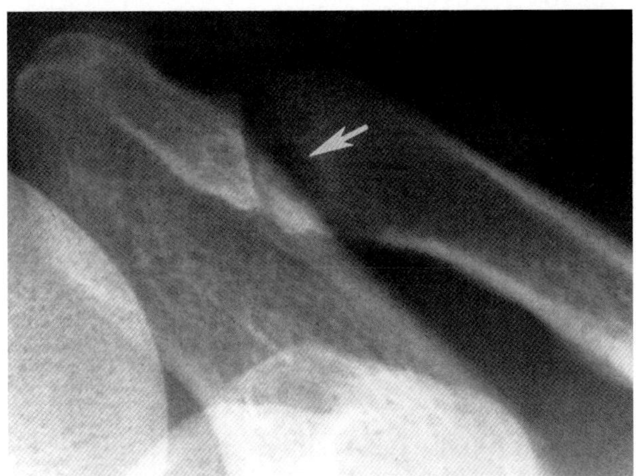
A

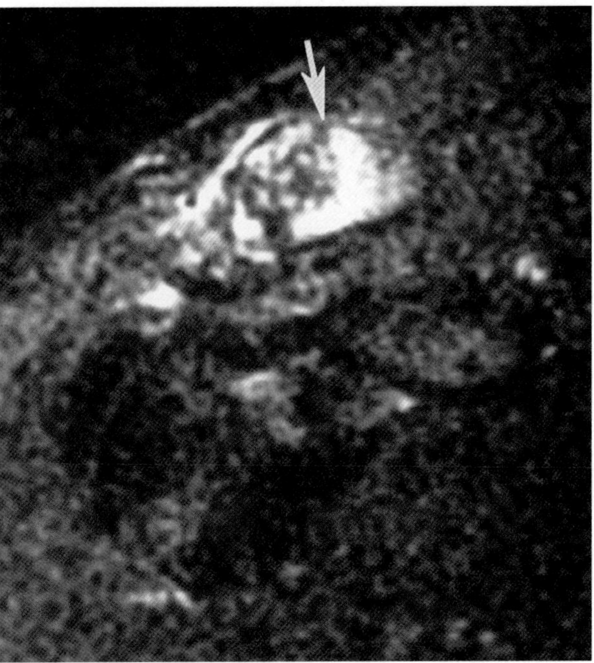
B

Fig. 9-48 Radiographic and magnetic resonance (MR) images of the injury sustained by a football player who fell on the point of the shoulder with ligament sprain. A: Radiograph several weeks later demonstrates irregular resorption of the distal clavicle (*arrow*) due to posttraumatic osteolysis. B: T2-weighted MR image demonstrates increased signal intensity in the distal clavicle.

## Pretreatment Imaging

Routine image projections of the shoulder or clavicle are usually adequate for detection of type III through VI injuries. Types I and II are more subtle and can be overlooked resulting in delayed diagnosis and reduced activity, especially in athletes (see Fig. 9-48). Weight-bearing images of both shoulders with 8 to 10 lb attached to each wrist can be obtained and compared to non–weight-bearing images. Patients should not be allowed to hold the weights because they can then voluntarily splint the shoulder resulting in an inaccurate study. The position of the clavicle in relation to the acromion and distance between the clavicle and the coracoid can be measured and compared. A difference of 5 mm in coracoclavicular distance when comparing the normal to the injured side indicates coracoclavicular ligament injury (see Fig. 9-49).

Low-grade injuries can also be evaluated with acromioclavicular arthrography using an anterior or superior approach.

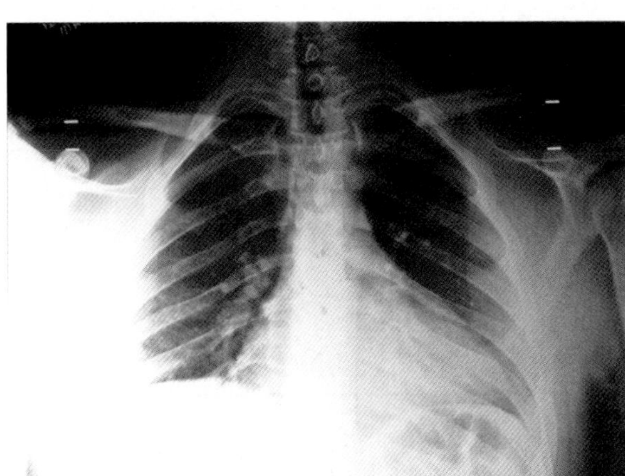

Fig. 9-49 Weight-bearing stress views of the acromioclavicular joints. Note the significant difference in coracoclavicular distance on the left (type V) separation compared to the normal right shoulder (*white lines*).

# Suggested Reading

Berquist TH. Diagnostic and therapeutic injections as an aid to musculoskeletal diagnosis. *Semin Interv Radiol.* 1993;10: 326–343.

Cofield RH, Berquist TH. The shoulder. In: Berquist TH. *Imaging of orthopaedic trauma*, 2nd ed. New York: Raven Press; 1992:579–657.

## Treatment Options

Most low-grade injuries (types I and II) can be managed with immobilization using a sling or brace until range of motion is tolerated in the shoulder. Weight bearing should be restricted for 6 to 12 weeks to avoid progression to a more significant injury. If symptoms do not improve or posttraumatic osteolysis is evident (Fig. 9-48) the distal clavicle can be resected. Resection should not exceed 10 mm of the distal clavicle.

Treatment of patients with type III injuries remains controversial with some favoring conservative and others operative repair. There is general agreement that patients with type IV to

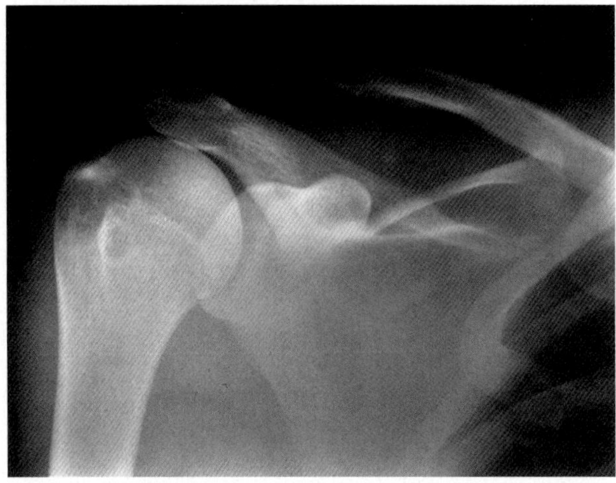
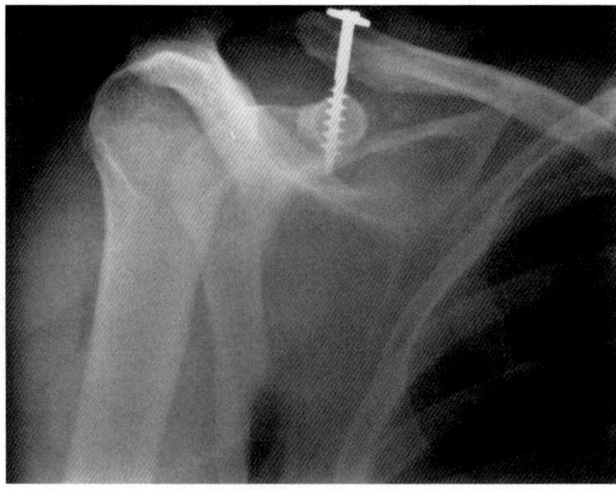

Fig. 9-50 A: Radiograph demonstrating a type V separation with superior elevation of the distal clavicle. B: The distal clavicle was resected and the clavicle fixed to the coracoid with a cancellous screw and washer.

VI injuries should be treated surgically. Repair of the ligaments or screw fixation of the clavicle to the coracoid has been used to stabilize the joint (see Fig. 9-50). Others advocate threaded Steinman pins. K-wire or cerclage wires have not proved to be successful due to migration or fracture. In some cases the distal clavicle is resected and the inferior acromioclavicular ligament used to repair the coracoclavicular ligaments.

## Suggested Reading

Cox JS. Current method of treatment of acromioclavicular joint dislocations. *Orthopaedics* 1992;15:1041–1044.

Eskola A, santavirta S, Viljakka H, et al. The results of operative resection of the lateral end of the clavicle. *J Bone Joint Surg.* 1996;78A:584–587.

Weaver HK, Dunn HK. Treatment of acromioclavicular injuries, especially complete acromioclavicular separation. *J Bone Joint Surg.* 1972;54A:1187–1194.

### Postoperative Imaging and Complications

Complications may be related to the initial injury or treatment. From an orthopaedic standpoint, associated fractures of the coracoid, clavicle, or acromion are not uncommon with advanced injuries (see Fig. 9-51).

Patients treated conservatively may have continued pain due to arthrosis or posttraumatic osteolysis (Fig. 9-48). Injections may help; however, the distal clavicle may have to be resected to relieve the symptoms. Also, extensive heterotopic ossification can occur in the region of the coracoclavicular ligaments (see Fig. 9-52).

Implant failure in surgically treated patients also occurs resulting in continued symptoms and arthrosis (see Fig. 9-53). In patients treated surgically, up to 59% may require additional surgery, up to 20% have fixation failure, and 3% demonstrate residual deformity. Infection is also more common in patients treated with operative intervention.

## Suggested Reading

Hootman JM. Acromioclavicular dislocation: Conservative or surgical therapy. *J Athl Train.* 2004;39:10–11.

Rockwood CA, Williams GR, Young DC. Acromioclavicular injuries. In: Rockwood CA, Green DP, Bucholz RW, et al., eds. *Fractures in adults*, 4th ed. Vol. I. Philadelphia: Lippincott-Raven; 1996:1341–1413.

# Sternoclavicular Dislocations

Sternoclavicular dislocations are uncommon, accounting for only 3% of shoulder-related dislocations. Significant trauma, usually applied through the shoulder, is required to disrupt this articulation. Posterolateral forces transmitted medially result in anterior subluxation or dislocation. Direct anterior trauma results in posterior dislocation. Posterior dislocations are rare and account for 5% of sternoclavicular dislocations.

Injuries are divided into three categories. Type I injuries are ligament sprains with partial tearing of the sternoclavicular ligaments. The injury is painful, but there is no instability. Type II lesions result in disruption of the sternoclavicular ligament with an intact costoclavicular ligament. Anterior or posterior subluxation may occur. Type III injuries result in disruption of both ligaments with dislocation.

## Suggested Reading

Allman FL. Fractures and ligamentous injuries of the clavicle and its articulations. *J Bone Joint Surg.* 1967;49A:774–784.

Biscos J, Nicholson GP. Treatment and results of sternoclavicular joint injuries. *Clin Sports Med.* 2003;22:359–370.

Nettles JL, Linscheid R. Sternoclavicular dislocations. *J Trauma.* 1968;8:158–164.

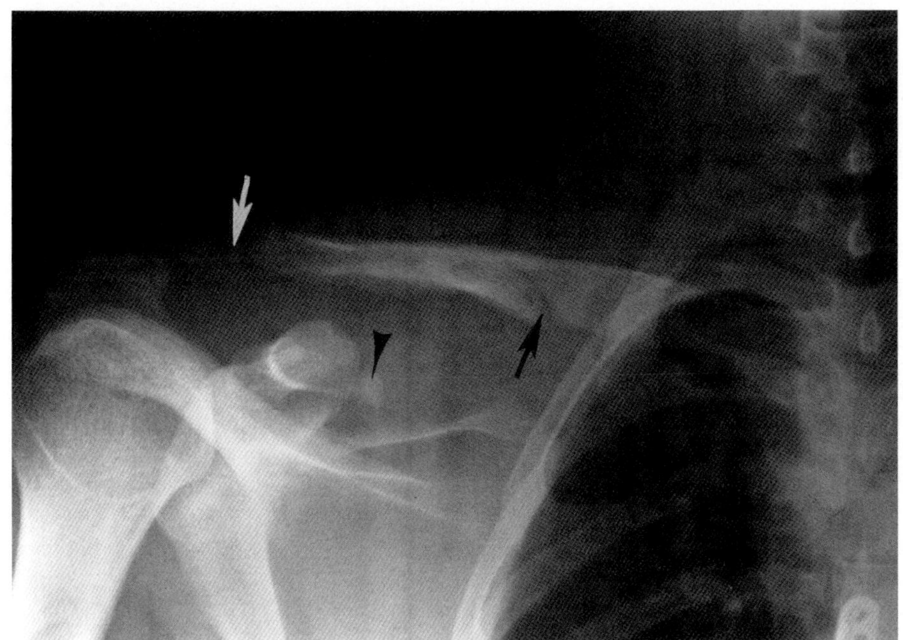

**Fig. 9-51** Radiograph of a type V separation with fractures of the mid clavicle (*black arrow*), distal clavicle (*white arrow*), and avulsion of the coracoid (*black arrowhead*).

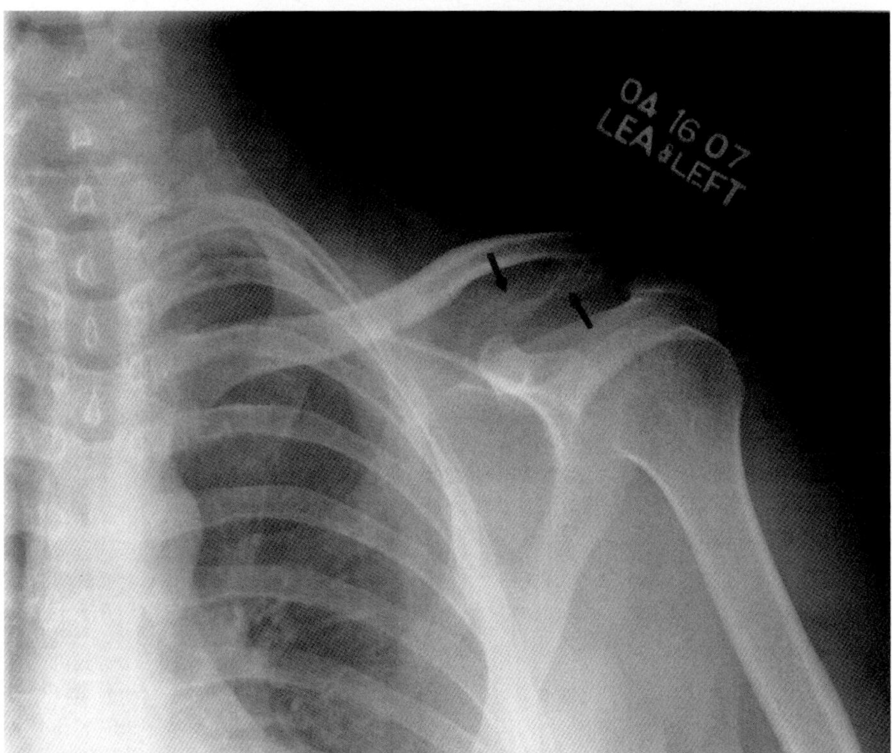


**Fig. 9-52** Heterotopic ossification in the coracoclavicular ligaments. Anteroposterior (AP) radiograph in a patient treated conservatively. There is disruption of the acromioclavicular and coracoclavicular ligament with unreduced separation and ossification in the coracoclavicular ligaments (*arrows*).

### Imaging of the Sternoclavicular Joint

Radiographic imaging of the sternoclavicular joint is difficult due to bony overlap. Multiple techniques have been attempted using oblique and angled views. Therefore, CT with reformatting has become the gold standard in patients with suspected sternoclavicular injury (see Fig. 9-54).

## Suggested Reading

Cofield RH, Berquist TH. The shoulder. In: Berquist TH. *Imaging of orthopaedic trauma*, 2nd ed. New York: Raven Press; 1992:579–657.

McCulloch P, Henley BM, Linnau KF. Radiographic clues for high energy trauma: Three cases of sternoclavicular dislocation. *AJR Am J Roentgenol.* 2001;176:1534.

### Treatment Options

Patients may have significant associated injuries that require immediate attention. Associated injuries are most common with posterior dislocations. Up to 25% of patients will have more serious injuries that require attention before dealing with the dislocation.

Treatment of anterior dislocations is generally conservative. However, ligament or soft tissue interposition may make reduction difficult to maintain. Follow-up CT studies are important to assess the joint alignment and exclude issues that may result in redislocation. Posterior dislocations must be evaluated (Fig. 9-54) to be certain that there are no associated mediastinal or intrathoracic injuries. Internal fixation is recommended when closed reduction under anesthesia fails and in patients with chronic posterior instability. Techniques for repair have been designed to reconstruct the ligamentous support. Tendon grafts, fascia, and synthetic materials have been used. Soft tissue anchors have been used in recent years. In the past, K-wires or threaded or smooth Steinman pins were used to hold reduction. These approaches have largely been abandoned due to problems with implants migrating into the chest.

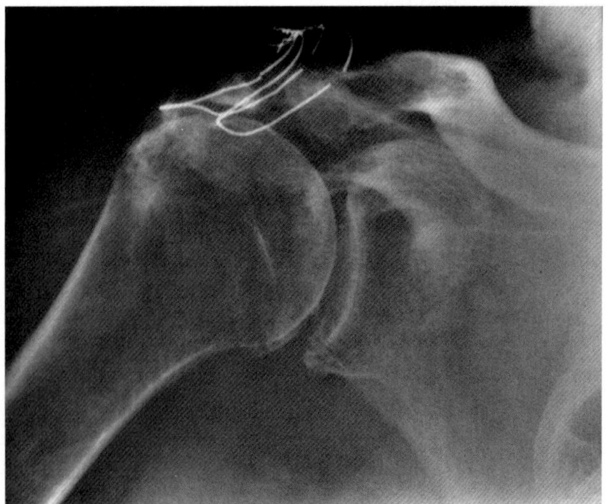

Fig. 9-53 Fixation of the acromioclavicular (AC) joint with cerclage wires. The wires have fractured. The joint is only slightly subluxed. There is interval advanced cuff arthropathy.

## Suggested Reading

Spencer EE, Kuhn JE. Biomechanical analysis of reconstructions for sternoclavicular joint instability. *J Bone Joint Surg.* 2004;86A:98–105.

### Imaging of Complications

Complications may be related to the joint or adjacent and distant structures in the case of high velocity trauma. Associated injuries are more common with posterior dislocations and include the following:

- Tracheal rupture
- Arterial or venous lacerations
- Subclavian arterial or venous occlusions
- Pneumothorax
- Chronic instability
- Chest wall deformity

Imaging of the articulation and associated potential complications is best accomplished with CT. Vascular injury may require conventional angiography (Fig. 9-54E). Postoperative evaluation can also be accomplished with CT even in the presence of orthopaedic hardware. Implant failure or migration can be evaluated with serial radiographs in most cases. If bioabsorbable anchors or synthetic devices are used MRI may be the preferred technique.

## Suggested Reading

Cofield RH, Berquist TH. The shoulder. In: Berquist TH. *Imaging of orthopaedic trauma*, 2nd ed. New York: Raven Press; 1992:579–657.

Lyons FA, Rockwood CA Jr. Migration of pins used in operations on the shoulder. *J Bone Joint Surg.* 1990;72A:1262–1267.

## Shoulder Arthroplasty

Glenohumeral joint replacement has become the technique of choice for patients with articular damage and pain that does not respond to more conservative measures. Currently, options include biological resurfacing, resurfacing of the humeral head, hemiarthroplasty, total joint replacement, and reverse shoulder prostheses.

### Indications and Preoperative Evaluation

The primary indication for shoulder arthroplasty is pain not responding to other conservative or surgical measures. Loss of function is also considered. The primary indications and contraindications are listed in the subsequent text.

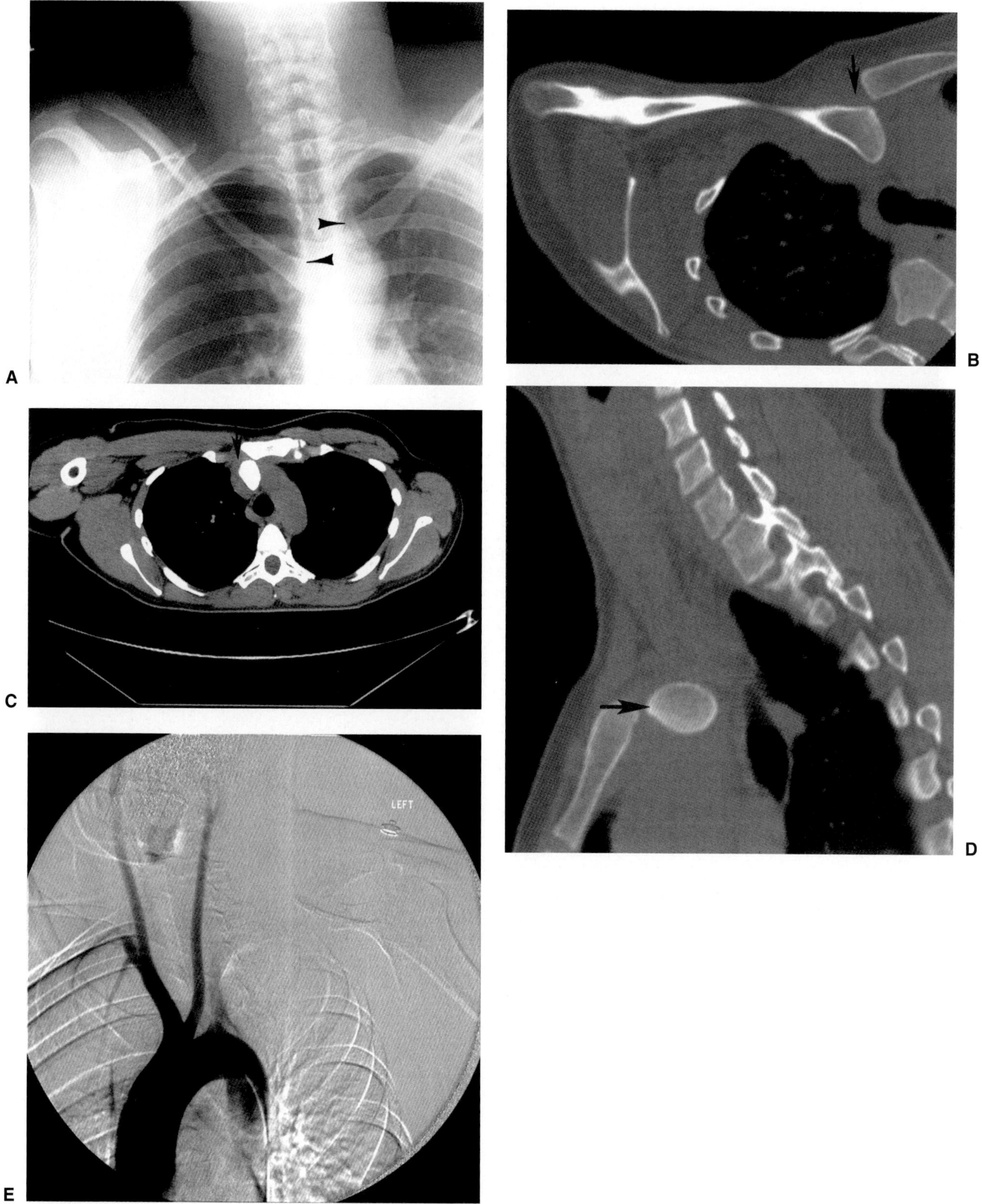


Fig. 9-54 Posterior sternoclavicular dislocation. A: Anteroposterior (AP) radiograph demonstrates asymmetry in the position of the medial clavicles (*arrowheads*). Axial computed tomography (CT) images with bone (B) and soft tissue (C) settings and sagittal reformatted image (D) demonstrate the posterior dislocation (*arrow*) clearly. The medial clavicle abuts the aorta and great vessels. Preoperative angiogram (E) shows no vessel laceration. (Courtesy of Miriam Mikhail, M.D., Flagler Hospital, St. Augustine, Florida.)

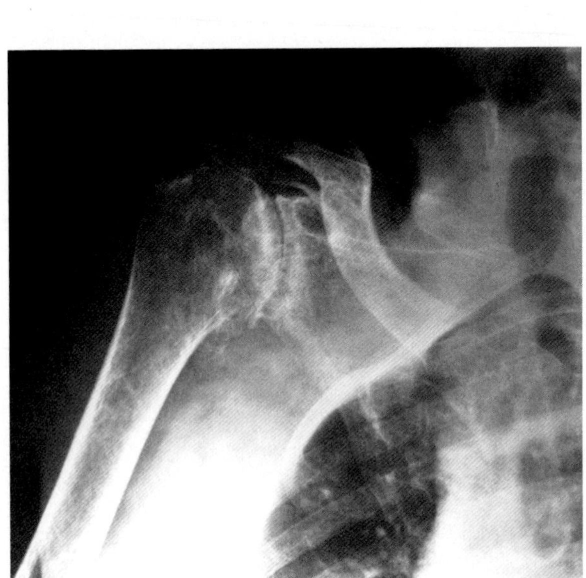


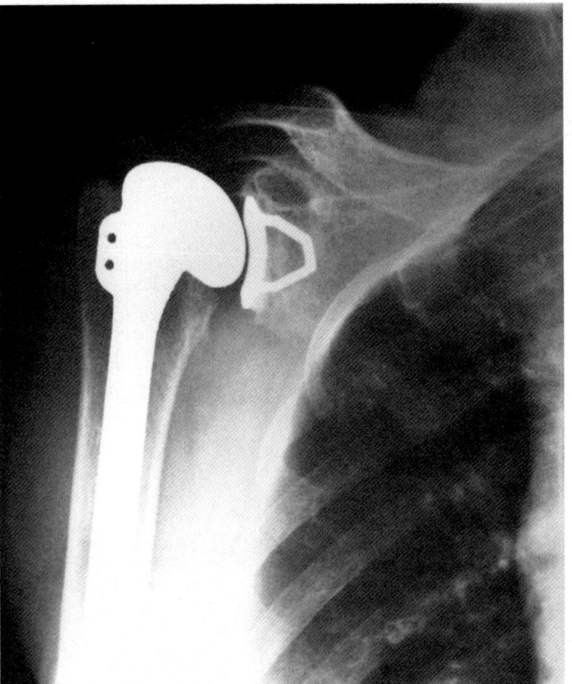


Fig. 9-55 Advanced osteoarthritis. A: Anteroposterior (AP) radiograph demonstrating marked joint space narrowing with small subchondral cysts in the humeral head and glenoid. B: Radiograph following total shoulder replacement.

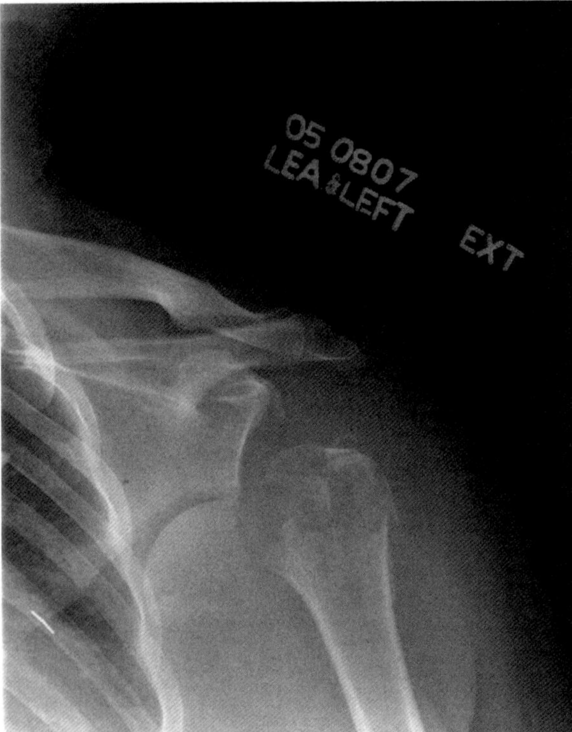


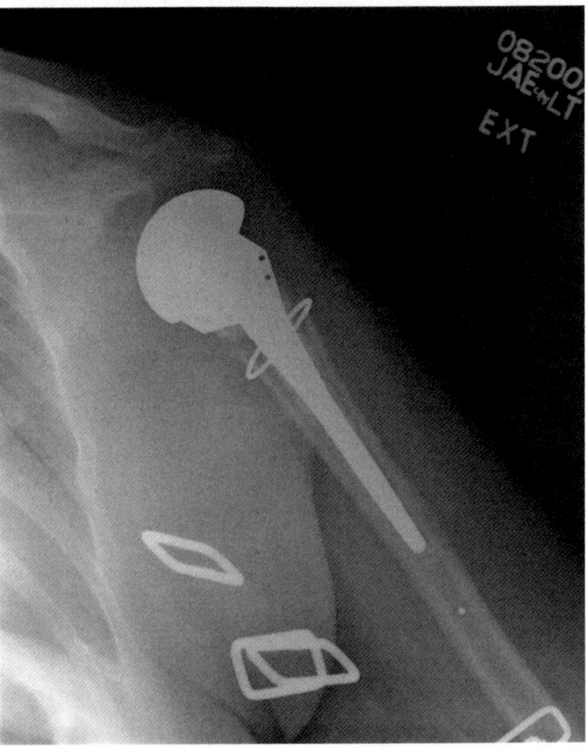


Fig. 9-56 Complex four-part proximal humeral fracture. A: Anteroposterior (AP) radiograph demonstrating the fracture with high risk for avascular necrosis of the humeral head, but normal appearing glenoid. B: Hemiarthroplasty was performed using a reverse shoulder humeral component and modular head with a single Dall-Miles cable around the proximal humerus.

**Indications for shoulder replacement**

Osteoarthritis
Rheumatoid arthritis
Traumatic arthropathy
Rotator cuff arthropathy
Avascular necrosis
Ankylosing spondylitis
Radiation necrosis

**Contraindications for shoulder replacement**

Infection
Neuropathic arthropathy
Neuromuscular disorders
Inadequate bone stock
Poor patient compliance (relative)
Uncontrolled seizure disorders (relative)

The prognosis and selection of repair technique varies with the extent of bone, joint, and soft tissue involvement. Clinical evaluation and image features are used to select the appropriate patients and approach to shoulder replacement.

There are numerous clinical scoring systems used to evaluate patients preoperatively and postoperatively. The Constant and Murley system is commonly used, reproducible, and can be performed in a matter of minutes. This 100-point system is based on pain (15 points), daily activities (20 points), range of motion (40 points), and strength (25 points). Points for pain are 0 if severe, 5 if moderate, 10 if mild, and 15 if there is no pain. Activities include work, recreation, and unaffected sleep.

Image features are also important. The extent of bone loss and articular or osseous deformity may be evident with routine radiographs of the shoulder (see Figs. 9-55 and 9-56). In some cases, CT is required to evaluate osseous changes of the

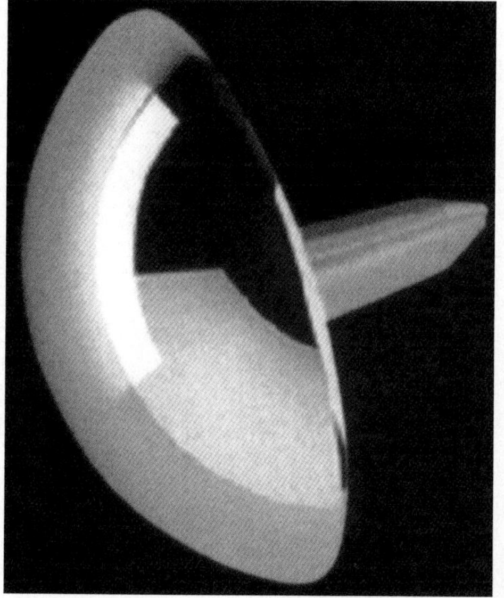
A

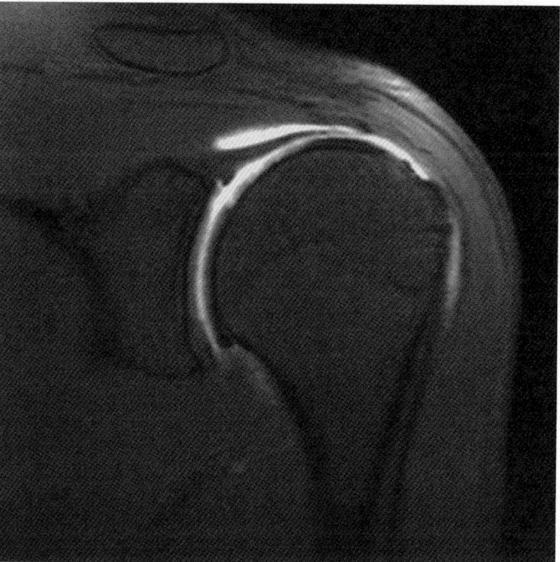
B

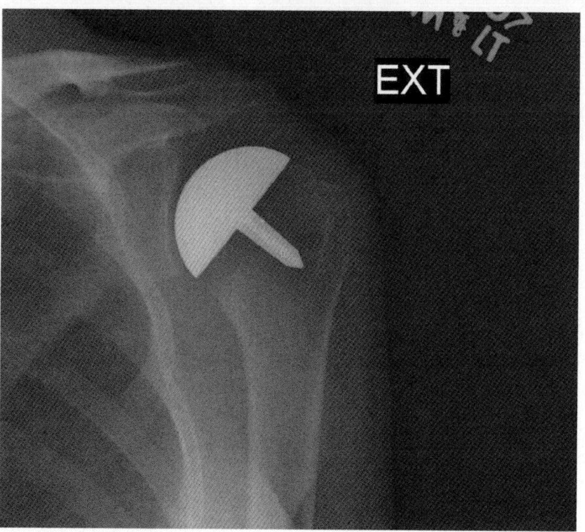

C

Fig. 9-57 Resurfacing arthroplasty in a patient with articular cartilage damage to the humeral head. A: Photograph of a resurfacing implant. (Courtesy of Tornier, Stafford, Texas.) B: Coronal fat-suppressed arthrogram image demonstrating grade III chondromalacia on the humeral head with normal glenoid articular cartilage. C: Anteroposterior (AP) radiograph following resurfacing arthroplasty.

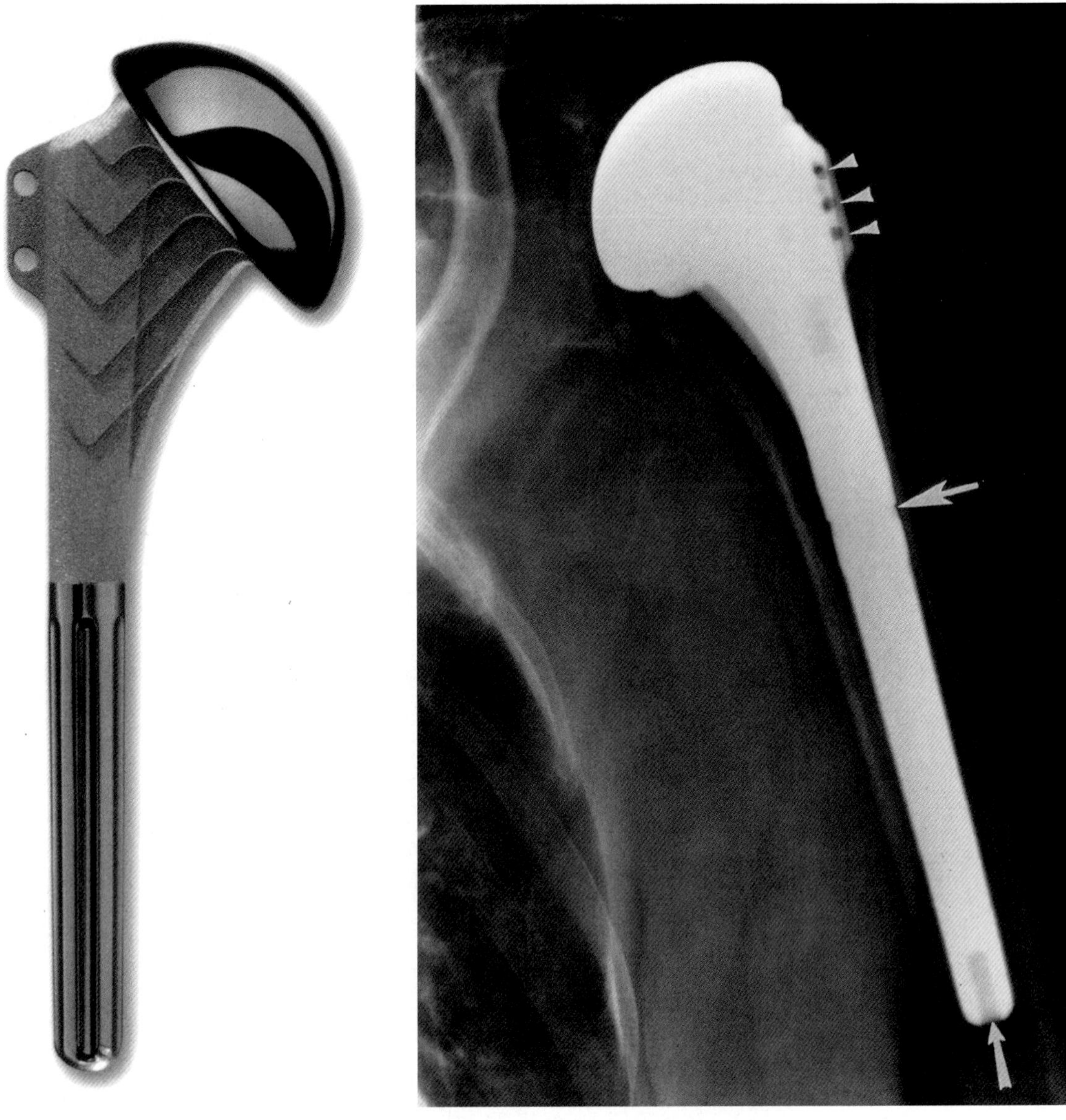


Fig. 9-58 A: Photograph of an Aequalis press fit humeral component with a grit blasted proximal surface and stair-step geometry of improved metaphyseal fixation. (Courtesy of Tornier, Stafford, Texas.) B: Anteroposterior (AP) radiograph of a different modular uncemented hemiarthroplasty. There are suture holes proximally (*arrowheads*), stem length (*arrow at intersection*) can be modified and there is a hollow tip (*arrow*) for a centralizer when the component is used with cement. The proximal portion is porous coated.

glenoid. MRI is useful for evaluation of soft tissues, the rotator cuff, labrum, and articular cartilage. Articular cartilage changes are especially important if resurfacing or hemiarthroplasty are considered (see Fig. 9-57). MR arthrography is most useful to evaluate subtle changes (Fig. 9-57A).

## Suggested Reading

Berquist TH, De Orio JK. The shoulder. In: Berquist TH. *Imaging atlas of orthopaedic appliances and prostheses*. New York: Raven Press; 1995:661–727.

Caniggia M, Fornara P, Franci M, et al. Shoulder arthroplasty. Indications, contraindications and complications. *Panminerva Med*. 1999;41:341–349.

Constant CR, Murley AHG. A clinical method of functional assessment of the shoulder. *Clin Orthop*. 1987;214:16–164.

Feldman F. Radiology of shoulder prostheses. *Semin Musculoskelet Radiol*. 2006;10:5–20.

### Treatment Options

Treatment options vary with patient age, gender, activity level, and associated comorbidities. Bone changes from prior trauma, arthropathy or surgical procedures, and soft tissue support are also important factors. Depending on these factors, surgeons may elect to perform soft tissue (biological) arthroplasty, humeral head resurfacing, hemiarthroplasty, or total joint replacement (see Figs. 9-58 to 9-60). Soft tissue glenoid resurfacing is not commonly performed. This technique has potential in young, athletically active patients with pain and reduced function not responding to more conservative approaches. This technique provides resurfacing of the glenoid using fascia lata, Achilles tendon allografts, or the joint capsule. The technique is combined with humeral hemiarthroplasty components.

## Suggested Reading


Berquist TH. Imaging of joint replacement procedures. *Radiol Clin North Am.* 2006;44:419–437.

Berquist TH, De Orio JK. The shoulder. In: Berquist TH. *Imaging atlas of orthopaedic appliances and prostheses*. New York: Raven Press; 1995:661–727.

Guery J, Favard L, Sirveaux F, et al. Reverse total shoulder arthroplasty. Survivorship analysis of eighty replacements followed for 5–10 years. *J Bone Joint Surg.* 2006;88A:1742–1747.

Krishnan SG, Nowinski RJ, Harrison D, et al. Humeral hemiarthroplasty with biological resurfacing of the glenoid for glenohumeral arthritis. *J Bone Joint Surg.* 2007;89A:727–734.

McFarland EG, Sanguanjit P, Tasaki A, et al. The reverse shoulder prosthesis: A review of features and imaging complications. *Skeletal Radiol.* 2006;35:488–496.

Wall B, Nove-Josserand L, O'Connor DP, et al. Reverse shoulder arthroplasty: A review of results according to etiology. *J Bone Joint Surg.* 2007;89A:1476–1485.


## Postoperative Evaluation and Complications

Following joint replacement procedures, patients are evaluated clinically and postoperative scores (Constant and Murley) are compared to preoperative data. Imaging plays an important role to provide a baseline for component position and evaluating potential complications that may develop. Routine shoulder images should include AP images in internal and external

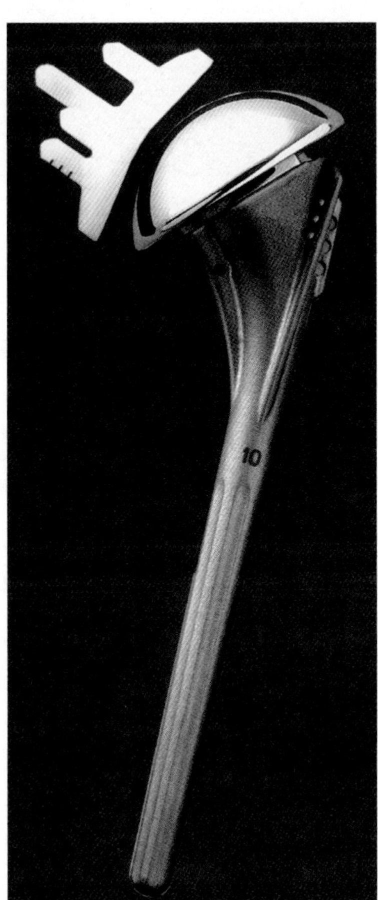


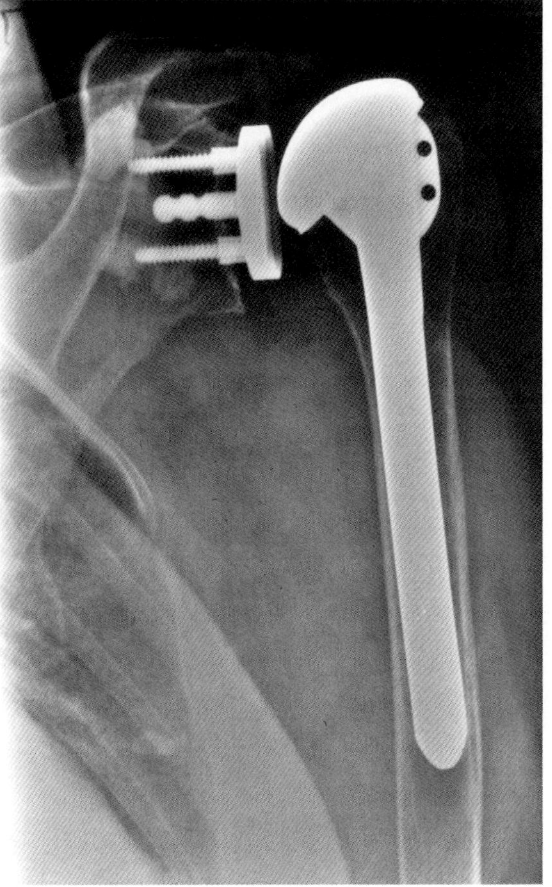


**Fig. 9-59** Total shoulder arthroplasty. **A:** DePuy Global Advantage shoulder arthroplasty system with a polyethylene glenoid component. The humeral component comes in six sizes with stem diameters for 6 to 16 mm. (Courtesy of DePuy, a Johnson and Johnson Company, Warsaw, Indiana.) **B:** Cofield shoulder with nonmodular humeral component and metal-backed polyethylene glenoid component. Anteroposterior (AP) **(C)** and axillary **(D)** views of a new generation modular Zimmer anatomic humeral component and a polyethylene glenoid component. (C and D Courtesy of Dr. Mark Broderson, M.D., Mayo Clinic Jacksonville.)

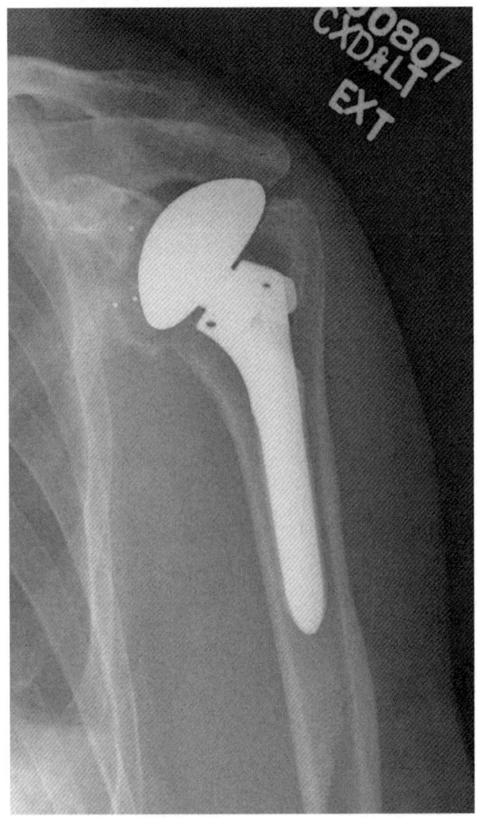


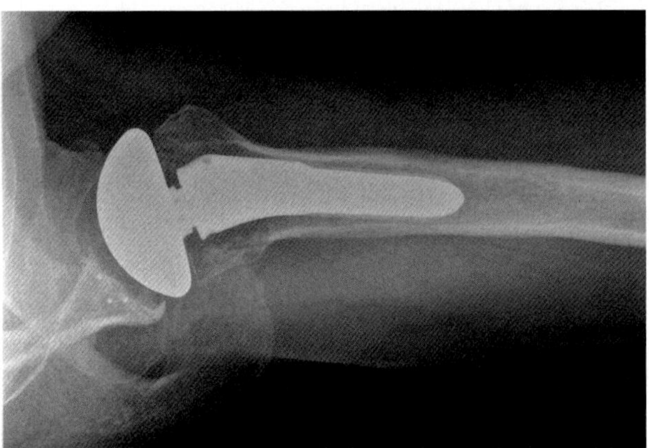


Fig. 9-59 (*Continued*)

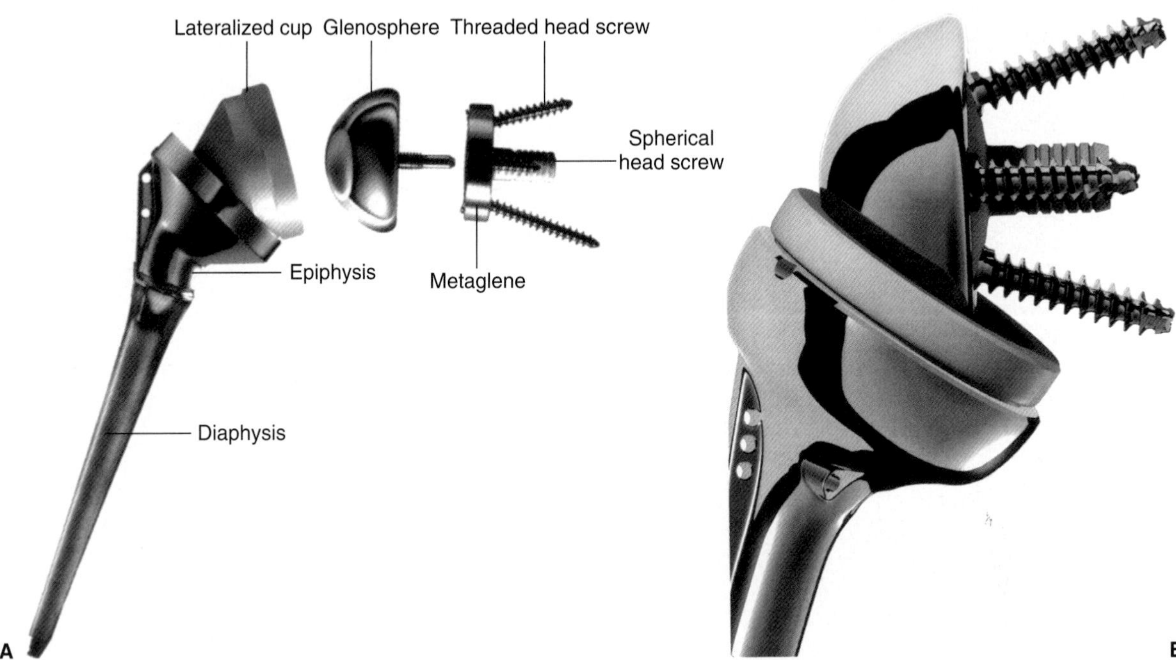


Fig. 9-60 Reverse shoulder prostheses. Reverse Delta CTA (**A**) and new reverse Delta Xtend (**B**). The Delta CTA has a humeral component, lateralized cup, glenosphere, metaglene, and glenoid screws. (Courtesy of DePuy, a Johnson and Johnson Company, Warsaw, Indiana.) **C:** Anteroposterior (AP) radiograph of a reverse Delta system. **D:** Encore reverse shoulder system. (Courtesy of Encore Medical Corporation, Austin, Texas.) **E:** Tornier Aequalis reverse shoulder system. (Courtesy of Tornier, Stafford, Texas.)

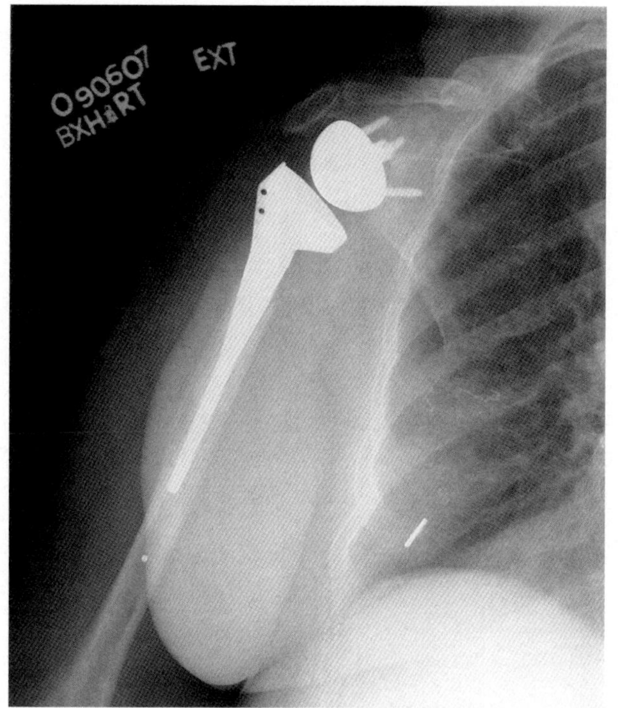


C

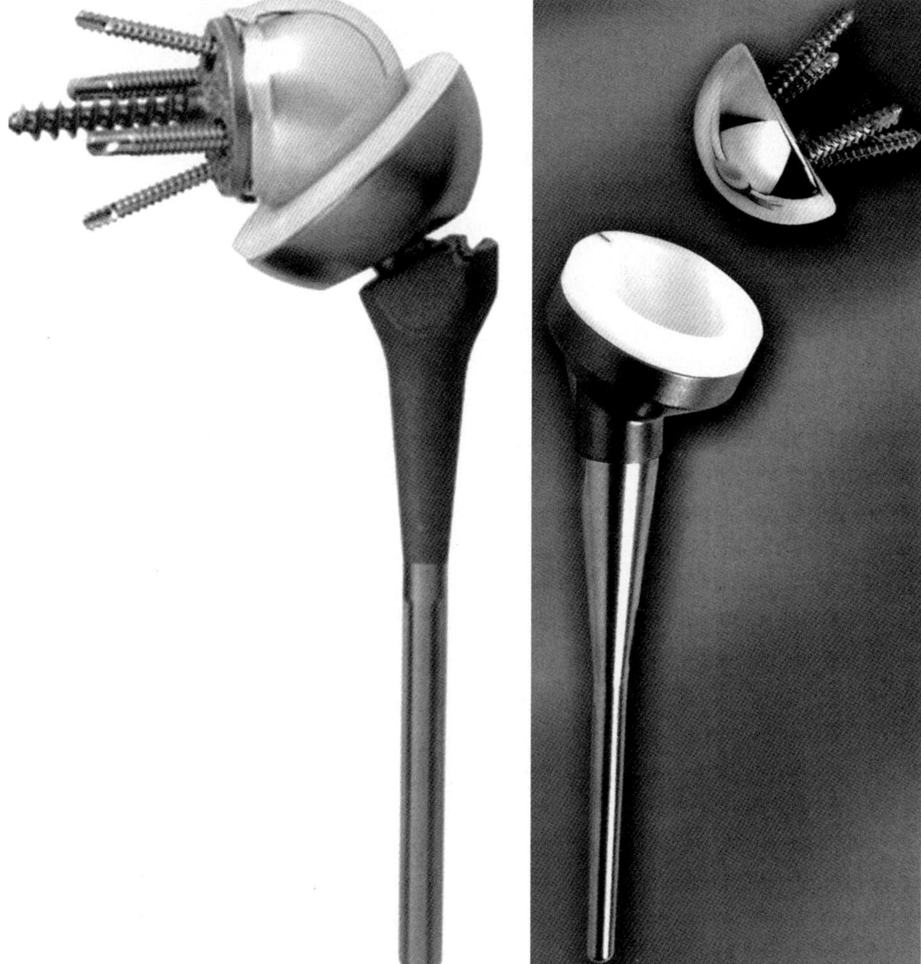

D

E

Fig. 9-60 (*Continued*)

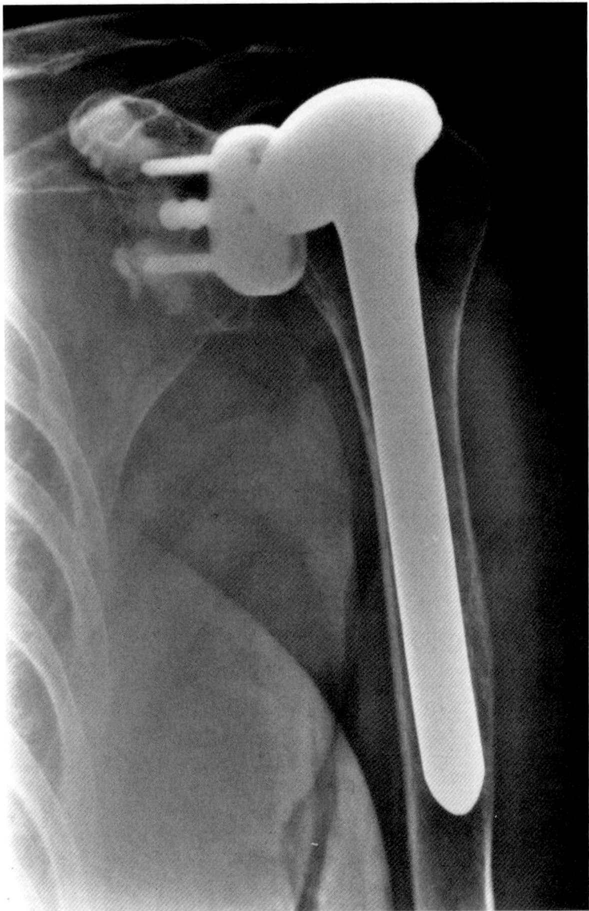


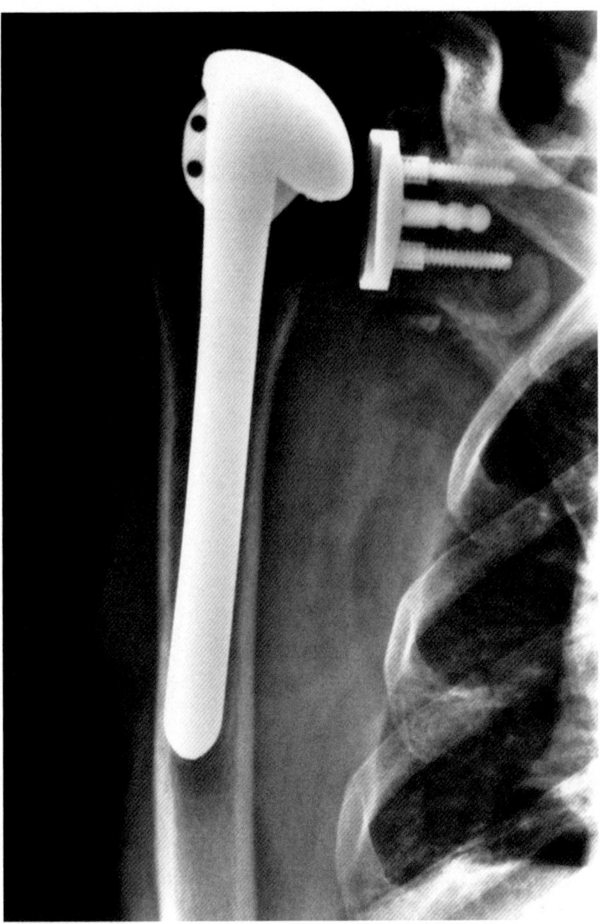


Fig. 9-61 Conventional radiograph (A) and fluoroscopically position (B) image following Cofield total shoulder replacement. The glenoid–bone interface is not clearly identified on the conventional image.

rotation, a true AP (patient rotated 40 degrees posteriorly), scapular Y or transthoracic view and an axillary projection. As with the knee, it may be difficult to accurately evaluate the glenoid interface and humeral component with conventional views. Ideally, the initial examination should be fluoroscopically positioned to avoid this problem (see Fig. 9-61). With cemented components the cement mantle should be uniform about both components. The humeral component cement mantle should blend with the cortex and extend several centimeters beyond the component with or without a cement restrictor. Ideally, there should not be cement voids about the component (see Fig. 9-62). The humeral component collar should be parallel to the bone cut proximally (see Fig. 9-63).

Complications following shoulder arthroplasty vary with the type of procedure, implants selected, and patient compliance.

## Component Loosening

Component loosening accounts for up to 39% of complications. Component loosening can be detected radiographically by the development of lucent lines at the bone–cement or component–bone interfaces, by component migration or shift and cement fracture on serial images. Component loosening is more common with glenoid than humeral components. Both all-polyethylene (Fig. 9-62) and metal back (Fig. 9-61) components have been used. Metal-backed uncemented components are more problematic in regard to loosening. The glenoid component loosens in 30% to 90% of cases radiographically over a 10- to 15-year follow-up (see Fig. 9-64). However, clinical loosening is much less common and revision surgery is required in only approximately 7% of patients.

Humeral component loosening is much less common (1% to 7%). Loosening is suggested radiographically (clinically at risk for loosening) by lucent zones exceeding 2 mm in three or more zones (see Fig. 9-65), component tilt, or subsidence. Humeral component subsidence (distal migration) occurs in up to 7% of patients. Serial radiographs are usually adequate for diagnosis of significant (2 mm) lucent lines, cement fracture, and component migration (Fig. 9-62). Lucent lines may also be evident about uncemented components. Shedding of the surface beads of mesh also indicates loosening (see Fig. 9-66).

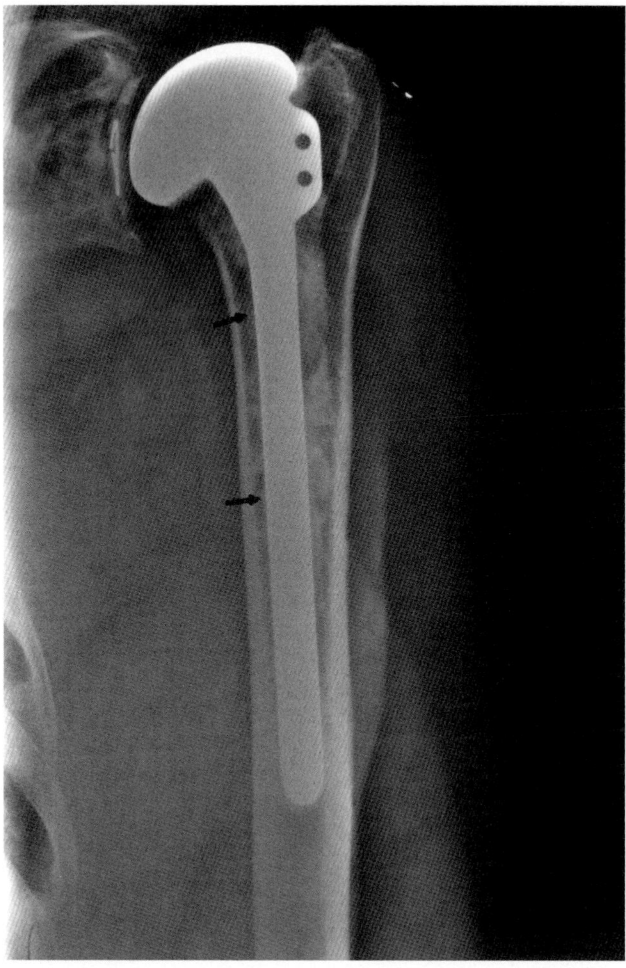

Fig. 9-62 Cemented total shoulder arthroplasty. There is no cement distal to the component and there are numerous voids medially (*arrows*).

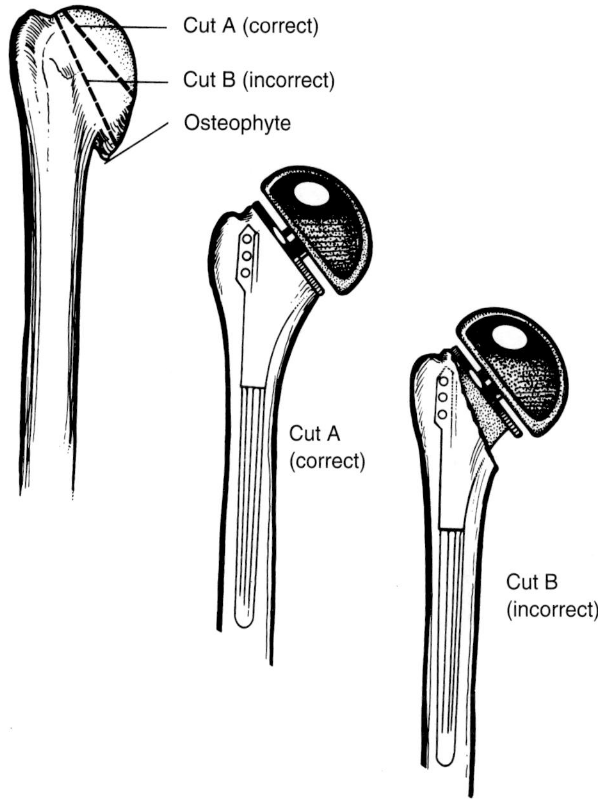


Fig. 9-63 Illustration of the proper bone cut and component alignment with the component collar parallel to the bone cut. (Courtesy of DePuy, a Johnson and Johnson Company, Warsaw, Indiana.)

Loosening may also be evaluated with radionuclide scans or positron emission tomography (PET). Subtraction arthrography is commonly performed in the hip, but less often used in the shoulder (see Fig. 9-67).

## Instability

Instability is the second leading cause of complications following shoulder arthroplasty, accounting for 30% of all complications. Instability may be anterior, superior, posterior, inferior, or multidirectional.

Anterior and superior instability account for 80% of postoperative instability cases. Anterior instability may be related to multiple soft tissue, component, and osseous issues. Humeral component rotation, anterior glenoid deficiency, and deficiency in the deltoid, anterior capsule, and subscapularis may all play a role. Tears of the subscapularis may be related to a component head that is too large, operative technique, or postoperative physical therapy.

Superior instability is common and related to a deficient rotator cuff and/or subacromial arch. Serial radiographs may demonstrate superior migration (see Fig. 9-68). Posterior instability may be related to posterior glenoid erosion, soft tissue deficiency, or excessive component retroversion. Inferior instability is most often due to failure to restore humeral length which can occur in patients undergoing joint replacement for proximal humeral fractures or neoplasms. Conventional arthrography is useful to address capsular anatomy and tears. MR images are usually significantly degraded by metal artifact resulting in suboptimal image quality. Stress maneuvers under fluoroscopy may be more accurate for evaluating the extent and directions of instability (see Fig. 9-69).

Dislocations occur in 1% to 7% of patients. This usually occurs in the postoperative period with range of motion beginning. Anterior dislocations are most common (see Fig. 9-70).

## Periprosthetic Fractures

Fractures may occur in the humerus or glenoid. Humeral fractures occur in approximately 1.8% of patients. They account for 11% of all postoperative complications. Intraoperative fractures may occur with reaming, improper component positioning, or manipulation of the extremity. Fractures that

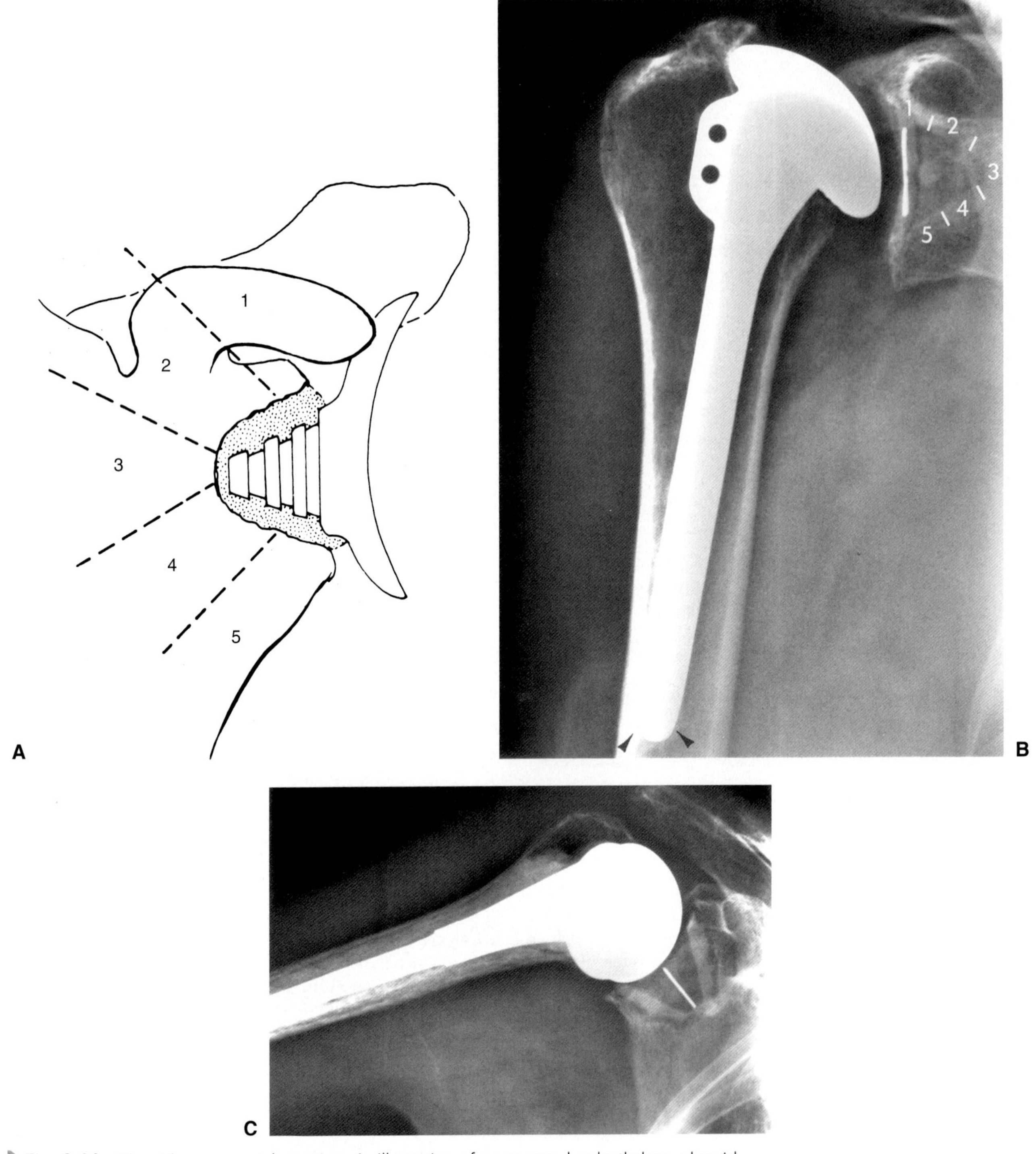


Fig. 9-64 Glenoid component loosening. A: Illustration of a cemented polyethylene glenoid component with the five zones superior to inferior used to describe lucent lines. B: Radiograph with the zones marked and no lucent lines at the bone–cement interface. The humeral component has subsided slightly (*arrowheads*). C: Fluoroscopically positioned image with a loose glenoid component and wide lucent lines in all five zones.

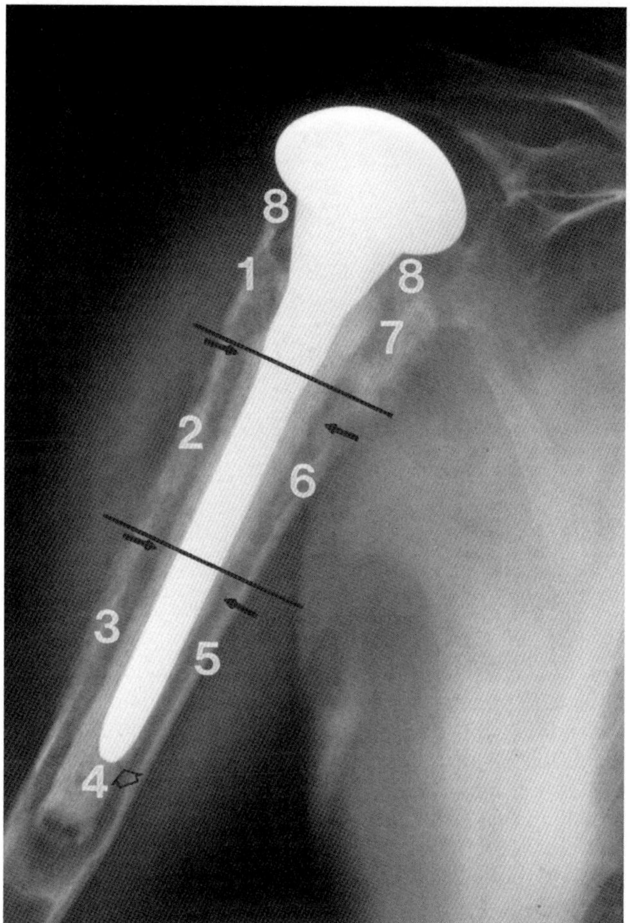


**Fig. 9-65** Humeral component loosening and infection. The humeral component is divided into eight zones for purposes of describing lucent lines at the bone–cement interface. Zone *8* is immediately below the head and zones *1* to *7* progress lateral to medial similar to femoral components in the hip. Anteroposterior (AP) radiograph demonstrates gross loosening with wide irregular lucency about the component (*arrows*) in all zones. There is also a cement fracture at the tip of the component (*open arrow*). There is cortical irregularity and periosteal reaction secondary to the infection.

occur proximal to the tip of the humeral component can be treated with cerclage wires or Dall-Miles cables. If the fracture is at the tip of the component a longer component should be used. The component should extend at least 5 to 6 cm beyond the fracture.

Postoperative fractures occur on average approximately 4 years following the procedure, but can occur at any time. They most commonly occur at the tip of the femoral component (see Fig. 9-71). Stress fractures can occur about the glenoid implants as well. Fractures may be treated conservatively or with internal fixation. The incidence increases in patients with osteopenia.

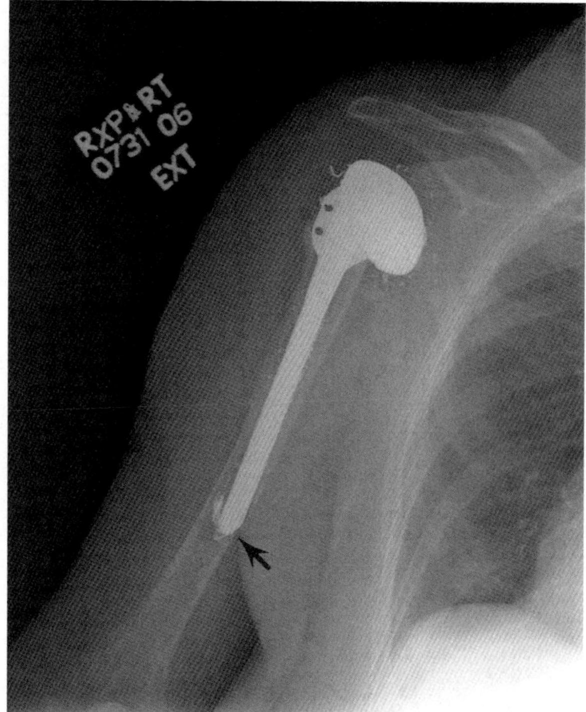

A

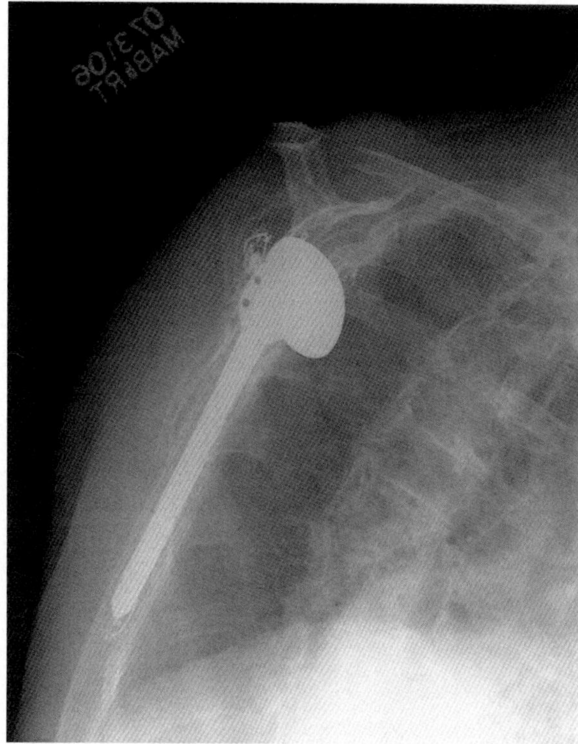

B

**Fig. 9-66** Loose uncemented component. Anteroposterior (AP) (**A**) and scapular Y (**B**) views demonstrate extensive shedding of surface particles. The tip of the humeral stem is breaking through the cortex (*arrow* in **A**).

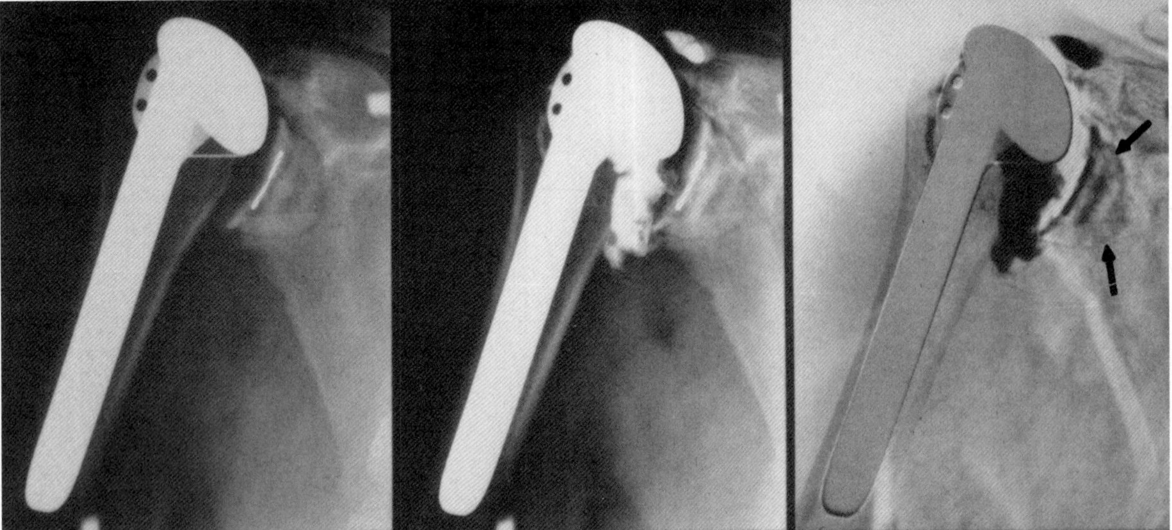

Fig. 9-67 Glenoid loosening. Scout, conventional, and subtracted arthrogram images demonstrating contrast extending about the glenoid component (*arrows*) due to loosening.

## Infection

The incidence of deep infection is reported at 0.7% in two series totaling 2,540 cases. The incidence of infections following revision surgery is higher approaching 4%. Up to 67% of deep infections occur within the first year following joint replacement. Predisposing factors include revision surgery, rheumatoid arthritis, systemic steroid therapy, obesity, and hematogenous spread from other common infections. Patient symptoms may be subtle, but pain is usually present. Radiographic changes may be absent (Fig. 9-71) or mimic loosening (Fig. 9-65). Positive laboratory tests including elevated white blood cell counts, erythrocyte sedimentation rates, and C-reactive protein are good indicators of infection. The most common organisms are *Staphylococcus aureus*, coagulase-negative Staphylococcus and *Propionibacterium acnes*.

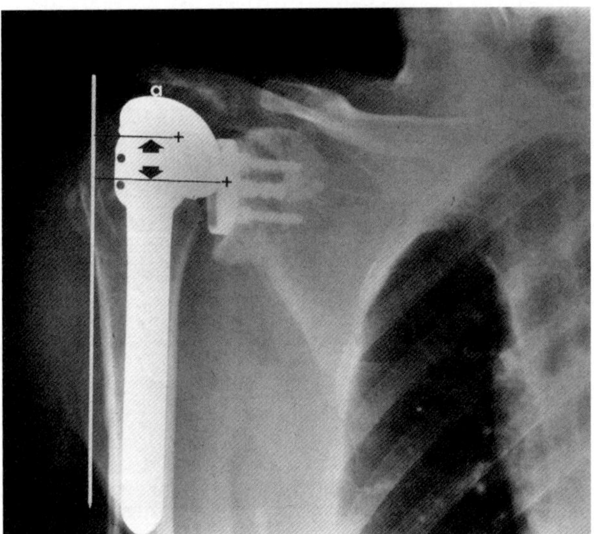

Fig. 9-68 Superior migration with reduced humeroacromial space (*a*). Follow-up evaluation can be more consistent by selecting the center of the glenoid (+) and the humeral head (+) and drawing lines (*black lines*) perpendicular to a line parallel to the humerus (*white line*). The distance between the lines can be compared on serial images.

Radiographs may be unimpressive or demonstrate signs of loosening (see Fig. 9-72 and also Fig. 9-65). Joint aspiration and subtraction arthrogram features may be useful. Demonstration of loosening, fistulous tracts, aggressive synovitis (see Fig. 9-73), and pocketing about the pseudocapsule are indicative of infection. Radionuclide scans are commonly used to identify infection. Unfortunately, uptake about implants can be variable when the infection occurs within the first year. Approaches include technetium Tc 99m methyl diphosphonate (MDP) scans that are positive with loosening, but uptake may appear more diffuse in cases of infection. Combination studies using Tc 99m MDP and indium-labeled white blood cells or technetium-labeled monoclonal antibodies or antigranulocytes improve the accuracy of confirming infection. Indium-labeled white blood cell scans are 84% to 96% sensitive and demonstrate specificities approaching 96%. PET imaging has also proved useful for evaluation of periprosthetic infections demonstrating sensitivities of 97% and specificities approaching 86%.

Once the diagnosis is established treatment must be aggressive. Depending on the virulence of the organism and extent of involvement, patients may be treated with debridement and intravenous antibiotics, implant removal with resection arthroplasty or component removal, and placement of antibiotic impregnated temporary implants with later revision (Fig. 9-72).

## Nerve Injuries

Nerve injuries to the brachial plexus or deltoid muscle dysfunction related to axillary nerve injuries occur in 1% to 2% of cases. Most resolve spontaneously although regional pain syndrome can occur. Radial nerve injury can occur with periprosthetic fractures at the junction of the mid and distal third of the humerus.

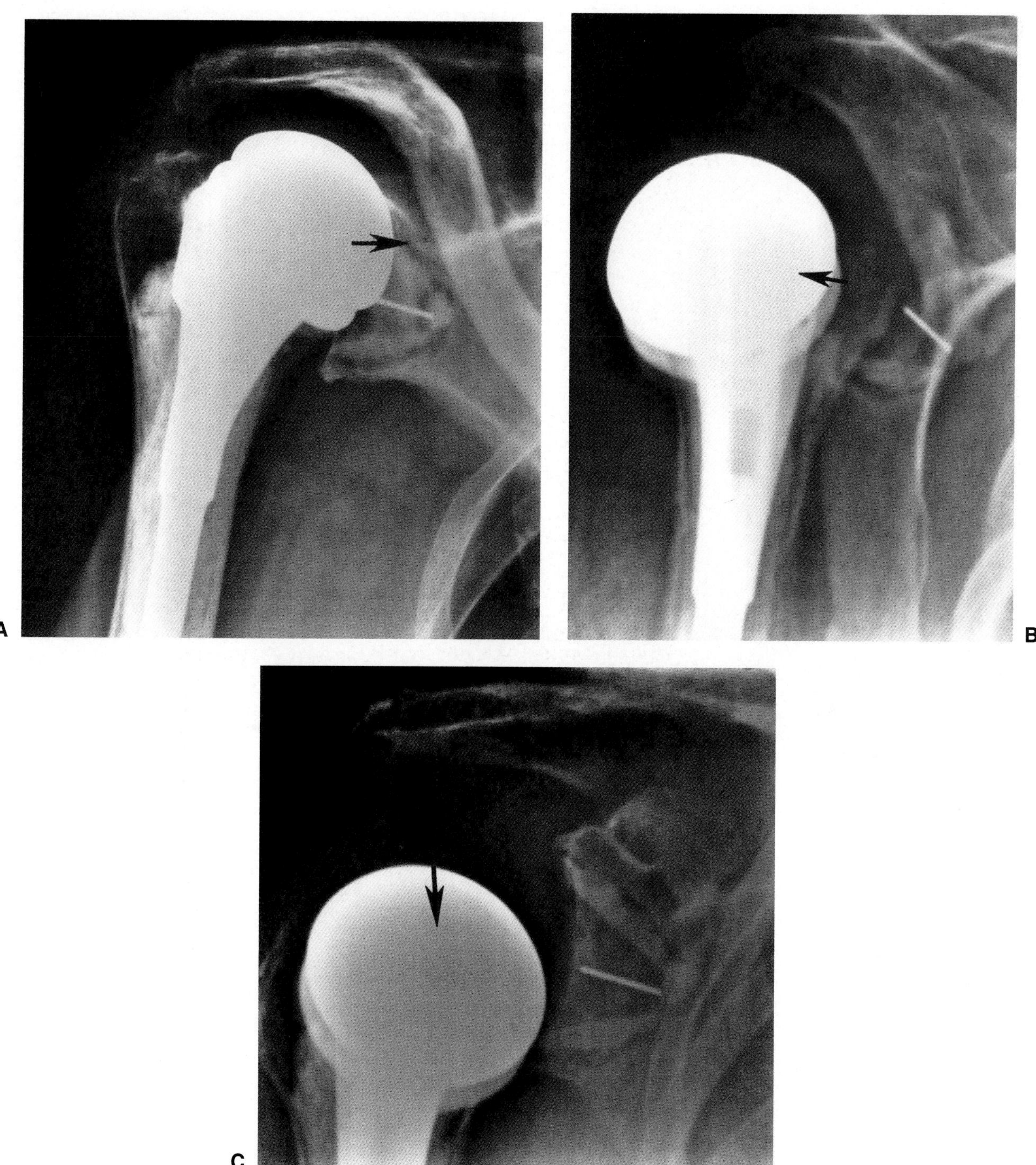


Fig. 9-69 Fluoroscopically positioned motion studies for instability and component position. There is anterior (A), posterior (B), and inferior (C) multidirectional instability and loosening of the glenoid component.

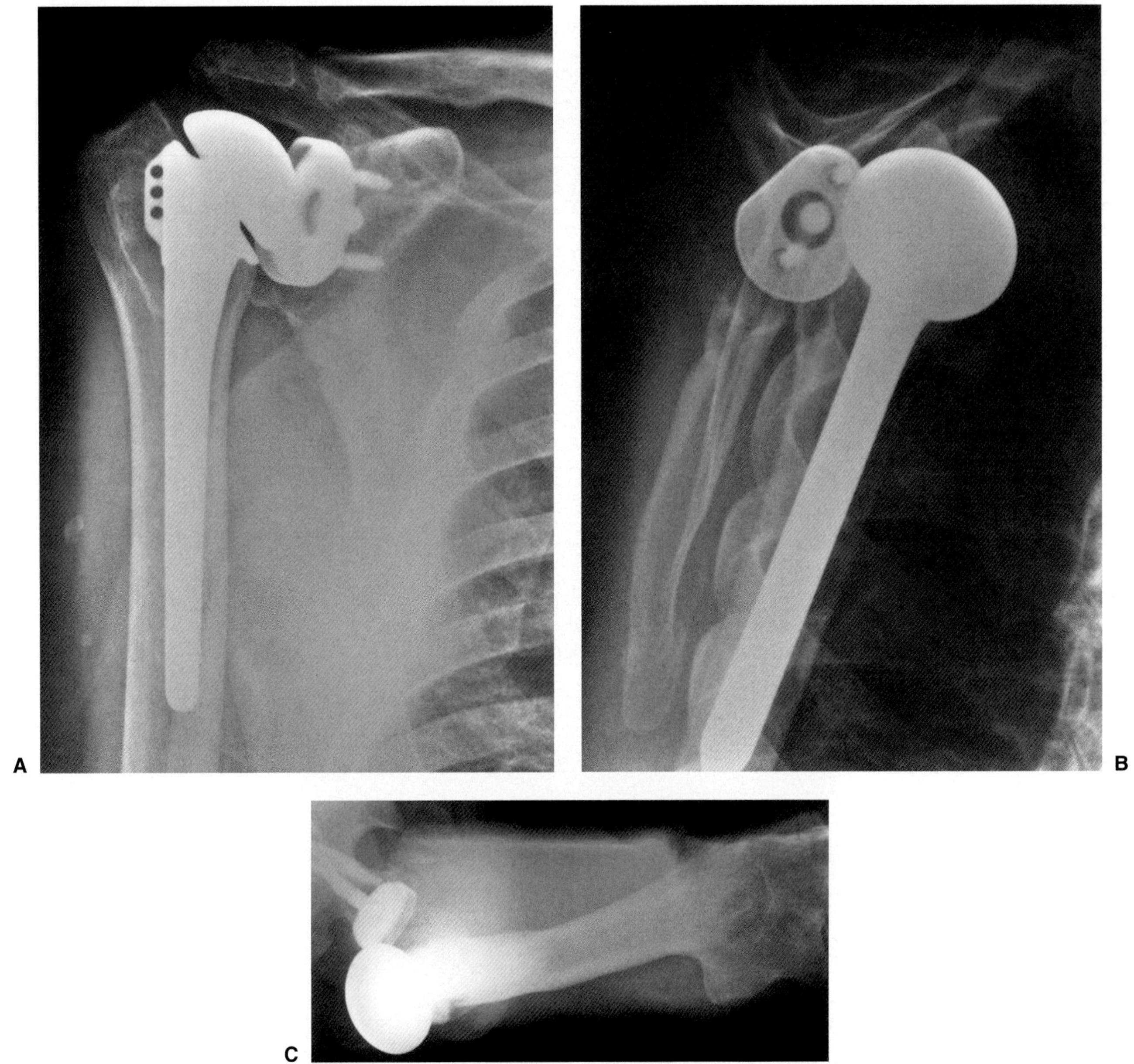

Fig. 9-70 Anterior dislocation. Anteroposterior (AP) (A), scapular Y (B), and axillary (C) views of an anterior dislocation.

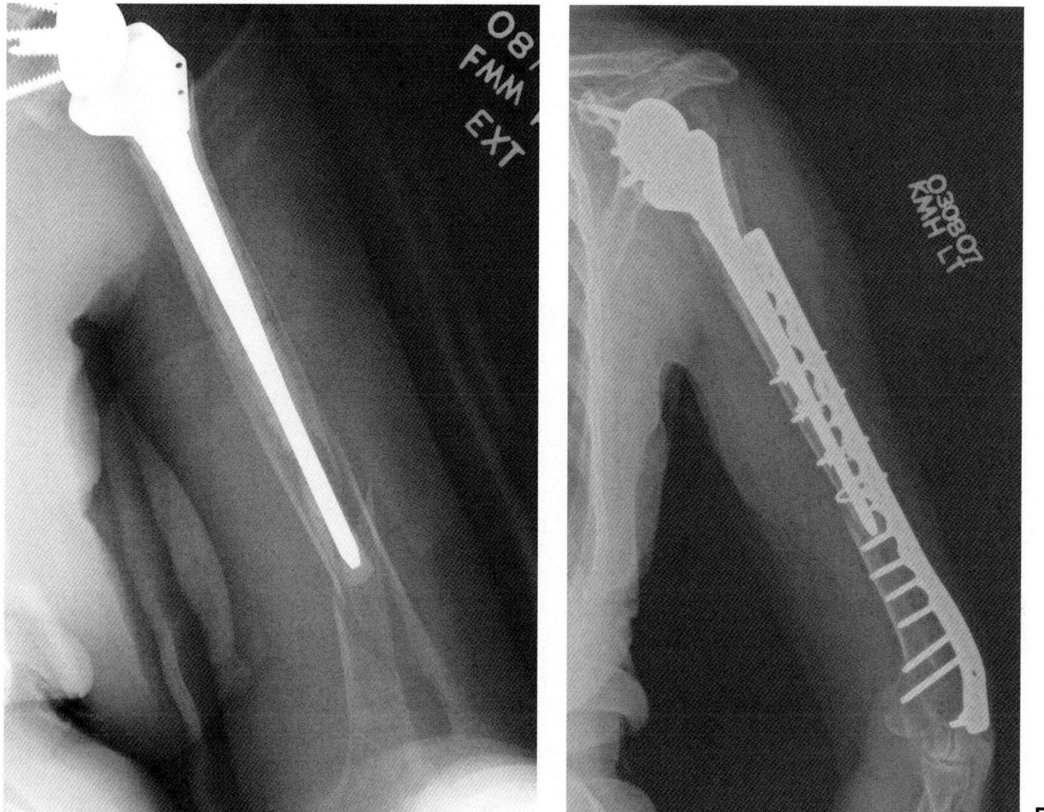


**Fig. 9-71** Periprosthetic humeral fracture. **A:** Radiograph demonstrates a reverse shoulder prosthesis with a comminuted fracture distal to the component tip. **B:** Radiograph following internal fixation with a low contact locking plate and Dall-Miles cables.

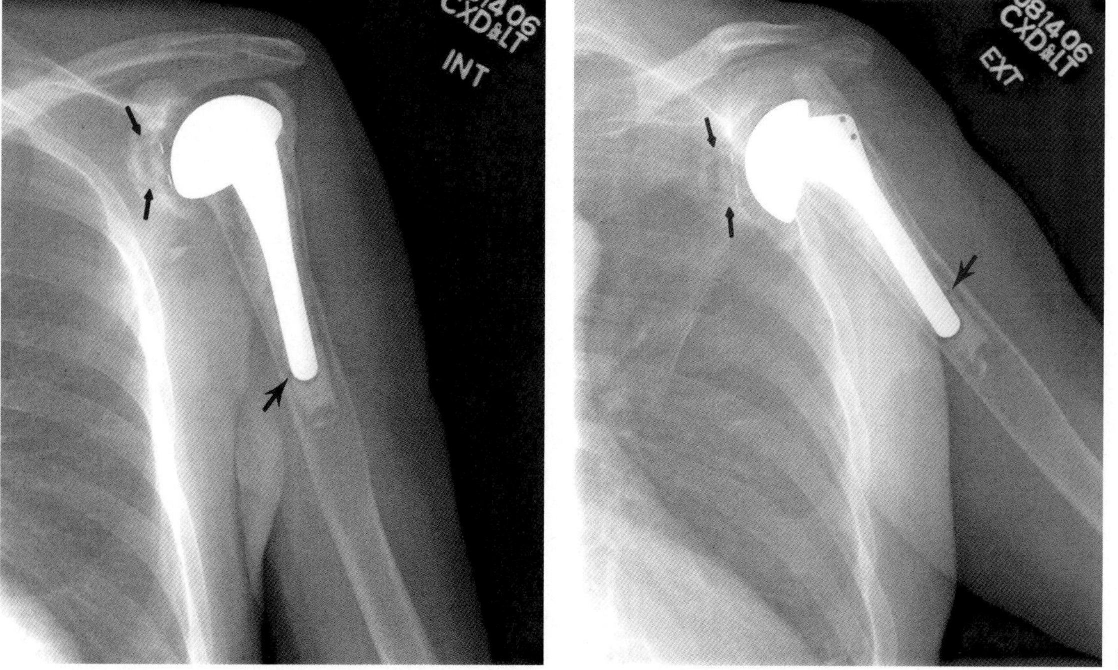


**Fig. 9-72** Periprosthetic infection. Radiographs (**A** and **B**) demonstrate signs of loosening of the glenoid component (*arrows*) with a cement fracture (*large arrow*) and lucency in zone 4 of the humeral component. **C:** Implants were removed resulting in proximal humeral fracture. An antibiotic-impregnated implant was placed until the infection cleared. **D:** The arthroplasty was later revised with a long stem cemented humeral component and reverse shoulder implant system.

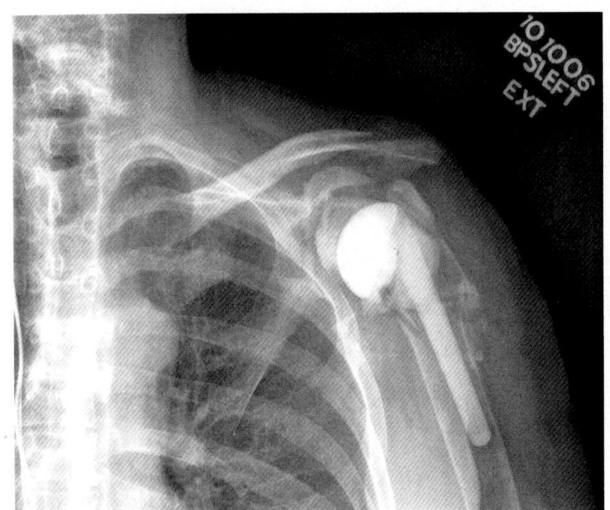


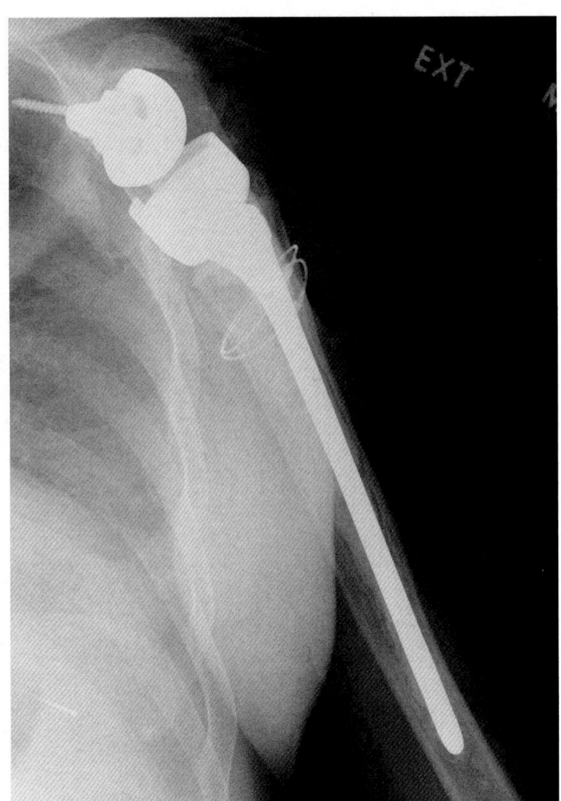


Fig. 9-72 *(Continued)*

## Reverse Shoulder Prostheses

Optimal results with these systems seem to be of use in patients with primary osteoarthritis and rotator cuff deficiency. Results in patients with prior proximal humeral fractures and when implants are used for revision are less favorable. Overall survival rates for reverse shoulder arthroplasty at 10 years approach 91%. Complications with the reverse shoulder systems can be similar to conventional shoulder arthroplasty. Complications occur in 20% of patients. This increases to 37% when implants are used for revision of primary arthroplasty. The incidence of infection is higher (4%), especially when used as revision of primary arthroplasty. The surgical technique is critical and complex resulting in problems beginning with component placement. Hematoma formation (21%) (also leads to increased rate of infection) and nerve injury are more common compared to conventional total shoulder replacements. Intraoperative fractures of the humeral shaft or tuberosities and glenoid are not uncommon, especially if a primary system has to be removed. The incidence of humeral fracture is 24% in this setting.

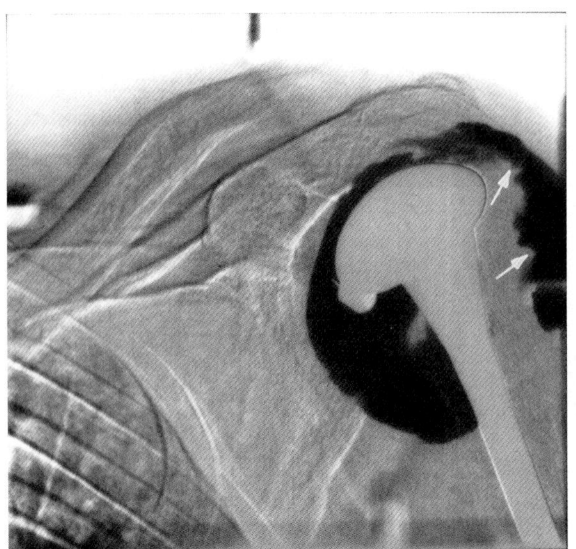

Fig. 9-73 Subtraction arthrogram demonstrating capsular distension and advanced synovitis (*arrows*) due to infection.

Postoperative radiographs should be carefully evaluated to determine the baseline component position. This can be accomplished with routine views noted earlier, but fluoroscopic positioning is more optimal especially for evaluation of the glenoid–metaglene interface (Fig. 9-60A). The glenoid should articulate properly with the humeral surface and screws should be appropriately placed within the scapula (see Fig. 9-74).

There are several other complications that are unique or more common with reverse shoulder implants. Dislocations occur in 7.5% of patients with primary reverse components and the rate is even higher for revision implants (see Fig. 9-75). Dislocation is usually related to soft tissue deficiency or improper implant placement. Soft tissue support can be enhanced with latissimus dorsi transfers combined with reverse shoulder placement.

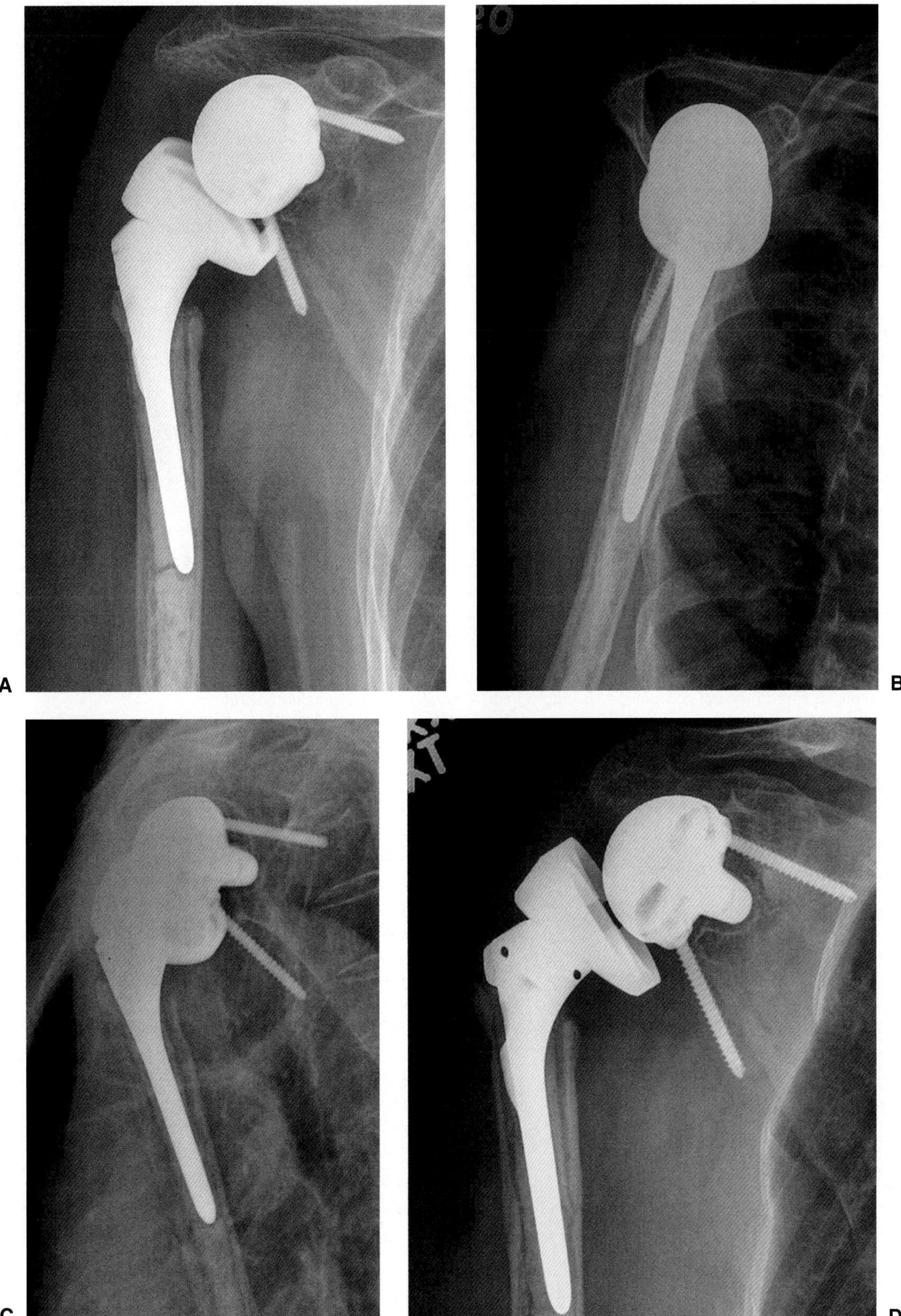


Fig. 9-74 Reverse shoulder prosthesis with radiographic features of loosening and misplaced inferior screw. Anteroposterior (AP) (A) and scapular Y (B) images show the displaced screw outside the scapula. There is also proximal bone loss along the medial humerus and a distal cement fracture suggesting loosening. Transthoracic (C) and true AP (D) images demonstrate lucency about the glenoid metaglene stem indicating glenoid loosening.

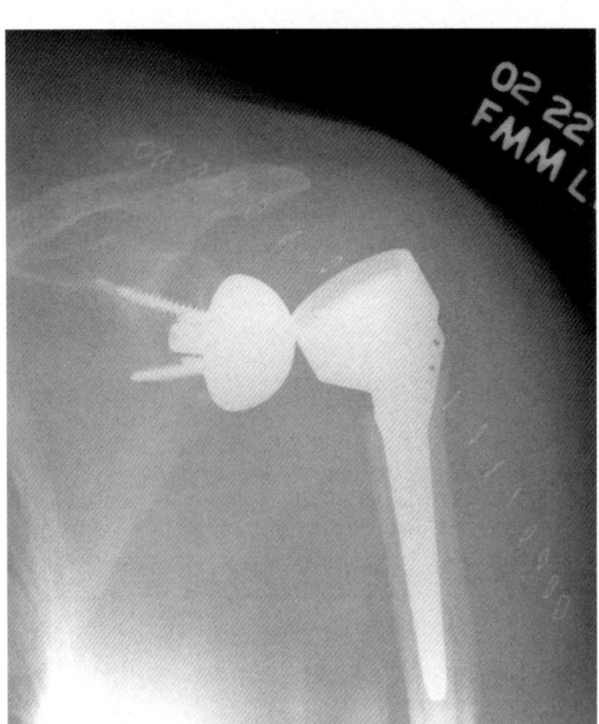


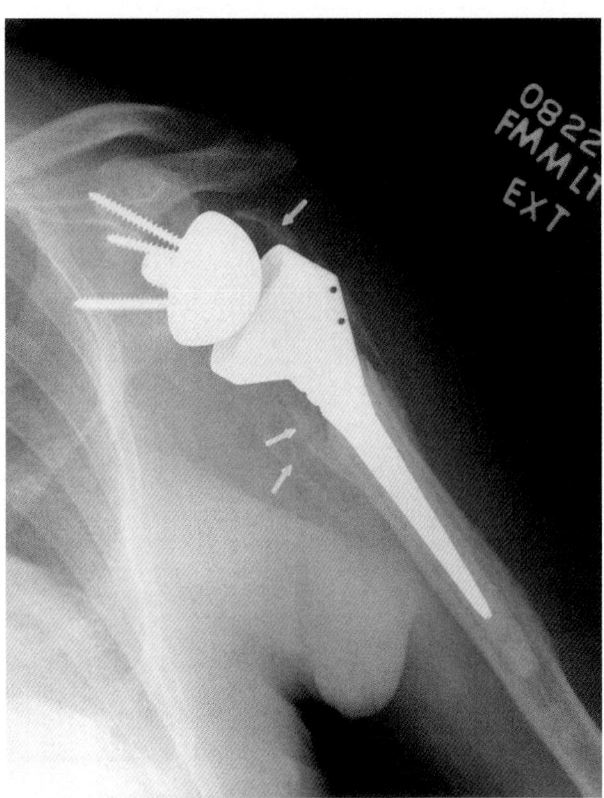


**Fig. 9-75** Dislocation of a reverse shoulder prosthesis. **A:** Anteroposterior (AP) radiograph demonstrates the dislocated humeral component. **B:** Radiograph several months later demonstrating considerable heterotopic ossification (*arrows*) in the soft tissue.

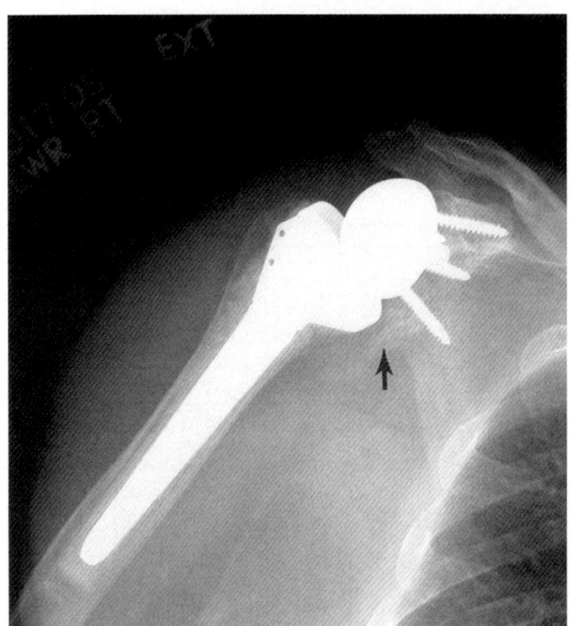


**Fig. 9-76** Radiograph demonstrating heterotopic ossification at the inferior glenoid neck (*arrow*) due to humeral component impingement.

Notching of the inferior scapula at the glenoid neck and secondary heterotopic ossification occur due to impingement of the humeral component edge on the glenoid (see Fig. 9-76). This finding commonly occurs and may affect the anterior or posterior glenoid. Therefore, axillary radiographs are necessary to determine the exact location along with properly (fluoroscopy is best) positioned AP radiographs. Notching occurs in up to 44% of patients. Changes are usually evident within the first 14 months of surgery. Notching can be graded using the Nerot system (see Fig. 9-77).

### NEROT CLASSIFICATION OF SCAPULAR NOTCHING IN REVERSE SHOULDER ARTHROPLASTY

| GRADE | DESCRIPTION |
|---|---|
| Grade 0 | No notch (Fig. 9-77A) |
| Grade 1 | Erosion of lateral pillar only (Fig. 9-77B) |
| Grade 2 | Lateral pillar erosion with sclerosis indicating instability (Fig. 9-77C) |
| Grade 3 | Erosion beyond inferior screw (Fig. 9-77D) |
| Grade 4 | Erosion of metaglene base, first sign of loosening (Fig. 9-77E) |

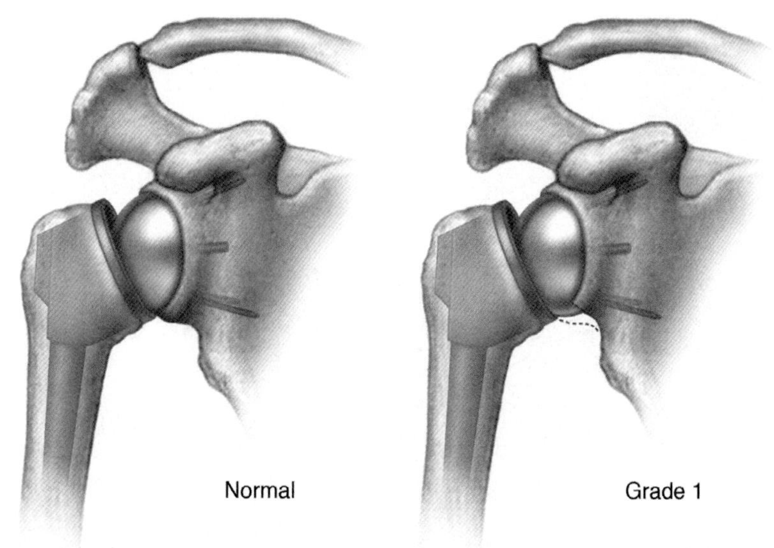


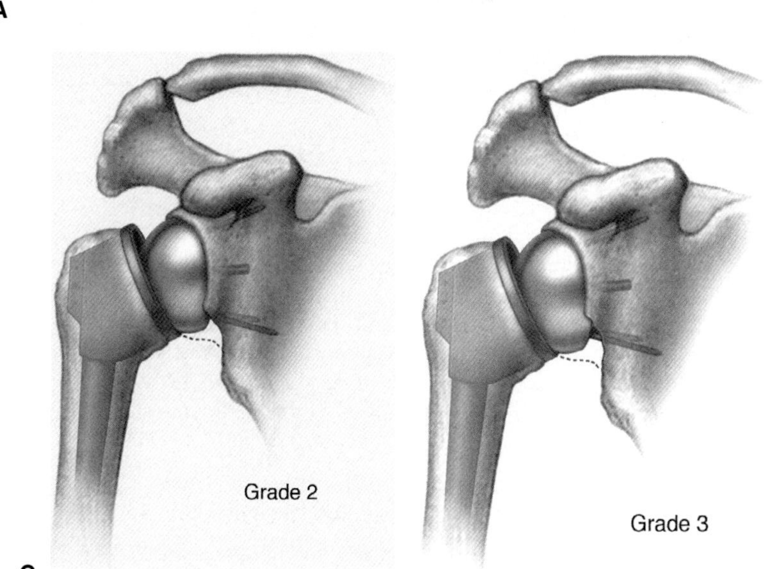


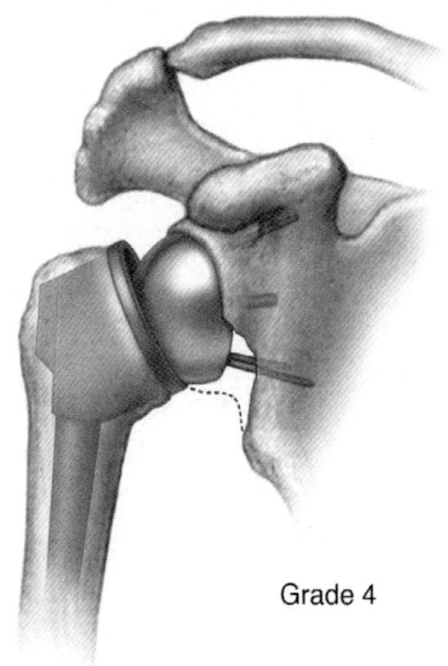


**Fig. 9-77** Illustration of scapular notching using the Nerot classification. **A**: Normal-appearing scapular notch and components. **B**: Grade 1—small notch (*dotted lines* show bone loss). **C**: Grade 2—notch with scapular condensation. **D**: Grade 3—erosion to inferior screw. **E**: Grade 4—more extensive erosion above screw; first sign of loosening.

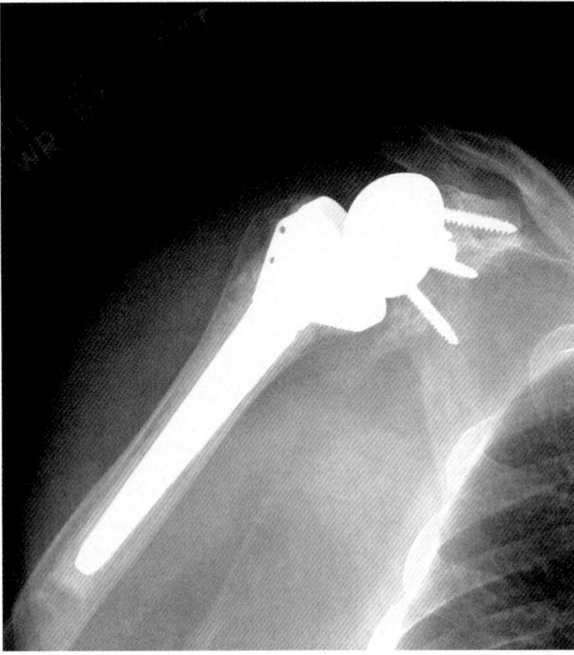

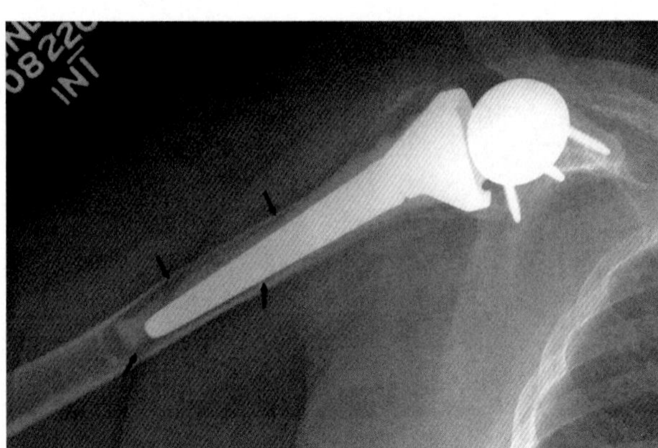

A B

**Fig. 9-78** Humeral component loosening with a reverse shoulder system. Radiographs in the early postoperative period (**A**) and 18 months later (**B**) demonstrating interval lucent areas in zones 2 to 5 (*arrows*).

Higher prosthesis-scapular neck angles are more often associated with notching. Placing the glenoid component slightly more inferiorly moves the humeral component slightly more distally so it does not impinge on the scapula.

Humeral component complications are similar to the conventional shoulder replacements and include subsidence, loosening (see Fig. 9-78), and periprosthetic fractures (Fig. 9-72). To date, these complications have been uncommon.

## Suggested Reading


Bohsali KI, Wirth MA, Rockwood CA. Complications of total shoulder arthroplasty. *J Bone Joint Surg*. 2006;88A: 2279–2293.

Feldman F. Radiology of shoulder prostheses. *Semin Musculoskelet Radiol*. 2006;10:5–21.

Gerber C, Pennington SD, Lingenfelter EJ, et al. Reverse Delta-III total shoulder replacement combined with latissamus dorsi transfer. *J Bone Joint Surg*. 2007;89A:940–947.

Guery J, Favard L, Sirveaux F, et al. Reverse total shoulder arthroplasty. *J Bone Joint Surg*. 2006;88A:1742–1747.

Matsen FA, Boileau P, Walch G, et al. The reverse total shoulder arthroplasty. *J Bone Joint Surg*. 2006;88A:660–667.

McFarland EG, Sanguanjit P, Tasaki A, et al. The reverse shoulder prosthesis: A review of imaging features and complications. *Skel Radiol*. 2006;35:488–496.

Roberts CC, Ekelund AL, Renfree KJ, et al. Radiologic assessment of reverse shoulder arthroplasty. *Radiographics*. 2007; 27:223–235.

Simovitch RW, Zumstein MA, Lohri E, et al. Predictors of scapular notching in patients managed with the Delta III reverse total shoulder replacement. *J Bone Joint Surg*. 2007; 89A:588–600.

Wall B, Nove-Josserand L, O'Connor DP, et al. Reverse total shoulder arthroplasty: A review of results according to etiology. *J Bone Joint Surg*. 2007;89A:1476–1485.

Wright TW, Cofield RH. Humeral fractures after shoulder arthroplasty. *J Bone Joint Surg*. 1996;77A:1340–1346.


### Revision Shoulder Arthroplasty

Total shoulder arthroplasty survival rates are 96% at 2 years, 92% at 5 years, and 88% at 10 years. As more procedures are being performed it is not surprising that the number of shoulder revisions has increased. Most primary arthroplasty failures are related to soft tissue deficiencies, poor bone stock, component wear, and infection (Figs. 9-66, 9-68, and 9-72). Revision shoulder arthroplasty may be required for resurfacing implants, hemi- and total shoulder implants. One of the primary indications for reverse shoulder prostheses is failed hemiarthroplasty with irreparable rotator cuff tears (see Fig. 9-79). Depending on the indication and patient status, longer stem humeral components and glenoid revision can also be used (Fig. 9-72D). In some cases, arthrodesis may be the only option.

Results correlate with the indications for the procedure. Patients revised because of glenoid deformity after hemiarthroplasty, humeral component loosening, or periprosthetic fractures have significantly better results compared to patients treated because of instability, cuff deficiency, or prior infections that tend to have less satisfactory results.

Imaging and complications are similar to those described earlier. However, infection rates are nearly twice as high compared to primary arthroplasty (4% compared to 0.7%).

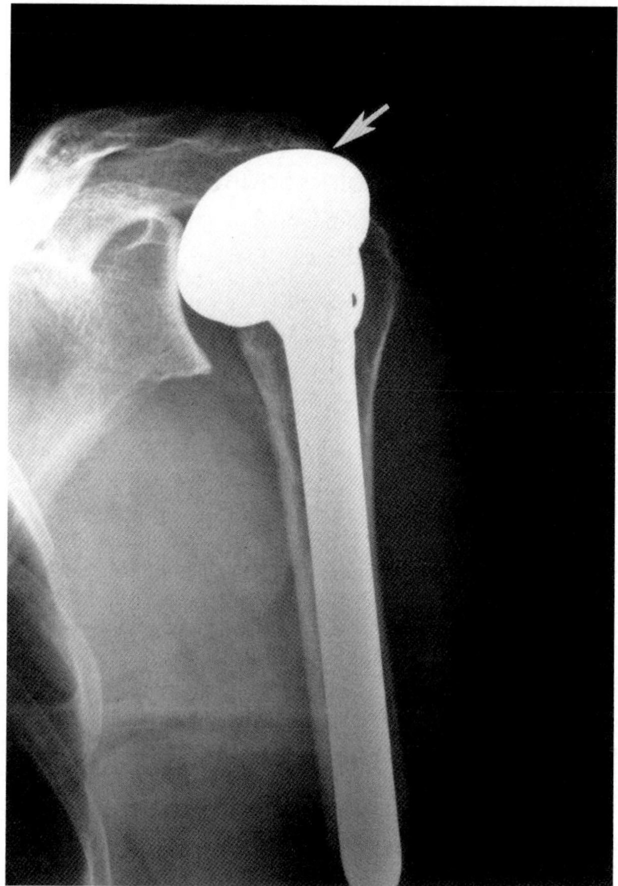

Fig. 9-79 Failed hemiarthroplasty with massive cuff tear and obliteration of the subacromial space (*arrow*).

## Suggested Reading

Dines JS, Feal S, Strauss EJ, et al. Outcome analysis of revision total shoulder replacement. *J Bone Joint Surg*. 2006;88A: 1494–1501.

# Shoulder Arthrodesis

Indications for shoulder arthrodesis include posttraumatic brachial plexus injuries, paralysis of the deltoid muscle, or other neuromuscular disorders about the shoulder, failed revision arthroplasty, instability, and tumor resection with limb sparing procedures. Shoulder arthroplasty is now more commonly performed in younger patients with bone preservation techniques. However, younger patients with the need to perform heavy manual labor may still be candidates for shoulder arthrodesis.

Selection of candidates for arthrodesis versus revision arthroplasty varies with each individual patient. Considerations include bone stock in the humerus and glenoid, soft tissue support, neural integrity, and infection.

Contraindications for shoulder arthrodesis are primarily related to loss of normal muscle function critical to a successful procedure. The trapezius, levator scapulae, serratus anterior, latissimus dorsi, and rhomboid muscles are critical to a successful outcome. Neuropathic arthropathy is also a contraindication because the incidence of nonunion and infection is unacceptably high.

Preoperative clinical and imaging evaluation is important. Radiographs may be adequate to evaluate bone stock. However, in patients with bone loss, CT is preferred to determine the feasibility and regions where bone grafting will be required.

## Suggested Reading

Clare DJ, Wirth MA, Groh GI, et al. Shoulder arthrodesis. *J Bone Joint Surg*. 2001;83A:593–600.

Safran O, Iannotti JP. Arthrodesis of the shoulder. *J Am Acad Orthop Surg*. 2006;14:145–153.

### Treatment Options

There are a number of treatment options and approaches for shoulder arthrodesis.

The appropriate position for fusion is important or dysfunction, winging of the scapula, and chronic pain may result. Most authors recommend that the humerus be in 15 to 20 degrees of abduction, 15 to 20 degrees of flexion, and 40 to 45 degrees of internal rotation such that the hand can reach the belt buckle and contralateral shoulder easily.

Arthrodesis can be accomplished with fusion of the glenohumeral joint or glenohumeral and acromiohumeral spaces. Extra-articular fusion involves fusion of the humerus and acromion, scapula, and clavicle without entering the glenohumeral joint. Intra-articular fusion preserves the rotator cuff tendons and fuses the glenoid to the humerus. Extra-articular

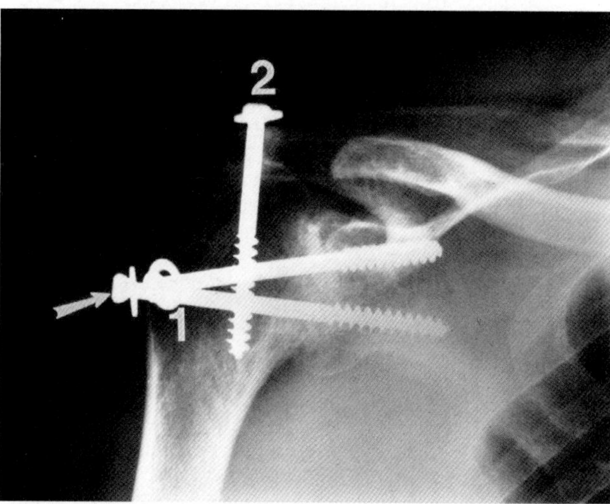


Fig. 9-80 Shoulder arthrodesis with cancellous screws and washers. Anteroposterior (AP) radiograph demonstrates two glenohumeral fixation screws (*1*) and acromiohumeral fixation (*2*). One of the glenohumeral screws projects into the soft tissues (*arrow*). The joint appears fused, but fluoroscopic positioning or computed tomography (CT) would be confirmatory.

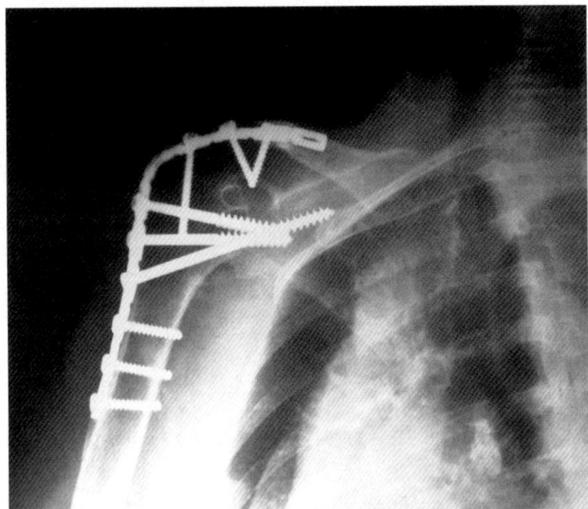

Fig. 9-81 Plate and screw arthrodesis. Anteroposterior (AP) radiograph demonstrates reconstruction plate and screw fixation with incorporation of the acromion and clavicle and long screws through the glenohumeral complex.

fusion is uncommonly performed as an isolated procedure in recent years.

Multiple fixation methods have been used including long cancellous screws (see Fig. 9-80), a variety of plate and screw combinations, (see Fig. 9-81) and external fixation.

## Suggested Reading

Clare DJ, Wirth MA, Groh GI, et al. Shoulder arthrodesis. *J Bone Joint Surg*. 2001;83A:593–600.

Nagano A, Okinaga S, Ochiai N, et al. Shoulder arthrodesis by external fixation. *Clin Orthop*. 1989;247:97–100.

Safran O, Iannotti JP. Arthrodesis of the shoulder. *J Am Acad Orthop Surg*. 2006;14:145–153.

### Postoperative Imaging and Complications

The goal of shoulder arthrodesis is to provide a functional painless shoulder. Over the years results have varied with primary indication, surgical approach, and method of fixation. In the early years only 25% of patients were free of pain following the procedure. This has improved to 67% to 75%. Functional improvement with ability to lift moderate to heavy weight and perform other daily functions occurs in 70% to 82%. Overall satisfactory to excellent results occur in up to 91% of patients with significant improvement (increases of 30 points) in Constant-Murley clinical scores.

Complications have been reported in up to 28% of patients. The most common complications include nonunion or pseudarthrosis, malposition, implant failure, fractures adjacent to the hardware, soft tissue irritation by implants due to their superficial position, and infection.

Nonunion has been reported in up to 20% of cases. However, except in patients with prior infection the rate is more likely in the 10% to 13% range. Diagnosis may be evident on serial radiographs (see Fig. 9-82). When radiographs are inconclusive, CT can be used to better define the presence of pseudarthrosis (Fig. 9-82B). Revision surgery with new implants and bone grafting is usually successful.

Fixation failure may occur with nonunion or result in soft tissue irritation requiring removal (Fig. 9-80). Serial radiographs are usually adequate to evaluate implants (see Fig. 9-83). Fluoroscopic positioning may be necessary to optimally evaluate implant position.

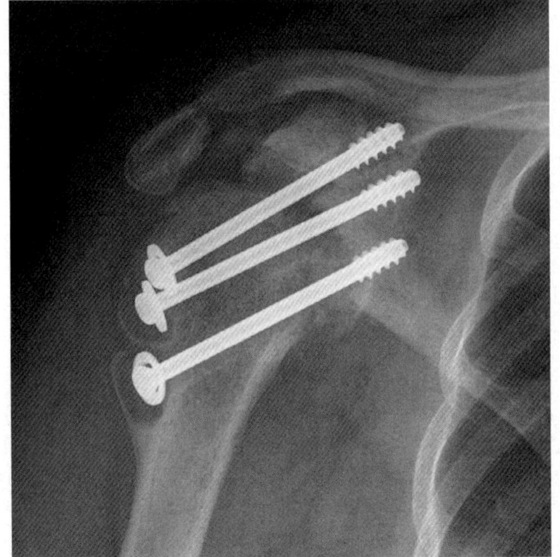

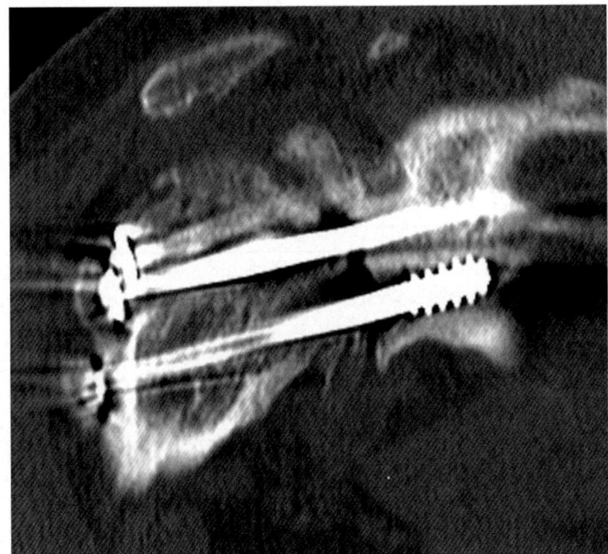

Fig. 9-82 Failed fusion with screw loosening. A: Anteroposterior (AP) radiograph demonstrates glenohumeral arthrodesis with three cannulated cancellous screws and washers. There is obvious lucency about the screws and the articulation does not appear fused. B: Coronal computed tomographic (CT) image shows no bony bridging of the joint.

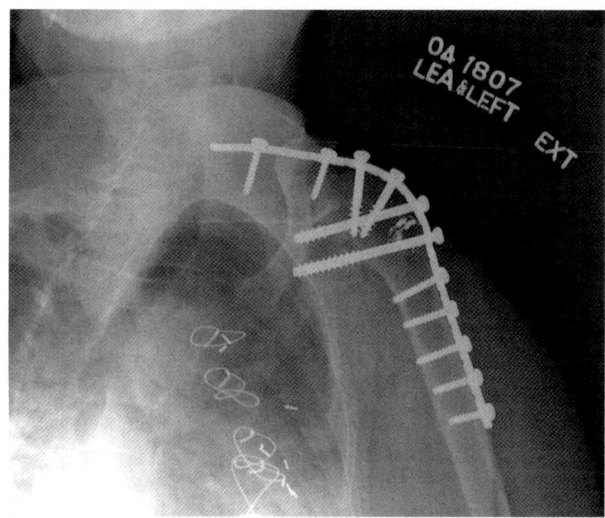


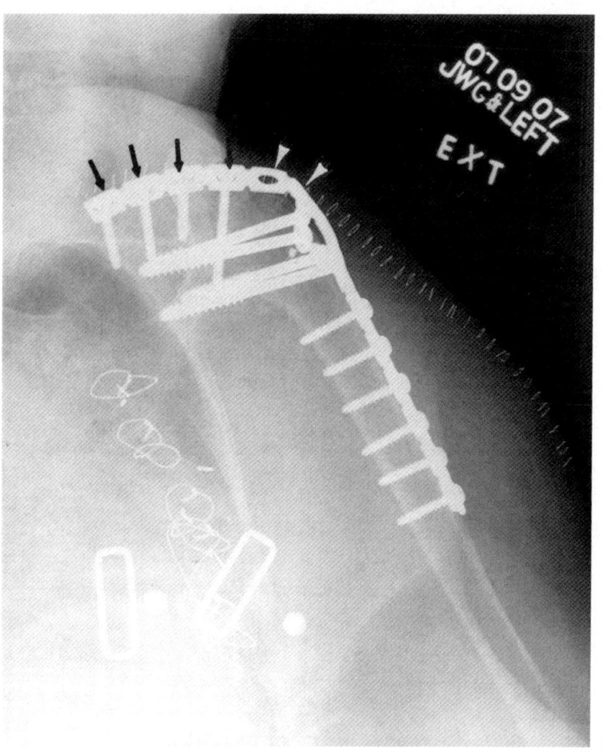


A B

Fig. 9-83 Implant failure. A: Anteroposterior (AP) radiograph following left shoulder arthrodesis with incorporation of the acromion and scapula. The scapular screws have pulled out with elevation of the plate. B: The plate was reattached with new screws proximally (*arrows*) and removal of the superior humeral head screws (*arrowheads*).

Fracture of the humerus or scapula adjacent to the implants occurs in up to 13% of patients. Fractures can be treated conservatively or with external fixation. If fractures are significantly displaced internal fixation is usually required. Serial radiographs are adequate for fracture detection and follow-up.

Infection occurs in up to 8% of cases. Radiographs may demonstrate bone loss or periosteal reaction. Fixation hardware loosening (Fig. 9-82) and nonunion are often present as well. Aspiration or radionuclide scans can be performed to isolate the organism and confirm the presence of infection. This usually requires hardware removal and aggressive antibiotic therapy similar to infected arthroplasty described earlier.

## Suggested Reading

Clare DJ, Wirth MA, Groh GI, et al. Shoulder arthrodesis. *J Bone Joint Surg*. 2001;83A:593–600.

Cofield RH, Briggs BT. Glenohumeral arthrodesis. Operative and long-term functional results. *J Bone Joint Surg*. 1979; 61A:668–677.

Ruhmann O, Schmolke S, bohnsack M, et al. Shoulder arthrodesis: Indications, technique, results and complications. *J Shoulder Elbow Surg*. 2005;14:38–50.

Safran O, Iannotti JP. Arthrodesis of the shoulder. *J Am Acad Orthop Surg*. 2006;14:145–153.

# 10 Humeral Shaft Fractures

Humeral shaft fractures account for 3% to 5% of all skeletal fractures. This chapter will focus on fractures of the shaft. Proximal humeral fractures were discussed in Chapter 9. Distal fractures including intra-articular fractures will be included in Chapter 11.

## Mechanism of Injury

There are several unique features of the humerus that present problems with fracture management. First, the humerus is the most freely movable osseous structure in the body. Scapulohumeral motion can exaggerate the already flexible range of motion in the humerus. Second, the humerus functions as a lever; therefore, nearly all stress to the bone is in tension from or is at an angle to the long axis of the bone. Weight-bearing and compression forces are not an issue with regard to fracture treatment. Finally, when the humerus hangs vertically it is influenced by gravity alone allowing realignment of the fracture fragments.

The location of the fracture in relation to the muscle attachments affects the displacement of fragments (see Fig. 10-1). Fractures of the proximal third (between the pectoralis and deltoid muscle insertions) result in medial displacement of the proximal fragment due to pectoralis major muscle forces (see Fig. 10-2). When fractures occur distal to the deltoid muscle attachment, the deltoid muscle forces cause abduction of the proximal fragment. The brachialis and biceps muscles cause proximal displacement of the distal fragment (see Fig. 10-3).

Direct trauma from blunt or penetrating injuries is the most common cause of humeral fractures. Transverse fractures are usually the result of bending forces. Spiral fractures occur due to a combination of bending and rotational forces. Compression forces acting on the humerus tend to affect the proximal or distal portions, but spare the diaphysis. Indirect forces, such as falling directly on the elbow or outstretched hand, vigorous

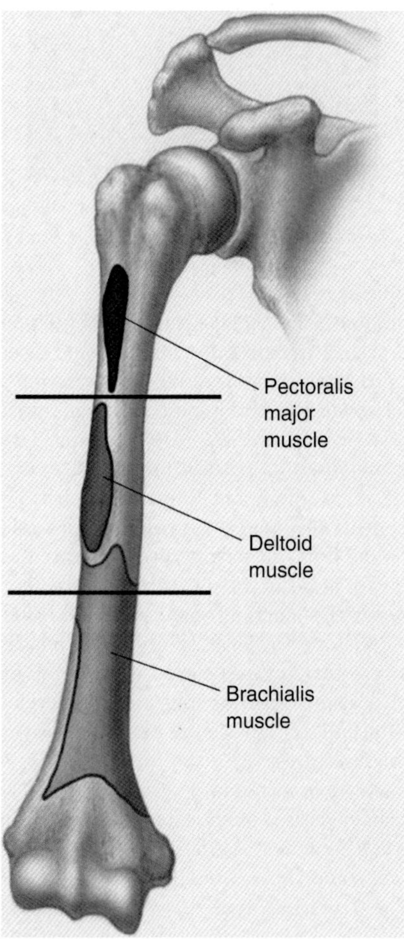


**Fig. 10-1** Illustration of the three segments of the humerus with muscle insertions affecting displacement. *Black lines* mark the junction of the proximal and middle thirds and middle and distal thirds. Fractures are described by their location as proximal, mid or distal or at the junctions of the proximal and middle thirds, or mid and distal thirds. Muscle forces displace the fragments differently depending on the location of the fracture.

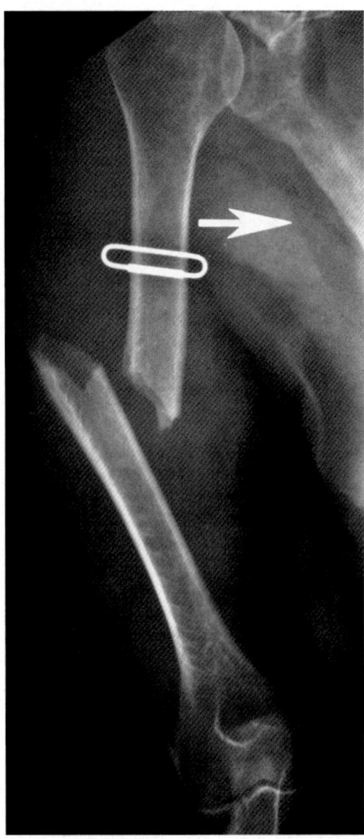

**Fig. 10-2** Fracture at the deltoid insertion with adduction of the proximal fragment due to pectoralis muscle forces (*arrow*).

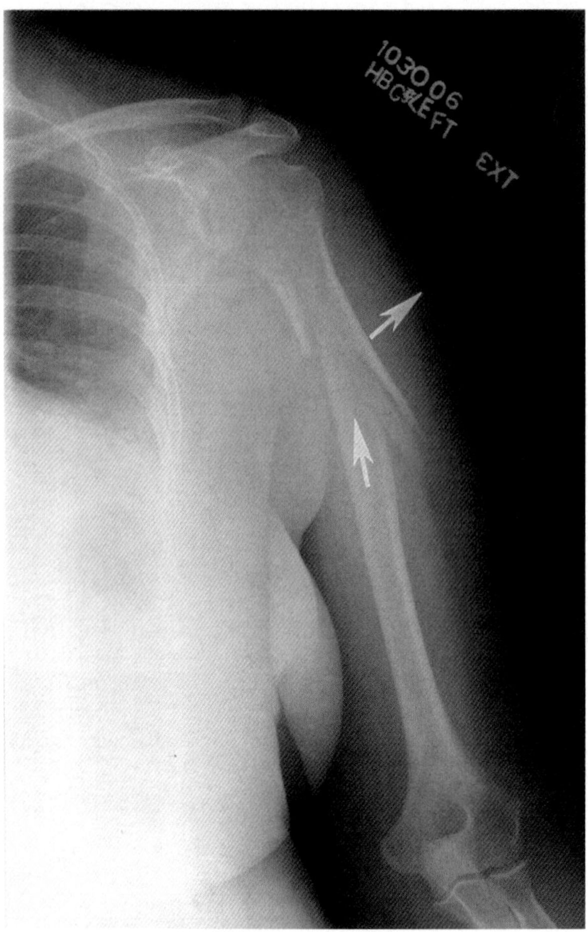


**Fig. 10-3** Fracture distal to the deltoid insertion with abduction (*arrow*) of the proximal fragment by the deltoid muscle and proximal displacement of the distal fragment (*arrow*) due to brachialis muscle forces.

throwing motions, and violent muscle contractions can also cause humeral shaft fractures. Fractures should be described by location as proximal, middle, distal, or at the junction of the proximal and middle thirds or middle and distal thirds (Holstein-Lewis fracture, see Chapter 2). Forty-three percent to 69% of fractures involve the mid shaft. Of these, 61% are transverse, 18% oblique, 17% spiral, and 4% comminuted or segmental. Thirty percent to 40% percent involve the proximal shaft and 10% to 16% the distal shaft. Fracture incidence has a bimodal distribution with peaks in the third and seventh decades.

Fractures at the junction of the mid and distal thirds are particularly difficult to manage. Injury to the nutrient artery at this level may contribute to delayed union or nonunion. The radial nerve is also at risk for injury at this level. Therefore, open reduction and fixation is more often required compared to more proximal fractures.

Open fractures occurred in 2% to 5% of cases. The severity of injury is classified based on the extent of soft tissue injury using the Gustilo and Anderson lassification listed in the subsequent text. Most are minor open wounds (72%), but 14% are more extensive type II and 14% type III open wounds.

## Classification

Most humeral shaft fractures are described by location and fracture line orientation or the degree of comminution. The AO (Arbeitsgemeinshaft fur Osteosynthesefragen)/Orthopaedic Trauma Association (OTA) classifications divide fractures into three large simple categories with multiple subcategories in each type.

**AO/OTA classification** (see Fig. 10-4)

- **Type A:** Simple, no comminution (63.3%) (Fig. 10-4A–C)
  - A1—simple spiral
  - A2—simple oblique
  - A3—simple transverse
- **Type B:** Wedge (butterfly) fragment (26.2%) (Fig. 10-4 D–F)
  - B1—spiral wedge
  - B2—bending wedge
  - B3—fragmented wedge
- **Type C:** Comminuted (10.5%) (Fig. 10-4G–I)
  - C1—spiral comminuted mid shaft
  - C2—segmental
  - C3—irregular shaft comminution

**Gustilo and Anderson classification for open fractures**

- **Type I:** Open fracture due to fragment penetration and minimal soft tissue damage, wound clean <1 cm (72%)
- **Type II:** Wound >1 cm without extensive soft tissue damage (14%)

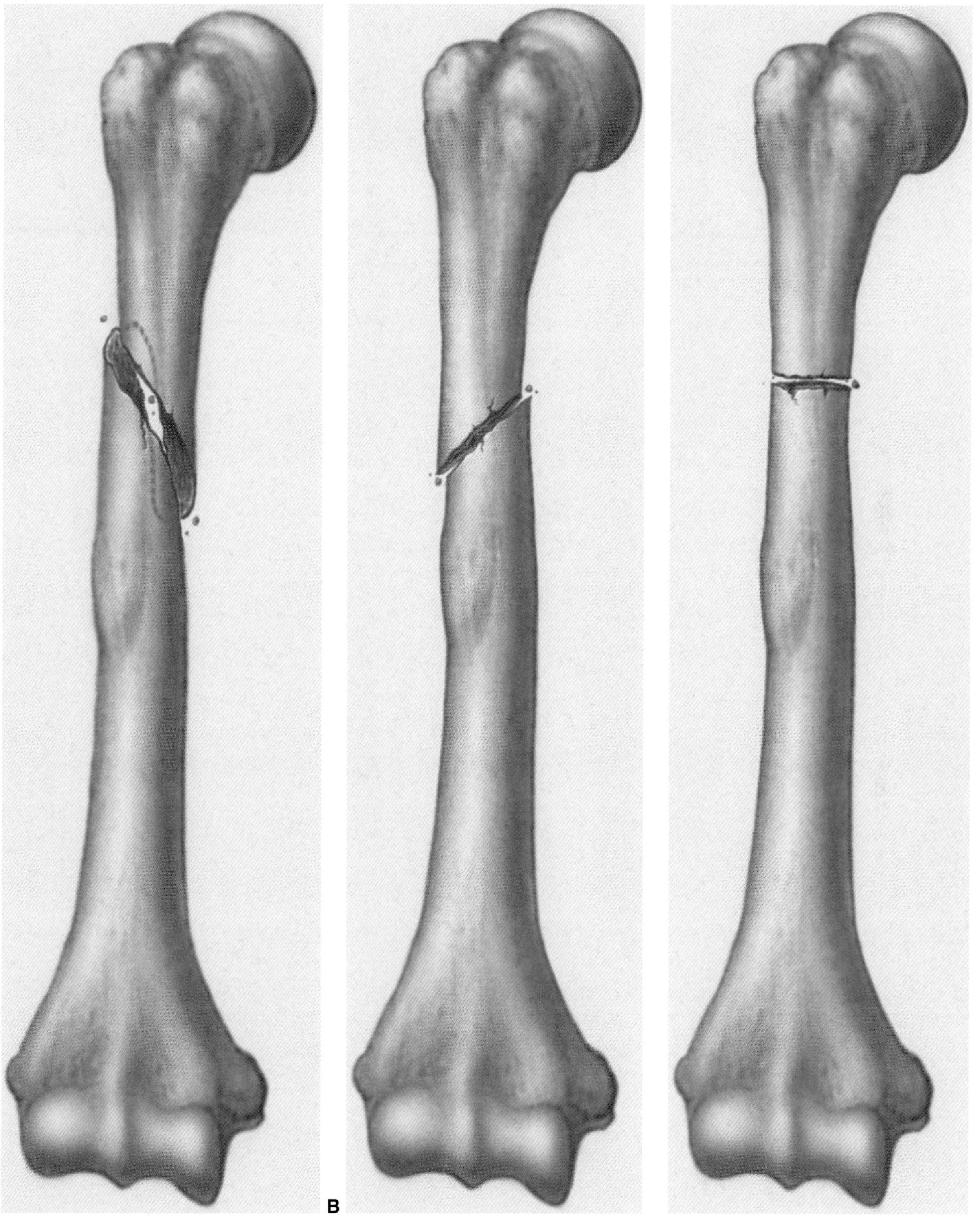


Fig. 10-4 Orthopaedic Trauma Association classification of humeral shaft fractures. Type A: diaphyseal simple. A: A1—spiral, B: A2—oblique, C: A3—transverse. Type B: humeral diaphyseal, wedge. D: B1—spiral wedge, E: B2—bending wedge, F: B3—fragmented wedge. Type C: humeral diaphyseal complex. G: C1—spiral comminuted, H: C2—segmental, I: C3—irregular shaft comminuted.

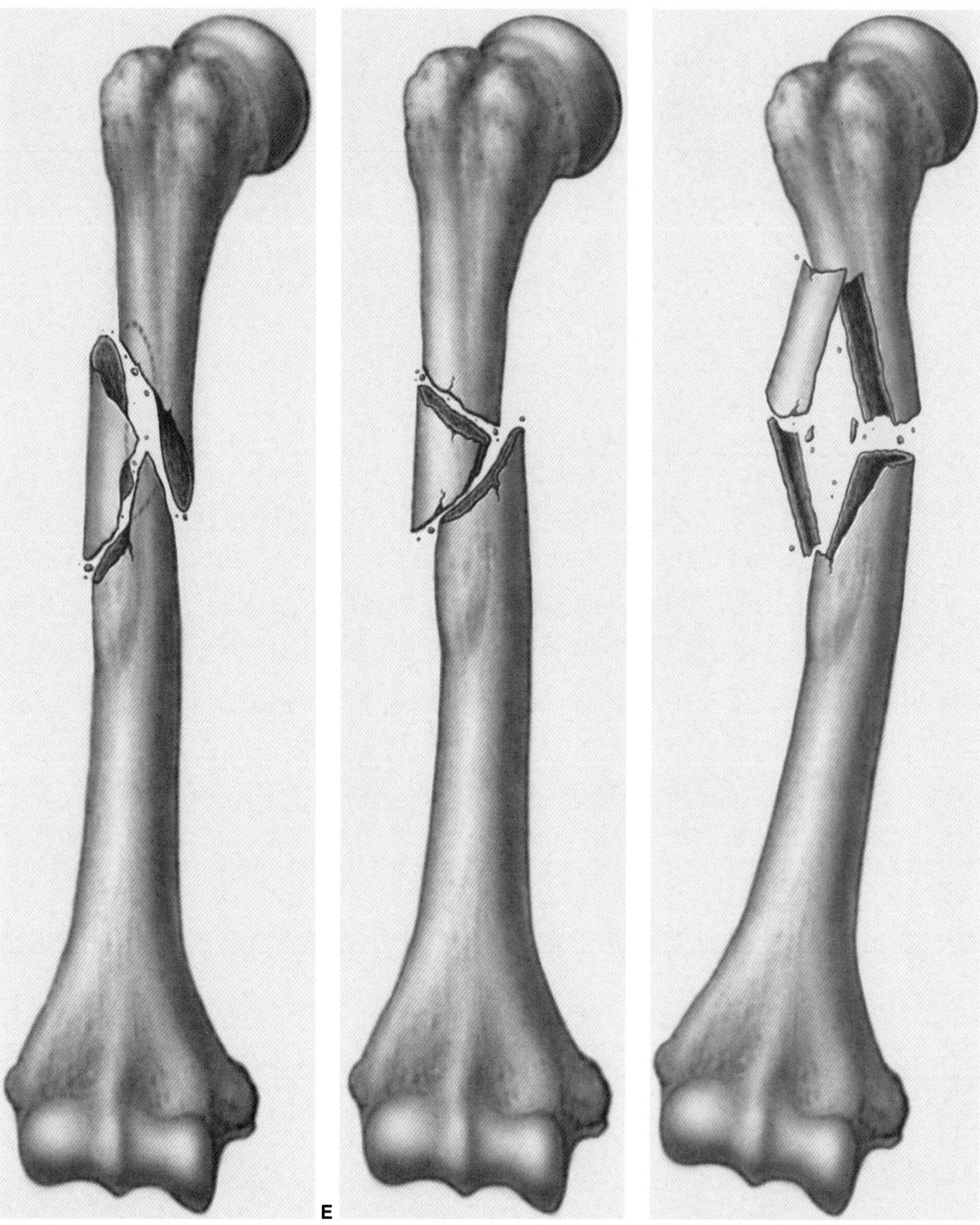


Fig. 10-4 *(Continued)*

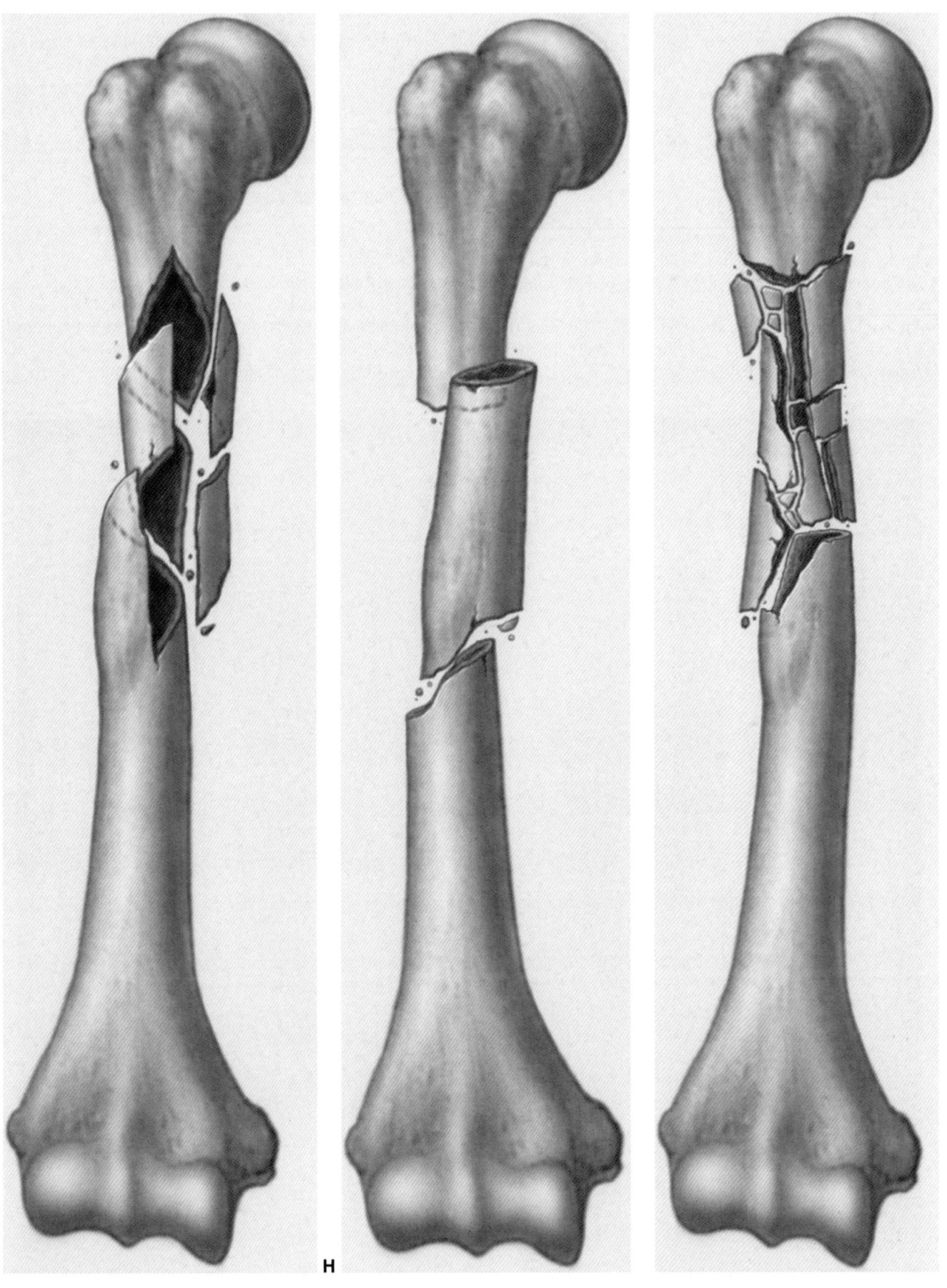


Fig. 10-4 (*Continued*)

**Type IIIA:** Extensive soft tissue damage with wound >10 cm, periosteum intact (7%)
**Type IIIB:** Periosteal stripping requiring wound coverage (7%)
**Type IIIC:** Same as IIIB, but with vascular injury requiring vessel repair (rare)

## Suggested Reading


Ekholm R, Adami J, Tidermark J, et al. Fractures of the shaft of the humerus: An epidemiological study of 401 fractures. *J Bone Joint Surg*. 2006;88B:1469–1473.

Ekholm R, Tidermark J, Tornkvist H, et al. Outcome after closed functional treatment of humeral shaft fractures. *J Orthop Trauma*. 2006;20:591–596.

Gustilo RB, Anderson JT. Prevention of infection in the treatment of one thousand and twenty-five fractures of the long bones. *J Bone Joint Surg*. 1976;58A:453–458.

Muller ME, Nazarian S, Koch P, et al. *The comprehensive classification fractures of long bones*. Berlin: Springer-Verlag New York; 1990.

Tytherleigh-Strong G, Walls N, McQueen MM, et al. The epidemiology of humeral shaft fractures. *J Bone Joint Surg*. 1998;80B:249–253.


### Imaging

Detection and classification of humeral shaft fractures can usually be accomplished with anteroposterior (AP) and lateral radiographs of the humerus. A transthoracic view is an excellent method of obtaining a lateral view at 90 degrees to the AP view. This is especially useful for fractures of the upper

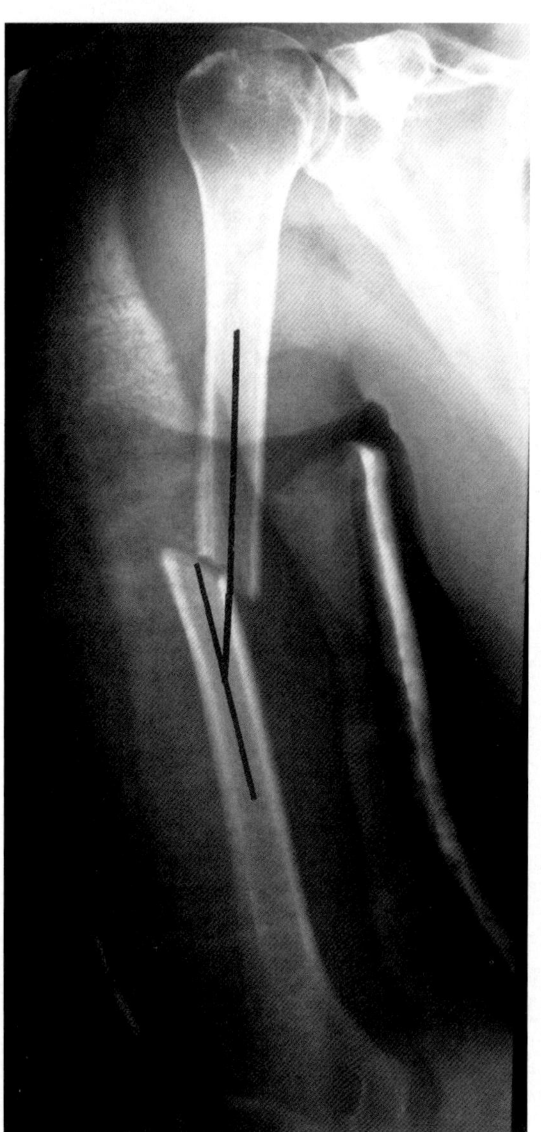

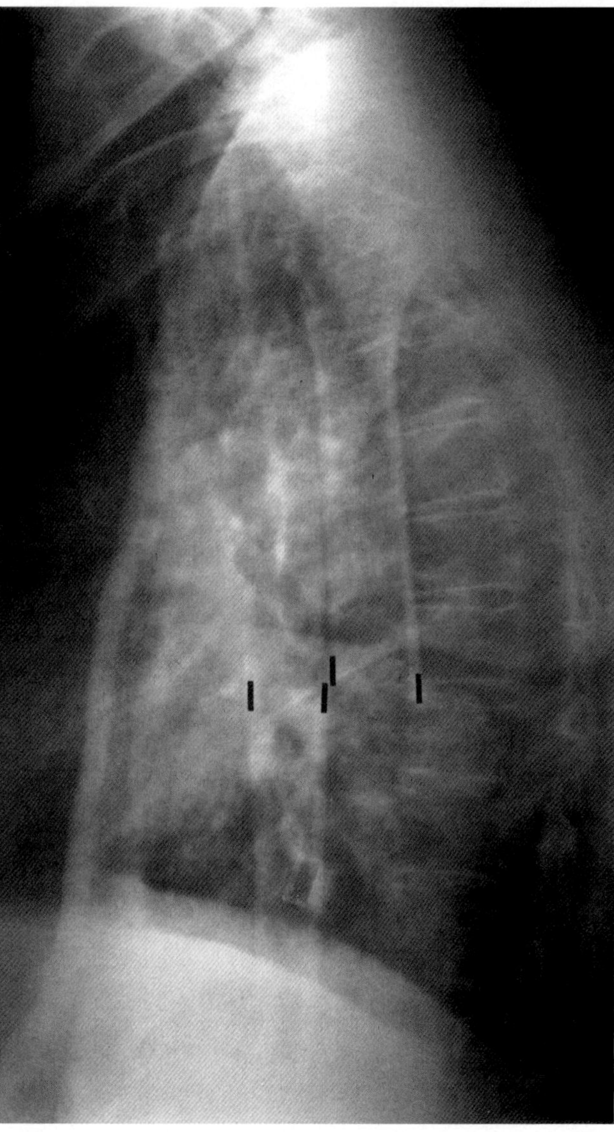

Fig. 10-5 Anteroposterior (AP) (A) and transthoracic (B) radiographs of a mid shaft fracture that appears laterally angulated on the AP projection. The transthoracic projection (B) demonstrates no bone apposition (*black lines*) of the fracture margins.

humerus (see Fig. 10-5). The shoulder and elbow need to be included on the images. Depending on the presence of other injuries, it is better to rotate the patient instead of turning the arm to obtain the two different views. Complex fractures (OTA type C) may require computed tomography (CT) or magnetic resonance imaging (MRI) for further evaluation. The former is useful for fragment position and MRI for subtle osseous changes or radial nerve injury. Complex open fractures (Gustilo and Anderson type IIIC) with vascular injury may require angiography to clarify the extent and location of vessel disruption or compression.

## Suggested Reading

Berquist TH. *Imaging of orthopaedic trauma*, 2nd ed. New York: Raven Press; 1992.

## Treatment Options

### Closed Reduction

Most closed fractures of the humeral shaft can be managed with conservative methods. Union rates of 90% have been reported with approximately 10% of patients requiring additional procedures (see Fig. 10-6). Multiple techniques have been used. These include a hanging cast, abduction humeral spica cast, functional braces, and Velpeau dressings. A functional brace comprises two halves, anterior and posterior, held together with Velcro straps. This approach is not effective with significant soft tissue injury or bone loss. In many cases a hanging cast is used initially for up to 3 weeks (see Fig. 10-7). Gravity assists with fracture reduction. After the initial therapy with the hanging cast, the cast is replaced with a functional brace. As soon as tolerated, the patient should begin range of motion exercises with the hand, wrist, elbow, and shoulder.

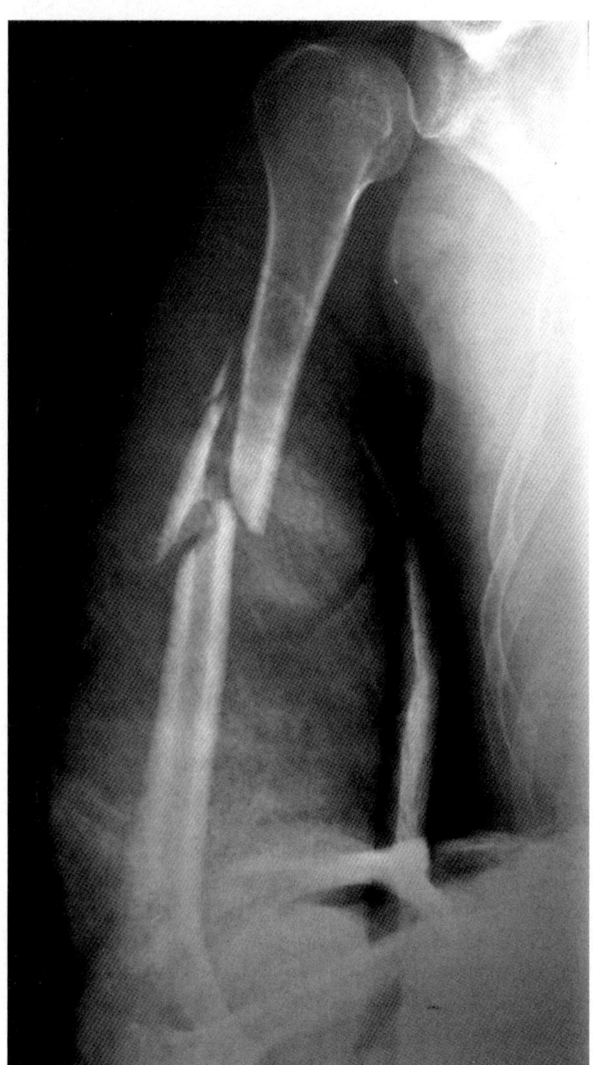


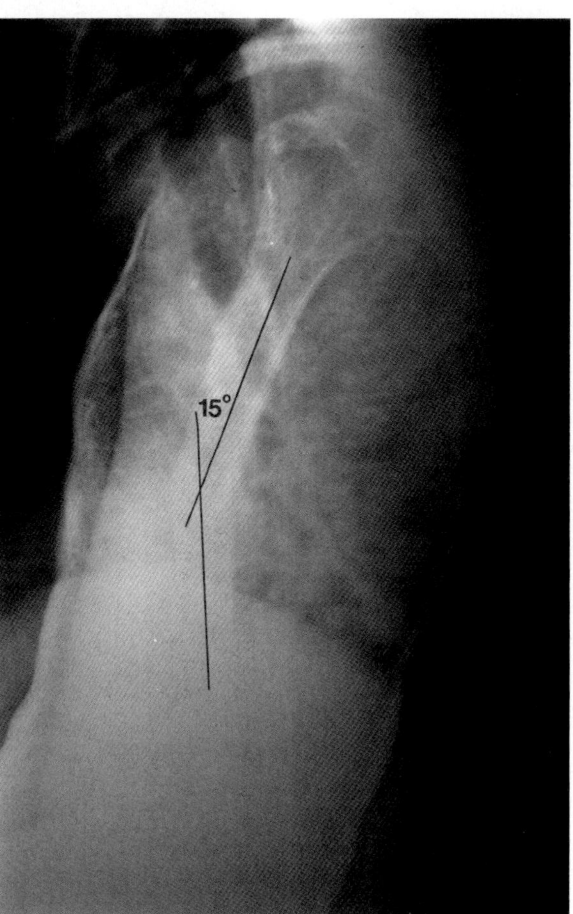


Fig. 10-6 Mid shaft wedge (butterfly) type B fracture. Anteroposterior (AP) (A) and lateral (B) radiographs in hanging cast, 1 month later (C) and healed at 4 months (D). There is minimal shortening and no significant angulation on the AP radiographs. The 15 degrees of anterior angulation on the original lateral is acceptable.

Fig. 10-6 (*Continued*)

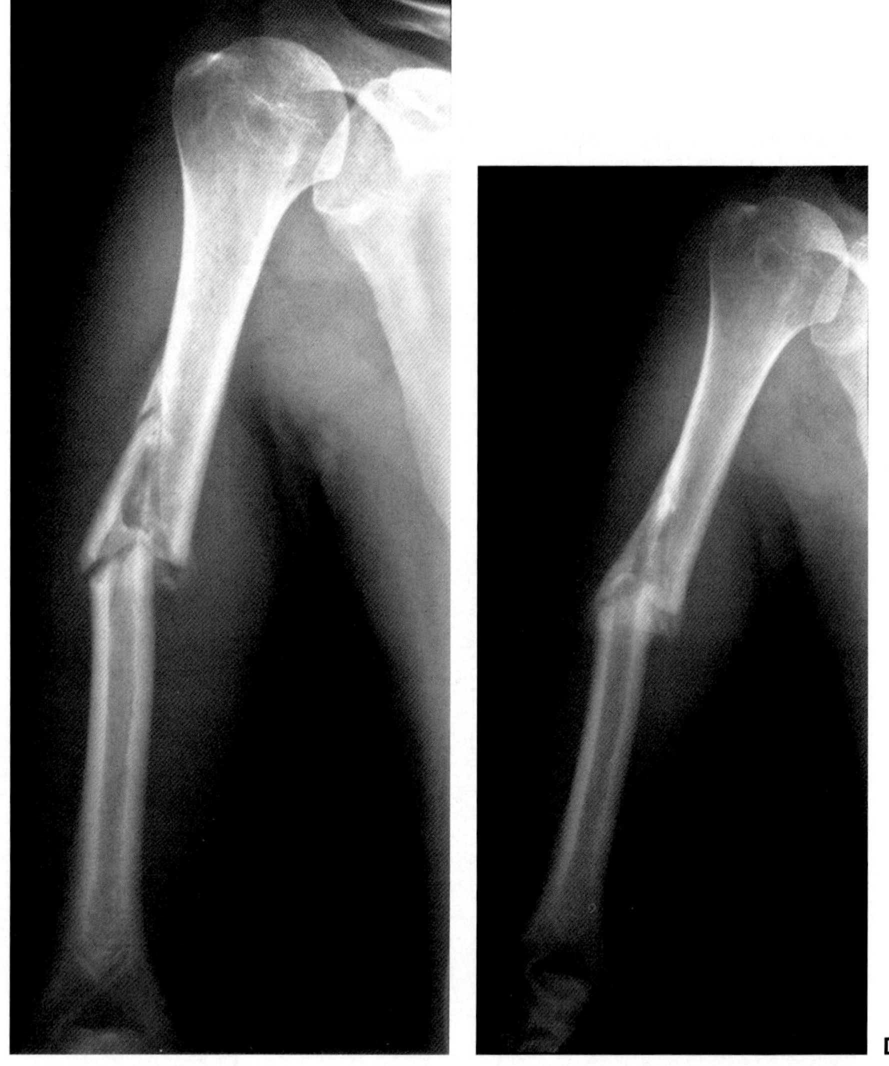

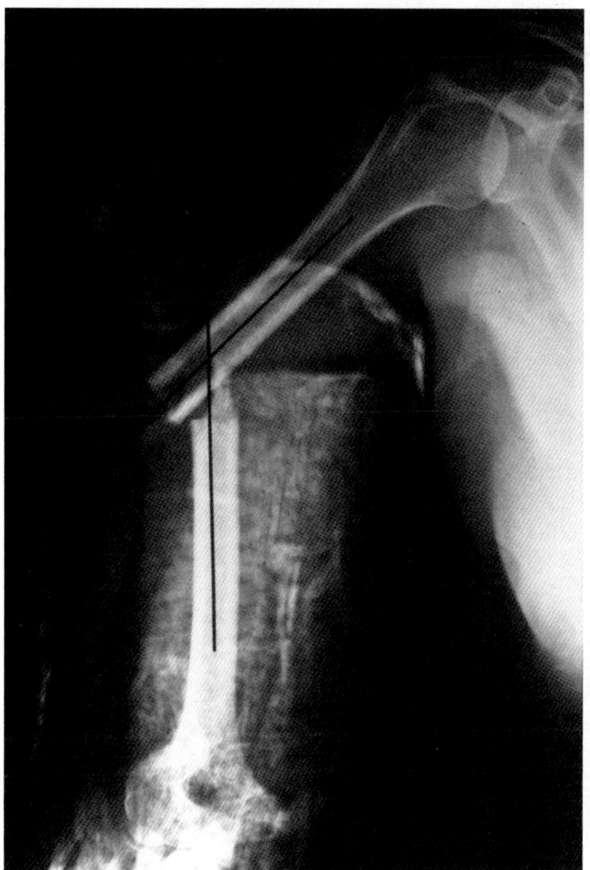


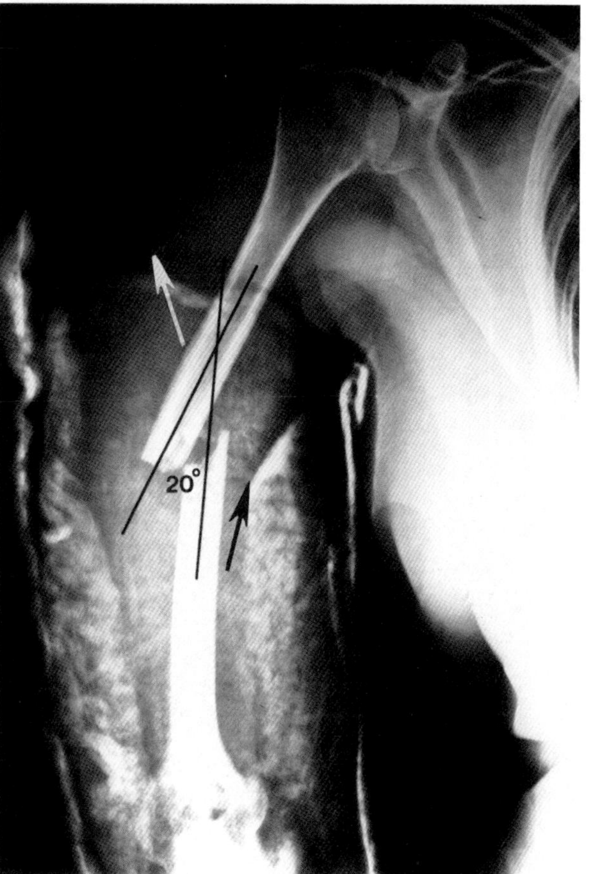


Fig. 10-7 Hanging cast. Initial radiograph (A) of a badly angulated mid shaft fracture placed in a hanging cast. At 3 weeks (B) the angular deformity has improved to 20 degrees. Deltoid muscle forces abduct the proximal fragment (*white arrow*) and the brachialis pulls the distal fragment proximally (*black arrow*).

Perfect alignment and apposition of the fracture fragments is not as essential as it would be with weight-bearing structures of the lower extremity. Anterior or posterior angulation of up to 20 degrees and varus or valgus angulation of up to 30 degrees is acceptable. Up to 3 cm of shortening may also be accepted.

## External Fixation

External fixation may be used in complex open injuries to allow wound access while stabilizing the fracture. A significant number of complex open fractures is related to gunshot wounds. Unilateral external fixators are commonly used for humeral fractures (see Figs. 10-8 and 10-9).

## Internal Fixation

Indications for internal fixation include the following:

- Failed closed reduction (see Fig. 10-10)
- Displaced transverse or short oblique fractures (Fig. 10-10)
- Long spiral fractures with displacement suggesting soft tissue interposition (see Fig. 10-11)
- Complex open fractures with neurovascular injury (may also use external fixation)
- Ipsilateral combined humeral and forearm fractures (floating elbow)
- Segmental fractures
- Fractures extending to the articular surface of the shoulder or elbow
- Pathologic fractures (8.5% of humeral fractures)

## Plate and Screw Fixation

Plate and screw techniques provide rigid fixation to control fracture fragments and the fracture gap (see Fig. 10-12). In past years, the major disadvantage was increased bone exposure with risk of periosteal blood supply and infection. New less compressive plates and less invasive stabilization systems (LISS) protect the periosteal vasculature. Lag screws or interfragmentary screws can also be placed (see Fig. 10-13). The

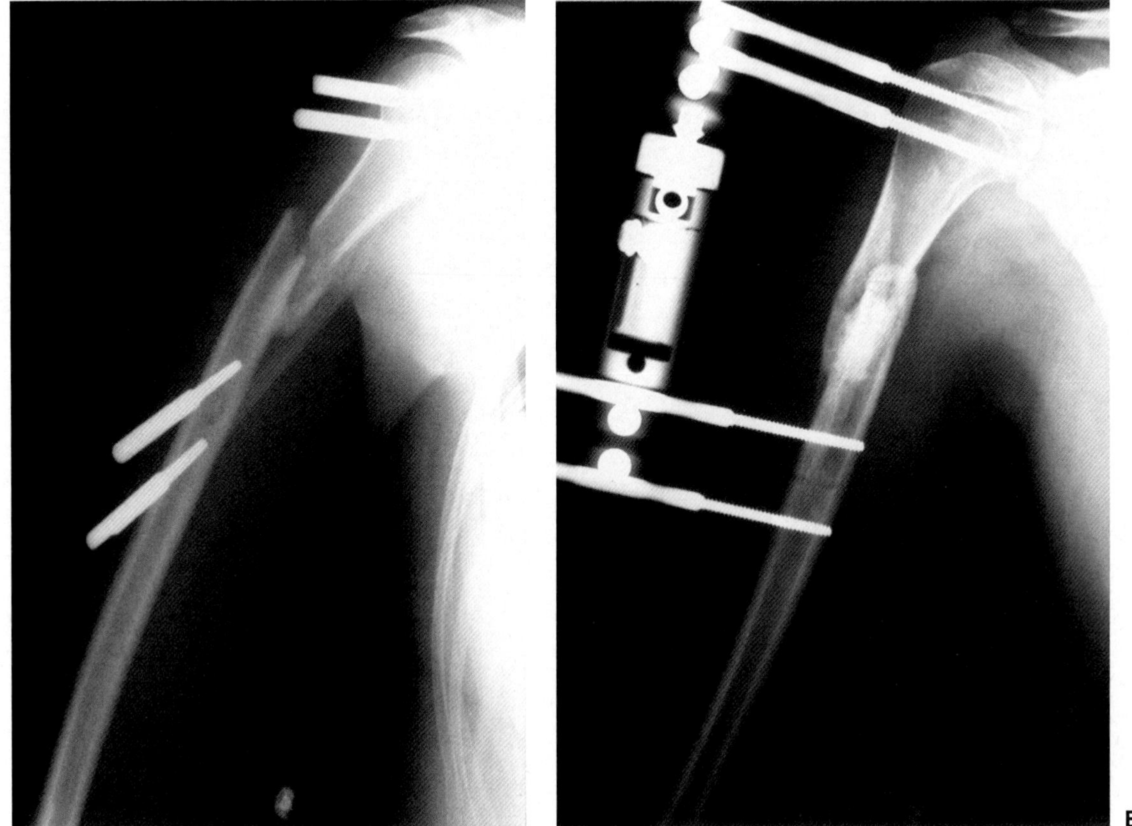


Fig. 10-8 Comminuted proximal shaft fracture reduced with external fixation. The pins (A) serve as handles to assist with reducing the fracture. Following application of the fixator (B) the alignment is improved although there is some shortening.

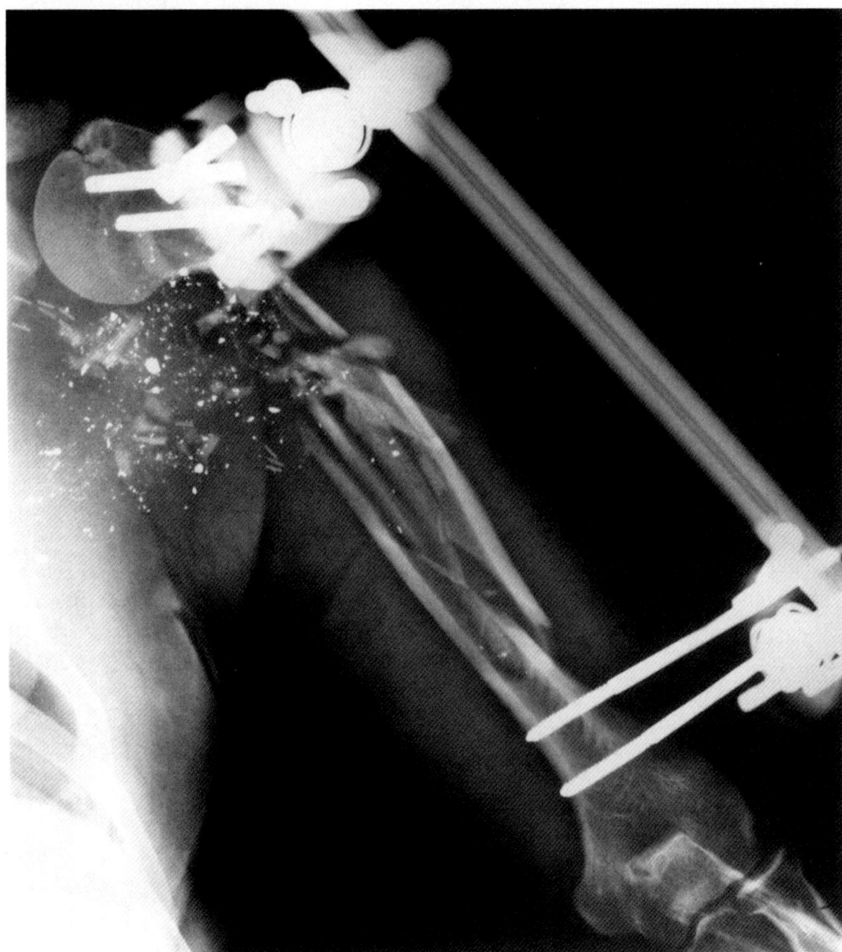

Fig. 10-9 Gunshot wound with shattering of the mid humerus. Alignment and length are maintained with a unilateral external fixator. There was considerable neurovascular injury in the axillary region with this type IIIC open wound.

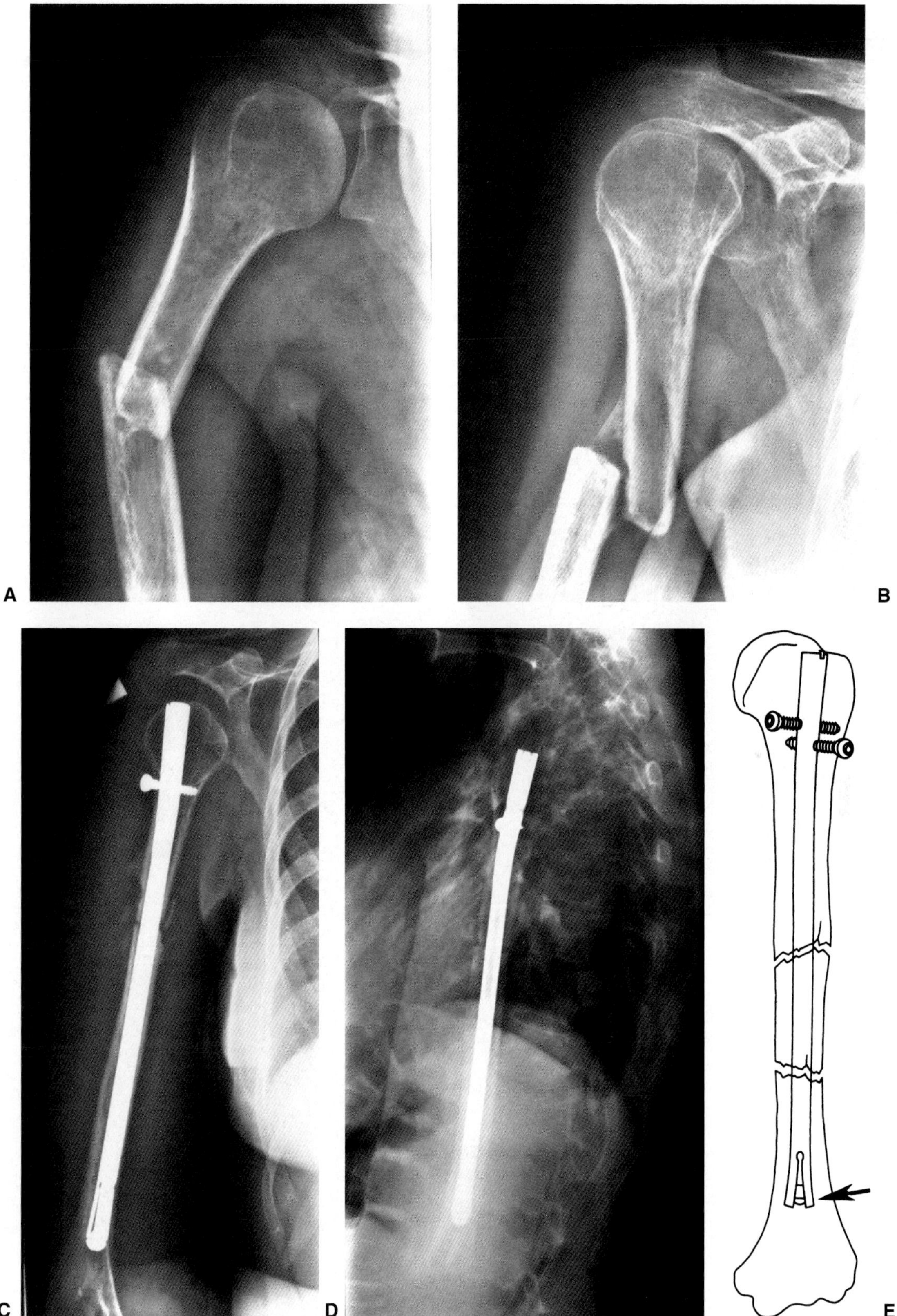


Fig. 10-10 Radiographs (A and B) of an ununited transverse proximal humeral shaft fracture. Anteroposterior (AP) (C) and transthoracic (D) images after intramedullary nail fixation using a Seidel nail. E: Illustration of Seidel locking nail with distal expander (*arrow*) and proximal screws to prevent fragment rotation. (Figure E Courtesy of Stryker, Howmedica, Osteonics, Allendale, New Jersey.)

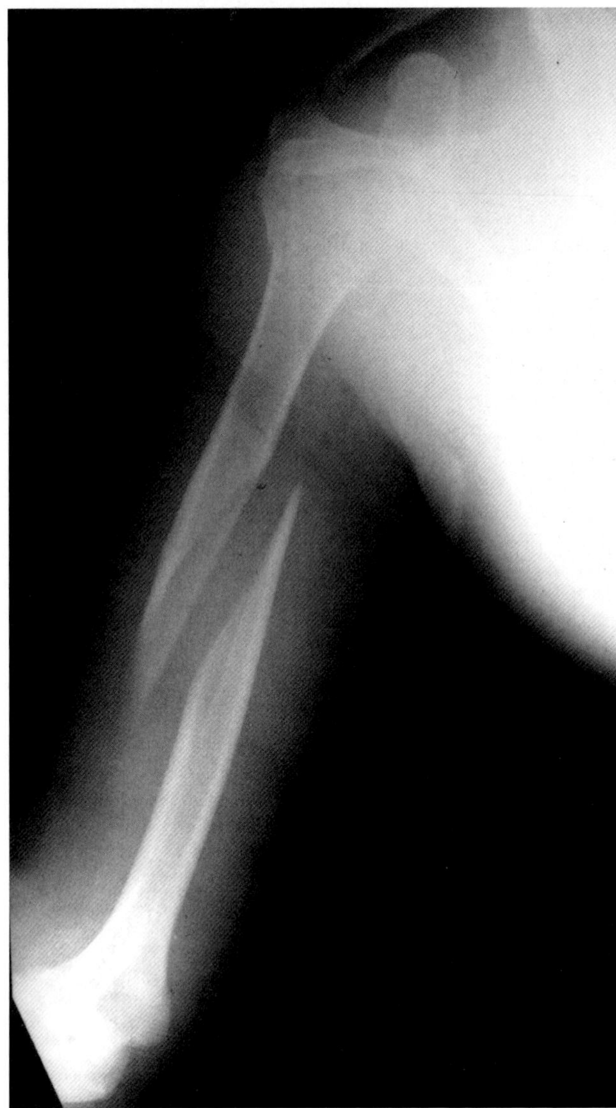

Fig. 10-11 Radiograph of a long spiral fracture with separation of the fragments due to soft tissue interposition.

need for bone grafting can be assessed at the time of surgery. In osteoporotic bone, methyl methacrylate can be used to enhance screw purchase (see Fig. 10-14).

## Intramedullary Nail Fixation

Intramedullary nails come in a variety of configurations. Potential advantages include less invasive technique with less blood loss, less subject to bending forces reducing implant failure, and less stress shielding than seen with plate and screw fixation. Currently, flexible Ender nails (see Chapter 2) are not commonly used. Locking nails with options for screws at each end for fragment stability or some other fixation method (Fig. 10-10) are more commonly used. Intramedullary nails can be inserted in an antegrade or retrograde manner depending on the fracture configuration and location. For use of these approaches, the fracture should be distal to the humeral neck and at least 3 cm proximal to the elbow. Care must be taken to select the proper length so that the nail does not enter the olecranon fossa and reduce elbow motion. The antegrade technique (see Fig. 10-15) is more commonly used. Using the antegrade technique, care must be taken to embed the nail below the rotator cuff (see Fig. 10-16). There is a higher incidence of shoulder pain and impingement with antegrade nail techniques. Care must also be taken not to injure the axillary nerve during proximal screw placement.

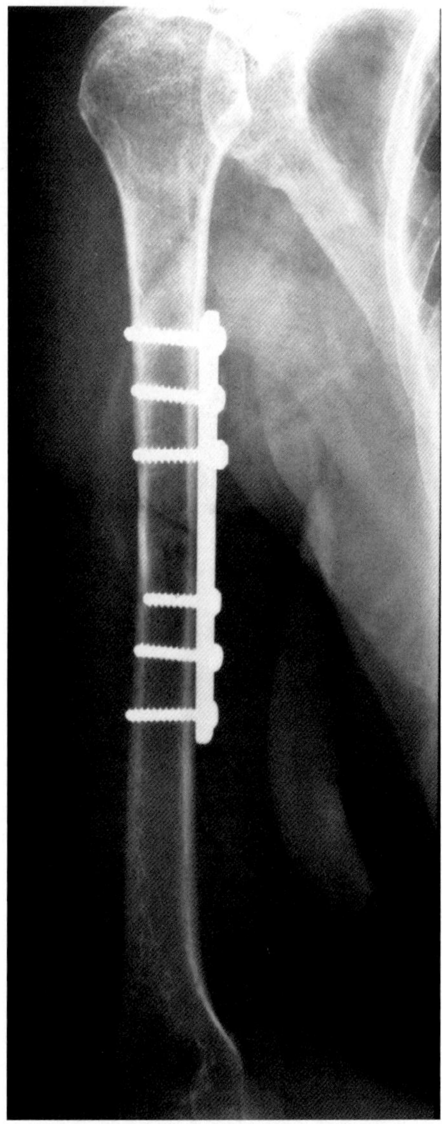


Fig. 10-12 Internal (A) and external (B) rotation radiographs of the humerus following conventional dynamic compression plate and screw fixation of an oblique mid shaft fracture.

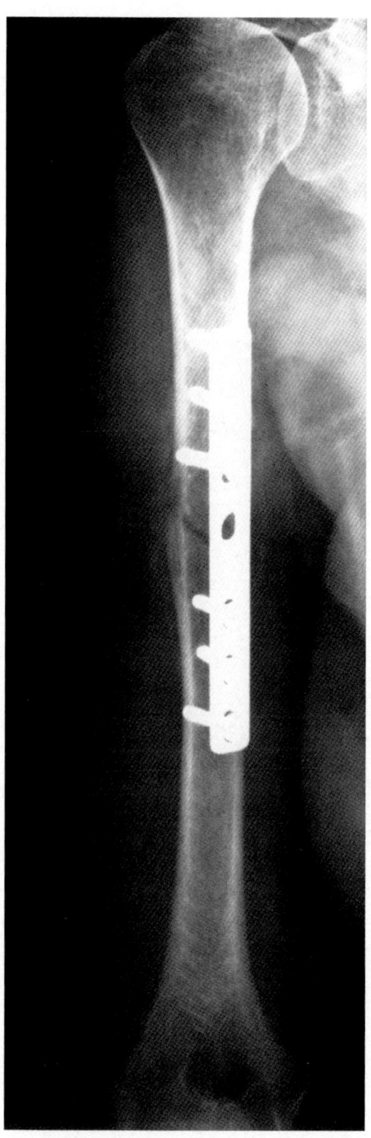


Fig. 10-12 *(Continued)*

## Suggested Reading


Crates J, Whittle AP. Antegrade interlocking nailing of acute humeral shaft fractures. *Clin Orthop*. 1998;350: 40–50.

Gregory PR, Sanders RW. Compression plating versus intramedullary fixation of humeral shaft fractures. *J Am Acad Orthop Surg*. 1997;5:215–223.

Lin J, Inoue N, Valdevit A, et al. Biomechanical comparison of antegrade and retrograde nailing of humeral shaft fracture. *Clin Orthop*. 1998;351:203–213.

VanderGriend R, Tomasin J, Ward EF. Open reduction and internal fixation of humeral shaft fractures. *J Bone Joint Surg*. 1986;68A:430–433.


## Complications

Complications vary with the extent of injury and method of treatment. Common complications include delayed union or nonunion, malunion, and infection. Radial nerve palsy occurs in 5% to 18% of patients, more commonly in fractures occurring at the junction of the mid and distal thirds of the humeral shaft (Holstein-Lewis fracture—see Chapter 2).

### Fracture Union

In most cases union is evident in 8 weeks. When the fracture is not healed in 3 to 4 months it is considered delayed union or nonunion >6 to 8 months. The overall incidence of nonunion is 1% to 15%. Factors associated with higher rates of nonunion include transverse fractures (Fig. 10-10), soft tissue interposition (Fig. 10-11), fracture distraction, infection, and poor vascular supply. The incidence also varies with treatment approach. Closed reduction has a 10% incidence of nonunion, although 90% respond to surgical intervention. The incidence of nonunion is 0% to 7% with plate and screw fixation and up to 6% with intramedullary nail techniques. Failed internal fixation can usually (40% to 60%) be treated with exchange intramedullary nailing (see Fig. 10-17). Radiographic features are characteristic and demonstrate no evidence of medullary bone crossing the fracture and lack of bridging callus. The fracture margins may be sclerotic with hypertrophic nonunion or atrophic with atrophic nonunion. CT with reformatting and three-dimensional (3-D) reconstructions is most useful to evaluate the status of callus formation and union (see Fig. 10-18).

### Deep Infection

The incidence of deep infection varies with the type of injury and treatment selection. The incidence is 2% with closed fractures. With open fractures, the incidence increases to 17%. Infection following intramedullary nailing is 3% to 5% and with plate and screw fixation 2% to 6%. In patients with open wounds, external fixation is often used for initial treatment (Gustilo and Anderson types II and III) and for more prolonged treatment with type IIIC open wounds. When external fixation is used (Figs. 10-8 and 10-9) pin tract infection is a concern. Irregular lucency along the fixation pins may be evident on radiographs. Serial radiographs may be useful for demonstrating nonunion with periosteal reaction due to infection (see Fig. 10-19). In most cases, further evaluation with CT, MRI, or radionuclide scans using combined Technetium Tc 99m and labeled white cells is required to confirm infection. Positron emission tomography (PET) has recently been used in patients with orthopaedic implants to evaluate infection.

### Implant Failure

Failure of the implants occurs in up to 7% of patients treated surgically. This may include nail or plate fracture and screw pullout or fracture. Serial radiographs are usually adequate for detection of implant failure (see Fig. 10-20 and also figs. 10-17 and 10-19).

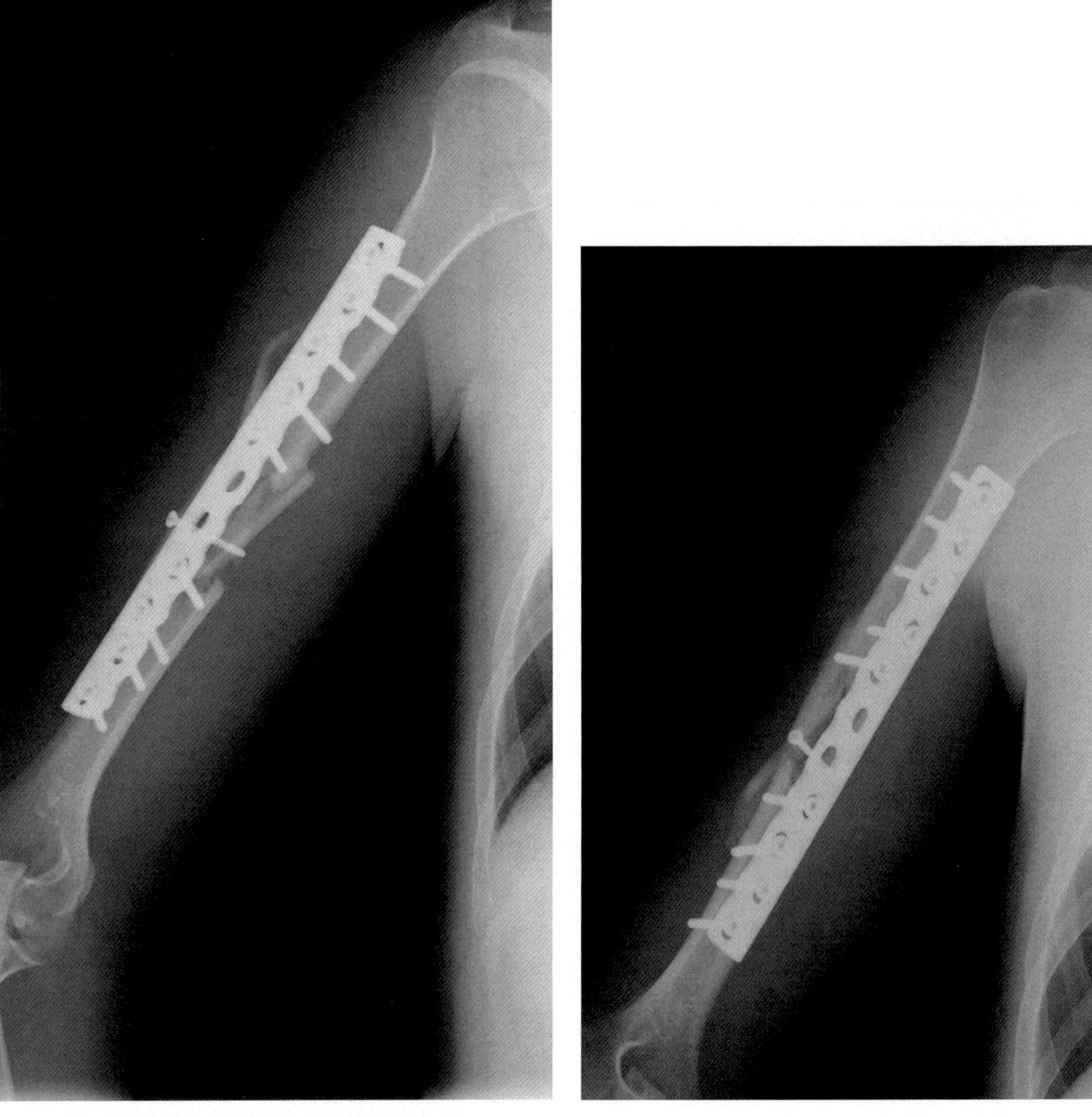


Fig. 10-13 Low-contact dynamic compression plate fixation. OTA C3 fracture of the humerus following plate and screw fixation (A) and 4 months later (B) with healing.

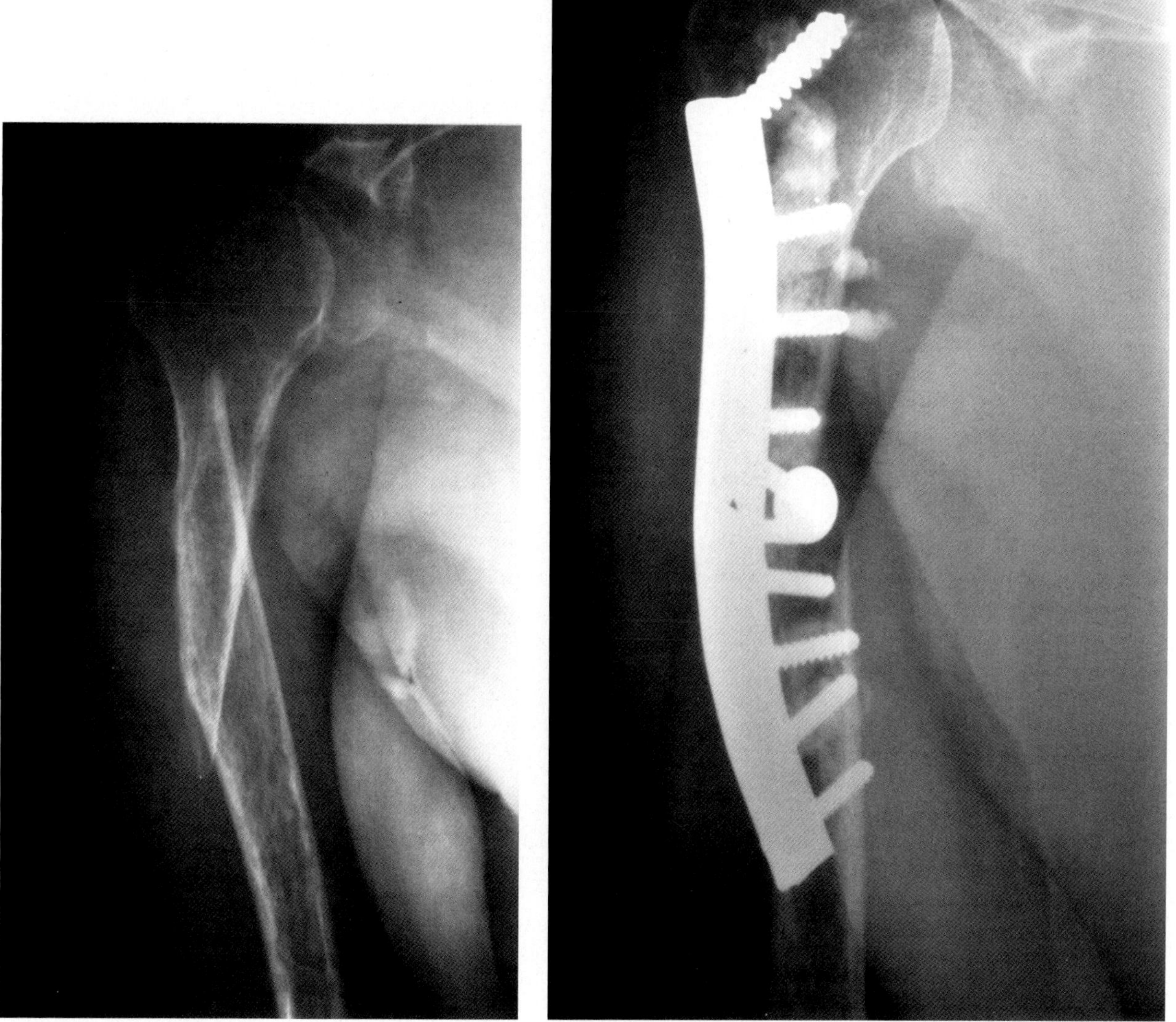


Fig. 10-14 A: Radiograph of an osteoporotic humerus fractured during a fall. B: Fracture fixation was achieved with plate and screw fixation using methyl methacrylate to improve screw purchase.

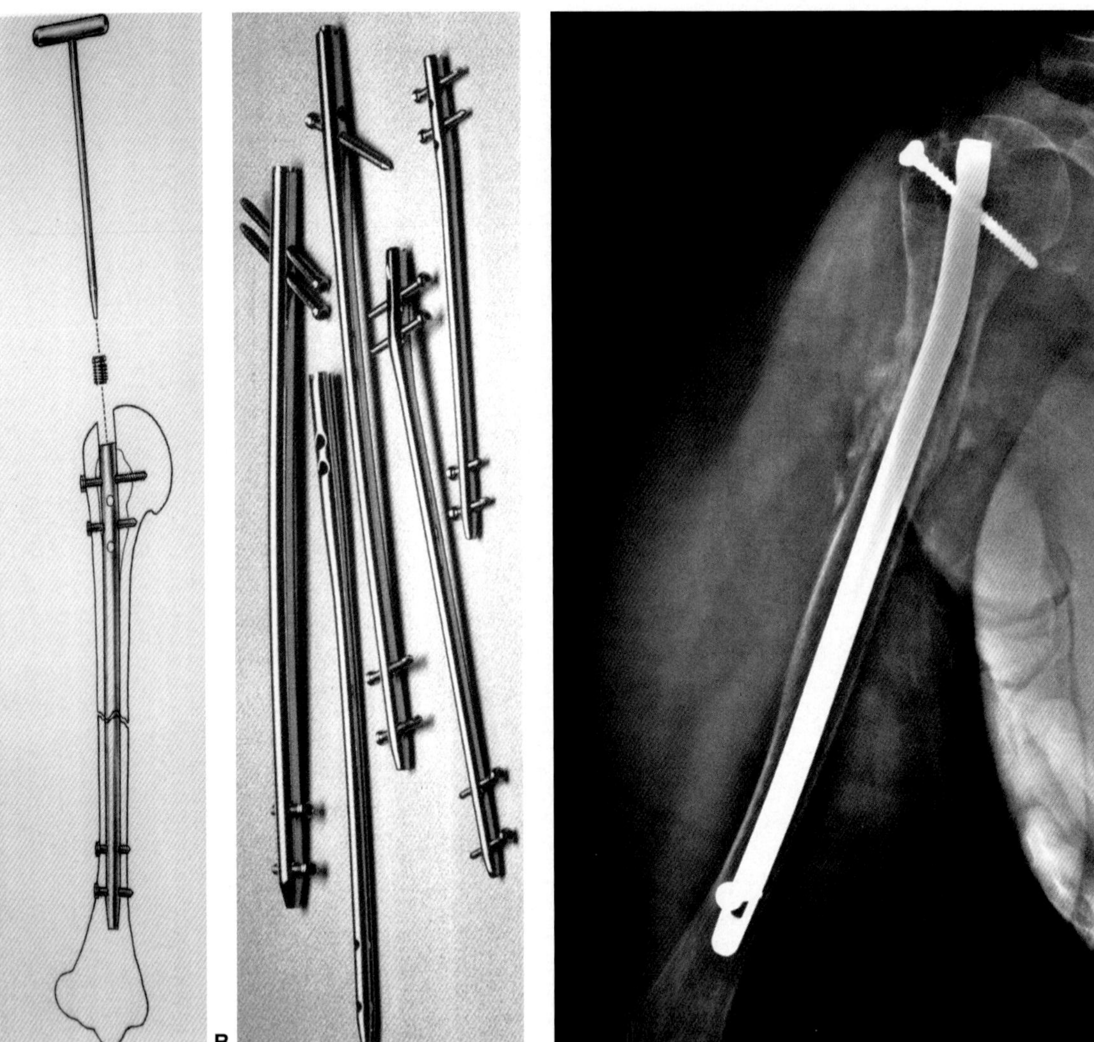


Fig. 10-15 Intramedullary nail techniques. A: Illustration of antegrade technique with proximal nail below the rotator cuff insertion and screw top to prevent fibrous ingrowth. B: Photograph of different interlocking nail configurations. (A and B Courtesy of Biomet, Warsaw, Indiana.) C: Radiograph following intramedullary nail fixation of a proximal humeral fracture.

## Neurovascular Complications

Nerve injury may occur at the time of injury or related to treatment. Radial nerve injuries occur in 5% to 10% of patients with humeral fractures, more commonly with those at the junction of the mid and distal thirds of the humerus (up to 18%). The radial nerve may also be injured during plate and screw fixation (0% to 5%) or when distal screws are placed with intramedullary locking nails. The axillary nerve is at risk when proximal screws are placed. The axillary nerve lies 5 to 6 cm distal to the acromial edge. Most nerve injuries are obvious due to fracture location and clinical examination. MRI is most useful for evaluating the anatomy and surrounding tissues about the nerves.

## Adhesive Capsulitis

Loss of range of motion can occur in the shoulder or elbow. Antegrade intramedullary nails are more commonly associated with shoulder pain and reduced motion. These findings are evident in 6% to 37% of patients. Arthrography with distension techniques may be useful for diagnosis and treatment in these cases.

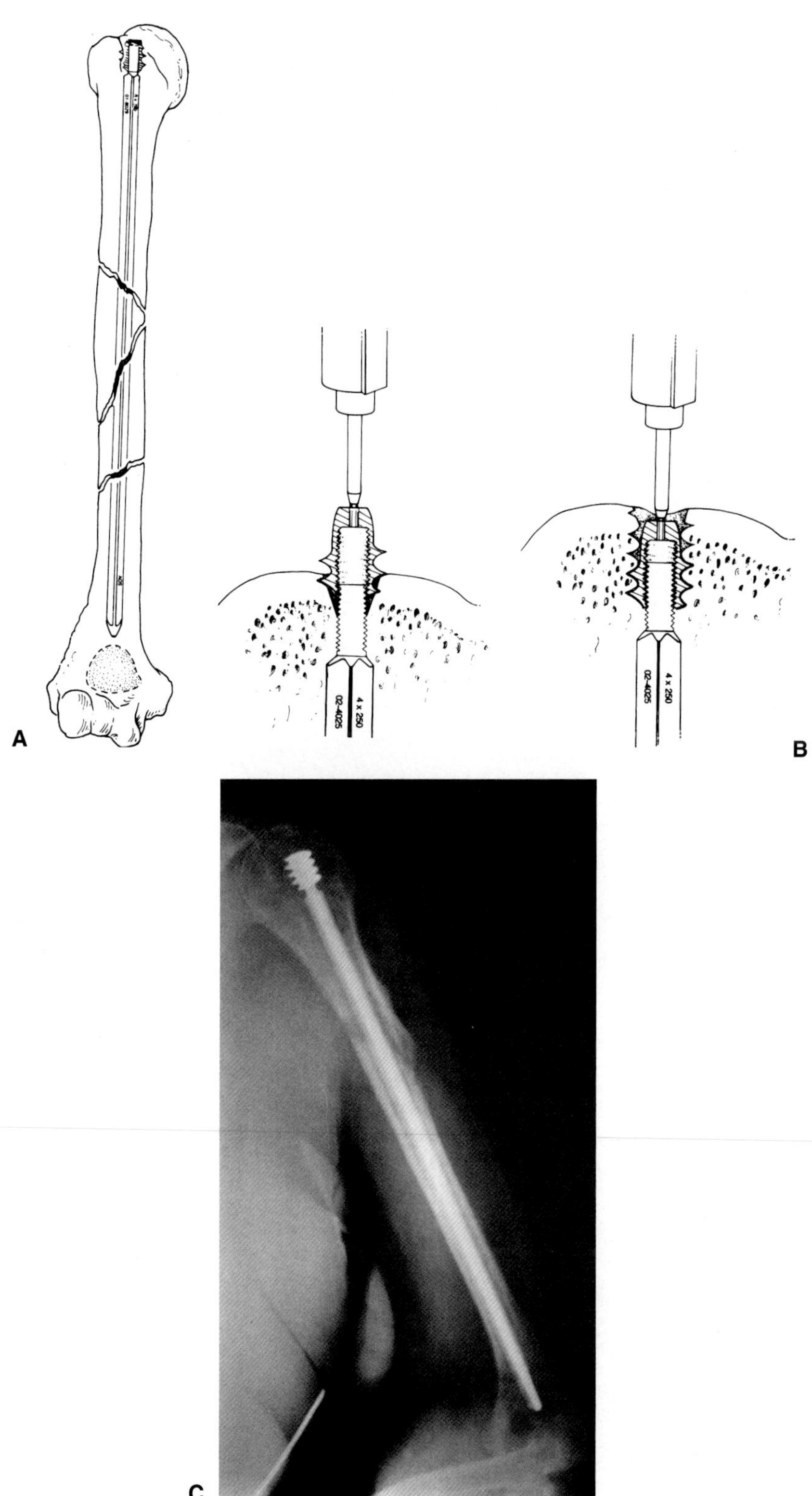


Fig. 10-16 A: Illustration of insertion of a True/Flex nail for treatment of a segmental mid shaft fracture. B: There is a proximal threaded cap that prevents migration and rotation. (Courtesy of Applied Osteosystems, Walnut Creek, California.) C: Radiograph following placement of a True/Flex nail.

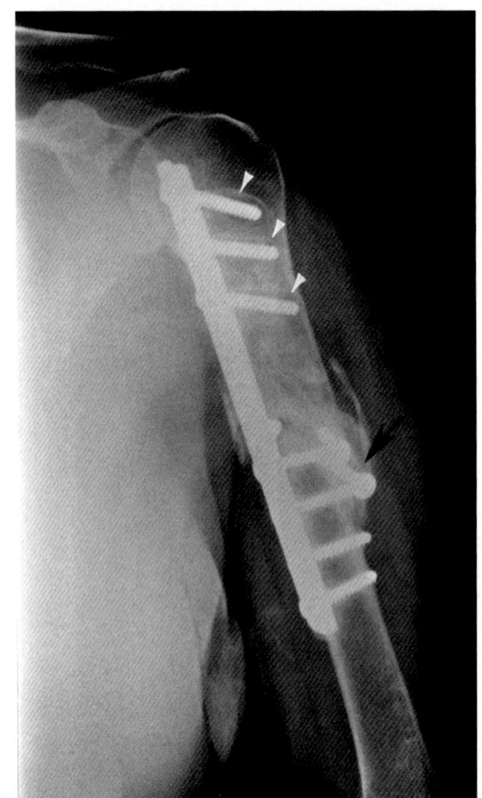

A

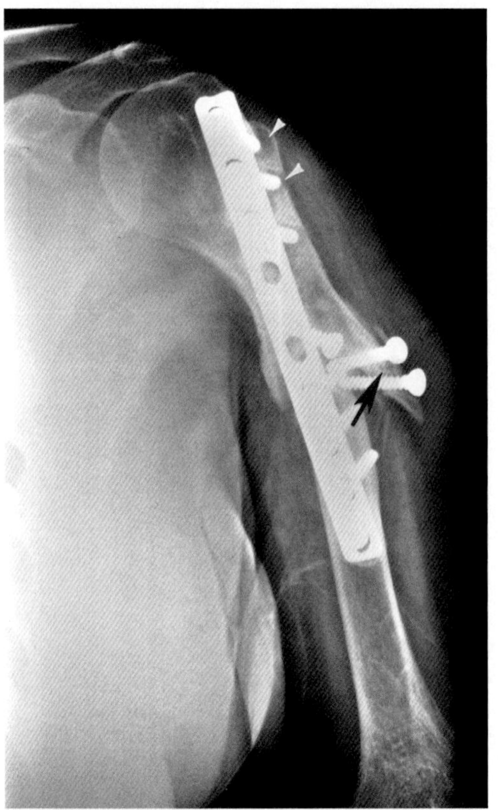

B

C

Fig. 10-17 Radiographs (A and B) of a proximal third humeral shaft fracture treated with plate and screw fixation with two lag or interfragmentary screws (*arrow*). There is lucency about multiple screws (*arrowheads*) due to implant failure. C: The plate and screws were replaced with a short locking nail which resulted in healing.

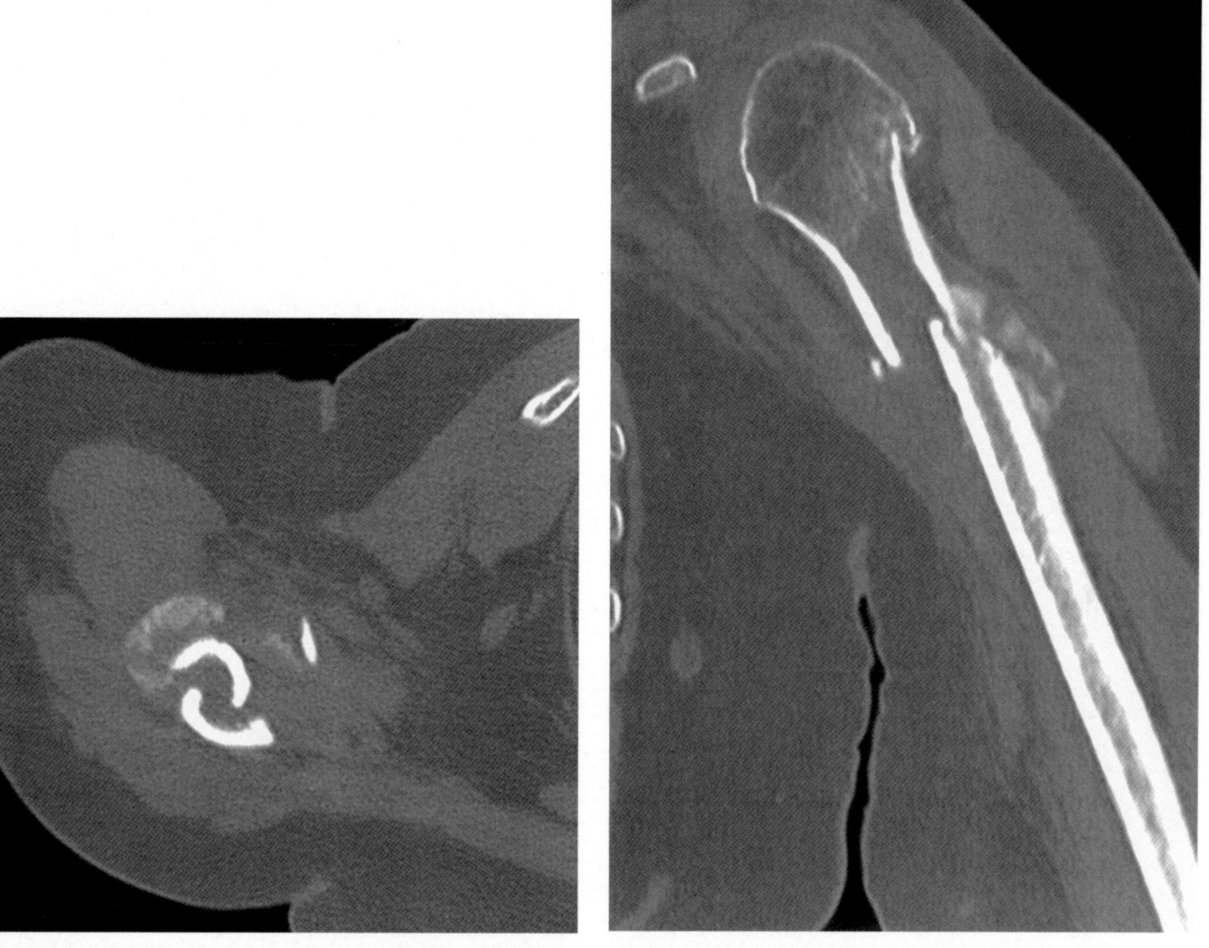


Fig. 10-18 Computed tomographic (CT) images in a patient with delayed union. Axial (A) and coronal (B) CT images demonstrate incomplete callus formation with little callus medially at 6 months.

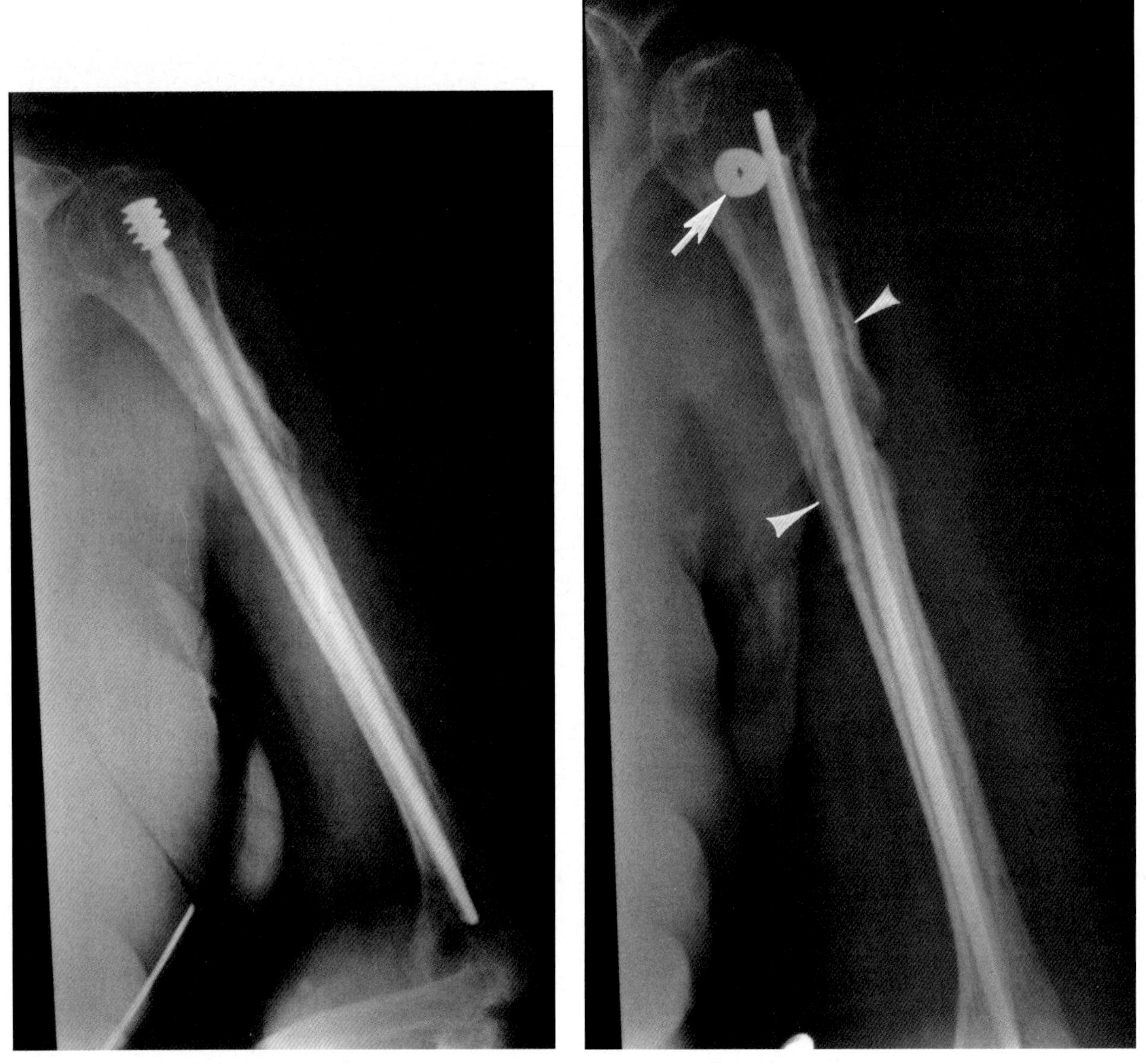


Fig. 10-19 A: Radiograph after intramedullary nail fixation with a True/Flex nail. B: Radiograph several months later demonstrates displacement of the fixation cap screw (*arrow*) and periosteal reaction (*arrowheads*) due to infection.

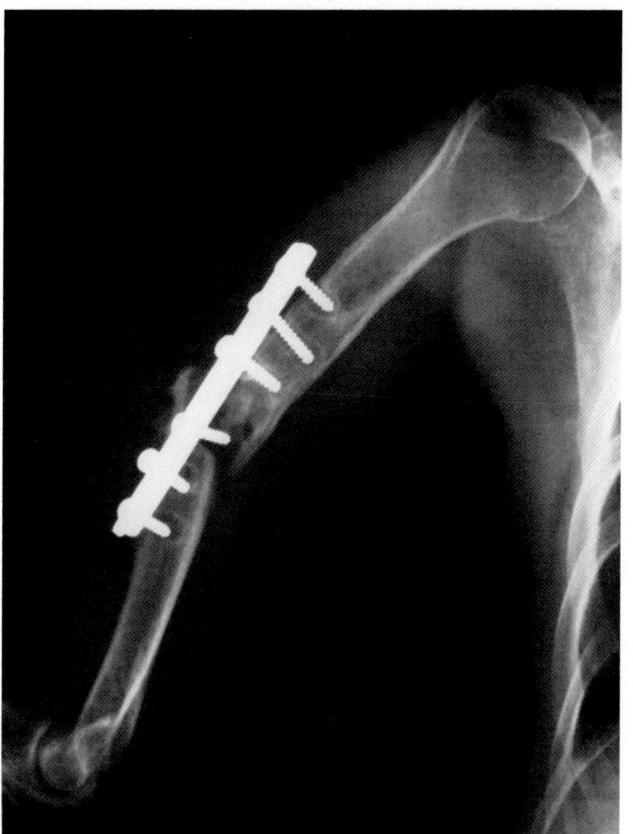

Fig. 10-20 Implant failure. Radiograph demonstrates a mid humeral fracture with bone loss at the fracture site and displacement of the plate and screws.

## Suggested Reading

Boyd HB, Lipinski SW, Wiley JH. Observations on nonunion of the shafts of long bones, with a statistical analysis of 842 patients. *J Bone Joint Surg*. 1962;43A:159.

Crates J, Whittle AP. Antegrade interlocking nailing of acute humeral shaft fractures. *Clin Orthop*. 1998;350:40–50.

Farragos AF, Schemitsch EH, McKee MD. Complication of intramedullary nailing for fractures of the humeral shaft: A review. *J Orthop Trauma*. 1999;13:258–267.

Gregory PR, Sanders RW. Compression plating versus intramedullary nail fixation of humeral shaft fractures. *J Am Acad Orthop Surg*. 1997;5:215–223.

Heim D, Herkert F, Hess P, et al. Surgical treatment of humeral shaft fractures–the Basel experience. *J Trauma*. 1993;35: 226–232.

Nepola JV, Seabold JE, Marsh JL, et al. Diagnosis of infection in ununited fractures. *J Bone Joint Surg*. 1993;75A:1816–1822.

Rosen H. The treatment of nonunions and pseudarthroses of the humeral shaft. *Orthop Clin North Am*. 1990;21:725–742.

Stern PJ, Mattingly DA, Pomeroy DL, et al. Intramedullary fixation of humeral shaft fractures. *J Bone Joint Surg*. 1984;66A: 639–646.

# 11 The Elbow

This chapter will review preoperative and postoperative imaging of elbow trauma, joint replacement procedures, and other common orthopaedic disorders for which implants are required.

## Trauma

Fractures and dislocations of the elbow can be complex and difficult to manage. This section reviews specific injuries to the distal humerus, radial head, and proximal ulna with emphasis on injuries that require orthopaedic fixation.

### Distal Humeral Fractures

Supracondylar fractures are extra-articular. Most of these injuries occur in children (80%). In children, intracondylar extension and physeal injuries are uncommon. Only approximately 6% of all physeal fractures involve the distal humerus. The second most common group involves insufficiency fractures in elderly patients with osteoporotic bone. Fractures of the elbow account for 7% of adult fractures. Overall, distal humeral fractures in adults account for only 3% of all skeletal fractures. In children, most injuries are related to significant falls or high-velocity injuries such as motor vehicle accidents. In more elderly patients, simple falls result in distal humeral fractures.

The distal humerus comprises medial and lateral columns with a transverse articular surface which includes the capitellum (anterior extension of the lateral column) and trochlea (see Fig. 11-1). Multiple classification systems have been used for distal humeral fractures. Classifications are designed to deal with the difficult reconstruction of the anatomic relationships.

Pediatric supracondylar fractures may be classified by the direction of the distal fragment. These fractures are the most common elbow fracture in children (60% to 80%). Most fractures are due to extension injury (98%) (see Fig. 11-2). Flexion injuries account for only 2% of supracondylar fractures.

Lateral condylar fractures account for 15% to 17% of pediatric elbow injuries. The metaphyseal fracture may enter the joint at the junction of the captellum and trochlea or more medially through the trochlea (see Fig. 11-3).

Fractures of the medial epiccondyle do not involve the articular surface. Most of these injuries (80%) occur during adolescence and are common in throwing athletes (see Fig. 11-4). Complex condylar fractures (T and Y configurations) are rare in children and account for <1% of pediatric elbow fractures (see Fig. 11-5).

Multiple classification systems have been used for distal humeral fractures in adults. These include the Riseborough and Radin classification developed in 1969, Mehne and Matta classification, AO (Arbeitsgemeinschaft fur Osteosynthesefragen), and in 1996 the Orthopaedic Trauma Association classification (see Fig. 11-6). The last system is more complex and based on fracture location and extent (extra-articular, partial articular, and complete articular). There are three groups with three major categories and subcategories in each (see Figs. 11-7, 11-8, 11-9, 11-10 and also Fig. 11-6).

**ORTHOPAEDIC TRAUMA ASSOCIATION CLASSIFICATION**

| TYPE | DESCRIPTION |
|---|---|
| A | Extra-articular (Fig. 11-6A to C) |
| A1 | Medial epicondyle avulsion (Fig. 11-7) |
| A2 | Simple extra-articular |
| A3 | Comminuted extra-articular |
| B | Partial articular (Fig. 11-6D to F) |
| B1 | Lateral condyle (Fig. 11-8) |
| B2 | Medial condyle |
| B3 | Frontal articular (Fig. 11-9) |
| C | Complex or complete articular (Fig. 11-6G to I) |
| C1 | Y or T intracondylar (Fig. 11-10) |
| C2 | Y or T with comminuted metaphysis |
| C3 | Y or T with comminuted articular surface |

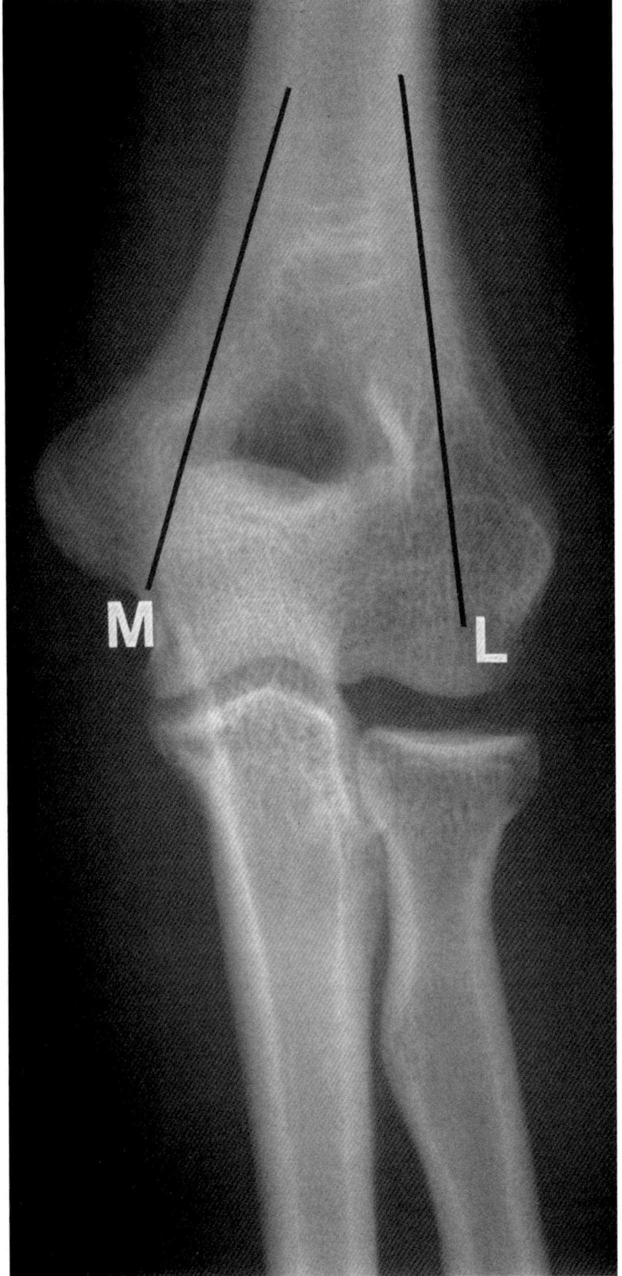


Fig. 11-1 Anteroposterior (AP) radiograph demonstrating the medial (*M*) and lateral (*L*) columns of the distal humerus with the central articular surface bordered by the columns.

## Suggested Reading

Davies MB, Stanley D. A clinically applicable fracture classification for distal humeral fractures. *J Shoulder Elbow Surg.* 2006;15:602–608.

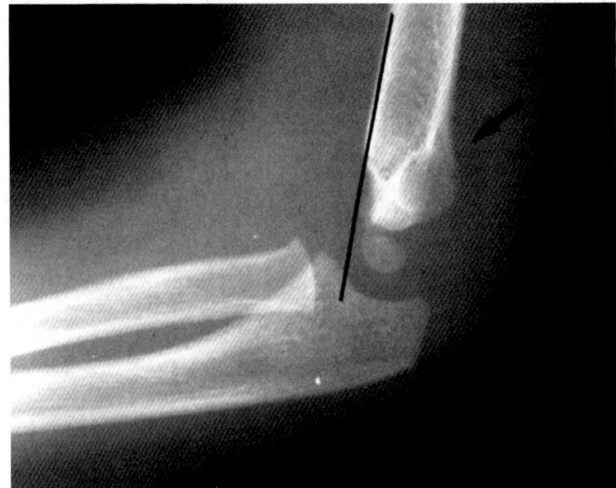

Fig. 11-2 Supracondylar extension fracture. Lateral radiograph demonstrating posterior displacement of the capitellum in relation to the anterior humeral line. There is a posterior fat pad sign (*arrow*).

Kasser JR, Beaty JH. Supracondylar fractures of the distal humerus. In: Beaty JH, Kasser JR, eds. *Rockwood and Wilkin's fractures in children*, 5th ed. Philadelphia: Lippincott Williams & Wilkins; 2001:577–624.

Orthopaedic Trauma Association Committee on Coding and Classifications. Fractures and dislocations compendium. *J Orthop Trauma*. 1996;10(Suppl):12–14.

## Radial Head Fractures

Radial head fractures account for 2% to 5% of all skeletal fractures, with 85% occurring in adults. In children, fractures of the metaphysis and physis are more common. Proximal radial fractures in children are most common between 8 and 12 years of age. Most fractures occur during a fall on the outstretched hand regardless of patient age.

The Mason classification is commonly used for isolated radial head fractures. This system is useful for treatment planning (see Fig. 11-11).

**MASON CLASSIFICATION FOR RADIAL HEAD FRACTURES**

| TYPE | RADIOGRAPHIC FEATURES |
|---|---|
| I | Undisplaced radial head or neck (Fig. 11-11A) |
| II | Radial head or neck with >2 mm displacement (Fig. 11-11B) |
| III | Severely comminuted head or neck fractures (Fig. 11-11C) |
| IV | Radial head fracture with associated dislocation (Fig. 11-11D) |

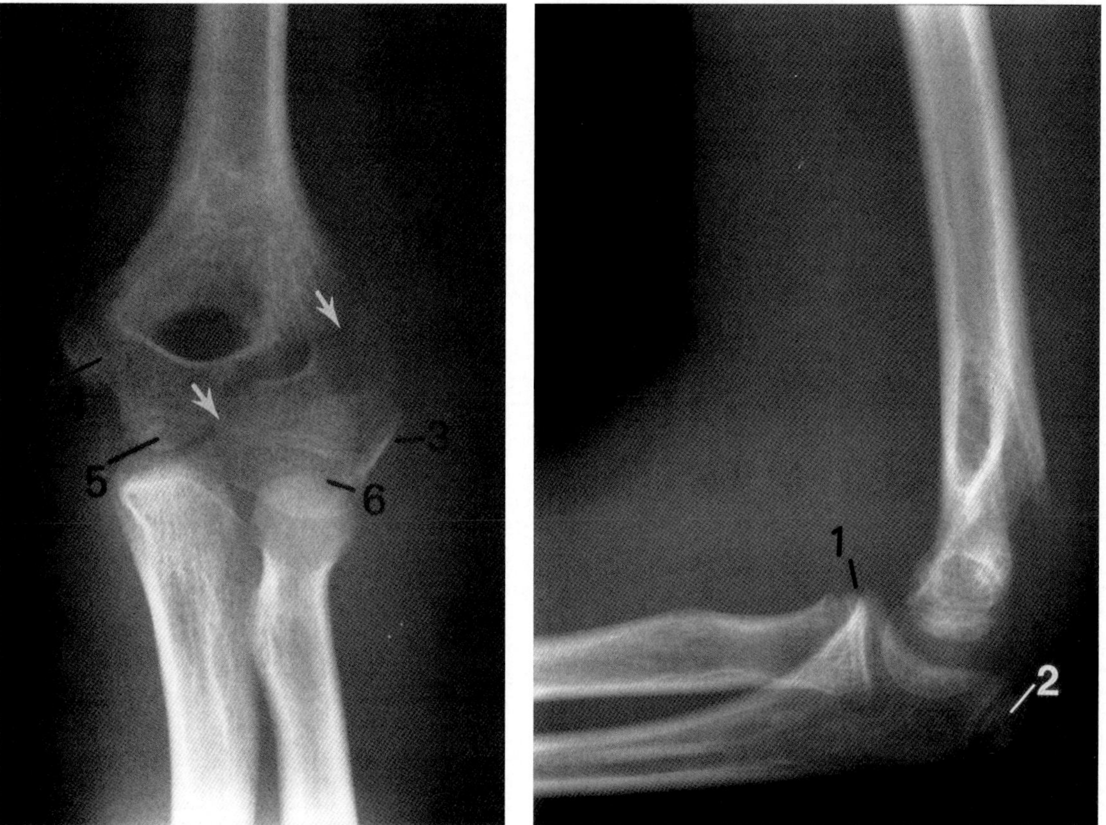


Fig. 11-3 Lateral (A) and anteroposterior (AP) (B) radiographs demonstrating a lateral condyle fracture entering the joint at the margin of the capitellar epiphysis (*arrows*). *1*-radial head epipysis, *2*-olecranon epiphysis, *3*-lateral epicondyle, *4*-medial epicondyle, *5*-trochlear epiphysis, *6*-capitellum.

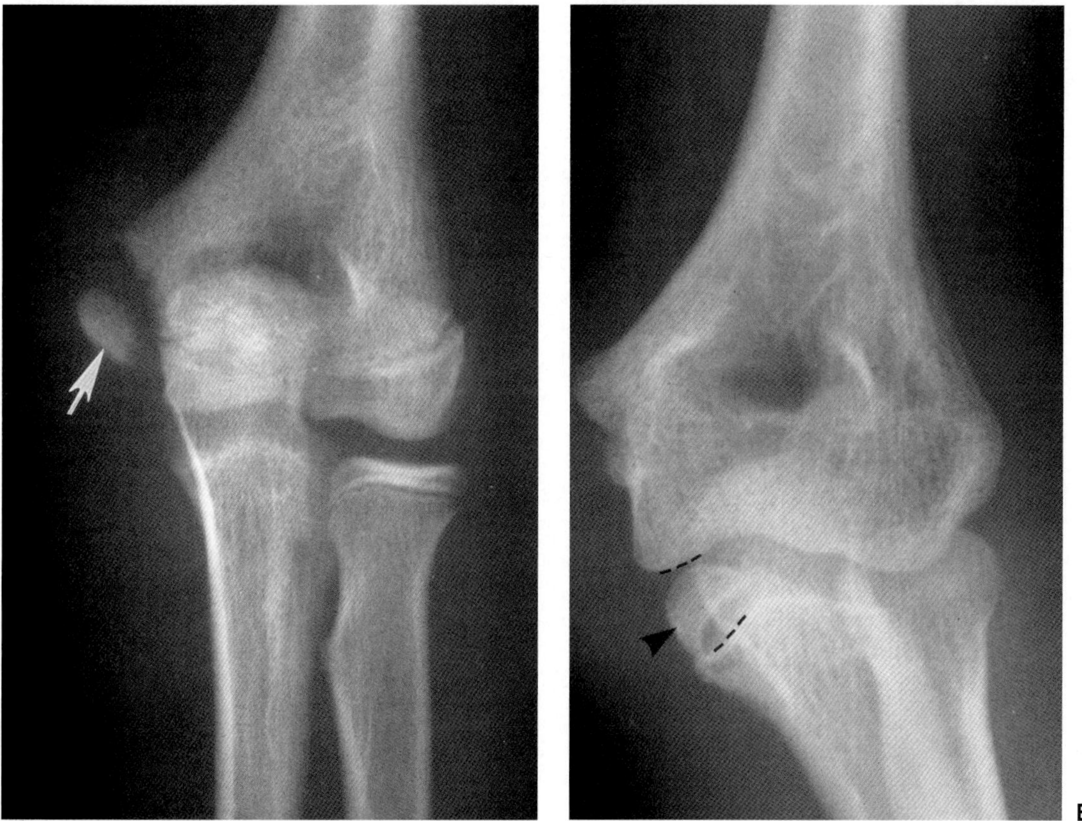


Fig. 11-4 Avulsion of the medial epicondyle. A: Anteroposterior (AP) radiograph demonstrates a displaced medial epicondylar epiphysis in a young baseball pitcher (*arrow*). B: AP radiograph of a different patient with the medial epicondylar epiphysis displaced into the joint (*arrowhead*) with widening (*broken lines*) of the joint space.

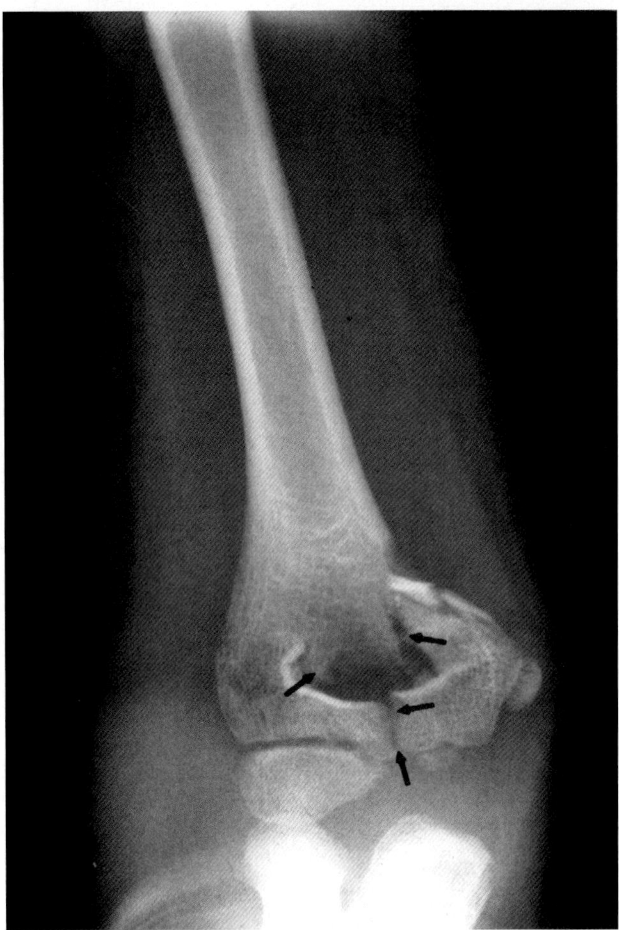

Fig. 11-5 Anteroposterior (AP) radiograph demonstrating a complex Y intracondylar fracture (*arrows*).

Radial head and neck fractures are commonly associated with other elbow fractures including coronoid, olecranon, and capitellar injuries. Up to 50% of capitellar fractures occur in association with radial head fractures. Associated ligament and neurovascular injuries are also common. Monteggia fractures classically demonstrate radial head dislocation with the proximal ulnar fracture. However, associated radial head and coronoid fractures are not uncommon.

## SUGGESTED READING

Beaty JH, Kasser JR. The elbow region: general concepts in the pediatric patient. In: Kasser JR, Beaty JH, eds. *Rockwood and Wilkins' fractures in children*, 5th ed. Philadelphia: Lippincott Williams & Wilkins; 2001.

Mason MB. Some observations on the fractures of the head of the radius with a review of 100 cases. *Br J Surg*. 1954; 42:123–132.

### Fractures of the Proximal Ulna

The proximal ulna is particularly susceptible to fracture due to its subcutaneous position. Most fractures are intra-articular which can alter joint function and stability (see Fig. 11-12). Fractures with disruption of the triceps fascial expansions tend to displace significantly (see Fig. 11-13). Most olecranon fractures occur from direct blows to the flexed elbow.

Several classification systems have been used. The Colton classification is commonly used and it is less complex than the Orthopaedic Trauma Association classification (see Fig. 11-14). The Mayo classification is similar, but based on the degree of comminution, displacement, and instability. Type I fractures are minimally undisplaced (separation ≤2 mm) with minimal comminution. These injuries account for 5% of olecranon fractures. Type II fractures are displaced, but stable and account for 85% of olecranon fractures. Type III fractures are displaced and unstable and may be comminuted. The type III fracture is associated with disruption of the medial collateral ligament, of the ulnar part of the lateral collateral ligament, or both. There is associated instability of the distal ulnar fragment.

**COLTON CLASSIFICATION FOR PROXIMAL ULNAR FRACTURES**

| TYPE | DESCRIPTION |
|---|---|
| I | Undisplaced (Mayo type I) |
| II | Avulsion with oblique or transverse fracture |
| III | Obique or transverse with articular involvement |
| IV | Comminuted |
| V | Associated dislocation (Mayo type III) |

## SUGGESTED READING

Colton CL. Fractures of the olecranon in adults. Classification and management. *Injury*. 1973;5:121–127.

Morrey BF. Instructional course lectures. Complex instability of the elbow. *J Bone Joint Surg*. 1997;79A:460–469.

### Coronoid Fractures

Isolated coronoid fractures are uncommon. Most are associated with other fractures or dislocations of the elbow. The incidence is 2% to 10% in association with posterior dislocations. Instability is common following coronoid fractures.

Regan and Morrey classified coronoid fractures into three types (see Fig. 11-15). Type I fractures are avulsions of the coronoid tip. Type II fractures involve ≤50% of the coronoid and type III fractures >50% of the coronoid. Subcategories are added to each type depending upon the lack of associated

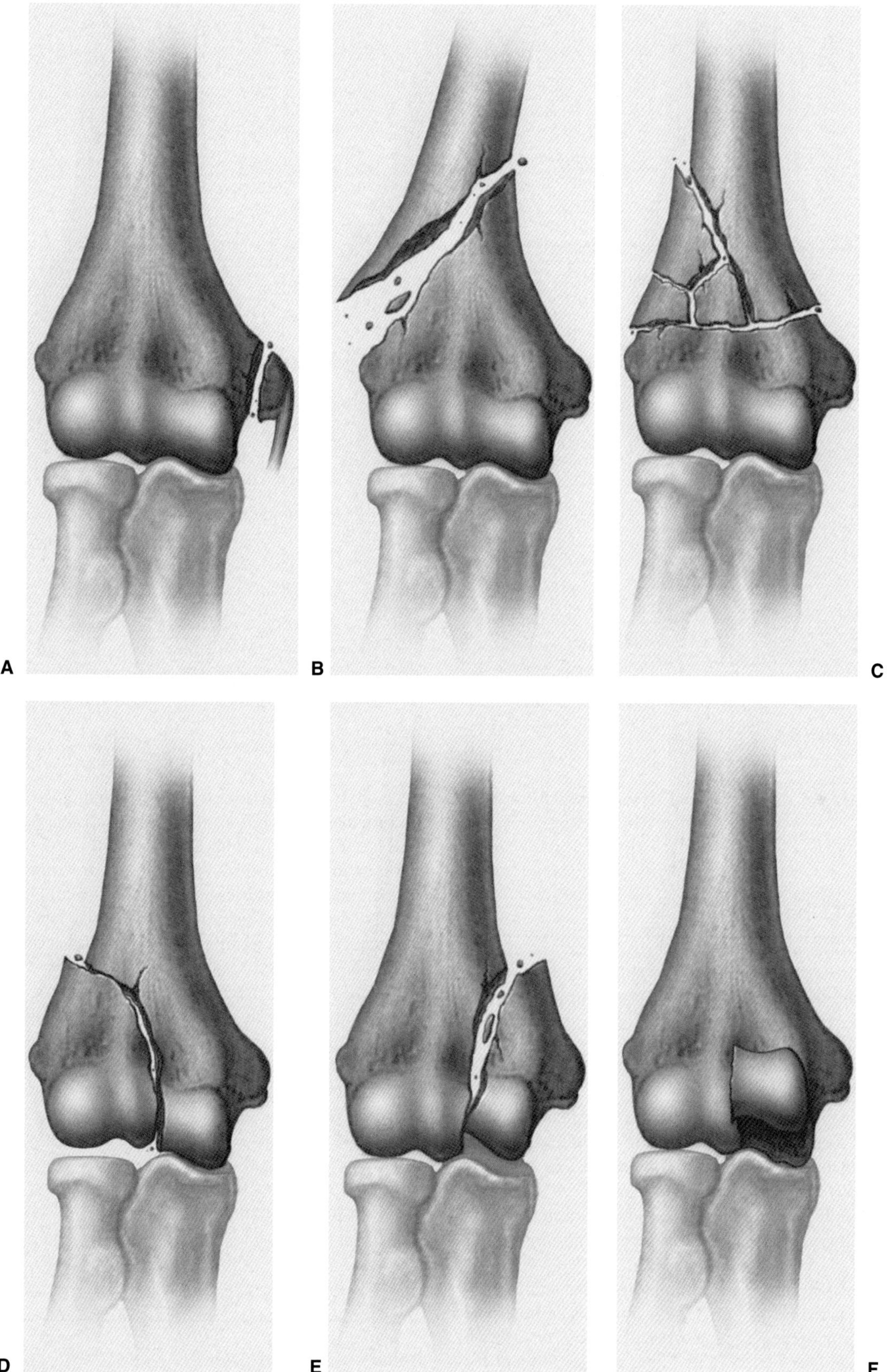


Fig. 11-6 Orthopaedic Trauma Association classification for distal humeral fractures. A: Type A1—medial epicondyle avulsion, B: Type A2—simple extra-articular, C: Type A3—comminuted extra-articular, D: Type B1—partial articular lateral, E: Type B2—partial articular medial, F: Type B3—partial articular frontal, G: C1—Y or T intracondylar, H: Type C2—Y or T with metaphyseal comminution, I: Type C3—Y or T with comminuted articular surface.

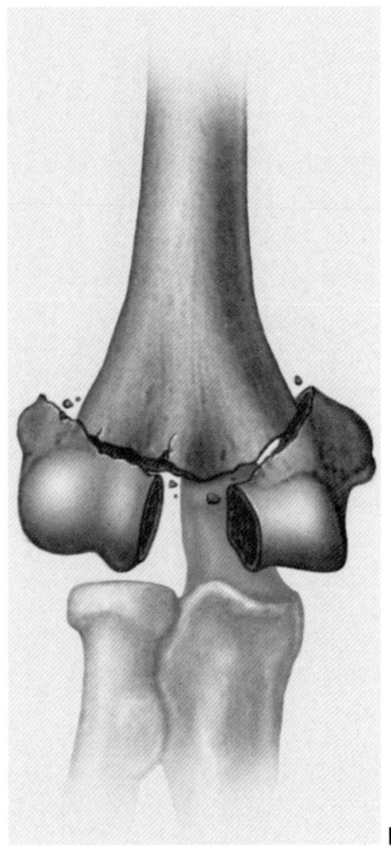

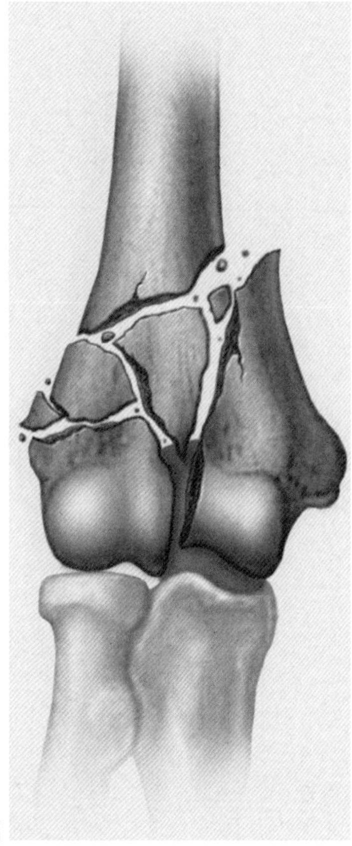

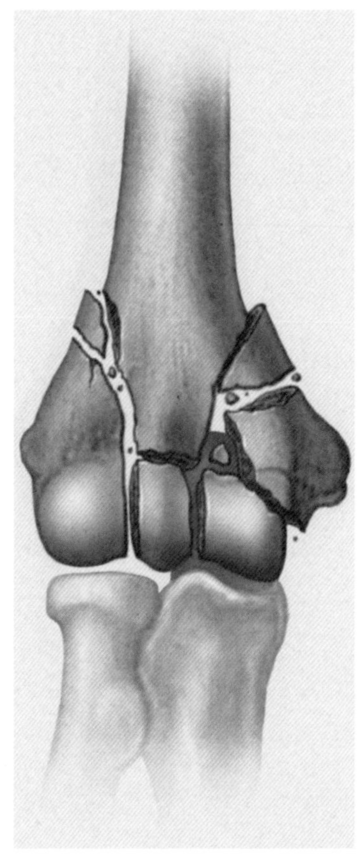


Fig. 11-6 *(Continued)*

dislocation (type A) or the presence of an associated dislocation (type B).

## Suggested Reading

Morrey BF. Current concepts in the treatment of fractures of the radial head, the olecranon and the coronoid. *J Bone Joint Surg*. 1995;77A:316–327.

### Monteggia Fractures

The Monteggia fracture accounts for 7% of proximal ulnar fractures and is associated with dislocation of the radial head. The injury is uncommon, accounting for only 0.7% of elbow injuries. Multiple mechanisms of injury have been described including a direct blow to the ulna, falls on the outstretched hand with the elbow flexed at impact, and hyperextension injuries of the elbow.

The Bado classification is commonly used for adult Monteggia fractures (see Fig. 11-16). Type I fractures demonstrate anterior angulation of the ulnar fracture and anterior dislocation of the radial head (see Fig. 11-17). These injuries account for 50% to 75% of Monteggia fractures. Type I injuries are also common in children. However, fractures are often incomplete. A greenstick fracture or bowing of the ulna may be the only ulnar features.

Bado type II fractures have posterior angulation of the ulnar fracture and posterior or posterolateral dislocation of the radial head (see Fig. 11-18). This injury is more common in adults and accounts for 10% to 15% of Monteggia fractures.

Bado type III injuries have metaphyseal ulnar fractures with lateral or antolateral dislocation of the radial head (Fig. 11-16C). This injury is also common in children and accounts for 6% to 20% of Monteggia fractures.

Bado type IV fractures have proximal fractures of the radius and ulna with anterior dislocation of the radial head (Fig. 11-16D). This is the most uncommon fracture, accounting for approximately 5% of Monteggia injuries.

Jupiter divided Bado type II fractures into four categories. Type IIA where the ulnar fracture involves the distal olecranon and coronoid, type IIB where the ulnar fracture is at the metaphyseal–diaphyseal junction distal to the coronoid, type IIC where the ulnar fracture is diaphyseal and type IID where the fracture extends into the proximal ulna.

## Suggested Reading

Bado JL. The Monteggia lesion. *Clin Orthop*. 1967;50:71–86.
Jupiter JB, Leibovic SJ, Bibbans W, et al. The posterior Monteggia lesion. *J Orthop Trauma*. 1991;5:395–402.
Letts M, Locht R, Weins J. Monteggia fracture-dislocations in children. *J Bone Joint Surg*. 1985;67B:724–727.

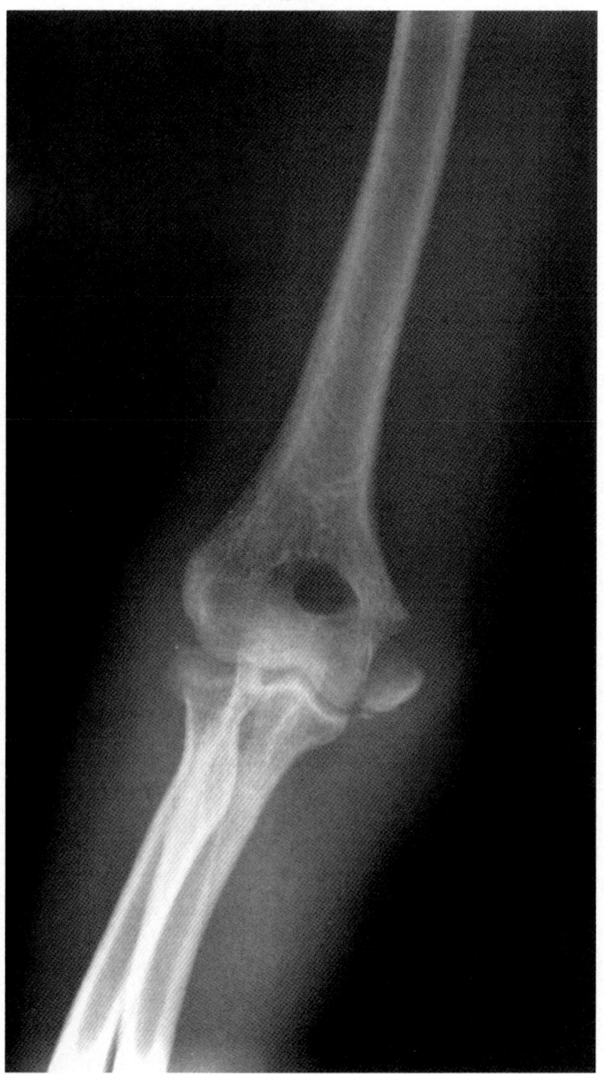

Fig. 11-7 Anteroposterior (AP) radiograph in an elderly adult with an avulsion of the medial epicondyle (OTA A1).

## Dislocations

Dislocations of the elbow are the most common dislocation in children and the second most common dislocation in adults. Most dislocations are posterior (see Fig. 11-19). Anterior dislocations are rare and usually occur in children. The mechanism of injury is a fall on the outstretched hand. The radius and ulna may also separate (divergent dislocation) with disruption of the interosseous membrane. This injury is the result of high-velocity trauma and is quite rare. Fractures are commonly associated dislocations. Fractures of the radial head and neck occur in 5% to 10%, epicondylar avulsions in 12%, and coronoid fractures in 10% of elbow dislocations.

## Suggested Reading

Cohen MS, Hastings H. Acute elbow dislocation: Evaluation and management. *J Am Acad Orthop Surg*. 1998;6:15–23.

O'Driscoll SW, Morrey BF, Korineck S, et al. Elbow subluxation and dislocation. A spectrum of instability. *Clin Orthop*. 1992;280:186–197.

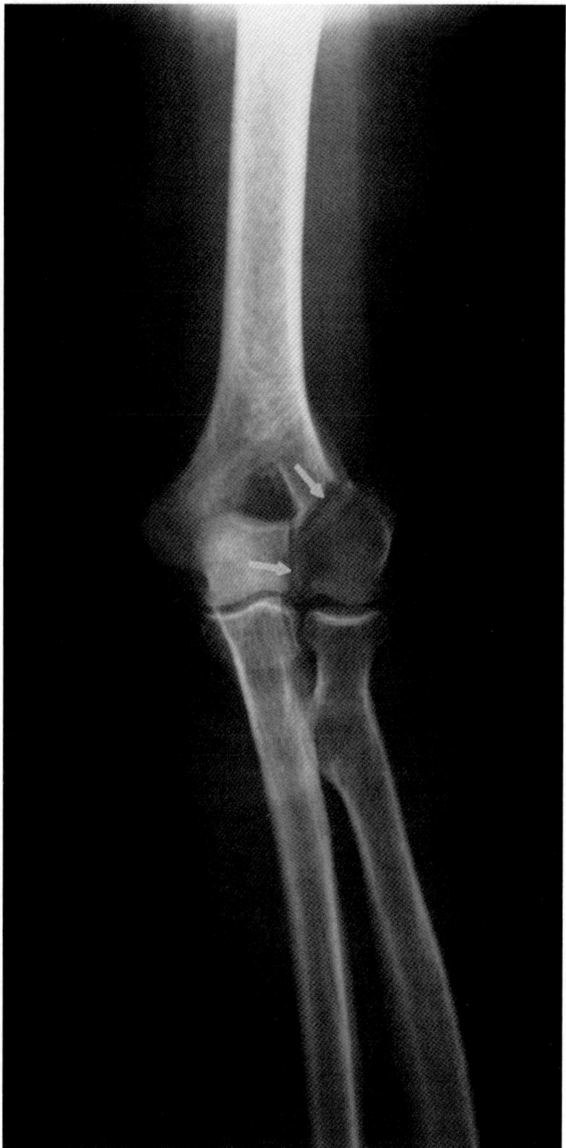

Fig. 11-8 Anteroposterior (AP) radiograph demonstrating a partial articular lateral condyle fracture (*arrows*) (OTA B1).

# Imaging of Elbow Injuries

Radiographs or computed radiographic (CR) images remain the primary screening technique for elbow fracture/dislocations. Anteroposterior (AP), lateral, and both oblique views account for routine trauma series. These views demonstrate alignment of the radial head with the capitellum regardless of the projection (see Fig. 11-20). The lateral view is useful for evaluating secondary signs of fracture such as displacement of the anterior and posterior fat pads. These structures are intracapsular, but

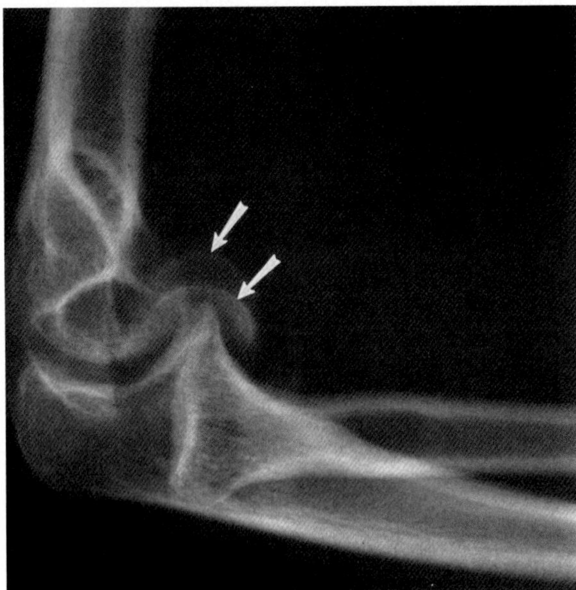

Fig. 11-9 Lateral radiograph demonstrating a partial articular frontal fracture (*white arrows*) (OTA B3).

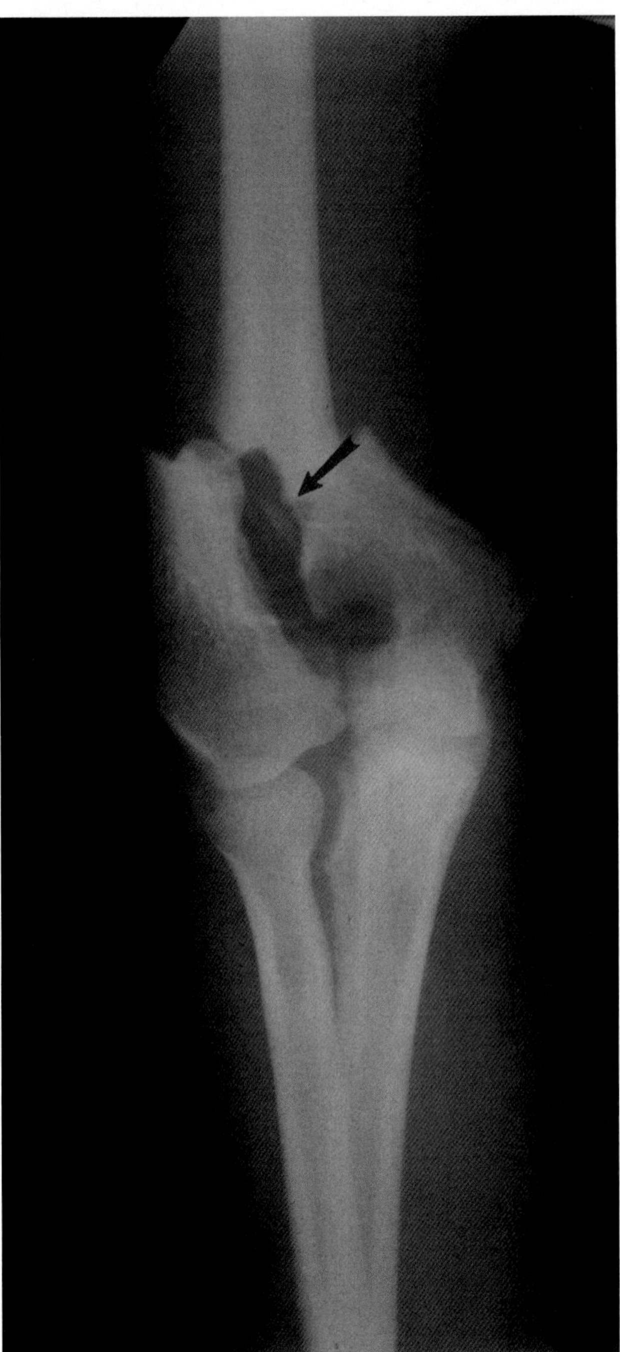

Fig. 11-10 Anteroposterior (AP) radiograph demonstrating a Y intracondylar fracture with subtle comminution of the metaphysic (*arrow*) (OTA C2).

extrasynovial (see Fig. 11-21). The anterior fat pad is normally visualized on the lateral view. The posterior fat pad is normally obscured within the olecranon fossa. When the anterior fat pad becomes elevated and the posterior fat pad (not normally visualized) is identified, a joint effusion is present and subtle fractures should be questioned (see Fig. 11-22). In children with posterior fat pads visualized on the lateral view, the incidence of fracture is approximately 90%. Cross-table lateral views may demonstrate a lipohemarthrosis, which also indicates an intraarticular fracture. The supinator fat stripe is also important to evaluate on the lateral view. Displacement or obliteration of this structure is common with fractures of the radial head and neck (Fig. 11-22). An abnormal fat stripe is also evident in 82% of other elbow injuries.

Additional views or fluoroscopically positioned spot images or stress views may also be obtained. However, currently, computed tomography (CT) is more commonly performed instead of additional radiographic views to clearly define the extent of the injury and evaluate subtle fractures following reduction of dislocations (see Figs. 11-23 and 11-24). In certain cases, magnetic resonance imaging (MRI) may be indicated to evaluate subtle fractures (see Fig. 11-25), neurovascular structures, the interosseous membrane, and for evaluating soft tissue compartments in patients with suspected compartment syndrome.

## Suggested Reading

Berquist TH, Trigg SD. The elbow. In: Berquist TH, ed. *Imaging atlas of orthopaedic appliances and prostheses*. New York: Raven Press; 1995:751–816.

Rogers SL, MacEwan DW. Changes due to trauma in the fat plane overlying the supinator muscle: A radiographic sign. *Radiology*. 1969;92:954.

Yousefzadeh DK, Jackson JH. Lipohemarthrosis of the elbow joint. *Radiology*. 1978;128:643–645.

## Treatment Options

Treatment options vary with the type and extent of injury and patient factors. Open reduction and internal fixation

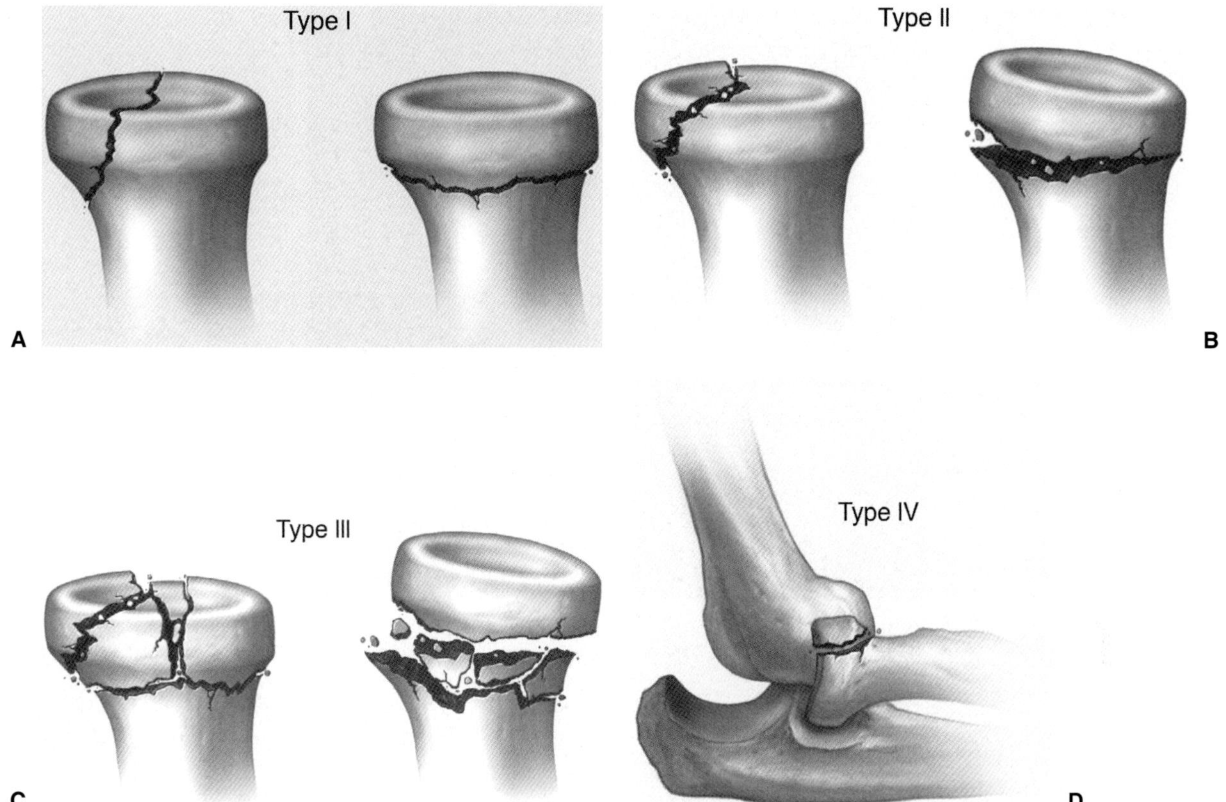


Fig. 11-11 Mason classification of radial head fractures. A: Type I—undisplaced radial head or neck fracture. B: Type II—radial head or neck fracture with >2 mm of displacement. C: Type III—comminuted radial head or neck fractures. D: Type IV—radial head fracture with associated dislocation.

is contraindicated in patients with advanced osteoporosis or significant bone loss, patients with neurologic deficit in the involved extremity, and in patients with significant health issues who cannot tolerate surgery. For purposes of discussion treatment of injury categories will be discussed separately.

## Distal Humeral Fractures

As noted in the preceding text, distal humeral fractures may be extra-articular (OTA type A), uniarticular (OTA type B), or complete articular (OTA type C). Unicondylar fractures may involve the medial or lateral column. These fractures are rare in adults and common in children. The lateral column is more frequently involved.

Stable undisplaced fractures may be treated with closed reduction and immobilization. External fixation with hinged or static techniques can be used for open wounds or in patients in whom stable reduction cannot be achieved.

Most displaced fractures require open reduction and internal fixation. Extra-articular fractures and stable unicondylar fractures may be treated with K-wire fixation or lag screws (see Figs. 11-26 and 11-27). Fractures involving the shaft may require plate and screw fixation.

Treatment of complete articular fractures (OTA type C) is more complex. Muscle forces act to displace and rotate the medial and lateral columns (see Fig. 11-28). Therefore, the columns and the distal articular surfaces must be stabilized. This can be accomplished with condylar and transverse K-wires or screws, medial and lateral plate, and screws using reconstruction plates (see Fig. 11-29) or locking plates (Fig. 11-27B), or Y plates (see Fig. 11-30). In certain cases, complex fractures of the distal humerus in older patients may be treated with elbow arthroplasty.

## Suggested Reading

Anglen J. Distal humeral fractures. *J Am Acad Orthop Surg.* 2005;13:291–297.

Cobb TK, Morrey BF. Total elbow arthroplasty as a primary treatment for distal humeral fractures in elderly patients. *J Bone Joint Surg.* 1997;79A:826–832.

Sanchez-Sotelo J, Torchia ME, O'Driscoll SW. Complex distal humeral fractures: Internal fixation with a principle-based parallel-plate technique. *J Bone Joint Surg.* 2007;89A: 961–969.

## Radial Head Fractures

The Mason classification for radial head fractures was reviewed in the previous section. Simple fractures (type I) are undisplaced and have no associated injuries. Type II injuries involve >30%

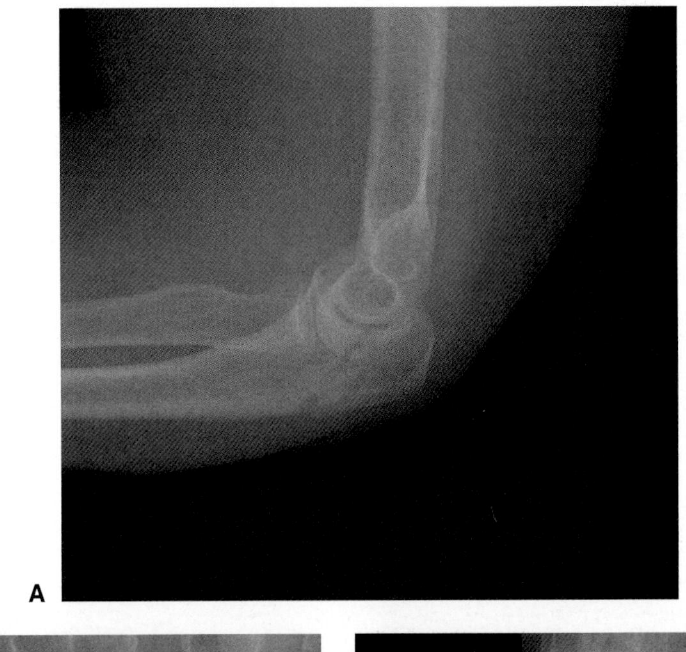

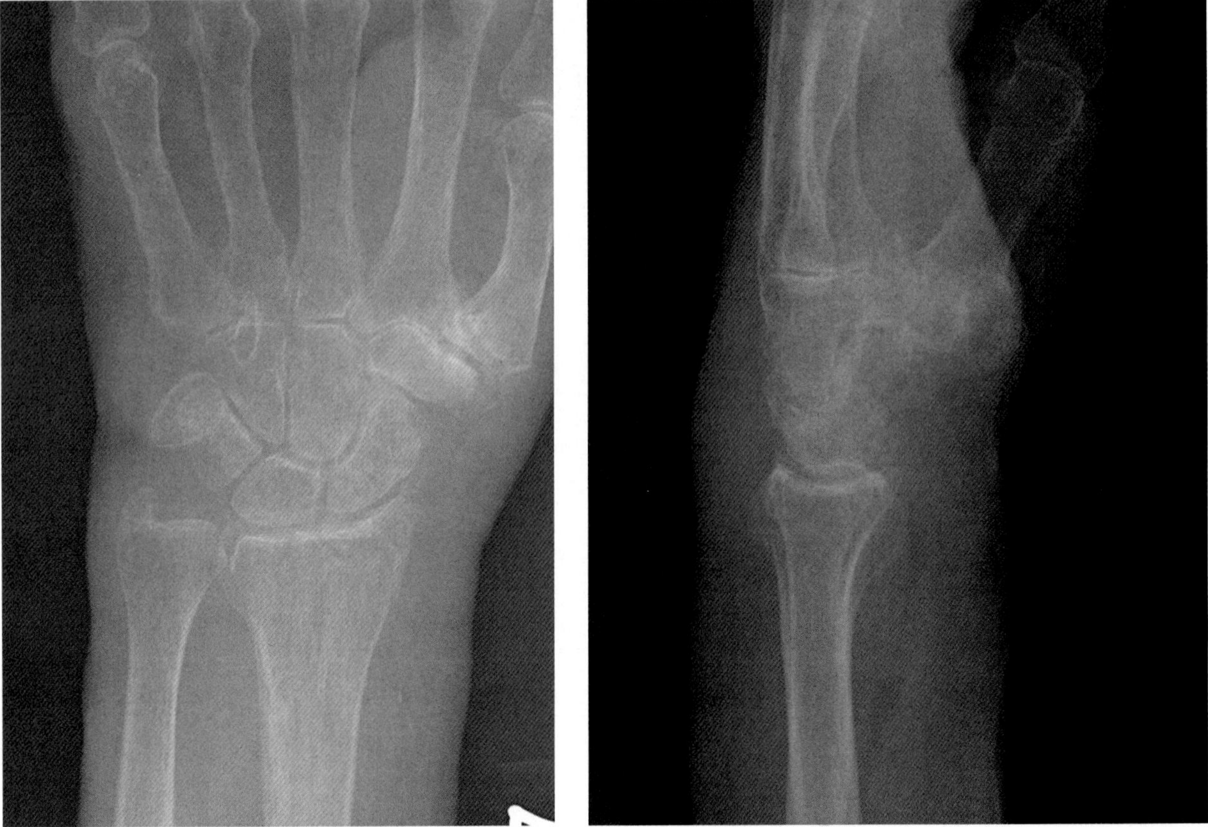

Fig. 11-12 Intra-articular fracture of the proximal ulna. A: Lateral radiograph demonstrating an undisplaced fracture of the ulna entering the joint space. Anteroposterior (AP) (B) and lateral (C) radiographs of the wrist demonstrate an associated impacted fracture of the distal radius.

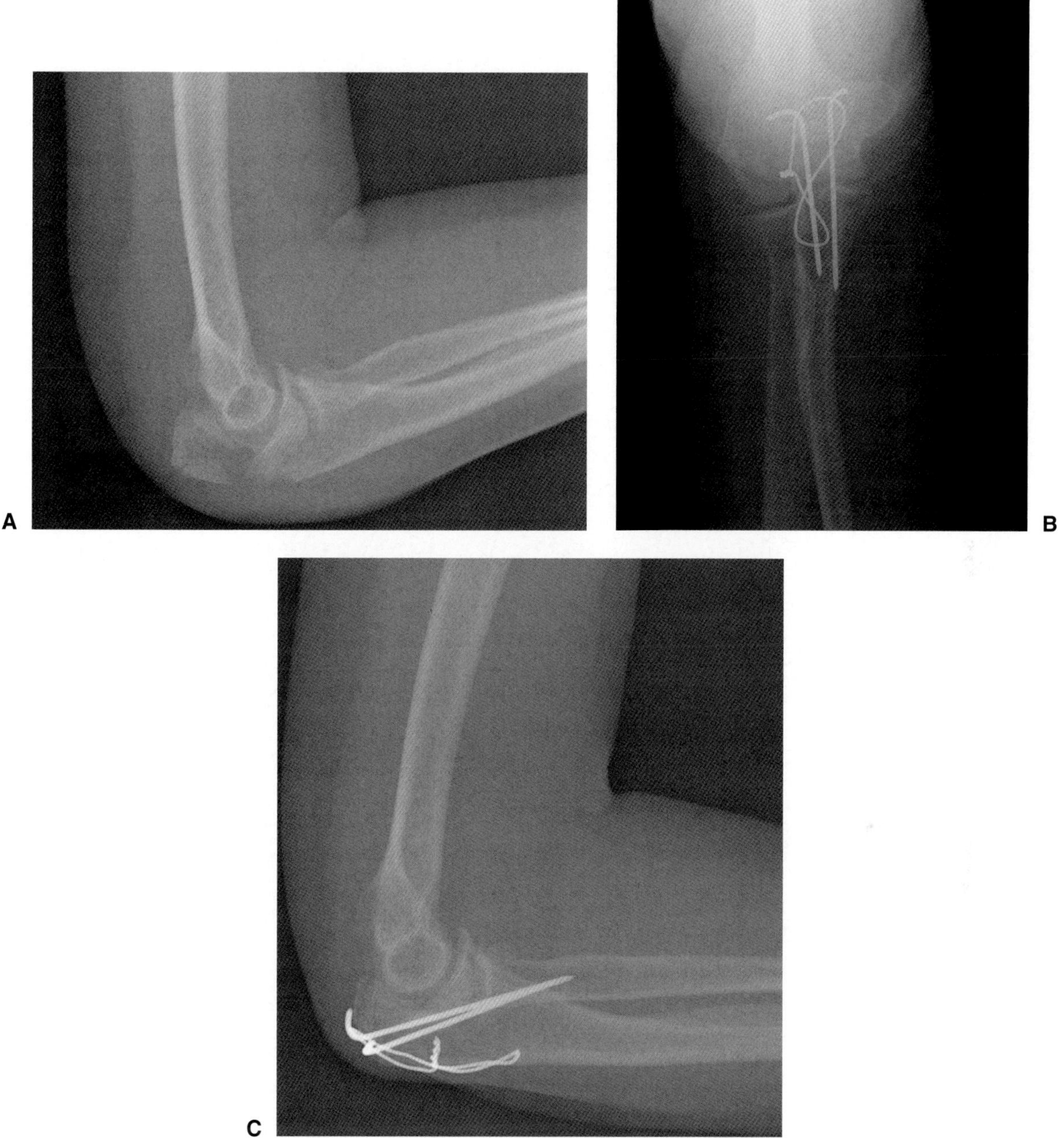


Fig. 11-13 Displaced olecranon fracture with disruption of the triceps fascia. A: Lateral radiograph demonstrating a significantly displaced olecranon fracture. Anteroposterior (AP) (B) and lateral (C) radiographs following reduction with K-wires and tension bands.

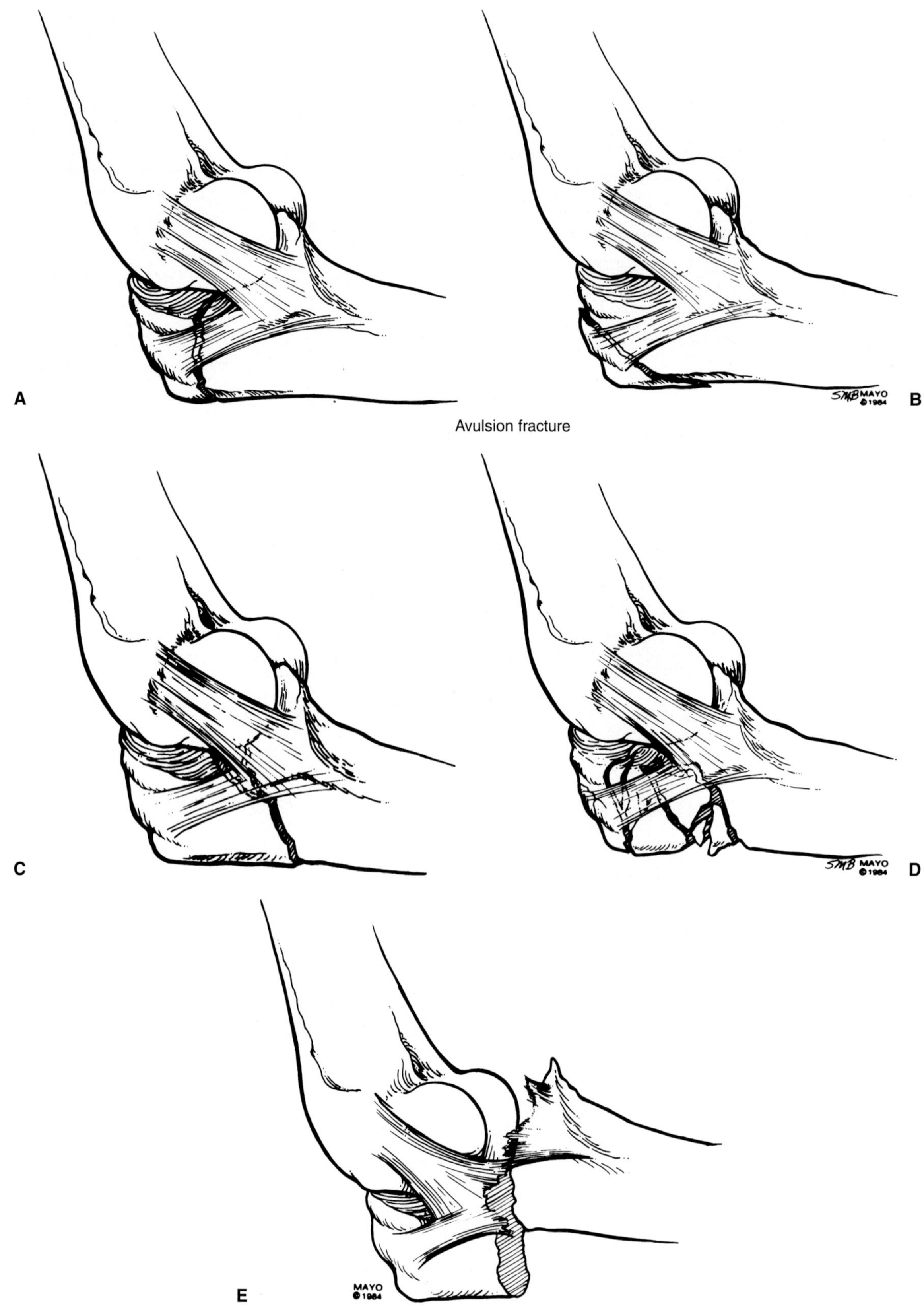


Fig. 11-14 A and B: Avulsion fractures which may (A) or may not (B) involve the joint space. B is a Colton type II injury. C: Transverse or oblique fractures involving the joint space (Colton type III). D: Comminuted fracture involving most of the olecranon process (Colton type IV). E: Ulnar fracture with displaced distal fragment (Colton type V, Mayo type III). (From Morrey BF. *The elbow and its disorders.* Philadelphia: WB Saunders; 1985.)

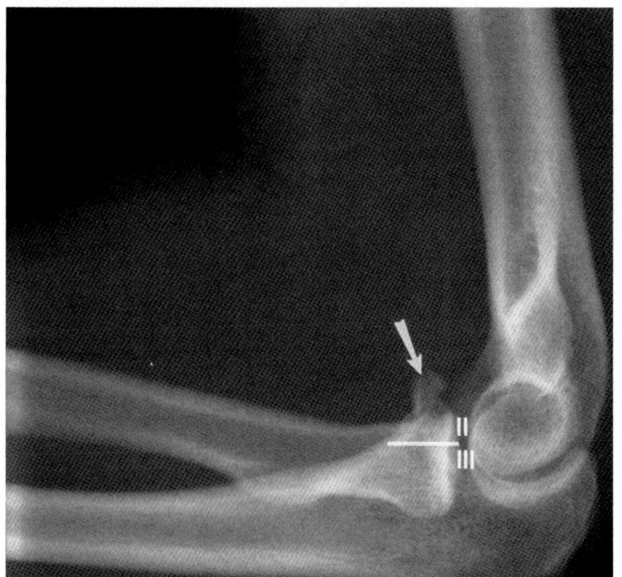


Fig. 11-15 Coronoid fracture classification of Regan and Morrey. Lateral radiograph demonstrating a type I avulsion of the coronoid tip (*arrow*). Type II fractures involve <50% of the coronoid (*white line*) and type III fractures involve >50% of the coronoid.

of the articular surface and type III injuries are comminuted. Simple type I fractures, without associated osseous or soft tissue injuries, are managed conservatively. The joint can be aspirated to decompress the hemarthoris.

Treatment of displaced fractures (type II) is more controversial. If there is good range of motion, the fracture can be treated with immobilization of the elbow and wrist for 2 to 3 weeks before beginning active range of motion. In younger patients, operative intervention should be considered if range of motion is not satisfactory following conservative management. Small lag screws can be placed to stabilize the radial head fragment and articular surface (see Fig. 11-31). If the radial neck is involved, a miniplate and screws can be used for fixation.

Type III comminuted fractures have been most often treated with resection of the radial head. However, in recent years good results have been obtained with open reduction and internal fixation (see Fig. 11-32).

Radial head fractures are associated with elbow dislocations (type IV) in 10% of patients. The elbow should be reduced and radial articular surface fully evaluated on radiographs or CT. Treatment is similar to isolated fractures, except type III fractures are more commonly treated with resection of the radial head. In patients with instability, radial head prostheses should be considered. Currently, titanium implants are more often used due to problems with earlier silicone implants (see Fig. 11-33).

## Suggested Reading

Ikeda M, Sugiyama K, Kang C, et al. Comminuted fractures of the radial head. *J Bone Joint Surg*. 2005;87A:76–84.

Morrey BF. Current concepts in the treatment of fractures of the radial head, the olecranon and coronoid. *J Bone Joint Surg*. 1995;77A:316–327.

### Fractures of the Proximal Ulna and Coronoid

Fracture classifications for the proximal ulna were reviewed in an earlier section. However, they are useful for treatment decisions. Undisplaced fractures (Mayo type I and Colton type I) are

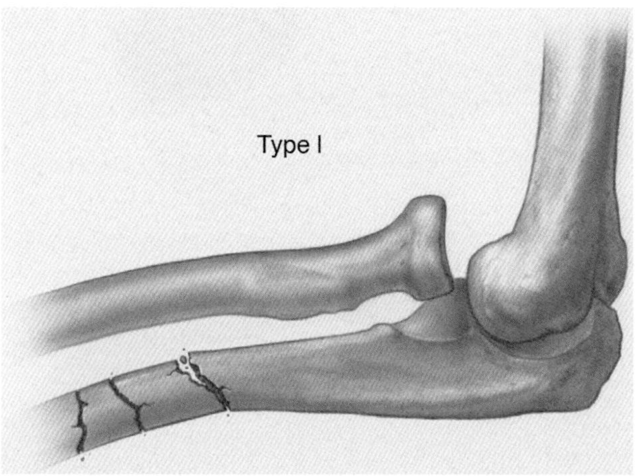


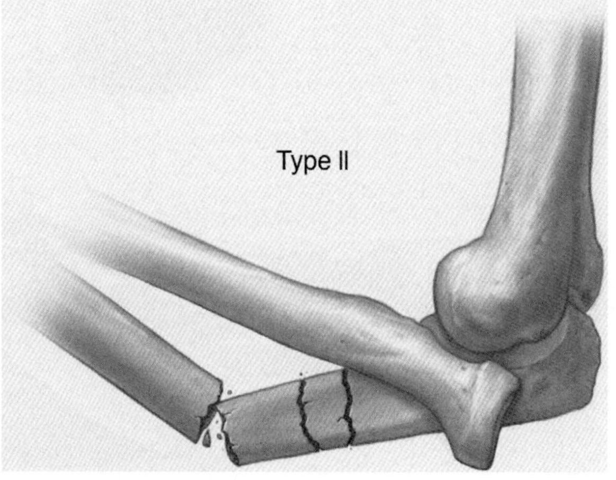


Fig. 11-16 Bado classification of Monteggia fractures. A: Type I—anterior angulation of the ulnar fracture with anterior dislocation of the radial head. B: Type II—posterior angulation of the ulnar fracture and posterior dislocation of the radial head. C: Type III—fracture of the ulnar metaphysic with anterolateral or lateral dislocation of the radial head. D: Type IV—fractures of both the radius and ulna with anterior dislocation of the radial head.

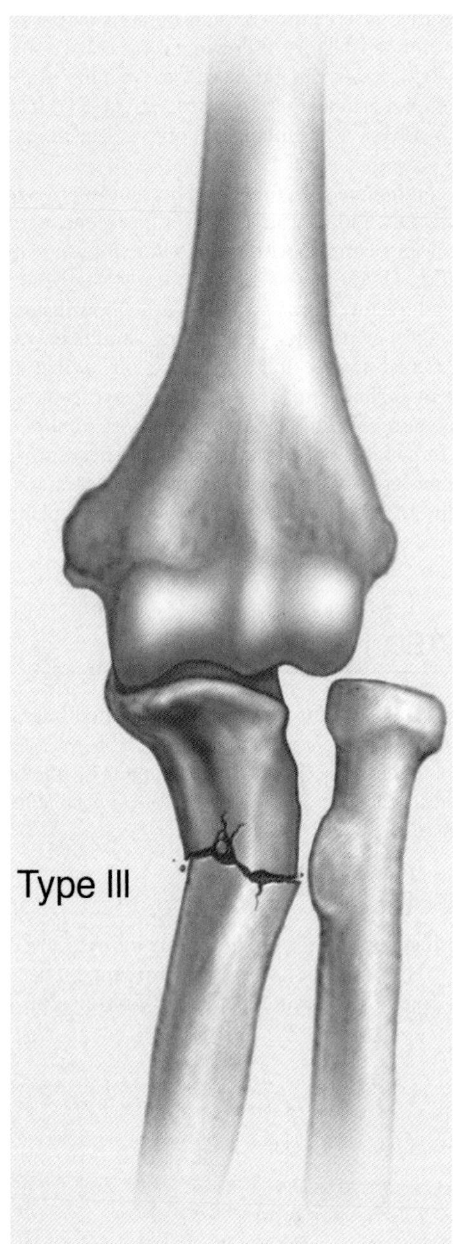


C

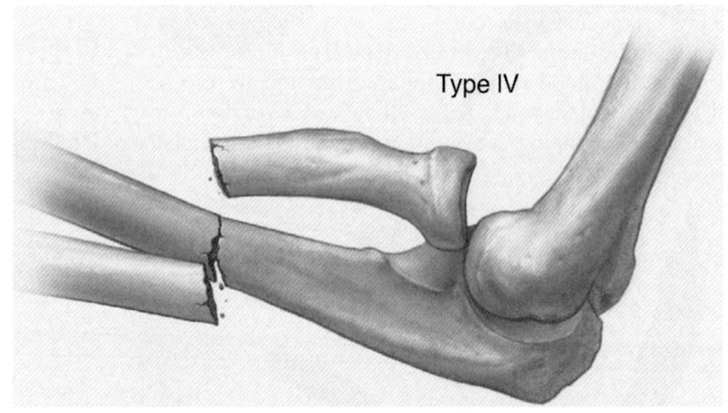


D

Fig. 11-16 *(Continued)*

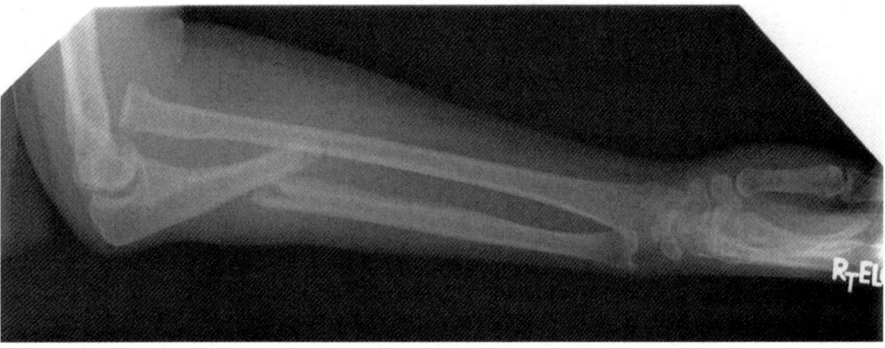


Fig. 11-17 Type I Monteggia fracture. There is an anteriorly angulated ulnar fracture with anterior dislocation of the radial head.

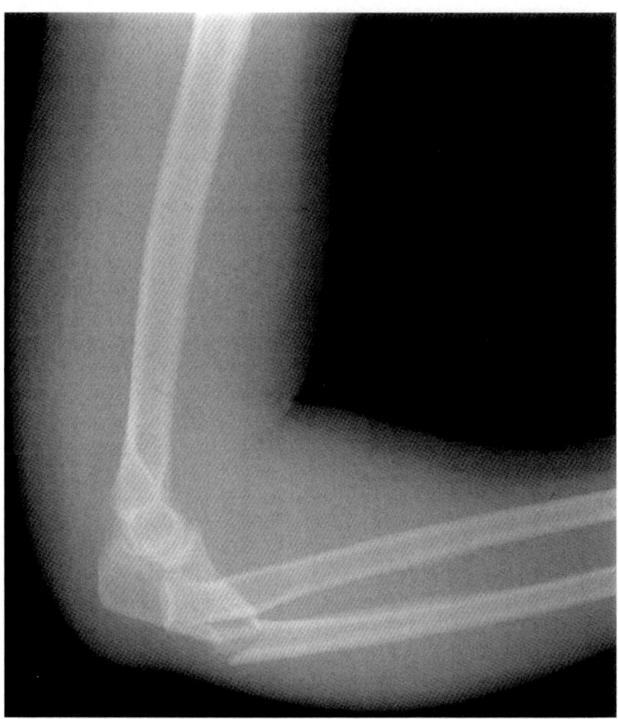

Fig. 11-18 Type II Monteggia fracture. There is a posterior angulation of the ulnar fracture with posterior dislocation of the radial head.

considered in a similar manner, whether simple or comminuted. Displaced fractures (separated by ≥3 mm) that have intact ligaments and no displacement of the distal ulna (Mayo type II) are placed in a different treatment category as are displaced fractures with an unstable distal ulnar fragment (Mayo type III, Colton type V) (Fig. 11-14).

Type I undisplaced fractures can be immobilized for 1 or more weeks with motion as tolerated by the patient (Fig. 11-12A). Stable displaced fractures (Fig. 11-13) are the most common olecranon fracture. These injuries are easily managed with K-wire and tension band fixation. A single cancellous screw can also be used. Cancellous screws are less likely to pull out and do not require removal. Type III fractures have ligament injury and require stabilization with plate and screw fixation (see Fig. 11-34).

Isolated type I and II coronoid fractures (Fig. 11-15) can be treated conservatively. Type III fractures that are not comminuted involve the entire coronoid and should be treated with open reduction and internal fixation. A distraction device is placed externally to reduce forces acting on the coronoid.

## Suggested Reading

Morrey BF. Current concepts in the treatment of fractures of the radial head, the olecranon and coronoid. *J Bone Joint Surg.* 1995;77A:316–327.

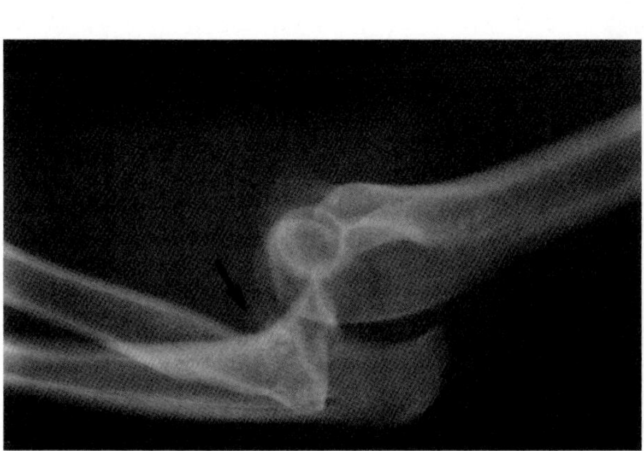



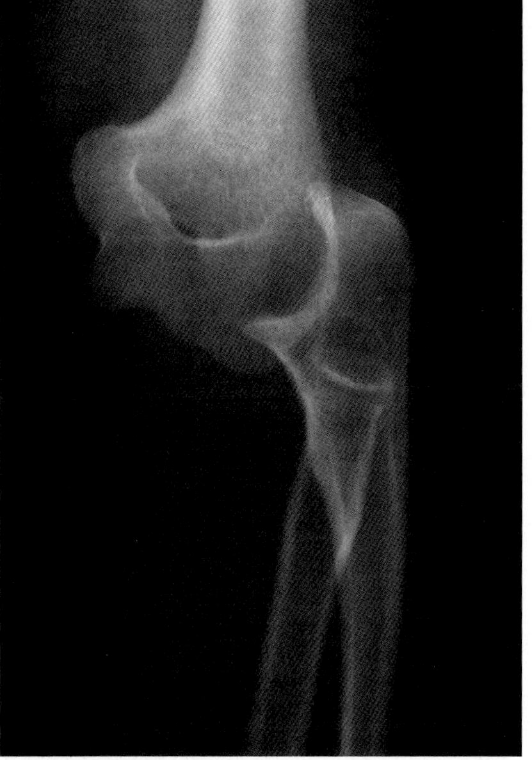



Fig. 11-19 Elbow dislocations. A: Lateral radiograph demonstrating a posterior dislocation with an associated osteochondral fracture of the capitellum (*arrow*). B: Frontal radiograph of a posterolateral dislocation.

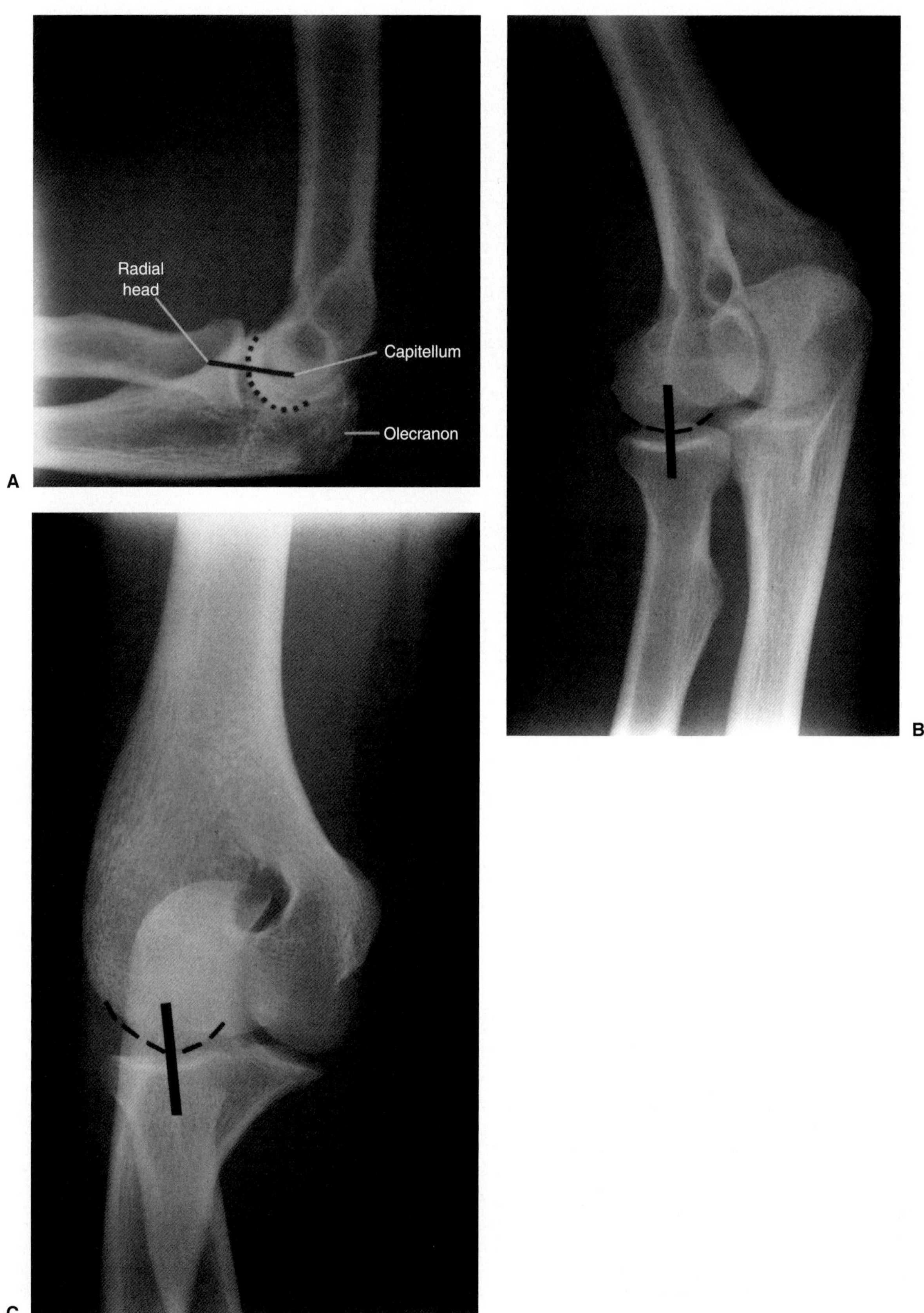


Fig. 11-20 Lateral (A), and oblique (B and C) radiographs demonstrating the alignment of the radial head (*black line*) with the capitellum (*broken lines*) regardless of the projection.

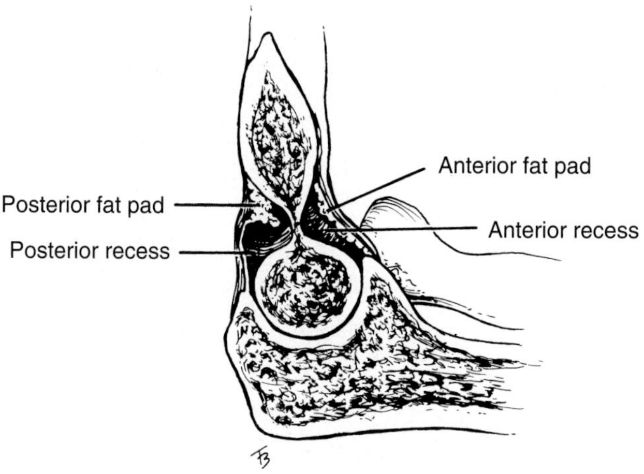


Fig. 11-21 Illustration of the anterior and posterior fat pads and recesses.

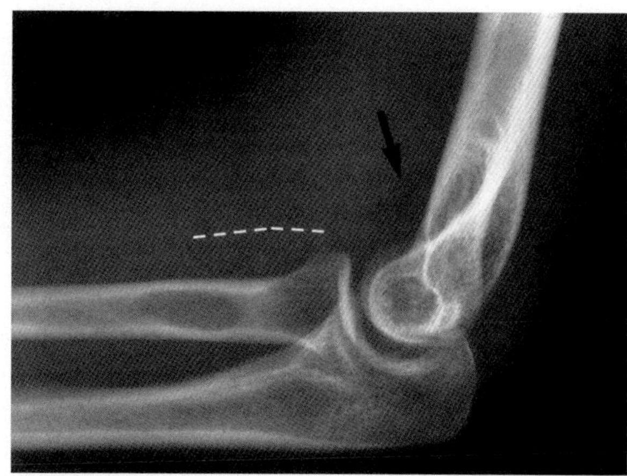

Fig. 11-22 Lateral radiograph in an adult with an occult radial head fracture. Both fat pads are displaced (*arrows*) and the supinator fat stripe (*broken line* demonstrates normal position) is obliterated.

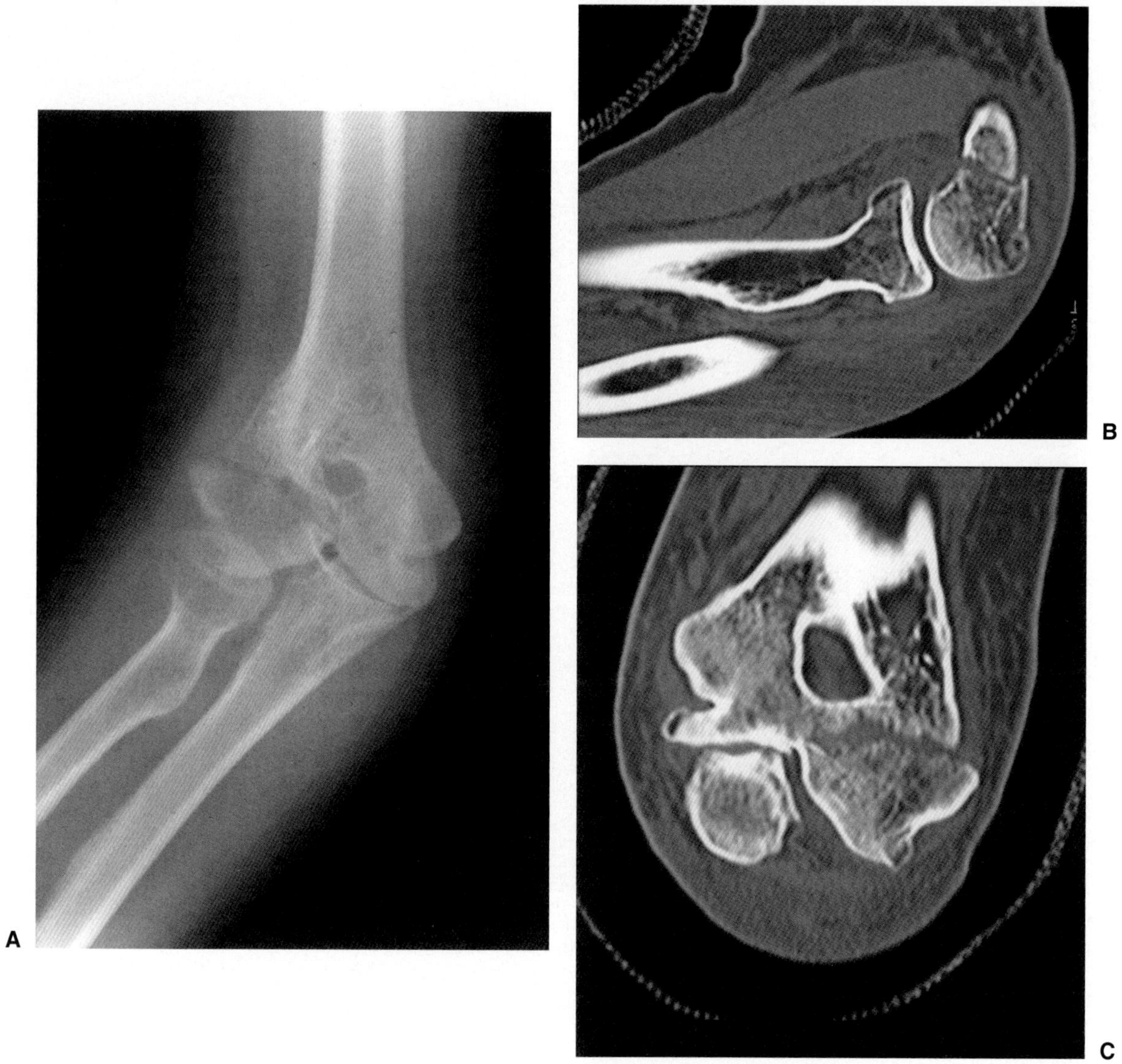

A

B

C

Fig. 11-23 Distal humeral fracture. **A:** AP radiograph of a lateral condylar fracture extending into the trochlear articulation (OTA B1). Sagittal (**B**) and coronal (**C**) reformatted computed tomographic (CT) images better demonstrate the fracture and degree of displacement.

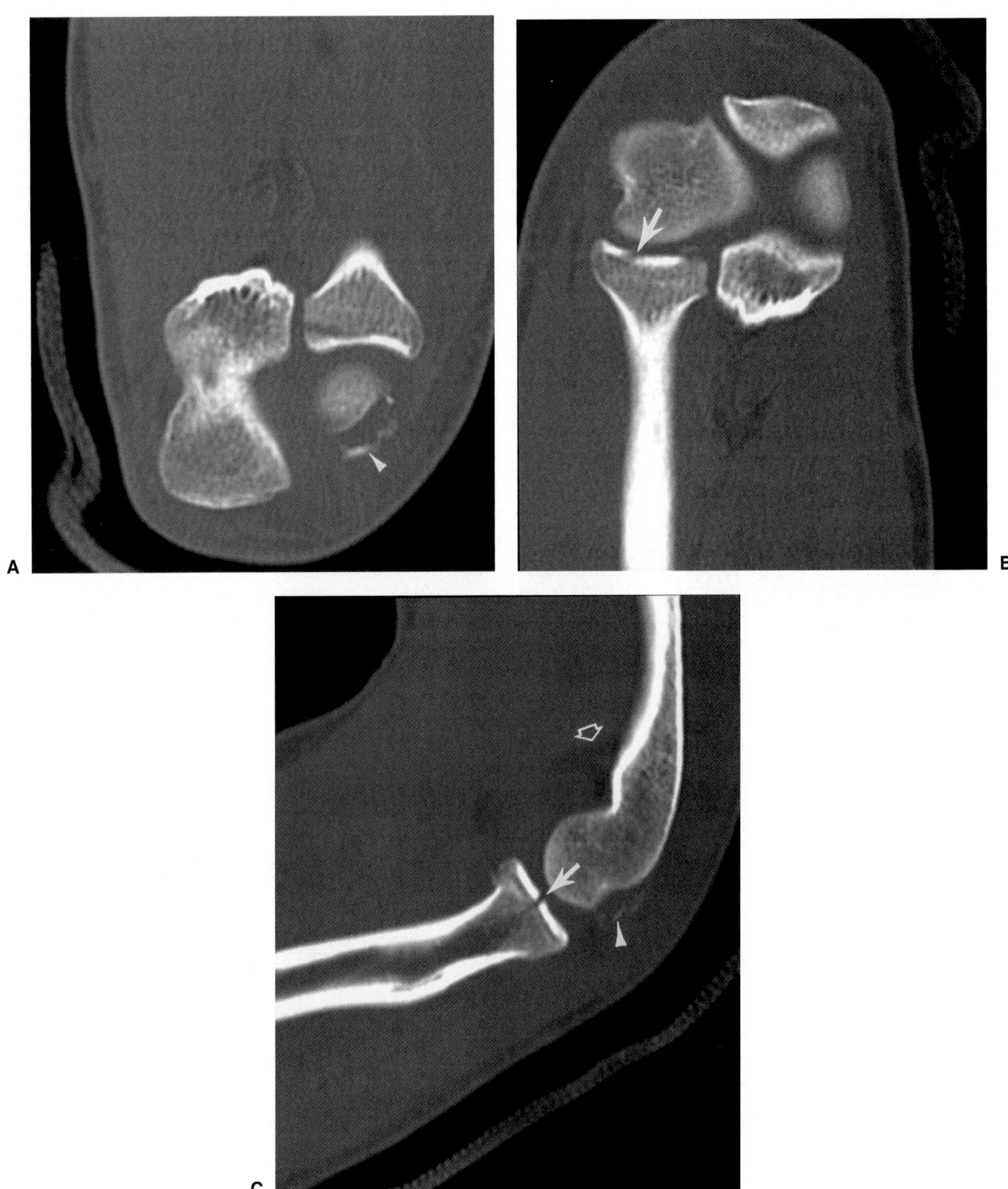


Fig. 11-24 Radial head fracture with capitellar osteochondral fragments. Axial (A), coronal (B) and sagittal (C) computed tomographic (CT) images demonstrate the radial head fracture (*arrow*) with multiple small capitellar fragments (*arrowhead*) and a displaced compressed anterior fat pad (*open arrow*).

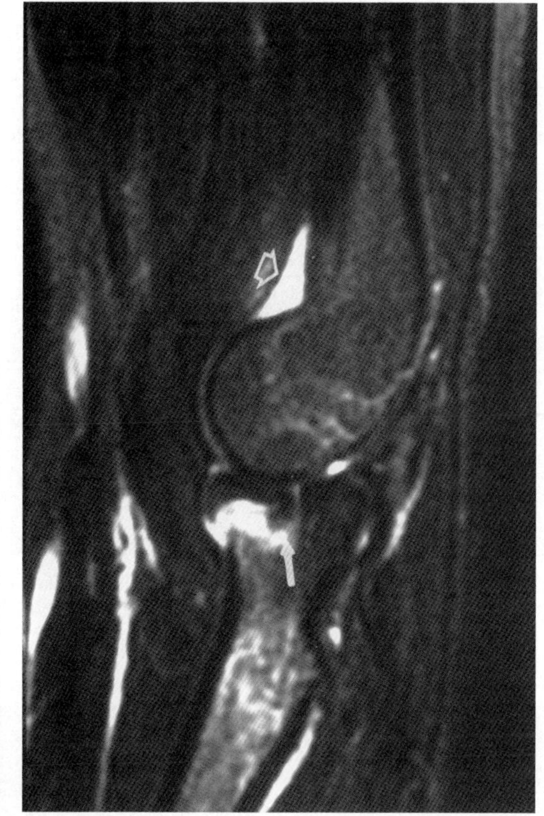
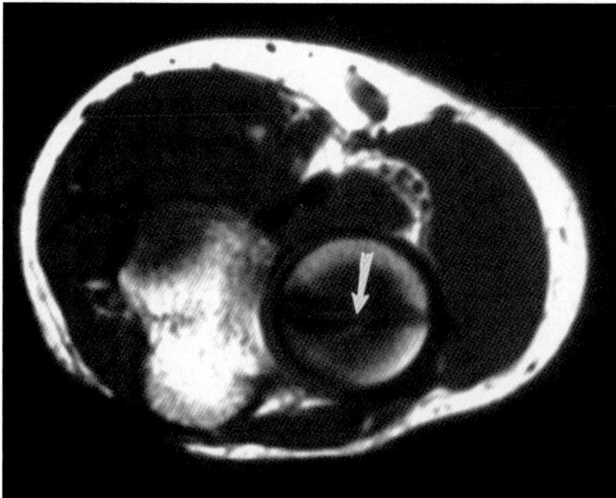

Fig. 11-25 Subtle fracture of the radial head. Axial T1- (A) and sagittal T2-weighted (B) images demonstrate a undisplaced radial head fracture (*arrow*) with displaced anterior fat pad (*open arrow*).

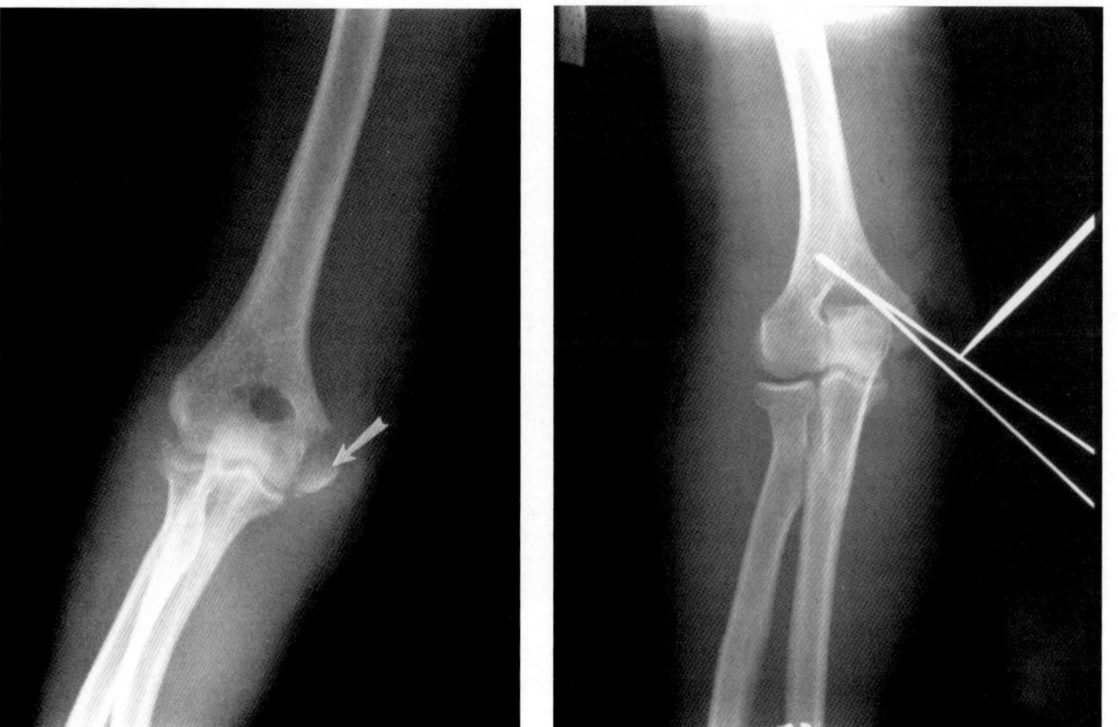

Fig. 11-26 Extra-articular displaced fracture of the medial epicondyle. A: Anteroposterior (AP) radiograph demonstrating a displaced medial epicondyle (*arrow*). B: Operative image during K-wire fixation with the fragment in excellent position.

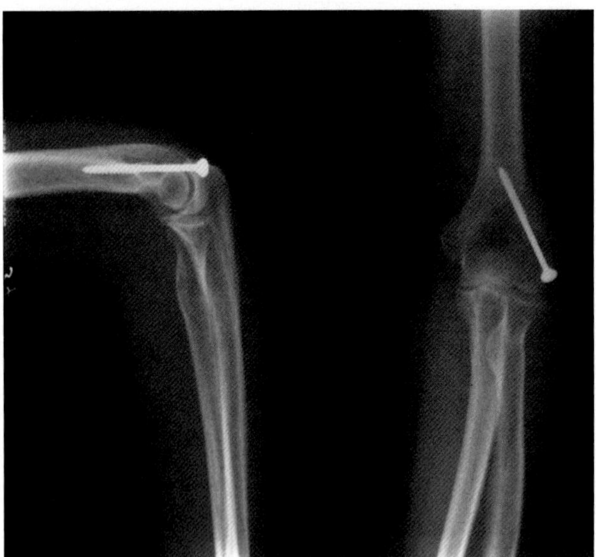

Fig. 11-27 Anteroposterior (AP) and lateral radiographs demonstrating a healed lateral unicondylar fracture (OTA type B1) treated with a single lag screw.

Morrey BF. Instructional course lectures. Complex instability of the elbow. *J Bone Joint Surg*. 1997;79A:460–469.

### Monteggia Fractures

Monteggia fractures (Figs. 11-17 and 11-18) can be treated with reduction of the radial head and, in most cases, internal fixation of the ulnar fracture with a dynamic compression plate or low contact compression plate (see Fig. 11-35). When there is an associated coronoid fracture, this can be addressed conservatively or with internal fixation if a large noncomminuted fragment is present. When ulnar fractures are more distal, an intramedullary nail is also an option for fixation.

## Imaging of Fracture Complications

Complications may be related to the initial injury or surgical intervention. Baseline radiographs or CT are important to provide guidance should complications occur following reduction

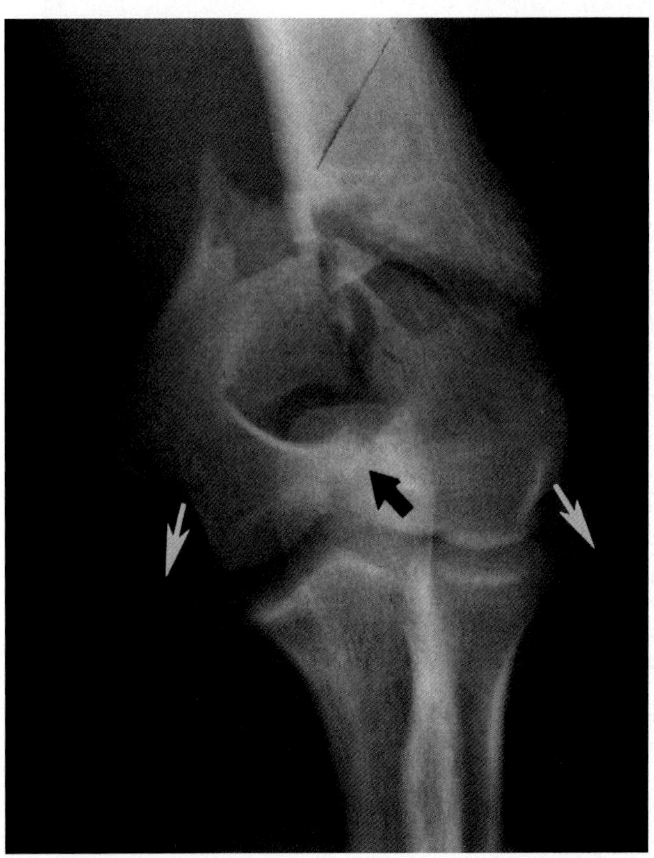

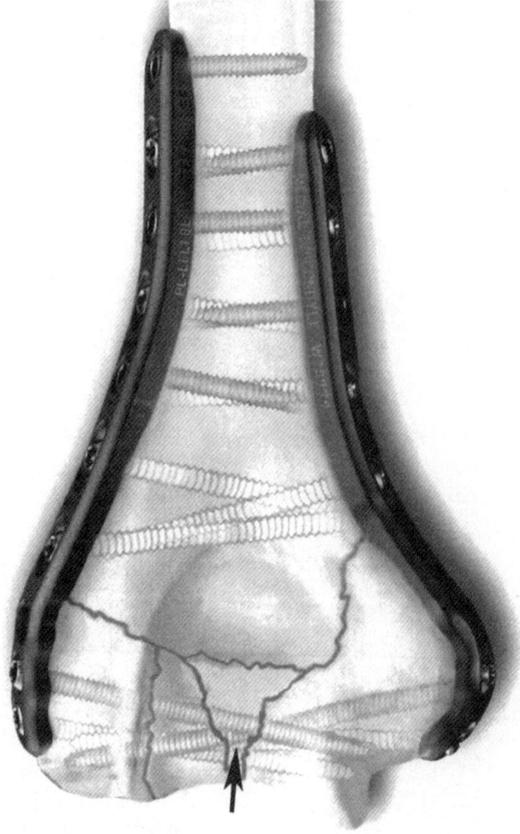

Fig. 11-28 Complete articular (OTA type C1) fracture. A: Anteroposterior (AP) radiograph demonstrates a T-type fracture entering the trochlea (*black arrow*). Muscle forces (*white arrows*) act to displace the fragments. This requires reconstruction of the medial and lateral columns and the articular surface. B: Illustration of Acumed Tap-Loc parallel plates that are precontured for the distal humerus and allow flexible angulation of the screws to secure the columns and articular surface (*arrow*). Threads in the plate for the locking screws can be created at the time of surgery. (Courtesy of Acumed, Hillsboro, Oregon.)

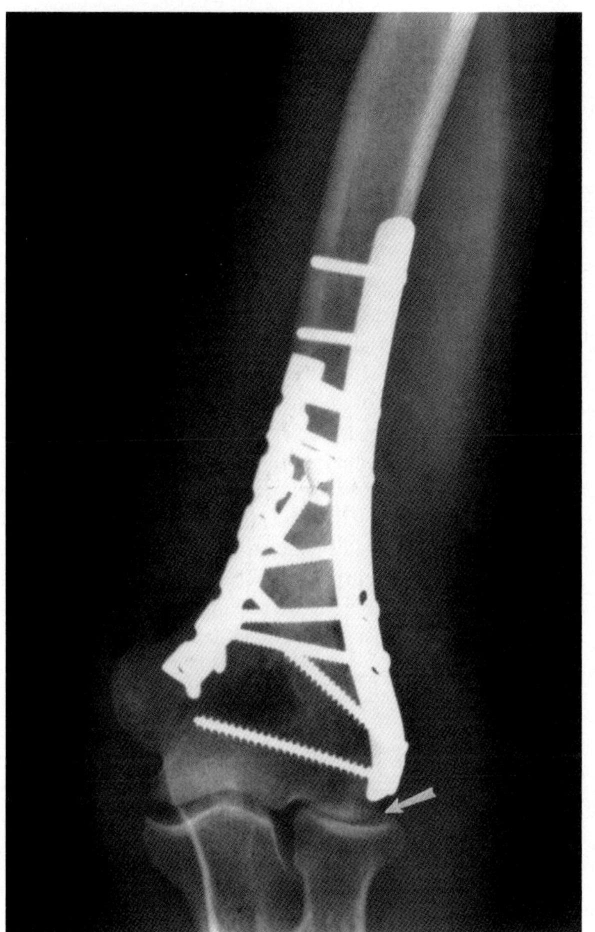


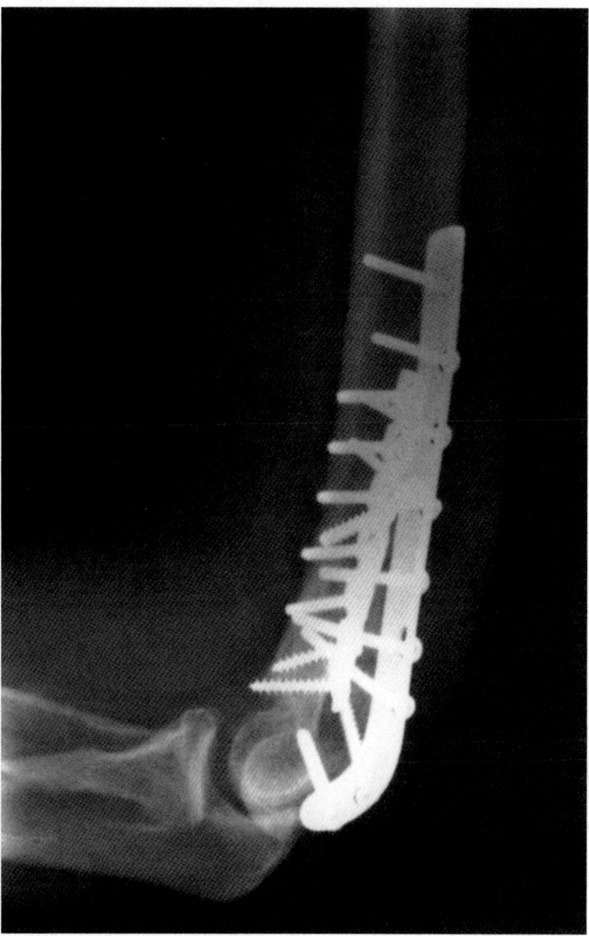


**Fig. 11-29** Medial and lateral plate and screw fixation. Anteroposterior (AP) (**A**) and lateral (**B**) radiographs demonstrate a healed complete articular fracture with notched reconstruction plate fixation of the medial column and a preshaped plate and screws for the lateral column. There is a transverse screw in the distal lateral plate for articular stabilization. Note the arthritic changes in the radiocapitellar articulation (*arrow*).

of elbow fracture/dislocations. In children with distal humeral fractures, the baseline position of the anterior humeral line and the Bauman angle should be noted and used in follow-up on serial radiographs (see Fig. 11-36).

## Soft Tissue Injuries

Soft tissue injuries may involve the ligaments and supporting structures, neurovascular structures, or be related to compartment syndrome. Neural injuries occur in 5% to 19% of elbow fracture/dislocations. The ulnar nerve and posterior interrosseous nerve are most commonly involved. The ulnar nerve may be injured with the initial injury, related to surgical procedures or related to compressive neuropathy following the surgery or trauma. Ulnar nerve injuries are most common following distal humeral fractures (12.3%) and olecranon fractures (6%) and occur in 10% of elbow dislocations.

The ulnar nerve passes through the arcade of Struthers which is 3 to 4 cm in length and 3 to 10 cm proximal to the medial epicondyle. The nerve then passes through the cubital tunnel before entering the forearm beneath the ulnar and humeral heads of the flexor carpi ulnaris (see Fig. 11-37). Injury may occur at any location. Postoperative nerve injury is usually related to traction neuropathy. Postoperative neuropathy may be related to scarring, adjacent implants, callus, or osteophytes (see Fig. 11-38) from posttraumatic arthrosis. Most neuropathies resolve over time, but chronic progressive changes may also occur. Ulnar nerve injuries are graded by McGowan as grade 1 to 3. Grade 1 represents an injury with no motor weakness, grade 2 neuropathies present with sensory loss and interrosseous muscle weakness in the hand, and grade 3 injuries have advanced motor weakness.

Other neural injuries may also occur. Radial and median nerve injuries may be related to fracture fragments or stretching. Both ulnar (3%) and posterior interrosseous (5%) nerve injuries have been noted in association with Monteggia fractures. In children the incidence is higher (8% to 17%). Regardless of the neuropathy the diagnosis is usually based on clinical and nerve conduction studies. MRI is useful if there is no significant adjacent metal fixation. Metal artifact may degrade images reducing the ability to follow the neural structures.

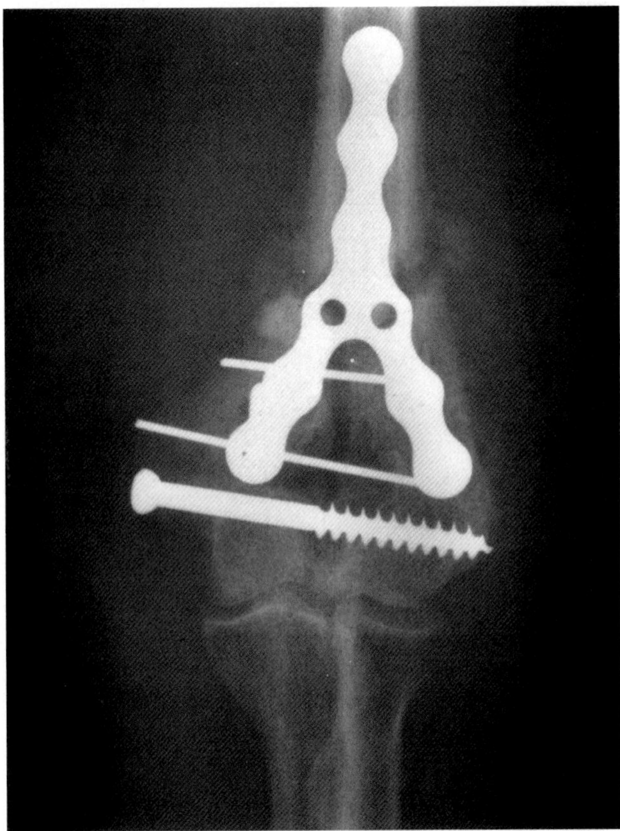

Fig. 11-30 Complete articular Y fracture of the distal humerus. There is a Y plate for fixation with two medial column K-wires and a distal cancellous screw for articular stabilization.

Vascular injuries include intimal tears, thrombosis, and lacerations. Angiography may be required for complete evaluation.

Ligament and soft tissue injuries can be evaluated clinically. Imaging studies include stress views (see Fig. 11-39), conventional, CT, or magnetic resonance (MR) arthrography. The last (see Fig. 11-40) is most useful in patients with prior fractures or dislocations treated with closed reduction.

### Osseous Complications

The more complex the fracture the more difficult the management, resulting in arthrosis in up to 85% of patients with OTA type C complete articular fractures of the distal humerus. Malunion and nonunion may also occur. Delayed union or nonunion is reported in 2% to 10% (see Fig. 11-41). Changes may be evident on serial radiographs. However, CT with reformatting is most useful, especially in the presence of fixation hardware. MRI is useful for evaluation of the physis and fracture healing in children.

Problems with hardware are common due to the superficial nature of the instrumentation, especially in patients with ulnar fixation. Hardware removal may be required in up to 58% of patients due to tissue irritation, nerve compression, or reduced forearm supination and pronation. Reduced motion may be related to wire or screw penetration of the ulna or radius and extending into the interosseous membrane or adjacent osseous structure. Changes may be evident on radiographs. However, CT is most useful to evaluate the exact position of screws and K-wires.

Infections occur in up to 7% of patients. Most are due to wound infection. However, deep infection is more problematic to diagnose and manage. Combined radionuclide studies or joint aspiration can be performed. Multiple approaches have been used including three-phase bone scans with technetium Tc 99m methylene-diphosphonate (MDP), technetium-labeled white blood cells, antigranulocyte antibody–labeledtechnetium, indium In 111–labeled white blood cells, and more recently, F-18 fluorodeoxyglucose positron emission tomographic (PET) imaging. Technetium-labeled white blood cells disassociate at a rate of 5% to 7% per hour following injection. This results in significant unwanted background activity. PET studies report sensitivities of 92% and specificities in the 97% range (Fig. 4-80). Indium In 111–labeled white blood cells remain the gold standard in the author's practice. Sensitivity ranges from 84% to 96% with specificity exceeding 96%.

MRI with constrast is also useful depending upon the extent of fixation hardware.

## Suggested Reading

Beaty JH, Kasser JR. The elbow region: general concepts in the pediatric patient. In: Kasser JR, Beaty JH, eds. *Rockwood and Wilkins' fractures in children*. 5th ed. Philadelphia: Lippincott Williams & Wilkins; 2001.

Helfet DL, Lloen P, Anand N, et al. Open reduction and internal fixation of delayed unions and nonunions of fractures of the distal part of the humerus. *J Bone Joint Surg*. 2003;85A:33–40.

Konrad GG, Kundel K, Oberst M, et al. Monteggia fractures in adults: Long-term results and prognostic factors. *J Bone Joint Surg*. 2007;89B:354–360.

Matthews F, Trentz O, Jacob AL, et al. Protrusion of hardware impairs forearm rotation after olecranon fixation. *J Bone Joint Surg*. 2007;89A:638–642.

Shin R, Ring D. The ulnar nerve in elbow trauma. *J Bone Joint Surg*. 2007;89A:1108–1116.

# Elbow Arthroplasty

Elbow replacement procedures have evolved over the years with continued improvement in implants and surgical techniques. Resection and interposition arthroplasties were preformed in the late 1800s primarily for tuberculosis. In the late 1940s, hinged implants were beginning to appear. Metal-hinged implants designed to be placed using cement were developed in the 1970s. Presently, multiple-hinged or constrained systems, linked semiconstrained, and unlinked or resurfacing implants are available. Alternative procedures, such as resection arthroplasy

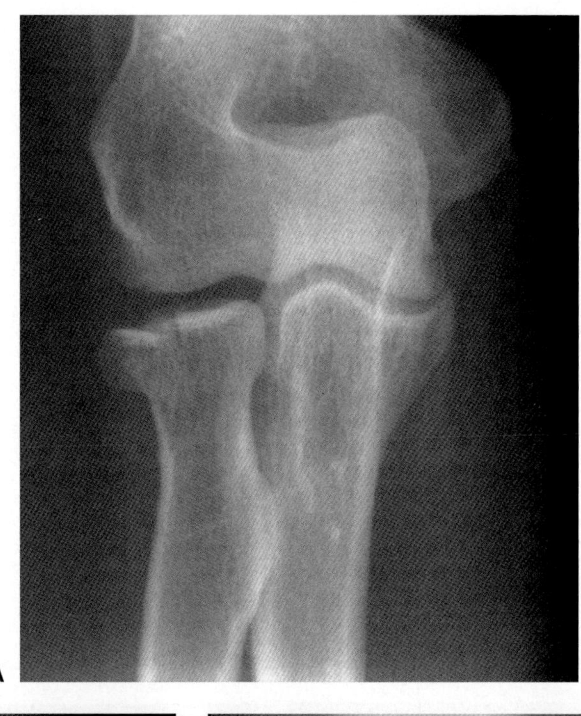

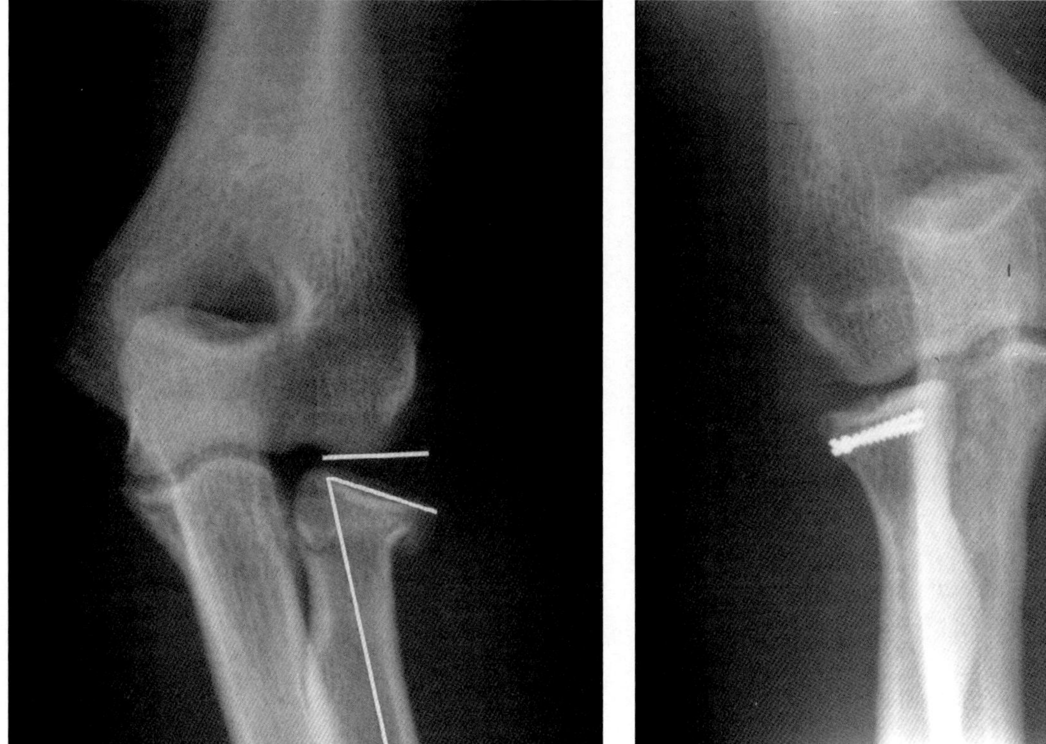

Fig. 11-31 Radiographs of displaced (Mason type II) fractures of the radial head (A) and neck (B). The radial head fracture (A) involves >30% of the articular surface and is displaced with an articular step-off. The radial neck fracture (B) is impacted and angulated with an incongruent articular surface (*lines*). C: The radial head can be internally fixed with miniscrews.

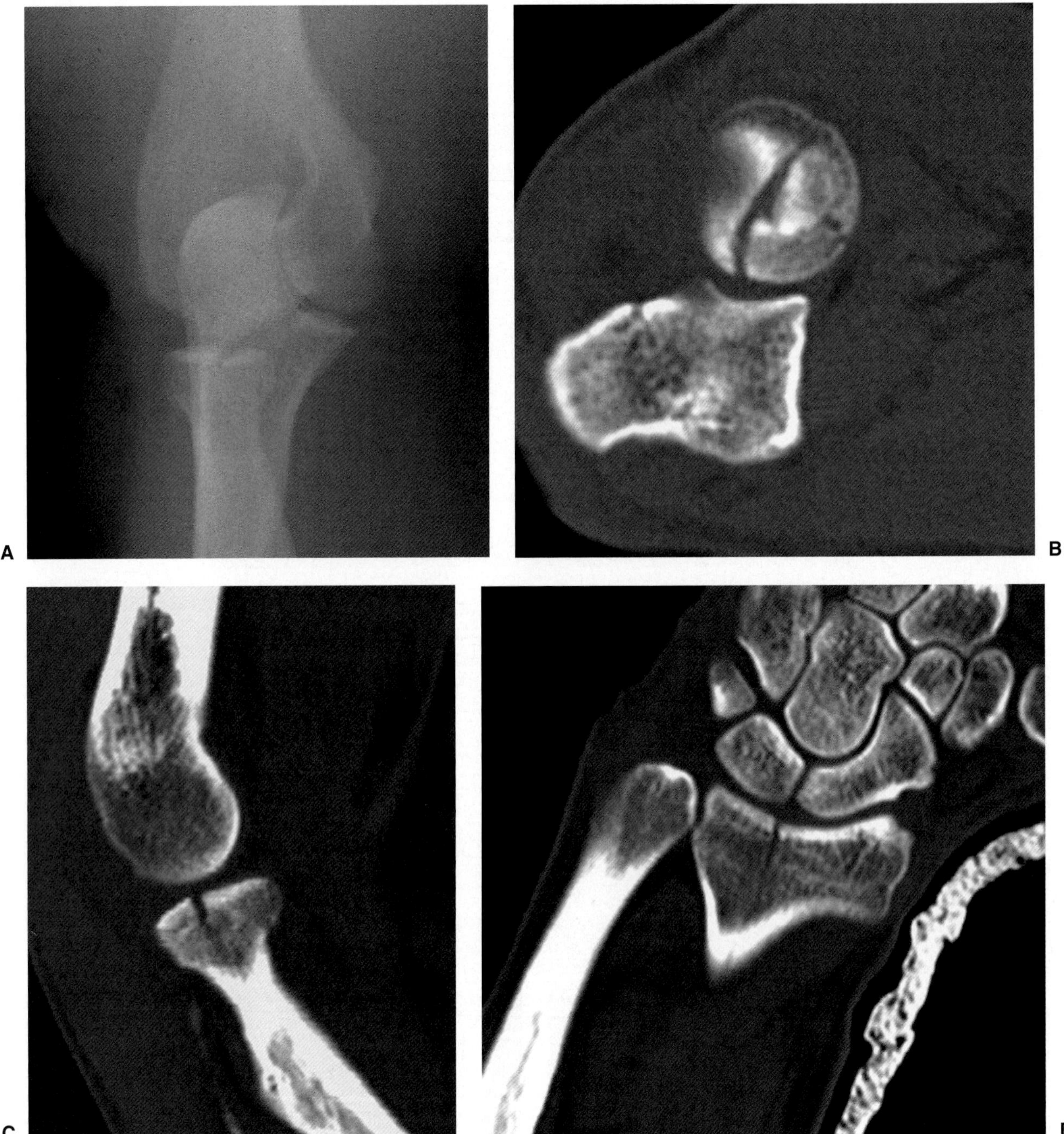


Fig. 11-32 A: Oblique radiograph demonstrates a radial head fracture with articular step-off. Axial (B) and sagittal (C) computed tomogaphic (CT) images demonstrate comminution of the radial head (Mason type III). The patient also complained of wrist pain. Coronal CT (D) demonstrates a longitudinal intra-articular fracture of the distal radius. In this case, the radial head fracture was treated with open reduction and internal fixation with miniscrews (E and F).

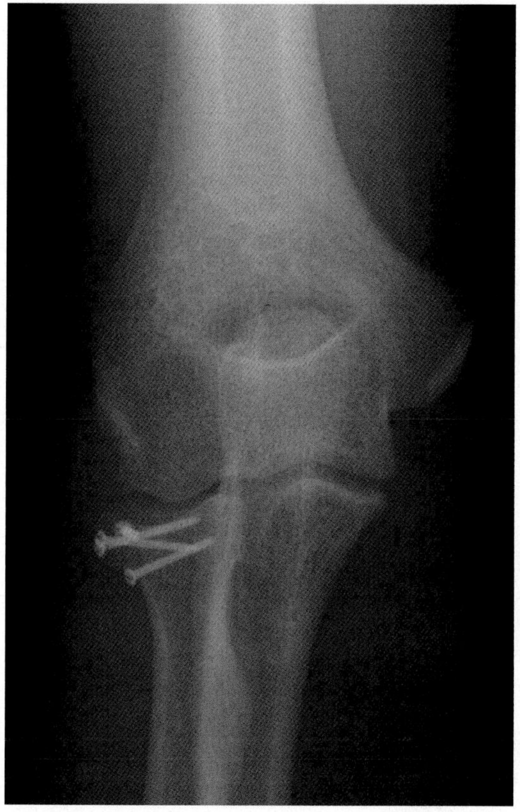


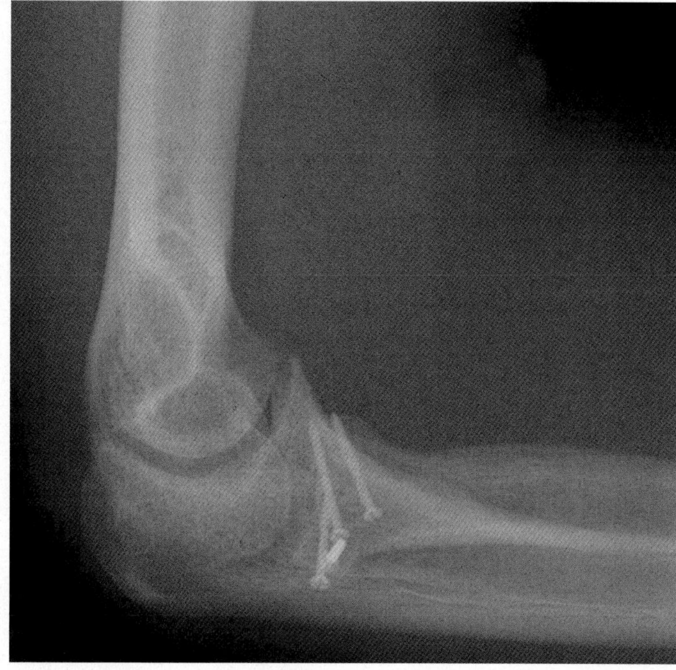


Fig. 11-32 *(Continued)*

and arthrodesis, are uncommonly performed now if elbow replacement arthroplasty can be performed.

The choice of implant and patient selection are based on clinical features (age, activity levels, associated comorbidities, neurologic function, and patient expectations) and image features. The degree of pain and function loss are major considerations.

## Suggested Reading

Coonrad RW. History of elbow arthroplasty. In: Inglis AE, ed. *American academy of orthopaedic surgery total joint replacement in the upper extremity*. St. Louis: Mosby; 1980:75–90.

Morrey BF, Adams RA. Semiconstrained arthroplasty for treatment of rheumatoid arthritis of the elbow. *J Bone Joint Surg*. 1992;74A:479–490.

Morrey BF, Bryan RS, Dobyns HJ, et al. Total elbow arthroplasty. *J Bone Joint Surg*. 1981;63A:1050–1063.

### Patient Selection

Elbow arthroplasty is considered when more conservative measures or prior surgery have been ineffective. The goals of elbow replacement surgery are to relieve pain, improve stability, and mobility. An arc of 30 to 130 degrees of motion will provide the necessary function. The primary indications for elbow arthroplasty are osteoarthritis, rheumatoid arthritis, and posttraumatic arthritis. Primary elbow arthroplasty can also be used in older patients with complex elbow fractures, specifically complete articular distal humeral fractures, and fracture nonunion. Contraindications include active infection, prior arthrodesis and paralysis, or neurologic function loss in the involved extremity. Patient age and compliance are important factors. In general, primary elbow replacement is reserved for older patients and interposition arthroplasty for younger patients.

Multiple clinical scoring systems have been used over the years to evaluate patients with elbow disorders. These clinical systems are useful for treatment decision making and posttreatment follow-up. Scoring systems include the Mayo Elbow Performance Index (MEPI), the disabilities of the arm, shoulder, and hand (DASH, Broberg and Morrey rating system), American shoulder and elbow surgeons (ASES), elbow evaluation instrument, and a general health status questionnaire (Short Form 36). At the author's institution, elbow surgeons prefer the MEPI or DASH systems. The Mayo system is one of the most commonly used nationwide. The index has a total score of 100 points (pain 45, ulnohumeral motion 20, stability 10, the ability to perform five different functional tasks 25). For example, a patient with no pain receives 45 points, moderate pain 15 points, and severe pain 0 points. The DASH

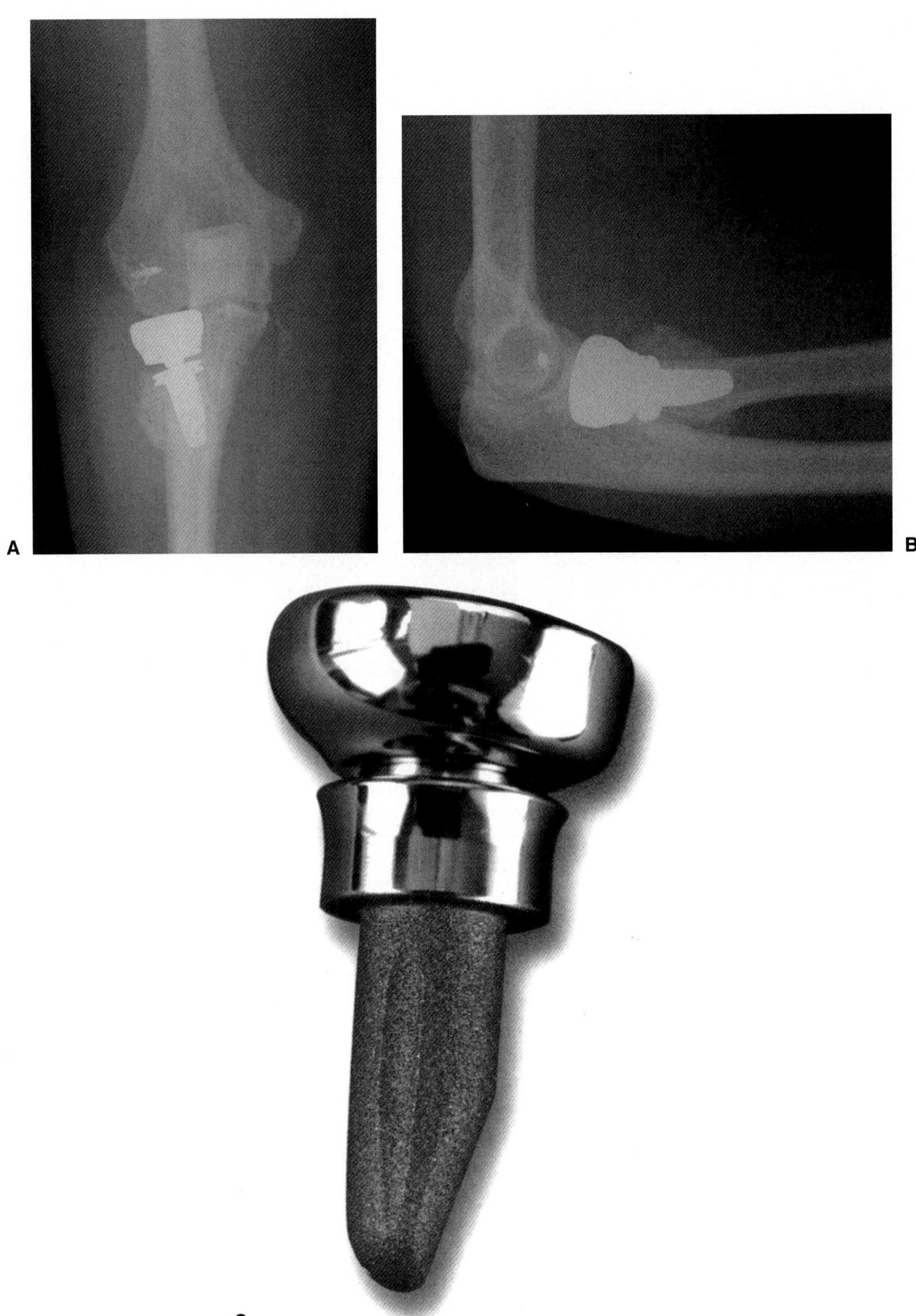


Fig. 11-33 Radial head fracture with associated instability. Anteroposterior (AP) (A) and lateral (B) radiographs demonstrate a radial head implant with proximal bone grafting. There is also a soft tissue anchor in the lateral epicondyle for associated ligament repair. C: Photograph on an Acumed Anatomic Radial Head System designed by Dr. Shawn O'Driscoll (Courtesy of Acumed, Hillsboro, Oregon).

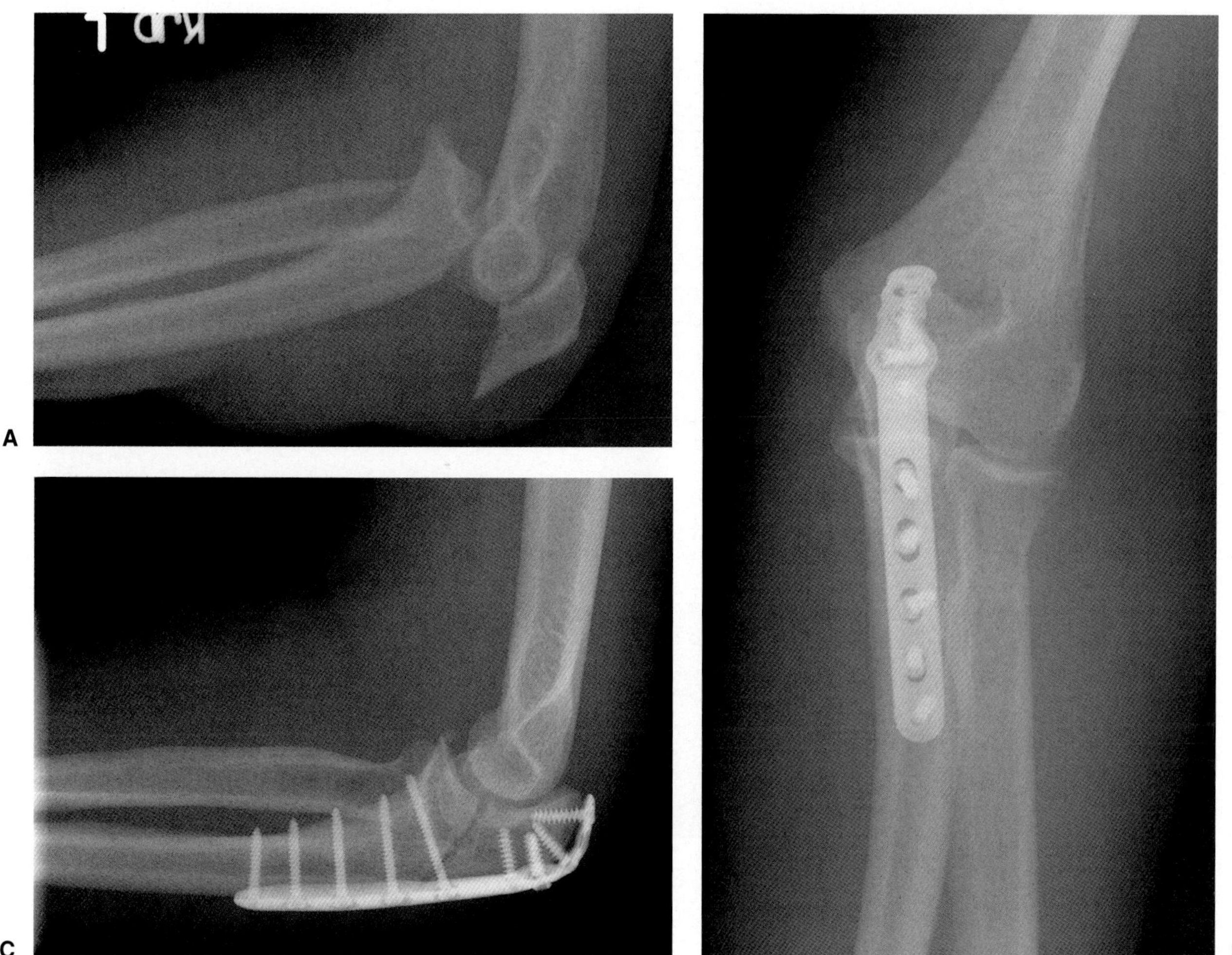

Fig. 11-34 A: Lateral radiograph demonstrating a displaced olecranon fracture with anterior displacement of the distal ulna and dislocation of the radial head. Anteroposterior (AP) (B) and lateral (C) radiographs following plate and screw fixation and reduction of the dislocation.

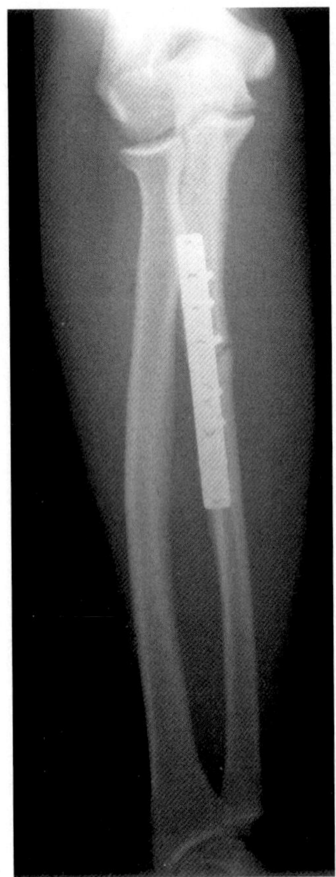

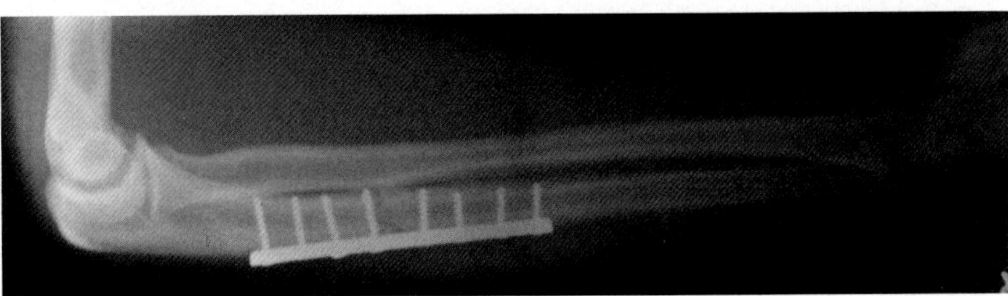

A B

Fig. 11-35 Anteroposterior (AP) (A) and lateral (B) radiographs following reduction of a Monteggia fracture. The radial head dislocation has been reduced and the ulnar fracture stabilized with a 3.5-mm dynamic compression plate and screws. Note there are four screws proximal and distal to the fracture.

system is a questionnaire containing 30 items. Twenty-one items evaluate difficulty performing certain tasks, five evaluate symptoms, and there are separate questions for social, work, sleep, and confidence issues. Scores range from 0 to 100 with higher numbers for poorer upper extremity function.

Preoperative imaging should include, at a minimum, AP and lateral radiographs of the elbow to include sufficient humerus and forearm for evaluation of bone deformities, marrow, and cortex in the region of the desired components. More of the humerus and forearm may need to be imaged in patients with prior surgery or trauma. Also, in this setting, the opposite extremity may need to be imaged for comparison purposes (length, angular deformity, etc.).

Additional studies including stress views for instability, CT for bone stock, and MRI for soft tissue abnormalities may also be required.

## Suggested Reading

Berquist TH, Trigg AD. The elbow. In: Berquist TH, ed. *Imaging atlas of orthopaedic appliances and prostheses*. New York: Raven Press; 1995:751–816.

Doornberg JN, Ring D, Fabian LM, et al. Pain dominates measurments of elbow function and health status. *J Bone Joint Surg*. 2005;87A:1725–1731.

Turchin DC, Beaton DE, Richards RR. Validity of observer-based aggregate scoring systems as descriptor for elbow pain, function and disability. *J Bone Joint Surg*. 1998;80A: 154–162.

## Component Selection

There are numerous elbow implants available. Selection depends upon the imaging and clinical evaluation, the implants that best meet the patient's situation and surgical experience and preference. The most important clinical features are the degree of pain, instability, and range of motion. Most systems relieve pain. Fully constrained hinged components are rarely used now due to the high incidence of loosening (see Fig. 11-42). Up to 42% demonstrate loosening in <2 years. Custom-designed fully constrained implants are used for limb-saving procedures with osseous neoplasms.

Resurfacing implants are designed to reproduce the anatomy of the normal sigmoid notch and condylar surface. Original designs were stemless, but currently most have humeral and ulnar stems of varing length. Resurfacing implants provide less

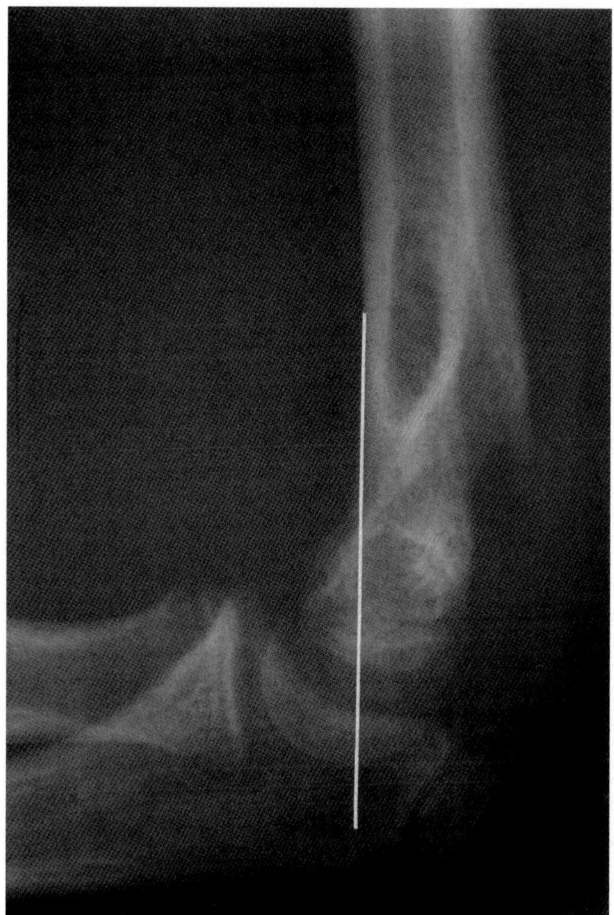
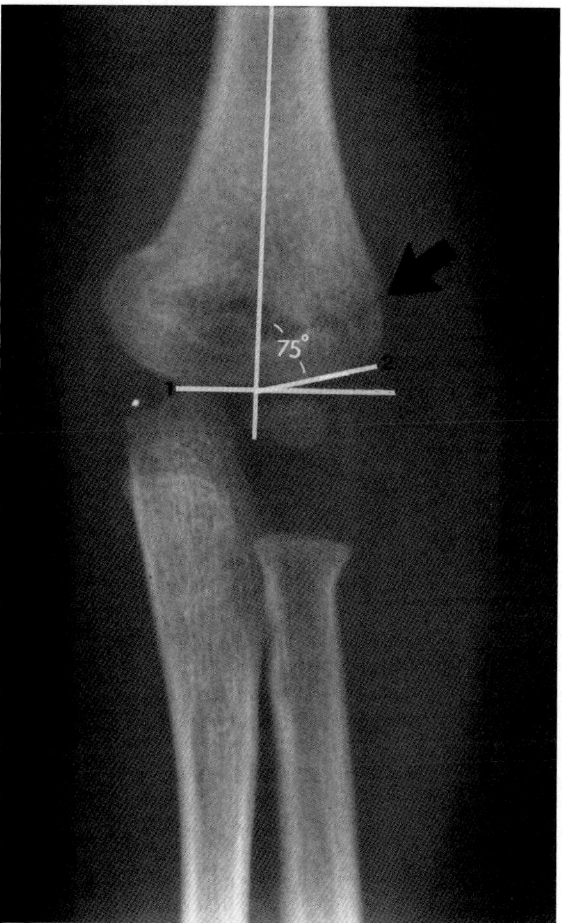


A B

Fig. 11-36 A: Lateral radiograph following a lateral condylar fracture. The anterior humeral line passes through the mid capitellum (normal middle third of the capitellum). B: Anteroposterior (AP) radiograph demonstrating Bauman's angle. The angle is formed by a line perpendicular to the humeral axis (1) and a second line along the lateral metaphysis (normal 70 to 75 degrees; both the normal and injured side should be evaluated for comparison).

stability in patients with preexisting instability (see Figs. 11-43 and 11-44).

Semiconstrained implants are commonly used and these designs were the result of unacceptably high failure rates for constrained implants. Also, resurfacing implants may not be useful in patients with bone loss and/or lack of adequate soft tissue support. Semiconstrained implants not only provide more stability but also sufficient axial and varus valgus motion to reduce problems with loosening. The most commonly used semiconstrained system at the author's institution is the Coonrad-Morrey prosthesis (see Fig. 11-45).

As noted in the preceding text (Fig. 11-32), radial head replacement can also be accomplished in patients with complex radial head fractures and instability.

## SUGGESTED READING

Ikavalko M, Lehto MUK, Repo A, et al. Souter-Strathclyde elbow arthroplasty: A clinical and radiologic study of 525 consecutive cases. *J Bone Joint Surg*. 2002;84B:77–82.

Mori T, Kudo H, Iwano K, et al. Kudo type-5 elbow arthroplasty in mutilating rheumatoid arthritis: A 5–11 year follow-up. *J Bone Joint Surg*. 2006;88B:920–924.

Shi LL, Zurakowskie D, Jones DG, et al. Semiconstrained primary and revision total elbow arthroplasty with use of the Coonrad-Morrey prosthesis. *J Bone Joint Surg*. 2007;89A: 1467–1475.

## Postoperative Imaging and Complications

Baseline radiographs following surgery should include AP and lateral projections at a minimum. The entire humeral and ulnar component and cement proximal and distal to the components must be included on the image. Ideally, the image should include approximately 2 cm distal or proximal to the implants and cement (see Figs. 11-46 and 11-47). In certain cases, fluoroscopic positioning is ideal to align the interfaces. These baseline images are important to evaluate potential complications on subsequent images. Component position or migration, bone graft status, lucent lines at the bone-cement or component bone interfaces, heterotopic ossification, and bone loss should all be evaluated on follow-up radiographs.

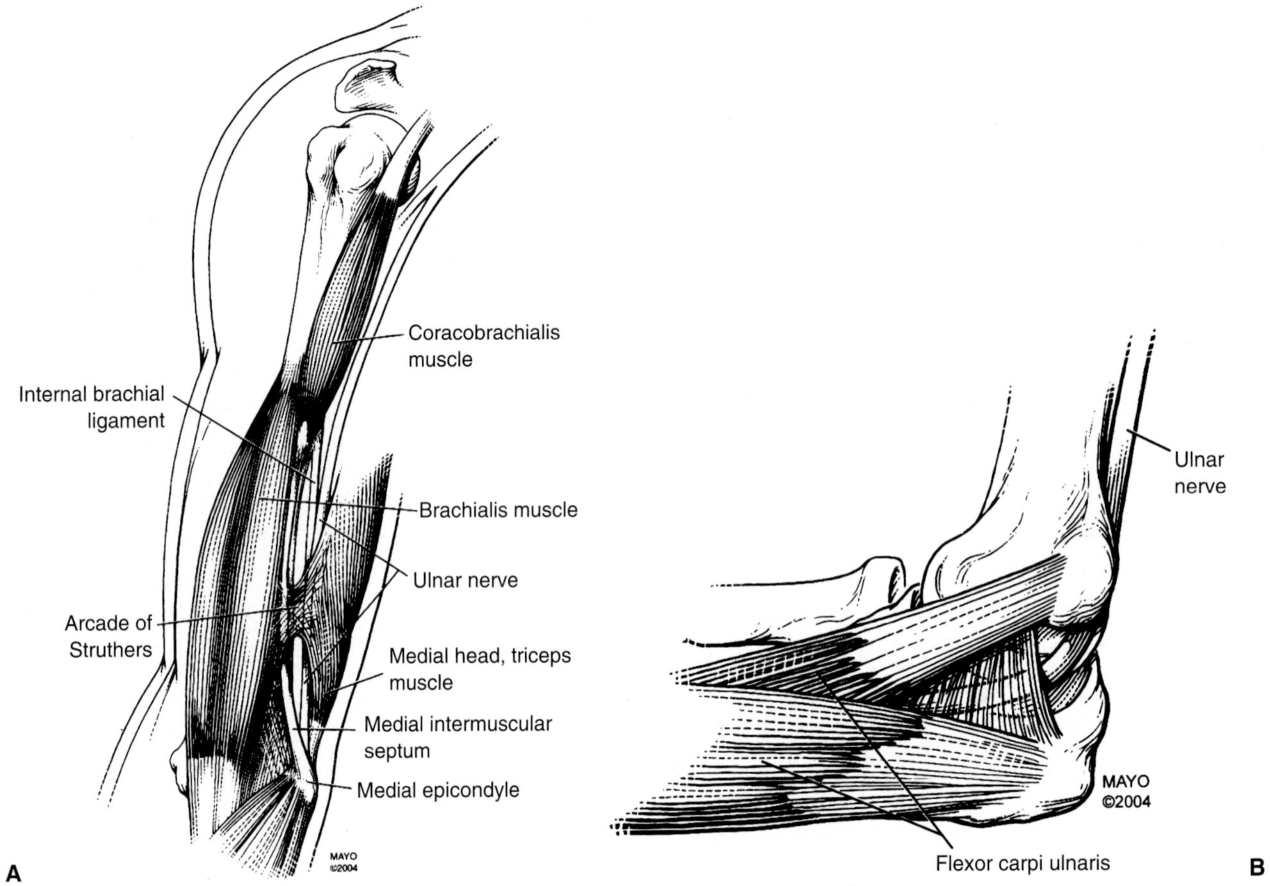

Coracobrachialis muscle
Internal brachial ligament
Brachialis muscle
Ulnar nerve
Arcade of Struthers
Medial head, triceps muscle
Medial intermuscular septum
Medial epicondyle
MAYO ©2004
A

Ulnar nerve
MAYO ©2004
Flexor carpi ulnaris
B

Fig. 11-37 Illustrations of the ulnar nerve as it passes through the arcade of Struthers to the medial epicondyle (A) and in the cubital tunnel as it passes into the forearm (B). (From Berquist TH. *MRI of the musculoskeletal system*, 5th ed. Philadelphia: Lippincott Williams & Wilkins; 2006.)

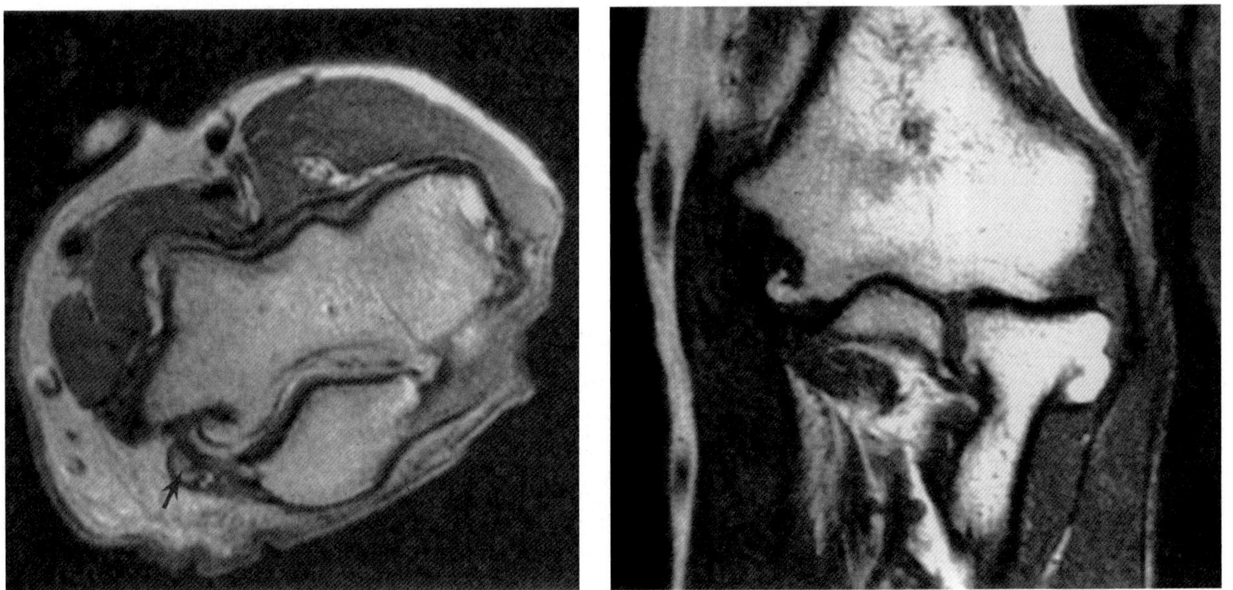


Fig. 11-38 Axial (A) and coronal (B) magnetic resonance (MR) images demonstrating prominent osteophytes compressing the ulnar nerve (*arrow*).

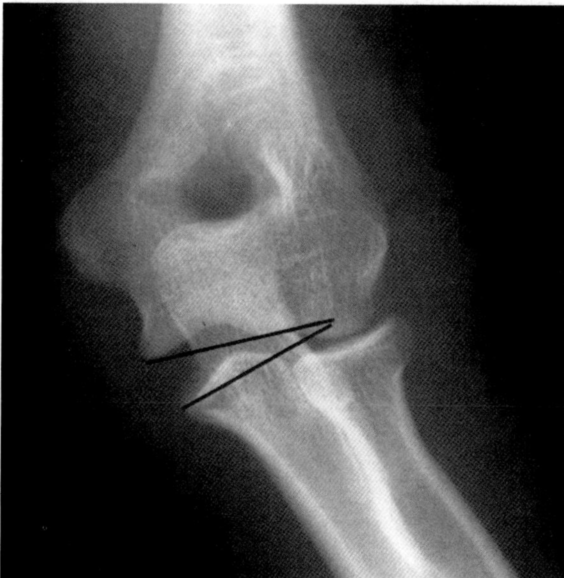

Fig. 11-39 Stress view of the left elbow demonstrating opening of the medial joint due to ligament disruption medially. Both elbows should be evaluated for comparison. The normal joint should not open >2 mm with varus and valgus stress.

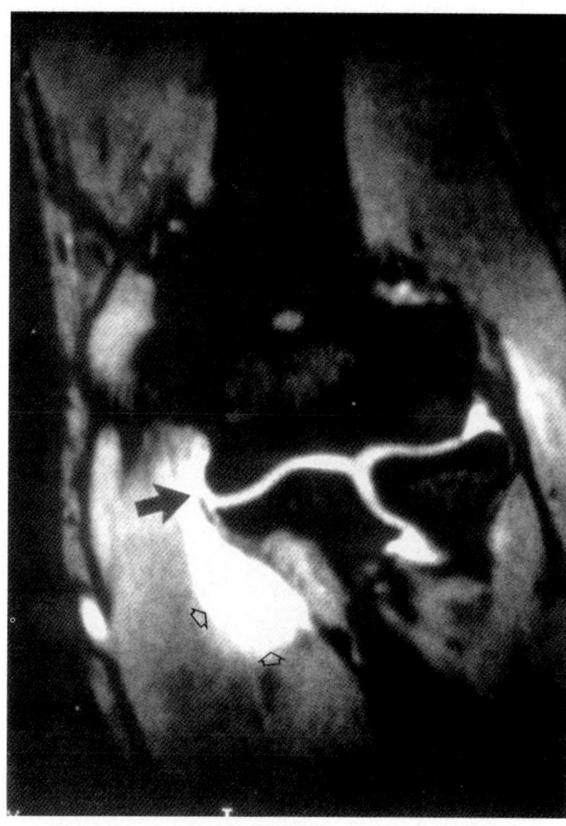

Fig. 11-40 Magnetic resonance (MR) image demonstrating a complete tear of the ulnar collateral ligament (*black arrow*) with a fluid collection distally (*open arrows*).

Complications following elbow arthroplasty may be related to the underlying disease process, type of implant, or surgical technique. The clinical outcome is not always adversely affected by the complication. The most significant complications are those that require implant removal, revision, or additional

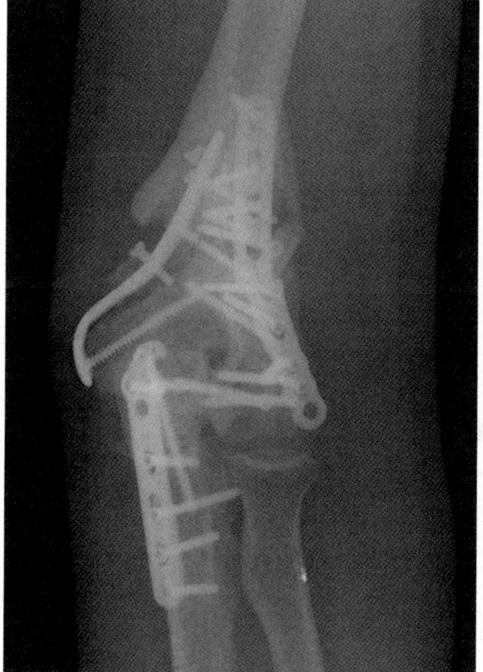

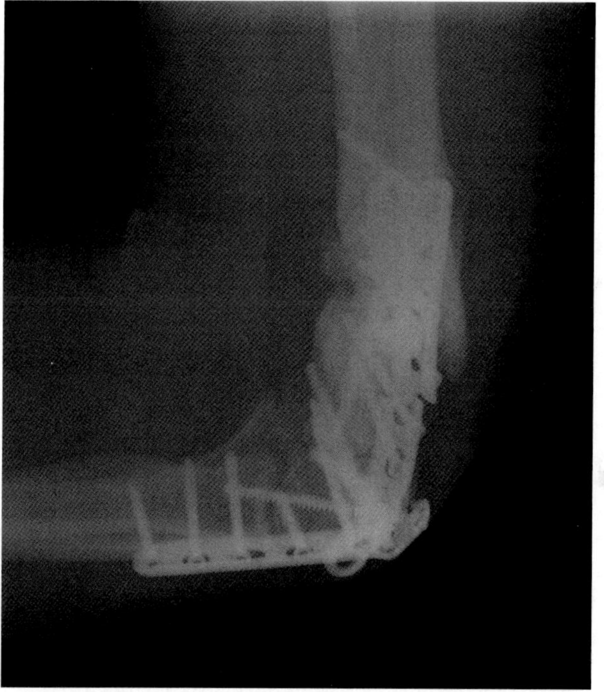

Fig. 11-41 Complex distal humeral fracture with nonunion. Anteroposterior (AP) (A) and lateral (B) radiographs demonstrate a hypertrophic nonunion with fractures of multiple screws, the lateral plate, and loosening of the medial plate.

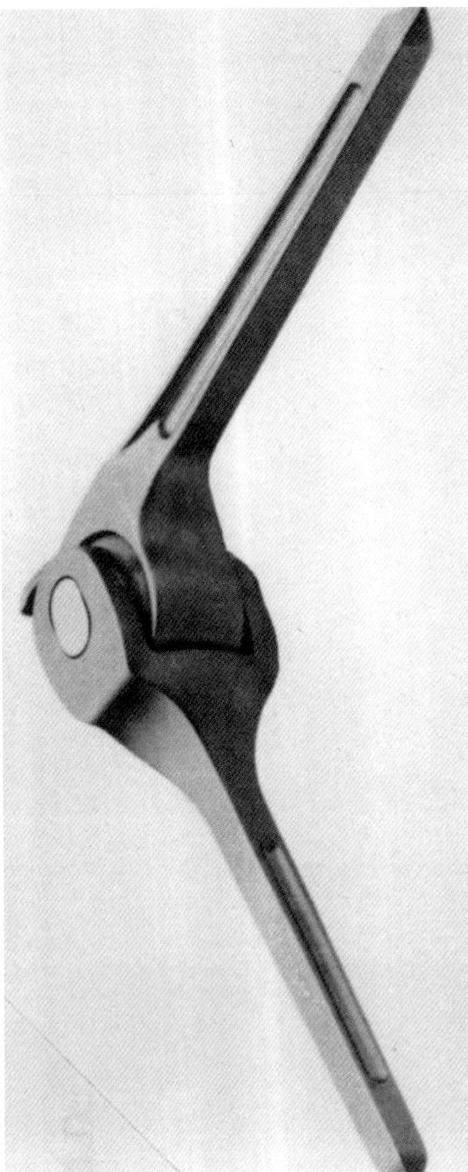

Fig. 11-42 Hinged elbow system. Illustration of the Schlein hinged prosthesis. (Courtesy of Howmedica, Rutherford, New Jersey.)

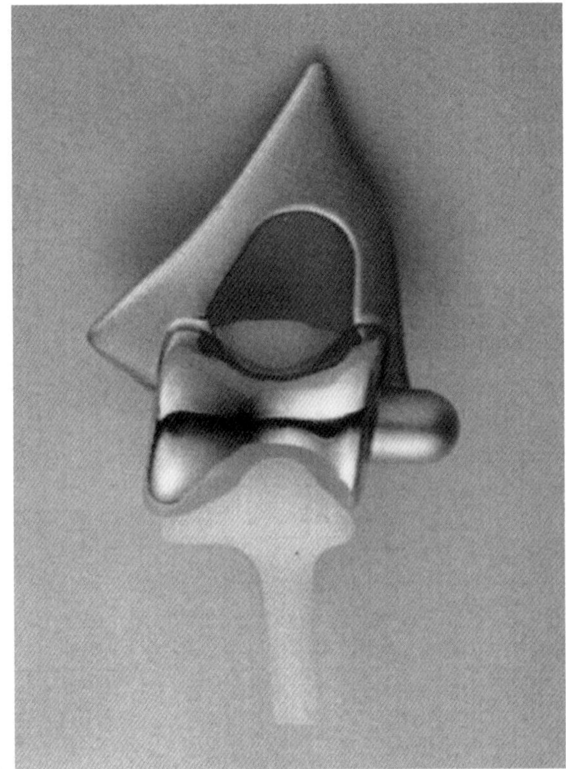

A

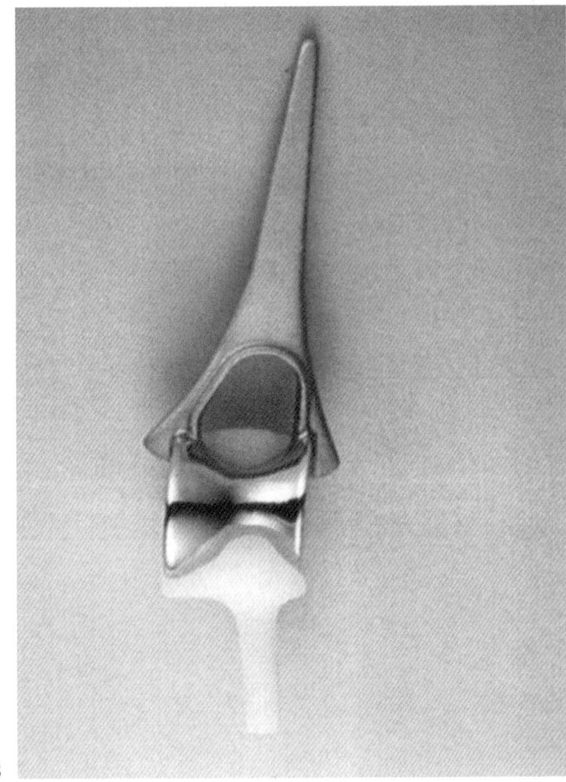

B

Fig. 11-43 Souter-Strathclyde anatomic resurfacing system. This system is commonly used in patients with inflammatory arthropathies such as rheumatoid arthritis. Stability is provided by retained ligaments. Humeral and ulnar components are not linked but closely congruent. Illustrations of the Souter-Strathclyde systems with a short (A) and longer humeral stem (B). (Courtesy of Stryker, Howmedica, Osteonics, Mahwah, New Jersey.)

procedures. Loosening, deep infection, instability and dislocation are the most common indications for revision surgery or implant removal.

Loosening was a common problem with hinged fully constrained components. During 5-year follow-up the incidence ranged from 25% to 42%. Loosening is much less common with resurfacing or semiconstrained implants. Radiographic signs of loosening may be evident in up to 17% of patients (Fig. 11-47). However, clinical loosening is much lower and is in the 2% to 6% range. Loosening is slightly more common for the humeral component compared to the ulnar component. Ulnar component loosening with semiconstrained implants may be related to impaction or pistoning of the anterior cement mantle about the proximal ulnar component against the anterior flange of the humeral component. This may be suspected on

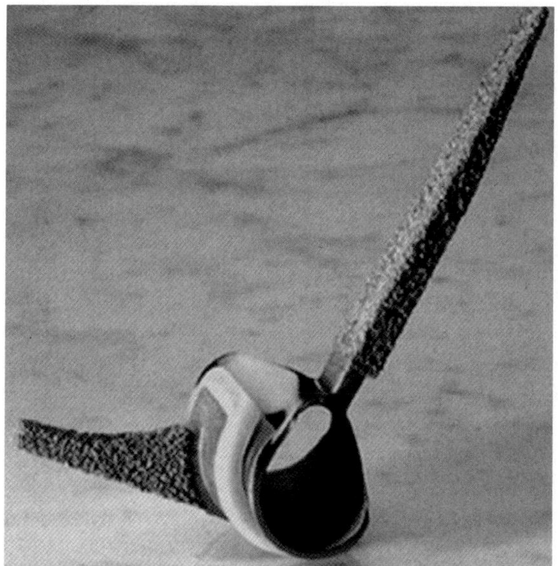

Fig. 11-44 Illustration of the Kudo 5 elbow system. Humeral and ulnar components are minimally invasive and can be used with or without cement. Cobalt–chrome components with polyethylene articular surface and titanium porous coating. (Courtesy of Biomet, United Kingdom.)

radiographs when there is varying degree of lucency between the ulnar component and cement mantle proximally (see Fig. 11-48). Signs of loosening on radiographs are similar to other joint replacements and include component migration, progressive lucent lines (>2 mm) at the bone-cement or metal-bone interfaces, cement fractures, and areas of osteolysis (see Fig. 11-49). Loosening may also be detected with radionuclide scans or PET. Arthrography is not as useful as in the hip for evaluating loosening.

Deep infection is a significant problem. In years past, deep infection was more common with elbow implants than any joint replacement procedure. Infection rates of 7% to 12% were reported. In recent years infection rates have decreased to 1% to 2%. Infections can be managed with irrigation and debridement if the components are well seated on images and at the time of surgery depending upon the organism. This technique has not been successful if the causative organism is *Staphyloccoccus epidermidis*. With more aggressive infections or when the implants are not well fixed, it is best to proceed with implant removal and revision arthroplasty following long-term antibiotic treatment or proceed to resection arthroplasty (see Fig. 11-50). Serial radiographs may demonstrate signs of loosening or periosteal reaction. Additional imaging studies or joint aspiration are most often required (Fig. 11-50). Radionuclide scans using combined agents are most successful.

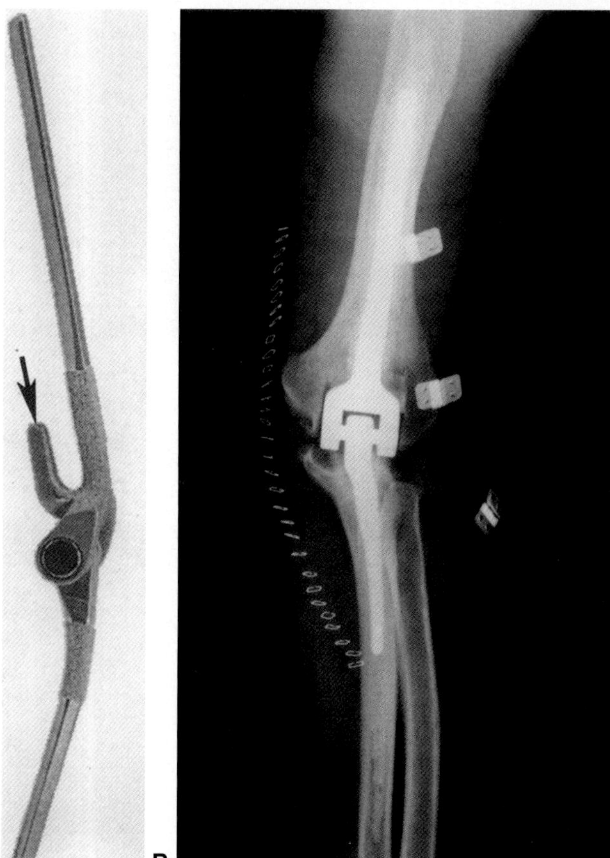


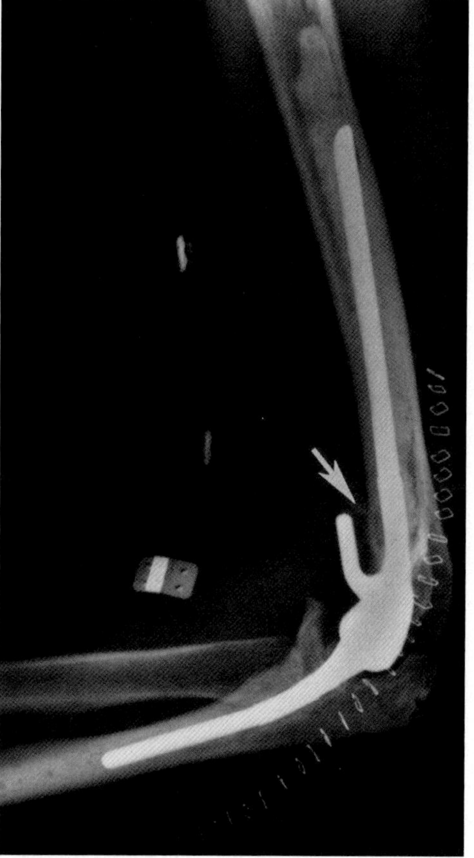


Fig. 11-45 Coonrad-Morrey total elbow replacement. A: Coonrad-Morrey elbow. There is a polyethylene link with an anterior extension (*arrow*). (Courtesy of Zimmer, Warsaw, Indiana.) Anteroposterior (AP) (B) and lateral (C) radiographs demonstrating a cemented Coonrad-Morrey total elbow. The radial head has been resected and there is bone graft (*arrow*) between the anterior extension and distal humerus.

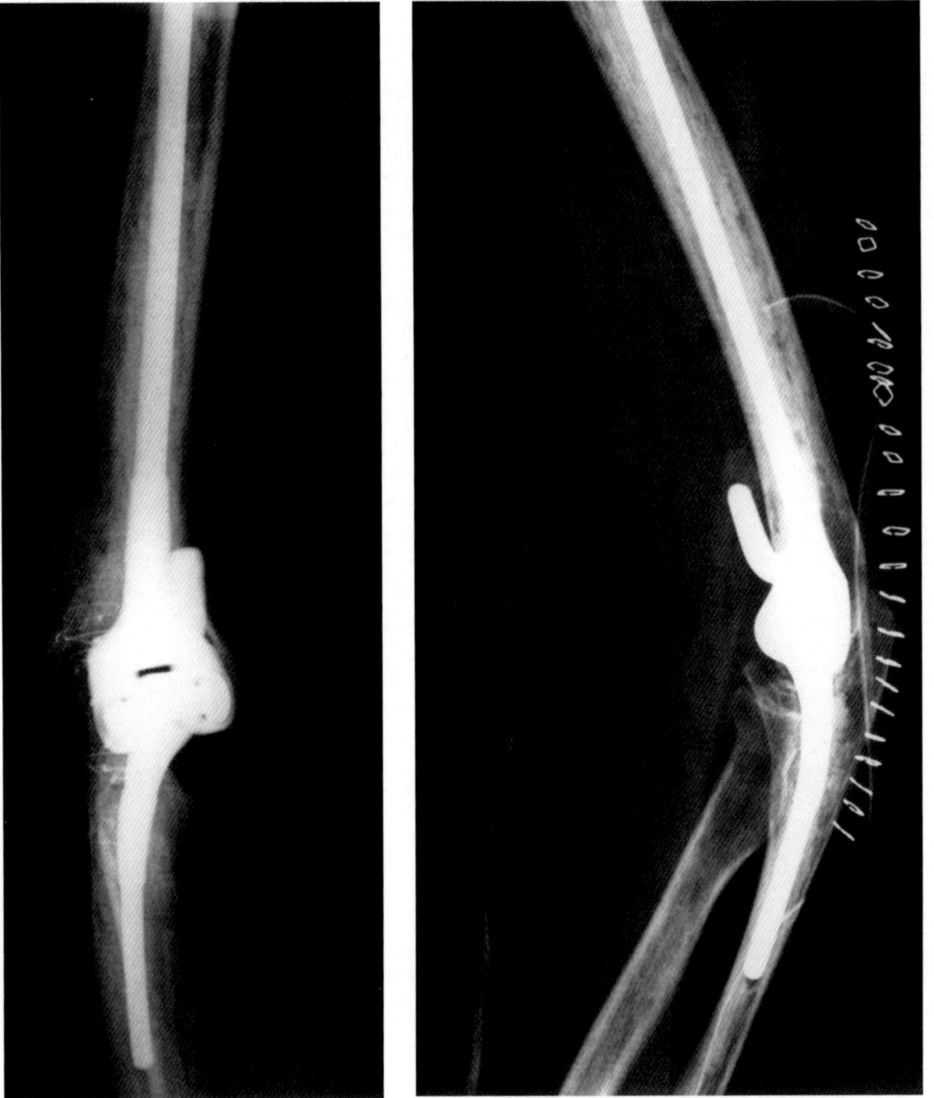

Fig. 11-46 Postoperative baseline radiographs. Anteroposterior (AP) (A) and lateral (B) radiographs following a Coonrad-Morrey semiconstrained athroplasty. The entire humeral component and all cement is not included on the image. The lateral view is improperly positioned. The images should be retaken when the patient can cooperate (note surgical drain still in place) using fluoroscopic guidance if necessary to assure a good baseline study.

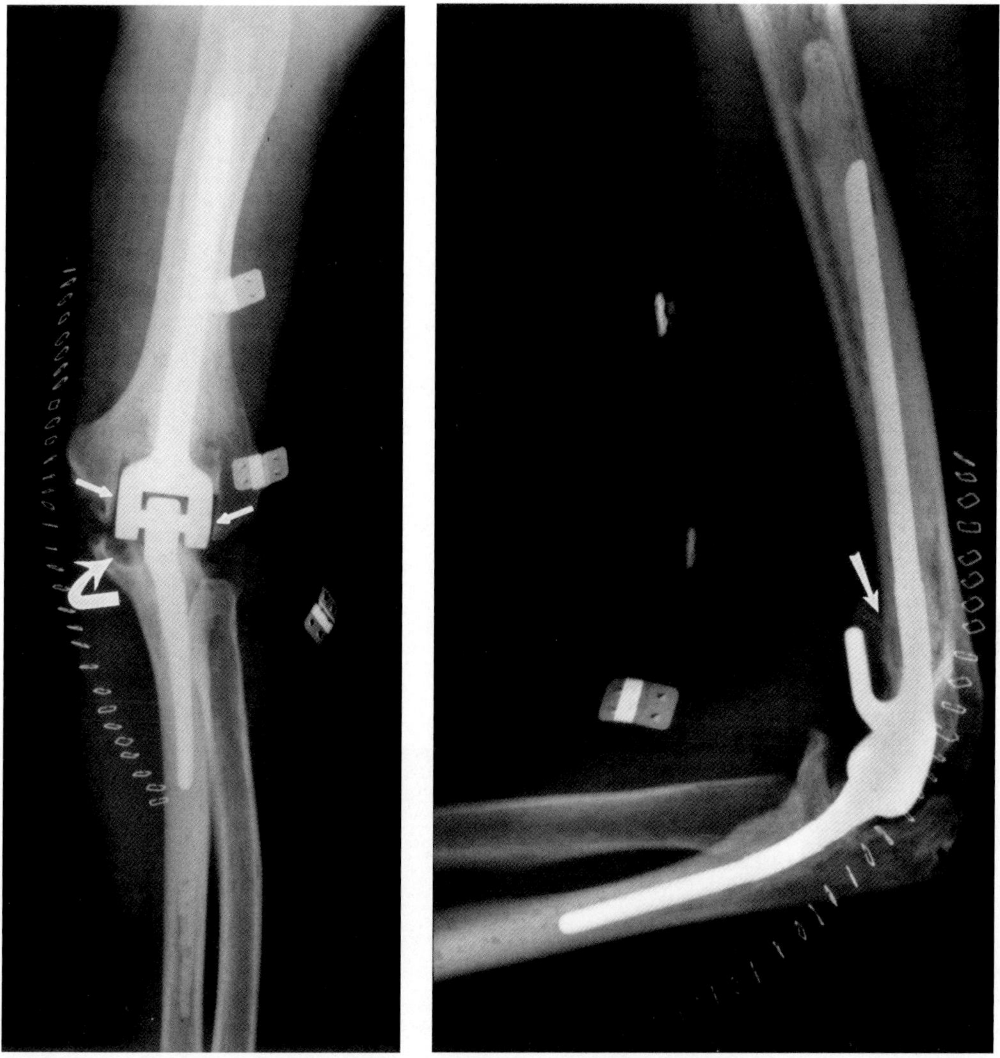


Fig. 11-47 Postoperative Coonrad-Morrey total elbow replacement. A: The anteroposterior (AP) radiograph demonstrates lucency adjacent to the distal humeral component (*arrows*) immediately following surgery that is of no significance. There is also a small area in the ulna with no cement (*curved arrow*) in the proximal ulna which should not be confused with osteolysis on later images. B: The lateral radiograph is better positioned compared to Figure 11-46B. Note the bone graft placed anteriorly (*arrow*). Both components are entirely included on the images and the cement is completely seen when combining the two images. Ideally, this should be accomplished on both images.

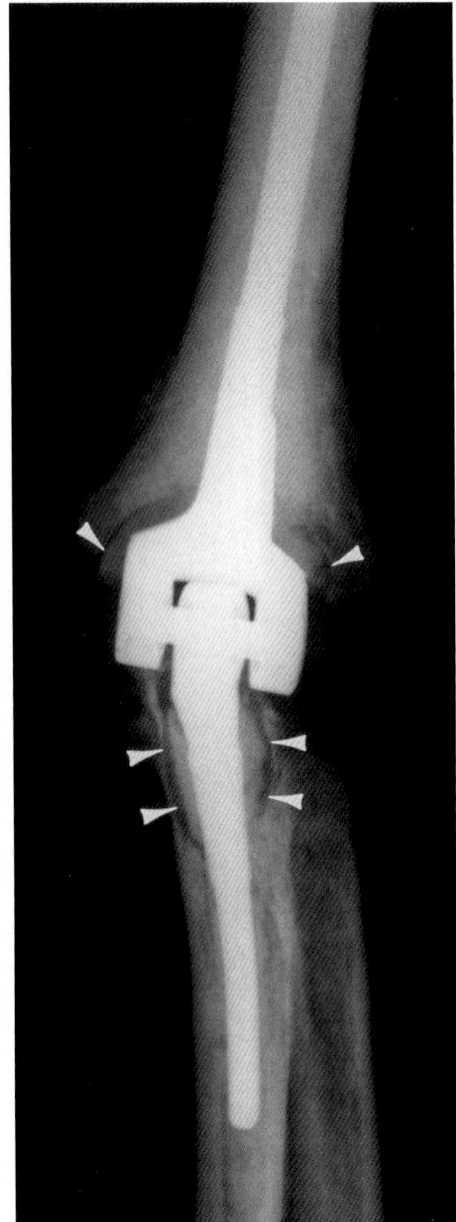


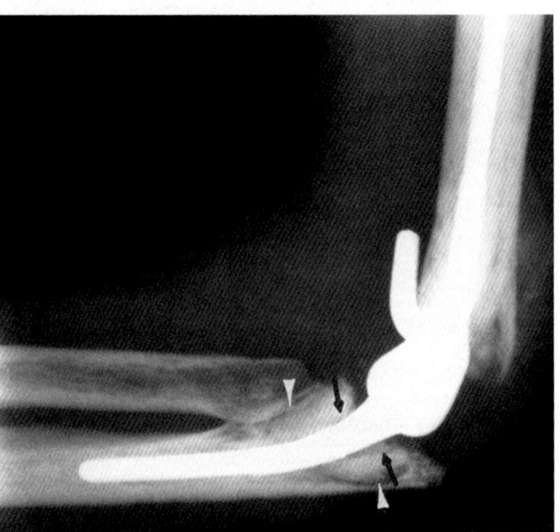


Fig. 11-48 Radiographic loosening without clinical loosening in an asymptomatic patient. A: Anteroposterior (AP) radiograph demonstrating lucency at the bone-cement interfaces of both components (*arrowheads*). B: The lateral radiograph demonstrates lucency at the bone-cement (*white arrowheads*) and metal-cement (*black arrows*) interfaces.

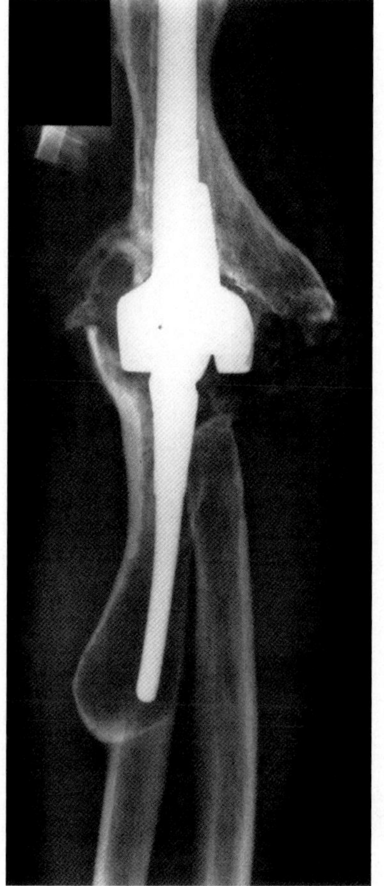


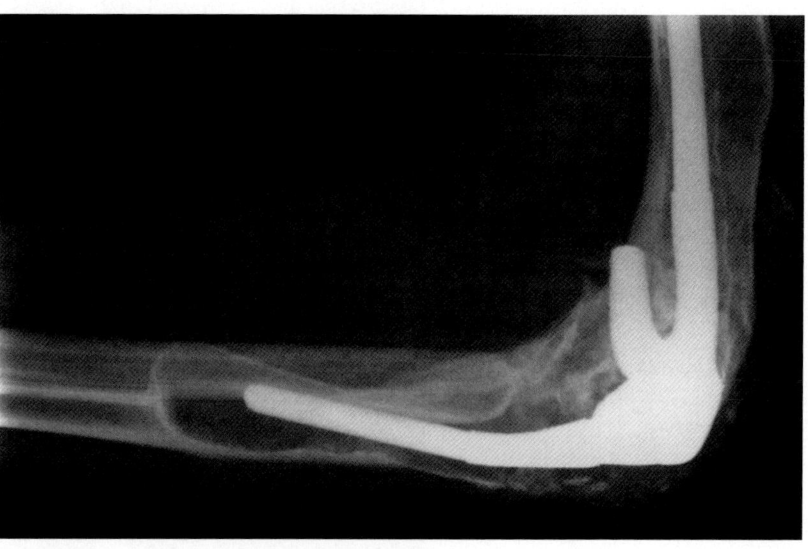


Fig. 11-49 Grossly loose ulnar component with toggling. Anteroposterior (AP) (A) and lateral (B) radiographs demonstrate gross loosening of the ulnar component with deformity of the cortex. There are more subtle changes along the humeral component with heterotopic ossification in the periarticular regions.

Multiple approaches have been used including three-phase bone scans with technetium Tc 99m MDP, technetium-labeled white blood cells, antigranulocyte antibody–labeled technetium, indium In 111–labeled white blood cells, and more recently, F-18 fluorodeoxyglucose PET imaging. Technetium-labeled white blood cells disassociate at a rate of 5% to 7% per hour following injection. This results in significant unwanted background activity. PET studies report sensitivities of 92% and specificities in the 97% range (Fig. 4-80). Indium In 111–labeled white blood cells remain the gold standard in the author's practice. Sensitivity ranges from 84% to 96% with specificity exceeding 96%.

Success of isolating the organism with joint aspiration is inconsistent, with accuracy ranging form 28% to 92%.

Instability is primarily a problem with resurfacing implants. Instability may be seen with subluxation or dislocation in 10% of patients with resurfacing implants (see Fig. 11-51). Revision arthroplasty is only required in approximately 20% of patients. Therefore, the overall incidence of surgical repair is only 1% to 5%. Instability may be evident on standard radiographs or stress images obtained under fluoroscopic control.

Implant failure may be due to component fracture, linkage failure, or cortical breakthrough by the component (see Fig. 11-52). Component fracture is uncommon (humeral component 0.65% and ulnar component 1.2%) and linkage failure or wearing of the bushing only occurs in approximately 3% of patients (see Fig. 11-53). Cortical breakthrough is more common with constrained implants (30%) compared to only 5% for semiconstrained components.

Neural injury is a fairly common problem. The ulnar nerve is most often involved. This is particularly common in patients with prior surgery or rheumatoid arthritis. Nerve injury may be related to traction or direct mechanical pressure during surgery, hematoma formation, or associated soft tissue swelling in the perineural tissues. The incidence of ulnar nerve injury has been reported to range from 2% to 26%. Fortunately, permanent neuropathy only occurs in 2% to 5% with the resolution of the neuropathy over a period of months in most patients.

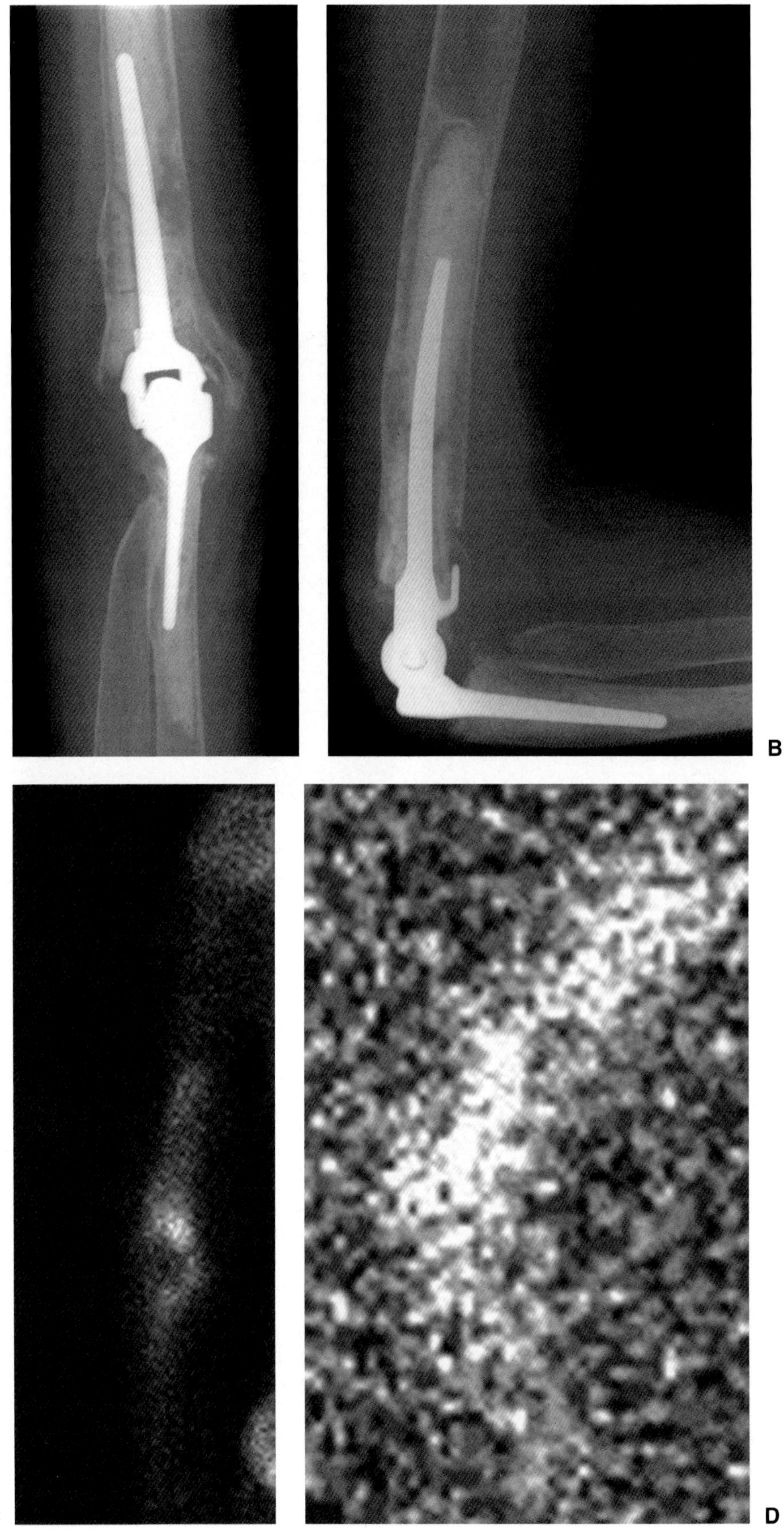


**Fig. 11-50** Infected elbow arthroplasty. Anteroposterior (AP) (**A**) and lateral (**B**) radiographs demonstrate soft tissue swelling and osteopenia with cortical thining. There is obvious loosening with wide lucent zones about the humeral bone cement interface and cement fractures. Technetium Tc 99m methylene-diphosphonate (MDP) (**C**) and indium In 111-labeled white blood cell scans (**D**) demonstrate increased tracer in the elbow and humerus due to infection. AP (**E**) and lateral (**F**) radiographs following implant removal and placement of antibiotic impregnated methacrylate beads. AP (**G**) and lateral (**H**) radiographs following reimplantation with long-stem components.

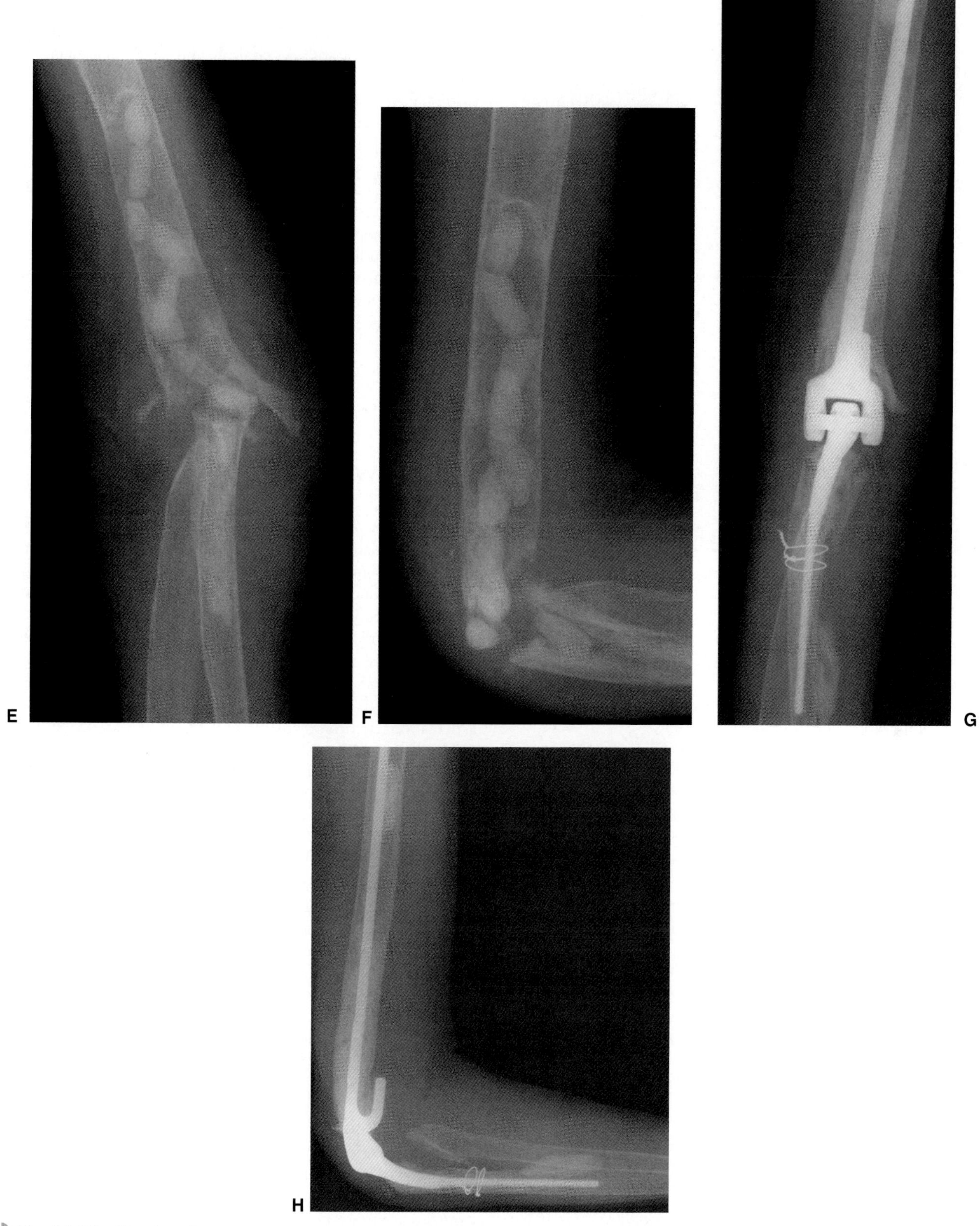


Fig. 11-50 *(Continued)*

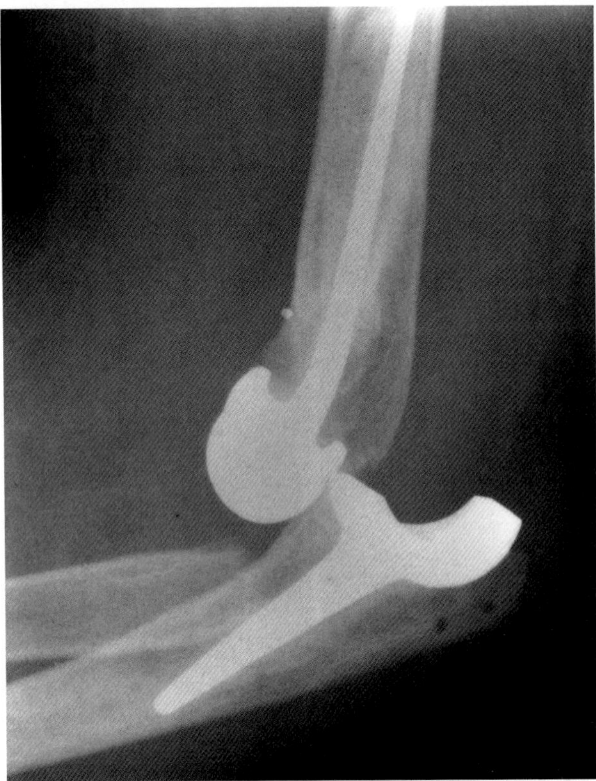

Fig. 11-51 Lateral radiograph demonstrating dislocation of an unlinked resurfacing arthroplasty.

Clinical and electromyographic (EMG) studies are most useful for diagnosis. MRI is optimal for evaluation of neural structures. However, metal artifact adjacent to the implants reduces the utility of this approach in most situations.

Additional complications include weakness of the triceps, heterotopic bone formation, and periprosthetic fractures. Heterotopic ossification is much less common compared to hip arthroplasty occurring in <1% of cases (Fig. 11-49). Periprosthetic fractures are more common occurring in up to 12% of patients. These complications are easily evaluated on serial radiographs.

Complications with revision arthtroplasty are similar. However, failure rates are slightly increased. Complications occur in roughly one third of cases requiring additional revision surgery in 16%, due to loosening, dislocation, and implant failures (see Fig. 11-54). Ulnar nerve injuries are also higher (13%) and intraoperative radial nerve injures occur in up to 7% during humeral component revision. Intraoperative fractures are also more common.

## SUGGESTED READING

Athwal GS, Morrey BF. Revision total elbow arthroplasty for prosthetic fractures. *J Bone Joint Surg*. 2006;88A:2017–2026.

Cheung EV, O'Driscoll SW. Total elbow prosthesis loosening caused by ulnar component pistoning. *J Bone Joint Surg*. 2007;89A:1269–1274.

Ikavalko M, Lehto MUK, Repo A, et al. Souter-Strathclyde elbow arthroplasty: A clinical and radiologic study of 525 cases. *J Bone Joint Surg*. 2002;84B:77–82.

Little CP, Graham AJ, Karatzas G, et al. Outcomes of total elbow arthroplasty for rheumatoid arthritis: Comparative study of three implants. *J Bone Joint Surg*. 2005;87A:2439–2448.

Morrey BF. Complications of elbow replacement surgery. In: Morrey BF, ed. *The elbow and its disorders*, 3rd ed. Philadelphia: WB Saunders; 2000:667–684.

Popovic N, Lemaire R, Georis P, et al. Midterm results with a bipolar radial head prosthesis: Radiographic evidence of loosening at the bone-cement interface. *J Bone Joint Surg*. 2007;89A:2469–2476.

Shi LL, Zurakowski D, Jones DG, et al. Semiconstrained primary and revision total elbow arthroplasty with use of the Coonrad-Morrey prosthesis. *J Bone Joint Surg*. 2007;89A:1467–1475.

# Elbow Arthrodesis

The elbow is the link between the shoulder and the hand. Fusion, especially in the presence of reduced shoulder motion, can result in significant functional loss. Presently, arthrodesis of the elbow is uncommonly performed due to improvements in primary and revision arthroplasty.

Indications for elbow arthrodesis include pain, instability, failed fracture fixation, failed elbow arthroplasty, marked deformity, and infection. Fusion may also benefit younger individuals with high-demand activities requiring a stable elbow articulation. Arthrodesis is difficult to achieve following failed total elbow replacement. Therefore, resection arthroplasty is more often used in these patients if further revision cannot be achieved (Fig. 11-52).

## Preoperative Imaging

Radiographs in the AP and lateral position are usually adequate to evaluate articular and bone changes. CT is useful to more fully evaluate bone stock before operative decision making and selection of the type of arthrodesis. Instability can usually be evaluated clinically, but on occasion stress views are useful for documentation.

## Treatment Options

The elbow is one of the most difficult articulations to fuse successfully. The extent of bone grafting, joint preparation, and fixation system varies with the preoperative diagnosis and image features. Rigid fixation should be achieved. Another dilemma is the degree of flexion for the fusion. The elbow is often fused in 90 degrees of flexion in males and 70 degrees in females as males are more likely to have more significant occupational

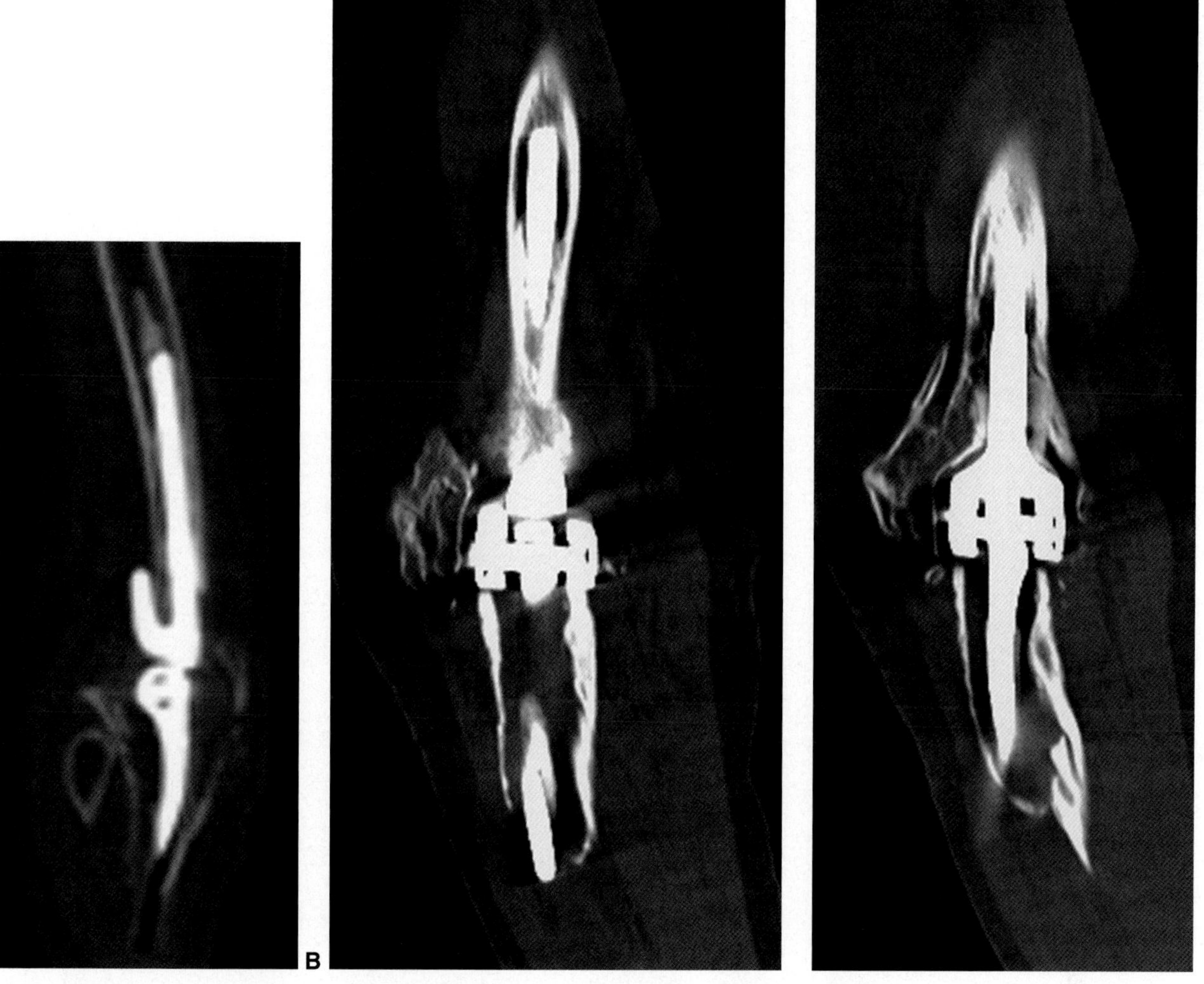


Fig. 11-52 Implant loosening with cortical breakthrough. Sagittal (A) and coronal (B and C) computed tomographic (CT) images of loose humeral and grossly loose ulnar components with cortical breakthrough in the ulna. Anteroposterior (AP) (D) and lateral (E) radiographs following revision with bone grafting of the ulna and soft tissue anchors.

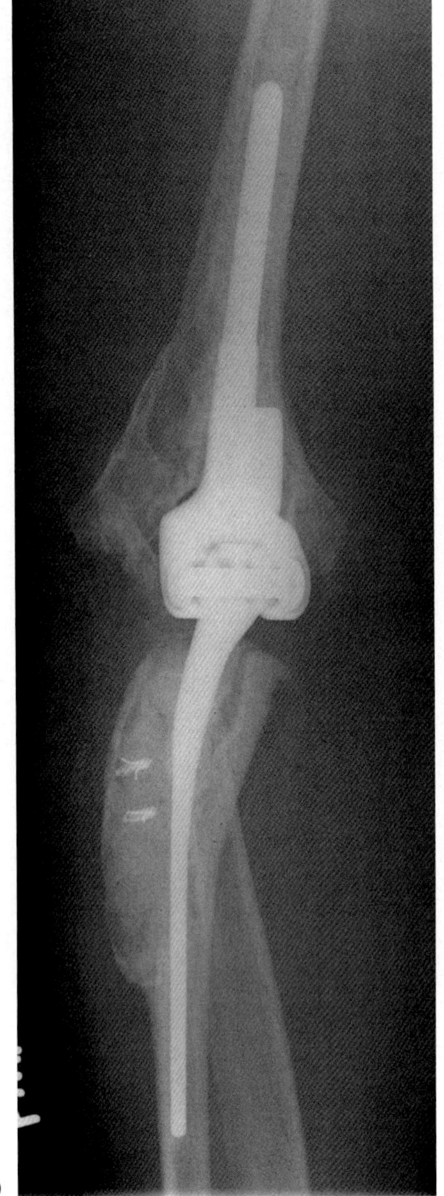

D

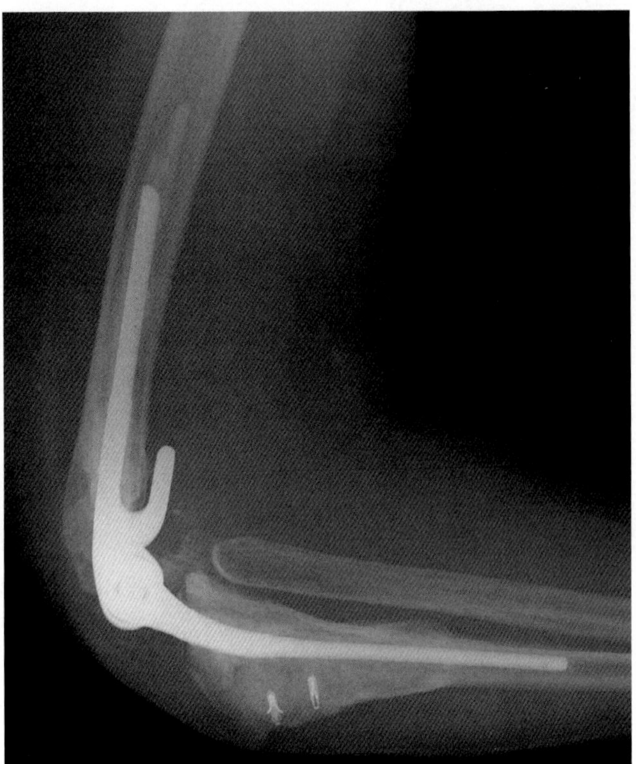

E

Fig. 11-52 *(Continued)*

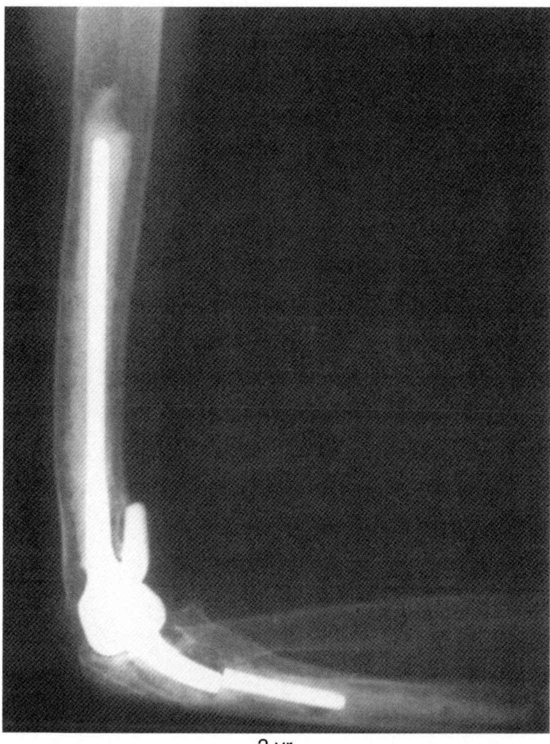


Fig. 11-53 Lateral radiograph demonstrating a fracture of the ulnar component 3 years following total elbow replacement. (From Morrey BF, Adams RA. Semiconstrained arthroplasty for treatment of rheumatoid arthritis of the elbow. *J Bone Joint Surg.* 1992;74A:479–490.)

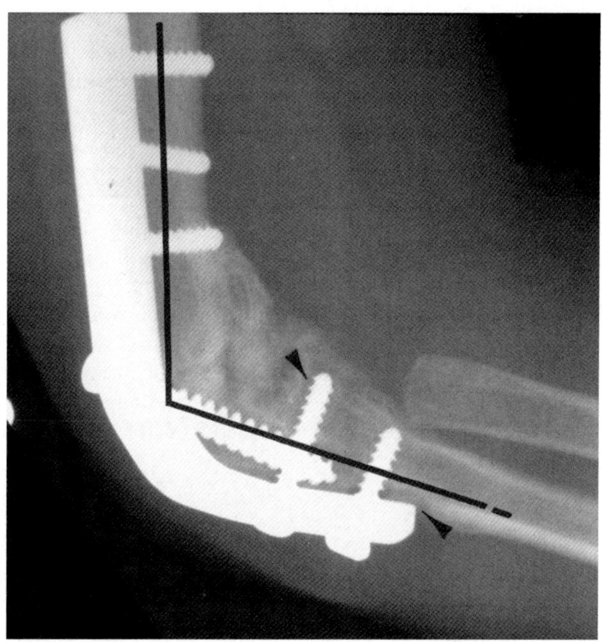

Fig. 11-55 Elbow arthrodesis with plate and screw fixation. The elbow is fused in 70 degrees (*black lines*) of flexion with resection of the radial head. There is lucency about the ulnar screws and distal plate suggesting motion and nonunion (*arrowheads*).

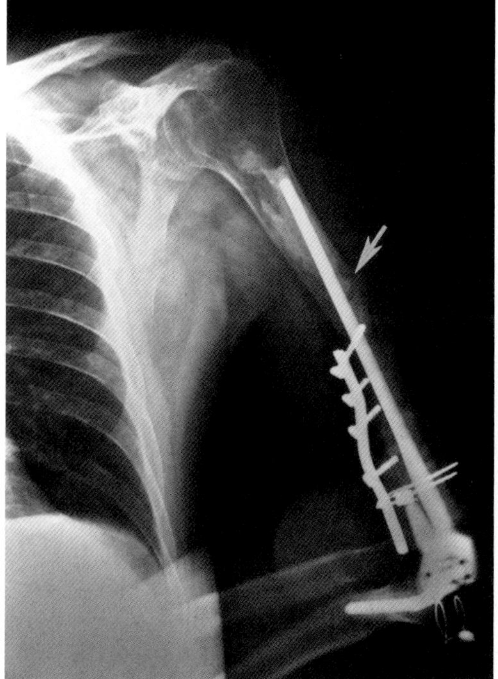


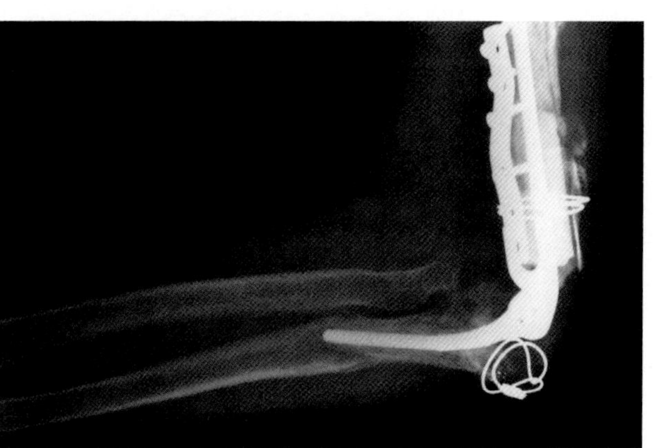


Fig. 11-54 Prior failed revision arthroplasty. Frontal radiographs of the humerus (A) and lateral radiographs of the elbow (B) demonstrating a long-stem humeral revision component with cortical defect from prior fracture (*arrow*) and cortical onlay bone graft with plate and screw and Dall-Miles cable fixation for intraoperative fracture and bone loss. There is a healed periprosthetic fracture at the tip of the ulnar component.

weight demands. External fixation can be used in the presence of infection. However, depending on the extent of bone loss, screw fixation or plate and screw fixation is most often employed (see Fig. 11-55).

### Postoperative Imaging and Complications

Data for this uncommonly performed procedure is not as extensive as for arthroplasty. Failure rates as high as 53% have been reported. Nonunion, implant failure (Fig. 11-55), fractures adjacent to the fusion site, and deep infection are the most common reported complications. Serial radiographs and CT are most useful to evaluate success of fusion and for fracture detection. As mentioned earlier, radionuclide scans 1 year following surgery are most successful for detection of deep infection.

## SUGGESTED READING

Bechenbaugh RD. Arthrodesis. In: Morrey BF, ed. *The elbow and its disorders*, 3rd ed. Philadelphia: WB Saunders; 2000: 731–737.

Figgie MP, Inglis AE, Mow CS, et al. Results of reconstruction of failed elbow arthroplasty. *Clin Orthop*. 1990;253: 123–132.

Hahn MP, Ostermann PA, Richter D, et al. Elbow arthrodesis and its alternative. *Orthopaedics*. 1996;25:112–120.

Rashkoff E, Burkhalter WE. Arthrodesis of the salvaged elbow. *Orthopaedics*. 1986;9:733–738.

Snider WJ, DeWitt HJ. Functional study for optimal position for elbow arthrodesis and ankylosis. *J Bone Joint Surg*. 1973; 55:1300–1308.

# 12 The Radius and Ulna

This chapter will focus on fractures of the radial and ulnar shafts. Monteggia and Galeazzi fractures will be included. Fractures of the radius and ulna may occur together or separately. Forearm fractures account for 10% to 14% of all skeletal fractures. The mechanisms of injury may be related to a direct blow, a fall on the outstretched hand, motor vehicle accidents, and gunshot wounds. Associated injuries of the elbow and wrist are fairly common. In a large series of adult forearm fractures, 75% involved both the radius and ulna, 15% the ulna alone, and 10% the radius alone. The incidence is also increasing in adolescents around the age of puberty when activities are increasing and bone turnover due to growth spurts is more active resulting in increased cortical porosity. In the last 30 years, the incidence of forearm fractures has increased 56% in adolescent females and 32% in males.

The incidence of fractures also varies with location in both the radius and ulna. In the ulna, 13% of fractures involve the proximal third, 59% the middle third, and 28% the distal third. In the radius, 21% involve the proximal third, 61% the middle third, and 18% the distal third. Clinical examination should include assessment of soft tissues for abrasions or open wounds and evaluation of neurovascular structure to rule out compartment syndrome.

Fracture eponyms for forearm fractures such as nightstick (isolated ulnar fracture), greenstick (incomplete bowing fracture), and microfracture were reviewed in Chapter 2. The Orthopaedic Trauma Association (OTA) classification will be used in this section to facilitate discussion of treatment. Classification of diaphyseal fractures includes simple (type A), wedge or butterfly (type B), and complex (type C). The OTA has added three subcategories to each and multiple subcategories (see Fig. 12-1). The latter group addresses variations in complexity and associated dislocations of the radial head or distal radioulnar joint.

## Orthopaedic Trauma Association Classification

### Type A: Simple

A1—simple ulna, radius intact
A2—simple radius, ulna intact
A3—simple fractures of both bones

### Type B: Wedge (butterfly fragment)

B1—wedge ulna, radius intact
B2—wedge radius, ulna intact
B3—wedge fractures of both bones

### Type C: Complex

C1—Complex ulna, simple radius
C2—Complex radius, simple ulna
C3—Complex fractures of both the radius and ulna

Two additional fractures are associated with articular dislocations. The Monteggia fracture (see Chapter 2) is a fracture of the proximal third of the ulna with an associated radial head dislocation. Monteggia fractures account for approximately 5% of forearm fractures. Type I Monteggia lesions (60%) present with anterior dislocation of the radial head and an ulnar fracture that is typically angulated anteriorly. Type II Monteggia lesions (15%) present with posterior or posterolateral radial head dislocation and the ulnar fracture is angulated more posteriorly (see Fig. 12-2). Type III lesions (20%) present with anterolateral or lateral dislocation of the radial head and an ulnar metaphyseal fracture (see Fig. 12-3). Type IV injuries (5%) present with anterior dislocation of the radial head and fractures of both the proximal radius and ulna.

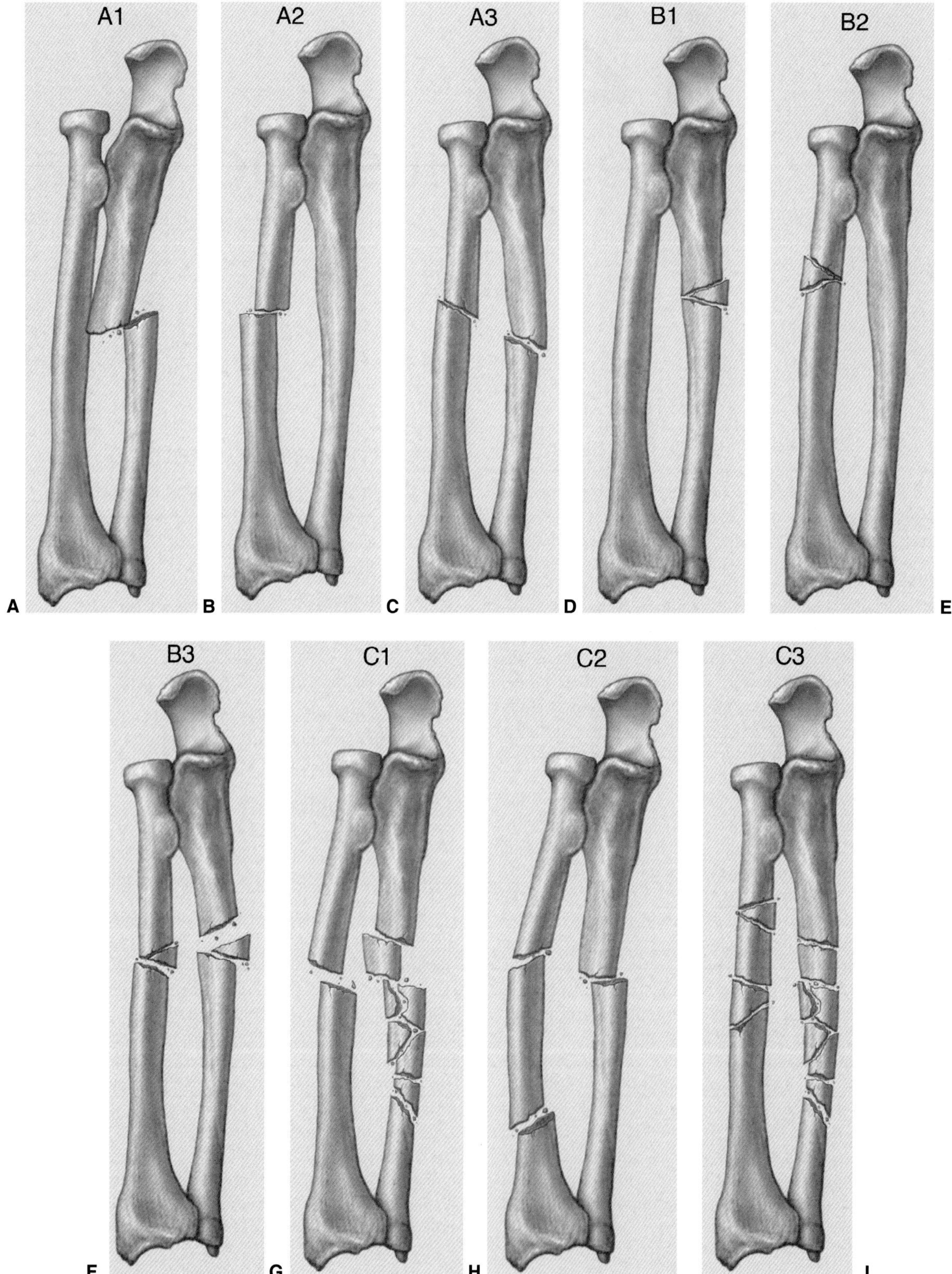


**Fig. 12-1** Orthopaedic Trauma Association classification for radius and ulna fractures. **A:** Type A1—simple ulna, radius intact. **B:** Type A2—simple radius, ulna intact. **C:** Type A3—simple fractures of radius and ulna. **D:** Type B1—wedge fracture of ulna, radius intact. **E:** Type B2—wedge fracture of radius, ulna intact. **F:** Type B3—wedge fractures of radius and ulna. **G:** Type C1—complex ulnar fracture with simple radius fracture. **H:** Type C2—complex radius fracture with simple ulna. **I:** Type C3—complex fractures of both the radius and ulna.

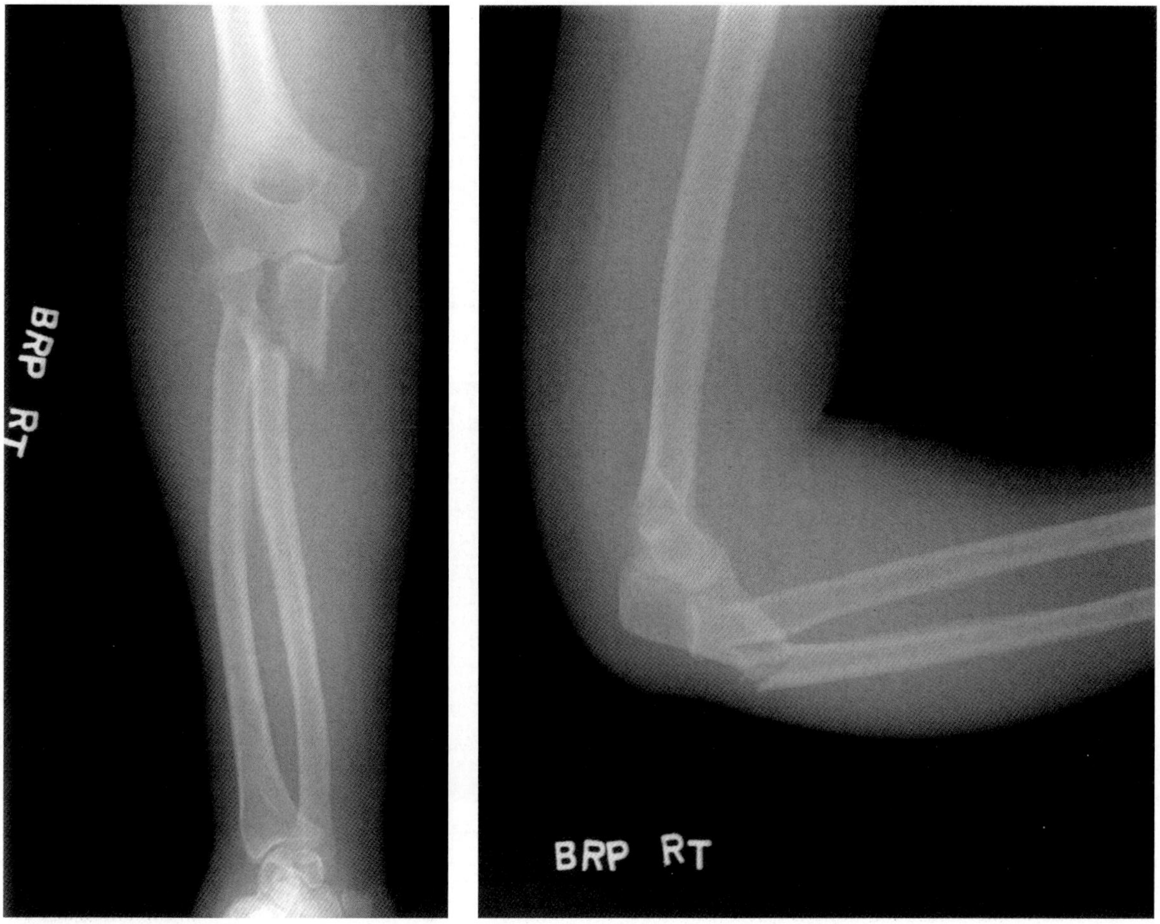

Fig. 12-2 Monteggia fracture. Anteroposterior (AP) (A) and lateral (B) radiographs of a type II fracture with posterior dislocation of the radial head and posterior angulation of the ulnar fracture.

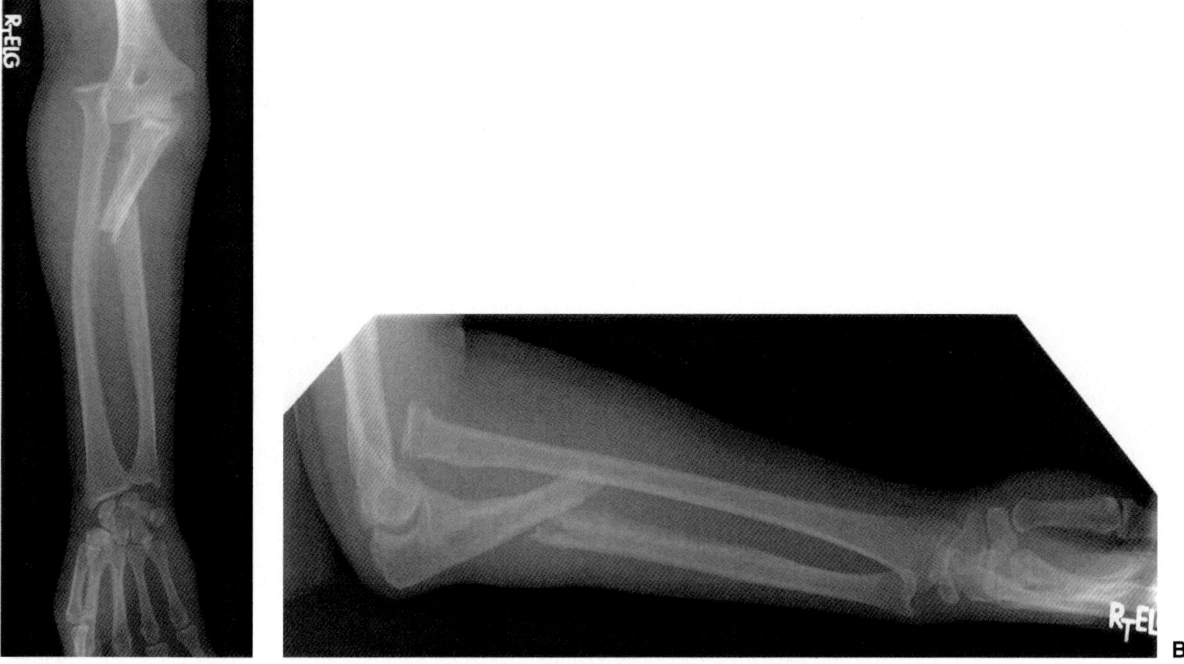

Fig. 12-3 Monteggia fracture. Anteroposterior (AP) (A) and lateral (B) radiographs of a type III lesion with anterolateral radial head dislocation and anterior angulation of the ulnar fracture.

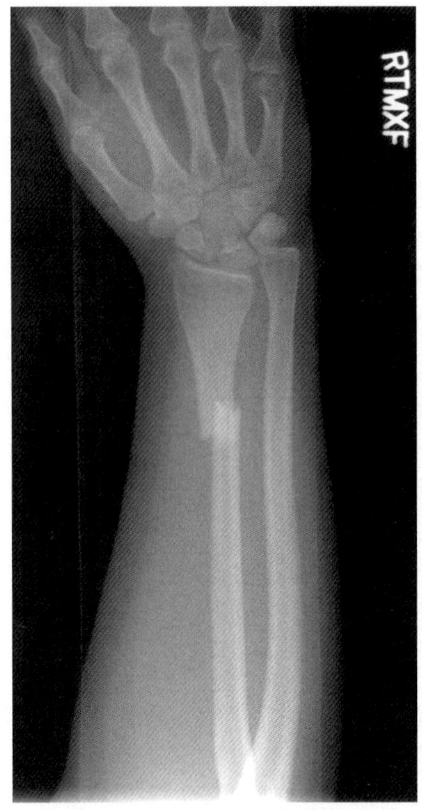


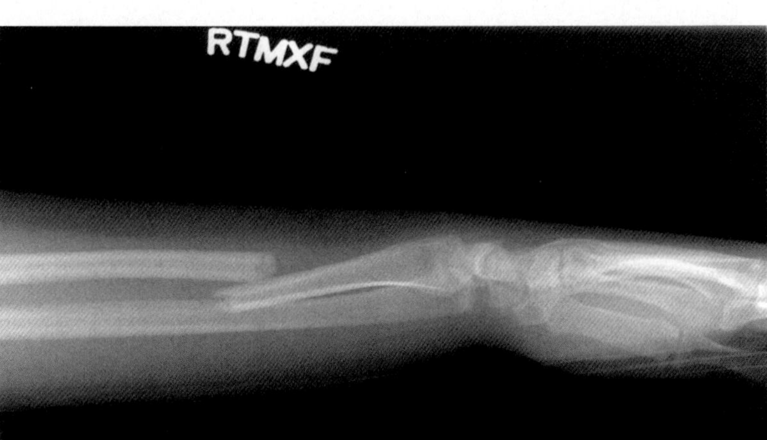


A B

Fig. 12-4 Galeazzi fracture. Anteroposterior (AP) (A) and lateral (B) radiographs of a distal radial fracture with dislocation of the distal radioulnar joint.

The Galeazzi fracture is a fracture of the distal radius with dislocation or subluxation of the distal radioulnar joint (see Fig. 12-4). This injury accounts for 5% to 7% of forearm fractures.

## Suggested Reading


Goldfarb CA, Ricci WM, Tull F, et al. Functional outcomes after fractures of both bones of the forearm. *J Bone Joint Surg.* 2005;87B:374–379.

Khosla S, Melton JL III, Dekutoske MB, et al. Incidence of childhood distal forearm fractures over 30 years. *JAMA.* 2003;290:1479–1485.

Orthopaedic Trauma Association Committee for Coding and Classification. Fracture and dislocation compendium. *J Orthop Trauma.* 1996;10:21–25.

Reckling FW, Cordell LD. Unstable fracture-dislocation of the forearm (Monteggia and Galeazzi lesions). *J Bone Joint Surg.* 1982;64A:999–1007.


## Imaging of Forearm Fractures

Radiographic evaluation is essential to evaluate the position, location, and type of fracture or fracture dislocation. Images must include the elbow and wrist. Anteroposterior (AP) and lateral views are obtained at a minimum. Oblique views may add additional information. The radiocapitellar relationship must be accurately evaluated. A line drawn through the mid radial head should intersect the capitellum regardless of the radiographic projection (see Fig. 12-5). Evaluation of the distal radioulnar joint is more difficult unless completely dislocated. Subluxation of the distal radioulnar joint may be difficult to evaluate on radiographs. In this setting, axial computed tomographic (CT) images in neutral, pronation, and supination will make the diagnosis. CT imaging can be performed after the other injuries are stabilized. Magnetic resonance imaging (MRI) is rarely indicated in the acute setting but may be helpful in patients with suspected compartment syndrome or interosseous membrane injury. Injury to the interosseous membrane may

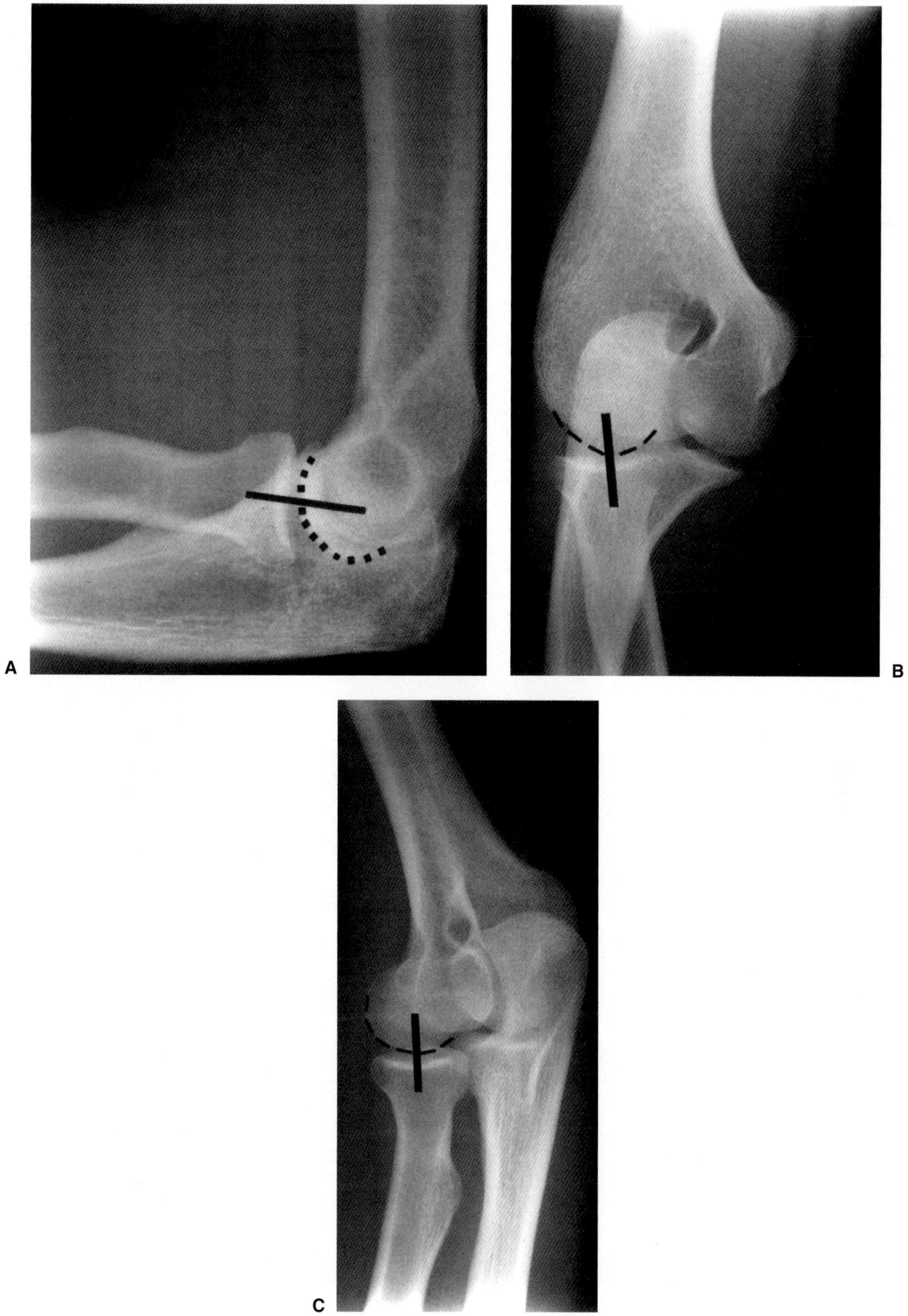

A B

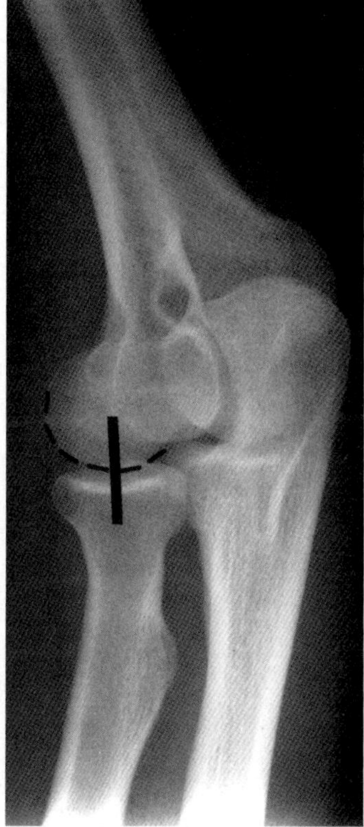

C

Fig. 12-5 Normal radiographic views of the elbow demonstrating the radiocapitellar line. Lateral (A) and both oblique views (B and C) show the line drawn through the mid radial head intersecting the capitellum in all projections.

result in long-term function loss. Therefore, early diagnosis and management is important.

## Suggested Reading


Berquist TH. *Imaging of orthopaedic trauma*, 2nd ed. New York: Raven Press; 1992.

McGinley JC, Roach N, Hopgood BC, et al. Forearm interosseous membrane trauma: MRI diagnostic criteria and injury patterns. *Skeletal Radiol.* 2006;35:275–281.


# Treatment Options

The goals of treatment are to restore alignment and length and preserve normal motion (pronation and supination). Although closed reduction can be successful in certain settings, internal fixation is most often required when both bones are involved.

## Closed Reduction

Undisplaced isolated fractures of the radius are rare due to the support and protection afforded by the forearm muscles. Isolated ulnar fractures (nightstick fractures) do occur. Undisplaced fractures of both the mid radius and ulna can be treated with closed reduction (see Fig. 12-6). However, closed reduction is typically reserved for isolated fractures of the ulna (nightstick or OTA A1) (see Fig. 12-7). Closed reduction can be accomplished with a long arm cast with the elbow flexed 90 degrees.

## Open Reduction and Internal Fixation

As noted earlier, undisplaced fractures in adults and children can be treated with closed reduction with a long arm cast and the elbow flexed 90 degrees. In children with displaced fractures and in adults, fractures are more often unstable which requires internal fixation. Surgical intervention should be performed within 24 hours when possible.

Indications for open reduction and internal fixation include the following:

All displaced diaphyseal fractures
Angulation exceeding 10 to 15 degrees
Monteggia fractures
Galeazzi fractures
Open fractures
Fractures with compartment syndrome

The goals of open reduction and internal fixation are to restore anatomic alignment and allow early motion to restore function. Accurate reduction of the normal radial bow and interosseous space is important to preserve function. Fracture fragments are frequently rotated, angulated, and encroach on the

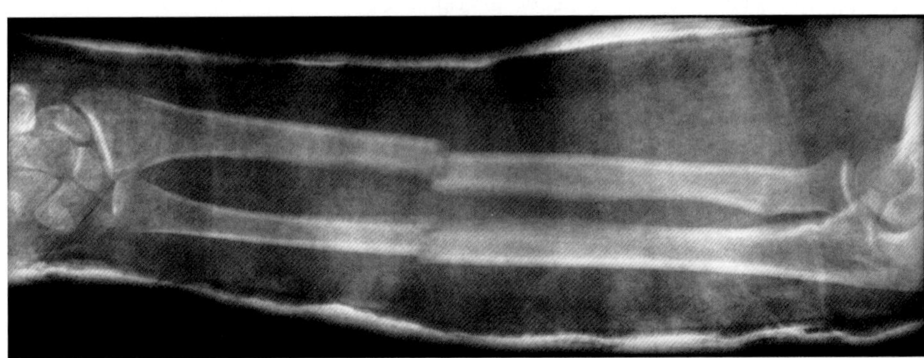

A

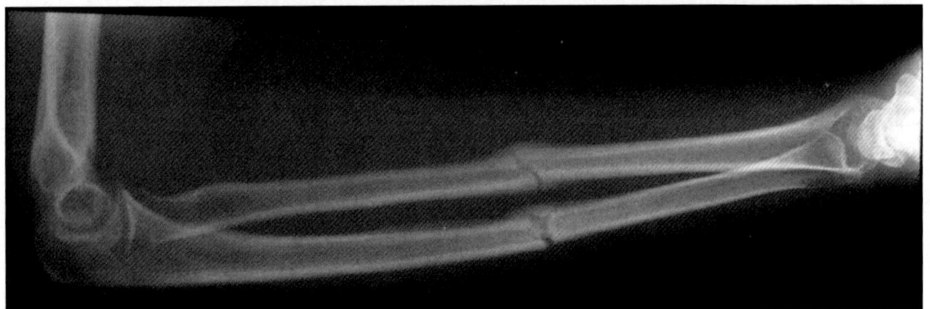

C

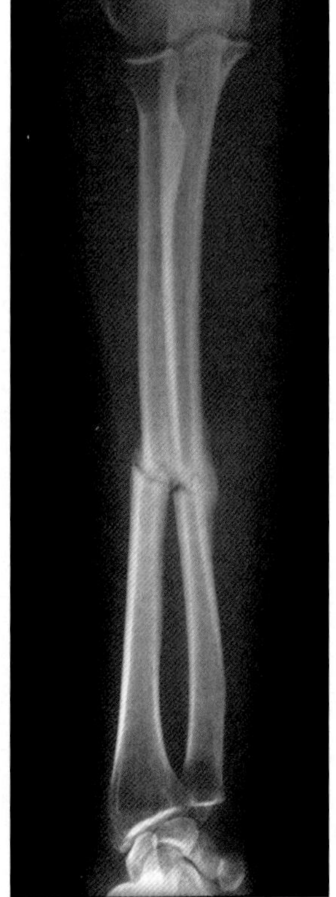

B

Fig. 12-6 Lateral (A) radiograph demonstrate slightly displaced fractures of the mid radius and ulna treated with a long arm cast and the elbow flexed 90 degrees. Anteroposterior (AP) (B) and lateral (C) radiographs 12 weeks later demonstrate bridging callus, although the fracture line is still visible.

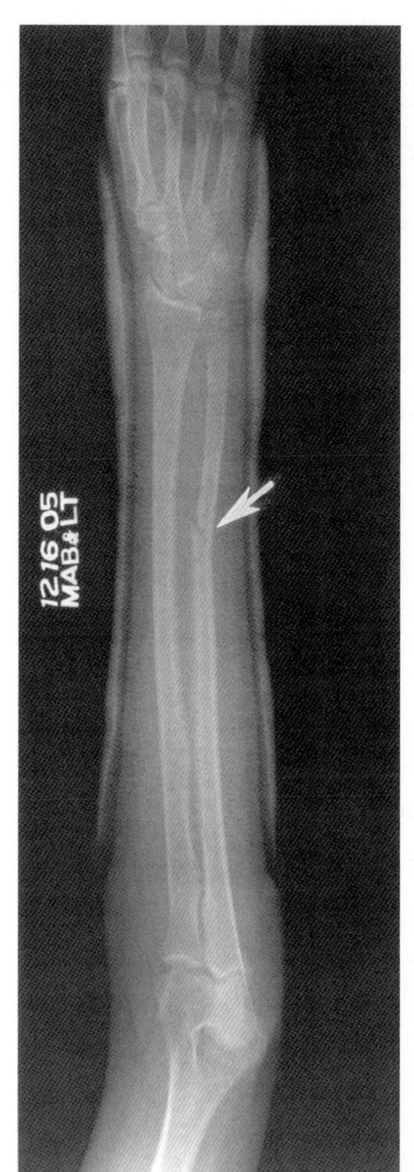

A

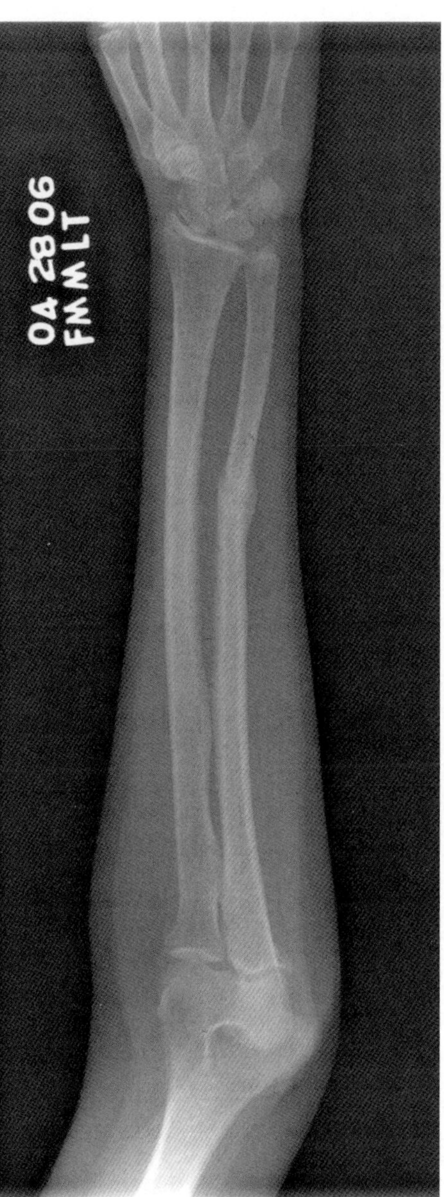

B

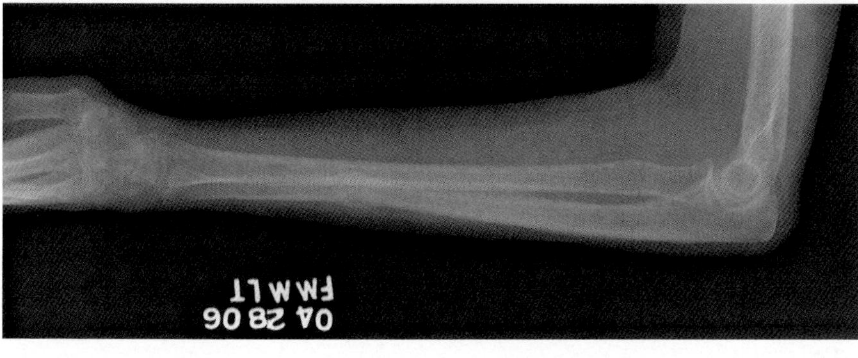

C

Fig. 12-7 Nightstick fracture. Anteroposterior (AP) (A) radiograph of the forearm with cast immobilization demonstrating a minimally displaced ulnar fracture (*arrow*). AP (B) and lateral (C) radiographs demonstrate the healed fracture.

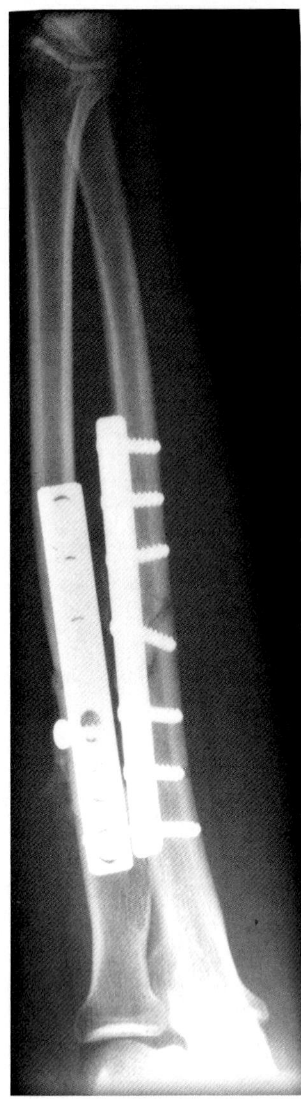

Fig. 12-8 Radiograph following dynamic compression plate and screw fixation of radius and ulnar fractures.

interosseous space. Generally fractures proximal to the pronator teres insertion on the radius cause supination of the proximal fragment. When fractures occur distal to the insertion of the pronator teres, the major forces of the biceps and supinator are neutralized so fragments are less likely to get displaced.

Internal fixation can be accomplished with 3.5 mm conventional dynamic compression plates (DCP) (see Fig. 12-8),

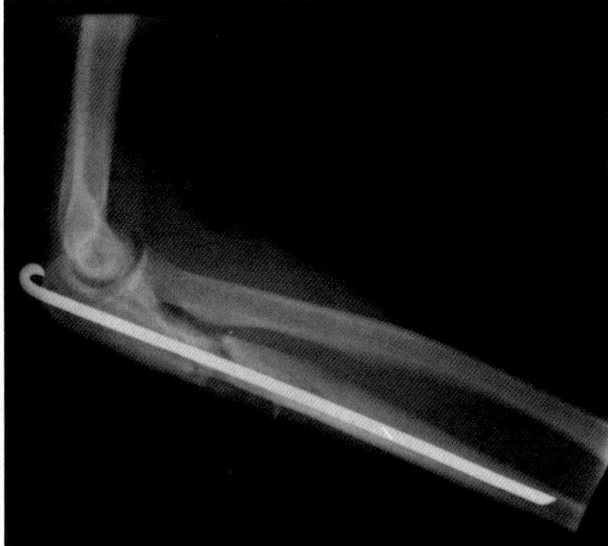

Fig. 12-10 Lateral radiograph demonstrating the use of a Rush rod for intramedullary nailing of a proximal ulnar fracture.

new low-contact dynamic compression plates (LC-DCP) (see Fig. 12-9), or intramedullary devices. When possible, four to six screws should be placed on either side of the fracture using compression plates. Bone graft can be added as necessary. Medullary nailing is better suited to ulnar fractures due to the straightness of the shaft compared to the radius which is bowed (see Fig. 12-10). Also, the radial canal narrows in the mid shaft limit the diameter of the intramedullary nail. In children, intramedullary nailing was introduced for displaced fractures in 1984. Indications for intramedullary nailing in children include inability to maintain reduction with closed methods, fracture angulation >15 degrees, malrotation >30 degrees, lack of fracture apposition (see Fig. 12-11), and loss of the interosseous space.

Pediatric Monteggia fractures can be treated with closed reduction using a long-arm cast. In adults, open reduction and internal fixation is performed. Delay in reduction of the radial head can lead to articular deformity and nerve injury. A 3.5-mm plate and screws are used to reduce the ulnar fracture. If the radial head is unstable, the elbow is splinted in supination which is the position of stability. Similarly, Galeazzi fractures are reduced with plate and screw fixation of the radius. Ideally, the distal radioulnar joint should be reduced and fixed with K-wires (see Fig. 12-12). If the distal radioulnar joint is stable it can be splinted in supination.

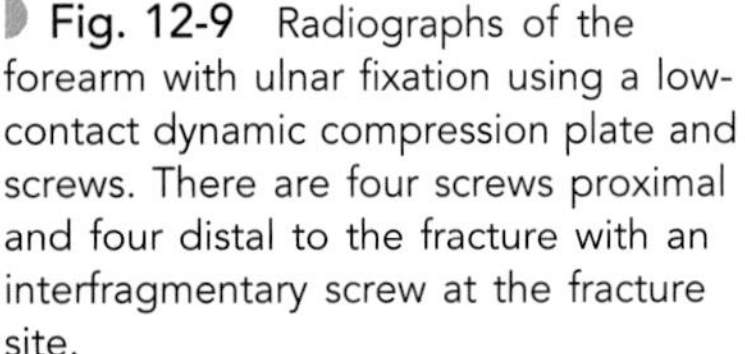

Fig. 12-9 Radiographs of the forearm with ulnar fixation using a low-contact dynamic compression plate and screws. There are four screws proximal and four distal to the fracture with an interfragmentary screw at the fracture site.

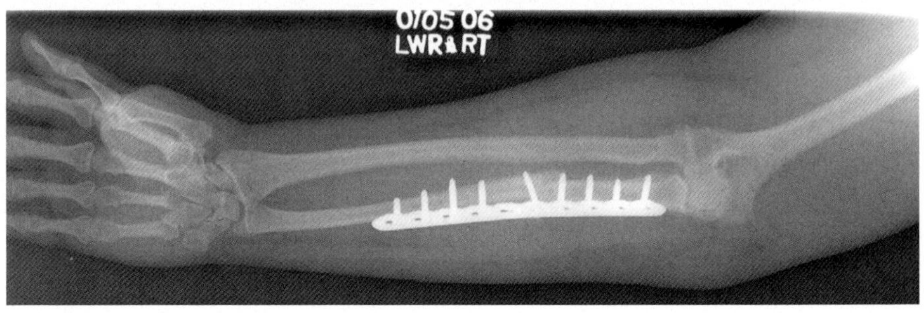

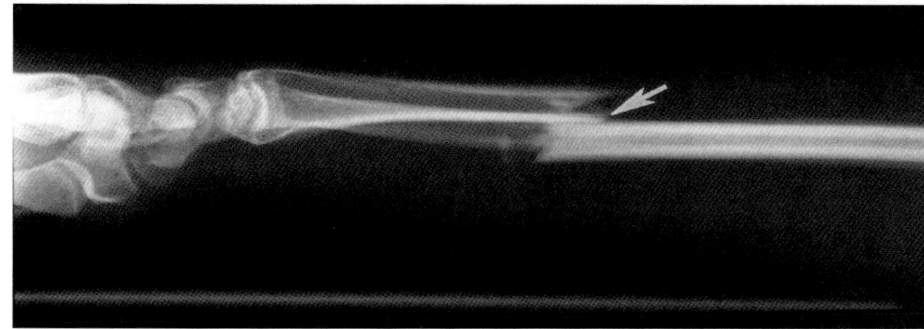

Fig. 12-11 Fractures of the mid radius and ulna with overlap and not fracture apposition (*arrow*) of the radius.

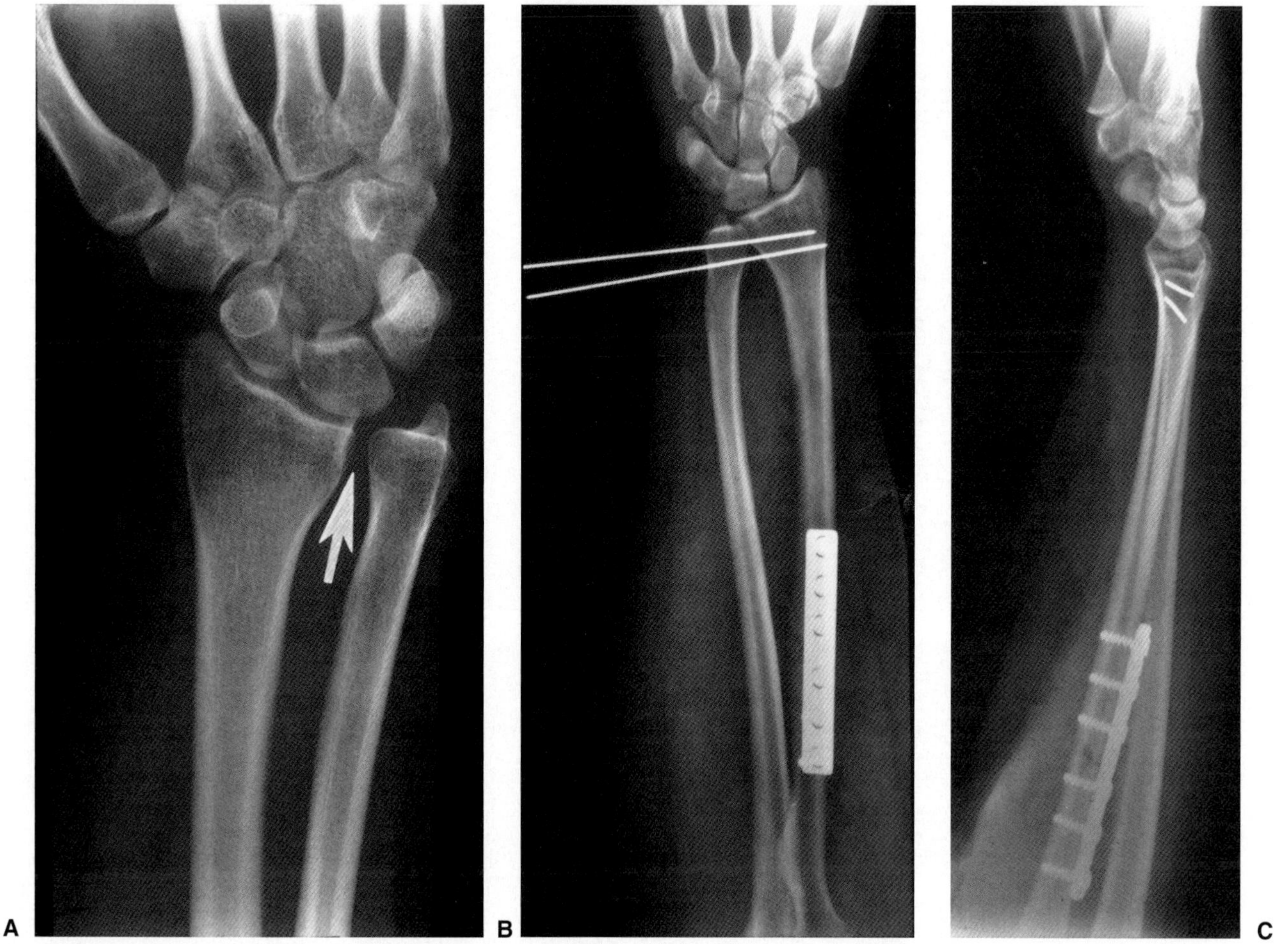

Fig. 12-12 A: Radiograph of the distal radioulnar joint with widening (*arrow*) associated with a radial fracture. Anteroposterior (AP) (B) and lateral (C) radiographs after plate and screw fixation of the radial fracture and K-wire fixation of the distal radioulnar joint.

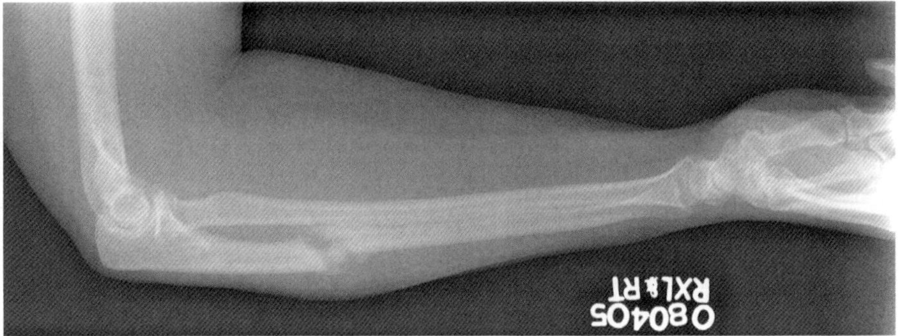

**Fig. 12-13** Lateral radiograph demonstrating nonunion of an ulnar fracture treated with closed reduction.

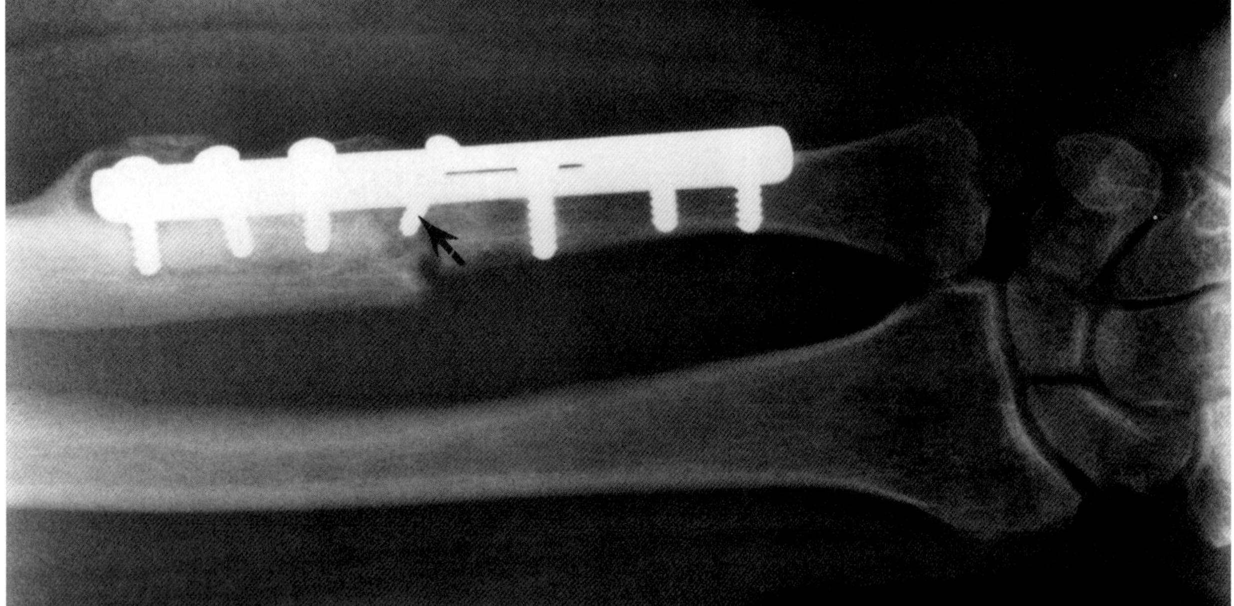

A

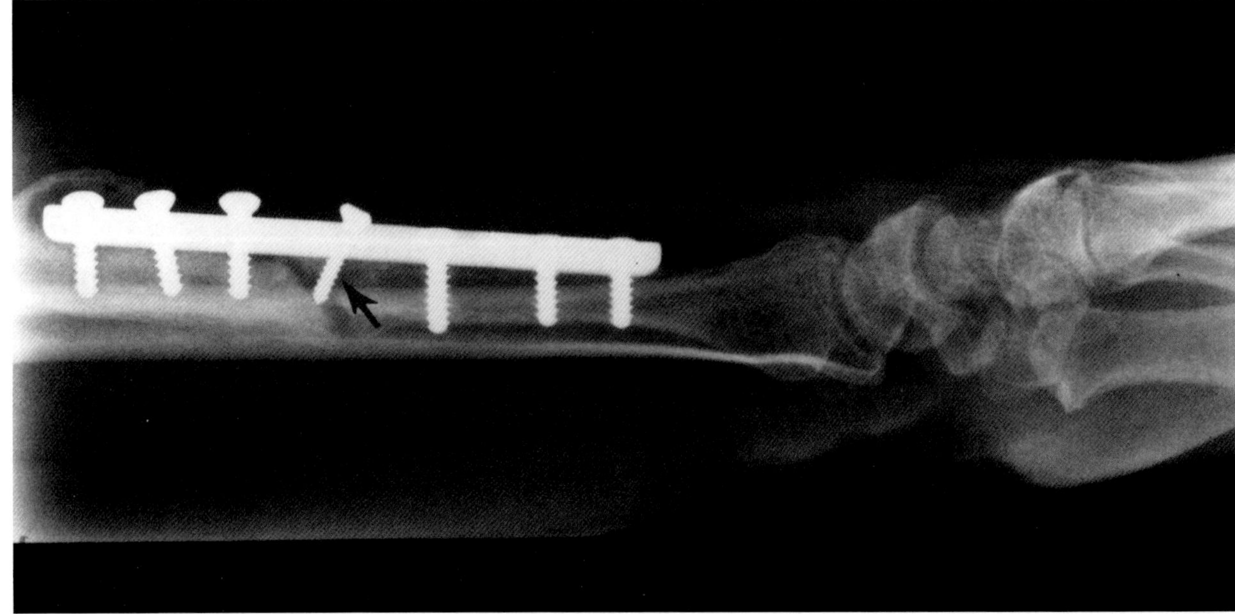

B

**Fig. 12-14** Posteroanterior (PA) (A) and lateral (B) radiographs demonstrate an ununited ulnar fracture with loosening of the plate. The lag screw (*arrow*) has pulled out.

## Suggested Reading

Anderson LD, Sisk D, Tooms RE, et al. Compression-plate fixation in acute diaphyseal fractures of the radius and ulna. *J Bone Joint Surg.* 1975;57A:287–297.

Bado JL. The Monteggia lesion. *Clin Orthop.* 1967;50:71–86.

Perron AD, Hersh RE, Brady WJ, et al. Orthopaedic pitfalls in the ED: Galeazzi and Monteggia fracture-dislocation. *Am J Emerg Med.* 2001;19:225–228.

## Imaging of Complications

Complications vary to some degree depending on category of injury (forearm diaphysis, Monteggia, Galeazzi). Functional outcome is related to the degree of reduction and ability to maintain forearm rotation and range of motion in the wrist and elbow. Treatment results can be categorized as follows:

**Excellent:** Fracture union with <10 degrees of loss of elbow and wrist motion and <25 degrees of loss of rotation

**Satisfactory:** Fracture union with <20 degrees of loss of elbow and wrist motion and <50 degrees of loss of rotation

**Unsatisfactory:** Fracture union with >30 degrees of motion loss in the wrist and elbow and >50 degrees of loss of rotation

**Failure:** Malunion, nonunion, or chronic osteomyelitis

Most complications occur with closed reduction (see Fig. 12-13). Fractures of the proximal radius and ulna result in permanent loss of rotation in 20% to 50% of patients.

Union typically occurs in 7 to 8 weeks. Union requiring longer than 3 months can be considered delayed union. Nonunion occurs in 12% of patients treated with closed reduction (Fig. 12-13), 7% of patients treated with intramedullary nails, and 2% to 3% of patients treated with plate and screw fixation (see Fig. 12-14). Serial radiographs may be sufficient for diagnosis. In certain cases, CT with reformatting is more useful for evaluating the degree of healing. Callus formation is often less obvious with rigid fixation with plate and screws.

Cross-union occurs in up to 11% of patients (see Fig. 12-15). The incidence is increased in patients with fractures at the same level, patients with high-velocity trauma, screws that extend too far beyond the cortex, and in patients with delayed operative treatment more than 2 weeks after injury. Cross-union results

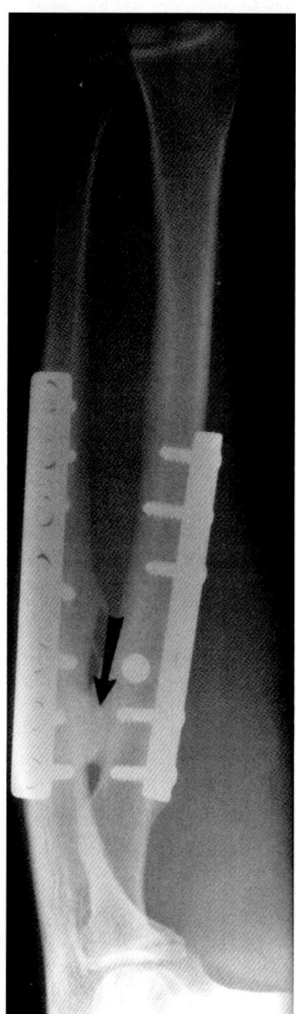


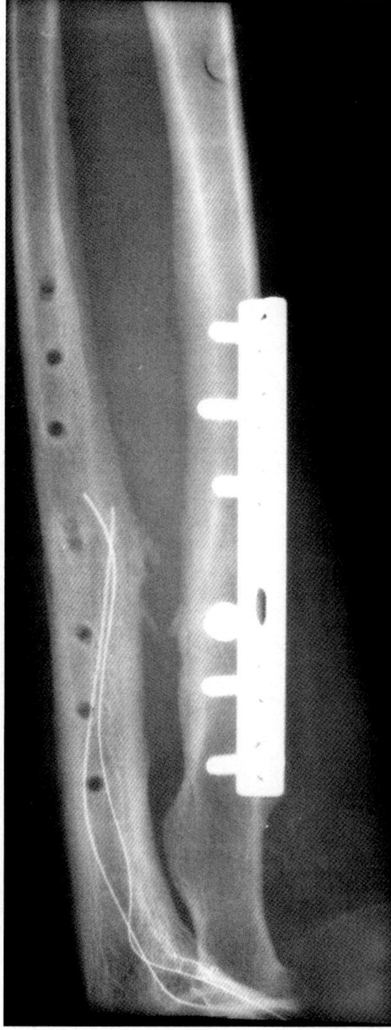


Fig. 12-15 **A:** Radiograph following plate and screw fixation of proximal forearm fractures with cross-union (bone formation across the interosseous membrane) (*arrow*). **B:** The ulnar plate was removed and the bony synostosis resected.

in limited, if any, rotational function. Radiographs (Fig. 12-15) may be diagnostic. Early changes are more easily appreciated with CT or MRI.

Nerve injuries may be transient or persistent. Injuries may be related to the initial trauma or surgical approach. Patients with Galeazzi fractures injure the anterior interosseous nerve, which results in loss of pinch due to paralysis of the flexor pollicus longus and flexor digitorum profundus. Patients with Monteggia lesions may injure the radial or ulnar nerves. Compartment syndrome is usually associated with complex injuries with extensive soft tissue damage. Associated nerve injury is not uncommon with compartment syndrome. The diagnosis may be made clinically in many cases. However, axial magnetic resonance (MR) images are useful to define the neural anatomy before exploration.

Refracture can occur following plate removal (see Fig. 12-16). The incidence is reported at 4% to 25%. Overall complications of plate removal are 10% to 20%.

Instability of the radial head or distal radioulnar joint is also a concern. Stress views of the elbow or CT evaluation of the

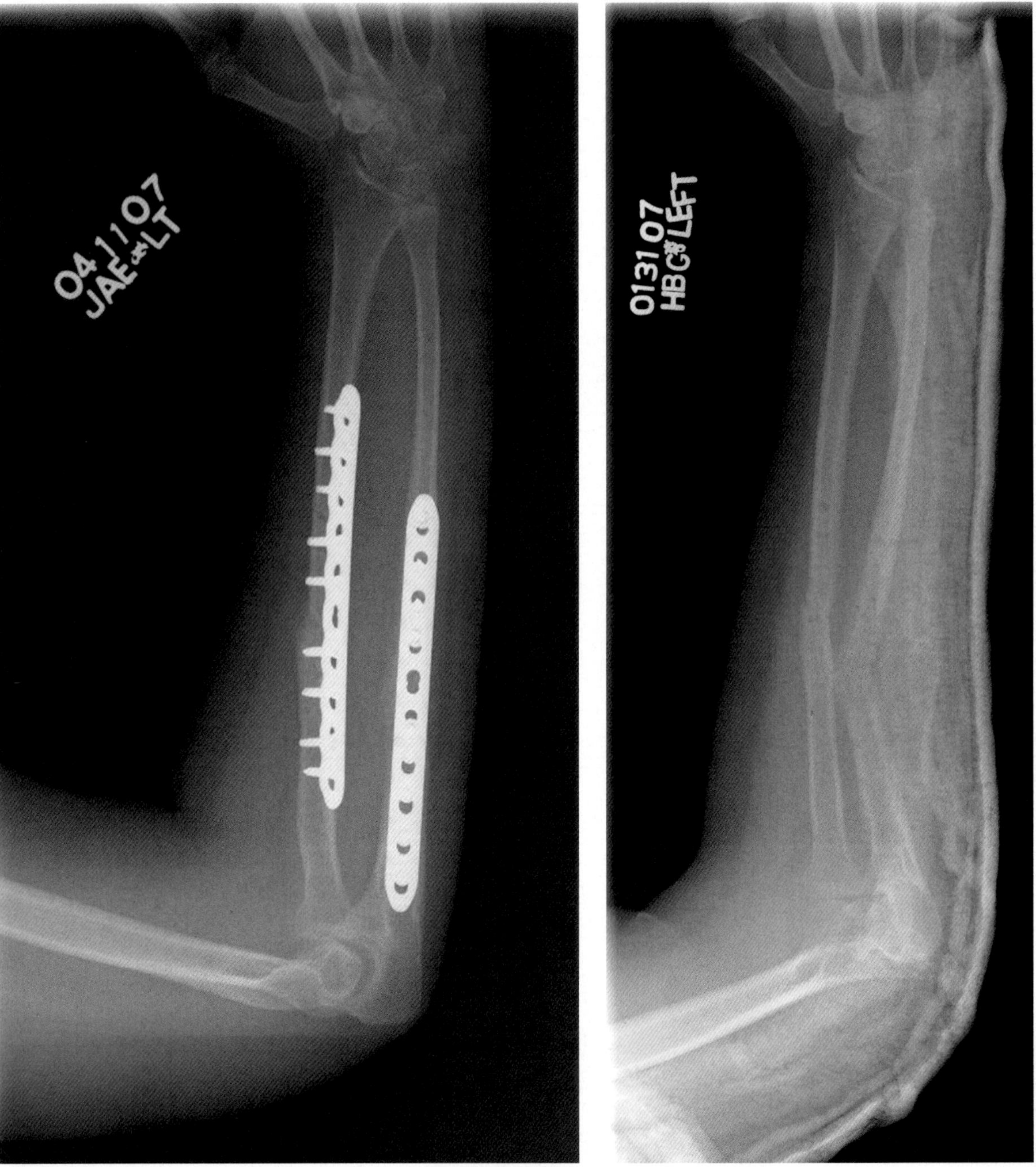


Fig. 12-16 Refracture following plate removal. A: Radiograph demonstrating plate and screw fixation of the radius and ulna. B: Following plate removal the ulna refractured requiring replating with bone graft.

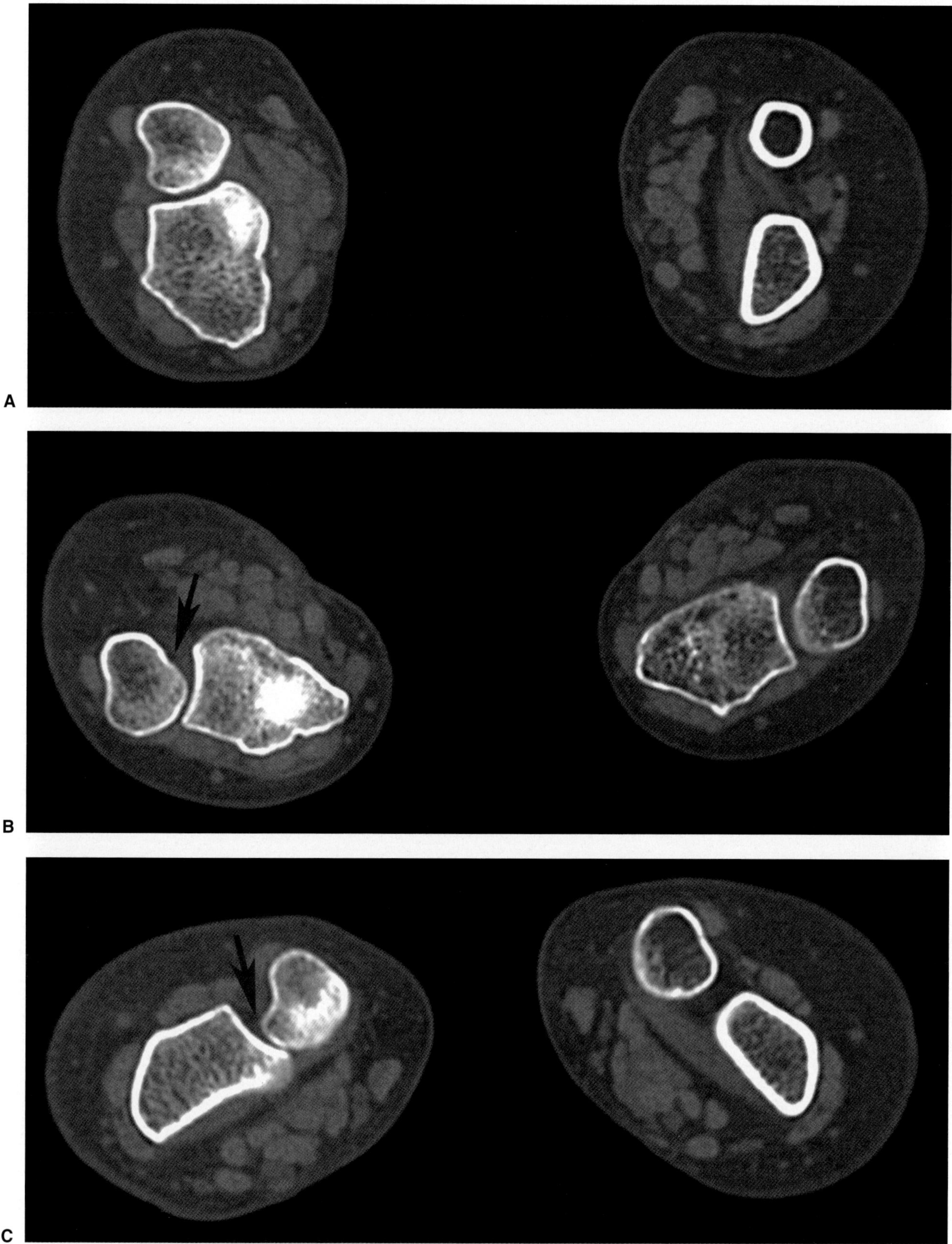


Fig. 12-17 Subluxation of the distal radioulnar joint. Axial computed tomographic (CT) images in neutral (A), pronation (B), and supination (C) demonstrate subluxation of the distal radioulnar joint (*arrow*).

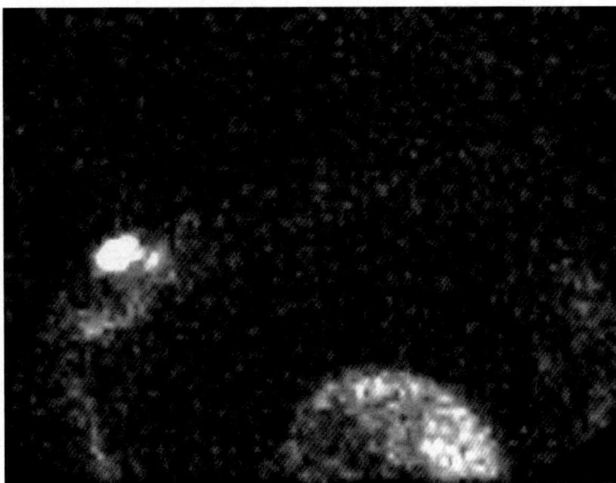

Fig. 12-18 Indium In 111–labeled white blood cell scan with the elbow flexed over the head demonstrating intense uptake in the proximal ulna due to an infected nonunion in a patient with plate and screw fixation.

distal radioulnar joint with the wrist in neutral, pronation, and supination will demonstrate the subluxation or dislocation (see Fig. 12-17).

Deep infection is more common with open wounds, but occurs in only approximately 0% to 3% of patients with closed fractures treated with internal fixation. Changes may be subtle radiographically. Radionuclide scans with indium-labeled white blood cells may be preferred over MRI in the presence of plate and screw fixation due to the image distortion in the area of potential infection (see Fig. 12-18).

## Suggested Reading

Anderson LD, Sisk D, Tooms RE. Compression-plate fixation in acute diaphyseal fractures of the radius and ulna. *J Bone Joint Surg*. 1975;57A:287–297.

Chapman MW, Gordon JE, Zissimos AC. Compression plate fixation of acute fractures of the diaphysis of the radius and ulna. *J Bone Joint Surg*. 1989;71A:159–169.

Jessing P. Monteggia lesions and their complication nerve damage. *Acta Orthop Scand*. 1975;46:601–609.

Jupiter JB, Ring D. Operative treatment of post-traumatic proximal radioulnar synostosis. *J Bone Joint Surg*. 1998; 80A:248–257.

Perron AD, Hersh RE, Brady WJ, et al. Orthopaedic pitfalls in the ED: Galeazzi and Monteggia fracture-dislocation. *Am J Emerg Med*. 2001;19:225–228.

# 13
# Hand and Wrist

The complex anatomy of the hand and wrist presents interesting imaging challenges regardless of the modality selected. Both detection and classification of pathology can be difficult. This chapter will focus on pre- and postoperative imaging of trauma, arthroplasty, and other common orthopaedic procedures used in the hand and wrist. Again, emphasis will be placed on procedures requiring orthopaedic implants or fixation devices.

## Trauma

Fractures and dislocations of the hand and wrist occur commonly. Common injury patterns, classifications, and methods of fixation will be discussed by anatomic region. Imaging of postoperative complications will be included with each major section.

### Distal Radius and Ulna

Fractures of the distal radius, with or without ulnar involvement, account for 15% to 25% of fractures in adults. There is a bimodal distribution with injuries due to high-velocity trauma in children and young adults and fractures due to minor falls in the elderly. The likelihood of sustaining a distal radial fracture is 6% in patients older than 80 years and 9% for white females older than 90 years. The mechanism of injury is a fall on the outstretched hand with varying degrees of osseous and soft tissue injury. Tears of the triangular fibrocartilage complex, scapholunate, and lunotriquetral ligaments are not uncommon. These injuries appear to be most common with radial fractures involving the lunate fossa. The importance of the radiolunate articulation has been emphasized by using a three-column approach. The lateral column is the osseous buttress of the wrist and includes the intracapsular ligaments. The intermediate column includes the radiolunate fossa and articulation that functions primarily for axial loading. The medial column functions for rotation and secondary load transmission. This column includes the triangular fibrocartilage complex (see Fig. 13-1).

#### Classification

There are numerous eponyms for fractures of the distal radius and ulna (see Chapter 2). Currently, these terms are less frequently used for describing fractures. It is more important to describe the relationships, degree and direction of displacement, and degree of comminution of the injury. Suspected soft tissue injuries should also be noted.

There have been numerous classification systems developed for the distal radius and ulna including the Mayo, Melone, Frykman, and AO (Arbeitsgemeinshaft fur Osteosynthesefragen) classifications. Classification systems should suggest treatment approaches, indicate prognosis, and demonstrate intra- and interobserver reliability. The Frykman classification is based on the extent of articular involvement and presence

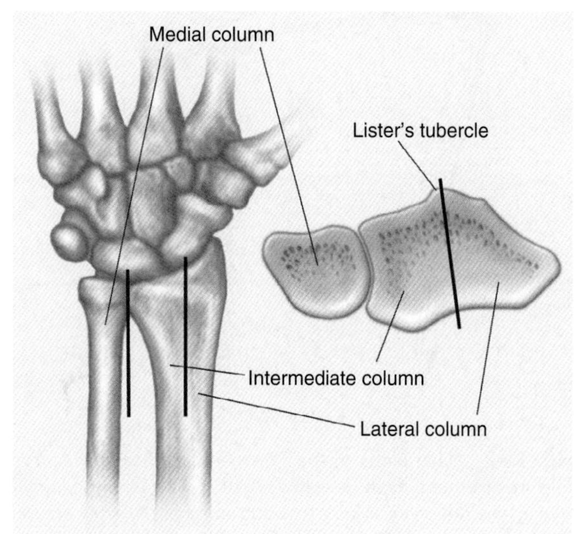


**Fig. 13-1** Illustration of the three columns of the wrist. The lateral column includes the lateral portion of the distal radius with the intracapsular ligaments; the intermediate column includes the medial portion of the radius, lunate fossa, and radiolunate articulation. This serves primarily for axial loading. The medial column includes the ulna and triangular fibrocartilage complex.

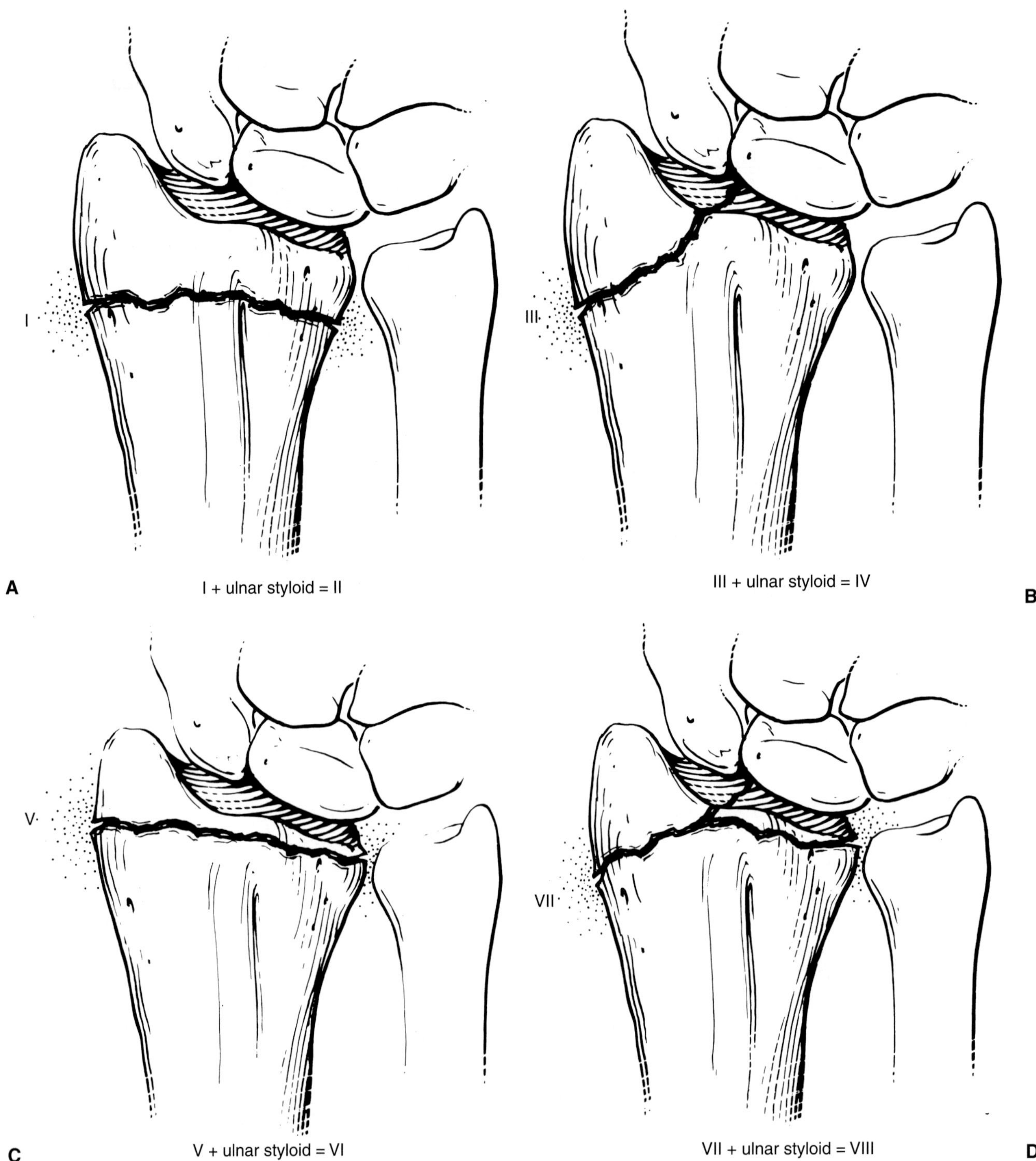


Fig. 13-2 Illustrations of the Frykman classification. A: Type I—extra-articular without ulnar styloid involvement, type II—extra-articular with ulnar styloid fracture. B: Type III—intra-articular involving the radiocarpal joint without an ulnar styloid fracture, type IV—same as type III with an ulnar styloid fracture. C: Type V—fracture involving the distal radioulnar joint without an ulnar styloid fracture, type VI—same as type V with an ulnar styloid fracture. D: Type VII—distal radial fracture involving both the radiocarpal and distal radiounlar joint without an ulnar styloid fracture, type VIII—same as type VII, but with an ulnar styloid fracture.

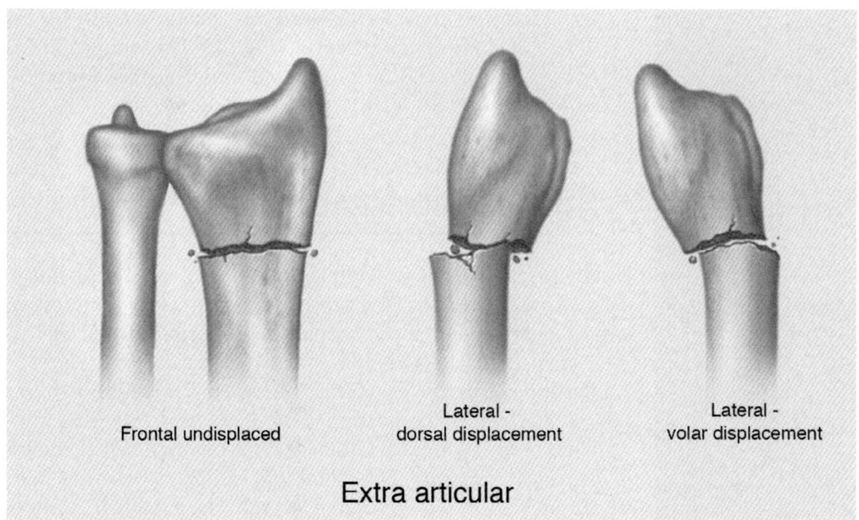


A

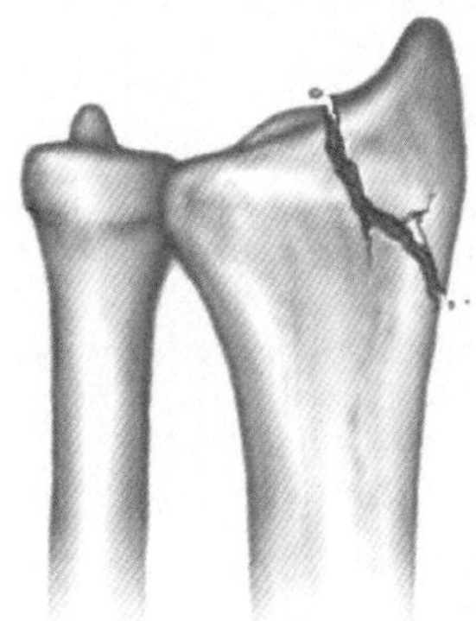

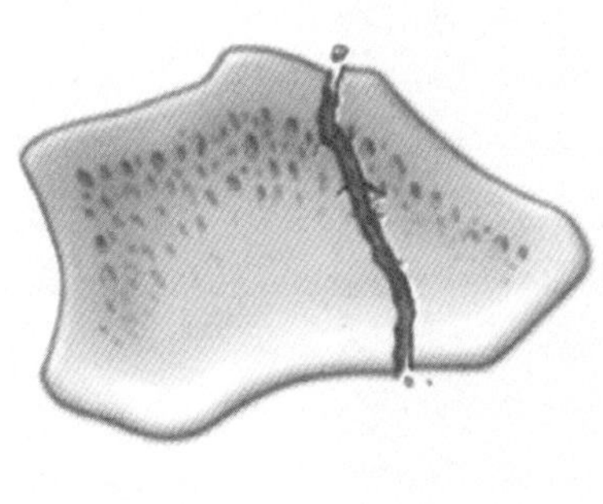

Simple articular

B

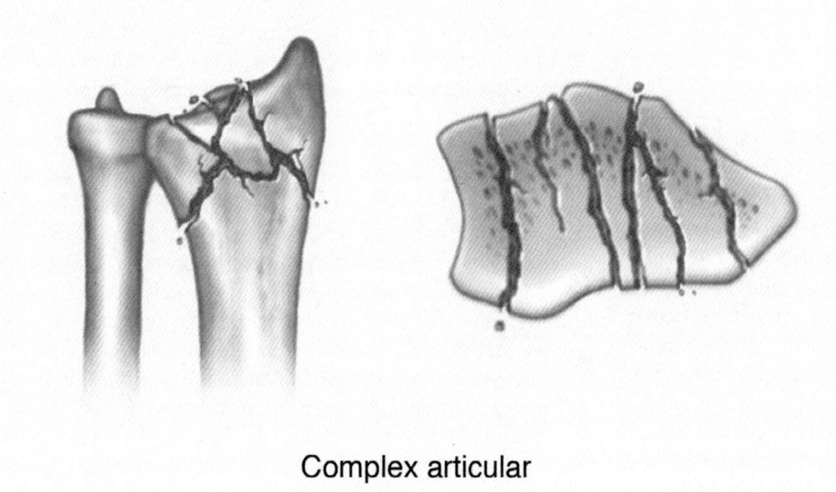


C

**Fig. 13-3** A: Illustration of extra-articular distal radial fractures. B: Illustration of simple articular distal radial fractures. C: Illustration of complex articular distal radial fractures. D: Radiograph of a simple articular fracture (*arrow*) entering the margin of the lunate fossa.

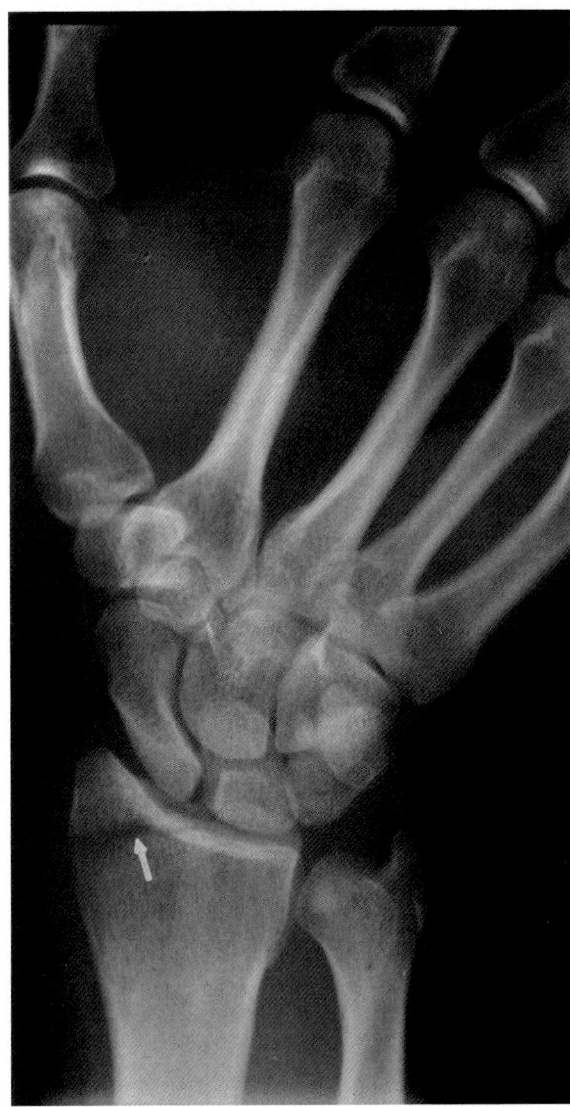


Fig. 13-3 *(Continued)*

or absence of an ulnar styloid fracture (see Fig. 13-2). This classification system does not address the direction and extent of displacement. The Mayo, Melone, and Association for Study of Internal Fixation (ASIF) systems consider the degree of comminution, degree of displacement, articular involvement, and mechanism of injury. The AO system considers extra-articular fractures. Type I, simple or partial articular type II, and complex or comminuted fractures are considered complete articular or type III. There are numerous subcategories for each type. The Mayo system is based on the degree of displacement and reducibility. For example, extra-articular fractures are subdivided into undisplaced (type I) and displaced (type II). Type III fractures are intra-articular and undisplaced and type IV are displaced articular fractures. Type IV is further subdivided based on being stable and reducible (type IVA), reducible and unstable (type IVB), and irreducible (type IVC). Studies using any of the above-mentioned systems fail to demonstrate highly reproducible inter- and intraobserver agreement for any of the classification methods discussed earlier. A more practical approach is to consider three major categories (see Fig. 13-3). These include extra-articular (Fig. 13-3A), simple articular (Fig. 3-13B and D), and complete articular (see Figs. 13-3C and 13-4).

## Suggested Reading


Andersen DJ, Blair WF, Steyers CM, et al. Classification of distal radius fractures: An analysis of interobserver reliability and intraobserver reproducibility. *J Hand Surg [Br]*. 1996;21A:574–582.

Barrett JA, Baron JA, Karagas MR, et al. Fracture risk in the US. Medicare population. *J Clin Epidemiol.* 1999;52:555–558.

Chen NC, Jupiter JB. Management of distal radial fractures. *J Bone Joint Surg*. 2007;89A:2051–2062.

Cooney WP III. Fractures of the distal radius. A modern treatment-based classification. *Orthop Clin North Am.* 1993; 24:211–216.

Flinkkila T, Nikkola-Sihto A, Kaarela O, et al. Poor interobserver reliability of AO classification of fractures of the distal radius. *J Bone Joint Surg*. 1998;80B:670–672.

Frykman G. Fractures of the distal radius including sequelae–shoulder hand-finger syndrome, disturbance of the distal radioulnar joint and impairment of nerve function. *Acta Orthop Scand Suppl.* 1967;108:1–55.

Geissler WB, Freeland AE, Savoie FJ, et al. Intracarpal soft-tissue lesions associated with fracture of the distal end of the radius. *J Bone Joint Surg*. 1996;78A:357–365.


### Imaging Techniques

Radiographic views of the wrist following trauma should include posteroanterior (PA), lateral, and at least one (we typically perform both) oblique. The scaphoid view is also frequently added. The forearm and elbow may also need to be imaged in patients with more proximal shaft fractures. Subtle fractures may be easily overlooked, especially in children and the elderly. Therefore, the pronator fat stripe should be carefully evaluated. If this structure is displaced or obliterated, it may be the only sign of a subtle distal radial fracture or physeal injury in a child (see Fig. 13-5). The navicular fat stripe will be reviewed in the carpal fracture section.

Additional studies may be required. Magnetic resonance imaging (MRI) may be useful in symptomatic patients without radiographic evidence of fractures (Fig. 13-5). MRI is also useful to evaluate associated or isolated soft tissue injuries in patients with wrist trauma. Once identified, computed tomography (CT) is often performed to properly classify the injury and provide a map for treatment planning (Fig. 13-4). CT images are reformatted in the coronal and sagittal planes. Three-dimensional reconstructions can also be obtained.

## Suggested Reading


Berquist TH, Trigg SD. Hand and wrist. In: Berquist TH, ed. *Imaging atlas of orthopaedic appliances and prostheses*. New York: Raven Press; 1995:831–921.

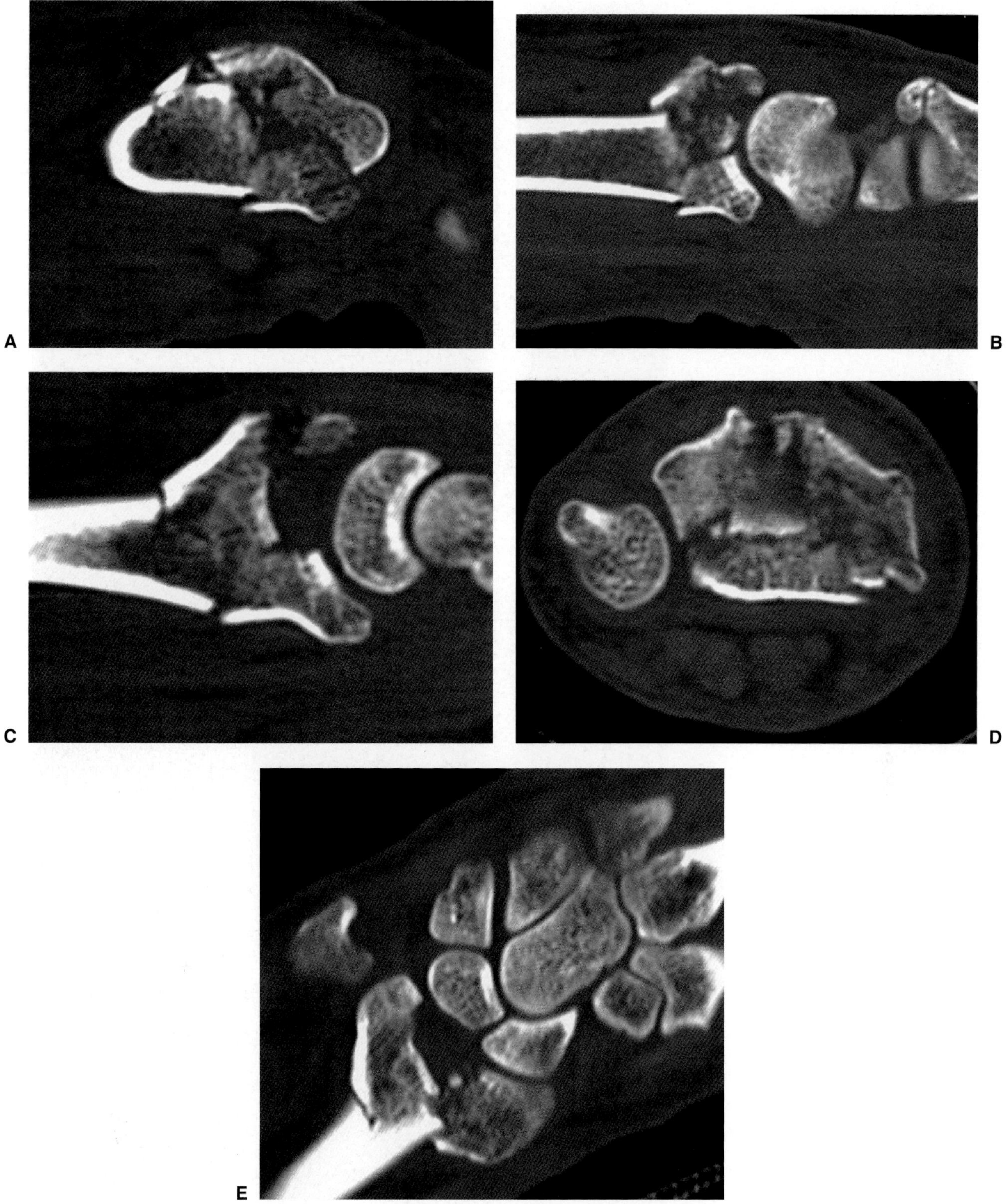


Fig. 13-4 Complete (complex) articular fracture. Sagittal (A to C), axial (D), and coronal (E) CT images of a complex distal radial fracture with dorsal impaction or the distal fragment (B), fragmentation of the radial styloid (A) and marked articular step off (C and E) of the lateral and intermediate columns. There is comminution of the metaphysis and articular surface (D).

**Fig. 13-5** Pronator fat stripe. Lateral radiograph (**A**) and sagittal T1-weighted magnetic resonance (MR) image (**B**) demonstrating the normal position and appearance of the pronator fat stripe (*arrows*). Lateral radiograph (**C**) in a patient with an occult distal radial fracture and a dorsal triquetral fracture (*arrowhead*). Note the displaced and partially obliterated fat stripe (*arrow*). Coronal T1- (**D**) and sagittal T2- (**E**) weighted images demonstrate the fracture (*arrows*) and displaced fat stripe (*open arrows*).

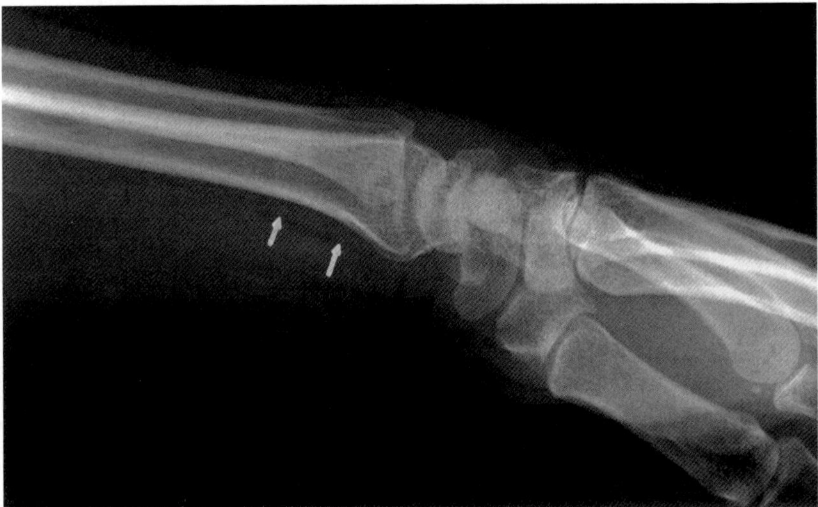


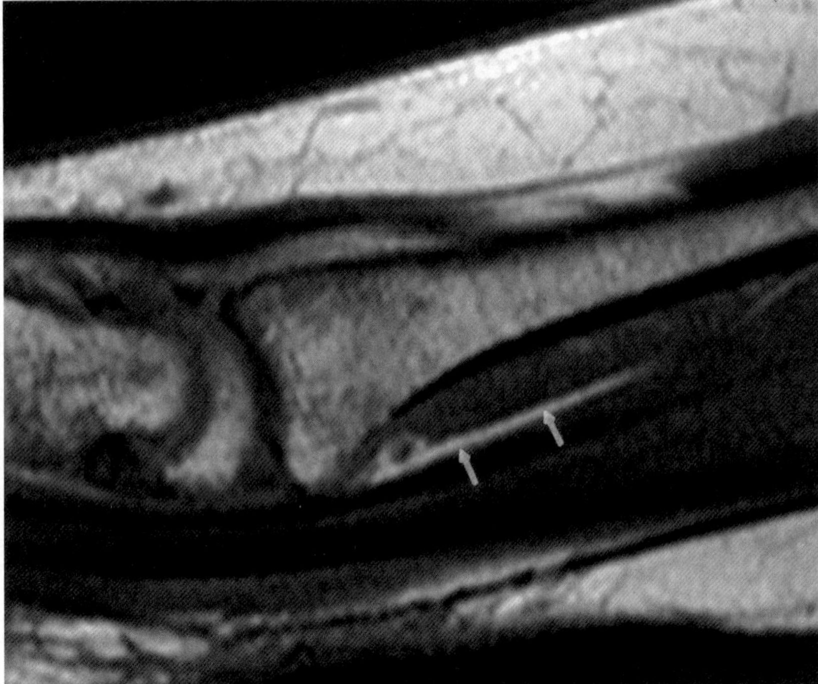


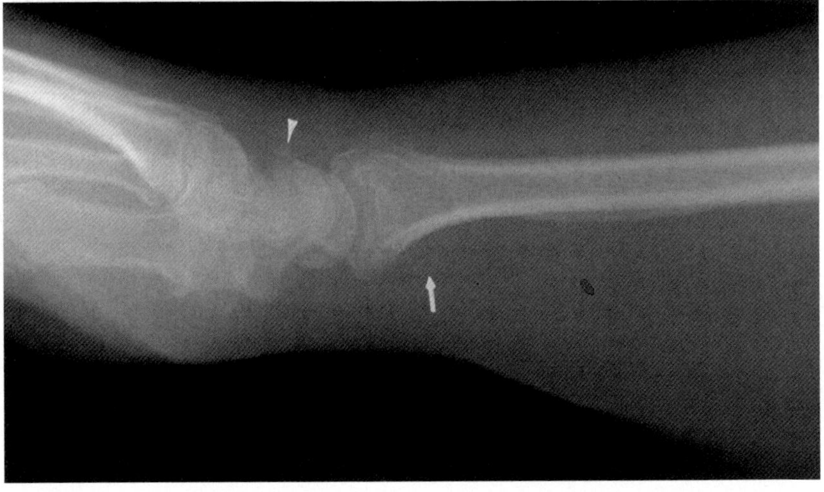

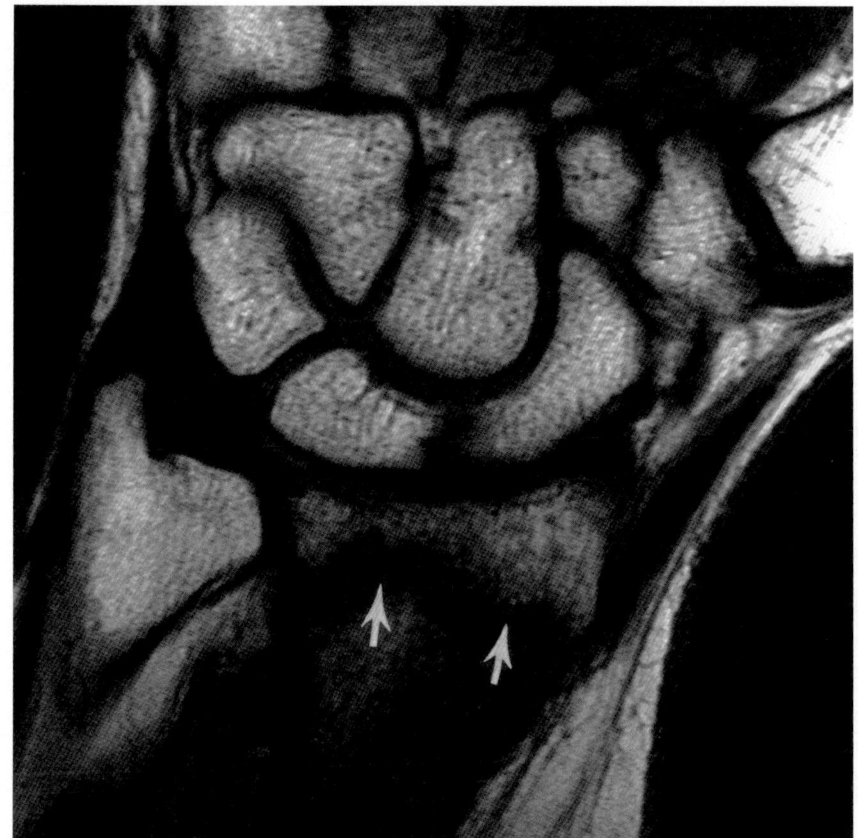


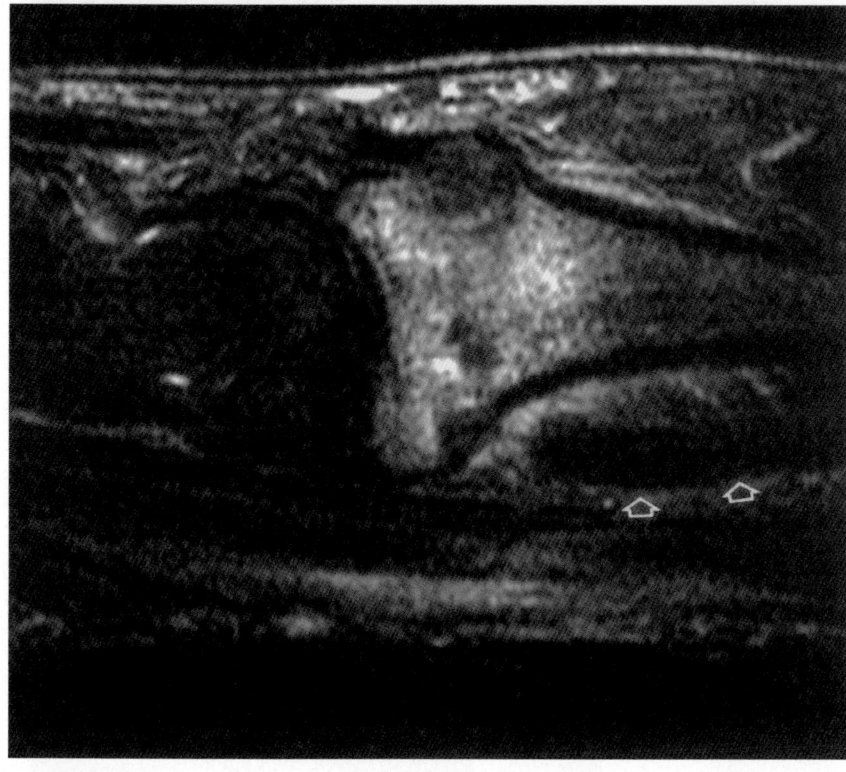


Fig. 13-5 *(Continued)*

## Treatment Options

Treatment options include closed reduction with cast immobilization, external, and internal fixation. Treatment goals include anatomic reduction, maintenance of radial length, and neutral ulnar length.

### Closed Reduction and Immobilization

Undisplaced extra-articular or simple articular fractures can be managed with closed reduction and cast immobilization. Circular or bivalved casts (see Chapter 2) may lead to compartment syndrome. Therefore, padded splints with the wrist in slight palmar flexion and neutral rotation are most often used. Displaced extra-articular or simple articular fractures can also be managed with closed reduction, but require fracture manipulation to achieve anatomic reduction. This may require finger traction before application of sugar-tong splints. Surgical intervention is indicated if reduction cannot be maintained as demonstrated on follow-up radiographs. In this setting, percutaneous pinning with K-wires or plate and screw fixation may be required.

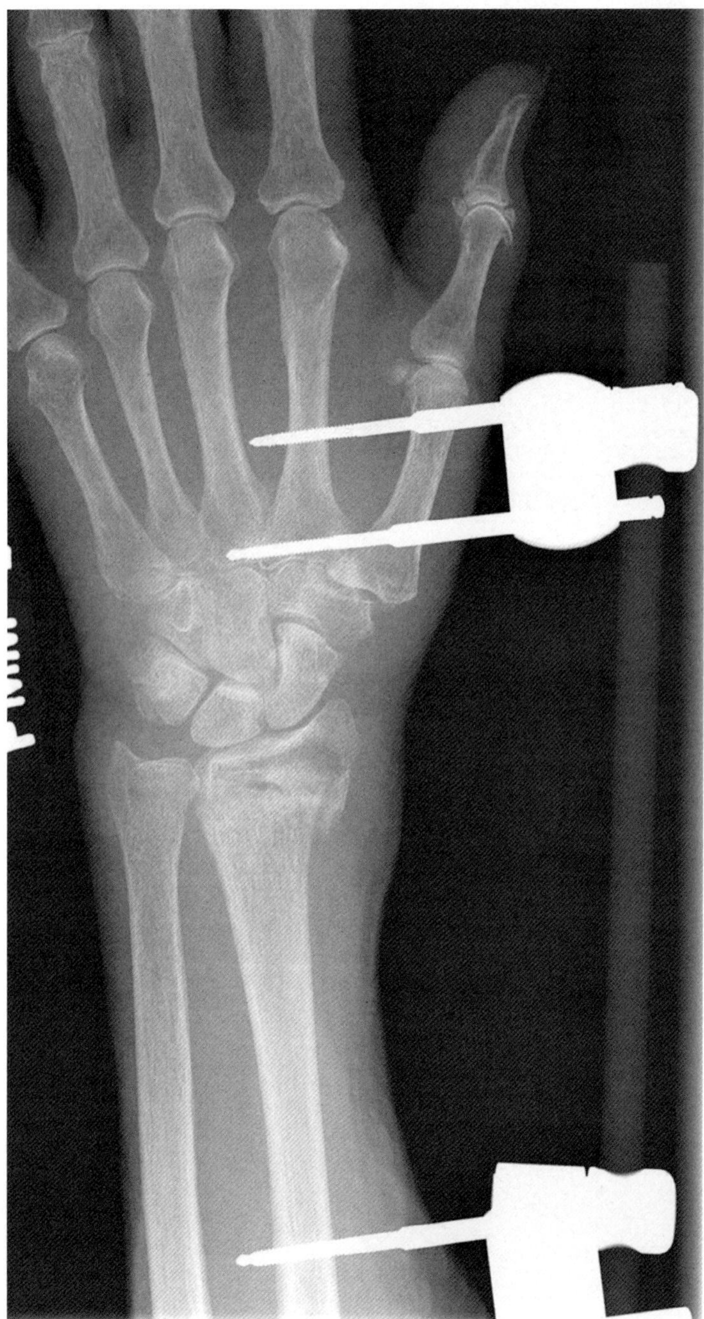


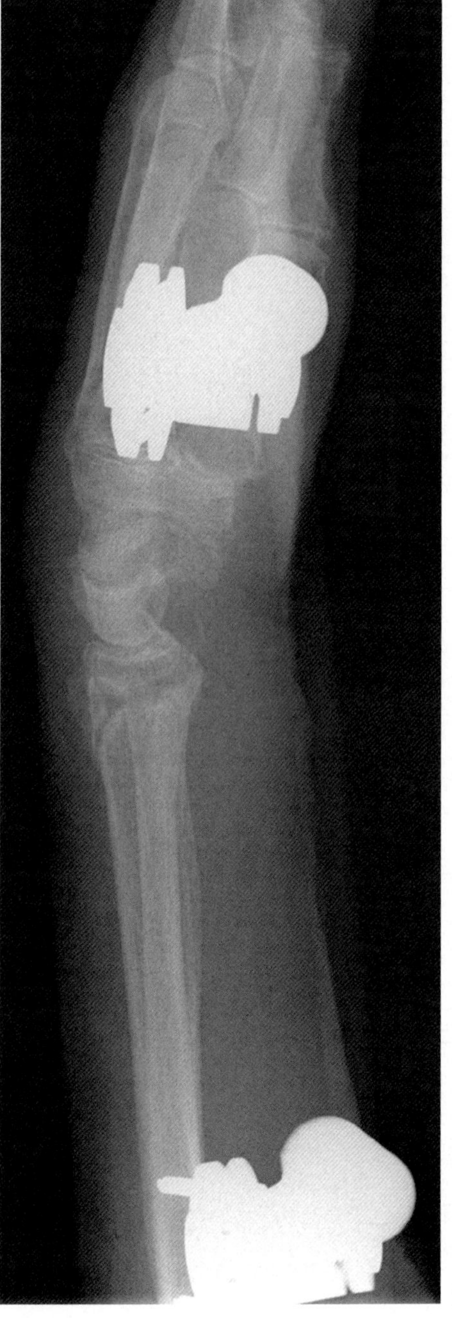


Fig. 13-6 Anteroposterior (AP) (A) and lateral (B) radiographs following external fixation of a complex distal radial fracture using a static fixation system with a radiolucent bar. The radial length is maintained, although there is slight reduction in the radial inclination angle.

## External Fixation

External fixation is useful for unstable distal radial fractures and provides a less invasive option to internal fixation. Static and dynamic devices along with radiolucent external fixators are available (see Figs. 13-6 and 13-7). Selection of the external fixation device is based on the perceived difficulty in maintaining radial length and alignment as well as surgical preference.

Initial fracture reduction can be accomplished with finger traction using 10 to 15 lb of weight. External fixation is then applied using four to five pins. Dynamic devices allow wrist motion, which should be started when tolerated to reduce stiffness and adhesive capsulitis following treatment.

## Internal Fixation

Internal fixation with open reduction is indicated for unstable fractures (does not adequately reduce with closed methods or reduction cannot be maintained). As noted earlier, percutaneous pins can be used for extra-articular fractures with dorsal or volar displacement and simple articular fractures (see Fig. 13-8). Volar plate and screw fixation is used when there is comminution of the metaphysis or there are multiple articular fragments (see Fig. 13-9).

Depressed central fragments in the lunate or scaphoid fossa should be evaluated with CT and repositioned using bone graft to reestablish the articular surface. Stabilization can be established with percutaneous pins or volar plate and screws.

A

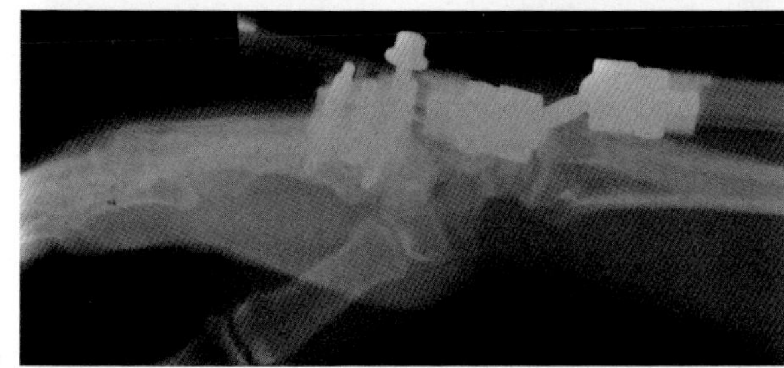

B

**Fig. 13-7** Anteroposterior (AP) (**A**) and lateral (**B**) radiographs following external fixation with a four-pin Orthofix external fixation system that allows motion at the wrist. The complex distal radial fracture is reduced with length and alignment maintained. There is also an ulnar styloid fracture.

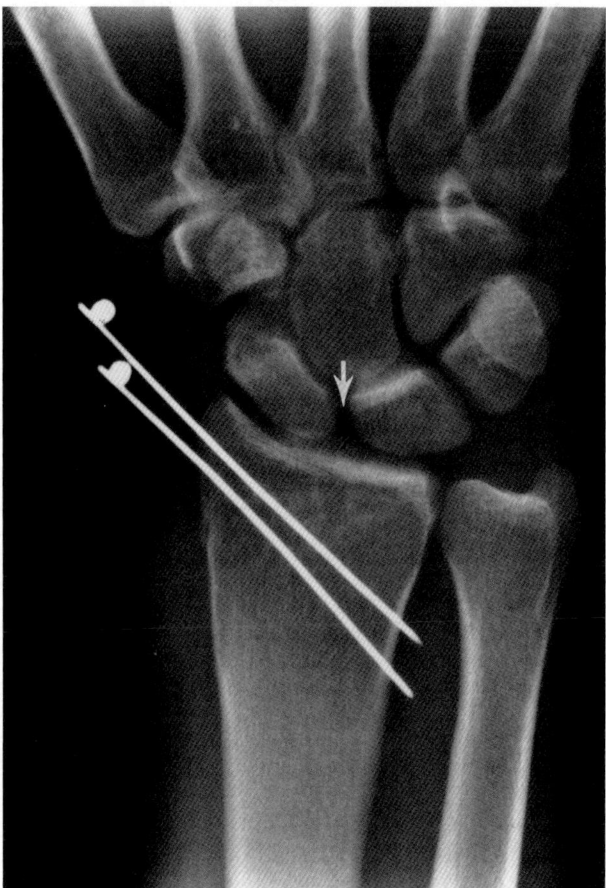

**Fig. 13-8** Posteroanterior (PA) radiograph following percutaneous pinning of an undisplaced radial styloid fracture with two K-wires. Note the widened scapholunate space (*arrow*) due to an associated scapholunate ligament tear. The fracture line had entered the lunate fossa.

## Suggested Reading


Chen NC, Jupiter JB. Management of distal radial fractures. *J Bone Joint Surg*. 2007;89A:2051–2062.

Chung KC, Watt AJ, Kotsis SV, et al. Treatment of unstable distal radial fractures with the volar locking plate system. *J Bone Joint Surg*. 2006;88A:2687–2694.

Thomas S, John C, Hohnny TP. Intra-articular distal radial fractures–external fixation or conventional closed reduction? *J Orthop*. 2007;4:39–43.

Werber KD, Raeder F, Brauer RB, et al. External fixation of distal radial fractures: Four compared to five pins: A randomized prospective study. *J Bone Joint Surg*. 2003;85A:660–666.


### Imaging of Distal Radial Fracture Complications

Postoperative radiographs should be consistently evaluated with certain features in mind. Radial length, alignment, articular deformity, radial inclination angle, palmar tilt, and findings that suggest associated ligament injury should all be assessed on each follow-up radiograph.

Radial length should be within 1 mm or the ulnar length, although some accept up to 5 mm of radial shortening (see Fig. 13-10). The normal radial inclination angle is 22 to 25 degrees. Following distal radial fracture, the fragments should be reduced to result in a radial inclination angle of 15 degrees or more (see Fig. 13-11). On lateral radiographs, the normal distal radial articular surface has a volar or palmar tilt of 11 to 12 degrees. Depending on the degree of dorsal or volar impaction, this angle can be increased, neutral, or reversed. Dorsal angulation of up to 15 degrees and increased volar tilt of 20 degrees are considered acceptable reductions (Fig. 13-11B). Articular deformity or step off should be <2 mm. This can be difficult to evaluate on radiographs. CT with reformatting (Fig. 13-4) is optimal for evaluation of articular fragments and involvement of three columns (Fig. 13-1).

Radial height and shift should also be evaluated (see Figs. 13-12 and 13-13). Radial height is measured by a line

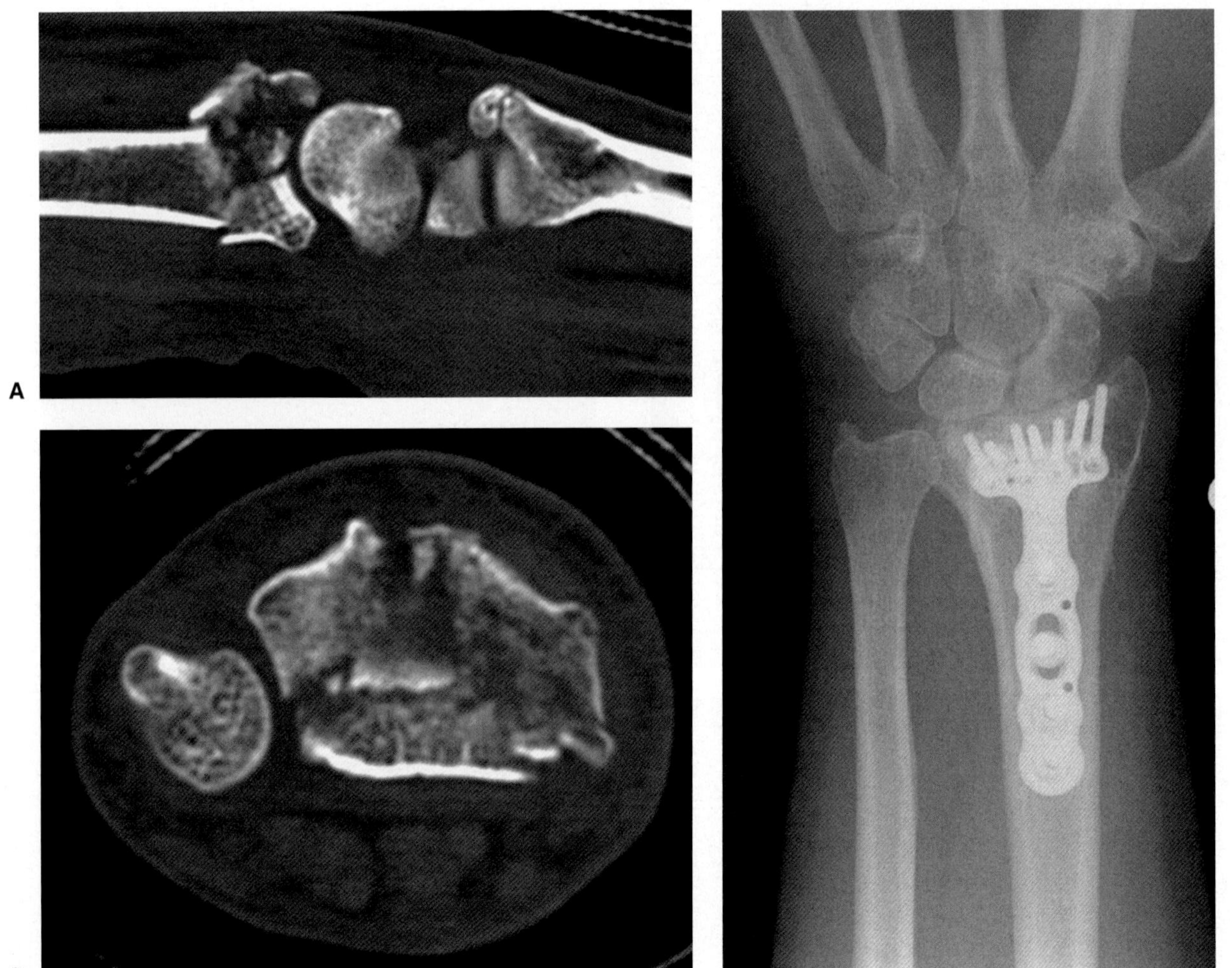


Fig. 13-9 Sagittal (A) and axial (B) computed tomographic (CT) images of a complex distal radial fracture involving the radiocarpal and distal radioulnar joints. Anteroposterior (AP) (C) and lateral (D) radiographs following reduction with a volar plate and screws. E: Acumed Acu-Loc targeted distal radius plate with locking screws. (Courtesy of Acumed, Hillsboro, Oregon.)

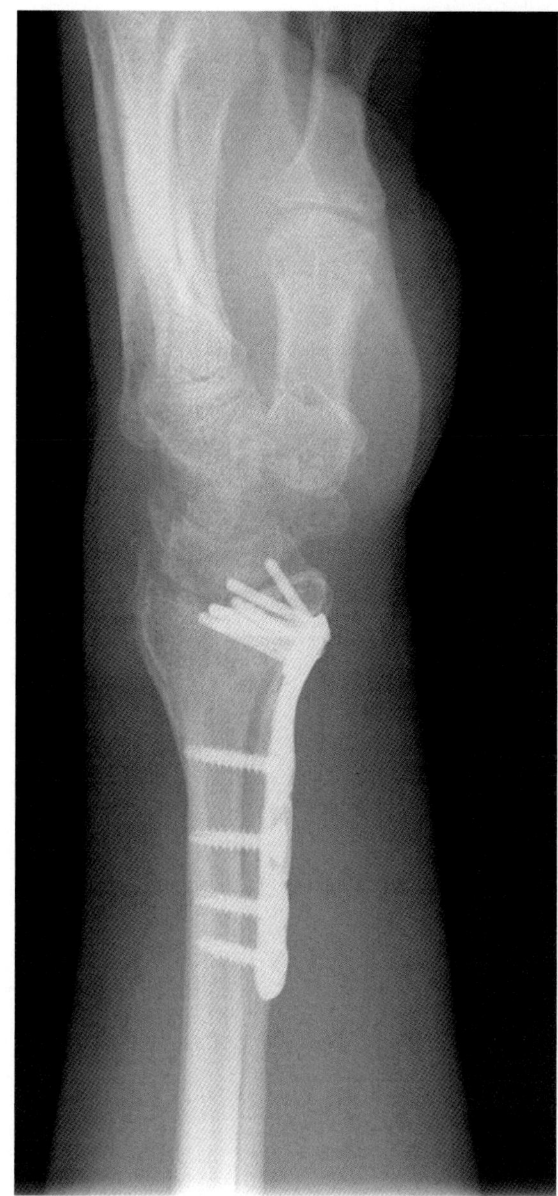
D

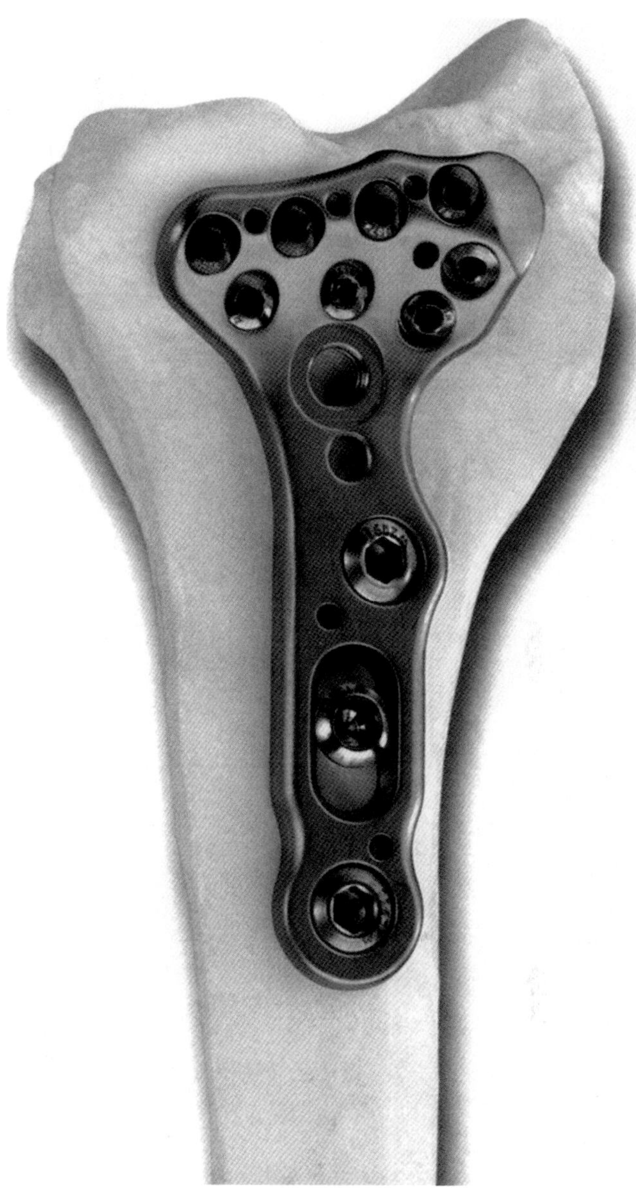
E

Fig. 13-9 *(Continued)*

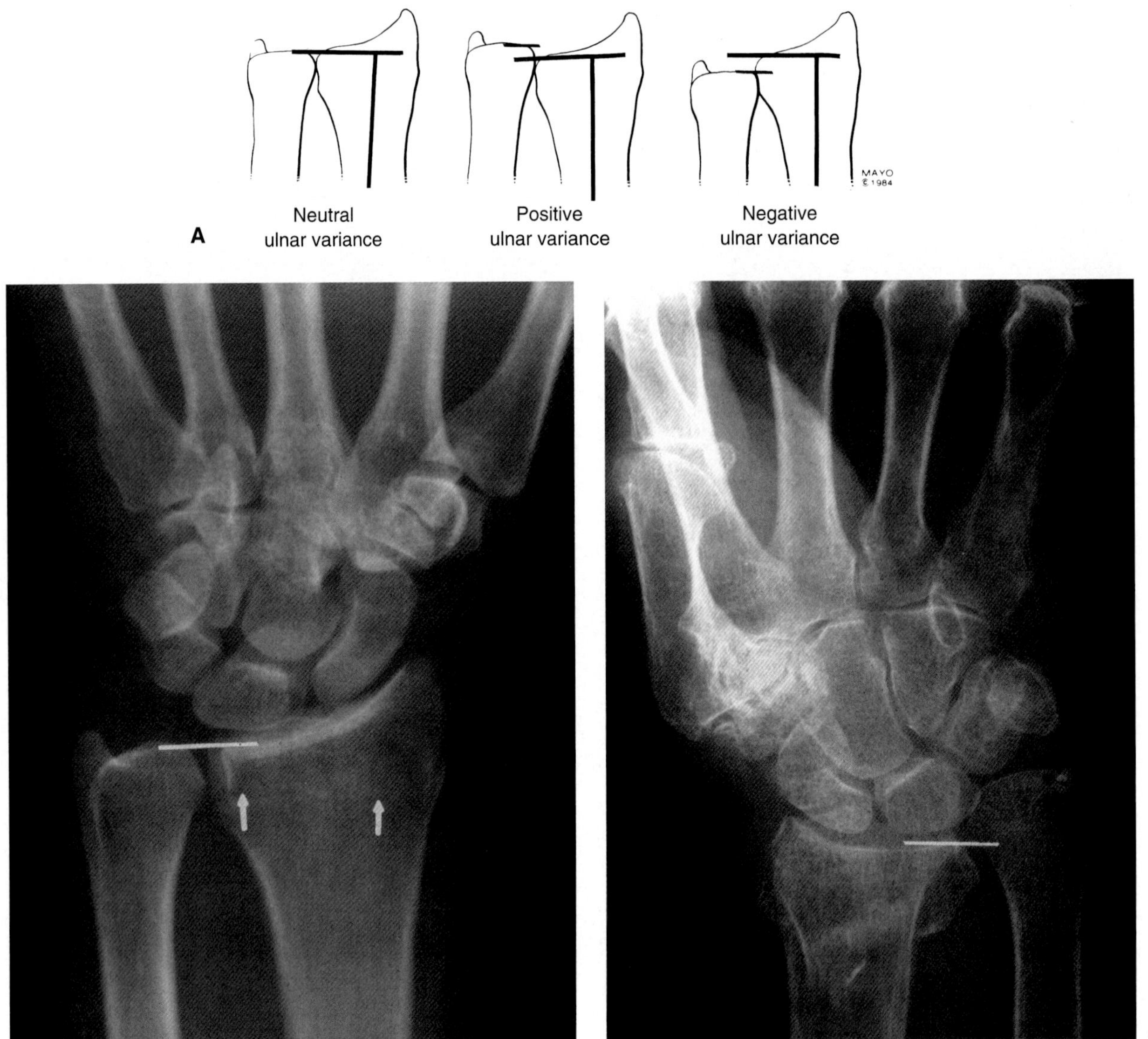


**Fig. 13-10** Radial length. **A:** Illustration of neutral, positive, and negative ulnar variance. **B:** Posteroanterior (PA) radiograph demonstrating a distal radial fracture (*arrows*) entering the distal radioulnar joint. Radial length (*line*) is maintained. **C:** Complex impacted distal radial fracture with marked loss of radial length (*line*) and >1 cm of ulnar positive variance.

perpendicular to the radial shaft and a parallel line along the radial styloid tip. This is normally 13.5 mm ± 3.8 mm (Fig. 13-12).

The carpal bones should be in normal position with parallel joint surfaces that normally measure approximately 2 mm. Asymmetry or widening, specifically at the scapholunate or lunotriquetral articulations, suggests associated ligament injury (Fig. 13-8). Fractures of the ulnar styloid or medial column and significant differences in radial and unlar length (Fig. 13-1) may be associated with triangular fibrocartilage complex injuries (Figs. 13-7 and 13-10C).

Complications related to distal radial fractures may be related to the injury or treatment method selected. Complications are common and classically divided into early and late complications (see Table 13-1).

Imaging of complications related to position of fragments (Figs. 13-10 to 13-13), loss of reduction, malunion, nonunion, and shortening (see Fig. 13-14) can be accomplished with serial PA and lateral radiographs. Nonunion can be more effectively evaluated with CT. CT can demonstrate the extent of callus, bone loss, and fragment position more easily than radiographs (see Fig. 13-15). Implant failure can also be effectively evaluated radiographically and with CT (see Figs. 13-15 and 13-16).

Osseous complications vary with treatment approaches. For example, the mean loss of radial length in patients with Colles' type fractures was 3 mm in patients treated with closed reduction. Dorsal angulation increased by 7 degrees in patients treated with closed reduction. Rigid fixation with external or internal fixation provides more stability.

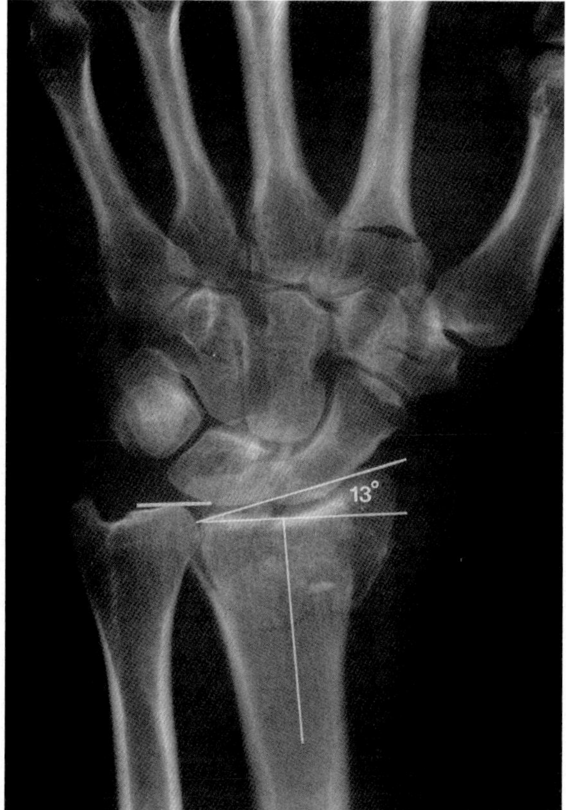


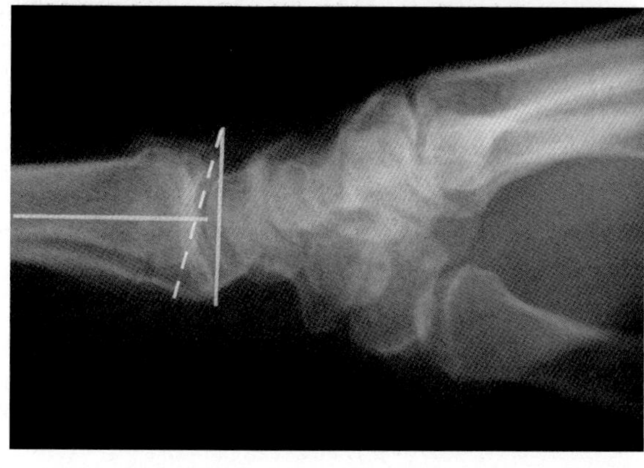


**Fig. 13-11** Radial inclination angle. **A:** Posteroanterior (PA) radiograph demonstrating an intra-articular fracture with loss of length (*ulnar line*) and a reduced radial inclination angle of 13 degrees (angle formed by a line perpendicular to the radial shaft and a line from the styloid tip to the ulnar margin of the distal radius, normal 22 to 25 degrees, acceptable ≥15 degrees). **B:** Lateral radiograph demonstrating dorsal impaction of the radius with neutral palmar tilt. *Broken line* demonstrates the normal palmar (volar) tilt of 11 to 12 degrees.

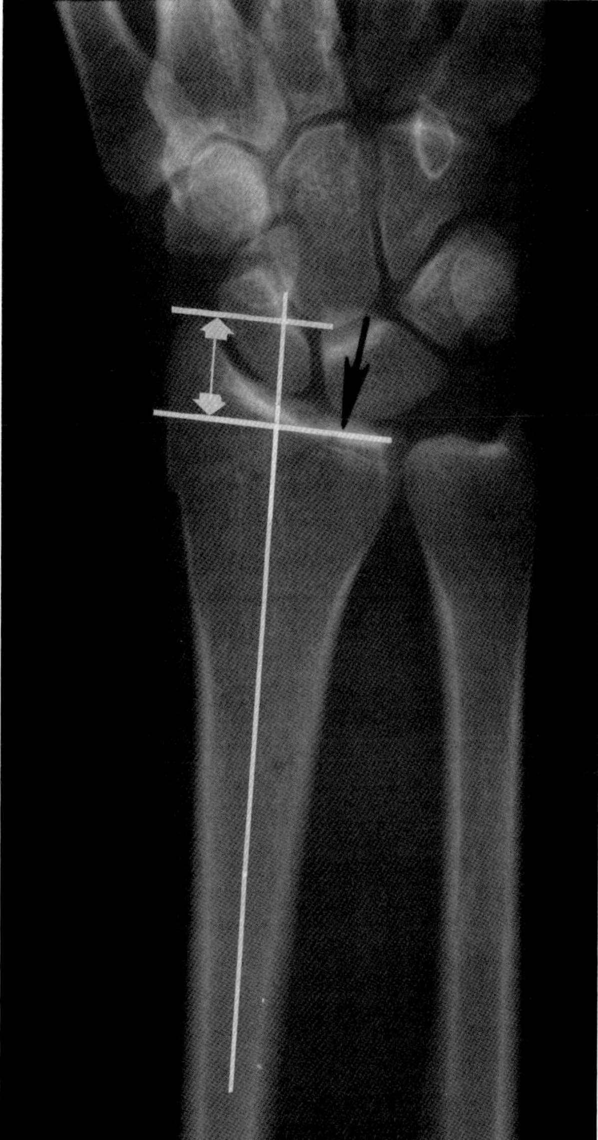

**Fig. 13-12** Radial height. Posteroanterior (PA) radiograph demonstrating a simple articular fracture (*arrows*) with measurement of radial height. A line is drawn perpendicular to the radial shaft at the ulnar articular margin of the distal radius. A second line is drawn parallel to this. The distance between the lines (*double arrow*) is the radial height (normal 13.5 mm ± 3.8 mm or 9.7 to 17.3 mm).

External fixation is associated with certain complications. Although often minor, complications occur in up to 67% of patients. Pin tract infections occur commonly (12% to 38%) but can usually be treated with local wound care and antibiotics. Sixteen percent of patients develop carpal instability and pin loosening occurs in 8% of patients. Imaging of these complications can usually be accomplished with serial radiographs. MRI or CT may be required to evaluate deep infection.

Volar plate fixation (Figs. 13-9 and 13-16) may cause irritation of the flexor carpi radialis and flexor pollicis longus. Dorsal screw prominence may result in extensor tendon irritation and retinacular scarring.

Ligament injuries are frequently associated with distal radial fractures. The scapholunate and lunotriquetral ligaments are most commonly involved. Scapholunate ligament injuries have been reported in up to 54% of patients with distal

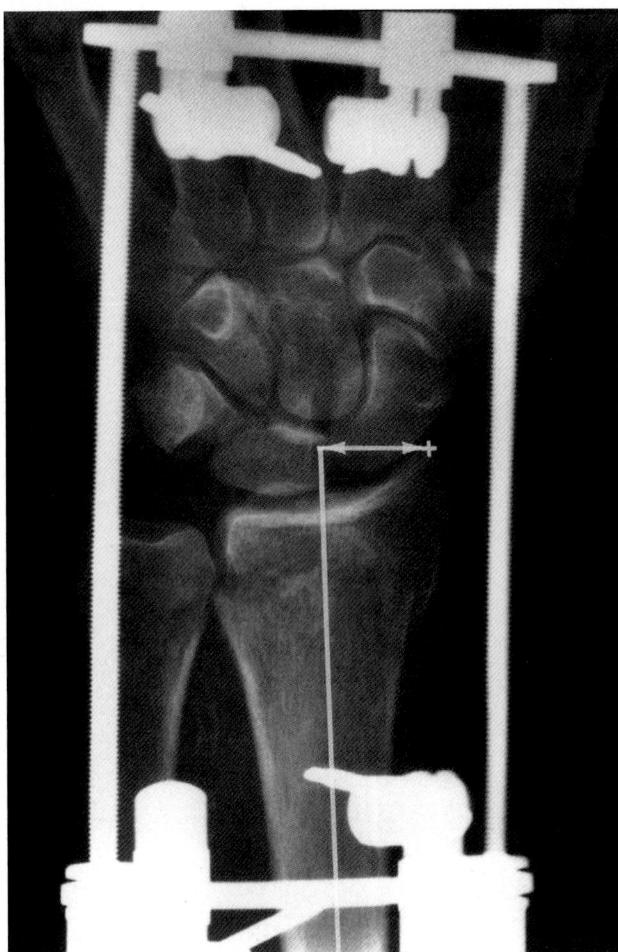

Fig. 13-13 Radial shift. This measures the offset of radial fragments from the central axis. Posteroanterior (PA) radiograph with external fixation of a distal radial fracture. The distance of a line down the center of the radial shaft to the styloid tip in this case measures the degree of shift. Displacement of >1 mm is considered significant.

radial fractures. Widening of the intercarpal joint spaces may be evident on radiographs (Fig. 13-8). More subtle injuries can be evaluated with motion studies using fluoroscopy and conventional or MR arthrography.

Neural injury may be related to the treatment approach or injury. Compressive neuropathies occur in the median nerve in 4%, and ulnar and radial neuropathies in <1% of patients treated with closed reduction. Transient paresthesias occur in 2% to 25% of patients. Soft tissue injuries (tendon rupture, tendon entrapment, compartment syndrome, and neural injuries) are optimally imaged with MRI. However, MRI may not be useful depending on the type and location of implants in relation to the structures in question. Subluxation of the distal radioulnar joint can be evaluated with CT in the axial plane with the wrist in neutral, pronation, and supination.

Complex regional pain syndrome or reflex sympathetic dystrophy can be evaluated with radiographs or three-phase bone scans (see Fig. 13-17). Arthrosis commonly occurs following distal radial fracture, especially those involving the

**Table 13-1**

DISTAL RADIAL FRACTURE COMPLICATIONS

| EARLY | LATE |
|---|---|
| Loss of reduction | Loss of reduction/malunion or nonunion |
| Dislocation/subluxation distal radioulnar joint | Shoulder-hand syndrome<br>Median nerve compression |
| Contusion, laceration, or entrapment of nerves, vessels, and tendons | Tendinitis or stenosing tenosynovitis<br>Contractures<br>Complex regional pain syndrome |
| Tendon rupture | Tendon rupture |
| Carpal tunnel syndrome | Loss of grip (radial shortening) |
| Compartment syndrome | Ulnar abutment syndromes |
| Carpal fractures | Arthrosis |
| Ligament injuries (scapho-lunate, lunotriquetral) | Adhesive capsulitis<br>Retinacular scarring |
| Pin tract infections | Pronator quadratus compartment syndrome or scarring |
| Pressure sores (cast immobilization) | |

joints. Radiocarpal and intercarpal changes can be easily followed with serial radiographs (see Fig. 13-18).

## Suggested Reading


Anderson JT, Lucas GL, Buhr BR. Complications of treating distal radius fractures with external fixation: A community experience. *Iowa Orthop J*. 2004;24:53–59.

Chen NC, Jupiter HB. Management of distal radial fractures. *J Bone Joint Surg*. 2007;89A:2051–2062.

Forward DP, Lindau TR, Melsom DS. Intercarpal ligament injuries associated with fractures of the distal part of the radius. *J Bone Joint Surg*. 2007;89A:2334–2340.

Hove LM. Nerve entrapment and reflex sympathetic dystrophy after fractures of the distal radius. *Scand J Plast Reconstr Surg Hand Surg*. 1995;29:53–58.

Hove LM, Soheim E, Skjeie R, et al. Prediction of displacement of Colles' fracture. *J Hand Surg [Br]*. 1994;19B:731–736.

Mann FA, Wilson AJ, Gilula LA. Radiographic evaluation of the wrist. What the surgeon want to know? *Radiology* 1992; 184:15–24.

Werber KD, Raeder F, Brauer RB, et al. External fixation of distal radial fractures: Four compared to five pins: A randomized study. *J Bone Joint Surg*. 2003;85A:660–666.

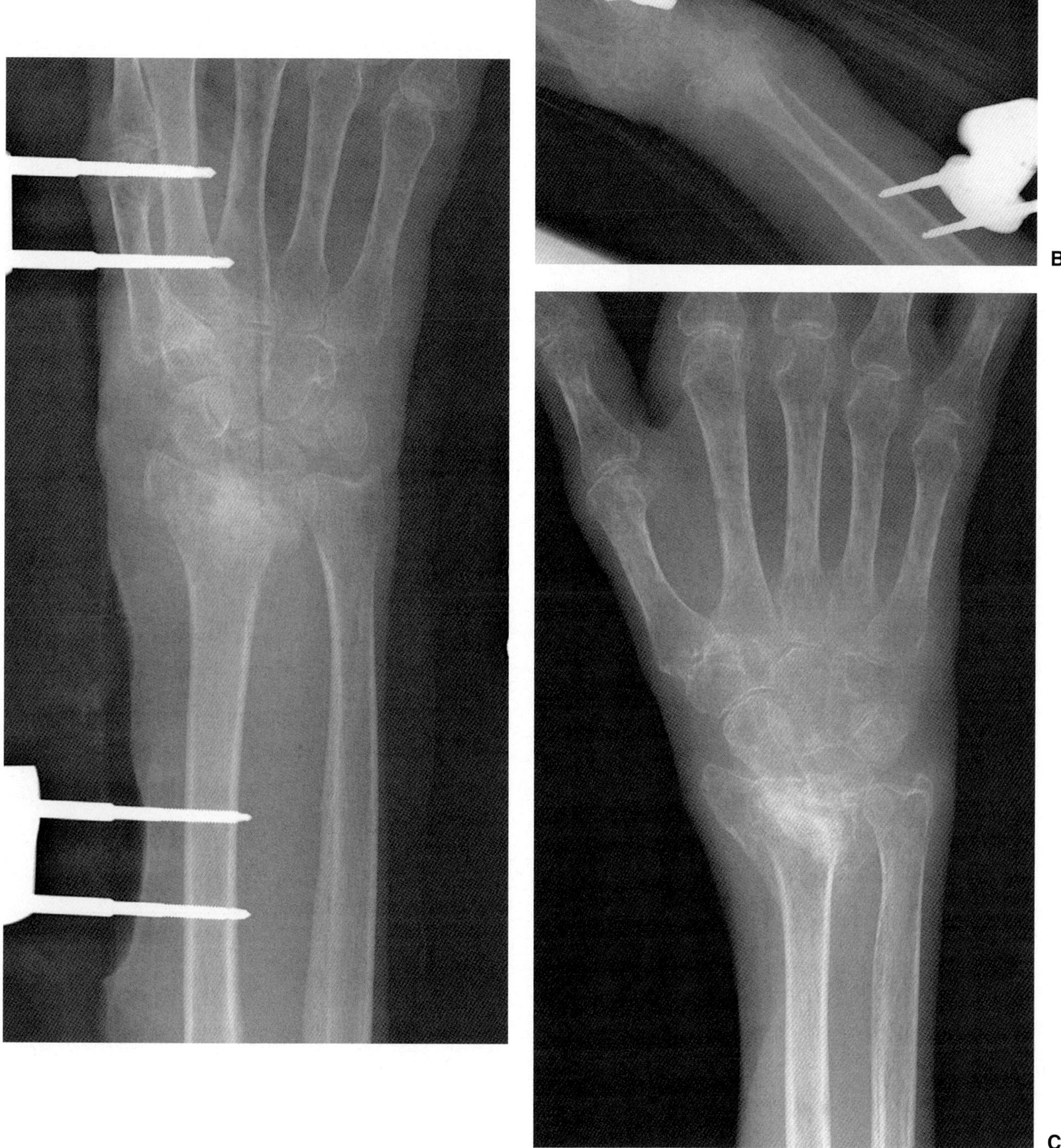


Fig. 13-14 Complex distal radial fracture with radial shortening treated with external fixation. Posteroanterior (PA) (A) and lateral (B) radiographs following external fixation demonstrate radial shortening with loss of radial inclination and height, carpal collapse, ulnar lunate abutment, and neutral palmar (volar) tilt. Radiographs following healing (C and D) demonstrate stable position with radiocarpal arthrosis and osteopenia.

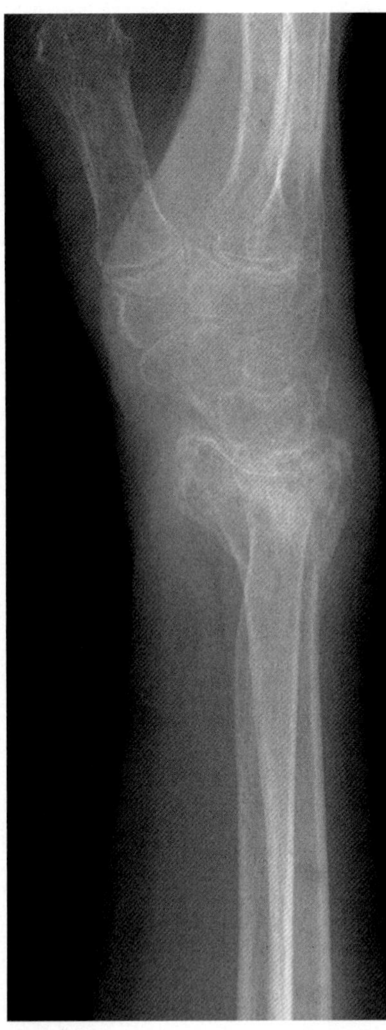


Fig. 13-14 *(Continued)*

### Carpal Fracture/Dislocations

The osseous and soft tissue anatomy of the wrist is complex. A complete discussion is beyond the scope of this text. However, key anatomic features are important to review. There are eight carpal bones (scaphoid, lunate, triquetrum, pisiform, trapezium, trapezoid, capitate, and hamate) that form two carpal rows. The scaphoid links the proximal and distal carpal rows. The proximal carpal row articulates with the radius and the second carpal row and the distal row articulates with the metacarpal bases. The joint spaces should be parallel and approximately 2 mm in width. Lines along the carpal bones on frontal radiographs (see Fig. 13-19) should form smooth arcs. With ligament injury and dislocation the arcs are interrupted. The carpal height can also be evaluated on the PA radiograph using two methods (see Fig. 13-20). The scapholunate relationship should be evaluated on lateral images (see Fig. 13-21). The neural and tendon relationships of the wrist are illustrated in Figure 13-22 and the complex ligament and triangular fibrocartilage complex anatomy in Figures 13-23 and 13-24.

#### Scaphoid Fractures

Scaphoid fractures are the most common carpal fracture accounting for 70% of carpal fractures and more than half of carpal injuries. Associated osseous and soft tissue injuries are not uncommon. Associated fractures occur in 5% to 12% of patients involving the radial styloid, triquetrum, capitate, and trans-scaphoid perilunate dislocations. Associated fractures of the radial head have been reported in 6% of patients. The mechanism of injury is a fall on the outstretched hand. Most injuries are sports related or occur with motor vehicle accidents. Patients present with pain and swelling. There is tenderness over the snuff box on the radial side of the wrist. Fractures can occur at any age, but males aged 20 to 30 years are affected most commonly.

Scaphoid fractures may involve the proximal, mid or distal scaphoid, or the tubercle (see Fig. 13-25). Most fractures (70%) involve the waist, 10% to 20% the distal pole, 5% to 10% the proximal pole, and 5% involve the tuberosity. Two classification systems are used for scaphoid fractures. The Russe classification is based on the orientation of the fracture line (see Fig. 13-26). The vertical oblique fracture is most susceptible to shearing forces, but accounts for only 5% of scaphoid fractures. Horizontal oblique fractures are subjected to compressive forces across the fracture site and transverse fractures have combined shearing and compressive forces.

The Herbert classification is based on stability and prognosis for delayed or nonunion. Fractures of the tubercle (type A1—Fig. 13-25, number 1) and incomplete fractures of the waist (type A2) are stable injuries. Type B includes acute unstable fractures. Type B1 is a distal oblique fracture, type B2 a fracture through the waist (Fig. 13-25, number 4), type B3 is a proximal pole fracture (Fig. 13-25, number 5), and type B4 injuries are trans-scaphoid perilunate fracture dislocations.

## SUGGESTED READING

Haisman JM, Rohde RS, Weiland AJ. Acute fractures of the scaphoid. *J Bone Joint Surg*. 2006;88A:2750–2758.

Herbert TJ. *Fractured scaphoid*. St. Louis: Quality Medical Publishers; 1990.

Nattass GR, King JW, McMurtry RY, et al. An alternative method for determination of carpal height ratio. *J Bone Joint Surg*. 1994;76A:88–94.

Russe O. Fracture of the carpal navicular. Diagnosis, non-operative treatment and operative treatment. *J Bone Joint Surg*. 1960;42A:759–768.

#### Imaging Techniques

Detection of scaphoid fractures may be accomplished with routine radiographs of the wrist. A special scaphoid view is typically added to the standard PA, lateral, and oblique images described in the prior section. The soft tissues and fat planes should be carefully evaluated along with the features described earlier. Specifically, the navicular fat stripe is a useful tool

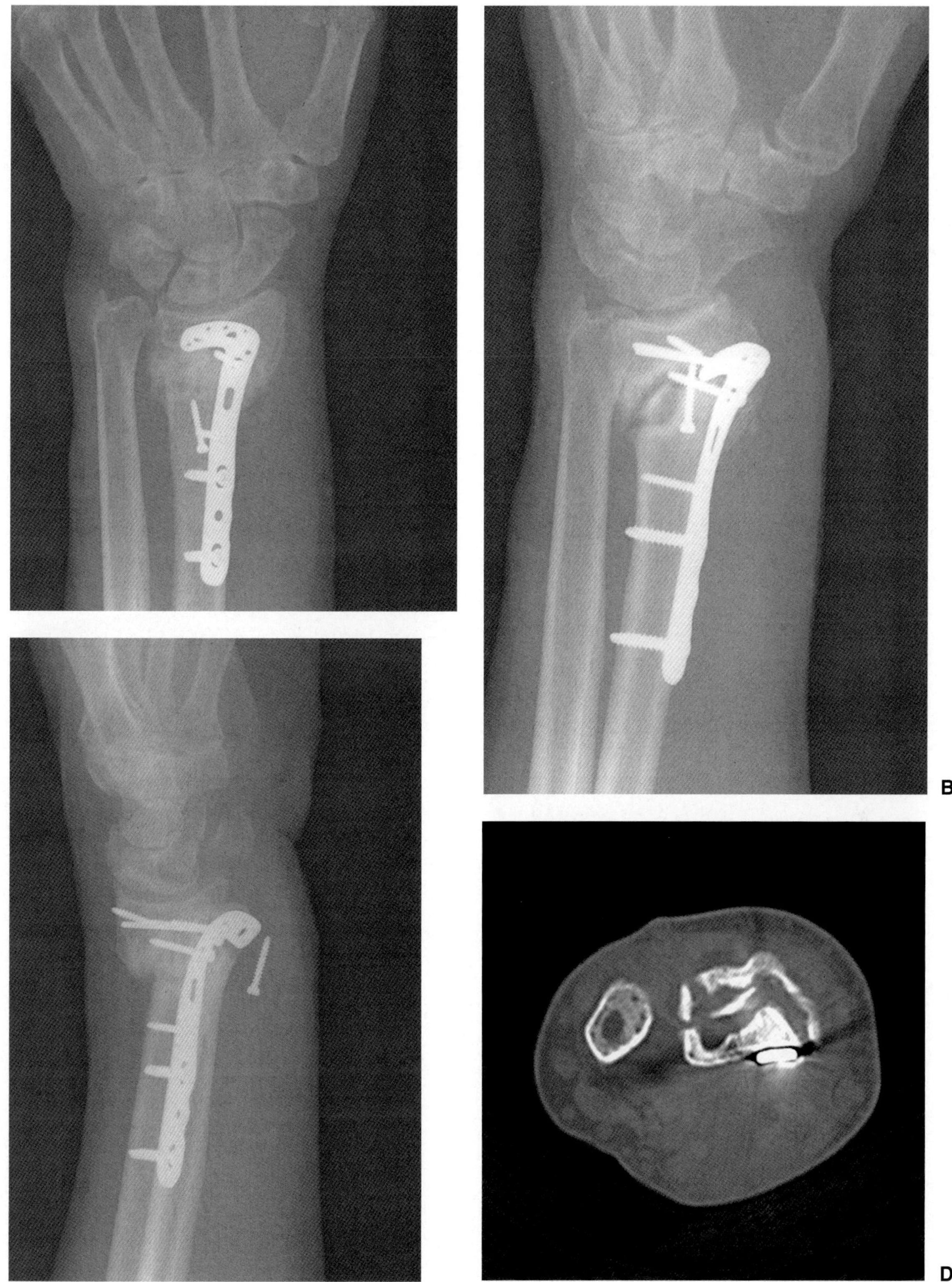


Fig. 13-15 Posteroanterior (PA) (A), lateral oblique (B), and oblique (C) radiographs of a distal radial fracture treated with volar plate and screw fixation. The fracture line is sclerotic indicating delayed union or nonunion and there is pull-out of one of the screws, which lies in the region of the flexor tendons and median nerve. Computed tomographic (CT) images in the axial plane (D to F) demonstrate bone loss with sclerosis of the main fragments and pull-out of the plate on the ulnar side. Sagittal (G and H) and coronal (I and J) reformatted images more clearly demonstrate the bone loss with a fragment in the area of nonunion and sclerosis at the margins of the main fragments.

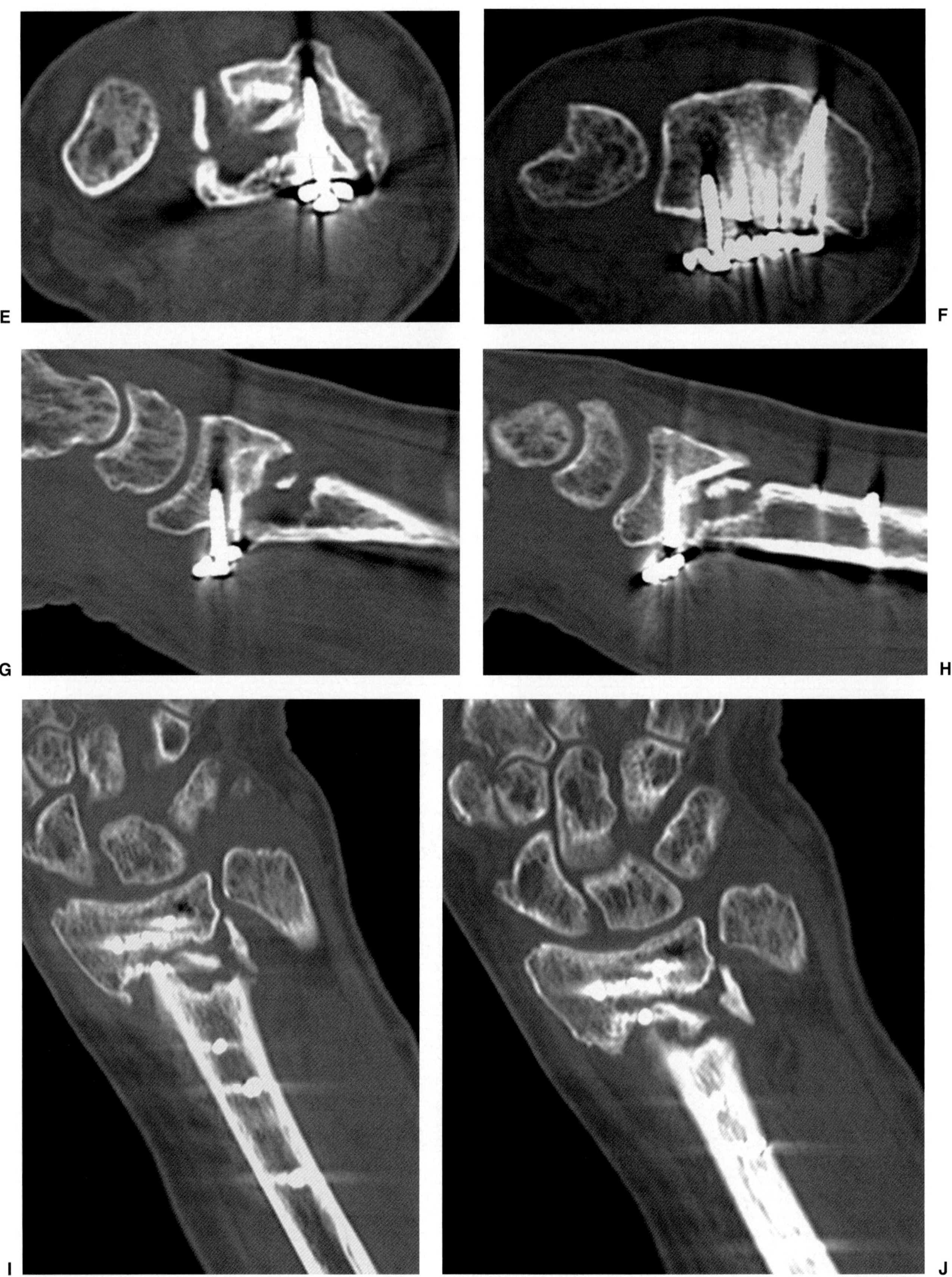


Fig. 13-15 *(Continued)*

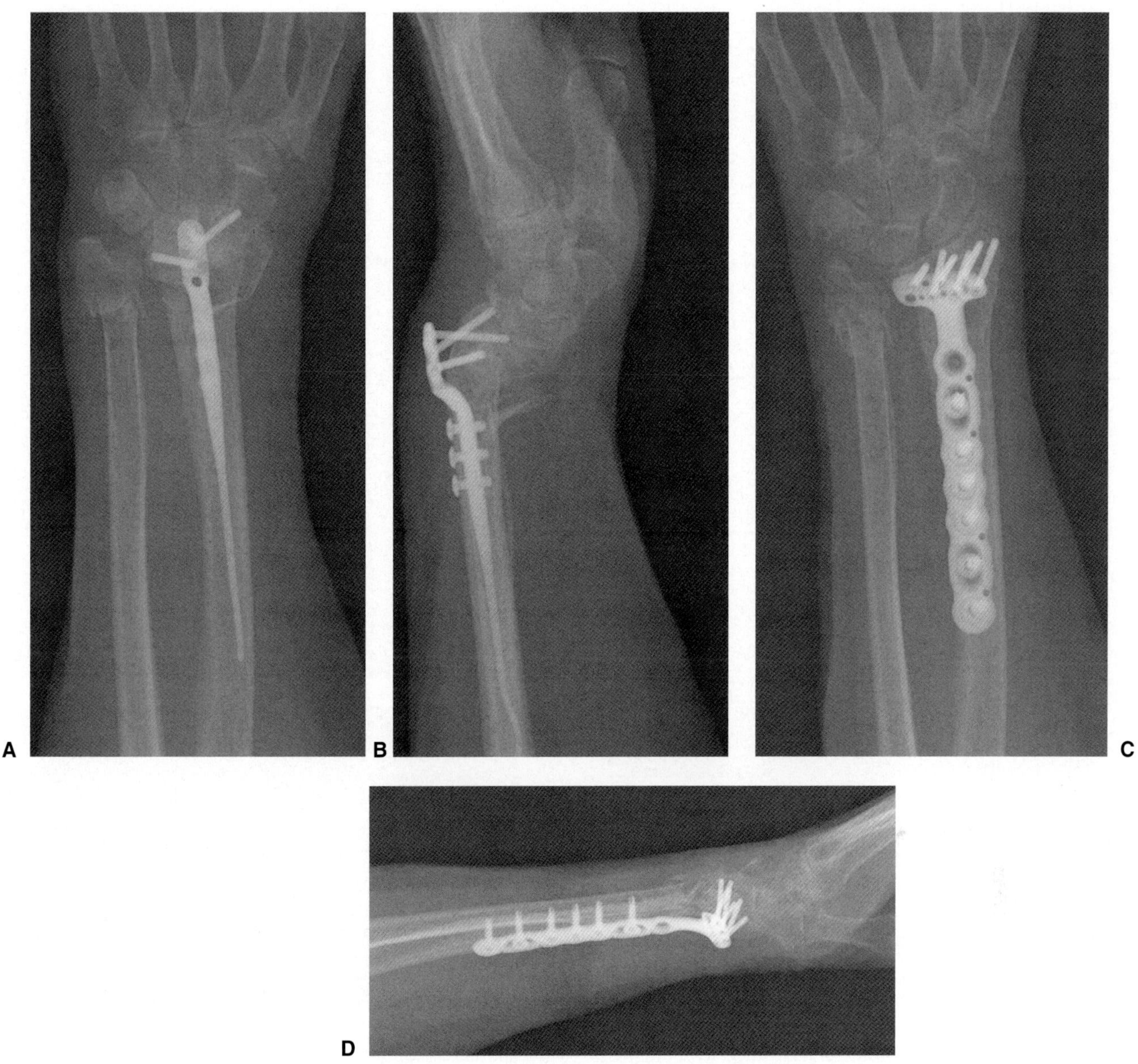


Fig. 13-16 Failed fixation. Posteroanterior (PA) (A) and lateral (B) radiographs demonstrating internal fixation of a distal radius fracture. There is also a distal ulnar fracture. The screws have pulled out of the distal radial fragment, which is now displaced volarly. PA (C) and lateral (D) radiographs following revision using a volar locking plate and screws. The distal radial fragment is realigned.

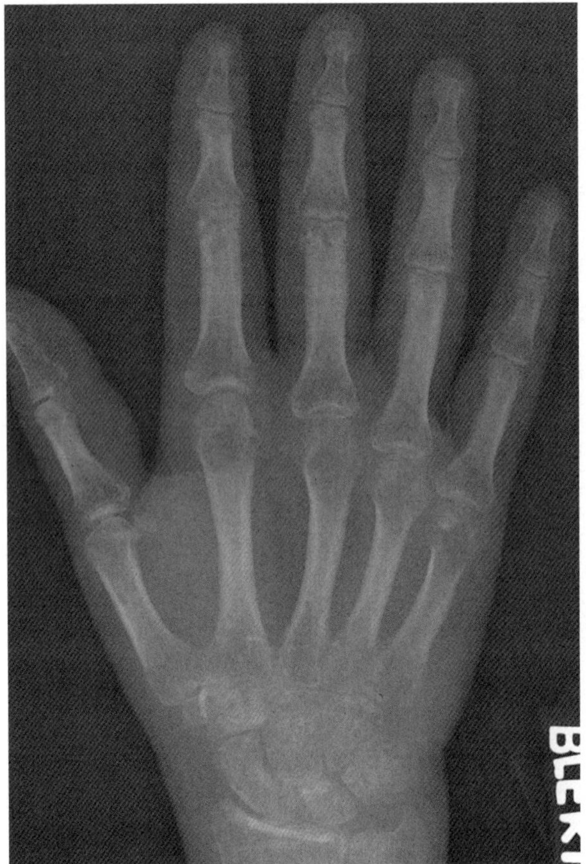


Fig. 13-17 Complex regional pain syndrome. Radiograph demonstrates marked osteopenia in the wrist and aggressive osteopenia about the articulations of the hand.

for detection of subtle scaphoid fractures. This fat plane lies between the radial collateral ligament and the tendon sheaths of the abductor pollicis longus and extensor pollicis brevis. Although the fat stripe is not consistently seen on radiographs in children, it is evident in 96% of adults. The fat plane is displaced or obliterated in 88% of radial-sided wrist fractures and 87% of scaphoid fractures (see Fig. 13-27).

Subtle fractures may go undetected. When radiographs are negative or the fat stripe is not clearly seen and when there is clinical suspicion for fracture, MRI can be obtained. CT is also more sensitive and specific compared to radiographs for detection of carpal fractures. In addition, CT is often performed to permit more accurate treatment planning (see Fig. 13-28).

## Suggested Reading

Berquist TH, Trigg SD. Hand and wrist. In: Berquist TH, ed. *Imaging atlas of orthopaedic appliances and prostheses*. New York: Raven Press; 1995:831–921.

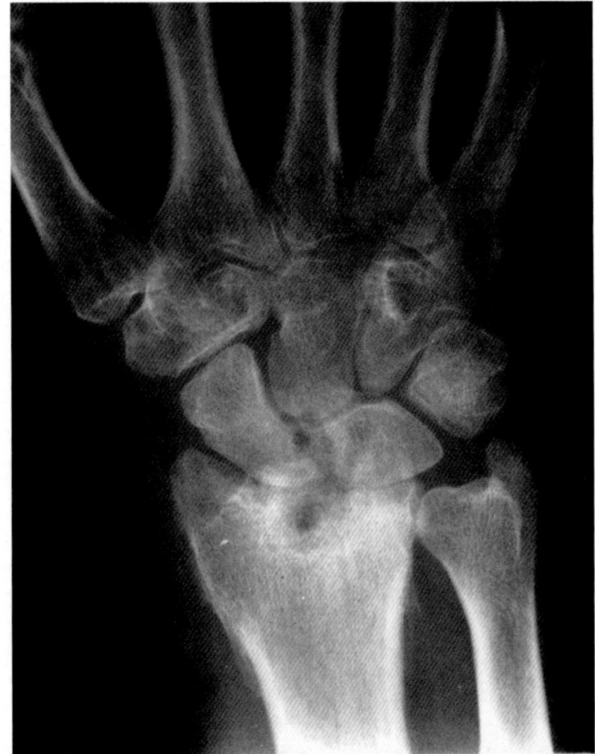
A

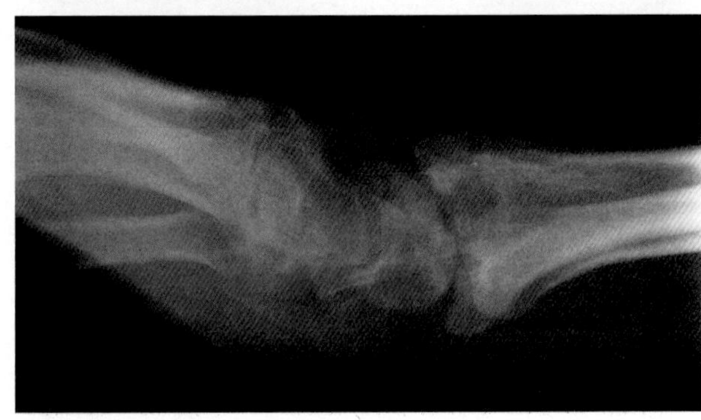
B

Fig. 13-18 Post-traumatic arthrosis. Posteroanterior (PA) (A) and lateral (B) radiographs following healing of an intra-articular fracture of the distal radius. There is advanced radiocarpal arthrosis with articular irregularity and joint space narrowing. There is also intracarpal arthrosis.

Terry DW, Ramin JE. The navicular fat stripe. A useful roentgen feature in evaluating wrist trauma. *AJR Am J Roentgenol*. 1975;124:25.

You JS, Chung SP, Chung HS, et al. The usefulness of CT for patients with carpal bone fractures in the emergency department. *Emerg Med J*. 2007;24:248–250.

### Treatment Options

Fracture management depends on patient factors and comorbidities, the type of fracture, and associated injuries. Fractures

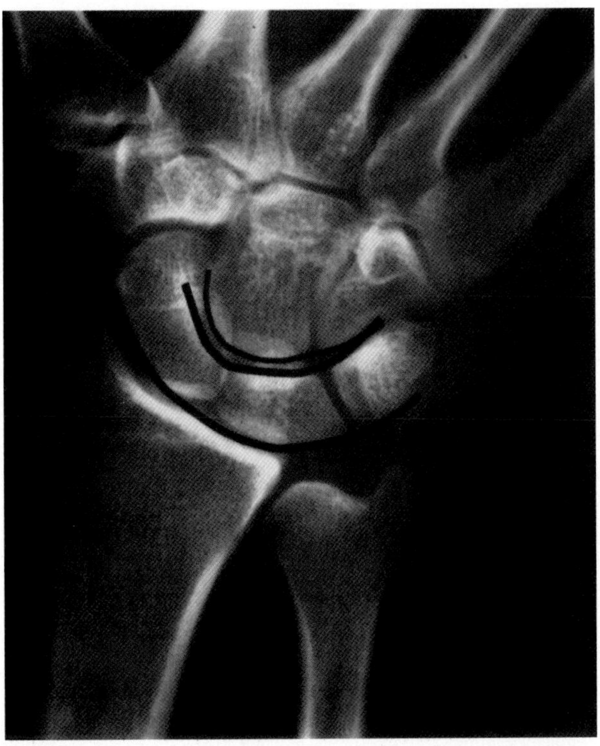
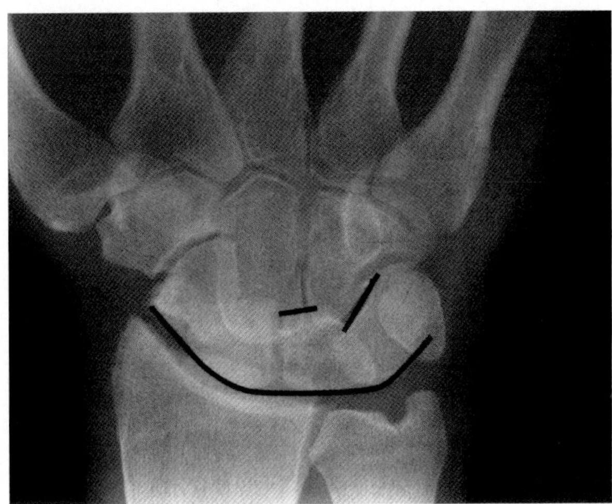

Fig. 13-19 Carpal relationships on the posteroanterior (PA) radiograph. A: Normal radiograph with smooth arcs (*curved lines*) formed by the articular surfaces of the carpal bones. B: The arcs are interrupted in this patient with a trans-scaphoid perilunate dislocation.

of the distal pole or tuberosity (Fig. 13-25, number 1) generally heal well, are likely related to vascularity, and can be managed with closed reduction and cast immobilization (long-arm or short-thumb spica) for 4 to 6 weeks.

Fractures of the waist may be managed with closed reduction and cast immobilization or internal fixation. CT (Fig. 13-28) is useful to evaluate displacement. Reformated coronal and sagittal images are obtained along the axis of the scaphoid. The fracture is displaced or unstable if there is >1 mm of cortical step off, angulation, or associated ligament injury. When the scapholunate angle exceeds 60 degrees and the radiolunate angle exceeds 15 degrees the fracture is considered displaced. The interscaphoid angle should not exceed 35 degrees (Fig. 13-28). Internal fixation using a Herbert screw or fully threaded Acutrak screw is used in this setting (see Fig. 13-29). Internal fixation provides the additional advantage in that the patient can begin motion earlier and the fracture is rigidly fixed so that loss of alignment is unlikely.

Fractures of the proximal pole should be treated with internal fixation. The approach and fixation used varies with the size of the proximal fragment. In recent years, percutaneous pinning over a guidewire placed down the axis of the scaphoid has become more popular. When combined with arthroscopy, the fracture site can be directly visualized during the procedure.

## Suggested Reading

Cooney WP, Dobyns JH, Linscheid RL. Fractures of the scaphoid: A rational approach to management. *Clin Orthop.* 1980;149:90–97.

Haisman JM, Rohde RS, Weiland AJ. Acute fractures of the scaphoid. *J Bone Joint Surg.* 2006;88A:2750–2758.

### Imaging of Complications

Scaphoid fractures present significant problems in management. Following diagnosis, imaging is important to assure that position is maintained and healing occurs. Delayed union and nonunion are common. Delayed union (failure to heal in 4 months) is even more common than nonunion and is evident in up to 30% of waist and proximal pole fractures. The incidence of nonunion is reported to range from 5% to 25%. Undisplaced fractures treated with cast immobilization heal in 90% of cases. The incidence of nonunion is higher with displaced fractures. Imaging is most easily accomplished with serial radiographs (see Fig. 13-30). However, CT is often required regardless of the treatment approach to evaluate position and healing more effectively (Fig. 13-29). MRI demonstrates low-intensity fracture margins with fluid signal intensity between the fragments when fractures are ununited (see Fig. 13-31). MRI is

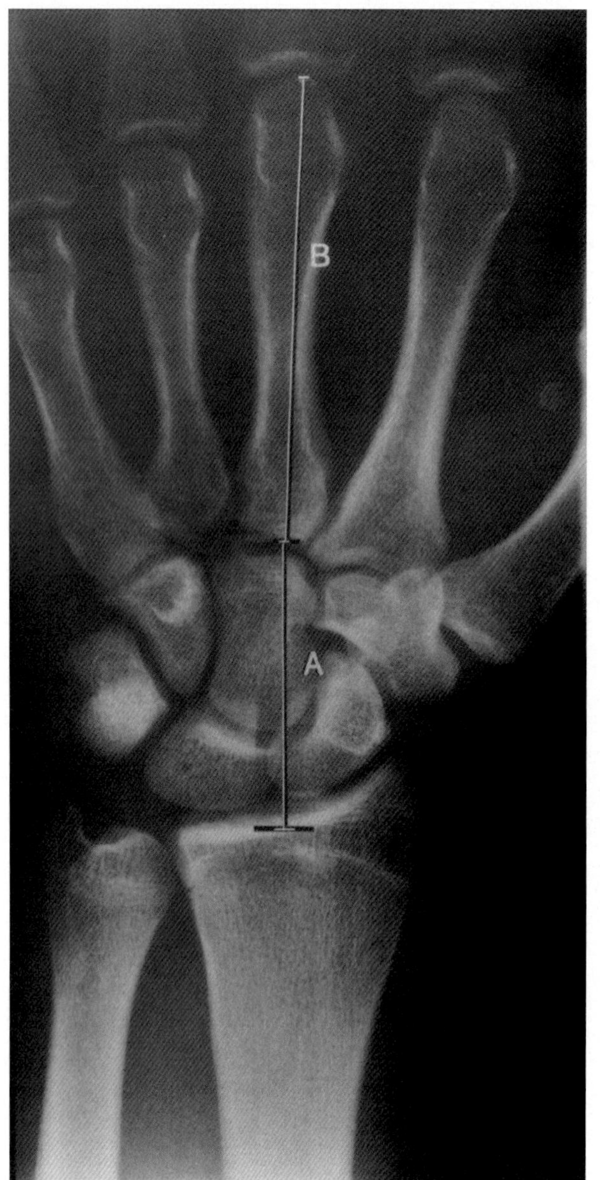


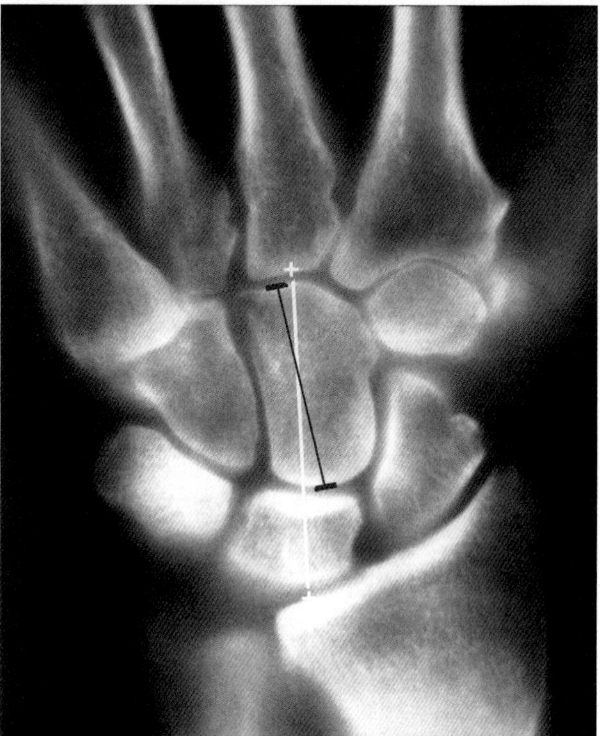

A B

Fig. 13-20 Carpal height. **A:** Carpal height ratio comparing the carpal height (*A*) to the length of the third metacarpal (*B*) (normal 0.54 ± 0.3). **B:** Modified method measured along the axis of the third metacarpal. The carpal height (*white line*) divided by the capitate height (*black line*) should be 1.57 ± 0.06.

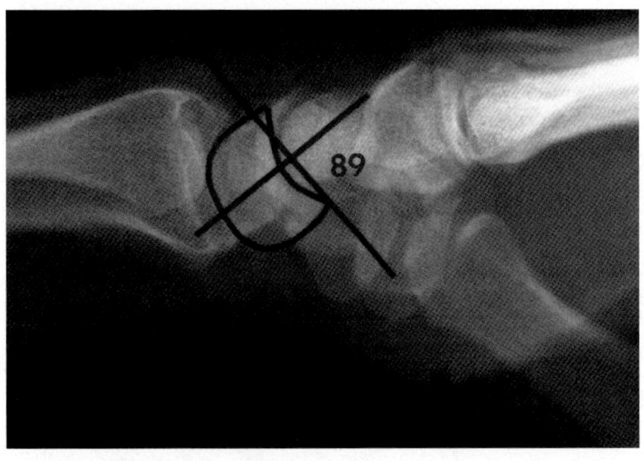


A

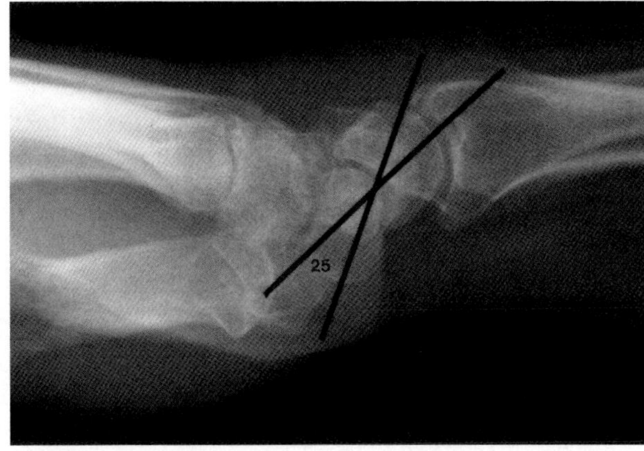


B

Fig. 13-21 Scapholunate angle. The normal scapholunate angle is 47 degrees with the wrist in neutral position. This can decrease to 30 degrees or increase to 60 degrees with radial or ulnar deviation. **A:** With dorsal intercalated segment instability (DISI) the angle increases (89 degrees in this case) and the lunate looks dorsally. **B:** With volar intercalated segment instability (VISI) the angle is decreased (25 degrees in this case) and the lunate is tilted in a palmar or volar direction.

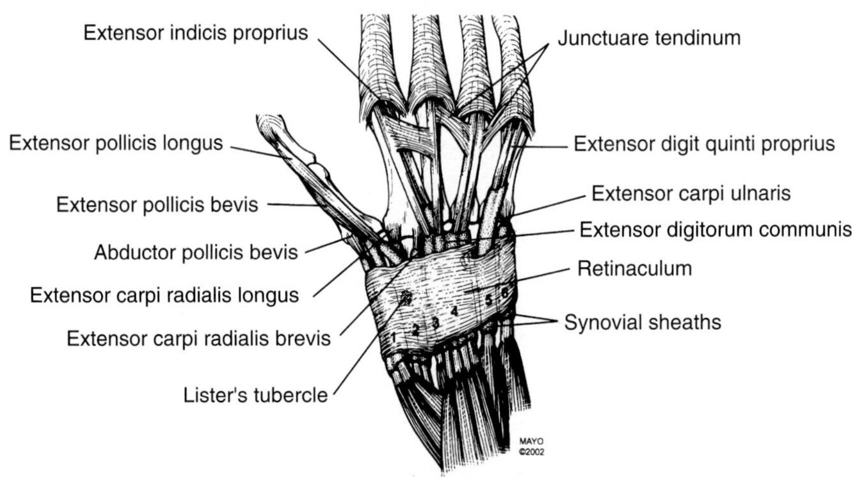


A

Tendon of flexor carpi radialis
Tendon of flexor pollicis longus
Abductor pollicis brevis
Median nerve
Tendon of palmaris longus
Ulnar artery
Palmar branch of ulnar nerve
Superficial branch of radial nerve
Abductor digiti minimi
Dorsal branch of ulnar nerve

B

Fig. 13-22 **A:** Illustration of the six dorsal extensor compartments and tendons. **B:** Illustration of the flexor tendons, carpal tunnel, and median and ulnar nerves. (From Berquist TH. *MRI of the hand and wrist.* Philadelphia: Lippincott Williams & Wilkins; 2003.)

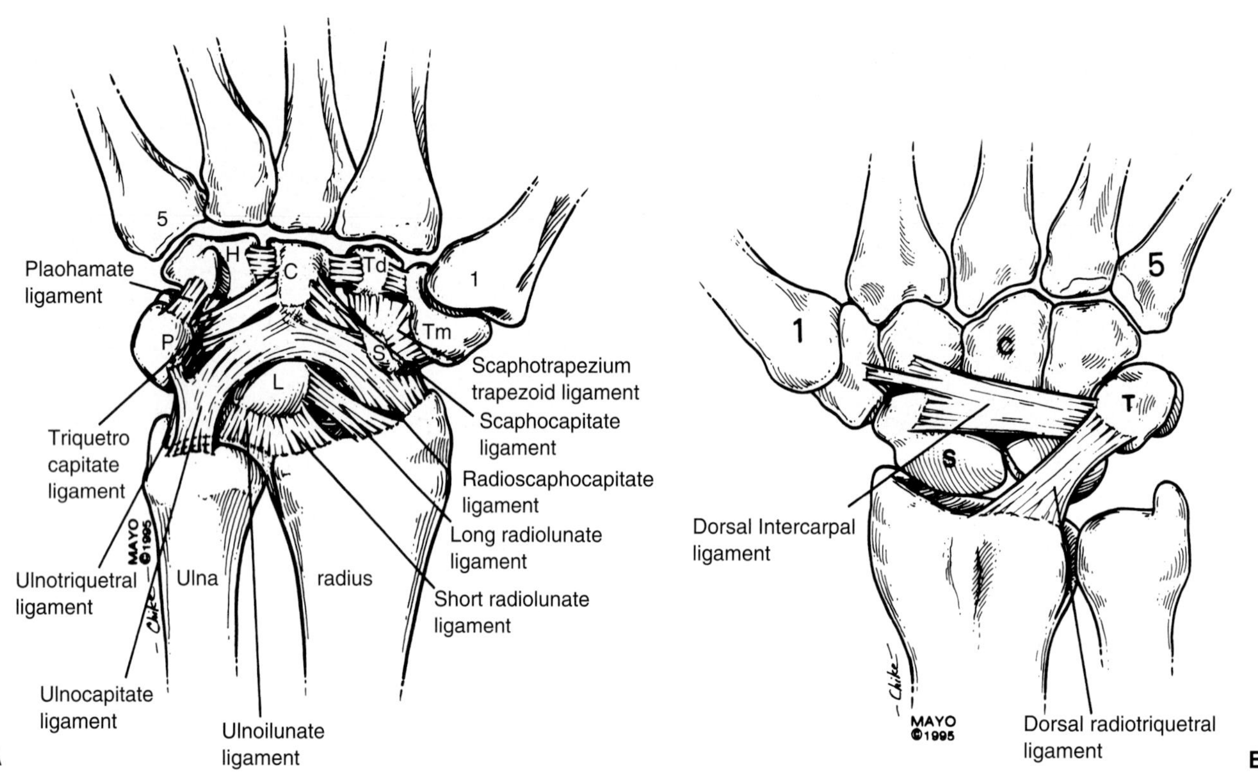


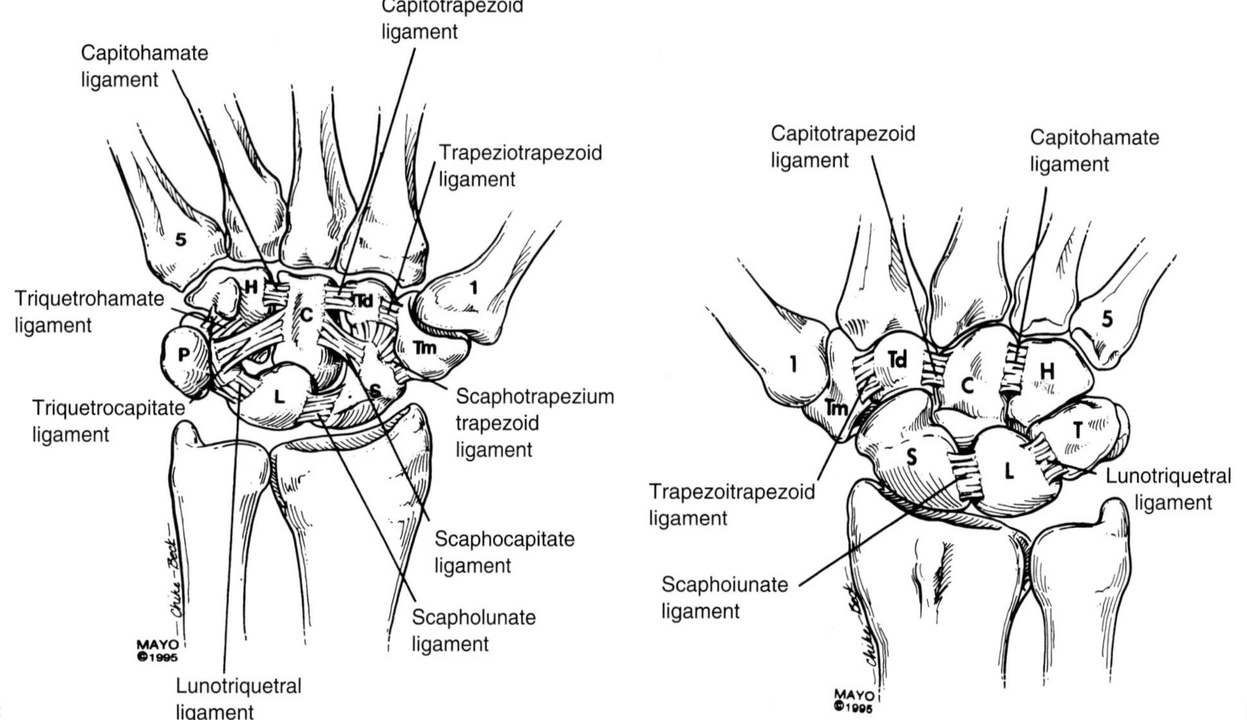


Fig. 13-23 Ligament anatomy of the wrist. Illustrations of the palmar (A) and dorsal (B) ligaments of the wrist. Illustrations of the palmar (C) and dorsal (D) intercarpal ligaments. *C*—capitate, *H*—hamate, *L*—lunate, *P*—pisiform, *S*—scaphoid, *T*—triquetrum, *Td*—trapezoid, *Tm*—trapezium, *1*—first metacarpal, *5*—fifth metacarpal. (From Berger RA. L-ligament anatomy. In: Cooney WP III, Linscheid RL, Dobyns JH, eds. *The wrist: diagnosis and operative treatment.* St. Louis: Mosby; 1998:72–105.)

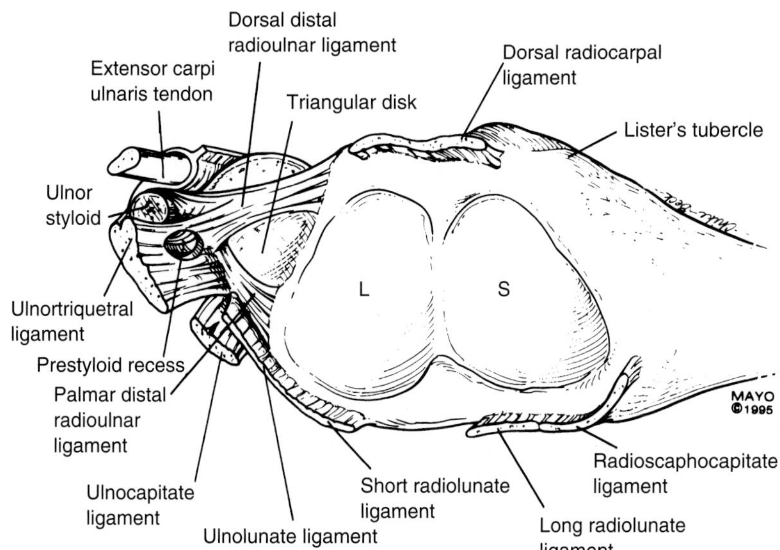


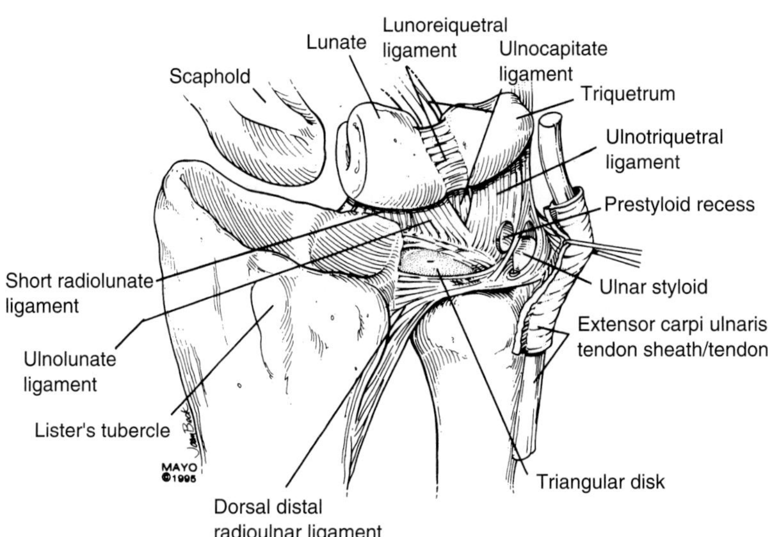


Fig. 13-24 A: Illustration of the distal radius (*L*—lunate fossa, *S*—scaphoid fossa), ligament attachments, and triangular fibrocartilage complex with radioulnar ligaments. B: Illustration of the ulnocarpal ligament complex and triangular fibrocartilage complex seen in the dorsal form. Note the relationship of the prestyloid recess and ulnotriquetral ligaments. (From Berger RA. L-ligament anatomy. In: Cooney WP III, Linscheid RL, Dobyns JH, eds. *The wrist: diagnosis and operative treatment.* St. Louis: Mosby; 1998:72–105.)

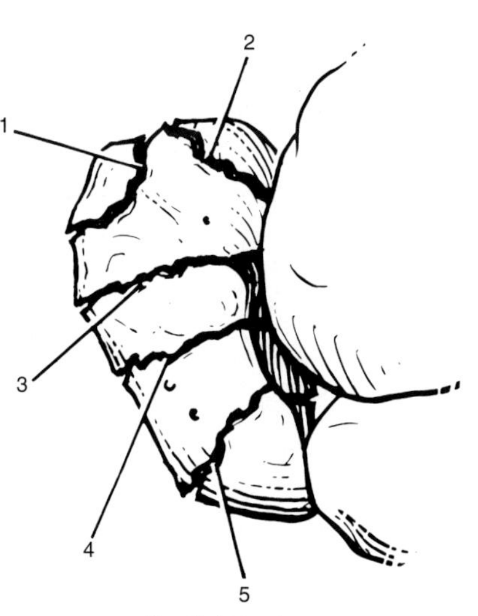


Fig. 13-25 Illustration of the locations for fractures of the scaphoid. *1*—tubercle, *2*—distal articular surface, *3*—distal third, *4*—waist, *5*—proximal pole.

optimal for evaluation in patients treated with closed reduction. In the presence of nonunion, internal repair with bone grafting may be required.

Avascular necrosis is reported to occur in 15% to 30% of scaphoid fractures, occurring most commonly with proximal pole fractures. Radiographs may demonstrate sclerosis and fragmentation of the proximal fragment (see Fig. 13-32). Both CT and MRI are more sensitive and can make the diagnosis earlier. However, over time it has become evident that neither modality is perfect. Signs suggesting avascular necrosis vary with the time between the injury and imaging. Abnormal signal intensity on MRI (see Fig. 13-33) and increased attenuation on CT images (see Fig. 13-34) may be reversible and do not always indicate impending osteonecrosis. Dynamic contrast-enhanced MR images with fat-suppressed T1-weighted sequences provide more effective evaluation of flow. This enhances the sensitivity and specificity for blood flow to the scaphoid and areas of necrosis.

Post-traumatic arthropathy is not uncommon, especially with nonunion or scaphoid fractures with associated osseous or soft tissue injury. Over time, carpal instability may also occur. In

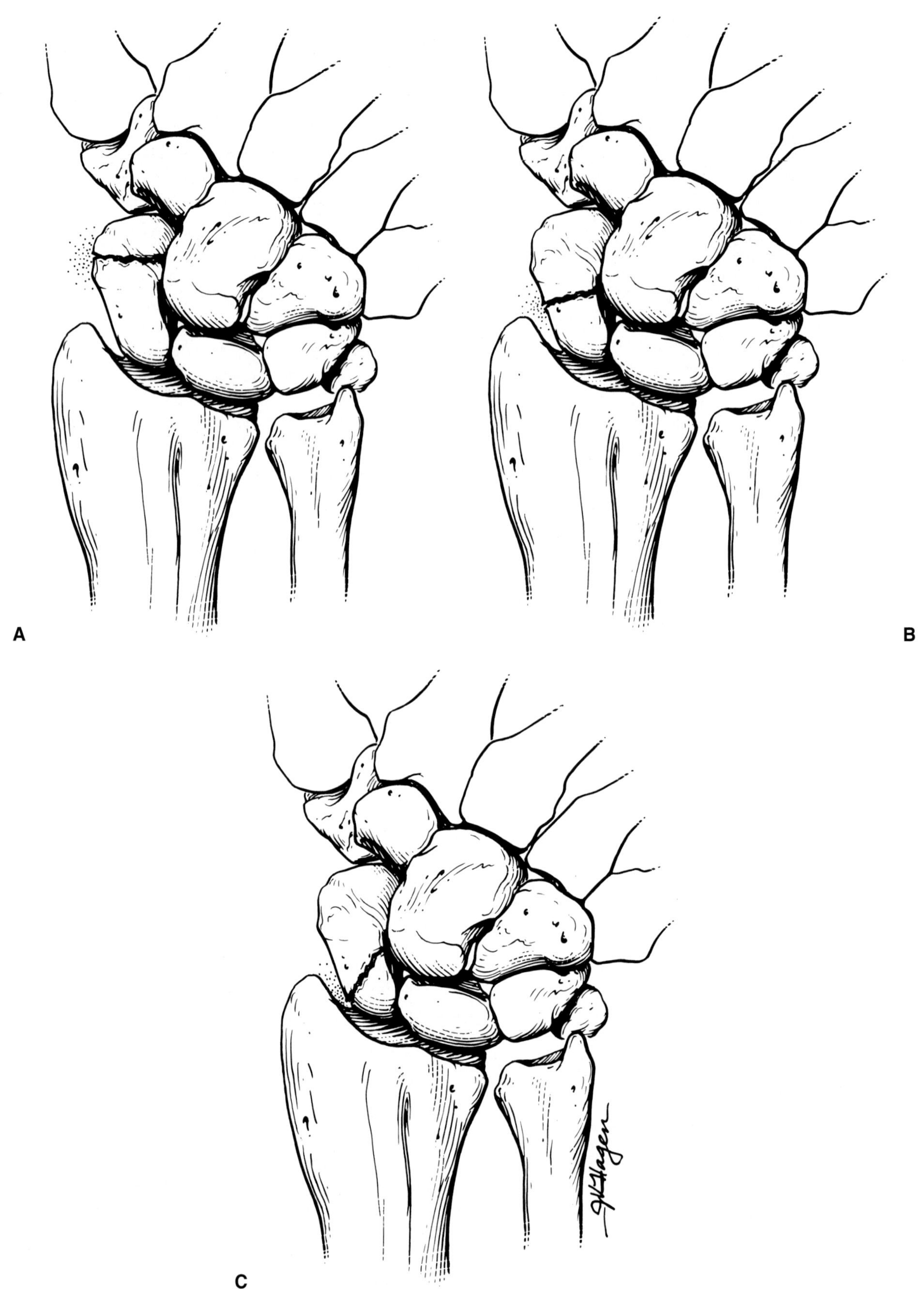

Fig. 13-26 Russe classification of scapoid fractures. A: Horizontal oblique. B: Transverse. C: Vertical oblique.

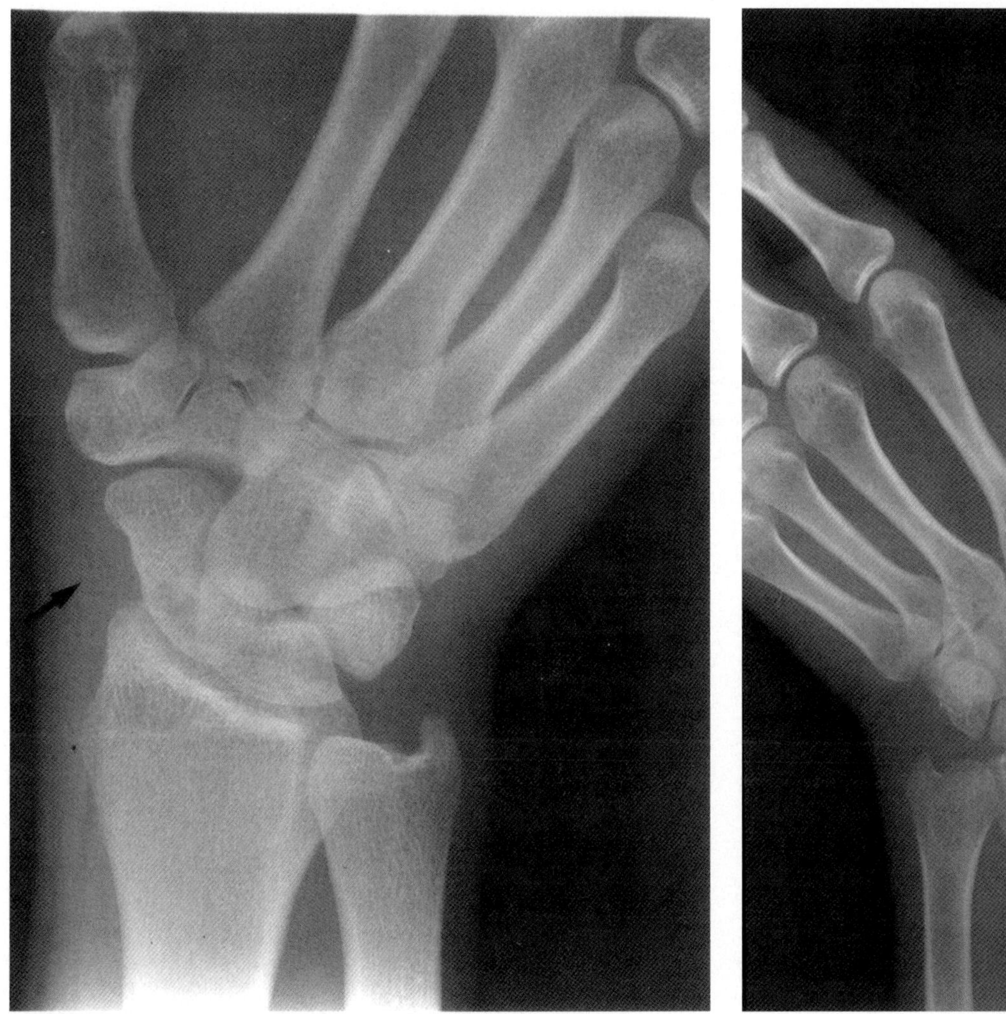
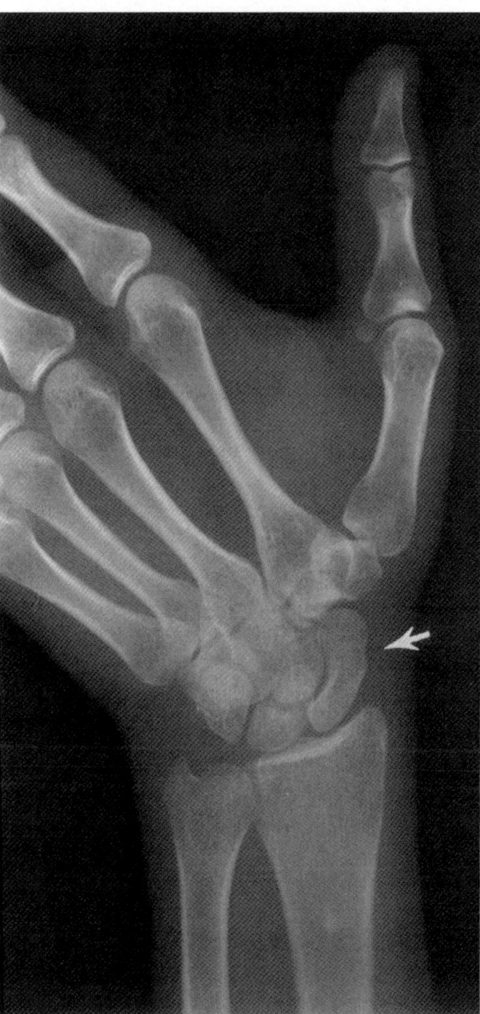

Fig. 13-27 Navicular fat stripe. A: Scaphoid view demonstrating a normal fat stripe (*arrow*). B: Occult scaphoid fracture with no visible fat stripe (*arrow*).

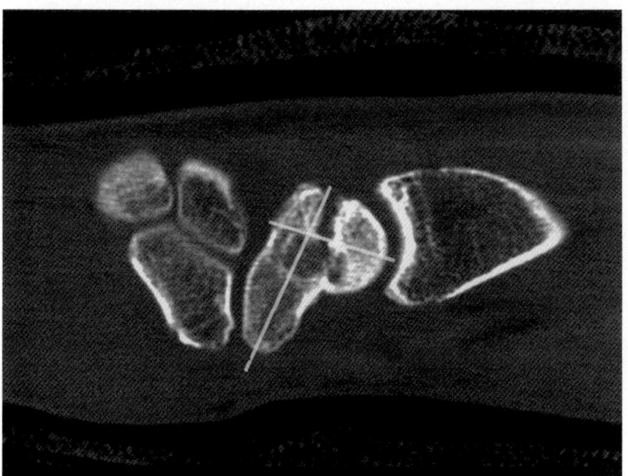

Fig. 13-28 Sagittal computed tomographic (CT) image demonstrating a scaphoid fracture with "humpback" deformity (*lines*).

patients with nonunion, this is termed *scaphoid nonunion advanced collapse* (SNAC). Serial radiographs are adequate for evaluation of joint and osseous changes. If fusion or surgical intervention may be indicated, MRI or CT are useful for more complete evaluation of cartilage and soft tissues. MR arthrography is optimal for evaluation of associated ligament and triangular fibrocartilage complex (TFCC) injuries.

## Suggested Reading

Cerezal L, Abascal F, Canga A. Usefulness of gadolinium-enhanced MR imaging in the evaluation of vascularity of scaphoid nonunions. *AJR Am J Roentgenol.* 2000;174:141–149.

Haisman JM, Rohde RS, Weiland AJ. Acute fractures of the scaphoid. *J Bone Joint Surg.* 2006;88A:2750–2758.

Mack GR, Bosse MJ, Gelberman RH, et al. The natural history of scaphoid non-union. *J Bone Joint Surg.* 1984;66A: 504–509.

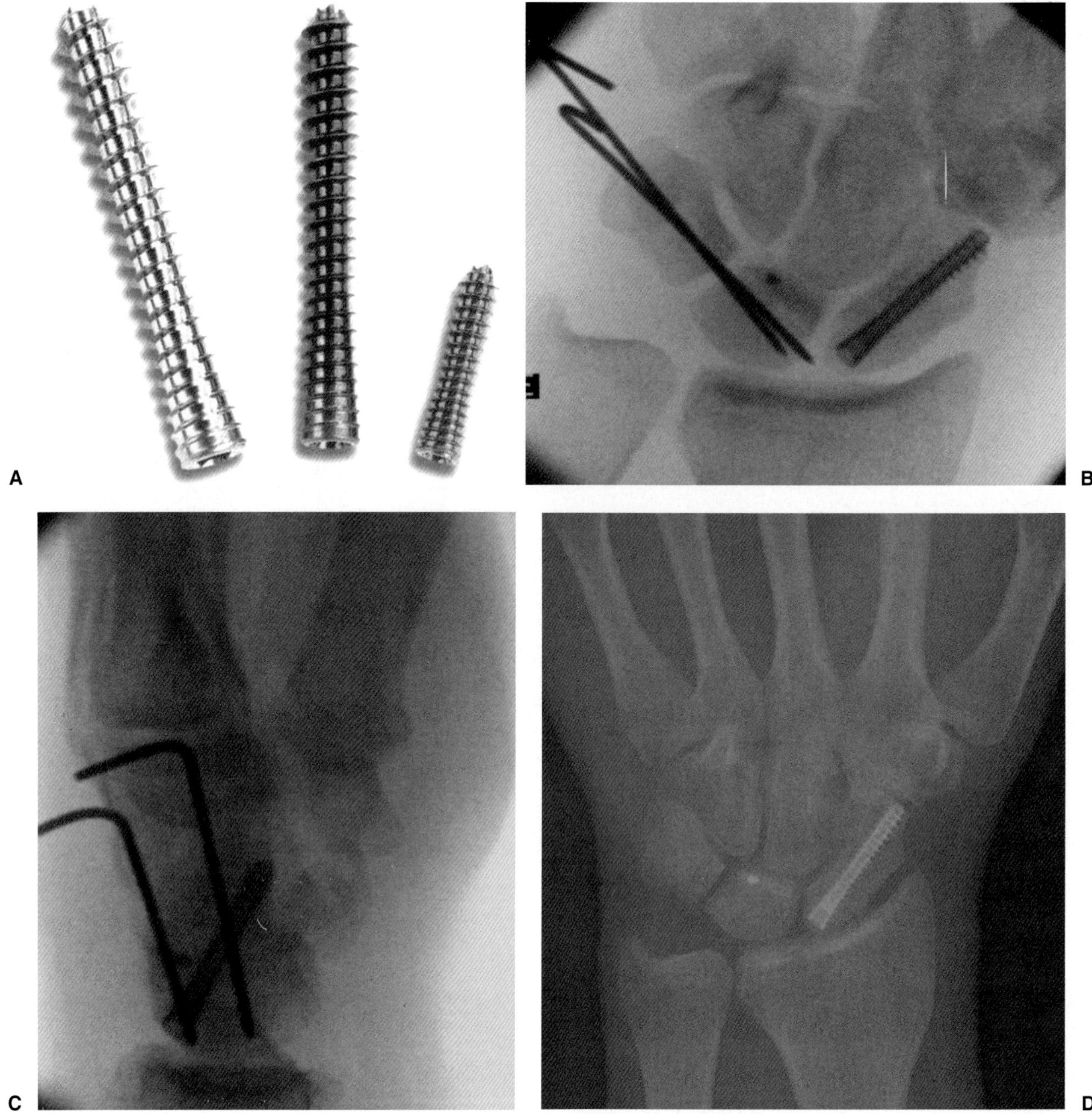


Fig. 13-29 Scaphoid fracture with Acutrak screw fixation. A: Acutrak screws. (Courtesy of Acumed, Hillsboro, Oregon.) Posteroanterior (PA) (B) and lateral (C) radiographs taken during screw fixation and ligament repair with K-wire fixation and a soft tissue anchor in the lunate. D: Follow-up PA radiograph following removal of the K-wires demonstrating fracture healing and normal carpal joint spaces. Soft tissue anchor in the lunate. Coronal (E) and sagittal (F) computed tomographic (CT) images demonstrate a healed fracture with no angular deformity. Note the previously nonvisualized distal radial fracture evident on the coronal CT image (E).

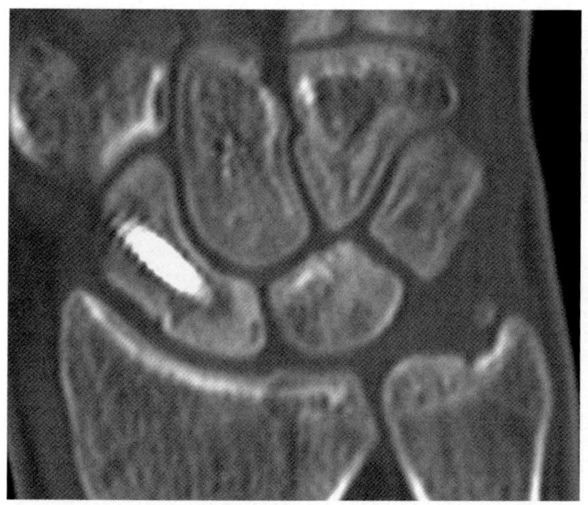

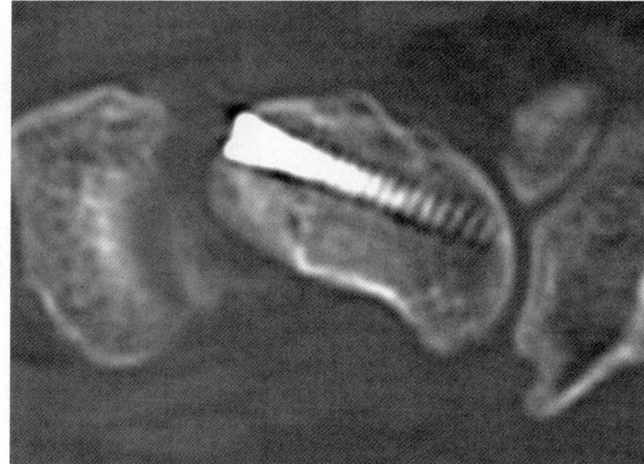

Fig. 13-29 *(Continued)*

Sakuma M, Nakamura R, Imaeda T. Analysis of proximal fragment sclerosis and surgical outcome of scaphoid nonunion by magnetic resonance imaging. *J Hand Surg [Br]*. 1995;20:201–205.

## Other Carpal Fractures

The incidence of fractures of carpal bones other than the scaphoid is much lower. The triquetrum is the second most commonly fractured carpal bone accounting for 14% of wrist injuries. The remaining carpal bones account for <5% of wrist injuries. The mechanism of injury is similar to scaphoid fractures and generally due to significant direct or indirect trauma. Triquetral fractures may result from a fall on the outstretched hand with extreme dorsiflexion or direct dorsal trauma. Lunate fractures may be related to direct trauma or chronic microtrauma and are classified based on the radiographic appearance. Stage I injuries present with normal radiographs. Stage II injuries demonstrate sclerosis of the lunate without collapse or fragmentation (see Fig. 13-35). Stage III injuries demonstrate collapse and fragmentation without (A) or with (B) fixed scapholunate dissociation. Stage IV lesions are similar to stage III, but with associated radiocarpal and midcarpal arthrosis.

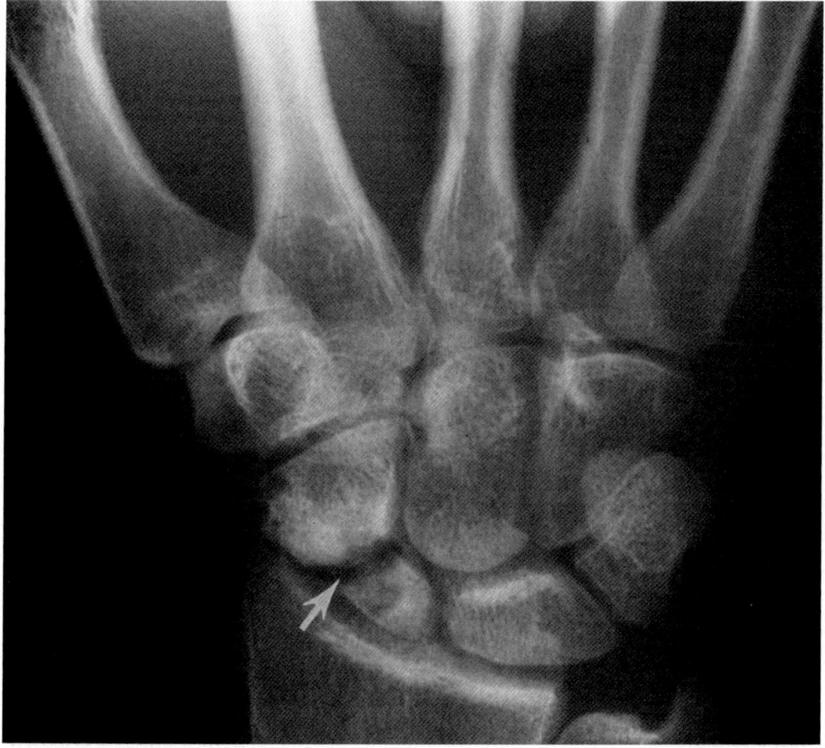

Fig. 13-30 Scaphoid nonunion. Posteroanterior (PA) radiograph demonstrating an ununited (*arrow*) scaphoid waist fracture.

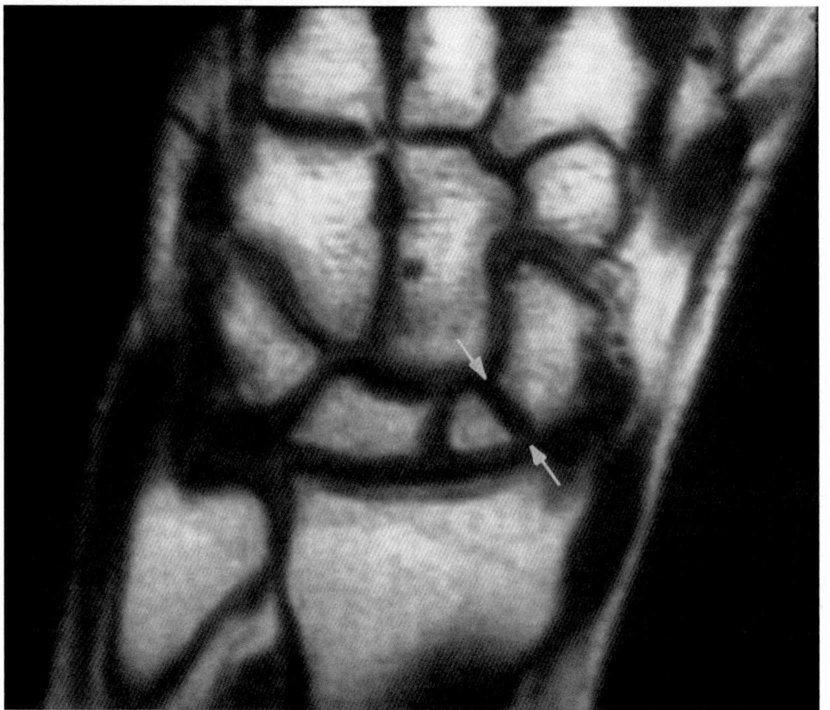

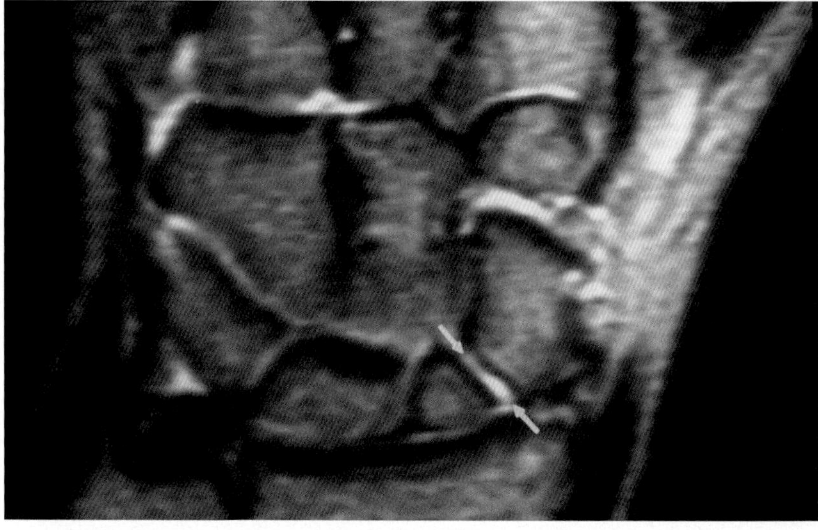

**Fig. 13-31** Scaphoid nonunion. T1- (**A**) and T2-weighted (**B**) magnetic resonance (MR) images demonstrate fluid signal intensity in the fracture line (*arrows*) due to nonunion.

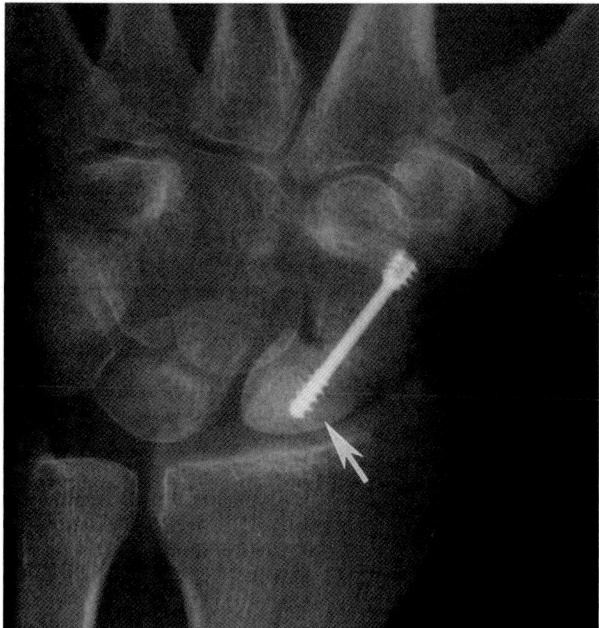

Fig. 13-32 Posteroanterior (PA) radiograph of the wrist following Herbert screw fixation of a proximal scaphoid fracture. The proximal fragment is sclerotic due to avascular necrosis.

Hamate hook fractures are usually related to racket sports, golf, or baseball with the handle impacting the palmar portion of the hand. Isolated capitate fractures are rare due to the central location in the wrist. Therefore, fractures are usually related to fracture dislocations with involvement of multiple carpal bones.

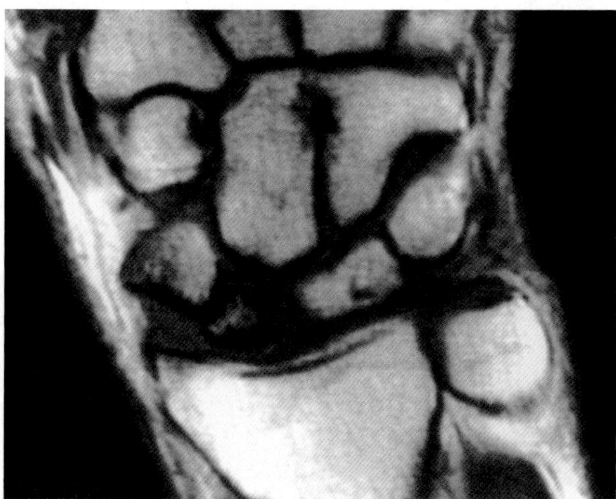

Fig. 13-33 Coronal T1-weighted magnetic resonance (MR) image in a patient with nonunion. The most proximal portion of the proximal pole has no signal intensity with fat signal intensity in the distal portion of the fragment. Is there loss of blood supply? The location of the fracture is more likely to result in loss of blood supply and the fracture line is vertical oblique resulting in increased shearing force at the fracture.

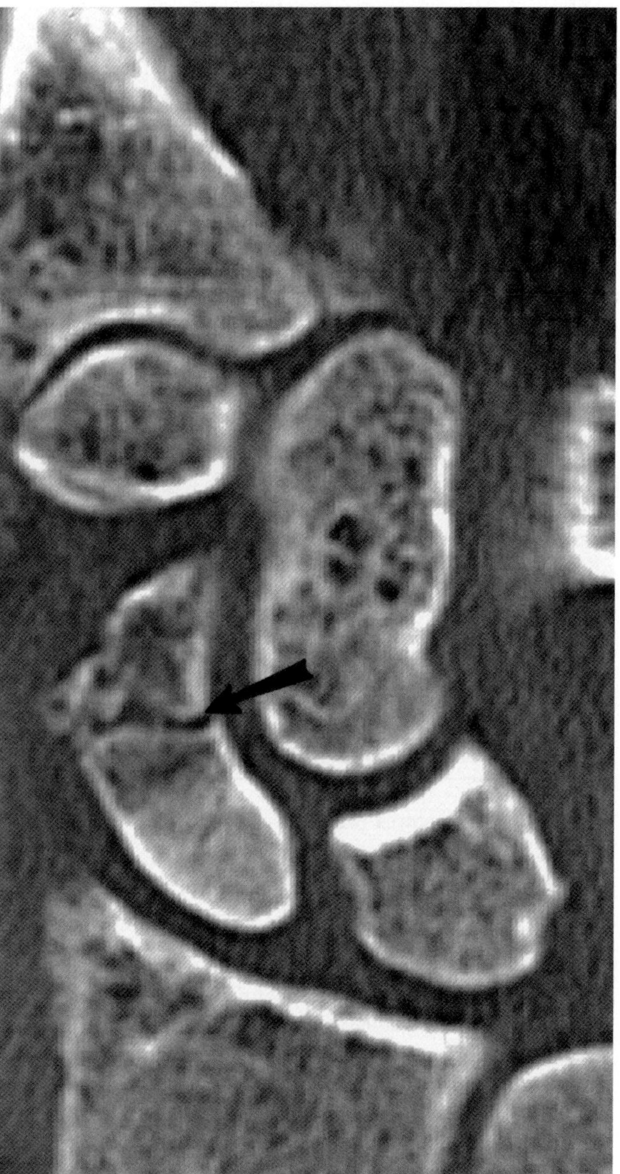

Fig. 13-34 Coronal computed tomographic (CT) image with a distal scaphoid fracture (*arrow*). There is increased attenuation in the proximal scaphoid. Location of the fracture suggests that this may be reversible.

Imaging is similar to other wrist injuries. Radiographs may be diagnostic. Triquetral fractures are usually dorsal and best identified on the lateral view (see Fig. 13-36). When symptoms suggest a hamate fracture, a carpal tunnel view is added to the normal PA, lateral, and oblique views of the wrist. CT with reformatting is frequently performed to fully evaluate the extent of the injury (see Fig. 13-37). Lunate fractures may be subtle. Depending on the location and mechanism of the fracture one must be concerned about avascular necrosis (see Fig. 13-38). Therefore, MRI may be the technique of choice to detect and classify the degree of injury (see Fig. 13-39).

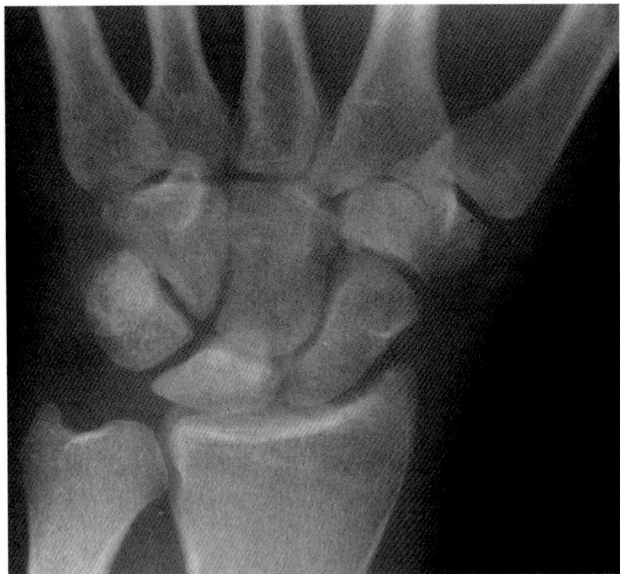

Fig. 13-35 Posteroanterior (PA) radiograph demonstrating sclerosis of the lunate without collapse or fragmentation (Lichtman stage II).

## Suggested Reading


Cohen MS. Fractures of the carpal bones. *Hand Clin.* 1997;13:587–599.

Gelberman RH, Bauman TD, Menon J, et al. The vascularity of the lunate and Kienbock's disease. *J Hand Surg [Br].* 1980;5:272–278.

Lichtman DM, Degnan GG. Staging and its use in the determination of treatment modalities of Kienbock's disease. *J Hand Surg [Br].* 1980;5:272–278.

Teisen H, Hjarbock J. Classification of fresh fractures of the lunate. *J Hand Surg [Br].* 1988;13B:458–462.


### Treatment Options

Most nonscaphoid carpal fractures can be managed with closed reduction and cast immobilization. There are exceptions for specific injuries. Lunate fractures are managed based on the stages described earlier. Conservative therapy with stress reduction is adequate for stages I and II. Revascularization with immobilization is contemplated for stage III disease (see Fig. 13-40). More aggressive therapy is required for stage IV depending on the patient's activity and pain levels. Options include lunate replacement, proximal row carpectomy, and arthrodesis.

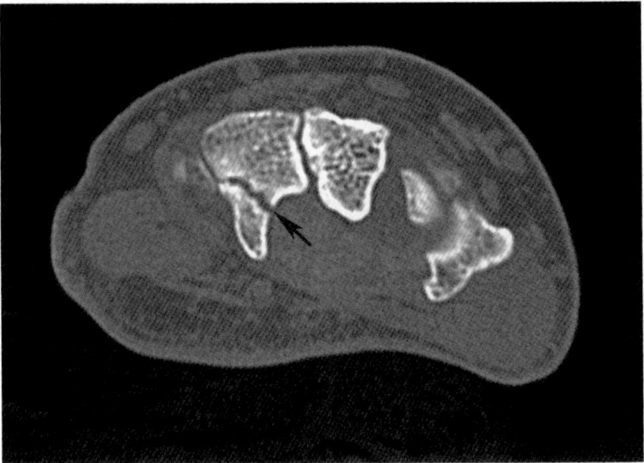

Fig. 13-37 Axial computed tomographic (CT) image demonstrating a fracture of the hamate hook (*arrow*).

Triquetral chip fractures (Fig. 13-36) and undisplaced body fractures can be treated with cast immobilization. However, displaced body fractures should be treated with percutaneous pins or open reduction and internal fixation.

Undisplaced fractures of the hook of the hamate or body can be treated conservatively. When displaced, internal fixation is performed using K-wires or screws. In some cases, the hamate fragment may have to be removed.

Capitate fractures are usually associated with other injuries such as an associated fracture of the scaphoid. In this setting, internal fixation with screws or K-wires is preferred.

Complications are similar to scaphoid fractures described earlier. Fracture union is easily evaluated with CT. MRI is useful for detection and follow-up of avascular necrosis which occurs in the proximal scaphoid, lunate, and capitate.

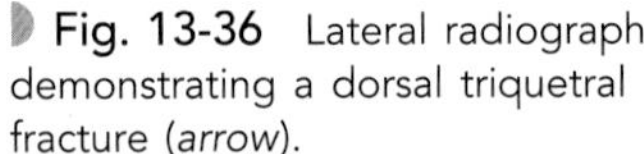

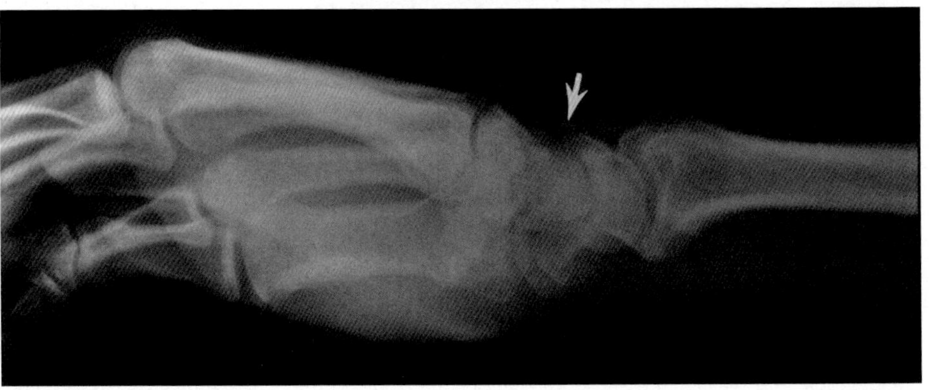

Fig. 13-36 Lateral radiograph demonstrating a dorsal triquetral fracture (*arrow*).

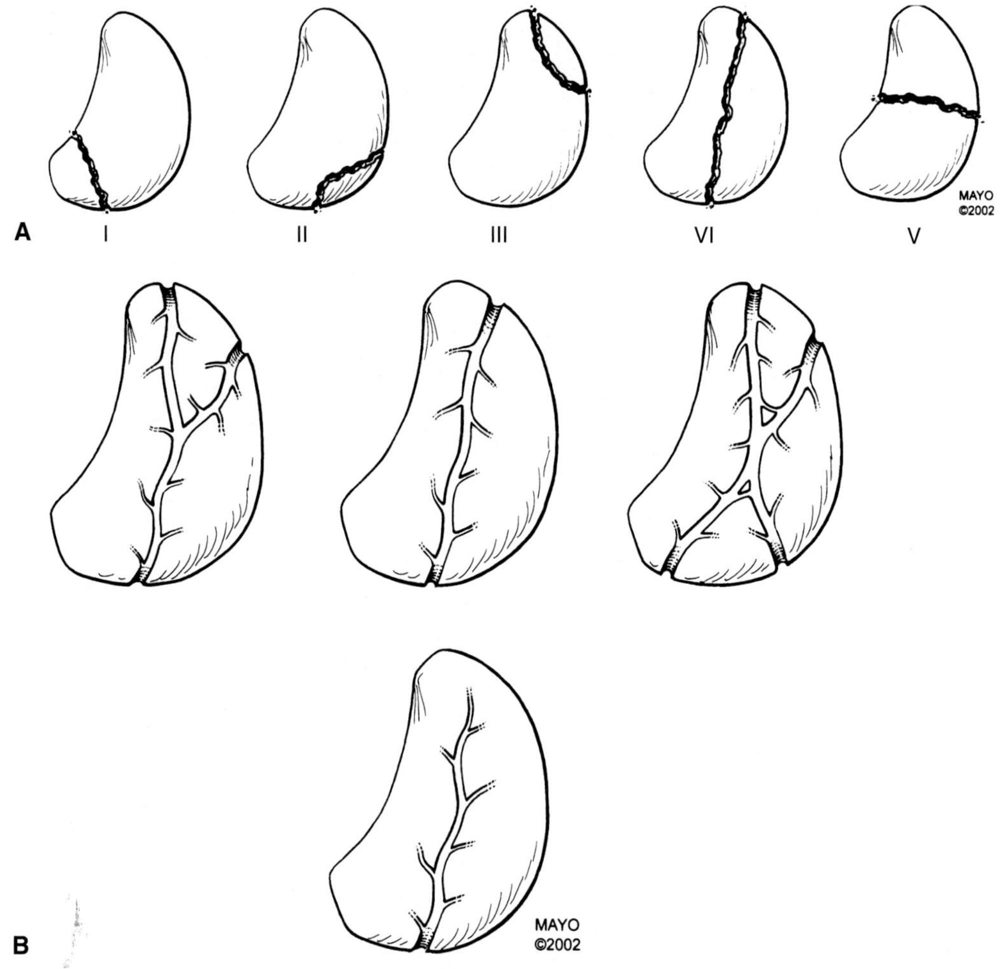


Fig. 13-38 A: Fracture patterns in the lunate: type I—palmar fracture, type II—chip fracture, type III—dorsal pole fracture, type IV—vertical fracture, type V—transverse fracture. B: Illustration of vascular patterns in the lunate. Bottom—single palmar vessel (8%). Top left—Y pattern with two dorsal and one palmar vessel (59%). Top middle—I pattern with single dorsal and palmar vessels (10%). Top right—X pattern with two dorsal and palmar vessels (23%). (From Berquist TH. *MRI of the hand and wrist.* Philadelphia: Lippincott Williams & Wilkins; 2003.)

## Suggested Reading

Barnaby W. Fractures and dislocations of the wrist. *Emerg Med Clin North Am.* 1992;10:133–149.

Cohen MS. Fractures of the carpal bones. *Hand Clin.* 1997;13:587–599.

Goldfarb CA, Yin Y, Gilula LA, et al. Wrist fractures: What the clinician wants to know. *Radiology* 2001;219:11–28.

Seitz WH, Papandrea RF. Fractures and dislocations of the wrist. In: *Rockwood and Green's fractures in adults*, 5th ed. Philadelphia: Lippincott Williams & Wilkins; 2001:749–799.

### Carpal and Carpometacarpal Dislocations

Dislocations of the carpal bones are complex injuries involving supporting ligaments, interosseous ligaments, and associated fractures. Injuries are usually due to falls on the outstretched hand with rotational or shearing forces. Multiple patterns have been described. The most common injury is the trans-scaphoid perilunate dislocation. The lunate and proximal scaphoid fragments may maintain the normal relationship with the distal radius. The distal scaphoid fragment and distal carpal row are displaced dorsally in most cases; volar dislocation can occur but volar displacement accounts for only 8% of trans-scaphoid perilunate dislocations (see Fig. 13-41).

Dorsal perilunate dislocations may also occur without an associated scaphoid fracture. Isolated dorsal or volar dislocations of the lunate may also occur (see Fig. 13-42). Isolated dislocations of the scaphoid and other carpal bones can occur, but they are rare.

Carpometacarpal dislocations may involve multiple articulations or occur alone. The latter usually involves the hamate-fifth metatarsal articulation (see Fig. 13-43). In most situations, there

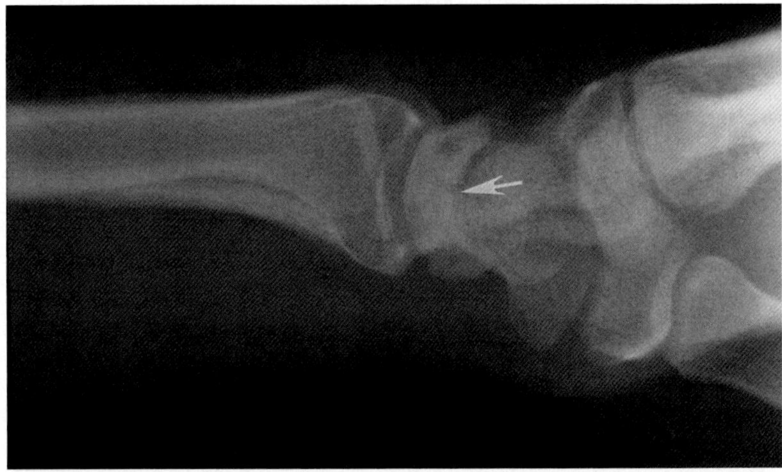

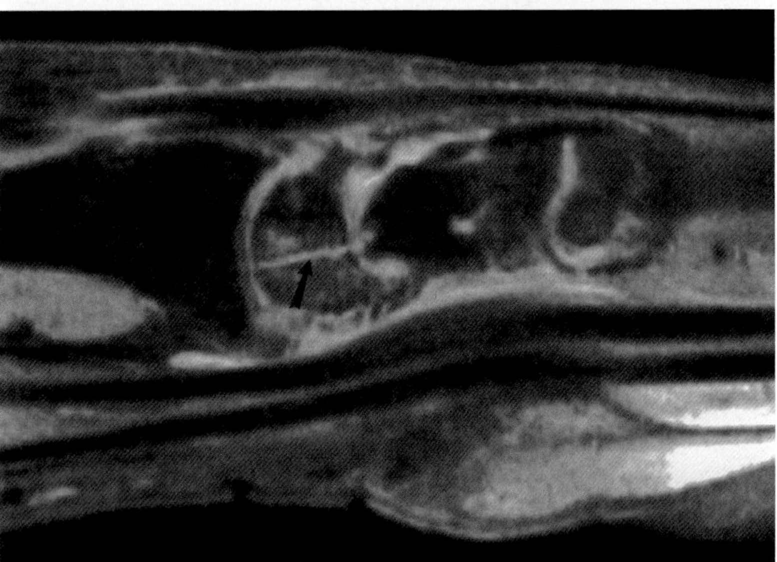

**Fig. 13-39** Lunate fractures. **A:** Lateral radiograph demonstrating compression and sclerosis of the lunate with a distal fracture line (*arrow*). **B:** Sagittal fat suppressed fast spin-echo T2-weighted magnetic resonance (MR) image demonstrating a fracture line (*arrow*) with normal marrow signal intensity.

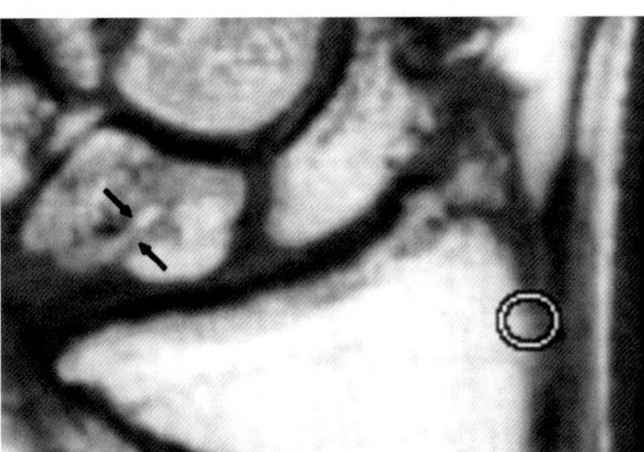

**Fig. 13-40** Revascularization for stage III Kienbock disease. T1-weighted magnetic resonance (MR) image 1 year after the procedure demonstrates normal marrow signal intensity. The graft entry site (*arrows*) is still visible.

are associated fractures of the carpal bones or metatarsal bases (see Fig. 13-44). CT is useful to fully evaluate the extent of osseous injury before treatment planning.

Treatment usually requires open reduction and internal fixation using K-wires, carpal screws (Herbert or Acutrak) for carpal fractures, and, in certain cases, external fixation systems in addition to the K-wires and screws (see Fig. 13-45).

Complications are similar to those described earlier with arthrosis, carpal instability, and avascular necrosis of the scaphoid, lunate, and capitate, all possible postreduction complications. Avascular necrosis of the proximal scaphoid occurs in up to 50% of trans-scaphoid perilunate dislocations.

Pin tract infections are common. Fortunately, deep infections are infrequent.

Soft tissue complications may be related to the type and extent of injury. Transient median nerve palsy occurs with volar lunate dislocation and trans-scaphoid perilunate dislocations. Follow-up imaging with CT is useful to assure stability of reduction for the fractures and carpal dislocations. On the

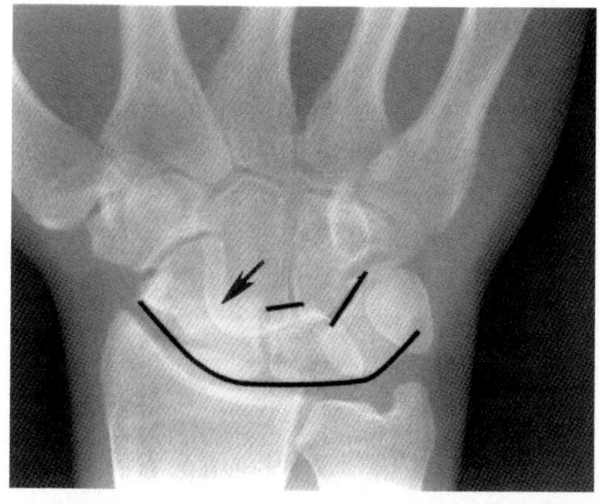

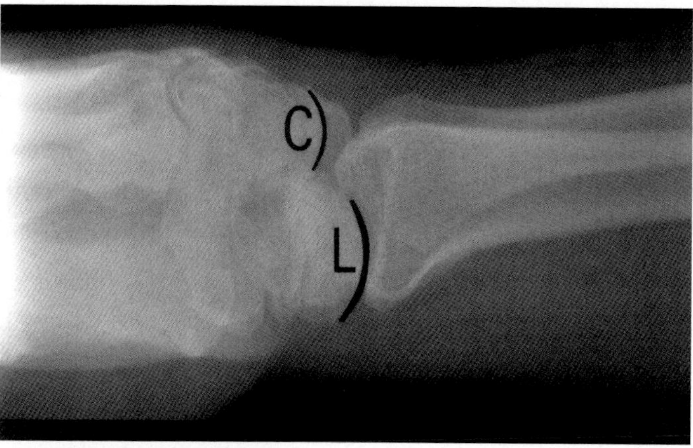


A B

Fig. 13-41 Dorsal trans-scaphoid perilunate dislocation. A: Posteroanterior (PA) radiograph demonstrates interruption of the arcs along the carpal rows with a fracture of the scaphoid waist (*arrow*). B: Lateral radiograph demonstrating dorsal dislocation of the capitate (*C*) and distal carpal row. The lunate (*L*) remains with the radial articulation.

basis of instrumentation, MRI is most useful for evaluation of avascular necrosis.

## Suggested Reading

Green DP, O'brien ET. Classification and management of carpal dislocations. *Clin Orthop*. 1980;190:227–235.

Herzberg G, Comtet JJ, Linscheid RL, et al. Perilunate dislocations and fracture dislocations: A multicenter study. *J Hand Surg [Br]*. 1993;18A:768–779.

Papadonikolakis A, Mavrodontidis AN, Zalavaras C, et al. Transscaphoid volar lunate dislocation: A case report. *J Bone Joint Surg*. 2003;85A:1805–1808.

Russell TB. Intercarpal dislocations and fracture/dislocations. A review of 59 cases. *J Bone Joint Surg*. 1949;31B:524–531.

Sides D, Laorr A, Greenspan A. Carpal Scaphoid: Radiographic pattern of dislocation. *Radiology* 1995;195:215–216.

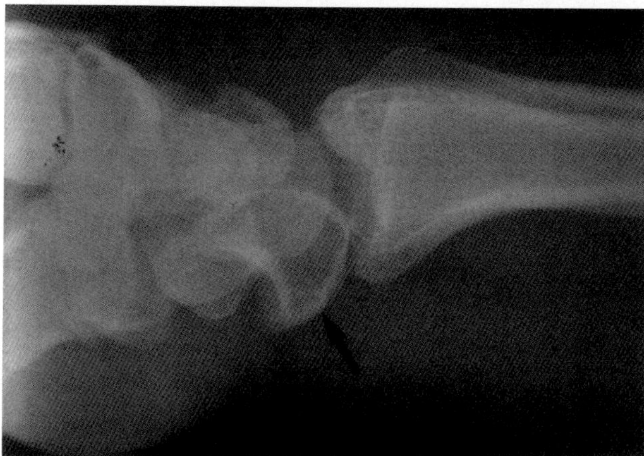

Fig. 13-42 Lateral radiograph demonstrating a volar lunate dislocation (*arrow*).

### Fractures and Dislocations of the Hand

Fractures and dislocations of the hand are common. Fracture of the phalanges account for 10% of all fractures. Metacarpal

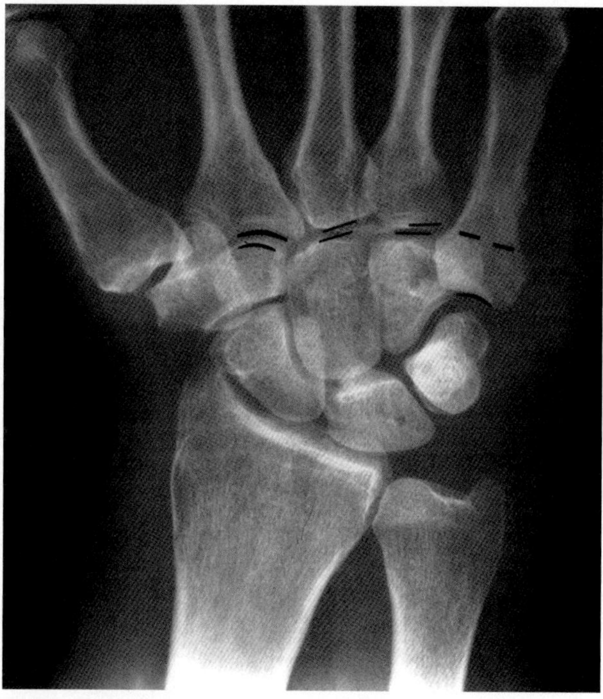

Fig. 13-43 Isolated dislocation of the fifth metacarpal base. *Lines* mark the normal carpometacarpal articulations for the two to four metacarpals. The fifth is dislocated dorsally and proximally. *Broken lines* mark the normal anatomic position.

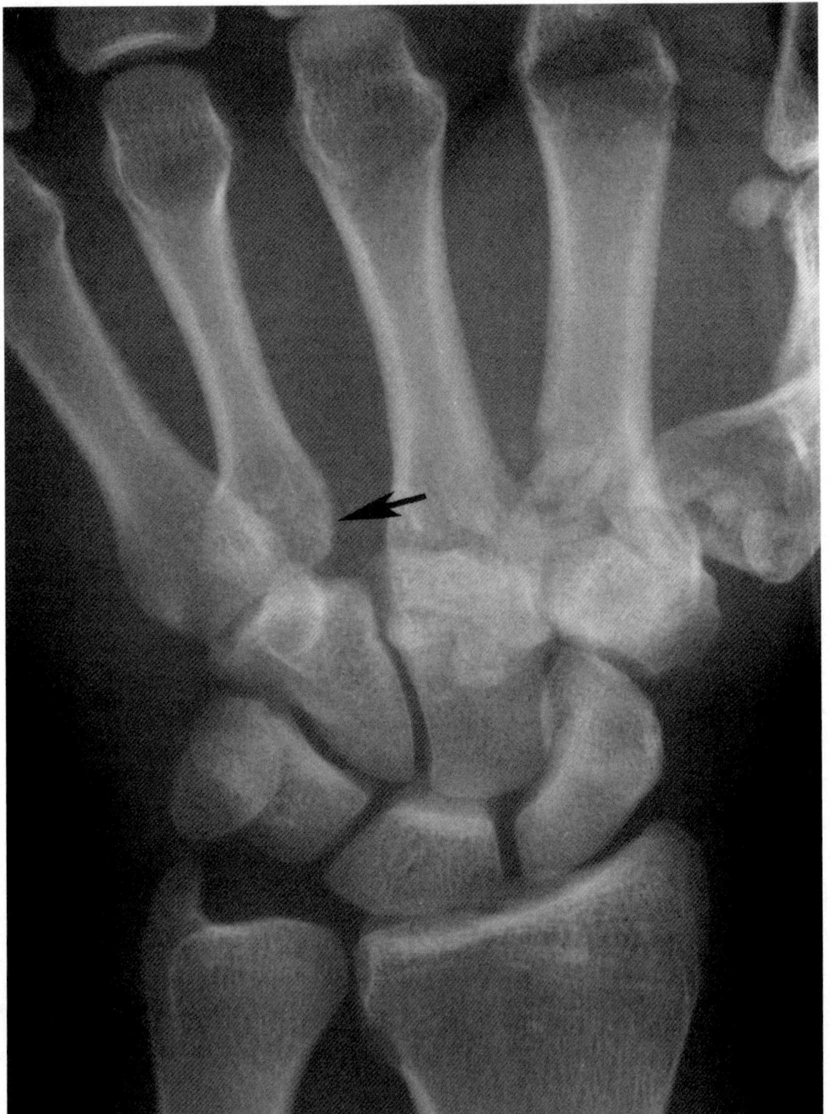

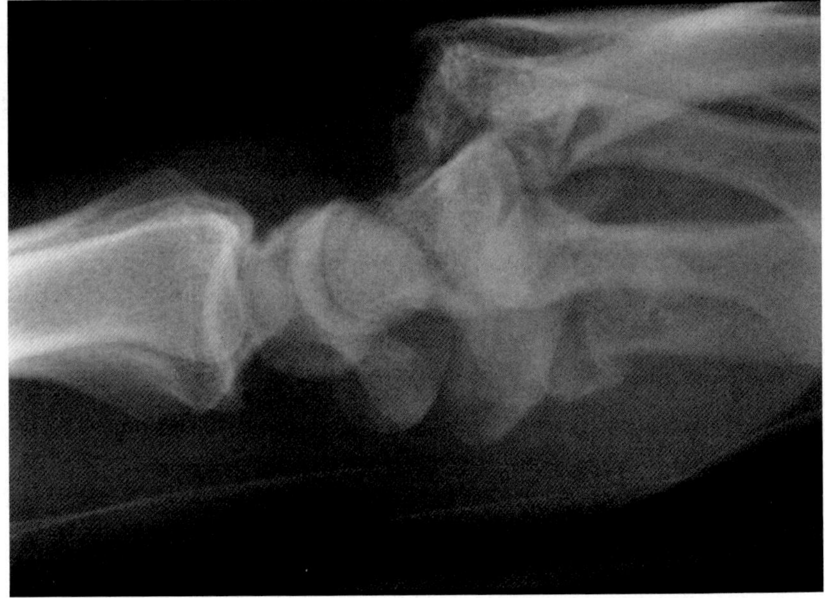

**Fig. 13-44** Complex fracture dislocation of the first through fourth metacarpal bases with associated fractures. Posteroanterior (PA) (**A**) and lateral (**B**) radiographs demonstrate the dorsal position of the metacarpal bases, multiple fracture fragments, and medial displacement of the fourth metacarpal base (*arrow*).

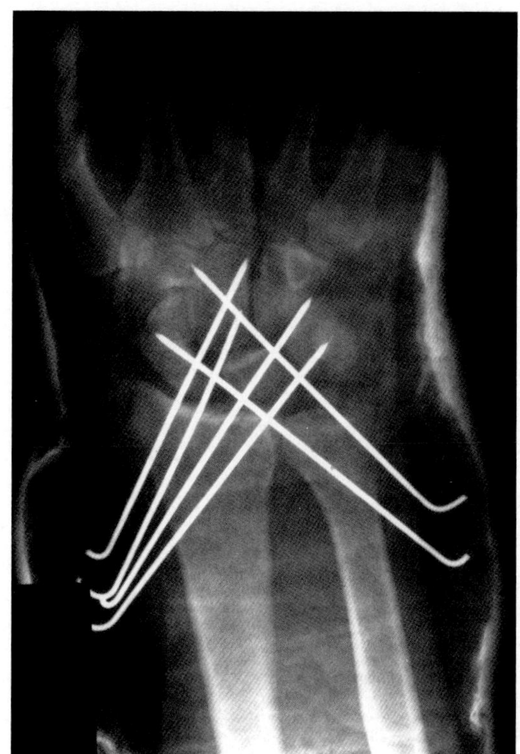


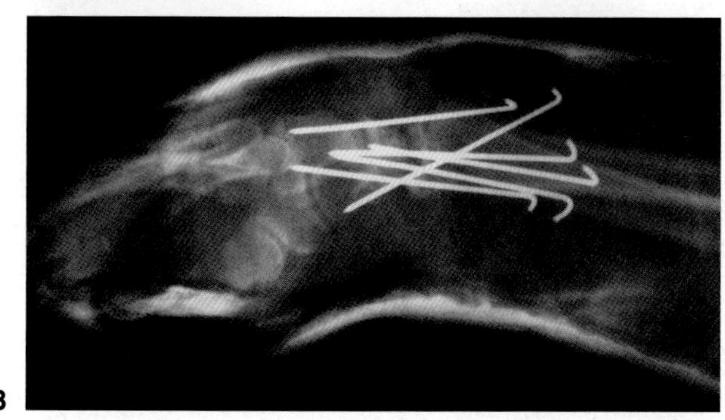


Fig. 13-45 Posteroanterior (PA) (A) and lateral (B) radiographs following K-wire reduction of a perilunate dislocation with cast immobilization.

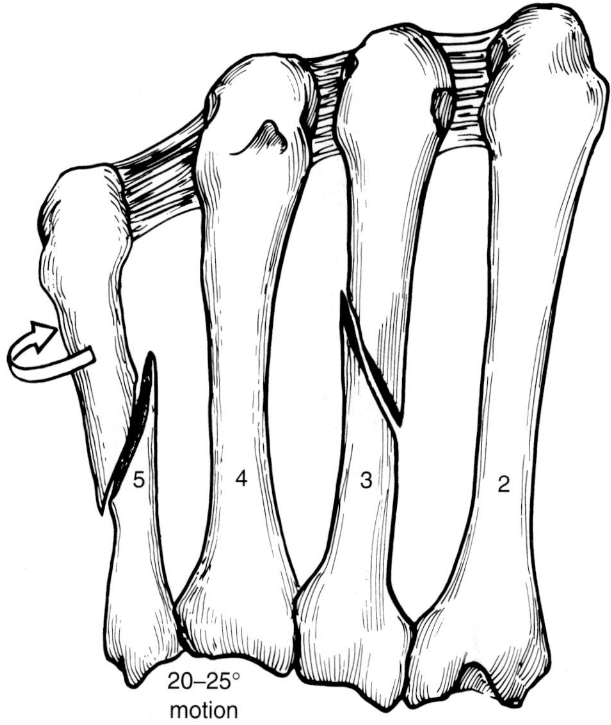


Fig. 13-46 Illustration of the second through fifth metacarpals with a spiral fracture and shortening of the fifth and spiral fracture and no shortening of the third. The transverse metacarpal ligament is stronger from the second to the third reducing the chances of shortening. There is essentially no motion at the second and third carpometacarpal articulations. The transverse ligament is more lax at the fourth and fifth that allows shortening to occur more easily. There is 20 to 25 degrees of motion at the bases of the fourth and fifth allowing some flexibility in treatment. (From Berquist TH. *Imaging of sports injuries.* Gaithersburg: Aspen Press; 1992.)

fractures account for 30% to 40% of fractures in the hand. The mechanism of injury may be direct or indirect trauma. Most can be managed conservatively. However, percutaneous pinning or open reduction and internal fixation are required in certain cases.

## Metacarpal Fractures

Metacarpal fractures are common and most frequently involve the fourth and fifth metacarpals. Owing to anatomic and treatment variations, we will discuss three fracture categories. These will include the thumb, mobile rays (fourth and fifth), and stable rays (second and third) (see Fig. 13-46).

**THUMB** The thumb is mobile, allowing more tolerance for rotation and angulation after fracture. However, pinch strength is critical so there is less room for error with fractures involving the carpometacarpal articulation. The cortex of the first metacarpal is thicker than the second through fifth metacarpals. Therefore, higher energy forces are required to cause fractures. Most fractures are due to axial loading.

Fractures of the first metacarpal most commonly involve the proximal articular surface (Bennett and Rolando fractures) followed by proximal extra-articular and transverse or spiral diaphyseal fractures. Fractures of the first metacarpal head and neck are uncommon.

Extra-articular fractures of the proximal first metacarpal may be transverse, oblique, or spiral. The muscles of the thenar region (adductor pollicis, abductor pollicis brevis, and flexor pollicis brevis) tend to flex and adduct the distal fragment.

The Bennett fracture is actually a fracture subluxation of the first carpometacarpal joint. The fracture is usually oblique with the volar (ulnar) fragment remaining in place due to the ulnar oblique ligament. The main fragment is displaced proximally by the abductor pollicis and flexor pollicis longus tendons (see Fig. 13-47).

The Rolando fracture is a T- or Y-shaped comminuted fracture of the base of the thumb. Fragment displacement similar to the Bennett fracture may also be evident (see Fig. 13-48).

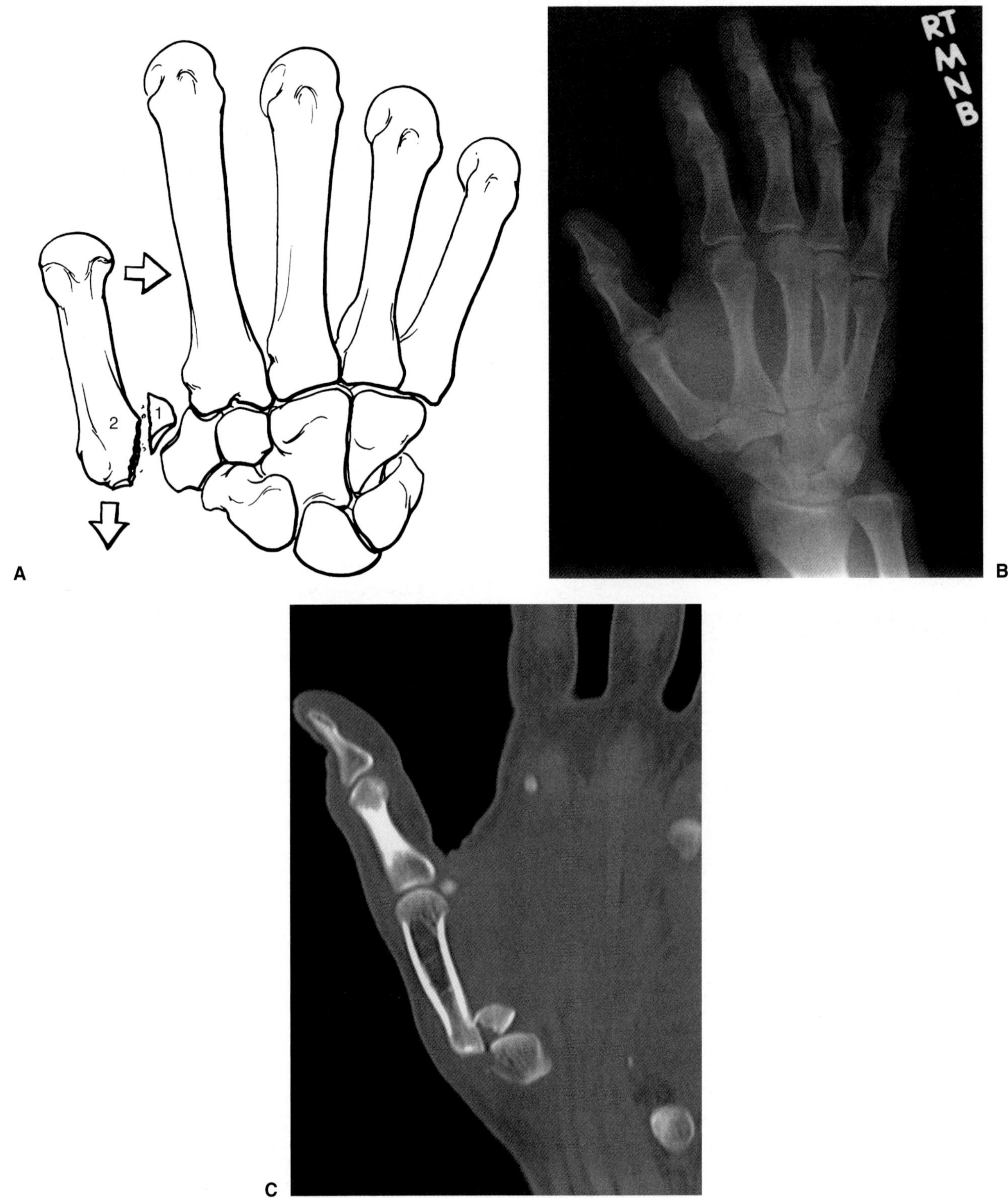


Fig. 13-47 Bennett fracture. A: Illustration of the Bennett fracture with the oblique fracture line and the small ulnar (volar) fragment (*1*) remaining in place due to the strong ulnar oblique ligament. The main fragment (*2*) is displaced proximally and flexed (*arrows*) by the abductor pollicis and flexor pollicis longus tendons. Radiograph (**B**) and coronal computed tomographic (CT) (**C**) images of a Bennett fracture.

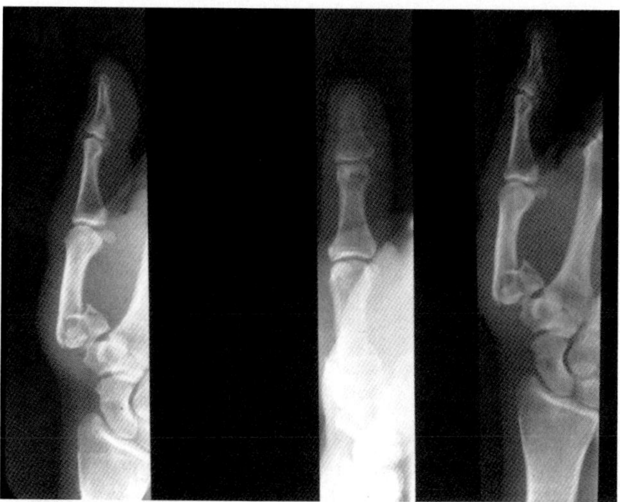

Fig. 13-48 Rolando fracture. Radiographs of the thumb demonstrating a Y-type fracture of the first metacarpal base. The main fragment is displaced similar to the Bennett fracture in Figure 13-47.

SECOND AND THIRD METACARPALS (STABLE RAYS) The second and third metacarpals are considered stable due to the lack of motion as the carpometacarpal joints (Fig. 13-46). This reduces the latitude for angular and rotational deformities that are acceptable after fracture compared to the thumb and mobile fourth and fifth metacarpals.

Fractures of the second and third metacarpals occur most commonly in the region of the neck (see Fig. 13-49). Muscle forces tend to angulate the distal fragment in a palmar direction. Transverse or spiral shaft fractures are less common. Spiral fractures have a tendency to rotate and shorten. Therefore, internal fixation may be required to maintain metacarpal length.

FOURTH AND FIFTH METACARPALS (MOBILE RAYS) Mobility at the fourth and fifth carpometacarpal joints allows more latitude for angulation in these metacarpals. However, excessive shortening, angulation, and malrotation are not acceptable. Fractures of the metacarpal necks and bases, especially the fifth, are common (Fig. 13-49). Proximal articular involvement is also most common with fifth metacarpal fractures. Transverse and spiral diaphyseal fractures are less common (see Fig. 13-50). Spiral fractures are prone to shortening and rotation when involving the fourth and fifth metacarpals.

Fractures of the fifth metacarpal neck (Boxer fracture) are common (see Fig. 13-51). Fractures are due to axial loading resulting in angular deformity with palmar displacement of the distal fragment. The lateral view is essential to evaluate the degree of angulation. Up to 40 degrees can be tolerated for fractures of the fifth metacarpal neck and 25 degrees for the fourth metacarpal neck.

## Phalangeal Fractures and Fracture/Dislocations

Phalangeal fracture dislocations are common. Phalangeal fractures account for more than 10% of all skeletal fractures. In younger patients the injuries are often sports related. In older individuals, injuries are more often due to falls, machinery accidents, and for the tuft, crush injuries. The flexor tendons are held in position by the pulley system along the finger (see Fig. 13-52). This effects fragment position, but injury to the

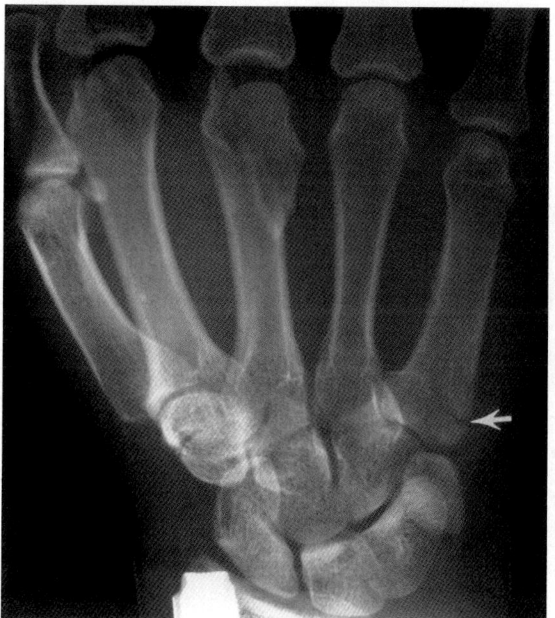


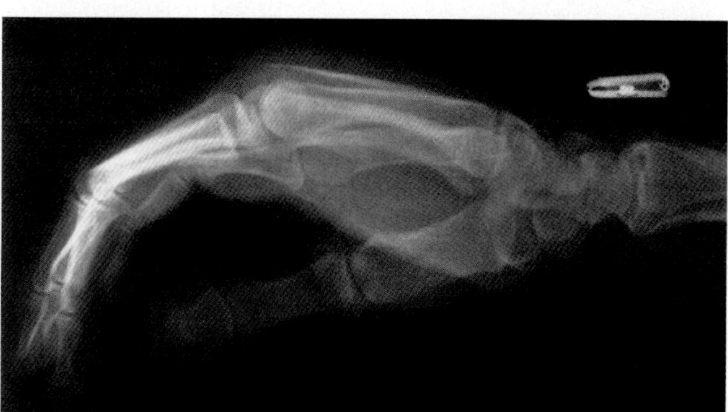


Fig. 13-49 Posteroanterior (PA) (A) and lateral (B) radiographs demonstrating oblique intra-articular fractures of the second and third metacarpal heads and necks with proximal displacement of the distal fragment of the third metacarpal resulting in significant articular deformity. There is also an undisplaced fracture at the base of the fifth metacarpal (*arrow*).

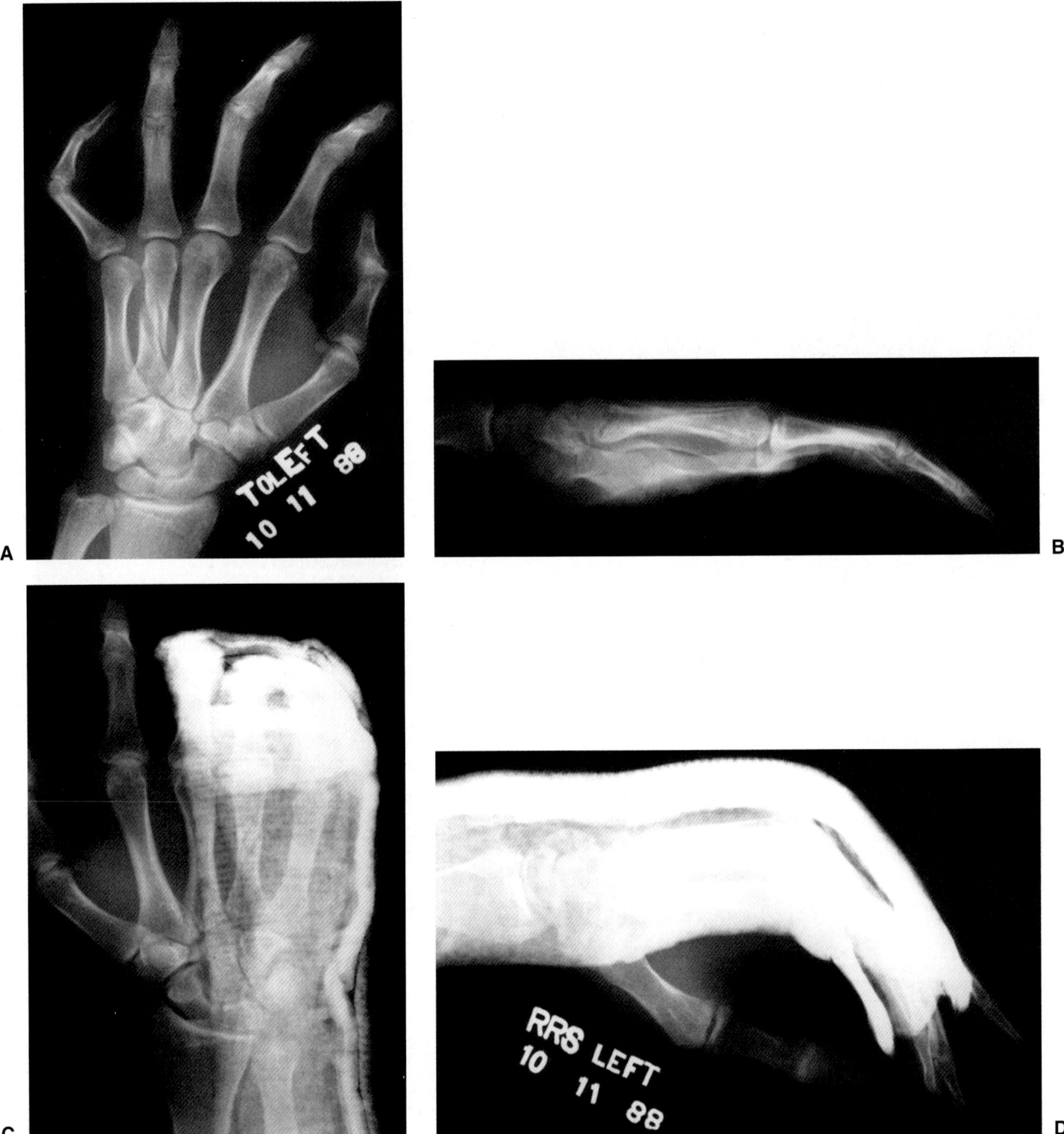


Fig. 13-50 Spiral fracture of the fourth metacarpal. Posteroanterior (PA) (A) and lateral (B) radiographs demonstrate a spiral fracture of the fourth metacarpal shaft with rotation and shortening. The fracture was reduced using finger traction and closed reduction with an ulnar splint (C and D). There is no angulation on the lateral view.

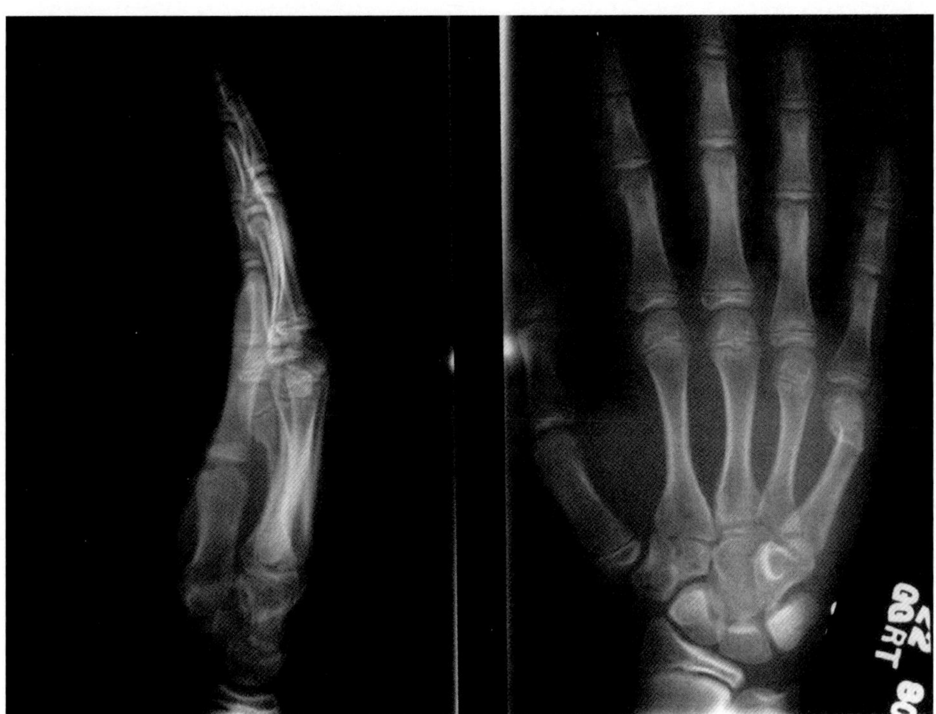

Fig. 13-51 Boxer's fracture. Lateral and posteroanterior (PA) radiographs demonstrate a fracture of the fifth metacarpal neck with palmar displacement of the distal fragment.

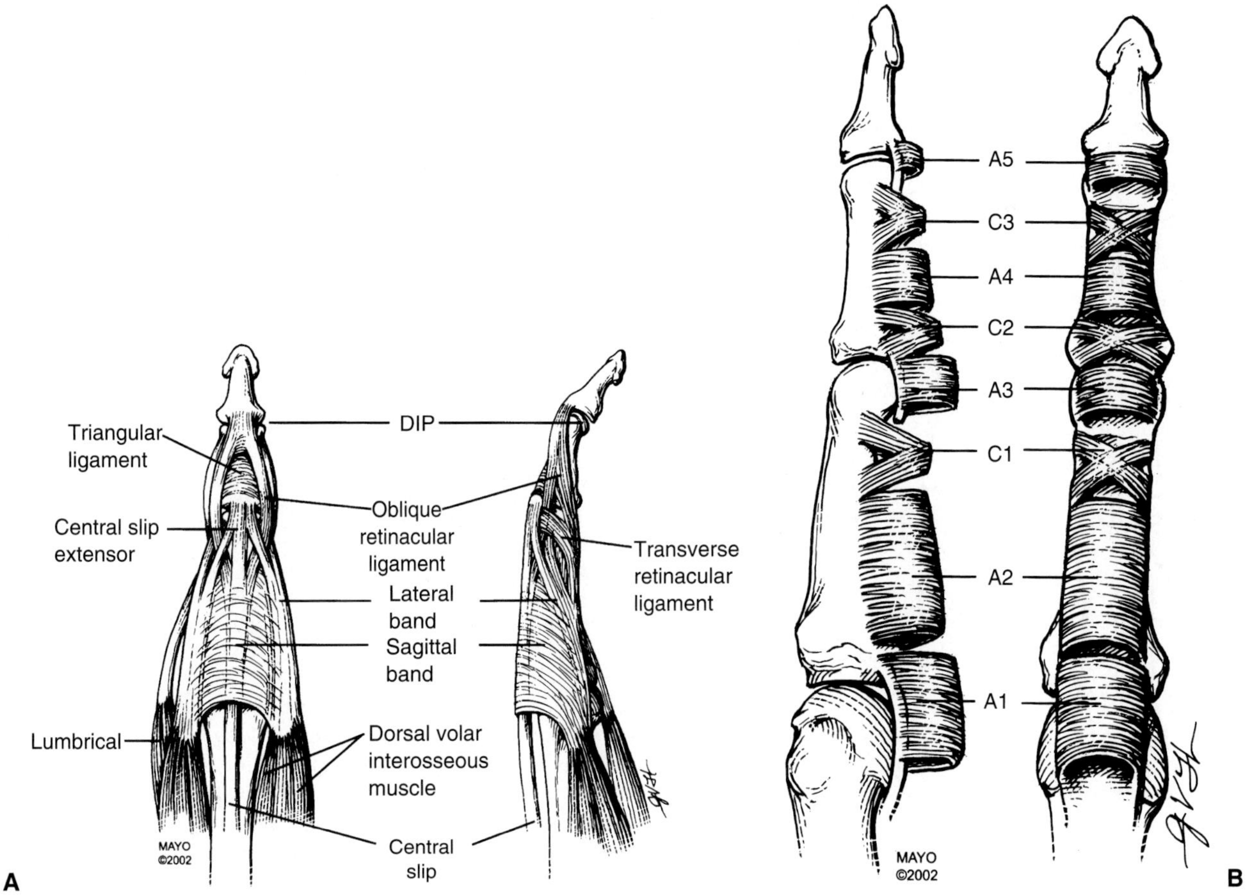

Triangular ligament
Central slip extensor
Lumbrical
DIP
Oblique retinacular ligament
Lateral band
Sagittal band
Dorsal volar interosseous muscle
Central slip
Transverse retinacular ligament
MAYO ©2002
A
A5
C3
A4
C2
A3
C1
A2
A1
MAYO ©2002
B

Fig. 13-52 Tendon anatomy of the fingers. A: Illustration of the relationships of the flexor and extensor tendons to the phalanges. B: Illustration of the pulley system for the flexor tendons and the relationships to the articular and phalangeal segments. (From Berquist TH. *MRI of the hand and wrist.* Philadelphia: Lippincott Williams & Wilkins; 2003.)

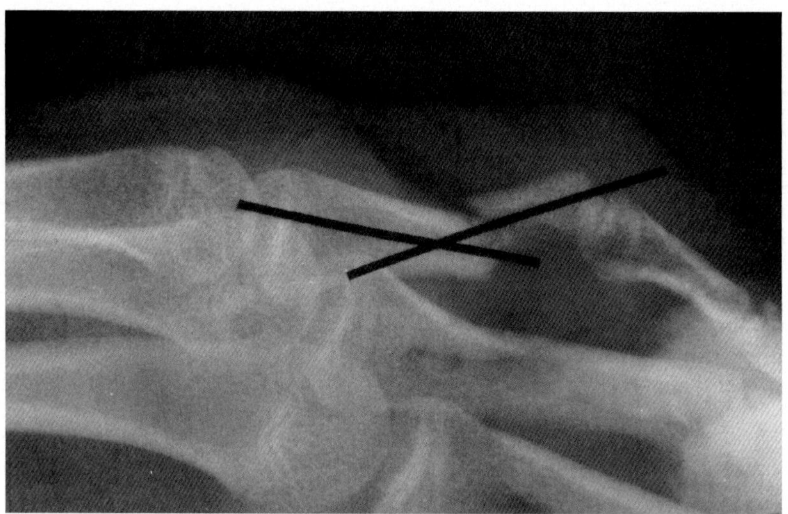

**Fig. 13-53** Lateral radiograph demonstrating a fracture of the proximal phalanx with apex volar angulation (*black lines*).

tendon sheath, tendons, and pulley system must also be kept in mind when imaging phalangeal injuries.

Fractures of the proximal phalanx are most common. In children, fractures at the base of the proximal phalanx are particularly common. Fractures of the diaphysis tend to angulate in a volar direction due to the deforming forces of the flexor and extensor tendons (see Fig. 13-53). Problems with malunion, shortening, and rotation tend to be more common with fractures of the proximal phalanx. Also, adhesions at the fracture site may cause tendon dysfunction. Fractures may also involve the articular surface. Unicondylar or bicondylar involvement may be present (see Fig. 13-54). Although these fractures may appear stable radiographically, they are frequently unstable clinically.

Fractures of the middle phalanx have similar patterns compared to the proximal phalanx. The most common middle phalangeal fracture is the volar plate of the proximal portion due to hyperextension of the joint (see Fig. 13-55). Diaphyseal fractures may angulate in a dorsal or volar direction depending on the relationship of the fracture to the sublimis tendon insertion. This tendon inserts along the proximal portion of the middle phalanx.

Fractures of the distal phalanx may be related to crush injuries. These fractures are usually stable. The mallet fracture or avulsion of the dorsal plate due to the extensor mechanism is more difficult to manage (see Fig. 13-56).

Dislocations of the phalangeal joints occur dorsally and may have associated articular fractures (see Figs. 13-57 and 13-58).

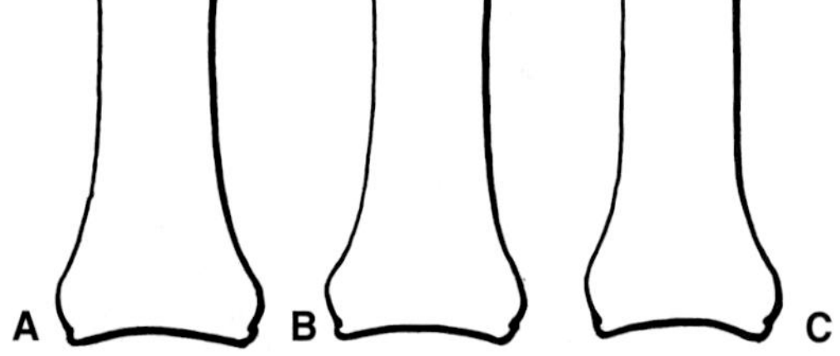

**Fig. 13-54** Illustration of articular fractures of the proximal phalanx. A—unicondylar, B—bicondylar, C—osteochondral shear fracture. (From Berquist TH. *Imaging of sports injuries*. Gaithersburg: Aspen Press; 1992.)

## Suggested Reading

Baratz ME, Divelbiss B. Fixation of phalangeal fractures. *Hand Clin*. 1997;13:541–555.

Green DP, Anderson JR. Closed reduction and percutaneous fixation of fractured phalanges. *J Bone Joint Surg*. 1973; 55A:1651–1653.

Lee SG, Jupiter JB. Phalangeal and metacarpal fractures of the hand. *Hand Clin*. 2000;16:323–332.

### Imaging of Hand Injuries

Imaging of the hand with PA, lateral, and oblique views will detect most fractures and fracture/dislocations of the metacarpals and phalanges (Fig. 13-50). When specific fingers are involved, they should be isolated to provide more optimal visualization of the anatomy (Fig. 13-55). CT is useful in selected cases to define the size and position of articular fragments before treatment planning (Fig. 13-47). MRI is capable of detecting subtle fractures in the hand and wrist and evaluating soft tissue structures as well. Conventional or MR arthrography is useful to evaluate articular and supporting anatomy following dislocations.

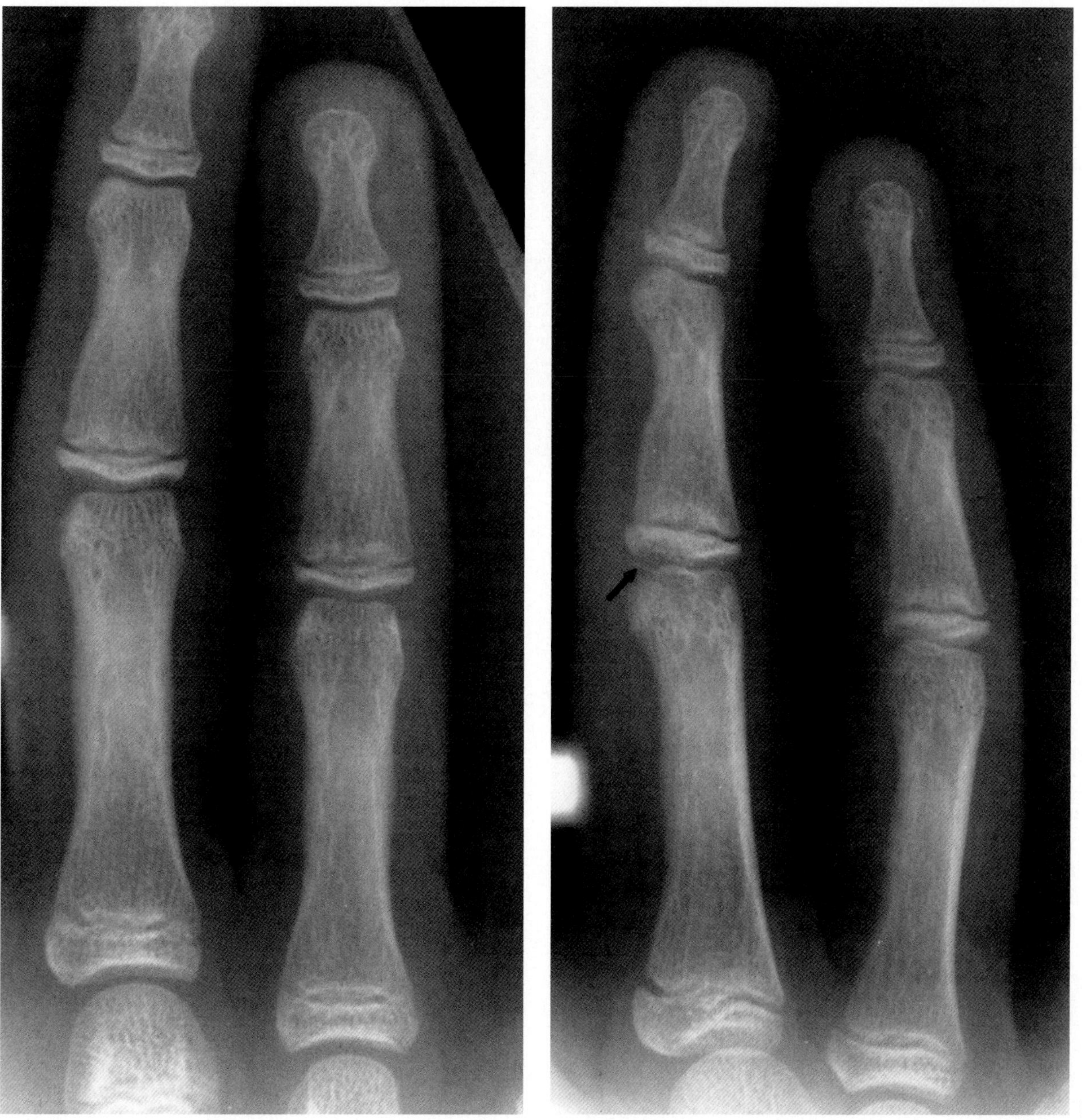


Fig. 13-55 Volar plate avulsion middle phalanx. Posteroanterior (PA) (A), oblique (B), and lateral (C) radiographs of the middle finger demonstrating an avulsion of the volar plate of the middle phalanx in an adolescent soccer player. The subtle fracture is best seen on the lateral view.

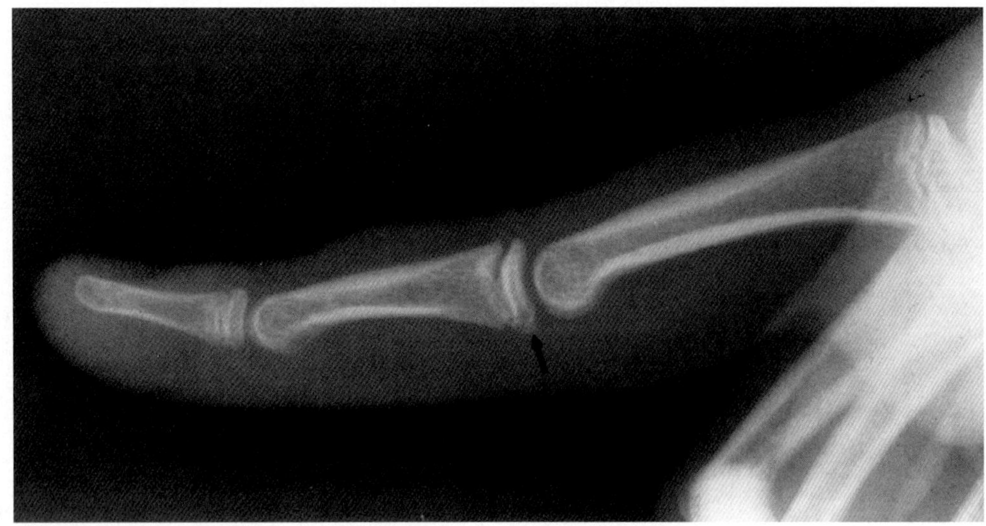


Fig. 13-55 *(Continued)*

## Suggested Reading

Berquist TH, Trigg SD. Hand and wrist. In: Berquist TH, ed. *Imaging atlas of orthopaedic appliances and prostheses*, ed. New York: Raven Press; 1995:831–921.

### Treatment Options

Treatment options vary with the type of hand injury and stability of the injury. In some cases percutaneous pinning or plate and screw fixation is performed initially, and in other cases surgical intervention is reserved for injuries where reduction cannot be maintained with conventional immobilization techniques (see Fig. 13-59).

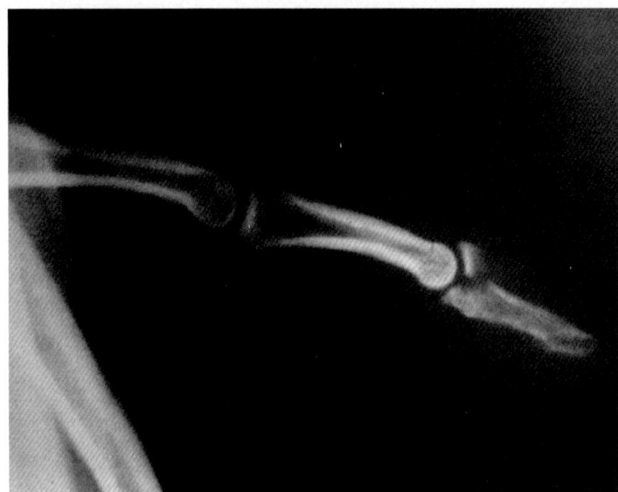

Fig. 13-56 Mallet finger. Lateral radiograph of the finger demonstrating a dorsal fracture of the distal phalanx with slight proximal displacement.

Fractures of the neck and diaphysis of the thumb can be treated conservatively if there is no significant displacement and <20 degrees of angulation. Spiral fractures tend to be less stable and may require percutaneous pinning. Articular fractures at the base of the thumb (Figs. 13-47 and 13-48). Reduction is difficult to maintain without internal fixation. K-wires are used percutaneously or with open reduction to attach the main fragment to the trapezium. Minifragment screws may also be used. It is not essential to include the small ulnar fragment with the K-wire fixation (see Fig. 13-60).

Fractures of the second and third metacarpals may be treated with closed reduction and cast immobilization (Fig. 13-50). Maintaining reduction can be difficult. It is important to preserve length and prevent rotation or angulation. Therefore, K-wires using the adjacent metacarpal for stability or miniplate and screw fixation are often required (see Fig. 13-61).

Fractures of the mobile rays (fourth and fifth) metacarpals can be managed with closed reduction in most situations. Fractures of the fifth metacarpal neck frequently angulate with the distal fragment displaced in a palmar direction. The lateral view can accurately measure the angular deformity. Angulation of <40 degrees can be accepted for fractures of the fifth metacarpal neck and 25 degrees for the fourth metacarpal neck. When angular deformities exceed this, K-wire fixation should performed (see Fig. 13-62). Spiral or oblique fractures of the fourth and fifth metacarpal shafts tend to shorten and rotate. This may require internal fixation with K-wires, multiple lag (interfragmentary) screws (see Fig. 13-63), or miniplate and screw fixation (see Fig. 13-64).

Treatment of phalangeal fracture/dislocations varies with the phalanx involved and whether there is articular involvement. Undisplaced phalangeal fractures and isolated dislocations can be treated with closed reduction in most cases (Fig. 13-57). Fractures of the phalangeal shafts may be angulated or reduction may be difficult to maintain (Fig. 13-53). In this setting, K-wire fixation is typically used. Unicondylar and bicondylar fractures

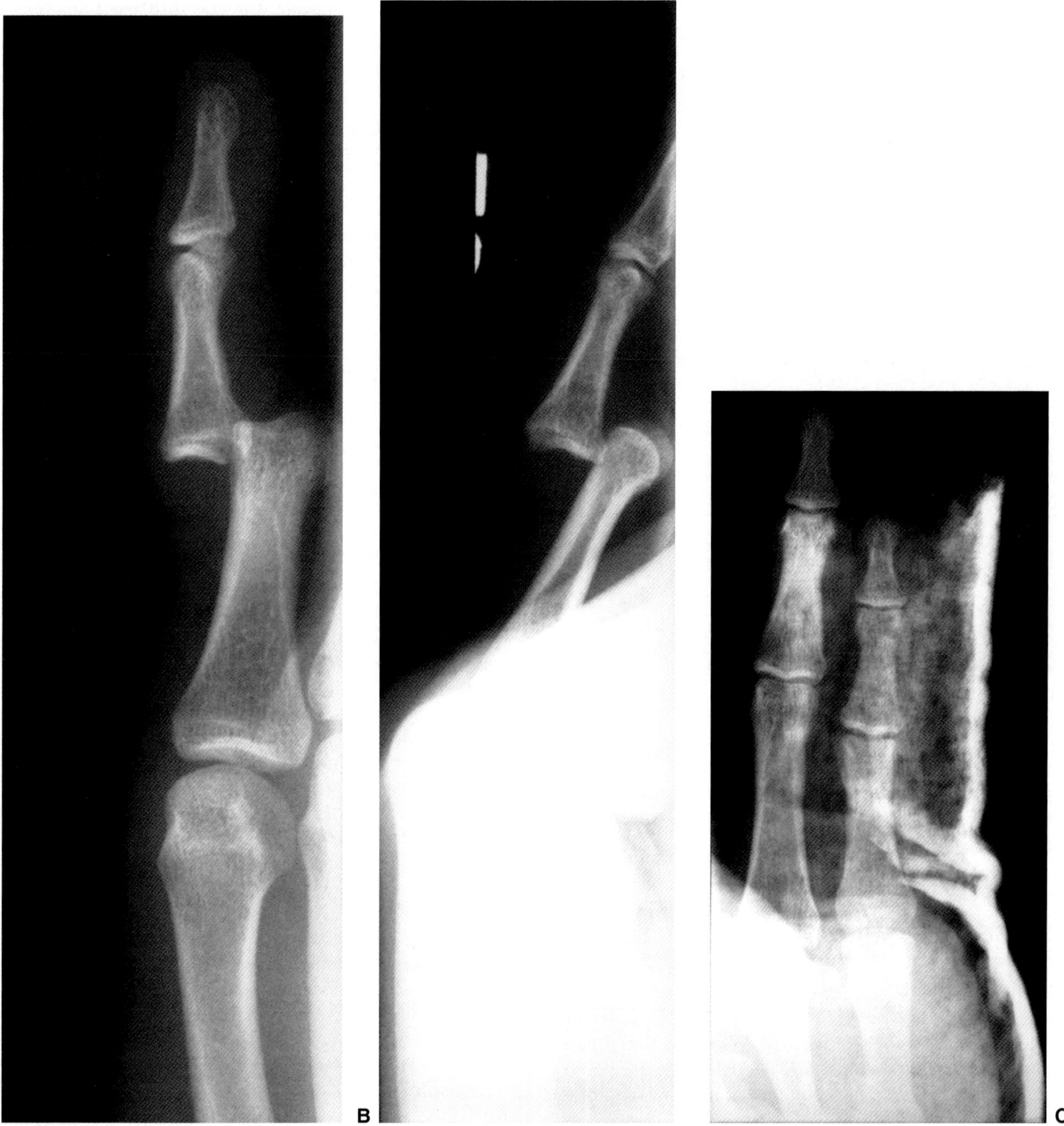


Fig. 13-57 Dislocation of the proximal interphalangeal joint. Posteroanterior (PA) (A) and lateral (B) radiographs demonstrate a dorsal medial dislocation of the fifth finger without associated fracture. C: Post reduction image with ulnar splint in place.

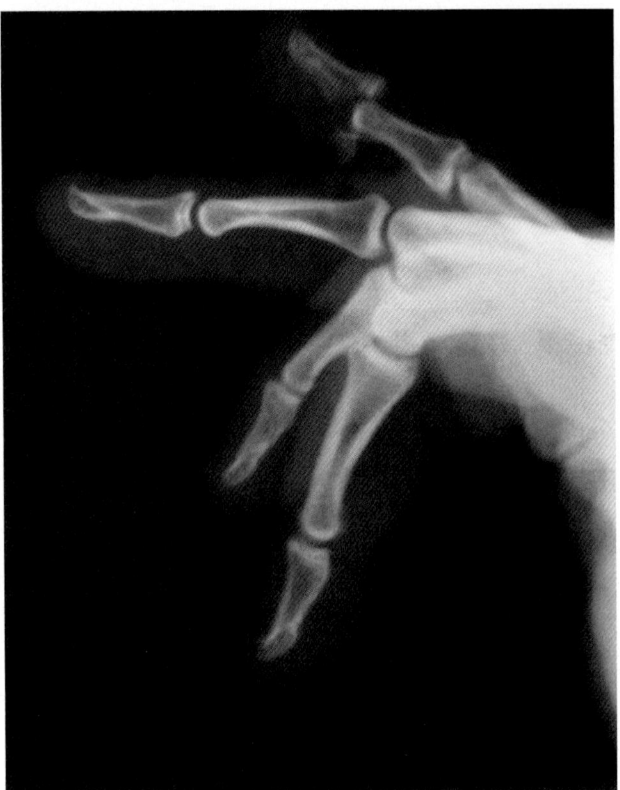

**Fig. 13-58** Lateral radiograph demonstrating a fracture dislocation of the distal interphalangeal joint.

(Fig. 13-54) also tend to displace. Therefore, K-wire or K-wire with tension band is used to maintain the articular surface (see Fig. 13-65).

## Suggested Reading

Ashkenaze DM, Ruby LK. Metacarpal fractures and dislocations. *Orthop Clin North Am*. 1992;23:19–33.

Beatty E, Light TR, Belsole RJ, et al. Wrist and hand injuries in children. *Hand Clin*. 1990;6:723–738.

Lee SG, Jupiter JB. Phalangeal and metacarpal fractures of the hand. *Hand Clin*. 2000;16:323–332.

### Imaging of Complications

Complications of metacarpal and phalangeal fractures and dislocations are similar to those described earlier. Fortunately, nonunion is rare. However, malunion, especially with rotational deformity, is more common. This may result in joint deformity and function loss. Osteotomy can be performed to restore alignment (see Fig. 13-66).

Arthrosis is also common following intra-articular fractures and dislocations. Post-traumatic arthrosis is usually adequately evaluated with serial radiographs. Additional studies with MRI may be useful to evaluate articular cartilage and associated capsular or tendon injuries.

## Suggested Reading

Creighton JJ, Streichen JB. Complications in phalangeal and metacarpal fracture management: Results of extensor tenolysis. *Hand Clin*. 1994;10:111–116.

Lee SG, Jupiter JB. Phalangeal and metacarpal fractures of the hand. *Hand Clin*. 2000;16:323–332.

# Hand and Wrist Arthroplasty

Arthroplasty of the wrist, hand, and thumb base has evolved as an alternative to arthrodesis. The wrist, hand, and thumb will be discussed separately.

## Wrist Arthroplasty

Wrist arthroplasty began to evolve soon after the introduction of total hip replacements. Most wrist arthroplasties are performed for rheumatoid disease as upper extremity involvement frequently drives the need for improved wrist function. In other arthropathies, the elbow and shoulder are frequently not involved, thereby reducing the need for wrist replacement surgery. In the ideal setting, patients considered for wrist arthroplasty should have bilateral painful arthropathy with relatively good soft tissue support and alignment. Patients with poor soft tissue support, such as lupus with marked joint laxity, are not good candidates for wrist replacement. Poor bone stock and previous arthrodesis make arthroplasty difficult, but they are not absolute contraindications.

Contraindications include neurologic dysfunction, paralysis, infection, or heavy-activity requirements. Patients who require walking assistance with a cane or crutches or need to lift weights >10 lb are not acceptable candidates.

Wrist function requires variable degrees of motion including flexion, extension, radial, and ulnar deviation. Various values have been paced on required motion over the years. The degree of flexion required has varied form 5 to 54 degrees, extension from 30 to 60 degrees, radial deviation 10 to 17 degrees, and ulnar deviation 15 to 40 degrees. The extensor carpi radialis brevis and longus tendons must be intact in order to provide satisfactory results following wrist arthroplasty. New implants allow 60 degrees of extension, 40 degrees of flexion, and 20 degrees of radial and ulnar deviation.

Preoperative evaluation includes clinical evaluation with the goal of relieving pain, increasing stability, and improving function following arthroplasty. A clinical scoring system similar to other joints is used for both pre- and postoperative assessment. There are multiple systems, but most evaluate balance, motion, pain relief, and strength. The system designed by Lamberta et al. is a 100-point system with 30 points for

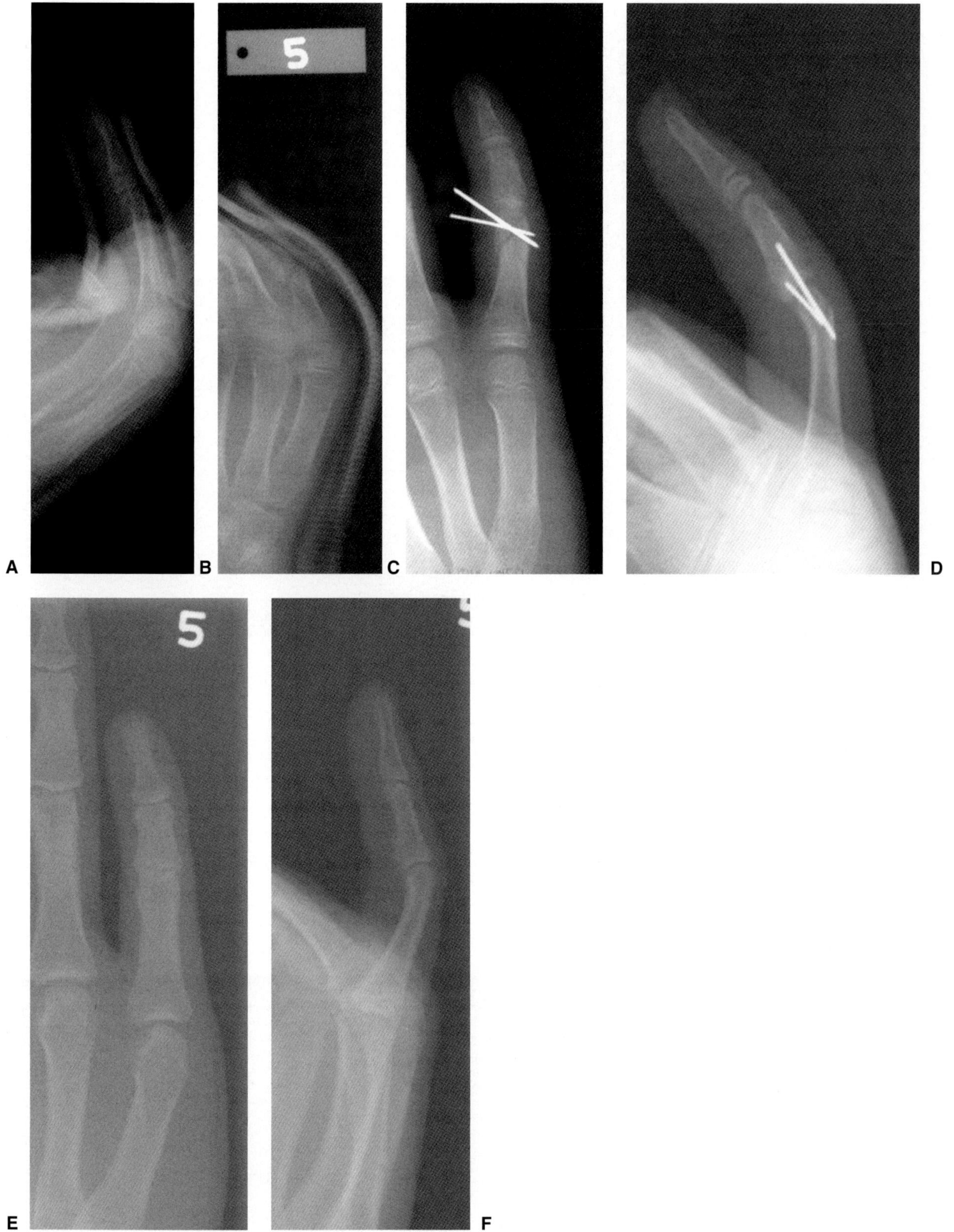


Fig. 13-59 Lateral (A) and oblique (B) radiographs of a minimally displaced fracture of the distal aspect of the proximal phalanx in a child. There was an attempt at cast immobilization. Anteroposterior (AP) (C) and lateral (D) radiographs following percutaneous pinning of the fragment. The fracture line was at the margin of the joint surface. AP (E) and lateral (F) radiographs following healing with no radiographic or functional deformity.

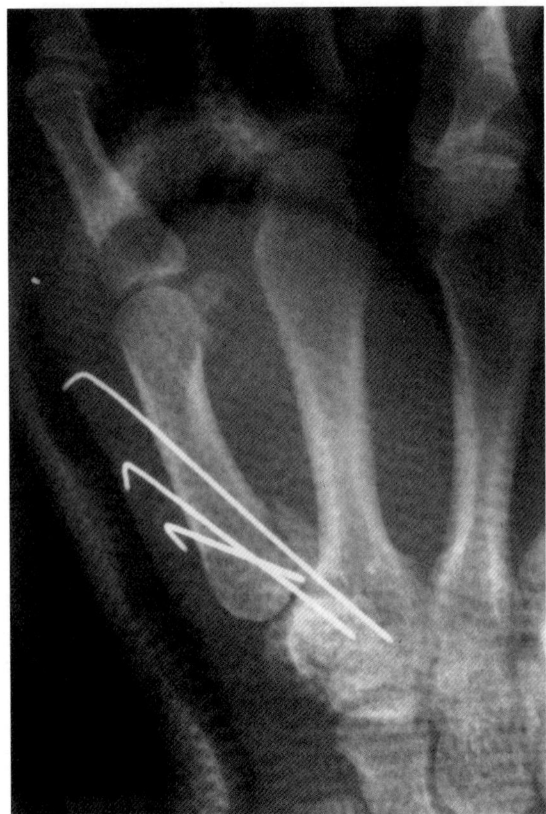


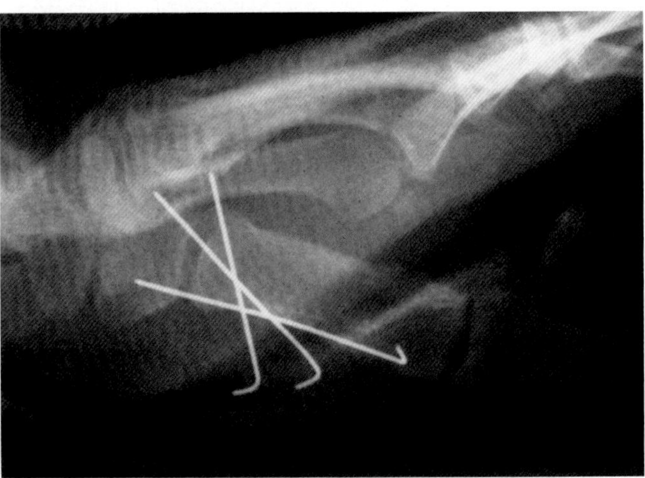


Fig. 13-60 Frontal (A) and lateral (B) radiographs following K-wire fixation of a Bennett fracture. The small ulnar fragment (*arrow*) is not included in the K-wire fixation. Cast immobilization.

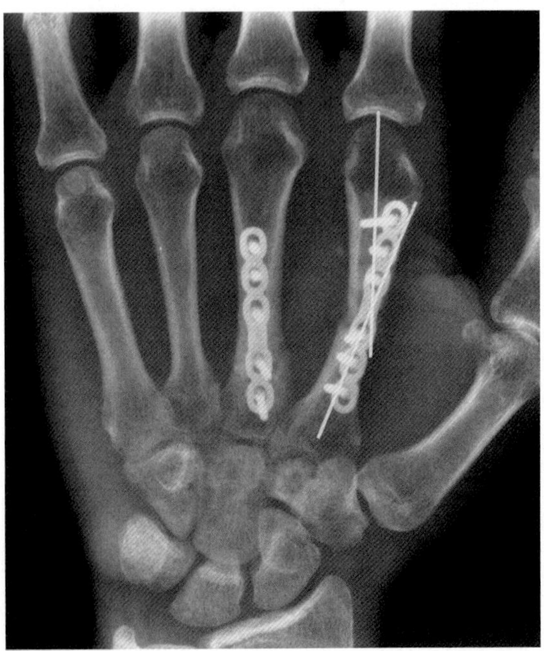


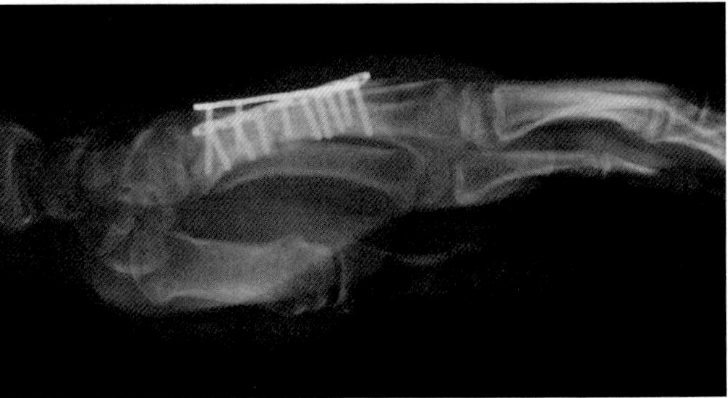


Fig. 13-61 Posteroanterior (PA) (A) and lateral (B) radiographs demonstrating miniplate and screw fixation of fractures of the proximal third and mid second metacarpal. There is residual angular deformity (lines) of the second metacarpal.

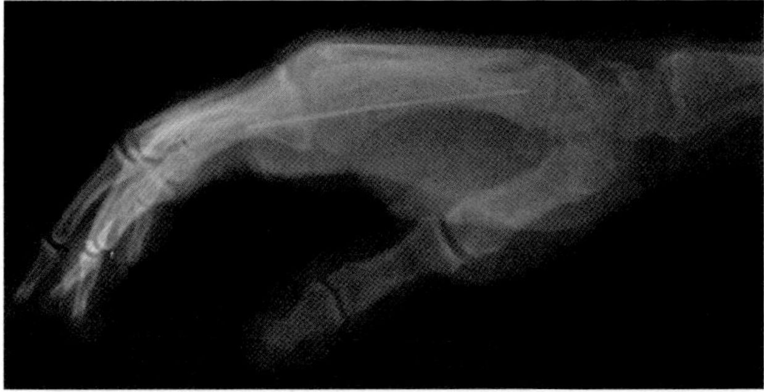

Fig. 13-62 Boxer's fracture. Lateral radiograph with K-wire fixation demonstrating anatomic alignment of a fracture with angular deformity exceeding 40 degrees before reduction.

balance (flexion-extension and radioulnar deviation), 25 points for the degree of motion in flexion and extension (70 to 90 degrees excellent or 25 points, 50 to 69 degrees good or 20 points, 15 to 49 degrees fair or 15 points, <15 degrees poor or 0 points), 35 points for pain relief (maximum of 35 points for no pain to 0 points for severe pain), and grip strength 10 points. Measurements are made clinically, but radiographs with maximum flexion, extension, and radial and ulnar deviation can also be used.

## Suggested Reading

Carlson JR, Simmons BP. Total wrist arthroplasty. *J Am Acad Orthop Surg*. 1998;6:308–315.

Lamberta FJ, ferlic DC, Clayton ML. Volz total wrist arthroplasty in rheumatoid arthritis. A preliminary report. *J Hand Surg [Br]*. 1980;5:245–252.

Takwale VJ, Nuttall D, Trail IA, et al. Biaxial total wrist replacement in patients with rheumatoid arthritis: Clinical review, survivorship and radiological analysis. *J Bone Joint Surg*. 2002;84(5):692–699.

Taljanovic MS, Jones MD, Hunter TB, et al. Joint arthroplasties and prostheses. *Radiographics*. 2003;23:1295–1314.

### Preoperative Imaging

Preoperative radiographs of the wrist include PA, lateral, and oblique views. Motion studies can be performed fluoroscopically

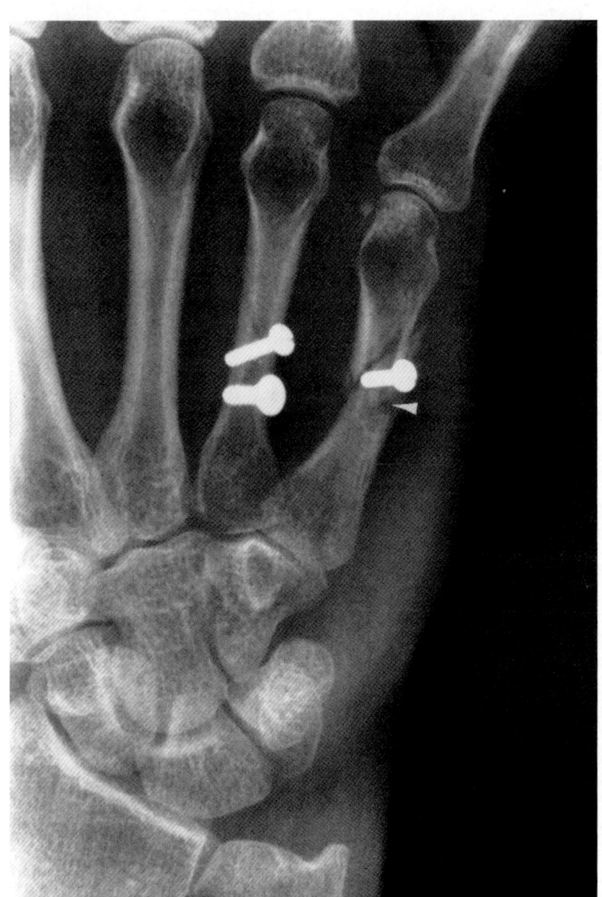

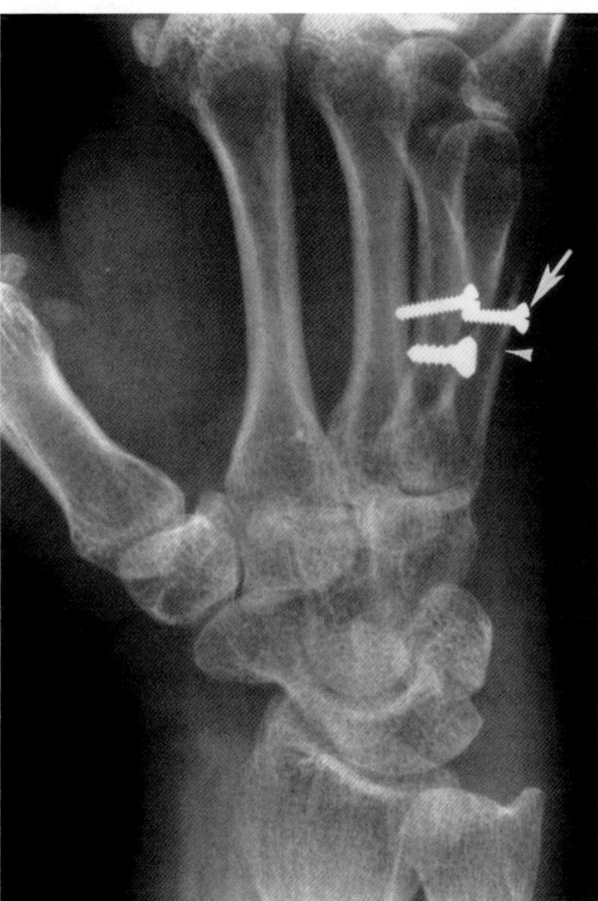

Fig. 13-63 Spiral fractures of the fourth and fifth metacarpals treated with multiple lag screws. Posteroanterior (PA) (A) and oblique (B) radiographs demonstrate excellent alignment and healing of the fourth metacarpal. The fifth metacarpal is angulated and the screw is pulling out of the distal fragment (*arrow*). A screw had been removed earlier (*arrowhead*) due to soft tissue irritation.

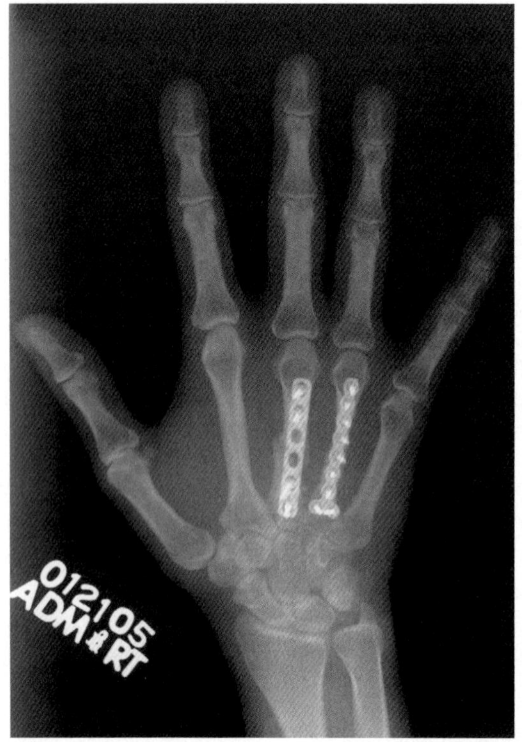


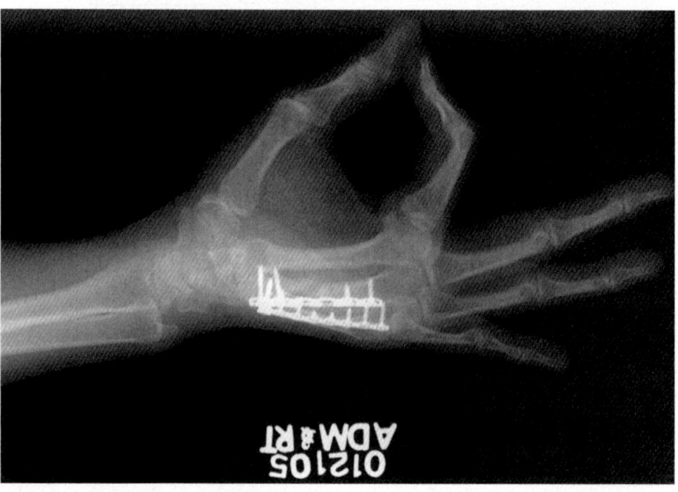


**Fig. 13-64** Fractures of the third and fourth metacarpals with miniplate and screw fixation. Posteroanterior (PA) (A) and lateral (B) radiographs demonstrate a healed fracture of the fourth metacarpal with delayed union of the third metacarpal fracture. There is hypertrophic callus with the fracture line still visible 8 months following the injury.

or using static images to obtain a baseline for the extent or flexion, extension, and radial and unlar deviation. These measurements are more frequently made clinically. Additional studies may also be required. CT with coronal and sagittal reformatting is used to evaluate bone stock. MRI can be used to evaluate soft tissue support and integrity of the key muscles required for successful wrist replacement surgery.

## Suggested Reading

Berquist TH, Trigg SD. Hand and wrist. In: Berquist TH, ed. *Imaging atlas of orthopaedic appliances and prostheses*. New York: Raven Press; 1995:831–921.

### Treatment Options

Wrist replacement approaches and implants have changed significantly over the years. In the late 1960s and 1970s, several designs were available. Swanson developed the silastic implant. Using this implant required resection of the distal radial articular surface and styloid and the distal ulna along with proximal row carpectomy. Implants were double stemmed and came in different sizes. The original implant had a Dacron core to increase strength and reduce rotary torque. Later designs have shorter stems with a metal grommet to protect the bony surfaces (see Fig. 13-67).

In the 1970s, Meuli and Volz developed a cemented system that used metal and polyethylene components. The Meuli implant had a distal cupped component with stems for the second and third metacarpals, a proximal trunnion for radial fixation, and a central polyethylene ball (see Fig. 13-68). The distal stems were later offset to facilitate centering of the wrist. The Mayo modification of the distal portion used a single dorsal stem to center wrist motion more accurately at the capitate head (see Fig. 13-69). Using the Meuli system, the radial styloid, distal ulna, scaphoid, lunate, triquetrum, and proximal capitate were resected.

The Volz system was similar and configured of cobalt-chromium alloy with an ultrahigh molecular weight polyethylene interface. This system was also later modified to have only one distal stem with small fixation pegs. Newergeneration systems have been developed to provide improved function and reduce bone loss. These include the Biax total wrist system (Depuy Orthopaedics, Inc., a Johnson and Johnson Company, Warsaw Indians), The Uni2 total wrist (Kinetikos Medical Inc. [KMI], Carlsbad, California) and the Avanta total wrist (Small Bone Innovations, Inc., Morrisville, Pennsylvania) (see Fig. 13-70). These systems provide increased stability and function with less bone resection including sparing the distal ulna.

Selected carpal replacement is also possible. The scaphoid and lunate are most often replaced using silastic implants. Indications include post-traumatic arthritis, avascular necrosis, and other arthropathies. Implants using elastomere (synthetic

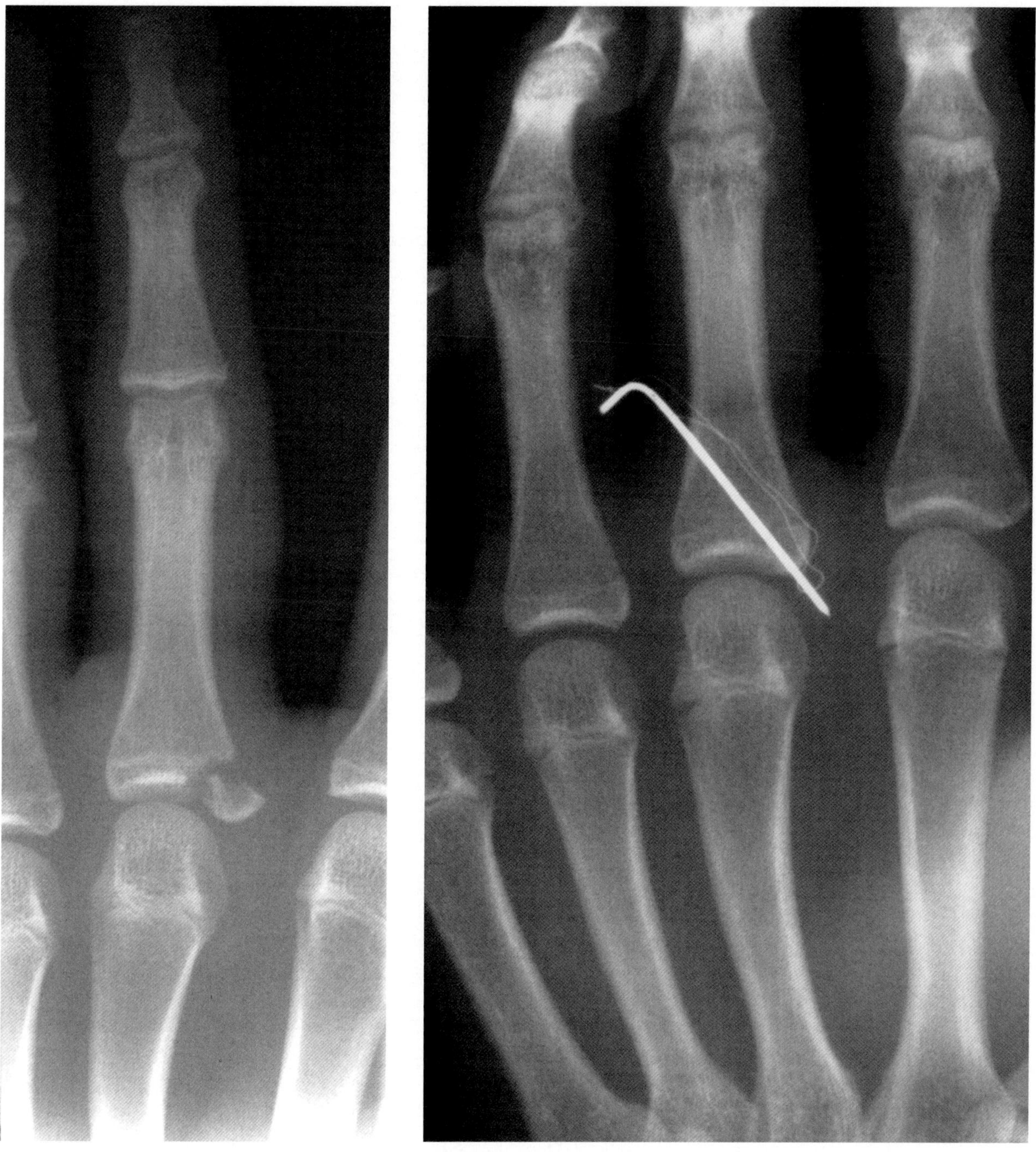

Fig. 13-65 Intra-articular fracture at the base of the third proximal phalanx (A) reduced and fixated with K-wire and tension band (B).

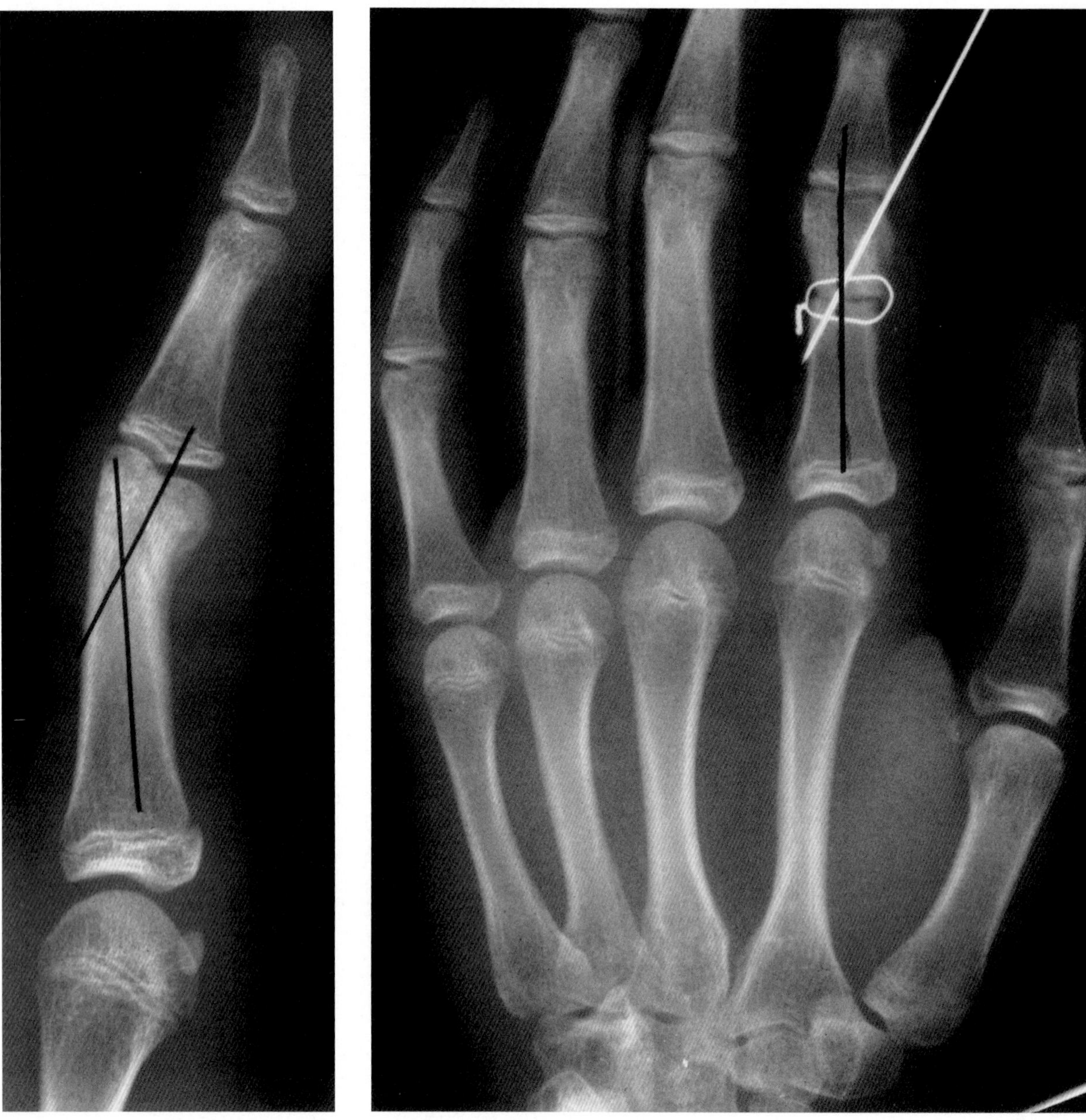


Fig. 13-66 Phalangeal malunion. A: Radiograph demonstrates angular and rotational deformity (*black lines*) after healing of a proximal phalangeal fracture. The proximal interphalangeal joint is incongruent with rotation of the proximal articular surface. B: Radiograph following midshaft osteotomy to correct the rotation and articular deformity.

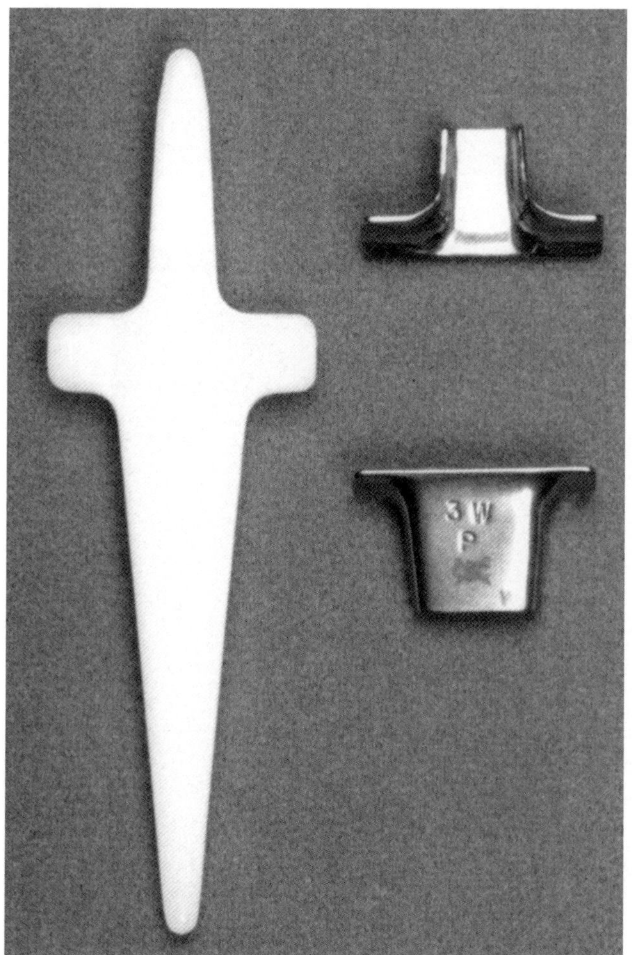


**Fig. 13-67** Swanson silastic implant with metal grommets for wrist arthroplasty. (Courtesy of Sutter, San Diego, California.)

rubber) and silicone or silastic (polymers) prostheses have been attempted. Silastic implants are most commonly used (see Fig. 13-71). These implants are obvious on radiographs and do not cause artifacts on MR images.

## Suggested Reading


Bechenbaugh RD. Total joint arthroplasty: The wrist. *Mayo Clin Proc.* 1979;54:513–515.

Carlson JR, Simmons BP. Total wrist arthroplasty. *J Am Acad Orthop Surg.* 1998;6:308–315.

Meuli HC. Arthroplasty of the wrist. *Clin Orthop.* 1980;149: 118–125.

Swanson AB. Flexible implant arthroplasty for arthritic disabilities of the radiocarpal joint. *Orthop Clin North Am.* 1973; 4:383–394.

Voltz RG. Total wrist arthroplasty. *Clin Orthop.* 1984;187: 112–120.


### Imaging of Postoperative Complications

Data regarding complications of wrist implants is less extensive compared to the hip and knee. Clinical evaluation including comparison with preoperative wrist scores is accomplished in addition to imaging studies. Initial PA and lateral radiographs are adequate for baseline position of the implants. Serial radiographs are also most useful in patients with suspected complications (Fig. 13-69). Additional studies may be indicated depending on the type of complications suspected.

Complications of wrist arthroplasty include loosening, infection, hematoma, soft tissue imbalance, tendon rupture, ulnar nerve compression, dislocation, implant failure, and fractures of the distal radius and metacarpals. Ulnar-sided symptoms may be related to ulnar impingement, ulnar stump instability in the case of ulnar resection, and pisiform impingement against the carpal base plate.

Failures are most commonly related to component positioning, fixation technique, and soft tissue imbalance. Proper placement is more difficult in the rheumatoid wrist.

When cement is used for fixation, the same problems described with the hip and knee can occur. Soft tissue imbalance is a major problem due to muscle deficiency, tendon imbalance, and tendon subluxation.

Early implants had high failure rates, especially the metacarpal components. Loosening occurred in 15% to 53% of patients (see Fig. 13-72). Second- and third-generation implants were designed to reduce loosening to 9% to 14%. However, loosening of metacarpal components remains high. A recent study of the Biax system using the modified longer stem noted 23% demonstrated some evidence of radiographic lucency about the distal stem without clinical evidence of loosening. At an average of 6.5 years, there were 19% failures (11/57). Most (8/11) were due to loosening of the distal component for a total incidence of loosening of 14%.

Fractures and dislocations can occur as well. Metacarpal fractures may occur during implant placement or later with component breakthrough (Fig. 13-72). Both osseous (see Fig. 13-73) and component fractures and dislocations (see Fig. 13-74) are easily detected with radiographs. The incidence of component fracture with silastic components is 8% during the first few years and increasing to 20% after 5 years. Implant fracture does not correlate completely with clinical failure. Metal implants rarely fracture, but more often break through the cortex (Figs. 13-72 and 13-73).

Isolatd carpal implants and silicone implants can cause painful synovitis. Silicone particle debris can result in a destructive inflammatory synovitis. Studies in patients with lunate replacement have demonstrated that 41% required removal due to development of painful silicone synovitis or cystic osteolysis from 1 to 18 years after placement. Radiographs may demonstrate fragmentation of the implant, lytic bone changes, cortical thinning, and soft tissue swelling. MRI demonstrates synovial inflammation with enhancement using gadolinium (see Fig. 13-75). Radionuclide bone scans also demonstrate intense uptake in the wrist (see Fig. 13-76). Although certain authors recommend implant removal and revision surgery or fusion, others have found success with conservative management.

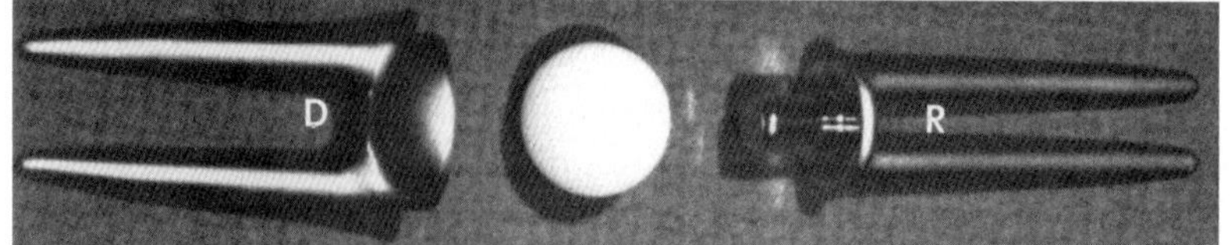


**Fig. 13-68** Meuli wrist implant. The distal cupped component (*D*) is positioned in the second and third metacarpals and the proximal trunnion (*R*) in the radius. (From Bechenbaugh RD. Total joint arthroplasty: the wrist. Mayo Clin Proc 1979; 54:513–515.)

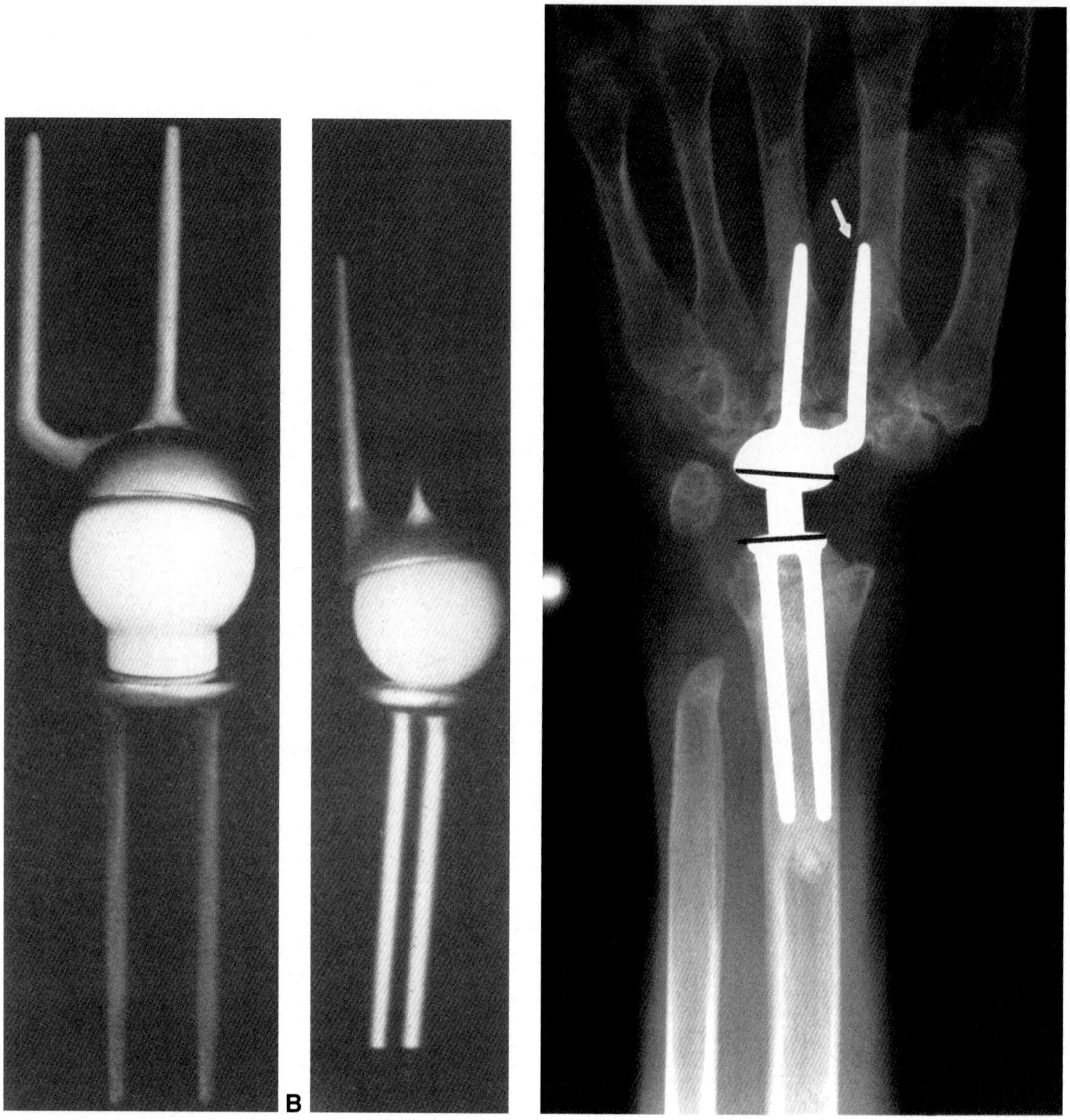

A B C

**Fig. 13-69** Meuli modification systems. **A:** Meuli modification with offset distal stems. **B:** Mayo modification of the distal position of the implant using a single stem dorsally to center wrist motion at the capitate head. (From Bechenbaugh RD. Total joint arthroplasty: The wrist. *Mayo Clin Proc.* 1979;54:513–515.) Posteroanterior (PA) **(C)** and lateral **(D)** radiographs of a Meuli modified implant with offset metacarpal stems. The second metacarpal stem is breaking through the cortex (*arrow*). The distal ulna is resected along with the scaphoid, lunate, triquetrum, and proximal capitate. Note the space between the proximal and distal components (*lines*). Two years later (**E** and **F**) the space between the components has changed (*lines*) and the polyethylene ball (*arrowheads*) has dislocated. The position of the second metacarpal stem (*arrow*) has not changed significantly.

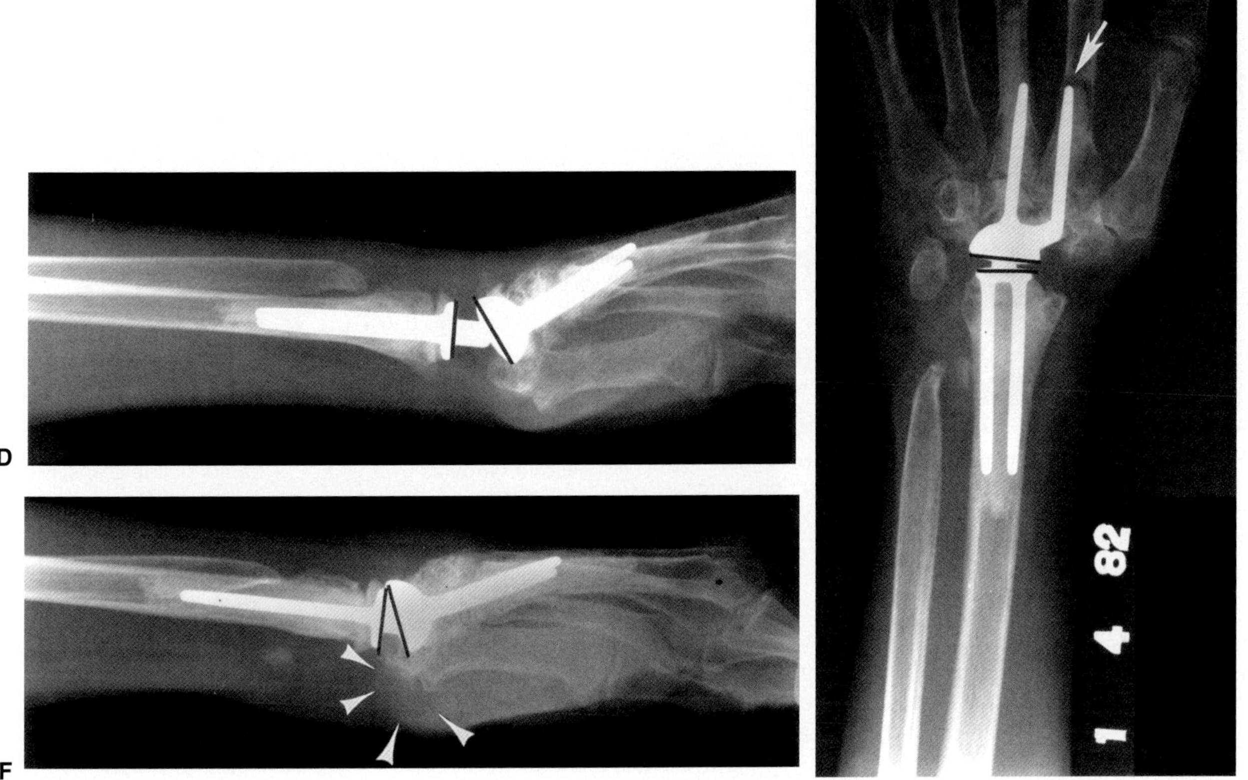


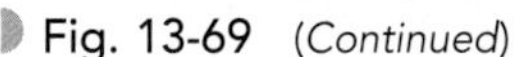
Fig. 13-69 *(Continued)*

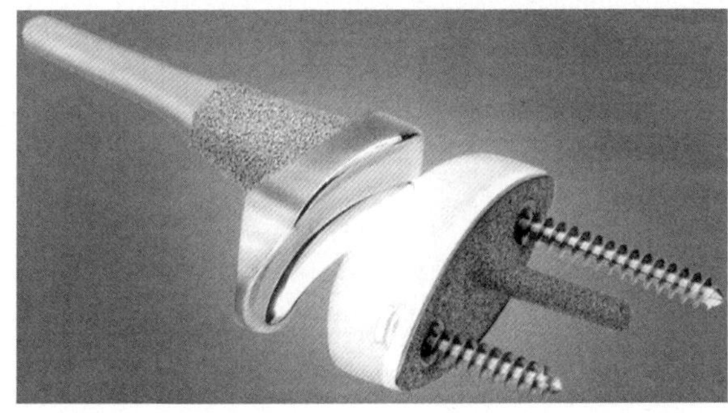


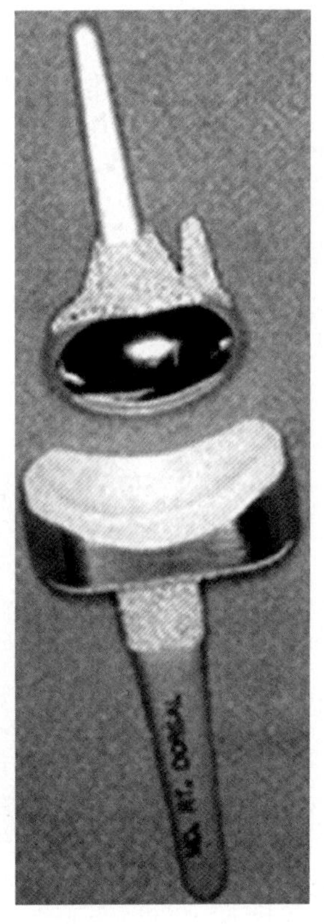


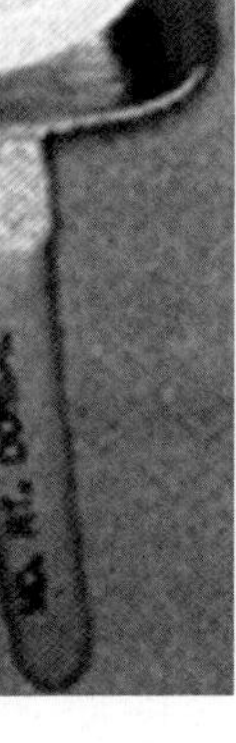

Fig. 13-70 New generation total wrist systems. **A:** Universal 2 total wrist provides improved motion and stability. The radial component is cobalt-chromium and the distal component titanium. The ulna does not need to be resected and palmar tilt is incorporated into the radial component. (Courtesy of Integra, San Diego, California.) **B:** Biax total wrist system. (Courtesy of DePuy, a Johnson and Johnson Company, Warsaw, Indiana.)

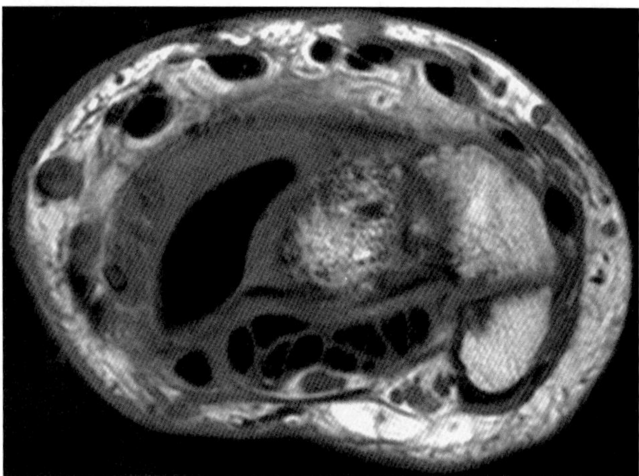

Fig. 13-71 Axial T1-weighted magnetic resonance (MR) image of a silastic scaphoid implant. The implant has low signal intensity with no associated artifact.

Table 13-2

WRIST ARTHROPLASTY COMPLICATIONS

| COMPLICATION | IMAGING APPROACHES |
|---|---|
| Soft tissue imbalance (20%–35%) | Motion studies, MRI |
| Loosening (9%–15%, new generation) | Serial radiographs |
| Dislocations (4%–10%) | Serial radiographs |
| Tendon ruptures (~6%) | MRI |
| Component/osseous fracture | Serial radiographs |
| Nerve compression (2%–5%) | MRI |
| Deep infection (1%–2%) | Radionuclide scans, MRI |
| Silicone synovitis | Radionuclide scans, MRI |
| Pisiform impingement | Fluoroscopic stress views |

MRI, magnetic resonance imaging.

Deep infection is uncommon (1% to 2%). Radiographic changes may be subtle. Aspiration is useful but often yields false-negative results. Combined radionuclide scans with Technetium Tc 99m and indium In 111–labeled white cells are still preferred, although newer isotope combinations and positron emission tomography (PET) are also in use.

Table 13-2 summarizes complications of wrist arthroplasty and imaging approaches.

## Suggested Reading


Berquist TH. Imaging of joint replacement procedures. *Radiol Clin North Am*. 2006;44:419–437.

Carlson JR, Simmons BP. Total wrist arthroplasty. *J Am Acad Orthop Surg*. 1998;6:308–315.


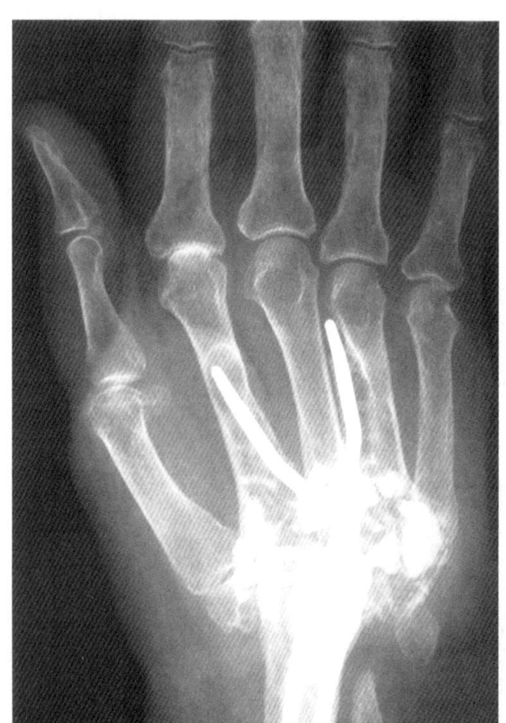

A

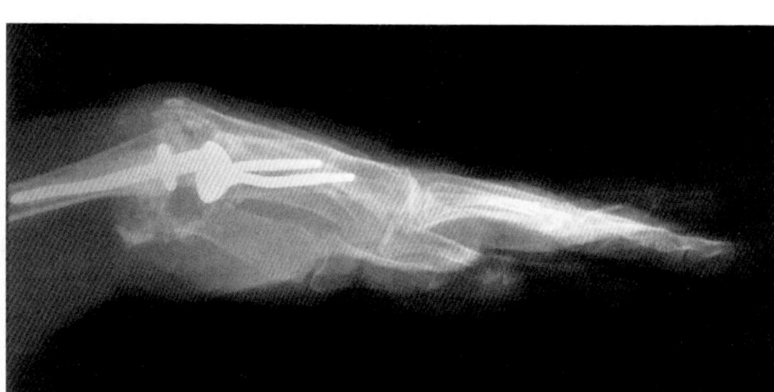

B

Fig. 13-72 Failed Meuli wrist arthroplasty. Posteroanterior (PA) (A) and lateral (B) radiographs demonstrate subluxation and impaction of the radius and metacarpals with gross loosening of the second metacarpal implant and breakthrough of the fourth metacarpal implant. The cement is grossly fragmented.

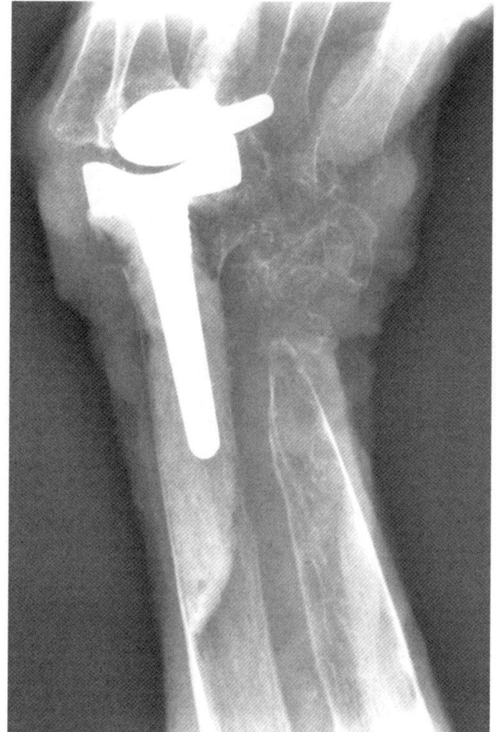

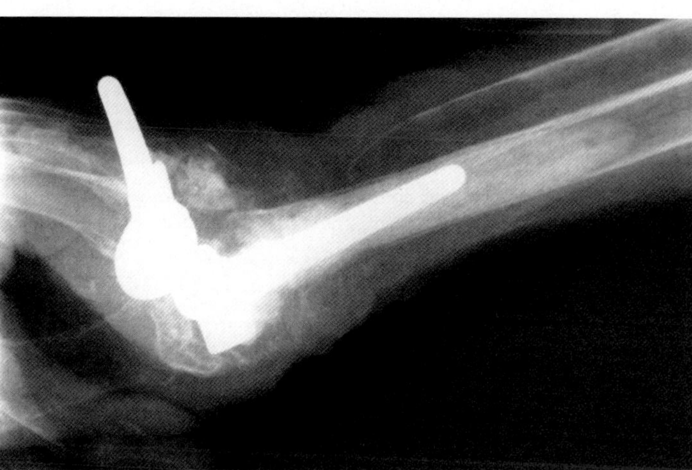

Fig. 13-73 Posteroanterior (PA) (A) and lateral (B) radiographs of a biaxial component with fracture of the distal component dorsally through the metacarpal.

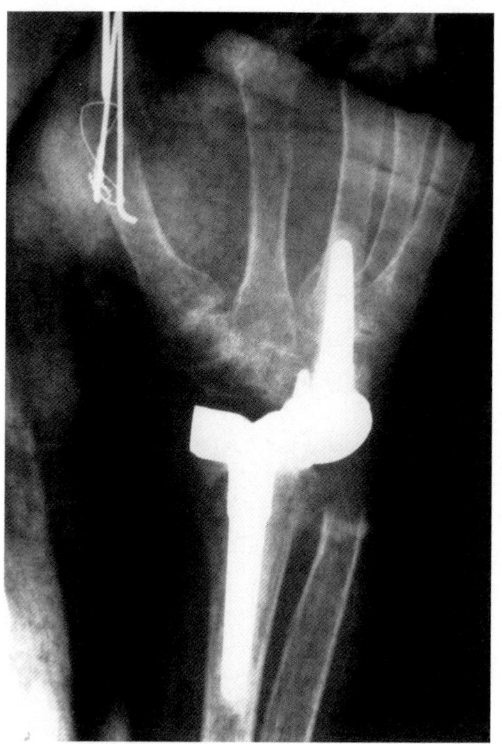

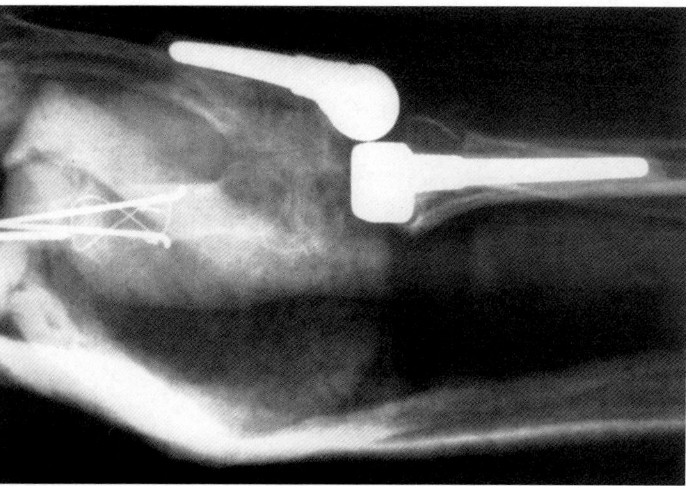

Fig. 13-74 Posteroanterior (PA) (A) and lateral (B) radiographs of a dislocated biaxial component. There has also been an arthrodesis of the thumb with K-wire and tension band fixation.

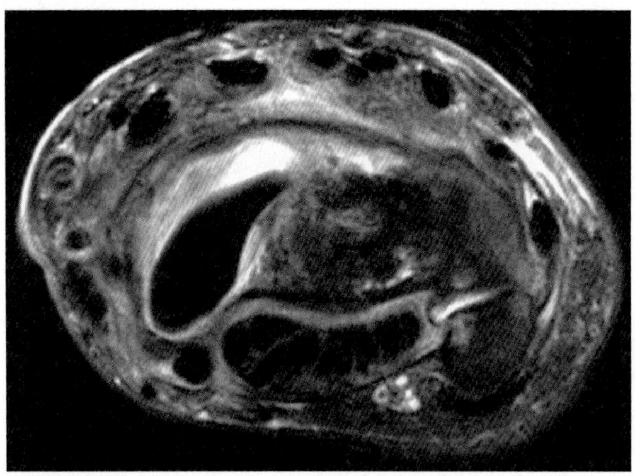
A

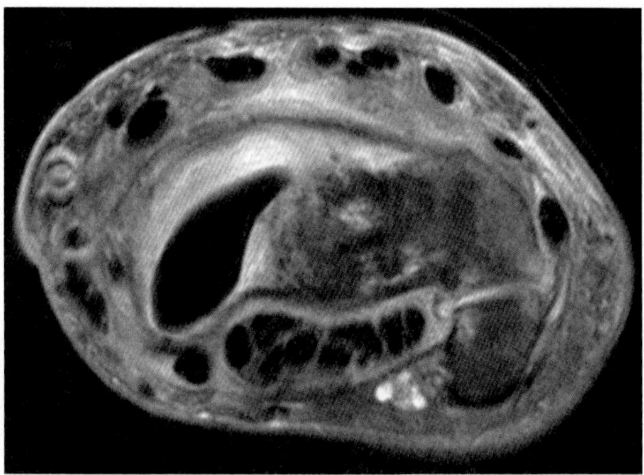
B

Fig. 13-75 Axial T2- (A) and contrast-enhanced fat-suppressed T1-weighted images (B) in a patient with a silastic scaphoid implant. There is inflammatory change in the synovium surrounding the implant due to synovitis.

Cobb RT, Bechenbaugh RD. Biaxial total-wrist arthroplasty. *J Hand Surg [Br]*. 1996;21A:1011–1021.

Johnson ST, Patel A, Calfee RP, et al. Pisiform impingement after total wrist arthroplasty. *J Hand Surg [Br]*. 2007;32A: 334–336.

Kaarela OI, Raatikainen TK, Torniainen PJ. Silicone replacement arthroplasty for Kienbock's disease. *J Hand Surg [Br]*. 1998;23B:735–740.

Murry PM, Wood MB. The results of treatment of synovitis of the wrist induced by particles of silicone debris. *J Bone Joint Surg*. 1998;80A:397–406.

Rizza M, Beckenbaugh RD. Results of biaxia total wrist arthroplasty with a modified (long) metacarpal stem. *J Hand Surg [Br]*. 2003;28A:577–584.

## Thumb Replacement Arthroplasty

Approximately 40% of adults are affected with osteoarthritis. The first carpometacarpal joint is one of the most frequent sites for osteoarthritis in the hand. Women older than 40 years of age are most commonly affected. Pain and loss of pinch strength can be disabling. Failed conservative therapy results in some type of surgical intervention in up to 20% of patients.

Rheumatoid arthritis also affects the trapezium and first metacarpal. However, other joints are more frequently affected in a similar manner.

Preoperative assessment includes clinical and imaging features. Clinical scoring described earlier and radiographic staging are used in patient selection. The Eaton classification is based on stability and radiographic changes (see Fig. 13-77).

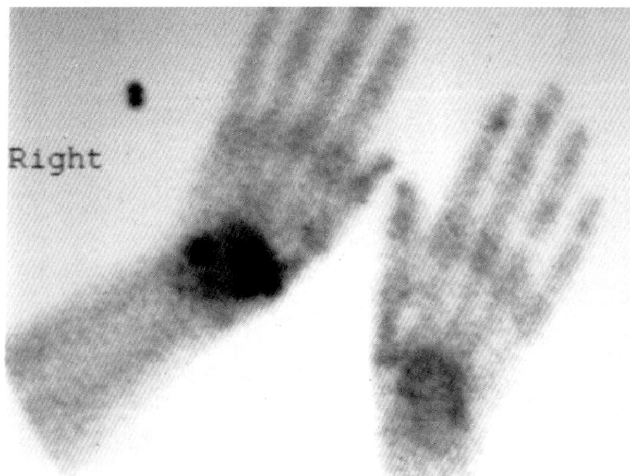


Fig. 13-76 Technetium-99m methyl diphosphonate (MDP) bone scan demonstrating intense uptake in the wrist 3 years following silicone implants due to silicone synovitis.

### EATON CLASSIFICATION

| STAGE | FEATURES |
|---|---|
| I | Radiographs normal<br>Pain, loss of pinch strength |
| II | Loss of joint space with lateral or dorsal subluxation<br>No clinical instability |
| III | More advanced joint changes with 75% subluxation<br>Clinical instability, pain, strength reduction |
| IV | Joint changes extend to scaphoid, trapezium and trapezoid articulations<br>Pain, instability, strength reduction |

# Suggested Reading

Eaton R, Lane L, Littler JW, et al. Ligament reconstruction for the painful thumb metacarpal joint: A long term assessment. *J Hand Surg [Br]*. 1984;9A:692.

Millender LH, Nalebuff EA, Amadio P, et al. Interposition arthroplasty for rheumatoid carpometacarpal disease. *J Hand Surg [Br]*. 1978;3A:533–541.

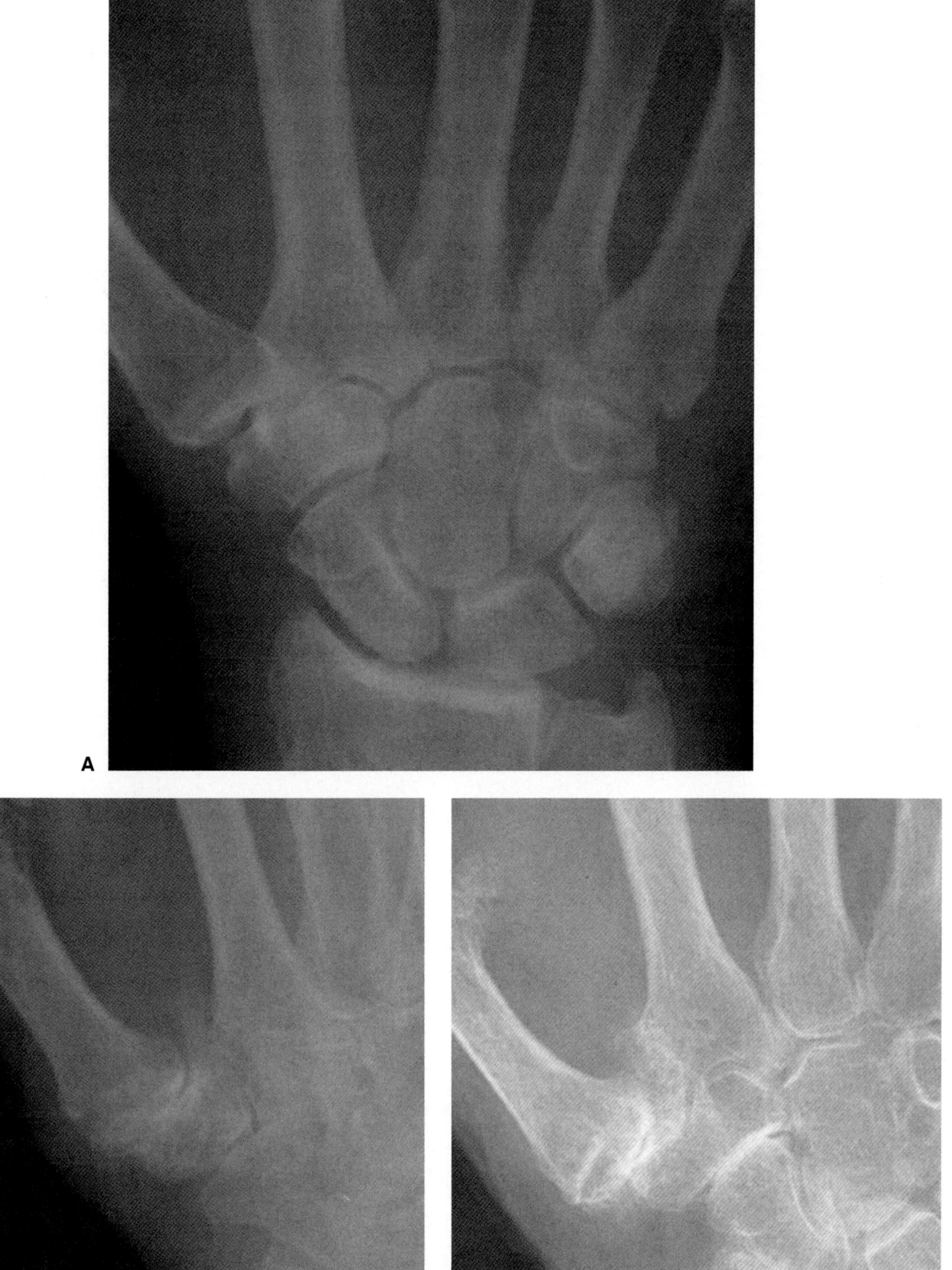


Fig. 13-77 Radiographic changes of the Eaton classification. A: Stage I—normal joint space. Posteroanterior (PA) radiograph demonstrating normal first carpometacarpal (CMC) and scaphoid-trapezium-trapezoid (STT) articulations. B: Stage II—joint space narrowing with slight subluxation. Radiograph demonstrates first CMC narrowing with mild subluxation. C: Stage IV—more advanced changes with STT involvement. Radiograph demonstrates advanced changes at the first CMC with subluxation and fragmentation and STT complex involvement.

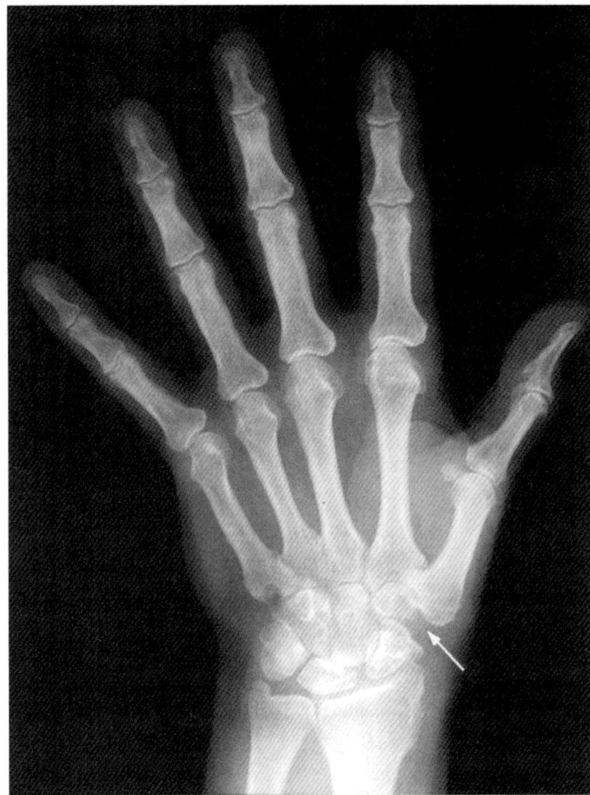


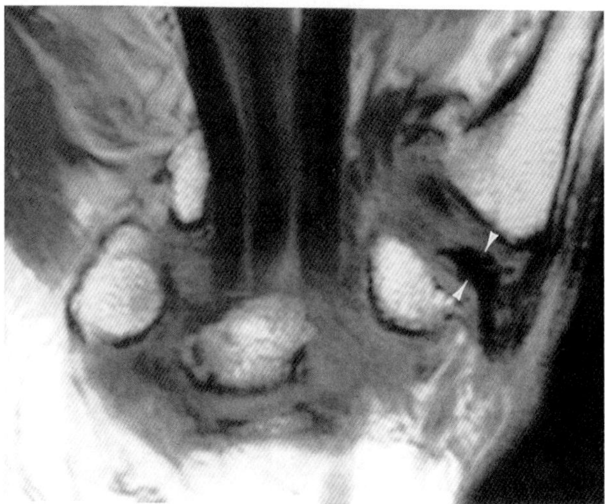


**Fig. 13-78** Trapezial resection and tendon interposition arthroplasty. **A:** Radiograph demonstrates resection of the trapezium (*arrow*). **B:** Coronal T1-weighted magnetic resonance (MR) image demonstrates the tendon interposition (*arrowheads*).

## Treatment Options

The goals of joint replacement procedures in the thumb are to relieve pain, improve function, and correct instability. Treatment approaches vary depending on the stage of disease. Arthroscopic debridement, arthroscopic capsulorrhaphy, interposition arthroplasty (tendon or silastic), osteotomy, resection arthroplasty, arthrodesis, and joint replacement procedures all play a role in patients requiring surgical intervention.

Treatment approaches remain controversial, but tend to vary with the stage of disease. Patients with stage I disease (normal joint space, pain with loss of pinch strength) are treated conservatively with nonsteroidal anti-inflammatory medications. Patients with stage II disease (joint space narrowing, mild subluxation, and loss of strength but no instability) can be treated with arthroscopic repair, interposition arthroplasty, or osteotomy (see Fig. 13-78). Numerous materials have been used for interposition arthroplasty including acellular dermal matrix allograft (GRAFT JACKET, Wright Medical Technology, Inc., Arlington Tennessee). Patients with more advanced disease (stage III or IV) may be treated with complete trapezial resection or joint replacement arthroplasty. Numerous modifications have been made over the years in implants used for the first carpometacarpal joint. Silicone implants are still available (see Fig. 13-79). Hemiarthroplasty with replacement of the base of the first metacarpal can be performed using polycarbon, titanium, or silastic implants. Resection of the trapezium with multiple implant configurations can also be performed. Total

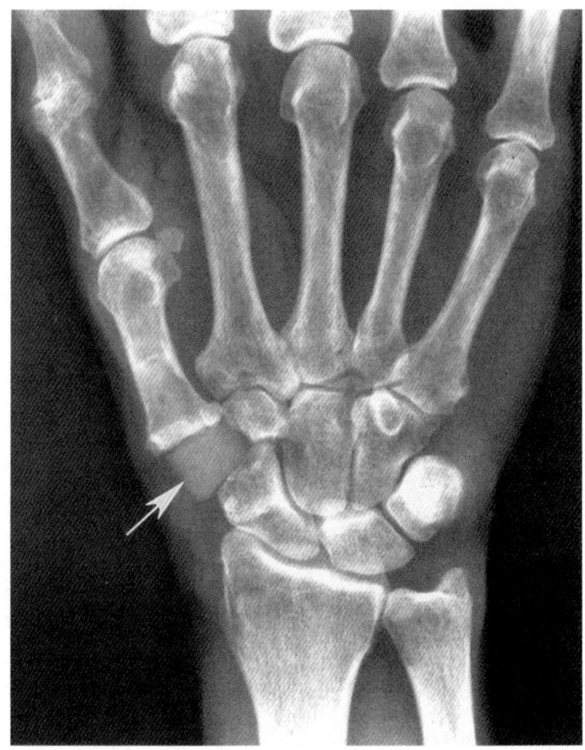

**Fig. 13-79** Radiograph demonstrating a silicone implant with resection of the trapezium.

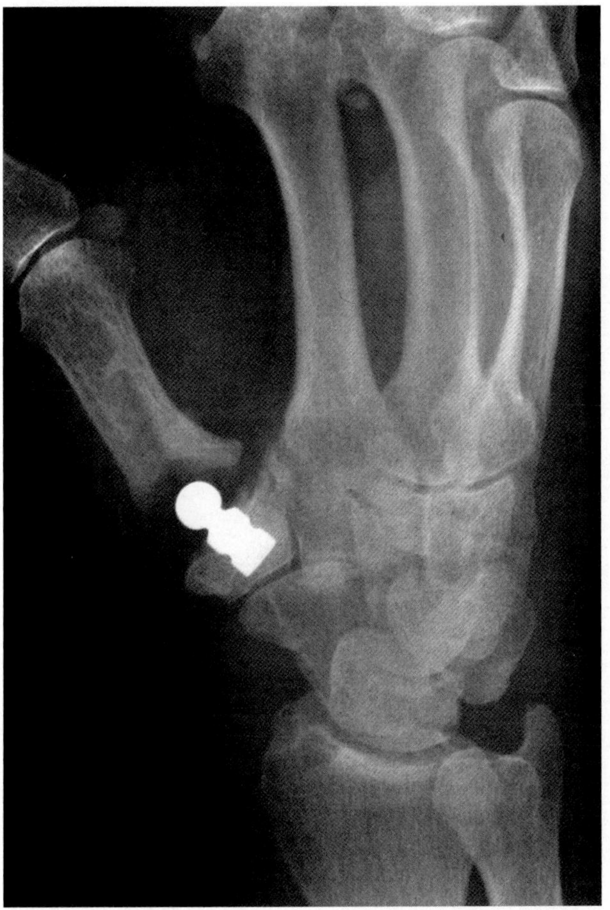

Fig. 13-80 Radiograph of the Mayo total joint replacement with components in the trapezium and first metacarpal.

joint replacement with implants placed in the trapezium and first metacarpal can also be performed (see Fig. 13-80).

## Suggested Reading

Adams JE, Merten SM, Steinmann SP. Arthroscopic interposition arthroplasty of the first carpometacarpal joint. *J Hand Surg [Br]*. 2007;32:268–274.

Badia A. Arthroscopy of the trapeziometacarpal and metacarpophalangeal joints. *J Hand Surg [Br]*. 2007;32A:707–724.

Eaton R, Lane L, Littler JW, et al. Ligament reconstruction for the painful thumb metacarpal joint: A long term assessment. *J Hand Surg [Br]*. 1984;9A:692.

Hartian BJ, Stern PJ, Kiefhaber TR. Thumb carpometacarpal osteoarthritis: Arthrodesis compared with ligament reconstruction and tendon interposition. *J Bone Joint Surg*. 2001; 83A:1470–1478.

Wilson JN, Bossley CJ. Osteotomy in the treatment of osteoarthritis of the first carpometacarpal joint. *J Bone Joint Surg*. 1983;65B:179–181.

Yoshinori OKA, Ikeda M. Silastic interposition arthroplasty for osteoarthrosis of the carpometacarpal joint of the thumb. *Tokai J Exp Clin Med*. 2000;25:15–21.

### Imaging of Complications

Improved motion, stability, and pain relief can be achieved with most trapeziometacarpal arthroplasty techniques. Patients report satisfactory or good results in 75% to 95% of cases. The large number of variations in procedures and implant designs suggests that the perfect technique is elusive. As with other arthroplasty techniques, baseline radiographs are an important first step. Fluoroscopic positioning is useful to align the interfaces of the bone, cement, and implants. Baseline MRI is useful for tendon interposition procedures.

Implant loosening is most common with total joint replacements (10% to 44%). Serial radiographs or CT are useful to evaluate loosening and implant failure. Silicone implants may also cause synovitis in up to 25% of patients. Changes related to silicone synovitis may be obvious on radiographs (see Fig. 13-81). However, contrast-enhanced MR images are most useful for demonstrating the extent of synovitis (see Fig. 13-82).

Fortunately, deep infection is uncommon. When infection is suspected (see Fig. 13-83), aspiration, radionuclide scans (>1 year after surgery), or MRI can be performed to confirm osteomyelitis.

## Suggested Reading

Adams JE, Merten SM, Steinmann SP. Arthroscopic interposition arthroplasty of the first carpometacarpal joint. *J Hand Surg [Br]*. 2007;32:268–274.

Fitzgerald RH, Kaufer H, Malikani AL. *Orthopaedics*. St. Louis: Mosby; 2002:1835–1836.

Hartian BJ, Stern PJ, Kiefhaber TR. Thumb carpometacarpal osteoarthritis: Arthrodesis compared with ligament reconstruction and tendon interposition. *J Bone Joint Surg*. 2001;83A:1470–1478.

Jennings CD, Livingstone DF. Convex condylar arthroplasty of the basal joint of the thumb: Failure under load. *J Hand Surg [Br]*. 1990;15A:573–581.

# Metacarpophalangeal and Interphalangeal Arthroplasty

There are multiple surgical approaches for arthropathies of the metacarpophalangeal and interphalangeal joints. Surgical options include synovectomy, resection arthroplasty, interposition arthroplasty, joint replacement, and arthrodesis (see Fig. 13-84).

Metacarpophalangeal joint replacement procedures are primarily performed on patients with rheumatoid arthritis with progressive, painful deformities (see Fig. 13-85). Numerous systems have been used including silicone-elastomer implants (see Fig. 13-86), metal-polyethylene implants (see Fig. 13-87), and pyrolytic-carbon implants (see Fig. 13-88). Some studies suggest that titanium metal implants demonstrate better bone integration compared to pyrocarbon implants.

The proximal interphalangeal joint has the greatest arc of motion of any finger articulations. Surgical reconstruction

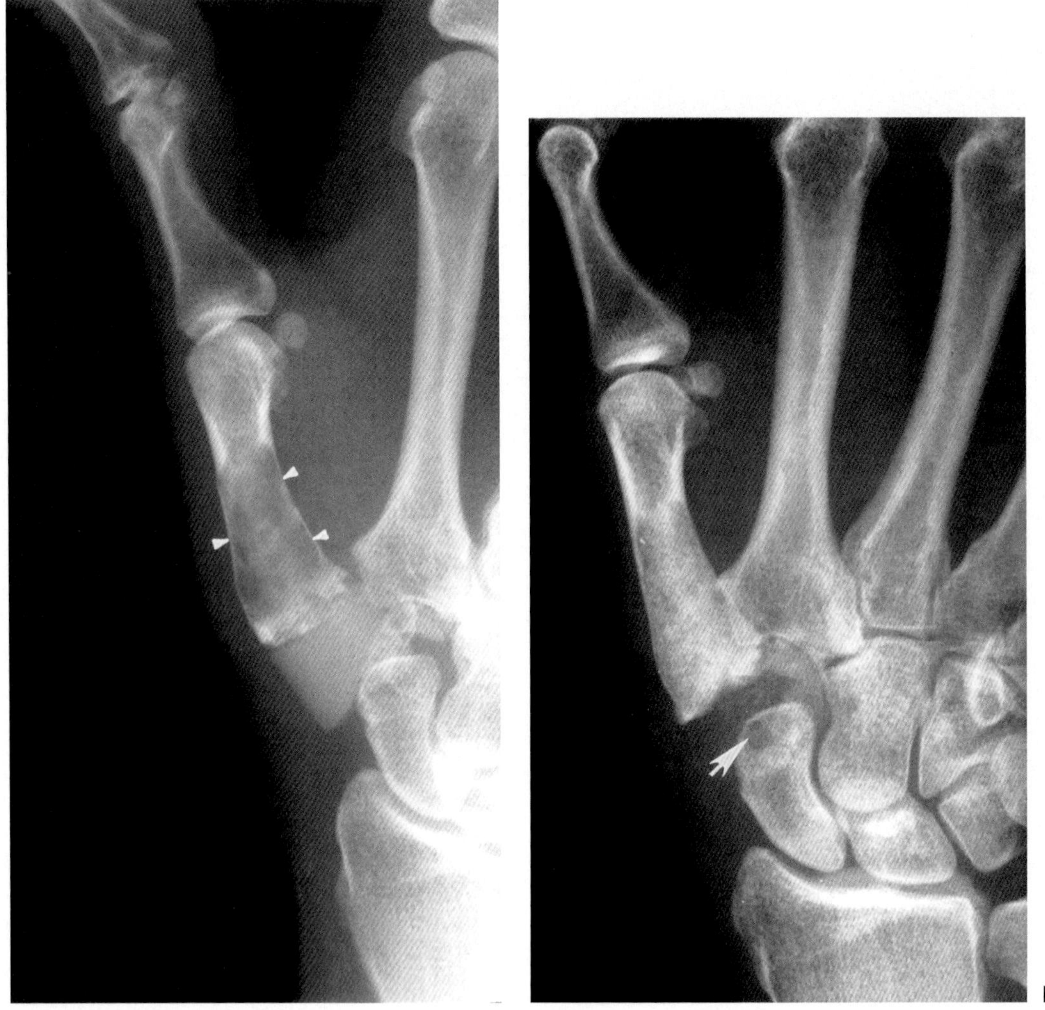


Fig. 13-81 Silicone synovitis. A: Radiograph of a silicone trapezial implant with aggressive bone loss in the first metacarpal and cortical thinning (*arrowheads*). B: The implant was removed and the first metacarpal defect filled with bone graft. There a persistent defect in the scaphoid (*arrow*) due to osteolysis.

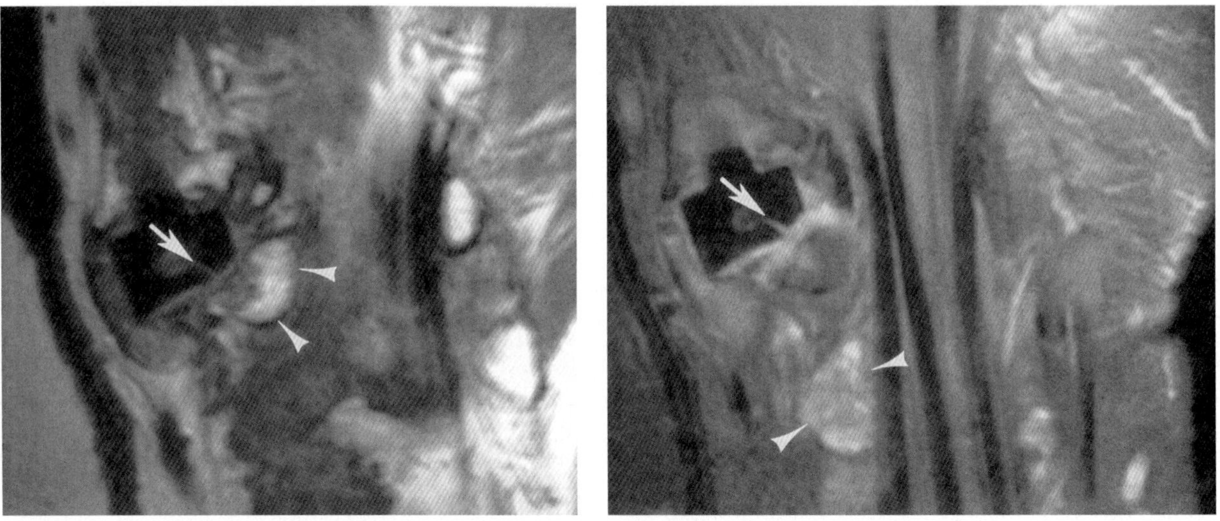


Fig. 13-82 Silicone synovitis. T2-weighted (A) and fat suppressed postcontrast T1-weighted (B) magnetic resonance (MR) images demonstrate a fracture (*arrow*) in the implant with synovitis (*arrowheads*).

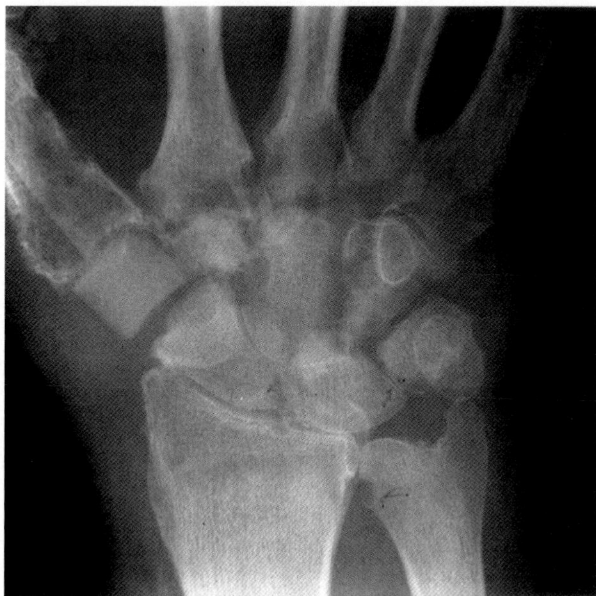

Fig. 13-83 Joint space infection and osteomyelitis. Radiograph demonstrates a joint replacement with aggressive bone destruction in the first metacarpal and erosions throughout the wrist due to infection.

is most often performed for inflammatory, degenerative, and post-traumatic arthritis. In most cases the options include arthroplasty or arthrodesis. Implants are configured similar to metacarpophalangeal arthroplasties described earlier (see Figs. 13-89 and 13-90).

## Suggested Reading

Cook SD, Beckenbaugh RD, Redondo J, et al. Long-term follow-up of pyrolytic carbon metacarpophalangeal implants. *J Bone Joint Surg*. 1999;85A:635–648.

Linscheid RL, Dobyns JH, Beckenbaugh RD, et al. Proximal interphalangeal joint arthroplasty with a total joint design. *Mayo Clin Proc*. 1979;54:227–240.

Millender LH, Nalebuff EA, Amadio P, et al. Interpositional arthroplasty for rheumatoid carpometacarpal joint disease. *J Hand Surg [Br]*. 1978;3A:533–541.

Rizzo M, Beckenbaugh RD. Proximal interphalangeal joint arthroplasty. *J Am Acad Orthop Surg*. 2007;15:189–197.

### Postoperative Imaging and Complications

Postoperative patient evaluation includes reviewing changes in the clinical scores, including pain and function, and baseline imaging. Radiographs are obtained in the PA, lateral, and oblique projections. Fluoroscopic positioning is usually not required unless the interfaces of the implants are not clearly defined on radiographs.

Serial radiographs are used to follow implant position, loosening, heterotopic ossification, ulnar drift, dislocation, subluxation, and implant fracture (Fig. 13-89). The Swanson silicone-elastomer arthroplasty has been most commonly used over the years (Fig. 13-85). Large series demonstrate pain relief in 98% of patients. Improvement in range of motion was less impressive. Component fractures occur in 5% and recurrent deformities in 6.5% (see Fig. 13-91). The revision rate is 10.9% after 1 year. Long-term follow-up (6.5 years) has demonstrated bone changes in 45% and the revision rate increased to 13%. Revision and arthrodesis are both options (Fig. 13-89).

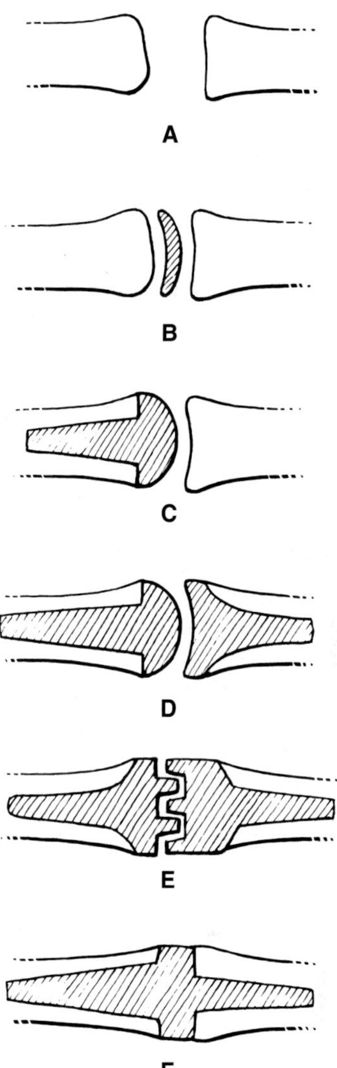


Fig. 13-84 Illustration of surgical interventions and arthroplasty of the hand. A: Resection arthroplasty. B: Interposition arthroplasty. C: Condylar replacement. D: Ball and socket replacement of both joint surfaces. E: Interlocking or hinged implants. F: Double stemmed silastic implants.

Pyrolytic carbon and titanium implants are also used. Data on pyrolytic carbon implants is more readily available. Follow-up data indicates lucency about the implants in 23% and subsidence in 64%, although implant stabilization usually occurs (Fig. 13-88). Survival rates are 70% over 15 years. Revision arthroplasty was required in 8%.

Deep infection is uncommon (1%) (see Fig. 13-92). Joint aspiration, radionuclide scans, or MRI with silicone-elastomer or pyrolytic-carbon implants can be used in this setting.

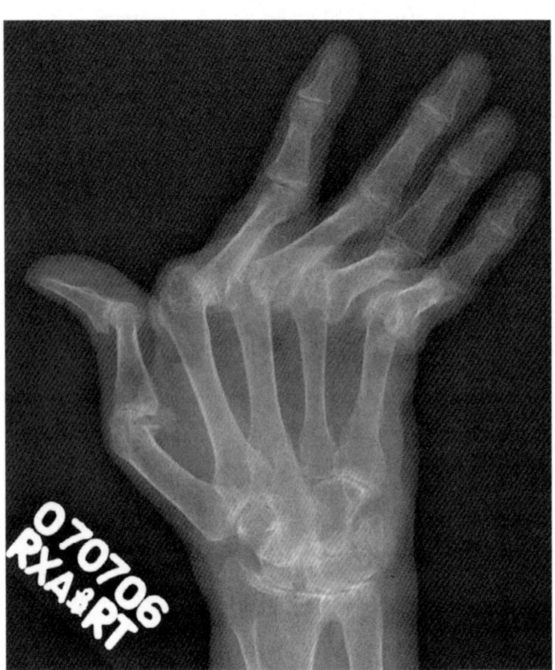


A

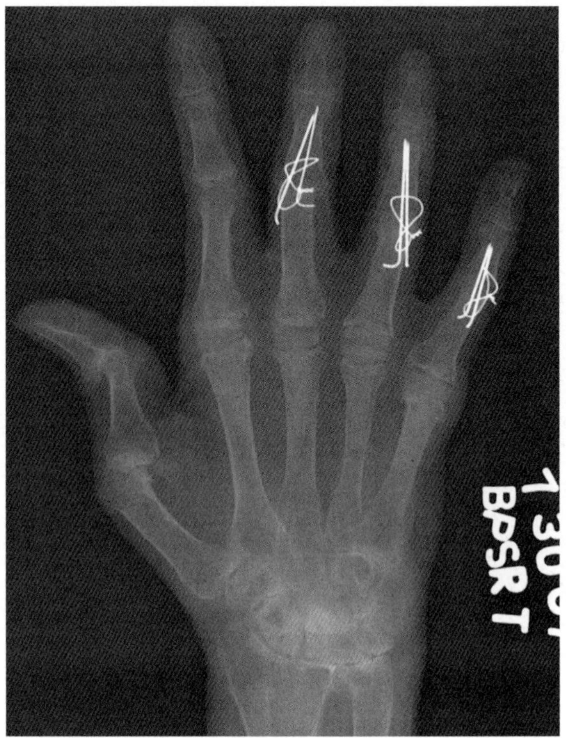

B

Fig. 13-85 Rheumatoid arthritis. A: Radiograph of the hand demonstrates advanced changes of rheumatoid arthritis with marked subluxations of the metacarpophalangeal (MCP) joints. B: Radiograph 1 year later after silicone-elastomer double-stemmed implants have been placed in the second through fourth MCP joints. There has been arthrodeses of the third through fifth interphalangeal joints with K-wire and tension band fixation.

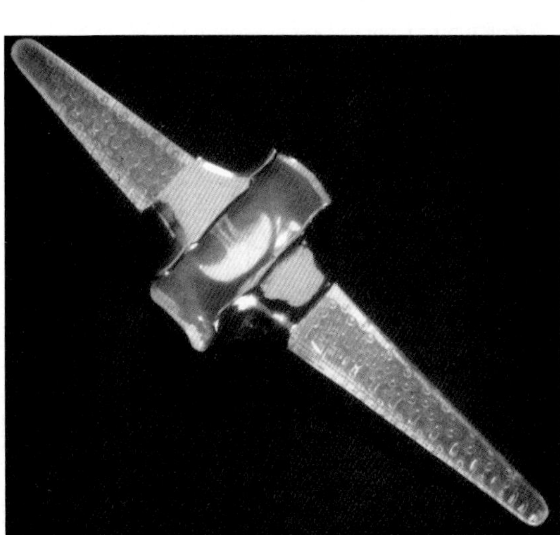

A

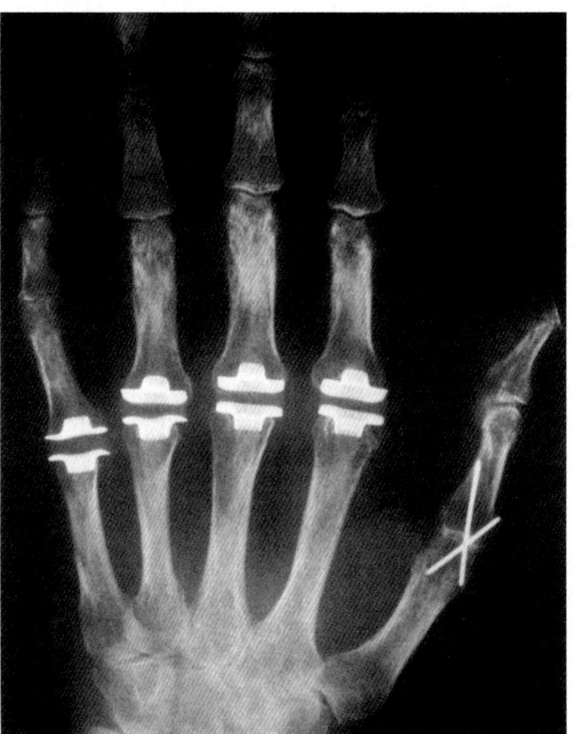

B

Fig. 13-86 Metacarpophalangeal (MCP) arthroplasty. A: Silastic Swanson implant with metal grommets. B: Radiograph following placement of Swanson implants in the second through fifth MCP joints with fusion of the first MCP joint. (Courtesy of Wright Medical Technology, Inc. Arlington, Tennessee.)

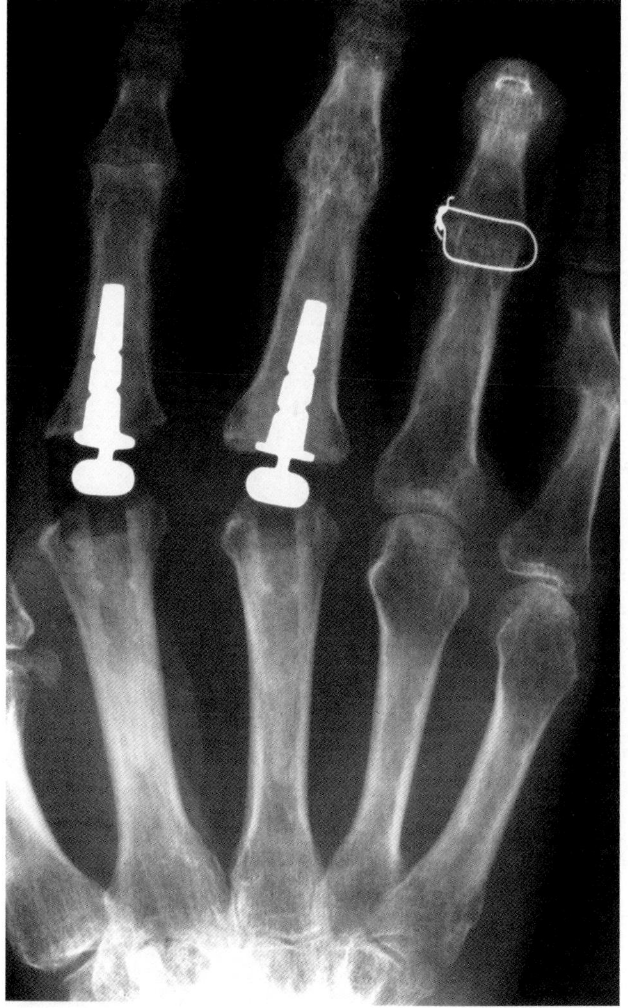

Fig. 13-87 Steffee arthroplasty with metal distal and proximal polyethylene components in the second and third metacarpophalangeal (MCP) joints. Fusion of the second through fifth proximal interphalangeal (PIP) joints.

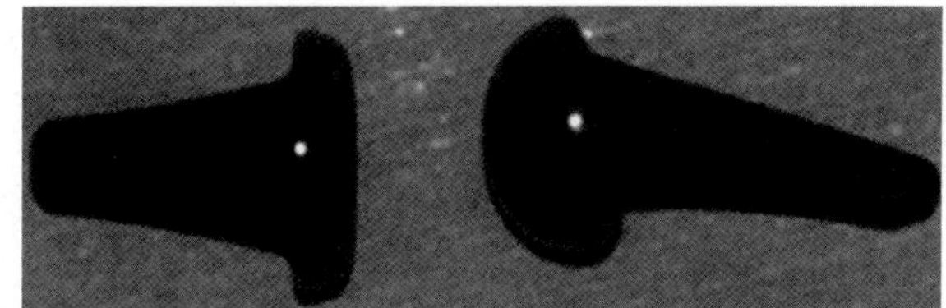

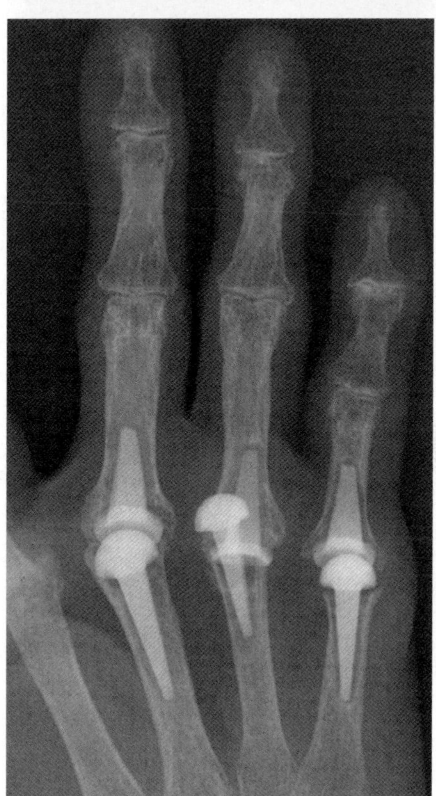

Fig. 13-88 Pyrolytic carbon implants. A: Pyrolytic carbon implants. (Courtesy of Ascension Orthopaedics, Austin, Texas.) B: Radiograph of the third through fifth metacarpophalangeal (MCP) joints with pyrolytic carbon implants. There is considerable lucency about the components, which is consistent with radiographic loosening. The fourth MCP joint has dislocated.

As with other silicone-elastomer implants described earlier, reactive synovitis can also occur (see Fig. 13-93). Lymphadenopathy and lymphoma have also been reported.

## Suggested Reading


Bravo CJ, Rizzo M, Hormel KB, et al. Pyrolytic carbon proximal interphalangeal joint arthroplasty: Results with minimum two-year follow-up evaluation. *J Hand Surg [Br]*. 2007;32A:1–11.

Cook SD, Beckenbaugh RD, Redondo J, et al. Long-term follow-up of pyrolytic carbon metacarpophalangeal implants. *J Bone Joint Surg*. 1999;81A:635–648.

Daecke W, Veyel K, Wieloch P, et al. Osseointegration and mechanical stability of pyrocarbon and titanium hand implants in a load-bearing *in vivo*model for small joint arthroplasty. *J Hand Surg [Br]*. 2006;31A:90–97.

Millender LH, Nalebuff EA, Amadio P, et al. Interposition arthroplasty for rheumatoid carpometacarpal joint disease. *J Hand Surg [Br]*. 1978;3A:533–541.

Rizzo M, Beckenbaugh RD. Proximal interphalangeal joint arthroplasty. *J Am Acad Orthop Surg*. 2007;15:189–197.

Takigawa S, Meletiou S, Sauerbier M, et al. Long-term assessment of Swanson implant arthroplasty in the proximal interphalangeal joint of the hand. *J Hand Surg [Br]*. 2004;29A:785–795.


## Arthrodesis

Arthrodesis is used to treat pain and instability in any of the joints in the hand and wrist. This technique, first performed in 1910, is still a useful alternative to joint replacement procedures described in the previous sections.

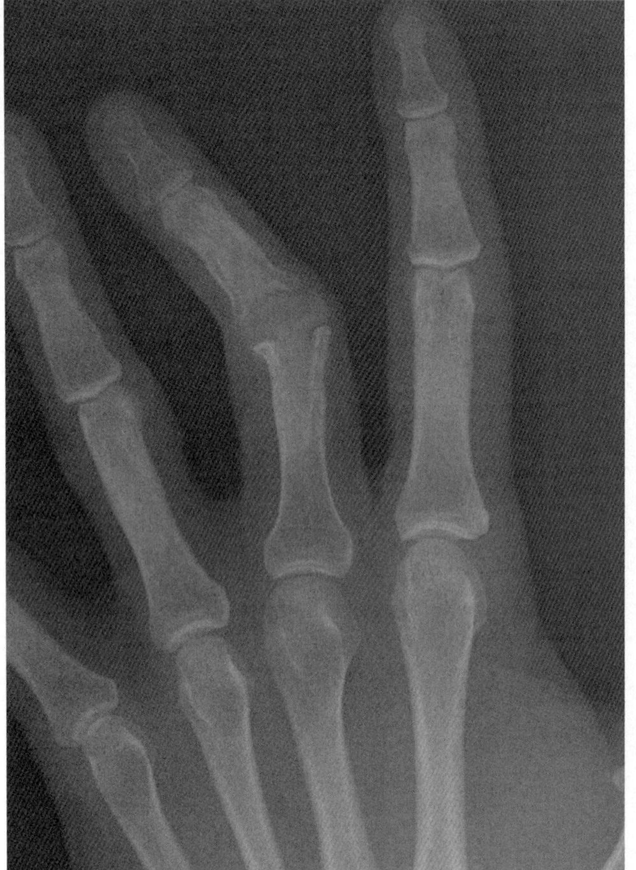
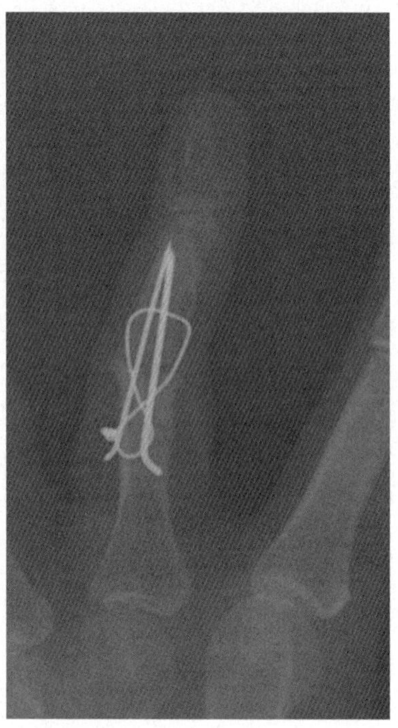

Fig. 13-89 Double-stemmed silicone-elastomer implant. A: Radiograph demonstrates angular deformity of the third proximal interphalangeal (PIP) joint. B: Radiograph following implant removal and arthrodesis with K-wires and tension band fixation.

Arthrodesis in the wrist may be partial or complete. Arthrodesis or fusion is most commonly performed for arthropathy (post-traumatic, osteoarthritis, rheumatoid arthritis), carpal instability, avascular necrosis, failed arthroplasty, and neoplasm.

Limited arthrodesis can be used in specific situations to preserve motion. This would include avascular necrosis of the lunate, arthropathy related to scapoid nonunion, carpal instability, or scapho-trapezial-trapezoid (STT) complex arthrosis (see Fig. 13-94). Midcarpal fusion can be performed in patients with carpal instability. This preserves motion in the radiocarpal joint. However, complete pain relief less frequently occurs with limited fusions compared to complete arthrodesis.

Wrist arthrodesis is contraindicated in patients with open growth plates, neuromuscular disorders, or paralysis and elderly patients with sedentary lifestyles.

Arthrodesis in the hand can be performed on the distal and proximal interphalangeal joints and metacarpophalangeal articulations. Indications include osteoarthritis, acute and chronic post-trauma deformities, inflammatory arthropathies, mallet finger deformities, and unrepairable tendon defects. The distal interphalangeal joint is commonly involved in patients with osteoarthritis. Although deformity is common, significant pain is less frequent. Therefore, arthrodesis is more often performed for cosmetic deformity and instability (see Fig. 13-95).

Pain and function loss are more often a problem in the proximal interphalangeal joint. Function is critical. Therefore, when possible, arthroplasty is preferred to arthrodesis. Arthrodesis is more commonly reserved for salvage of a failed arthroplasty (Fig. 13-89). Arthrodesis of the metacarpophalangeal joint is less commonly performed for functional reasons and usually reserved for isolated joints.

## Suggested Reading

Carroll RE, Hill NA. Small joint arthrodesis in hand reconstruction. *J Bone Joint Surg*. 1969;51A:1219–1221.

Clayton ML, Ferlic DC. Arthrodesis of the arthritic wrist. *Clin Orthop*. 1984;187:89–93.

Jebsen PJ, Adams BD. Wrist arthrodesis: Review of current technique. *J Am Acad Orthop Surg*. 2001;9:53–60.

Leibovic SJ. Arthrodesis of the interphalangeal joints with headless compression screws. *J Hand Surg [Br]*. 2007;32A: 1113–1119.

Murry PM. Current status of wrist arthrodesis and arthroplasty. *Clin Plast Surg*. 1996;23:385–394.

Tomaino MM, Miller RJ, Burton RI. Outcome assessment following limited wrist fusion: Objective wrist scoring versus patient satisfaction. *Contemp Orthop*. 1994;28:403–410.

## Preoperative Imaging

Radiographs of the wrist (PA, lateral, oblique) and hand (PA, lateral, and oblique) may be adequate for surgical planning. Fingers should be isolated on the lateral view to obtain optimal images. CT is particularly useful to more accurately evaluate bone stock and bone defects (see Fig. 13-96). Preoperative MR images can be useful for evaluation of neurovascular structures and tendon position and deficiency (see Fig. 13-97). However, clinical evaluation is often adequate for evaluation of range of motion, deformity, and instability.

# Suggested Reading

Berquist TH, Trigg SD. Hand and wrist. In: Berquist TH, ed. *Imaging atlas of orthopaedic appliances and prostheses*. New York, Raven Press, 1995:831–921.

## Treatment Options

Treatment options vary with the anatomic region, etiology, and extent of bone loss. In the wrist, options include midcarpal

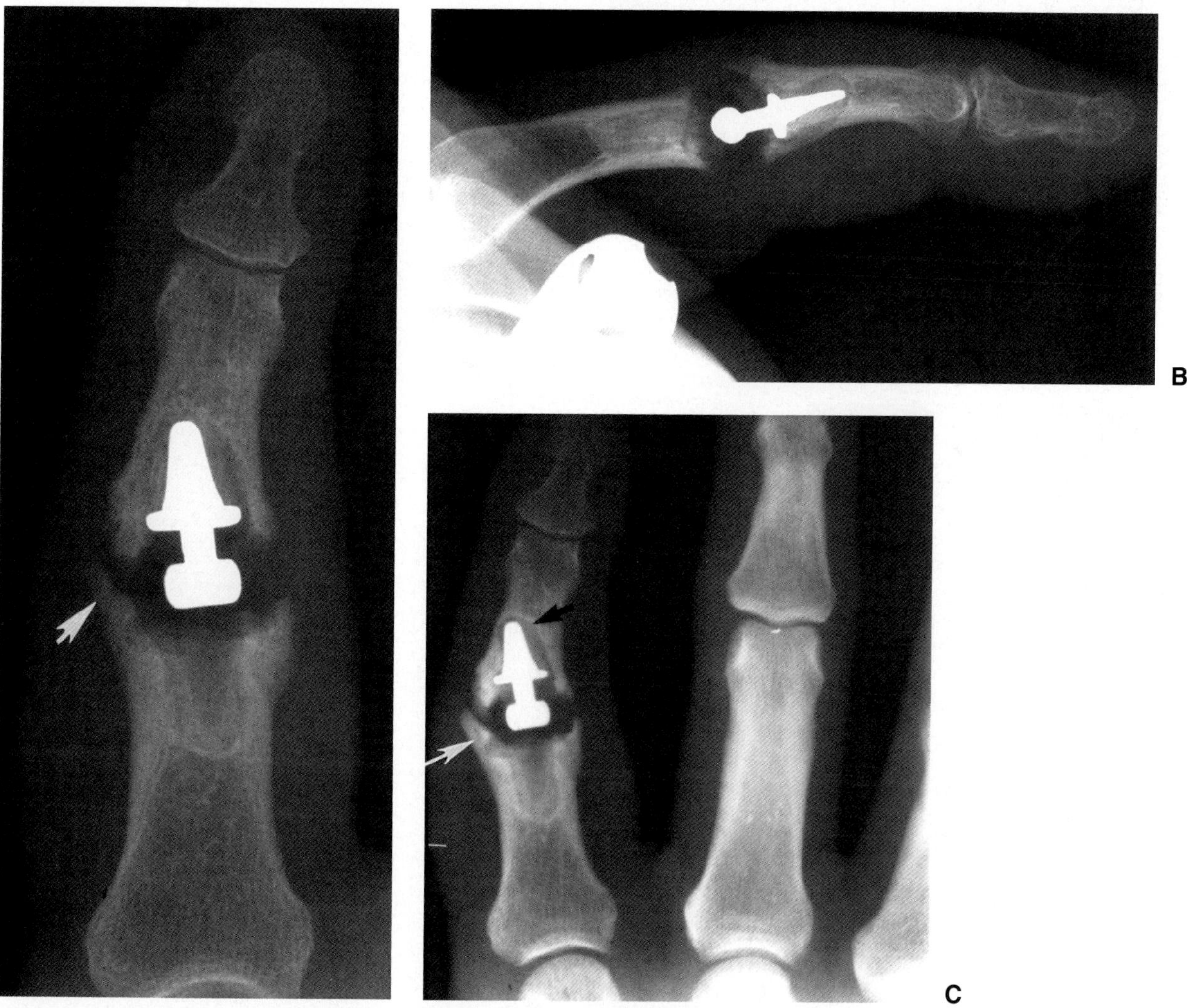


**Fig. 13-90** Mayo implant with proximal polyethylene and distal cobalt–chromium cemented components. Posteroanterior (PA) (**A**) and lateral (**B**) radiographs demonstrate heterotopic ossification (*arrow*), ulnar drift of the middle phalanx with tilt of the distal stem toward the radial cortex. **C:** Radiograph 1 year later shows the distal stem eroding through the cortex (*black arrow*) and component loosening. There is progression of ulnar drift of the middle phalanx and increasing heterotopic ossification (*white arrow*). (From Linscheid RL, Dobyns JH, Beckenbaugh RD, et al. Proximal interphalangeal joint arthroplasty with a total joint design. *Mayo Clin Proc.* 1979;54:227–240.)

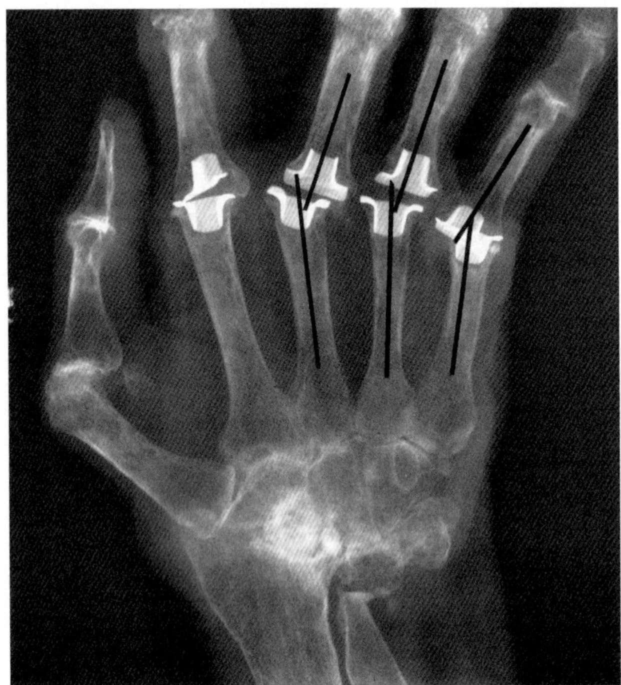

Fig. 13-91 Follow-up radiograph on a patient with silicone-elastomer metacarpophalangeal (MCP) arthroplasties in the second through fourth MCP joints with grommets. There is recurrent ulnar drift in the third through fifth MCP joints (*lines*).

fusion, partial arthrodesis (Fig. 13-94), and total arthrodesis. Partial arthrodesis techniques are not effective in patients with rheumatoid arthritis. Partial arthrodesis can be used for carpal instability, lunate avascular necrosis, scaphoid nonunion, and selected carpal arthropathies.

In patients with total fusion, it is important to include the radius, scaphoid, and its articulations with the lunate, radius, and capitate and the capitate with the trapezoid and lunate articulations and the third carpometacarpal articulations. The surgical approach and technique vary with the extent of bone loss, articular deformity, and patient requirements. In many cases, the wrist is fused with 10 to 30 degrees of extension and slight ulnar deviation to improve grip and function. Fixation devices have changed over the years. External fixation is less commonly used currently. Internal fixation can be accomplished with intramedullary devices (see Fig. 13-98), staples, plate and screws (see Fig. 13-99), and K-wire and tension band (see Fig. 13-100) techniques. Currently, a dorsal wrist arthrodesis plate with larger screws in the distal radius and smaller screws distally is used to avoid metacarpal fractures (see Fig. 13-101). Iliac cancellous or cortical bone graft is added as necessary for total and partial wrist fusions.

Fusion of the interphalangeal articulations can be accomplished with multiple approaches as well. Again, the extent of bone loss and need for bone graft play a significant role in selecting the surgical techniques. The degree of flexion varies with the patient requirements. K-wire and tension band fixation is commonly used for proximal interphalangeal arthrodesis

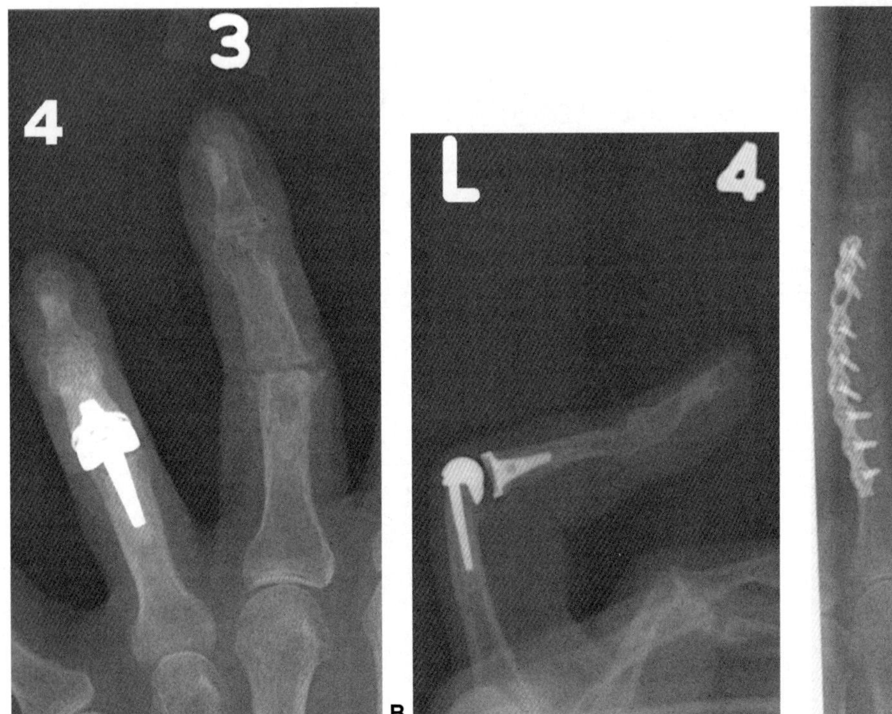


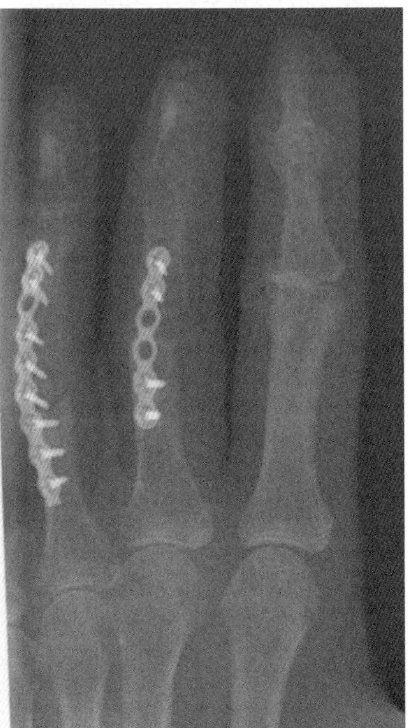


Fig. 13-92 Deep infection following interphalangeal arthroplasty. A: Posteroanterior (PA) and lateral (B) radiographs following removal of the third interphalangeal arthroplasty components and flexion deformity of the fourth interphalangeal joint. C: Radiographs following arthrodesis with miniplate and screw fixation following treatment of the infection.

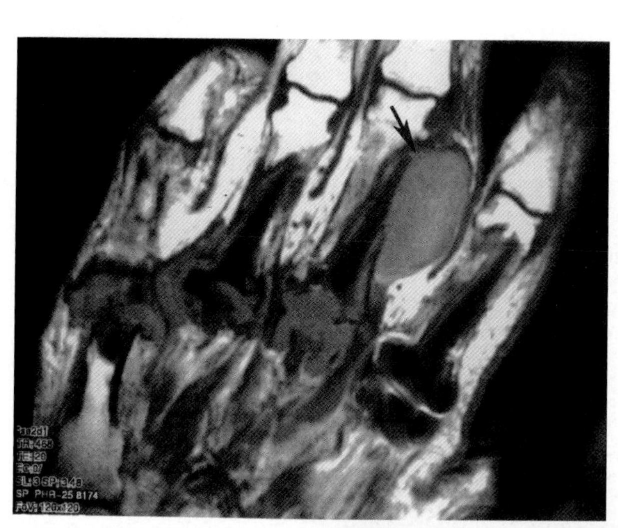

A

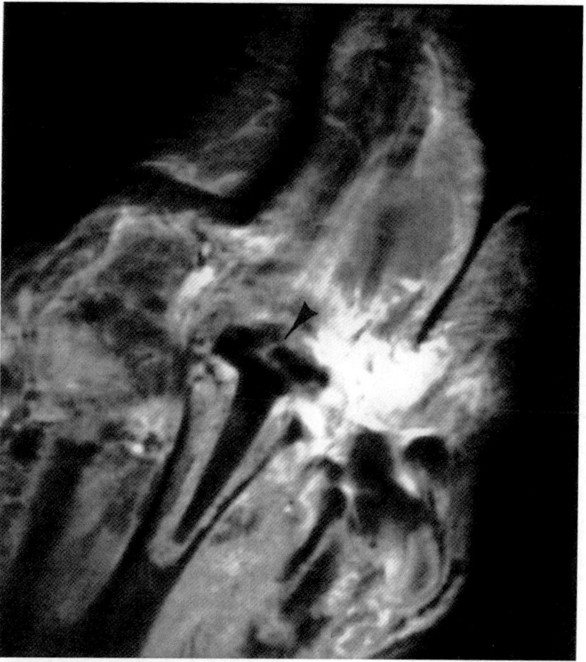

B

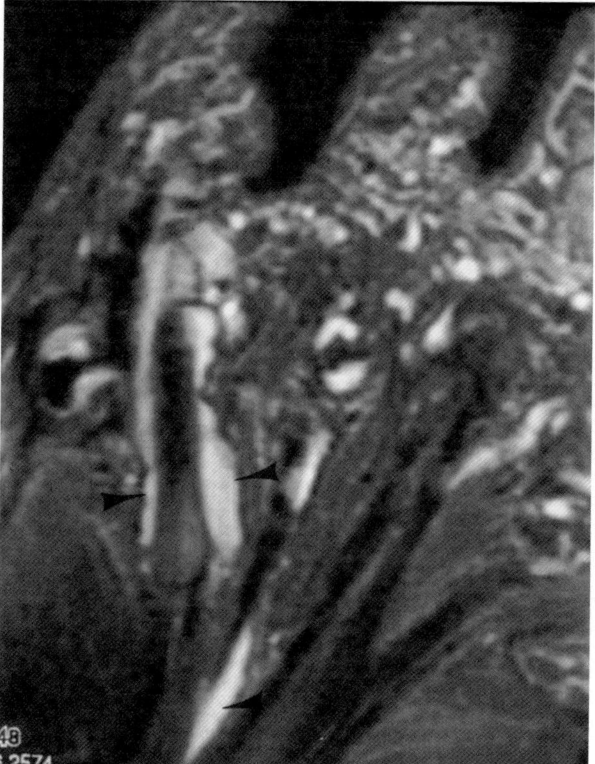

C

Fig. 13-93 Silicone-elastomer implants in the second through fifth metacarpophalangeal (MCP) joints with aggressive synovitis. A: T1-weighted coronal magnetic resonance (MR) image demonstrates extensive abnormal signal intensity about the implants with breakthrough of the third and a large reactive granuloma (*arrow*). T2-weighted coronal images (B and C) at different levels demonstrate synovitis extending into the tendon sheath (*arrowheads* in C) and a fracture of the implant (*arrowhead* in B) with adjacent synovitis.

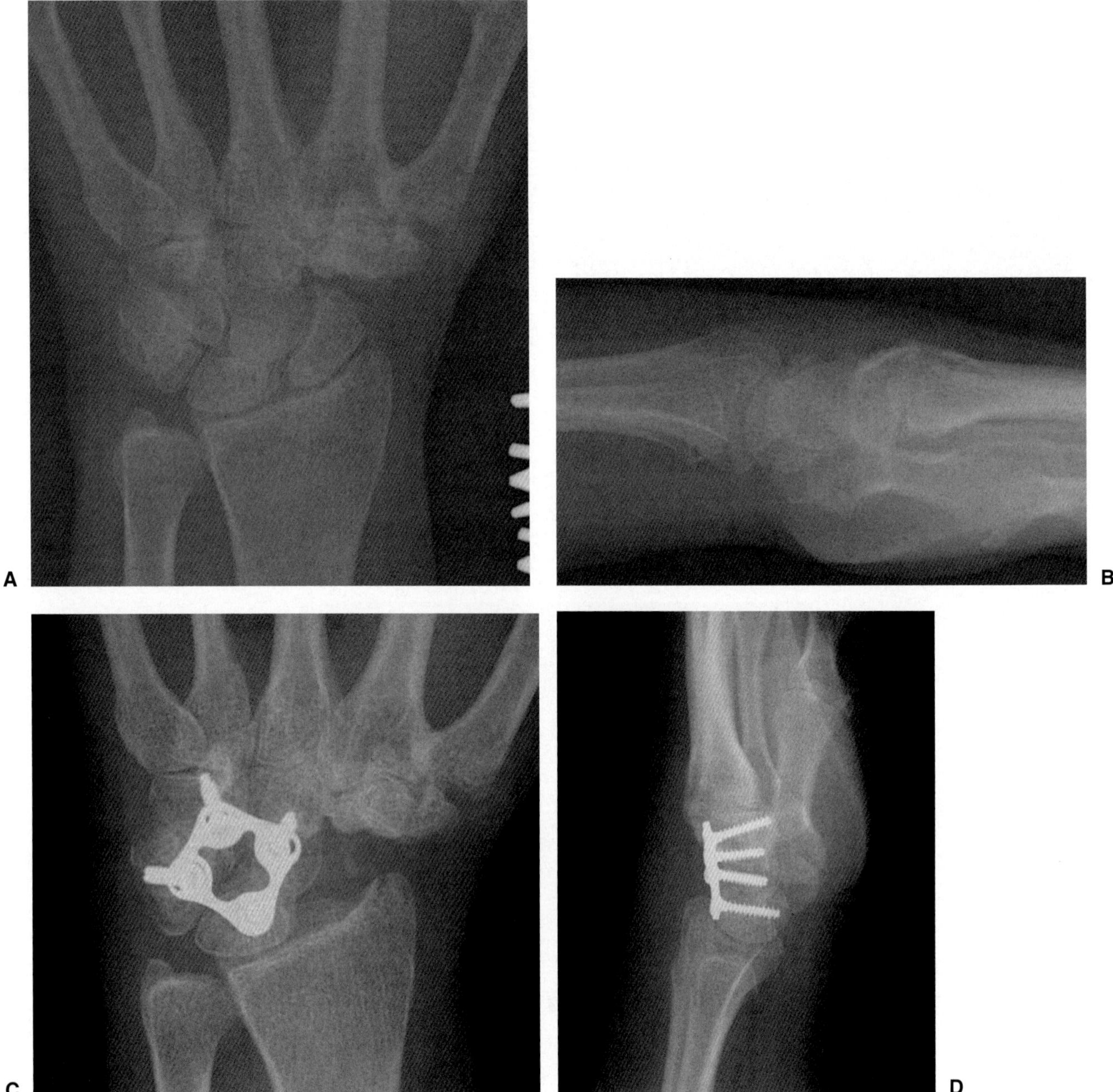

**Fig. 13-94** Carpal instability with partial arthrodesis. Posteroanterior (PA) (A) and lateral (B) radiographs demonstrating carpal collapse with dorsal intercalated segment instability. There is partial resection of the distal scaphoid and trapezium. PA (C) and lateral (D) radiographs following arthrodesis of the capitate, hamate, lunate, and triquetrum with a four-corner plate and screws.

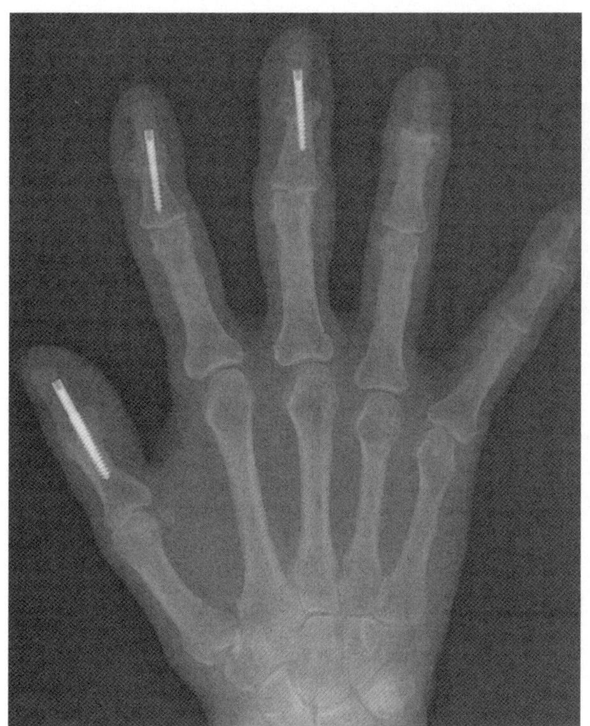

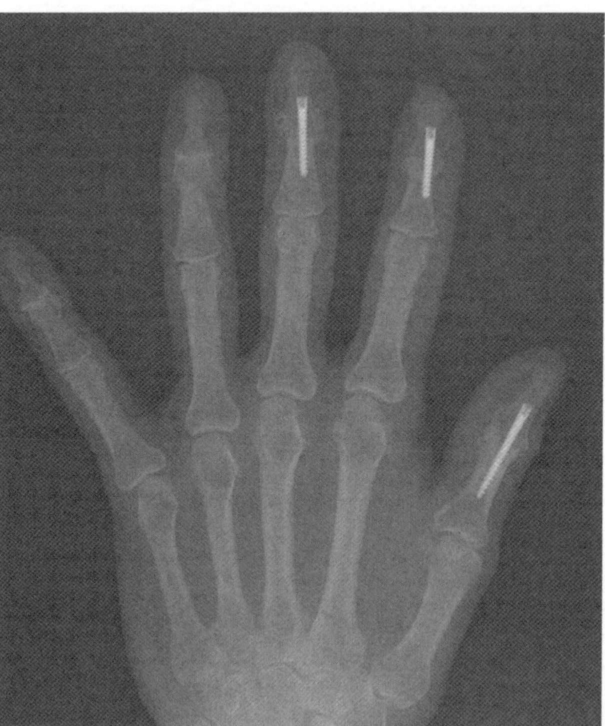

Fig. 13-95 Distal interphalangeal arthrodesis. Posteroanterior (PA) radiographs of the right (A) and left (B) hands following headless tapered Acutrak compression screw arthrodesis of the first through third distal interphalangeal joints bilaterally.

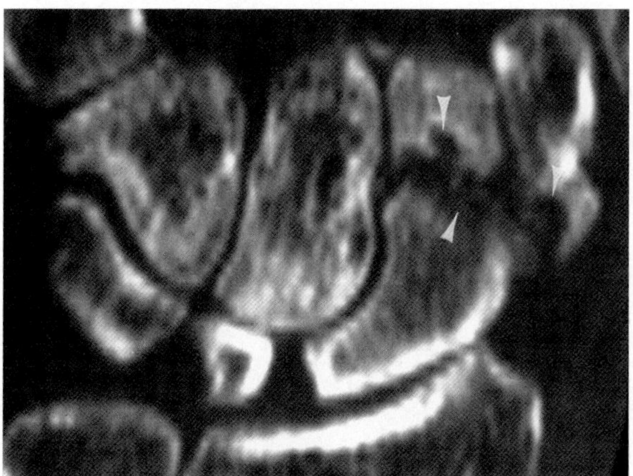

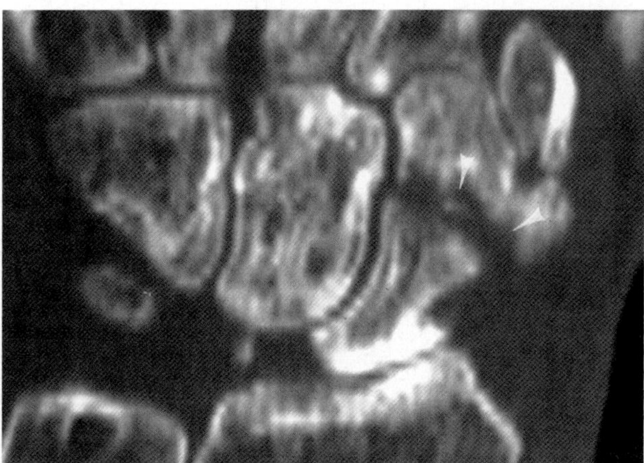

Fig. 13-96 Coronal computed tomographic (CT) images (A and B) demonstrating extensive bone loss and cyst formation in the scapho-trapezial-trapezoid articulations (*arrowheads*) and scapholunate joint space widening.

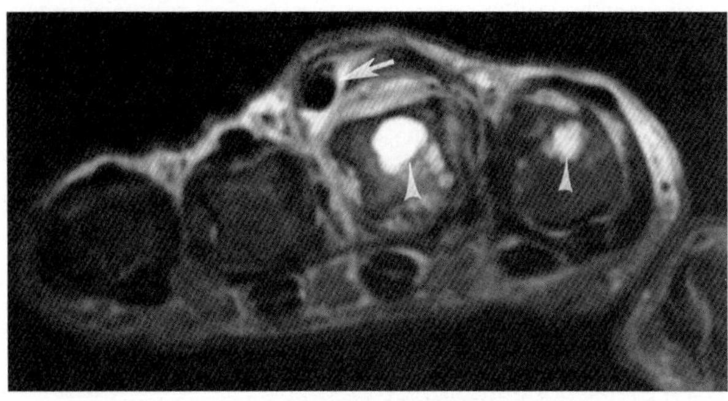
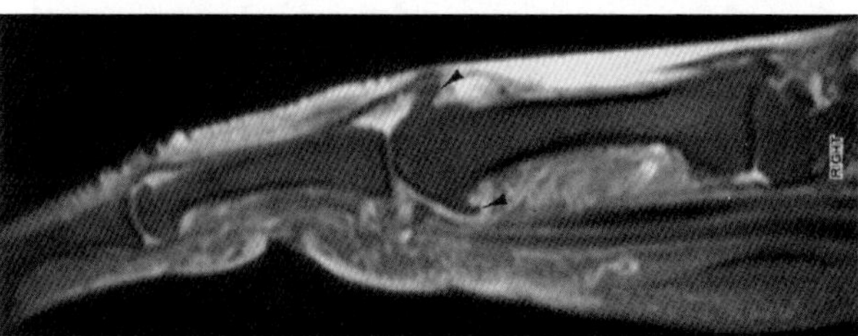

A B

Fig. 13-97 A: Axial fat suppressed T2-weighted fast spin-echo images demonstrate geodes in the metacarpal heads (*arrowheads*) and dislocation of the extensor tendon (*arrow*). B: Sagittal image using the same pulse sequence as in (A) demonstrating osteophyte formation at the metacarpophalangeal joint (*arrowheads*) with displacement of the extensor tendon. The flexor tendons are normal.

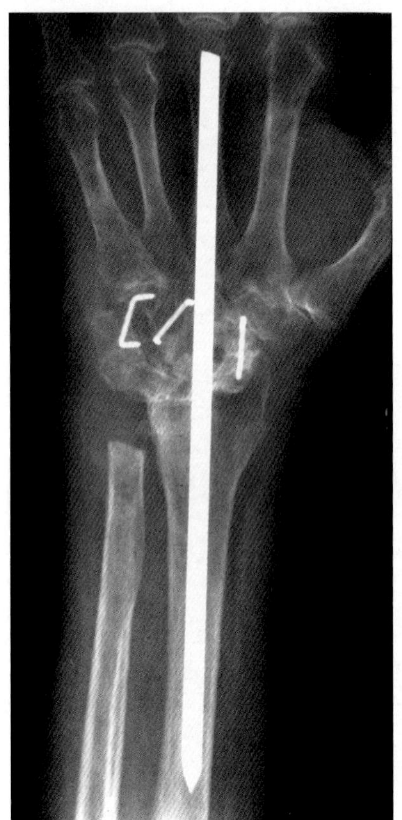
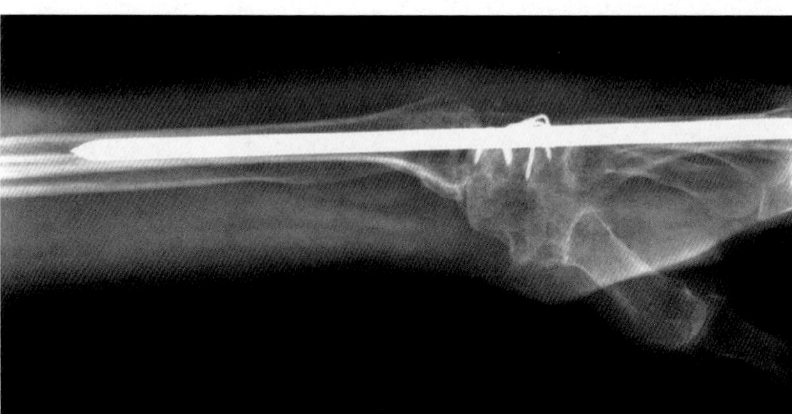

A B

Fig. 13-98 Wrist arthrodesis. Posteroanterior (PA) (A) and lateral (B) radiographs following total arthrodesis with an intramedullary nail extending from the radius through the third metacarpal. There are three carpal staples for carpal bone fusions and the distal ulna has been resected. The wrist is in neutral position.

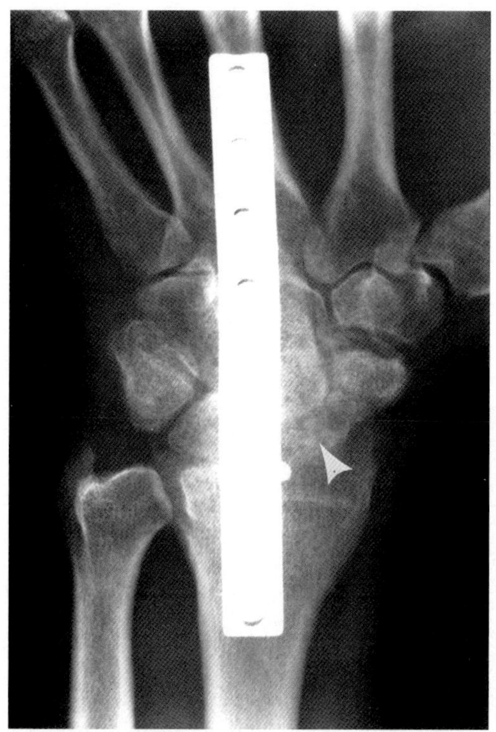
A

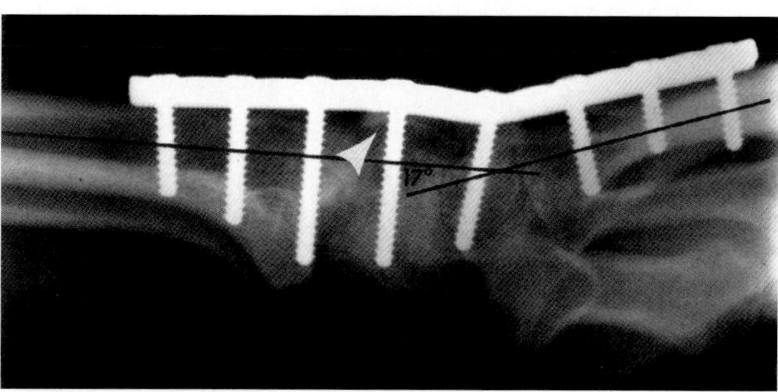

B

Fig. 13-99 Posteroanterior (PA) (A) and lateral (B) radiographs following arthrodesis with dorsal dynamic compression plate and screw fixation. The wrist is fused in 17 degrees of extension with bone graft (*arrowhead*) dorsally and radially.

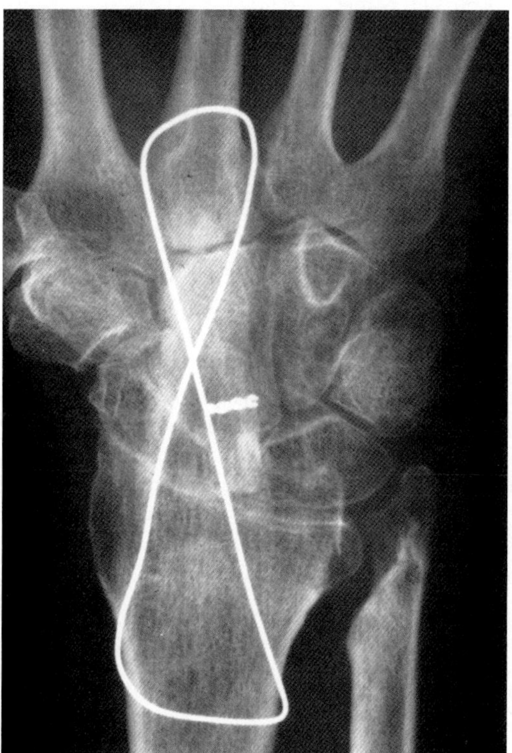
A

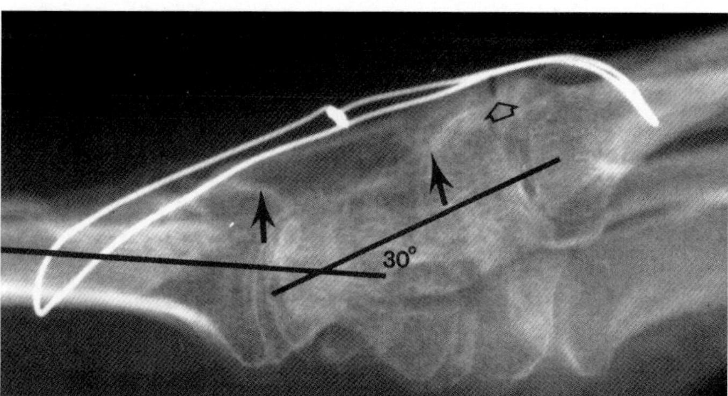

B

Fig. 13-100 Posteroanterior (PA) (A) and lateral (B) radiographs following total wrist arthrodesis with dorsal cortical bone graft and tension band from the radius through the third metacarpal. The bone graft is placed dorsally (*arrows*) from the radius to third metacarpal base and is solidly incorporated except at the base of the third metacarpal (*open arrow*). The wrist is fused in 30 degrees of extension.

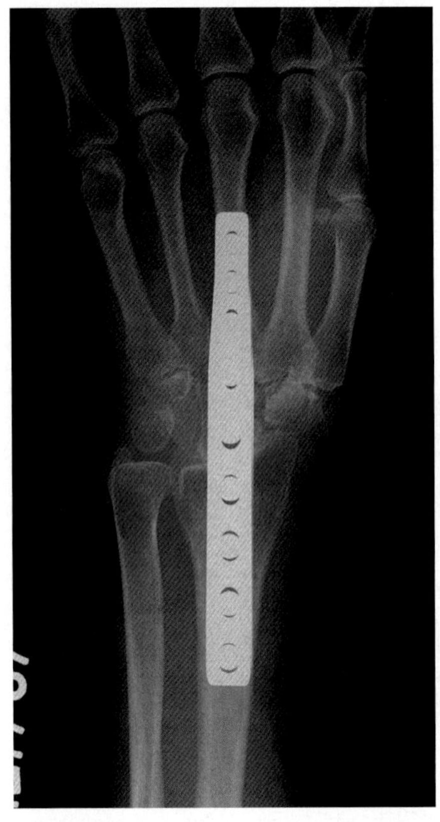

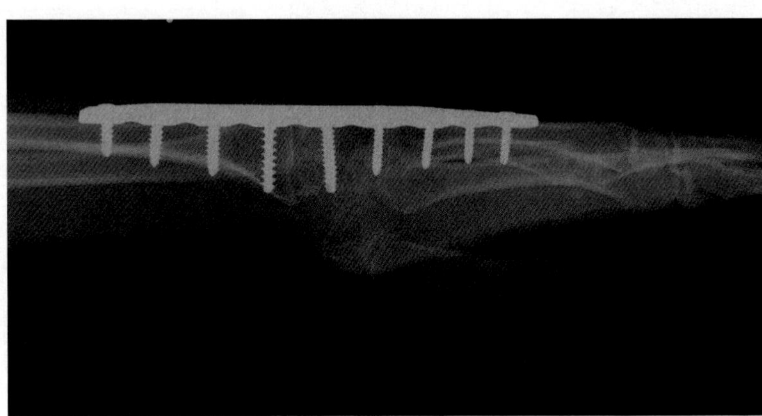

Fig. 13-101 Posteroanterior (PA) (A) and lateral (B) radiographs following proximal row carpectomy and dorsal compression plate and screw fixation. Note the smaller length and caliber of the distal screws to prevent metacarpal fractures. The wrist is fused in neutral position.

(Figs. 13-85 and 13-89). Other options include headless compression screws (Fig. 13-96) and titanium plate and screw fixation (see Fig. 13-102 and also Fig. 13-92).

## Suggested Reading

Carroll RE, Hill NA. Small joint arthrodesis in hand reconstruction. *J Bone Joint Surg*. 1969;51A:1219–1221.

Jebsen PJ, Adams BD. Wrist arthrodesis: Review of current technique. *J Am Acad Orthop Surg*. 2001;9:53–60.

Leibovic SJ. Arthrodesis of the interphalangeal joints with headless compression screws. *J Hand Surg [Br]*. 2007;32A: 1113–1119.

Murry PM. Current status of wrist arthrodesis and arthroplasty. *Clin Plast Surg*. 1996;23:385–394.

### Imaging of Postoperative Complications

Complications following arthrodesis vary with the technique and anatomic location. Pseudarthrosis or nonunion, implant failure, and soft tissue irritation resulting in removal of the implants can occur with all procedures. Carpal tunnel syndrome may follow wrist fusion.

Pseudarthrosis following metacarpophalangeal and interphalangeal arthrodesis was reported in 5% of 635 articulations. This was most commonly observed in patients treated with arthrodesis for spastic paralysis and rheumatoid arthritis. Pseudarthrosis can usually be treated successfully with revision arthrodesis. Malpositioning (rotation) may also require revision of the fusion. Arthrodesis in the proximal interphalangeal using headless compression screws (Fig. 13-95) resulted in union in 98% with an incidence of pseudarthrosis of up to 2%. Nonunion with K-wire technique approaches 21%, with K-wire and tension band 4.5%, and Herbert screws 0%. The highest nonunion rates with compression screws occur in patients with psoriatic arthritis followed by rheumatoid arthritis. Infection is uncommon with interphalangeal arthrodesis.

Although patient satisfaction is high following wrist arthrodesis, complications are not uncommon. Minor and major complications occur in up to 18% of patients.

**Complications of wrist arthrodesis**

- Pseudarthrosis/nonunion
- Soft tissue irritation from fixation devices
- Tendon adhesions
- Carpal tunnel syndrome
- Complex regional pain syndrome
- Wound healing
- Persistent pain

Implant failure and osseous changes can be followed with serial radiographs (Fig. 3-101). Fracture at the end of fusion plates has been reported resulting in plate removal by some

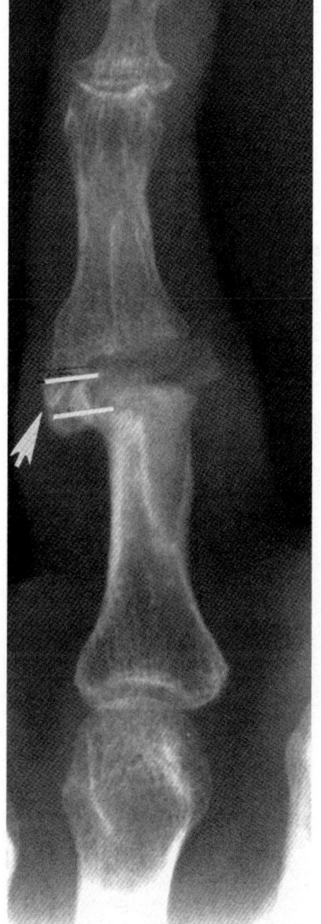
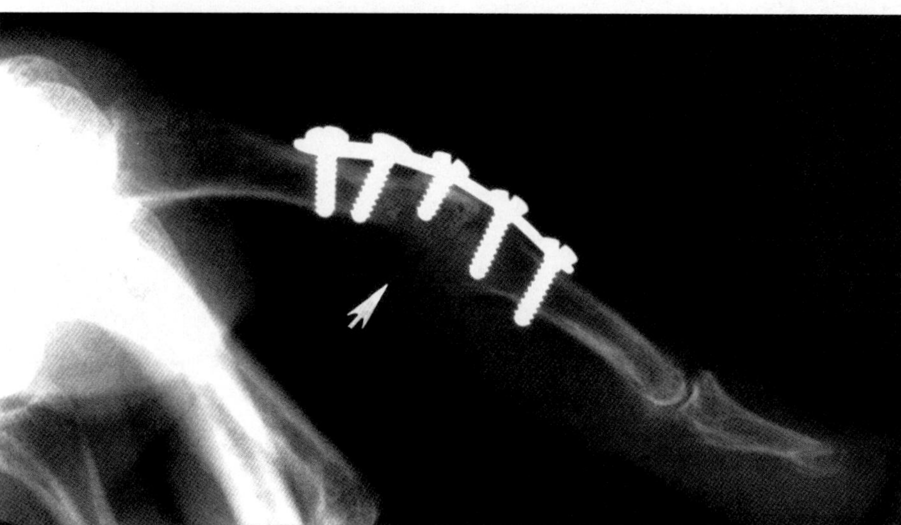

Fig. 13-102 Failed interphalangeal silicone-elastomer arthroplasty. A: Posteroanterior (PA) radiograph demonstrates incongruency of the joint with heterotopic ossification (*arrow*). B: Lateral radiograph following dorsal plate and screw fixation with iliac bone graft (*arrow*).

surgeons once the fusion is solid. Pseudarthrosis or nonunion is best evaluated with thin section CT with reformatted images in the coronal and sagittal planes.

Tendon adhesions and carpal tunnel syndrome may be diagnosed with laboratory studies (electromyography [EMG]) and clinical evaluation. MRI can be used depending on the extent and type of metal. Tendon sheath evaluation can be accomplished with MRI or tendon sheath injections. The latter allows injection of anesthetic to confirm the source of pain and aspiration to exclude infection. Radionuclide imaging is useful for infection and complex regional pain syndrome.

## Suggested Reading

Bansky R, Racz N. The use of titanium miniplates in arthrodesis of the interphalangeal joints and metacarpal neck fracture. *Bratisl Lek Listy*. 2005;106:287–290.

Clendenin MB, Green DP. Arthrodesis of the wrist-complications and their management. *J Hand Surg [Br]*. 1981; 6A:253–257.

Leibovic SJ. Arthrodesis of the interphalangeal joints with headless compression screws. *J Hand Surg [Br]*. 2007;32A: 1113–1119.

Tomaino MM, Miller RJ, Burton RI. Outcome assessment following limited wrist fusion: Objective wrist scoring versus patient satisfaction. *Contemp Orthop*. 1994;28:403–410.

Vicar AJ, Burton RI. Surgical management of the rheumatoid wrist-fusion or arthroplasty. *J Hand Surg [Br]*. 1986; 11A:790–796.

## Osteotomies

Osteotomies are frequently performed on the osseous structures of the hand, distal radius, and ulna and carpal bones. Fractures of the hand are among the most common skeletal fractures. Malunion can result in significant functional loss and cosmetic deformity. Fractures involving the articular surface may lead to early arthrosis. Malunion may result in excessive angulation, rotation, or shortening and most commonly occurs in the phalanges (Figs. 13-53 and 13-66). Angular deformity may occur with rotational deformity in the proximal and middle

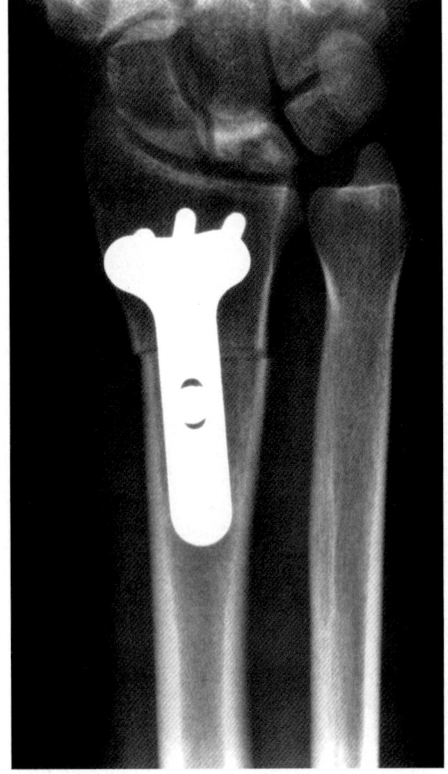


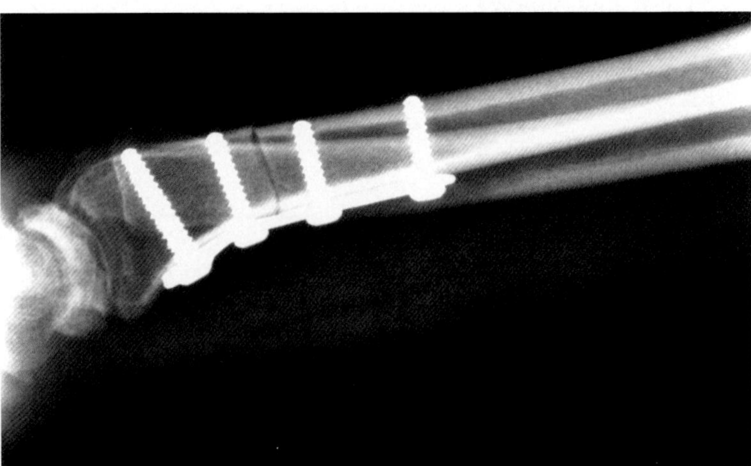


**Fig. 13-103** Radial shortening osteotomy for Keinbock disease. Posteroanterior (PA) (**A**) and lateral (**B**) radiographs demonstrate avascular necrosis of the lunate. The radius was shortened and internally stabilized with a volar plate and screws.

phalanges. Functional issues are most likely when angulation exceeds 25 to 30 degrees.

Transverse metacarpal fractures can angulate dorsally resulting in cosmetic and functional deformity. Shortening and rotation are more common with spiral fractures of the fourth and fifth metacarpals (Figs. 13-46 and 13-50).

In the wrist, malunion most often occurs with scaphoid fractures (Figs. 13-28 and 13-32). This can result in carpal instability. Osteotomies can also be performed on the distal radius and ulna for purposes of articular realignment. Additional indications include avascular necrosis of the lunate, ulnar positive variance with impaction syndrome, premature closure of physeal fractures, and congenital disorders such as Madelung deformity.

Imaging of malunion or other deformities treatable with osteotomy can be accomplished with routine radiographs (see Fig. 13-103). CT may be required to provide more optimal assessment of osseous structures such as the scaphoid (Fig. 13-28) and the degree of articular deformity. MRI can be useful to exclude associated soft tissue or tendon disorders. MR arthrography is especially useful in patients with ulnar positive variance and abutment syndromes. In this setting, the triangular fibrocartilage complex, articular cartilage, and associated ligaments can be assessed preoperatively (see Fig. 13-104).

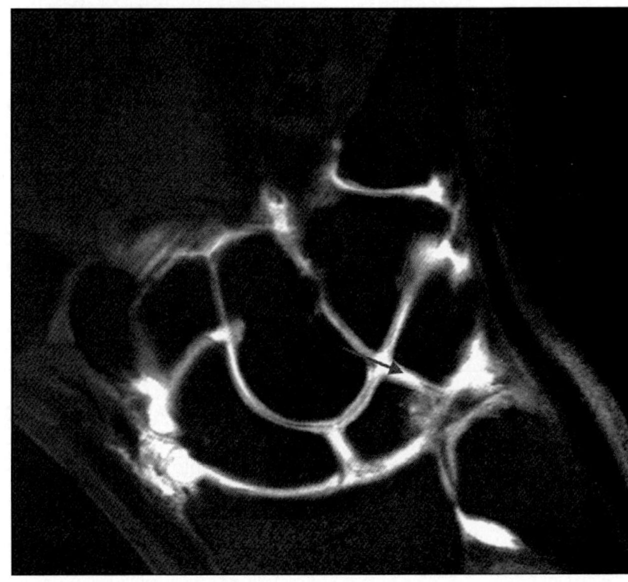

**Fig. 13-104** Ulnar lunate abutment syndrome. Coronal fat-suppressed T1-weighted arthrogram image demonstrating edema in the lunate (*arrow*) and contrast in the intercarpal joint (*upper arrow*) due to a lunotriquetral ligament tear.

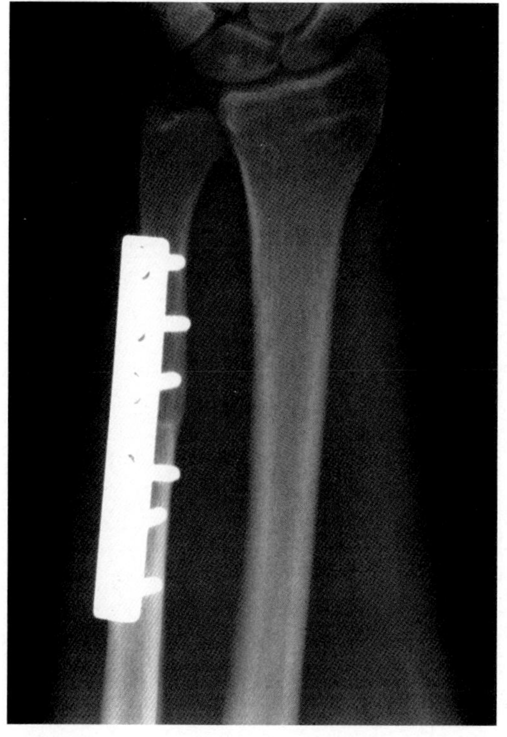
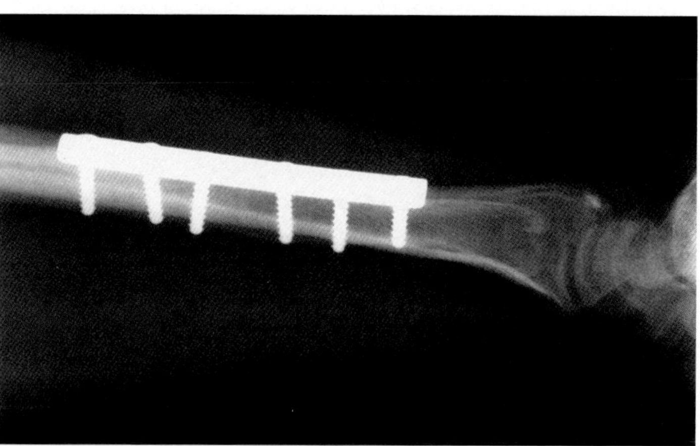

Fig. 13-105 Ulnar shortening osteotomy. Posteroanterior (PA) (A) and lateral (B) radiographs following ulnar shortening with a healed transverse osteotomy with plate and screw fixation.

## Suggested Reading

Berquist TH, Trigg SD. Hand and wrist. In: Berquist TH, ed. *Imaging atlas of orthopaedic appliances and prostheses*. New York: Raven Press; 1995:831–921.

Gollamudi S, Jones WA. Corrective osteotomy of malunited fractures of the phalanges and metacarpals. *J Hand Surg [Br]*. 2000;25A:439–441.

Reis FB, Katchburian MV, Faloppa F, et al. Osteotomy of the radius and ulna for Madelung deformity. *J Bone Joint Surg*. 1998;80B:817–824.

Ring D. Malunion and nonunion of the metacarpals and phalanges. *J Bone Joint Surg*. 2005;87A:1380–1388.

Seffar P. Ulna oblique osteotomy for radius and ulnar length inequality: Technique and applications. *Tech Hand Upper Ext*. 2006;10:47–53.

### Treatment Options and Complications

Treatment options vary with the anatomic location and indication. Osteotomies may be transverse, oblique, or step shaped and vary with the situation. Shortening osteotomies are designed to reduce the length of a bone (see Fig. 13-105). Lengthening can be accomplished with bone graft, either uniform or wedge, to vary the configuration as necessary. Fixation can be accomplished with K-wires, cerclage wires (Fig. 13-66), or plate and screw fixation (Figs. 13-103 and 13-105).

Complications include nonunion, loss of correction, implant failure, neurovascular injury, and infection. Serial radiographs are adequate for evaluation of the implants and loss of correction. CT is most effective to follow healing if there is question of delayed union or nonunion. MRI is most effective for evaluation of soft tissue complications. Suspected infection can be imaged using MRI or radionuclide scans as described earlier.

## Suggested Reading

Berquist TH, Trigg SD. Hand and wrist. In: Berquist TH, ed. *Imaging atlas of orthopaedic appliances and prostheses*. New York: Raven Press; 1995:831–921.

Ring D. Malunion and nonunion of the metacarpals and phalanges. *J Bone Joint Surg*. 2005;87A:1380–1388.

VanHeest A. Wrist deformities after fracture. *Hand Clin*. 2006; 22:113–120.

# 14 Musculoskeletal Neoplasms

Musculoskeletal neoplasms are treated with surgical excision, radiation therapy, chemotherapy, and combination therapeutic approaches. This chapter will focus on orthopaedic approaches to treatment of neoplasms. Emphasis will be placed on the role of imaging in detection and classification and postoperative monitoring.

## Preoperative Evaluation

Decisions regarding the approach to musculoskeletal neoplasms may be relatively simple in the case of a localized benign lesion or more complex. The therapeutic decisions may be more complex depending on the histology, location, bone and soft tissue involvement, and patient factors such as age, general health status, activity, and prognosis. Limb-saving procedures, often with extensive reconstruction, are usually considered when the lesion is located in a region that allows complete resection with wide surgical margin. This would require a 6-cm margin for bone and soft tissue sarcomas. Preoperative chemotherapy is often used preoperatively in conjunction with limb-saving procedures.

Limb-saving procedures are usually contraindicated in patients with neurovascular encasement, which would result in functional impairment in the extremity following resection, and in patients with significant pathologic fractures that may result in dissemination of tumor cells. Lower extremity procedures may compromise growth in an immature skeleton. However, new prosthetic designs and other surgical options do not totally exclude limb-saving procedures in children in whom the growth plate may be at risk. Additional considerations for limb-saving procedures include the risk of local recurrence, long-term survival, functional outcome compared to amputation, psychological benefit, and immediate and delayed morbidities of the surgical procedure.

Preoperative assessment includes multiple clinical and imaging factors. Enneking et al. developed a functional system for pre- and postoperative evaluation that scored 7 categories (0 to 5 points) for a total of 35 points. The categories included motion, pain, stability, deformity, strength, functional activity, and emotional acceptance.

Lesion identification may be accomplished with radiographs or other imaging modalities. Once identified, multiple approaches are used to identify the type of lesion and extent of involvement. This may be initiated with lesion biopsy, followed by additional imaging for staging if the lesion is malignant. Planning the biopsy requires close communication with the orthopaedic surgeon so that the needle path can be resected along with the tumor during the procedure. In addition, knowledge of the anatomic compartments is essential when planning bone or soft tissue biopsies (see Fig. 14-1). Inappropriate needle approaches can unnecessarily contaminate compartments that could interfere with the planned limb-saving procedure. Biopsies are most often performed using computed tomographic (CT) guidance, but ultrasonography or fluoroscopy can also be used to guide needle placement (see Fig. 14-2).

Tumor staging typically involves the lesion (T), grade (G), nodal involvement (N), and metastasis (M). Thorough and accurate staging requires the use of multiple imaging modalities. Multiple staging systems have been used. Enneking et al. proposed a staging system in 1980 that incorporated prognostic factors of local recurrence and metastasis, included surgical implications and provided guidelines for adjuvant therapy. Malignant bone lesions were staged based on grade, inter- and extraosseous extent, and whether there was associated metastasis. This system was later endorsed by the Musculoskeletal Tumor Society (MSTS) and the American Joint Committee on Cancer (AJCC). The MSTS staging system remains the most commonly used system (see Table 14-1).

Using the MSTS system, low-grade bone lesions are considered stage I and high-grade lesions stage II. Metastases

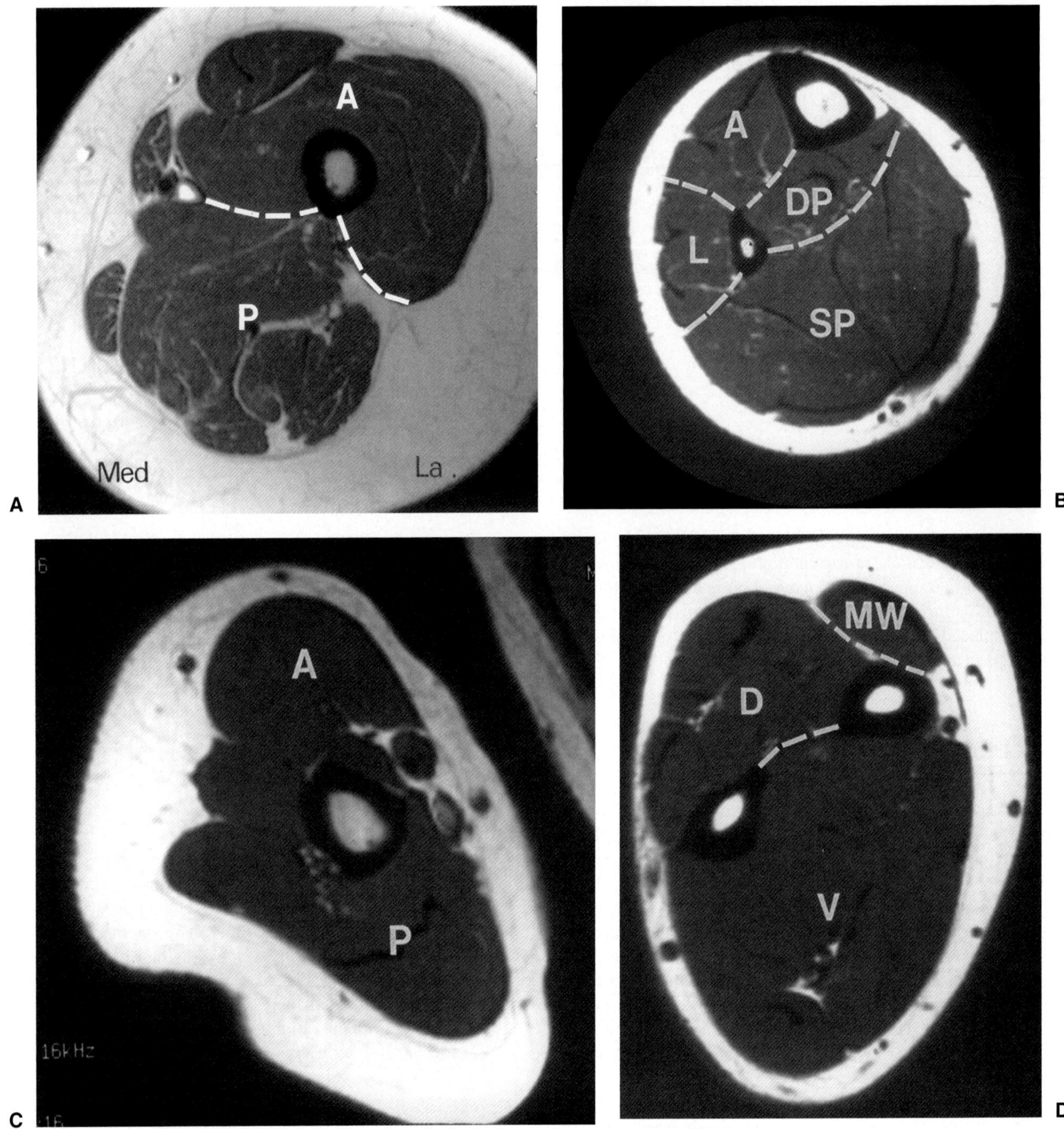


Fig. 14-1 Compartmental anatomy. A: Thigh divided into anterior (*A*), posterior (*P*), and medial compartments. The anterior compartment contains the quadriceps and sartorius muscles; the posterior compartment contains the semimembranosus, semitendinosus, and biceps group; and the medial compartment the adductors and gracilis muscles. B: The calf is divided into anterior (*A*), lateral (*L*), superficial posterior (*SP*), and deep posterior (*DP*) compartments. The anterior compartment contains the extensors hallucis longus and digitorum longus and the tibialis anterior. The lateral compartment contains the peroneus brevis and longus. The superficial posterior compartment contains the gastrocnemius and soleus and the deep posterior compartment the tibialis posterior, flexor hallucis longus, and flexor digitorum longus. C: The arm is divided into anterior (*A*) and posterior (*P*) compartments. The anterior compartment contains the biceps brachii and brachialis, and the posterior compartment the triceps. D: The forearm is divided into the volar (*V*), dorsal (*D*), and mobile wad (*MW*). The volar compartment contains the flexor muscle groups, pronator teres, and palmaris longus and the dorsal compartment the extensor muscle groups and abductor pollicis longus. The mobile wad contains the brachioradialis and extensor carpi radialis longus and brevis.

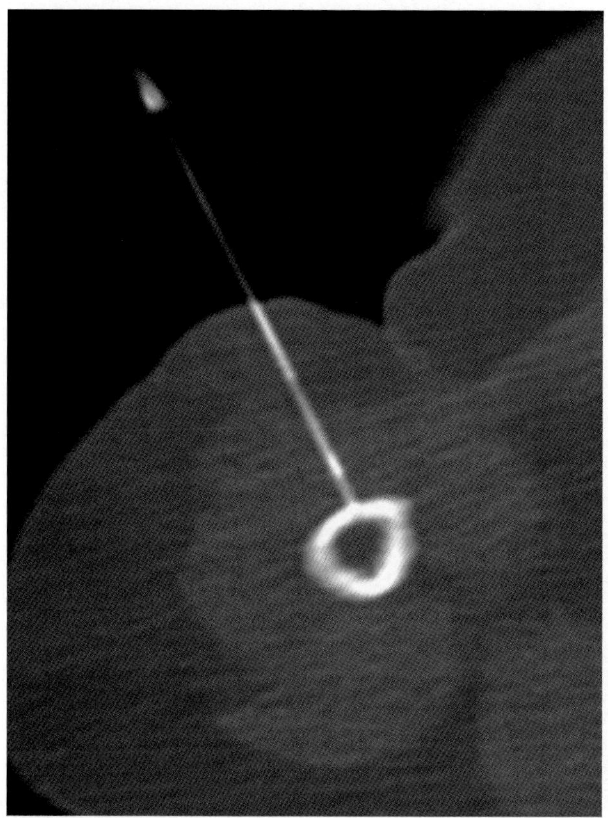

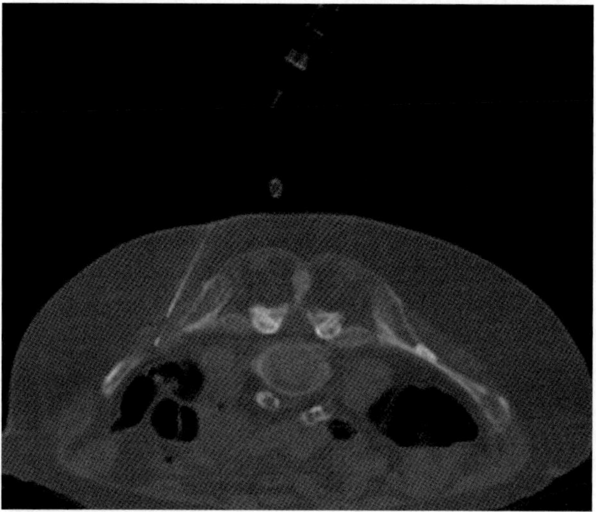

Fig. 14-2 Needle biopsy. Computed tomography (CT)-guided needle biopsies of the humerus (A) in a patient with lymphoma. The needle enters through the anterior compartment. CT-guided biopsy (B) of an iliac lesion entering posteromedially.

are considered stage III regardless of the histology. The stages are subdivided based on local extent. Lesions confined to bone are substage A (intracompartmental). Lesions that extend through the cortex into the soft tissues are substage B (extracompartmental).

Imaging of primary skeletal or soft tissue lesions and potential metastasis requires multiple modalities to optimize staging. Over the years accuracy has greatly improved with the additions of CT, magnetic resonance imaging (MRI), and positron emission tomographic (PET) imaging. To assist the clinician, the radiologist must identify all of the following features so that they can be correlated with the staging system:

**Imaging features for tumor staging**

- Tumor location and size (greatest diameter)
- Intra- or extracompartmental
- Soft tissue involvement
- Joint involvement
  - Neurovascular displacement or encasement
- Skip lesions
- Local and distant metastasis

Table 14-1

STAGING OF MALIGNANT MUSCULOSKELETAL NEOPLASMS

| STAGE | GRADE | SITE | METASTASIS |
|---|---|---|---|
| I | | | |
| IA | G1 | T1 | No metastasis |
| IB | G1 | T2 | No metastasis |
| II | | | |
| IIA | G2 | T1 | No metastasis |
| IIB | G2 | T2 | No metastasis |
| III | G1 or G2 | T1 or T2 | Metastasis |

G1, low grade histologically; G2, high grade histologically; T1, intracompartmental; T2, extracompartmental.

# Primary Skeletal Lesions

Radiographs or computed radiographic (CR) images are still useful for detection of benign and malignant skeletal lesions. Radiographic features are extremely useful for characterizing the aggressiveness of the lesion (see Fig. 14-3). In addition, CT is useful in patients with subtle lesions, soft tissue calcification, tumor matrix, and thin cortex (see Fig. 14-4). MRI with contrast is most useful for evaluation of local bone, soft tissue compartment, and neurovascular involvement. The bone and soft tissue anatomy for at least 6 cm about the lesion should be

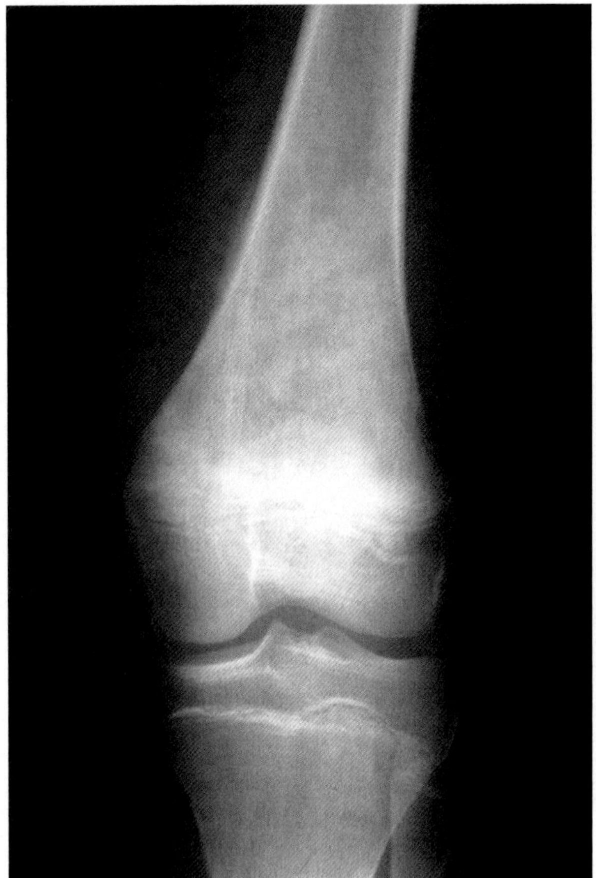


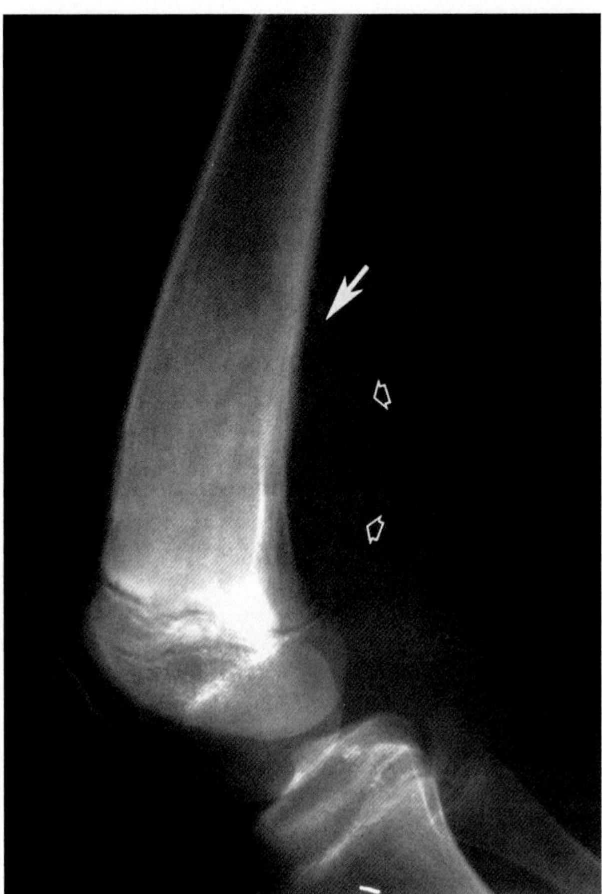


**Fig. 14-3** Osteosarcoma. Anteroposterior (AP) (A) and lateral (B) radiographs of the distal femur demonstrating a mixed lytic and sclerotic lesion with periosteal reaction and a Codman triangle (*arrow*) on the lateral view. There is also a large posterior soft tissue mass (*open arrows*).

evaluated to assess the ability to perform and extent of resection for limb-saving procedures.

For skeletal lesions, the entire structure (i.e., entire femur and proximal and distal articulations) should be included on the image for operative planning and to exclude skip lesions (see Fig. 14-5). Images should be obtained in at least two planes using T1- and T2-weighted sequences. Additional imaging with short T1 inversion recovery (STIR) may be indicated in some cases. Post–contrast-enhanced (gadolinium) images are routinely obtained unless there is a history of allergy or renal compromise. The same approach should be used postoperatively to establish a baseline for patient follow-up (see Fig. 14-6).

Angiography may be necessary in some cases to define neovascularity and vascular displacement or encasement (see Fig. 14-7). Angiography can also be used preoperatively to deliver chemotherapy and embolize tumor vessels.

## Soft Tissue Neoplasms

Radiographs demonstrate bone changes and soft tissue calcification. Fatty lesions may also be evident on radiographs. MRI is the technique of choice for detection and local staging of soft tissue lesions. Certain benign lesions such as lipomas, myxomas, hemangiomas, and cysts have characteristic appearances, which may obviate the need for biopsy or surgical intervention (see Fig. 14-8). Malignant or indeterminate lesions are evaluated using T1- and T2-weighted conventional or fast spin-echo sequences with or without fat suppression. Gadolinium-enhanced T1-weighted images are also obtained. Two image planes are necessary to fully evaluate the extent, compartment, and neurovascular involvement (see Fig. 14-9). Dynamic gadolinium techniques may be of value for differentiating benign from malignant lesions. Angiography is not often performed, but can be used for indications noted earlier.

## Metastasis

Radionuclide bone scans with technetium Tc 99m methylene-diphosphonate (MDP) have long been the standard for detection of skeletal metastasis. With a few exceptions (myeloma, aggressive lytic lesions) this technique is still useful (see Fig. 14-10). MRI can be used for axial skeleton screening with axial and sagittal spine images and coronal images of the pelvis and hips using T1-weighted and/or STIR images. PET,

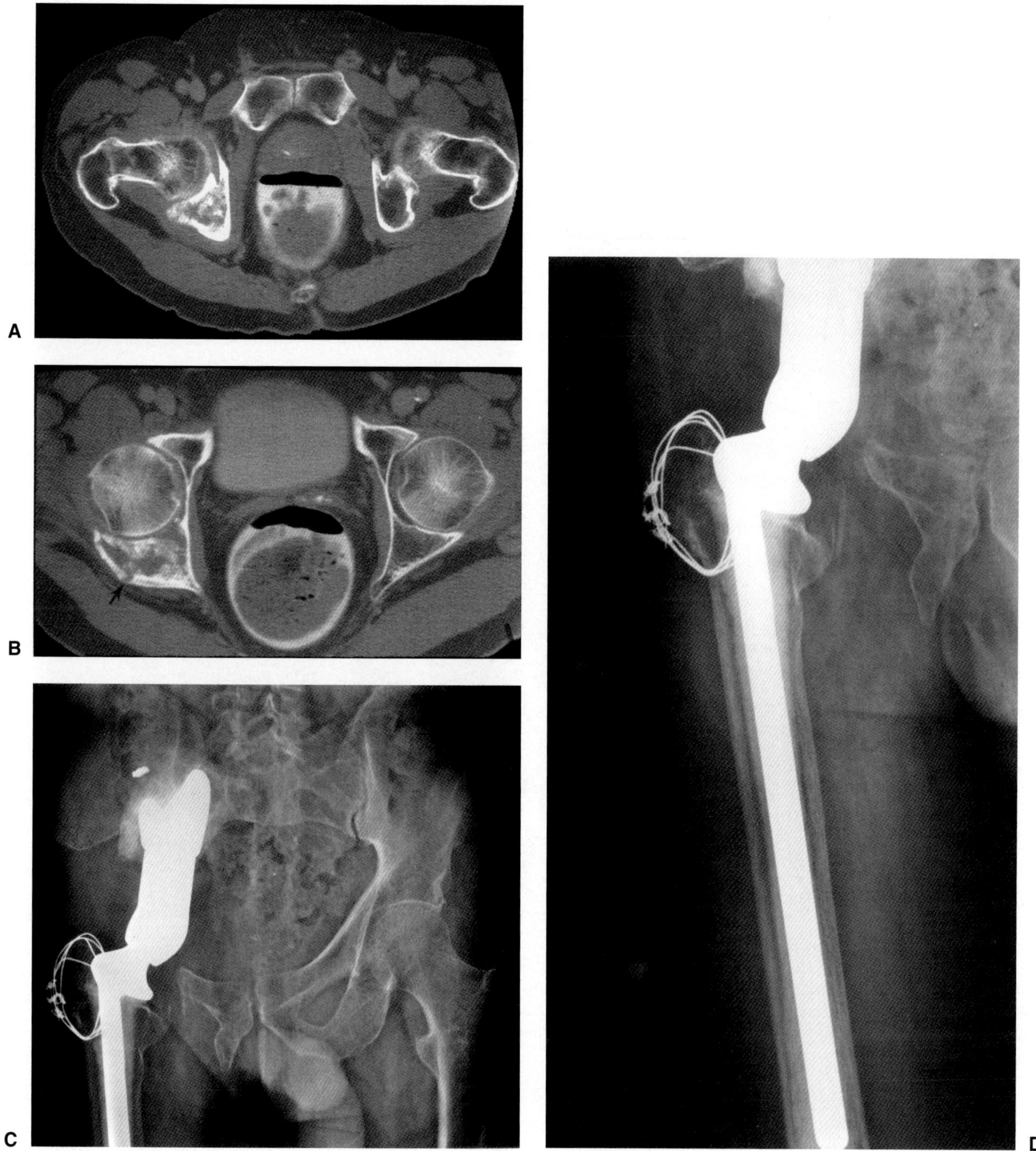


Fig. 14-4 Chondrosarcoma. Axial computed tomographic (CT) images (A and B) demonstrating a lesion in the right acetabulum with matrix characteristic of chondrosarcoma and a pathologic fracture (*arrow*). The patient was treated with wide excision and reconstruction using a saddle prosthesis (C and D).

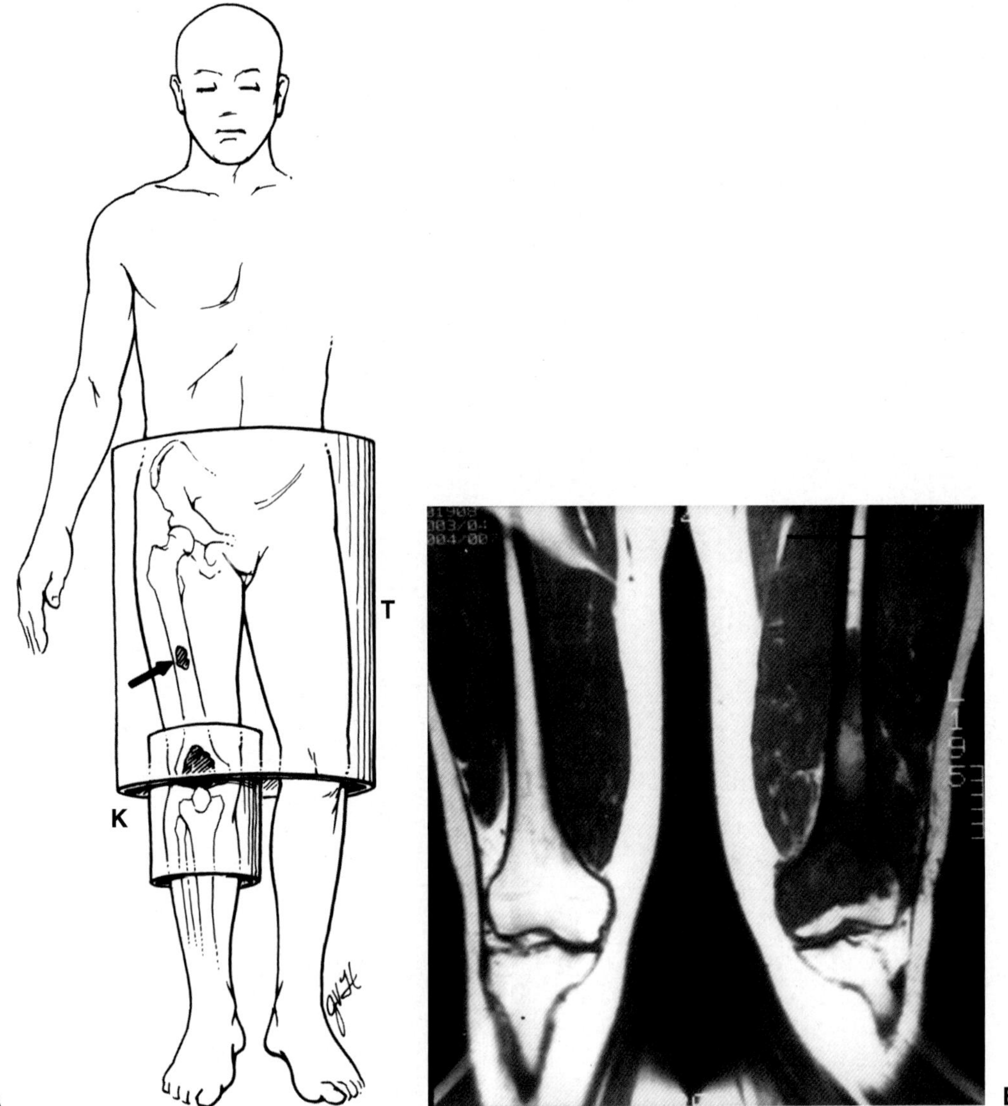


Fig. 14-5 Magnetic resonance (MR) imaging of skeletal neoplasm. **A:** A larger torso coil (*T*) and field of view is required to include the entire osseous structure. This allows operative planning and avoids overlooking skip lesions (*arrow*) more proximally. In most cases, a smaller knee coil (*K*) would be used to improve resolution. **B:** Distal femoral sarcoma demonstrated on a T1-weighted image. The entire femur is not included. At least 5 to 6 cm of normal tissue is required for limb-saving purposes (*line*).

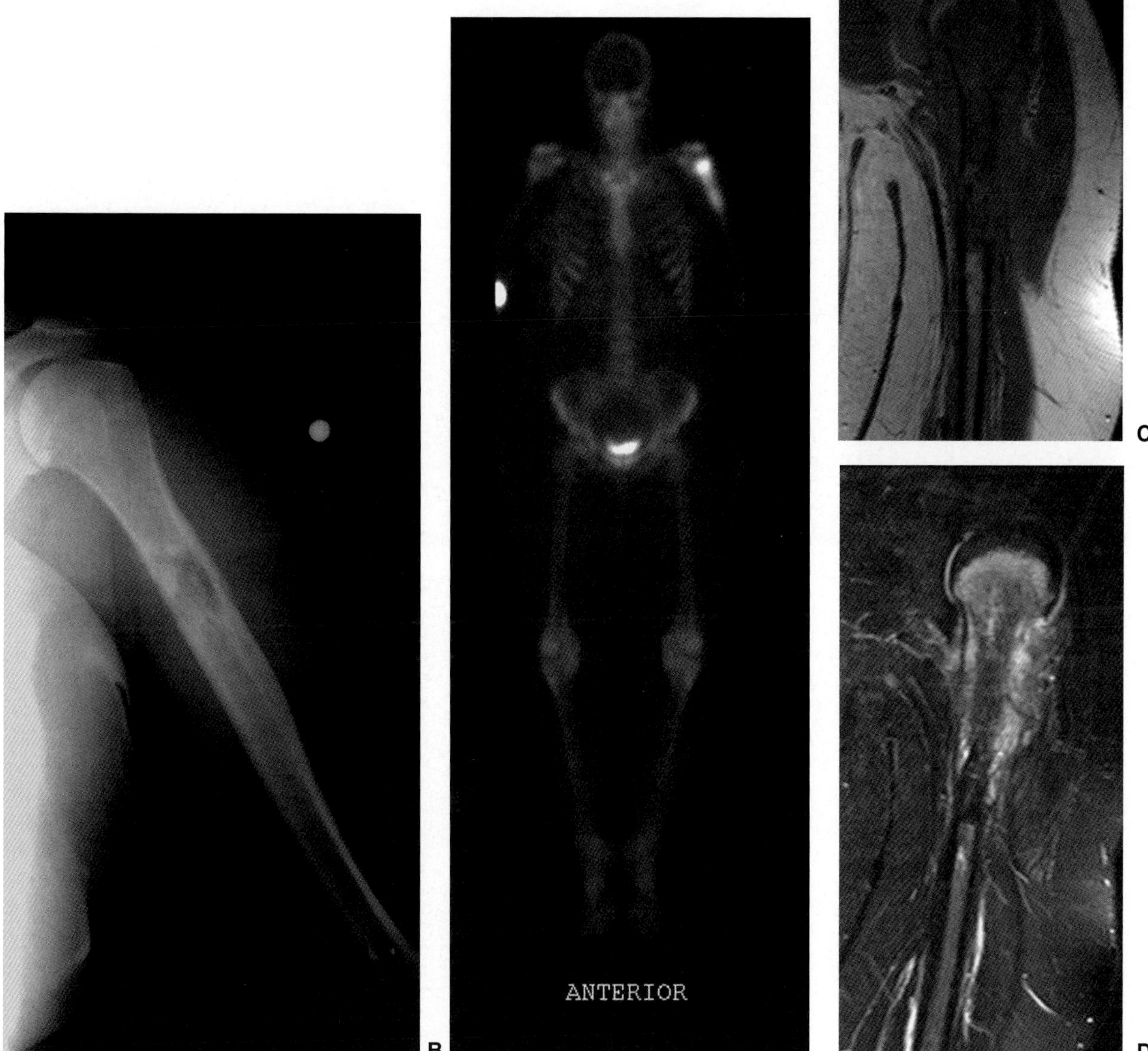


Fig. 14-6 High-grade osteosarcoma. A: Radiograph demonstrates a destructive lesion in the upper humerus with periosteal reaction. B: Technetium Tc 99m methylene-diphosphonate (MDP) whole body bone scan demonstrates intense uptake in the proximal humerus with no distant metastasis. Coronal T1 (C) and short T1 inversion recovery (STIR) (D) images and axial T1-weighted (E), T2-weighted (F), and postcontrast (G) images clearly demonstrate the extent of the tumor. H: Specimen radiograph of the resected proximal humerus. I: The patient was treated with a long stem hemiarthroplasty component and proximal allograft with cortical bone graft at the allograft–humeral junction.

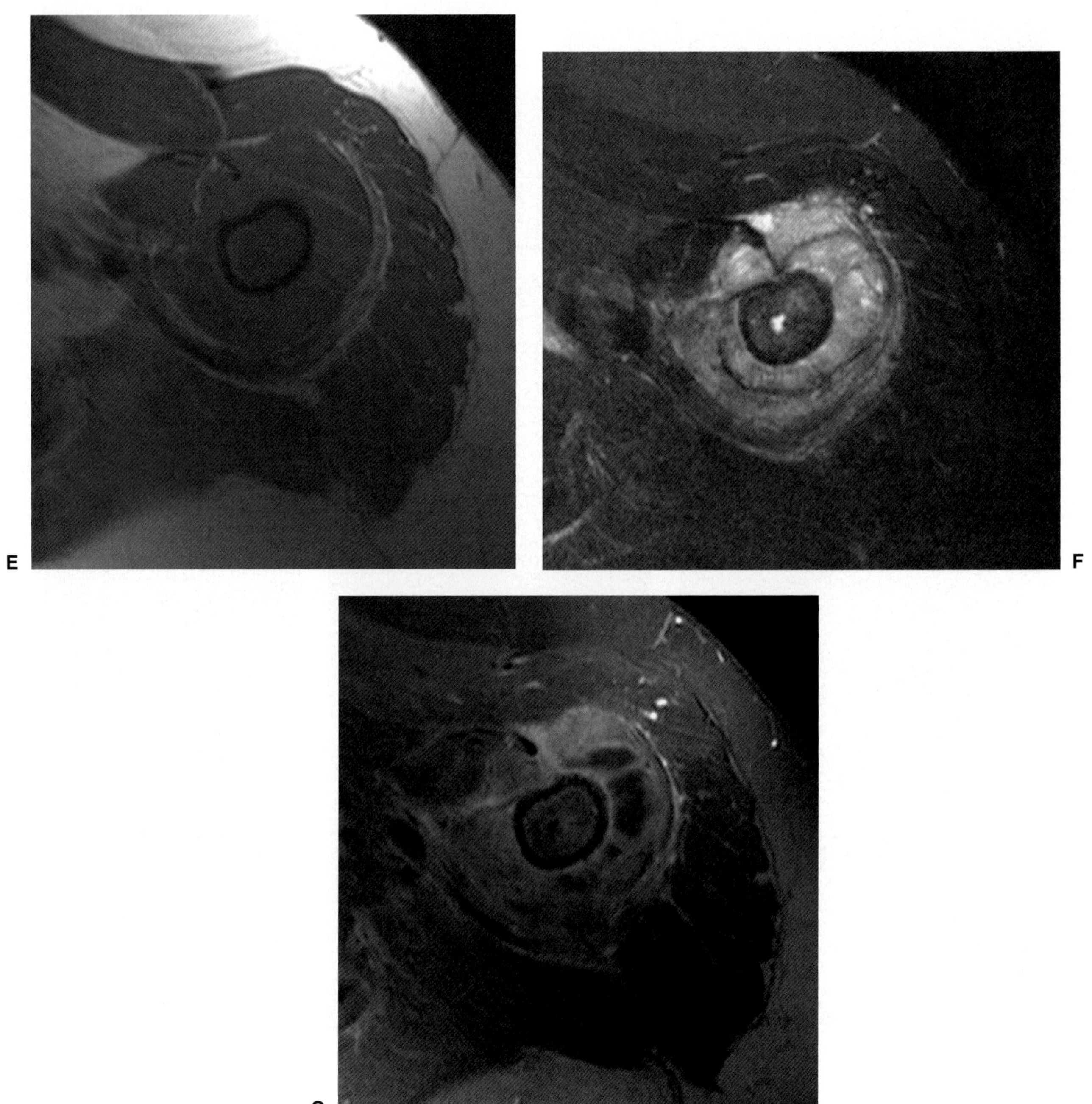


Fig. 14-6 *(Continued)*

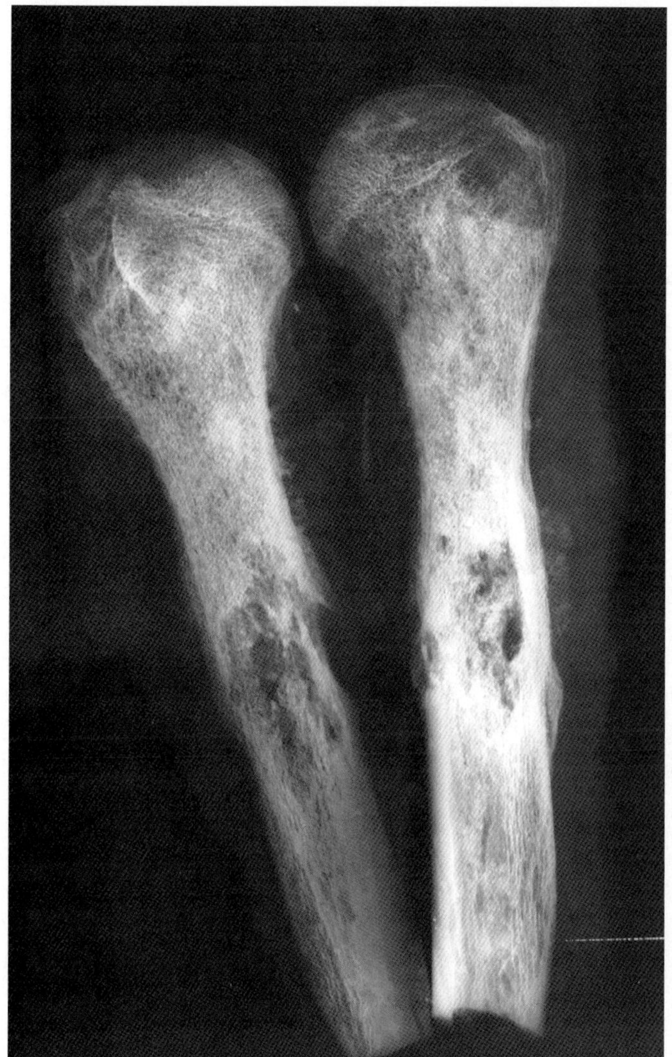
H

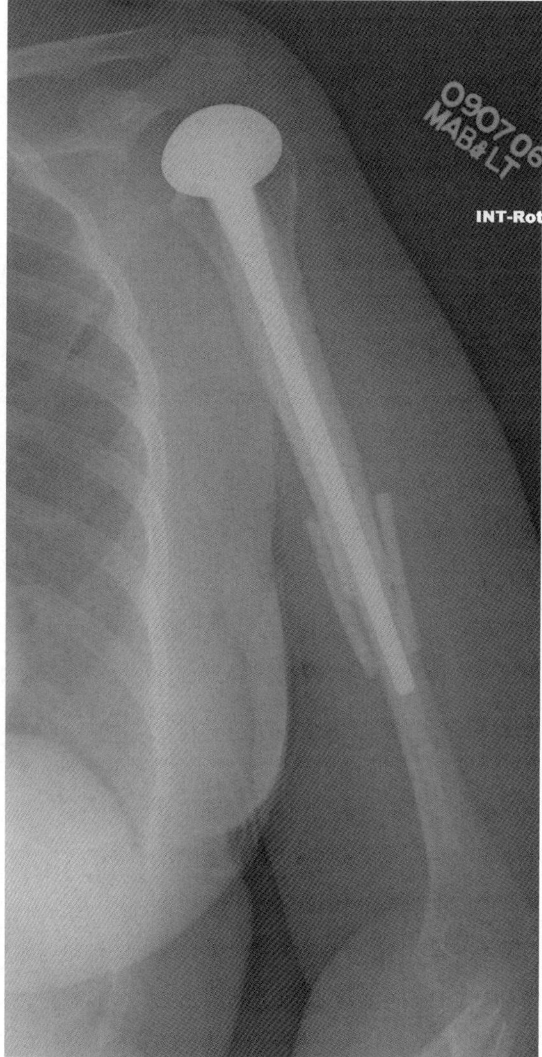

I

Fig. 14-6 *(Continued)*

especially PET/CT, plays an important role in tumor staging (see Fig. 14-11).

## Suggested Reading

Bancroft LW, Peterson JJ, Kransdorf MJ, et al. Compartmental anatomy relevant to biopsy planning. *Semin Musculoskelet Radiol.* 2007;11:16–27.

Enneking WF. Staging of musculoskeletal neoplasms. *Skeletal Radiol.* 1985;13:183–194.

Heck RK, Peabody TD, Simon MA. Staging of primary malignancies of bone. *Cancer J Clin*. 2006;56:366–375.

Liu PT, Valadez SD, Chiver FS, et al. Anatomically based guidelines for core needle biopsy of bone tumors: Implications for limb-sparing surgery. *Radiographics* 2007;27:189–206.

Peabody TD, Gibbs CP, Simon MA. Evaluation and staging of musculoskeletal neoplasms. *J Bone Joint Surg*. 1998;80A: 1204–1218.

Stacy GS, Mahal RS, Peabody TD. Staging of bone tumors: A review with illustrative examples. *AJR Am J Roentgenol.* 2006;186:967–976.

Tateishi U, Yamaguchi U, Seki K, et al. Bone and soft-tissue sarcoma: Preoperative staging with Fluorine 18 Fluorodeoxyglucose PET/CT and conventional imaging. *Radiology* 2007;245:839–855.

# Treatment Options

Limb-saving procedures for bone lesions are indicated in the following circumstances:

- Tumor in the axial skeleton or extremity
- Margins amenable to surgical resection
- Only moderate soft tissue extension
- Neurovascular structures intact
- Metastasis absent or can be resected
- Patient in good general health

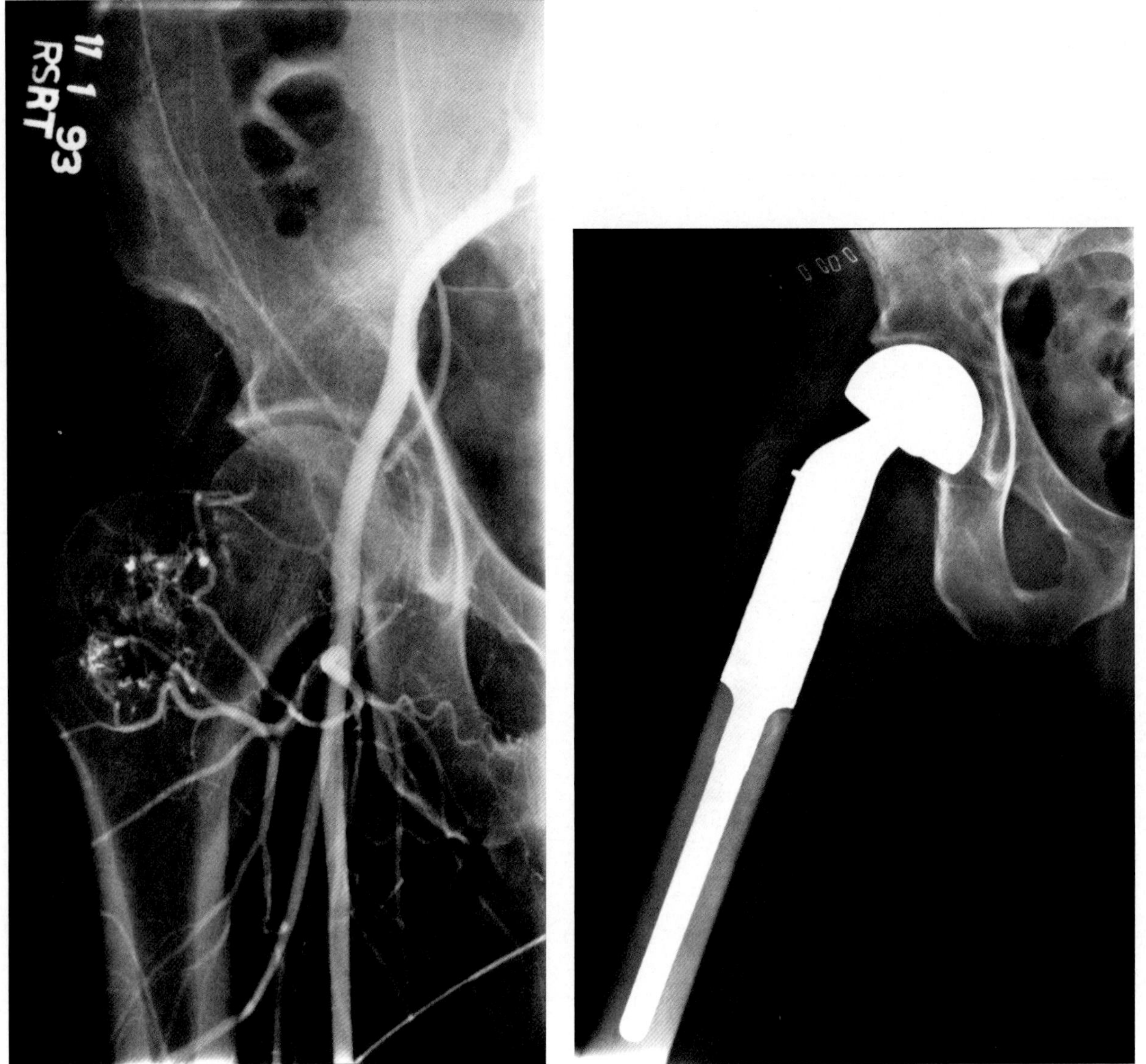


Fig. 14-7 A: Preoperative angiogram demonstrating neovascularity in a malignant tumor in the proximal femur. B: The proximal femur was resected and a custom bipolar prosthesis was inserted.

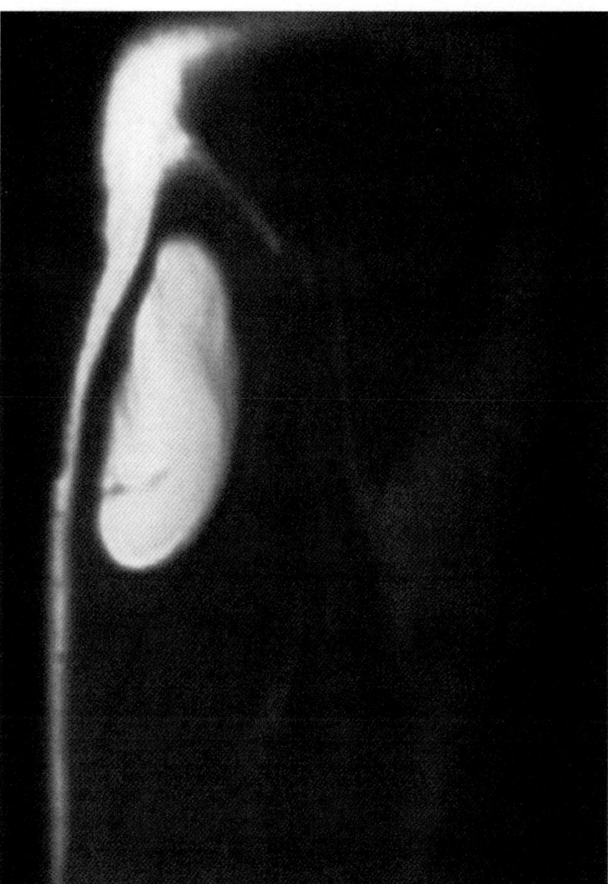

Fig. 14-8 Benign lipoma. Coronal T1-weighted magnetic resonance (MR) image of the proximal arm demonstrating the characteristic appearance of a benign lipoma with a few well-defined fibrous septae.

Contraindications include the following:

- Neurovascular encasement
- Surgery would lead to functional impairment
- Significant pathologic fracture with tumor cell dissemination
- Poorly placed biopsy incisions (relative contraindication)

Treatment options vary with the site, tumor histology, extent of the lesion, and patient comorbidities. In some cases, implants used for fracture treatment or conventional arthroplasty can be used (Fig. 14-10). This section will focus on techniques used for limb-saving procedures.

## Bone Grafts

Bone grafts are used for many situations in orthopaedic practice. Bone graft materials include autografts (cortical or cancellous bone obtained from the patient), allografts (cadaver grafts), and synthetic materials.

Autografts may be cortical, cancellous, or marrow aspirates. Grafts are usually obtained from the iliac crest, fibula, ribs, or adjacent sites in the tibia and radius. Multiple configurations can be used including intact segments, bone morsels, blocks, or paste. Larger segments may be used as vascular or nonvascularized grafts. Autographs are more often used in lesions that are curetted and require smaller amounts of bone replacement. The advantage of autografts is the presence of osteogenic bone-forming cells without autoimmune concerns. Disadvantages include donor site complications and the lack of large segment availability except for fibular grafts.

Allografts are commonly used for limb-saving procedures. Grafts may be intercalary (replaces a segment of long bone), osteoarticular (replaces a bone segment with the joint surface), used as part of an arthrodesis, or as an allograft/prosthesis composite. Allografts provide larger segments compared to autografts for replacement of resected segments of long bone (see Figs. 14-12 and 14-13). These grafts are often used in combination with prostheses and cortical on-lay bone grafts (Fig. 14-6). Allografts do not have the same osteogenic properties as autografts. Therefore, the adjacent fibrous and granulation tissue provides the osteogenesis for incorporation. Considerations regarding allograft usage include cost, host immune response, and inconsistent incorporation or fusion with the native bone. Disease transmission, although possible, is rare due to the processing of allograft segments. Other complications of allografts include infection, fracture, and lack of incorporation.

Synthetic substitutes include demineralized bone matrix, ceramics, and composite materials. Demineralized matrix is obtained by acid extraction of cortical or cancellous bone resulting in a mixture of noncollagenous proteins, bone growth factors, and collagen. This substance causes osteoinduction to stimulate bone healing. This material is not readily visible on radiographs and does not provide the rigidity of other graft materials or methacrylate.

Ceramic materials such as calcium sulfate, tricalcium phosphate, hydroxyapatite in various combinations produce a framework for osteogenesis, but lack osteogenesis properties. This synthetic substitute is radiopaque and visible on radiographs.

Composite materials include both demineralized matrix and ceramic elements providing a matrix and osteoinductive properties. Demineralized matrix can be combined with cancellous allograft providing similar properties (see Fig. 14-14).

Methyl methacrylate can also be used as a bone substitute following curettage of focal, typically benign lesions (see Fig. 14-15). It is also used with orthopaedic implants for diaphyseal lesions. This substance provides immediate stability when placed in the marrow defect created by tumor removal.

## Suggested Reading

Beaman FD, Bancroft LW, Peterson JJ, et al. Imaging characteristics of bone graft materials. *Radiographics* 2006;26: 373–388.

Delloye C, Banse X, Brichard B, et al. Pelvic reconstruction with a structural pelvic allograft after resection of a malignant bone tumor. *J Bone Joint Surg*. 2007;89A:579–587.

Ortiz-Cruz E, Gebhardt MC, Jennings C, et al. The results of transplantation of intercalary allografts after resection of tumors. *J Bone Joint Surg*. 1997;79A:97–106.

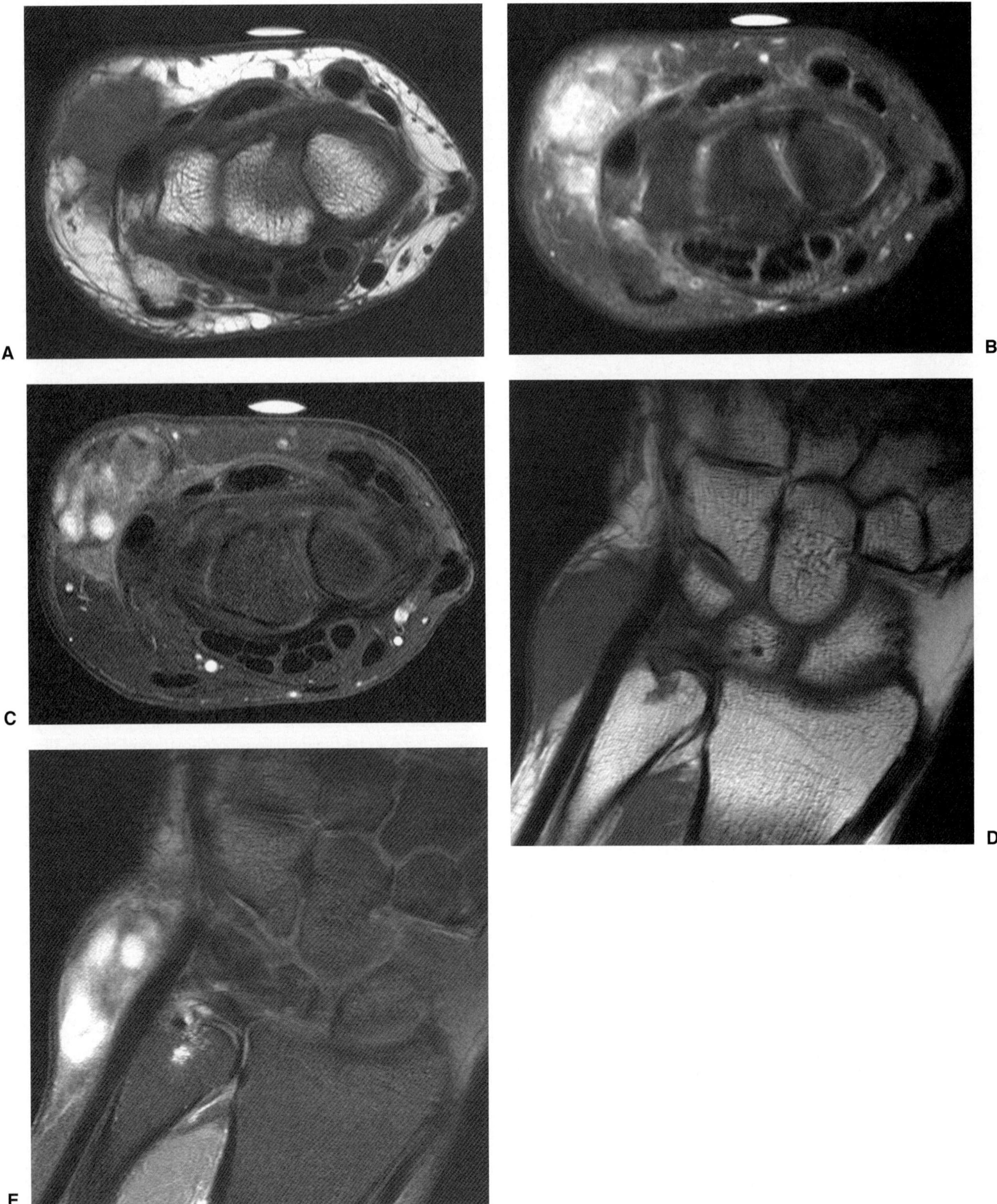


Fig. 14-9 Spindle cell sarcoma. Axial T1-weighted (A), T2-weighted (B), and postcontrast (C) fat-suppressed T-weighted images and coronal T1- (D) and postcontrast fat-suppressed T1-weighted (E) images demonstrate the lesion with irregular enhancement.

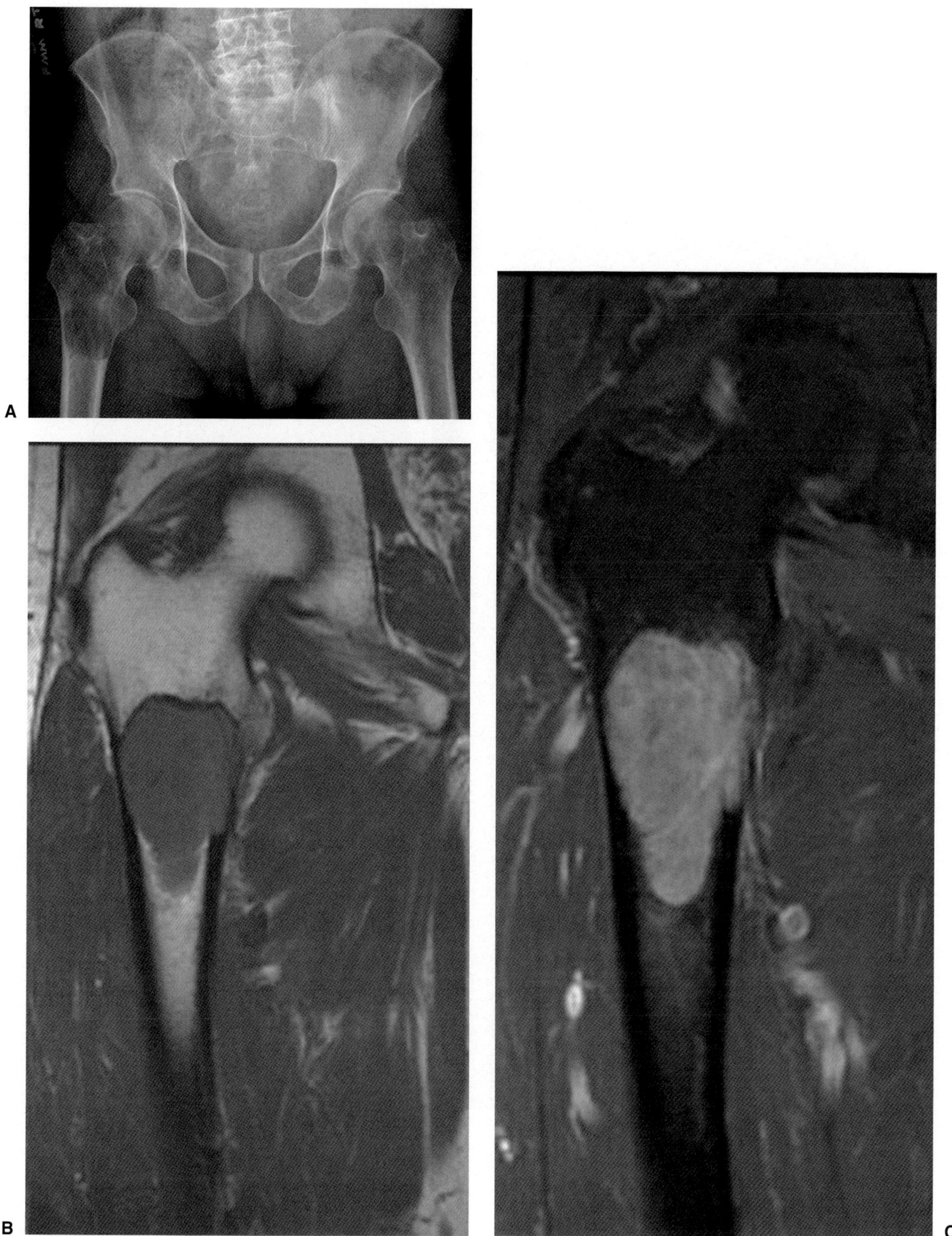


Fig. 14-10 Plasmacytoma of the proximal femur. **A:** Radiograph demonstrates a lytic destructive lesion in the proximal diaphysis with marked cortical thinning placing the femur at risk for pathologic fracture. Coronal T1- (**B**) and contrast-enhanced fat-suppressed T1-weighted images (**C**) clearly demonstrate the lesion. **D:** Technetium Tc 99m methylene-diphosphonate (MDP) bone scan shows a small photopenic area in the region of the tumor. The patient was treated with a static intramedullary nail (**E** and **F**).

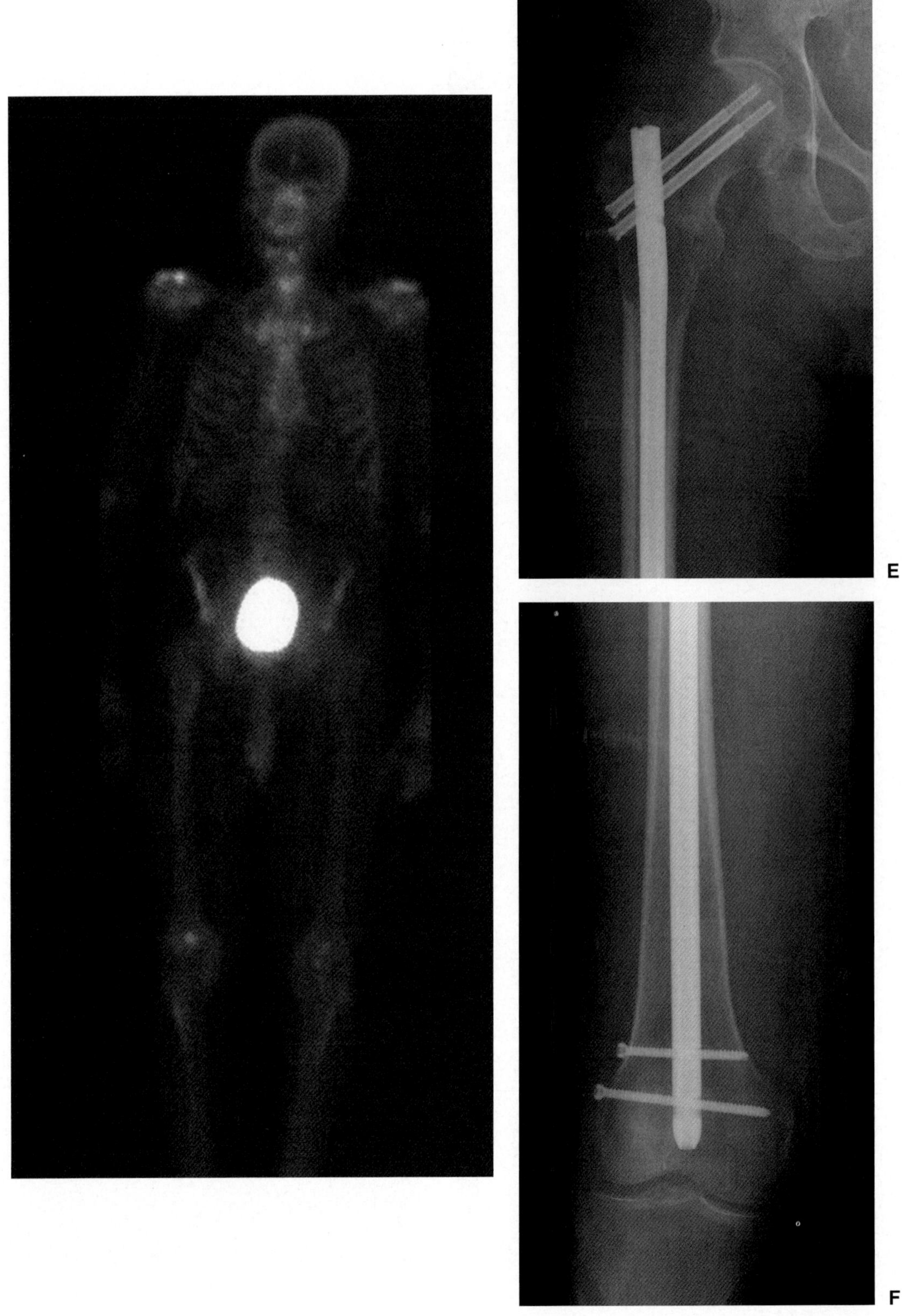


Fig. 14-10 *(Continued)*

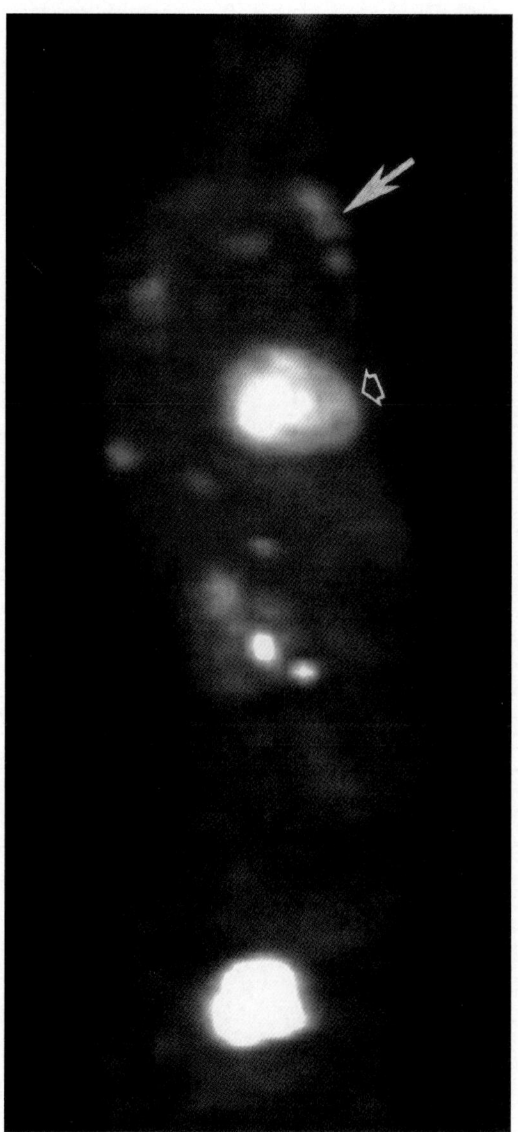

Fig. 14-11 Sternal metastasis. Sagittal positron emission tomographic (PET) image demonstrating sternal metastasis (*arrow*). Note the usual cardiac uptake (*open arrow*).

Patel SR, Miller PR, Gross M, et al. Massive bone allografts for limb salvage. *AJR Am J Roentgenol.* 1997;168:543–546.

Stevenson S, Qing Z, Davy DT, et al. Critical biological determinants of incorporation of non-vascularized cortical bone grafts. *J Bone Joint Surg.* 1997;79A:1–16.

### Custom Prostheses and Spacers

Many bone tumors involve the metaphysis and epiphysis. Therefore, joint prostheses or customized joint prostheses are commonly considered for limb-saving procedures (Fig. 14-7). Allograft-prosthesis composites may also be used (see Fig. 14-16).

In the upper femur and hip, lesions are approached based on tumor extent, patient age, level of activity, and prognosis. In certain cases, such as pathologic fractures, intramedullary nailing may be used alone (see Fig. 14-17). Prosthetic-allograft replacement is often used in the proximal femur (Fig. 14-16). Lesions involving the acetabulum may be treated with saddle prosthesis (see Fig. 14-18) or pelvic allograft reconstruction. Treatment is difficult due to the high complication rate. However, recent studies with allograft reconstruction have provided good results, especially in young patients. Complete femoral replacement is not commonly performed and is usually reserved for failure of more conventional components, major bone loss, or infection (see Fig. 14-19).

Neoplasm in the distal femur and proximal tibia can be managed with a number of custom prostheses (see Fig. 14-20). Hinged and rotating hinged components are commonly used (see Figs. 14-21 and 14-22). Component survivals of 72% at 5 years and 64% at 7 years have been reported. More constrained implants tend to have a higher incidence of loosening. Infection is also more common with custom or revision systems.

Shoulder and humeral reconstructions for limb-saving procedures may require resection of the scapular and upper humerus (see Fig. 14-23). Tumors of the proximal humerus are often treated with hemiarthroplasty (see Fig. 14-24). Resection and allograft are also options (see Fig. 14-25). Diaphyseal lesions may be treated with graft material (see Fig. 14-26) or custom spacers (see Fig. 14-27).

Spine procedures for neoplasms are most commonly performed for local solitary lesions or metastasis resulting in vertebral destruction and neural compromise or instability. The goals of spinal instrumentation are to reduce pain, improve stability, and decompress neural structures. The same systems described in Chapter 3 are used for tumor procedures. Short segment devices with either corpectomy and cages or bone graft and anterior or anterior and posterior instrumentation are employed. The exact instrumentation used depends on the spinal level or levels involved, patient status, and comorbidities and surgical preferences (see Figs. 14-28 to 14-30).

## Postoperative Imaging and Complications

Complications (minor and major) have been reported in 30% to 90% of patients for limb-saving procedures compared to 41% for amputation. Imaging following limb-saving procedures or other stabilization or reconstructive procedures is essential to evaluate fixation, graft incorporation, and detect recurrence or metastatic disease. Complications vary with the location (upper extremity, lower extremity, pelvis, or spine), type and extent of procedure, and the implants or grafts utilized. Most structural changes can be detected with serial radiographs. Baseline magnetic resonance (MR) studies with static or dynamic gadolinium are useful to better evaluate tumor recurrence at a

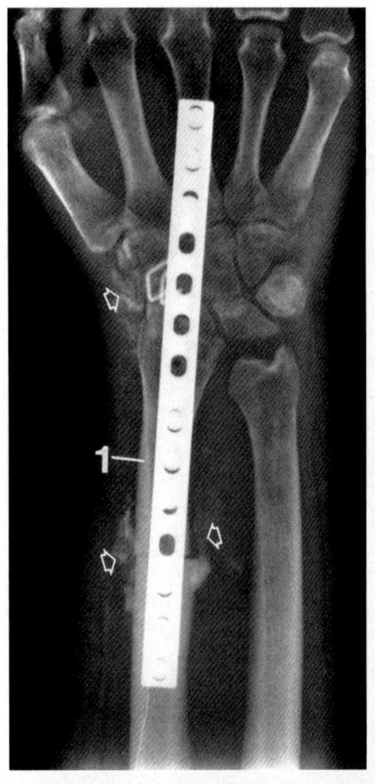


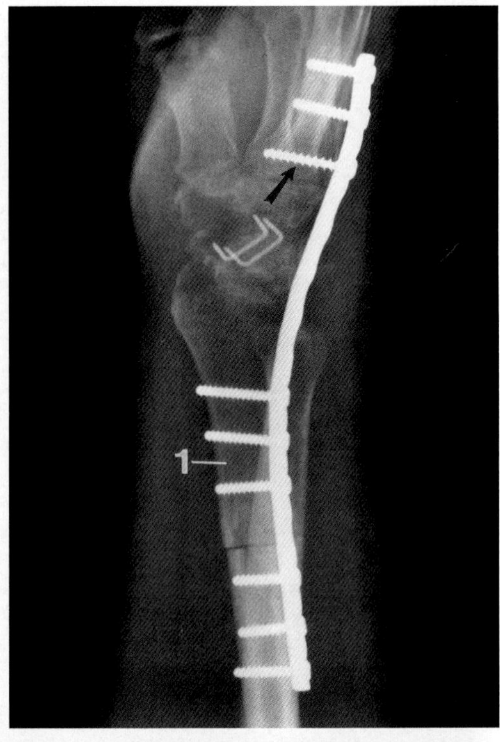


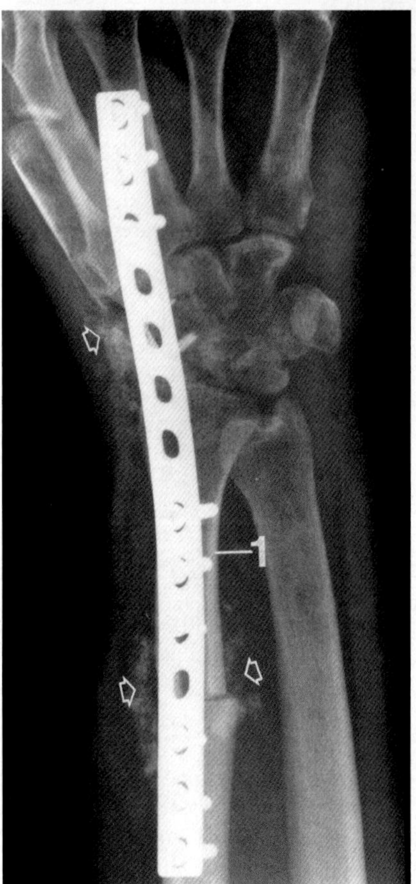


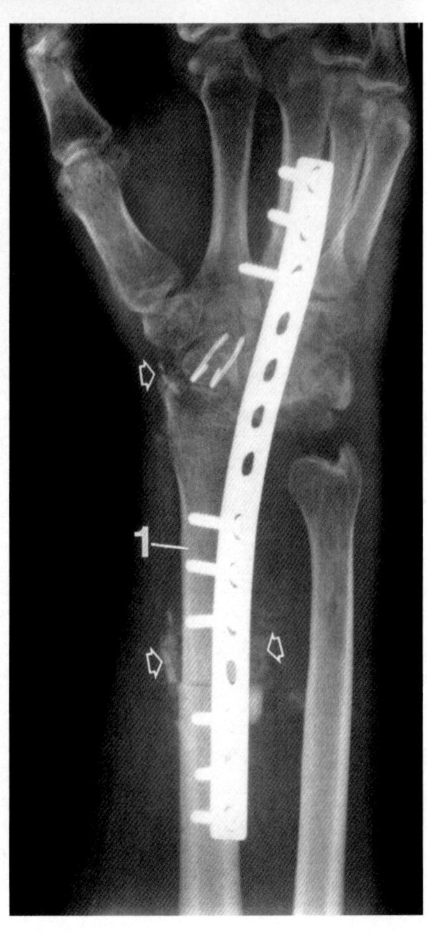


**Fig. 14-12** Allograft for treatment of an aggressive giant cell tumor of the distal radius. Posteroanterior (PA) (**A**), lateral (**B**), and oblique (**C** and **D**) radiographs of the distal forearm demonstrate resection of the distal radius with fibular allograft (*1*) fused to the radial remnant and metacarpals with a 14-hole dynamic compression plate with cortical screws. Note one cancellous screw (*arrow*) distally. Two staples fuse the distal allograft to the carpal bones. There is morcelized bone graft (*open arrows*) at the allograft-radius and allograft-carpal junctions to facilitate union.

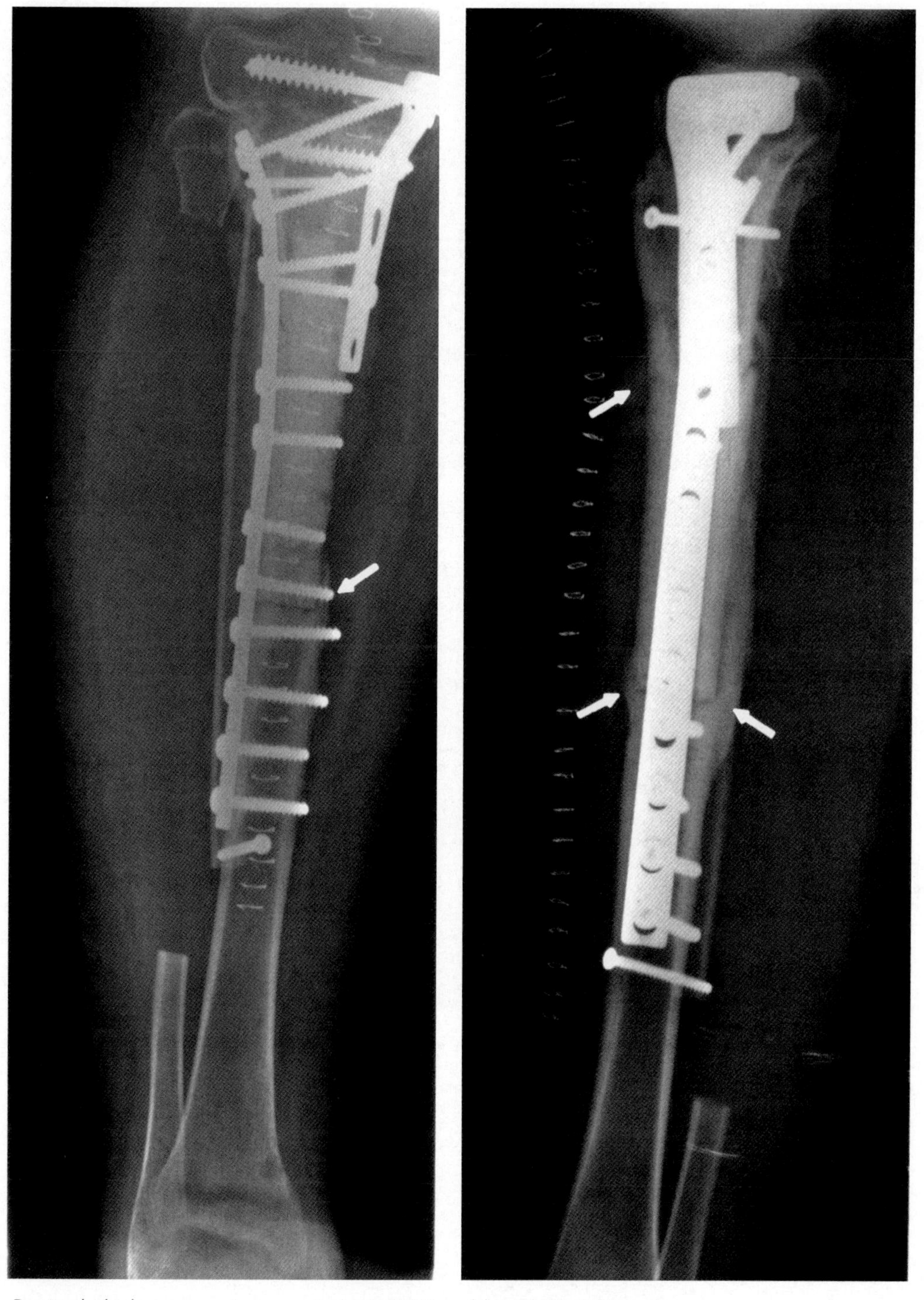


Fig. 14-13 Proximal tibial sarcoma. Anteroposterior (AP) (A) and lateral (B) radiographs following resection of a proximal tibia segment with allograft positioned and fixed with double plates and screws. A fibular autograft has also been fused to the native proximal and distal tibia with proximal and distal fixation screws. The allograft is incorporating proximally and distally (*arrows*).

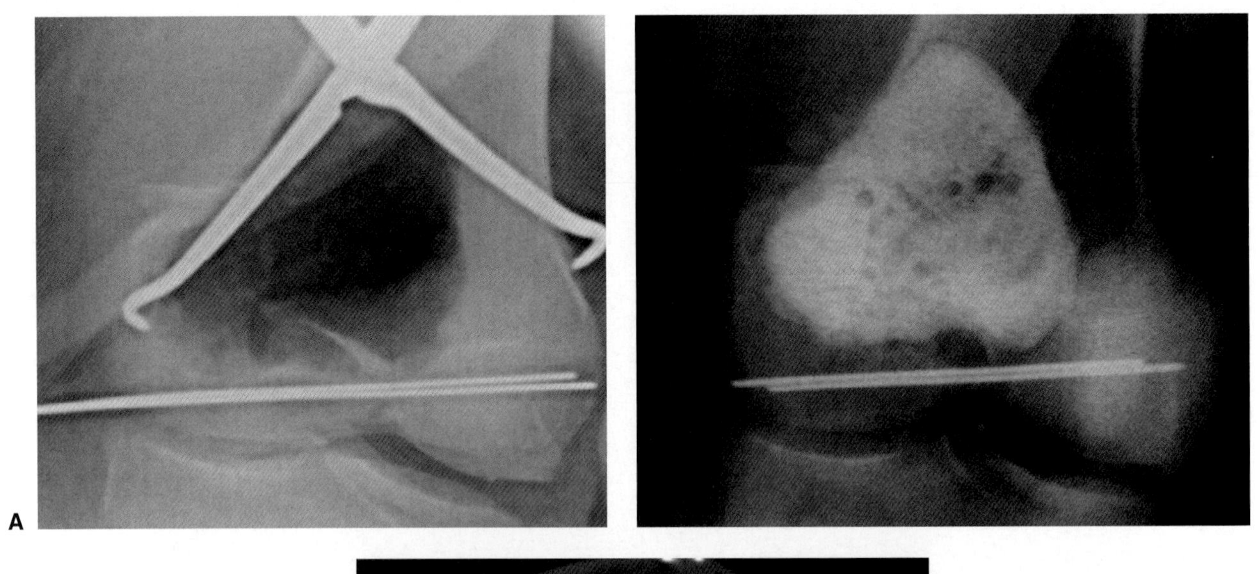


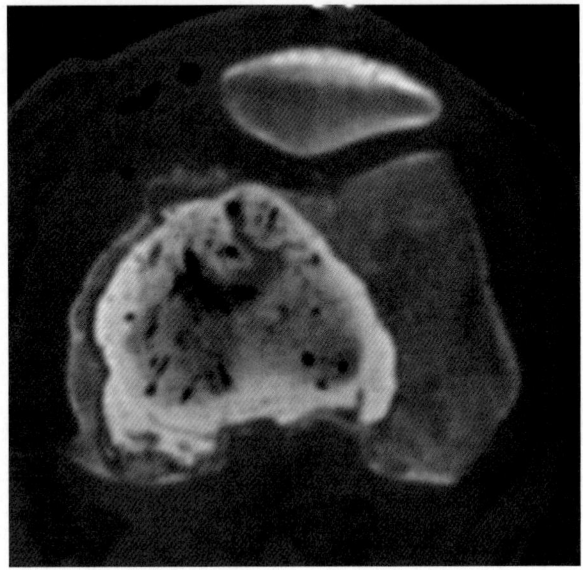


**Fig. 14-14** Giant cell tumor of the distal femur. **A:** Operative image following curettage with an intra-articular defect treated with K-wires. The area was packed with a composite of cancellous allograft and demineralized matrix demonstrated on radiograph (**B**) and computed tomography (CT) (**C**).

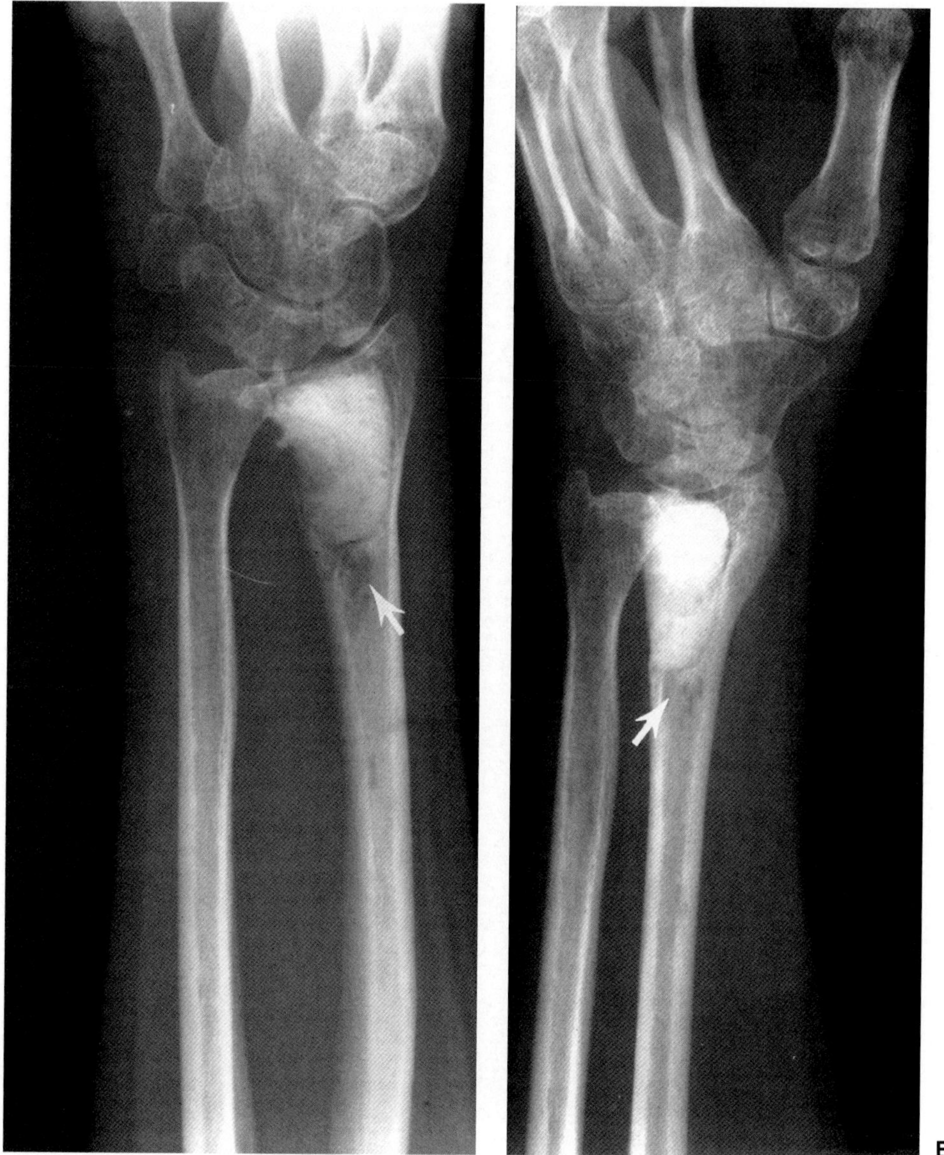


Fig. 14-15 Giant cell tumor of the distal radius. Posteroanterior (PA) (A) and oblique (B) radiographs following curettage and methyl methacrylate packing. There is irregular permeative change (*arrow*) proximal to the lesion indicating recurrence. PA (C) and lateral (D) radiographs following distal radial resection with fibular allograft with eight-hole compression plate for fixation. The distal allograft is fixed to the ulna with a K-wire.

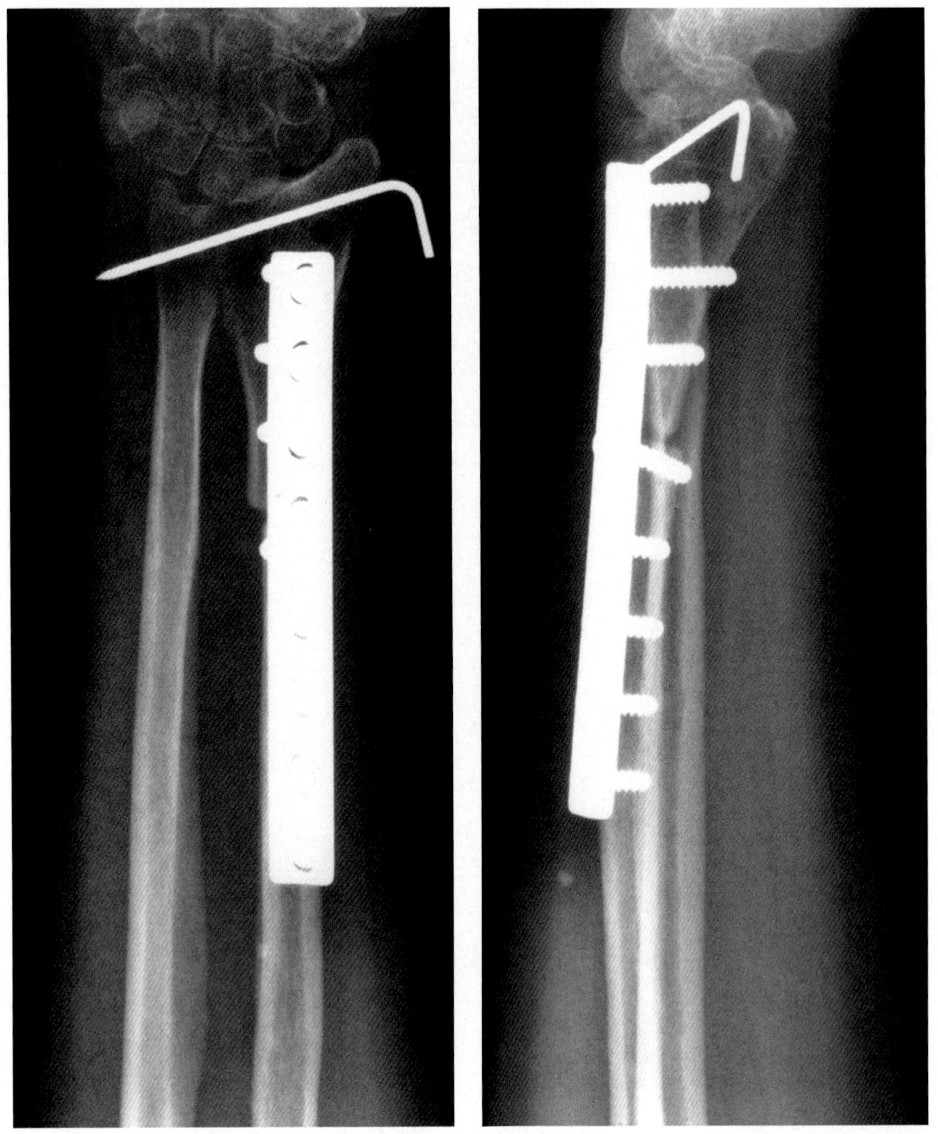


Fig. 14-15 *(Continued)*

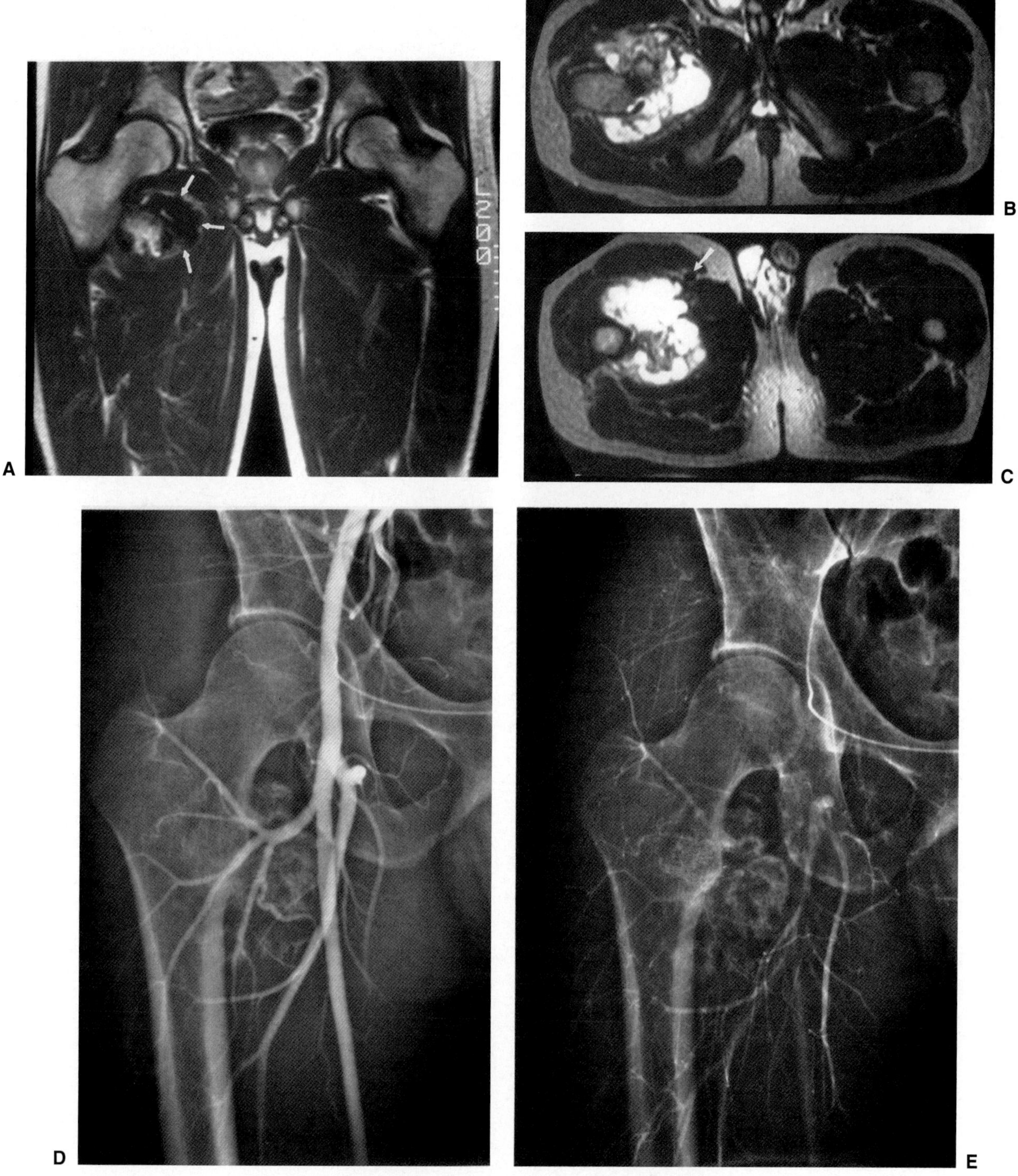

**Fig. 14-16** Chondrosarcoma with soft tissue extension. Coronal T1-(**A**) and axial T2-weighted (**B** and **C**) magnetic resonance (MR) images demonstrate a degenerated osteochondroma with medial extension which appears to displace (*arrow* in **C**) the vascular structures. Angiograms during the early (**D**) and late (**E**) phases demonstrate a normal superficial femoral artery that was easily separated from the tumor at surgery. The medial and posterior branches were encased. The profunda was displaced but not encased. **F–H:** The tumor was resected with clear margins and treated with a proximal femoral allograft (*white arrows*), bipolar implant with long femoral stem, with cortical autograft placed at the junction of the allograft, and native femur fixed with Dall-Miles cables (*distal black arrow*). There is also a Dall-Miles cable-claw system (*upper black arrow*) proximally.

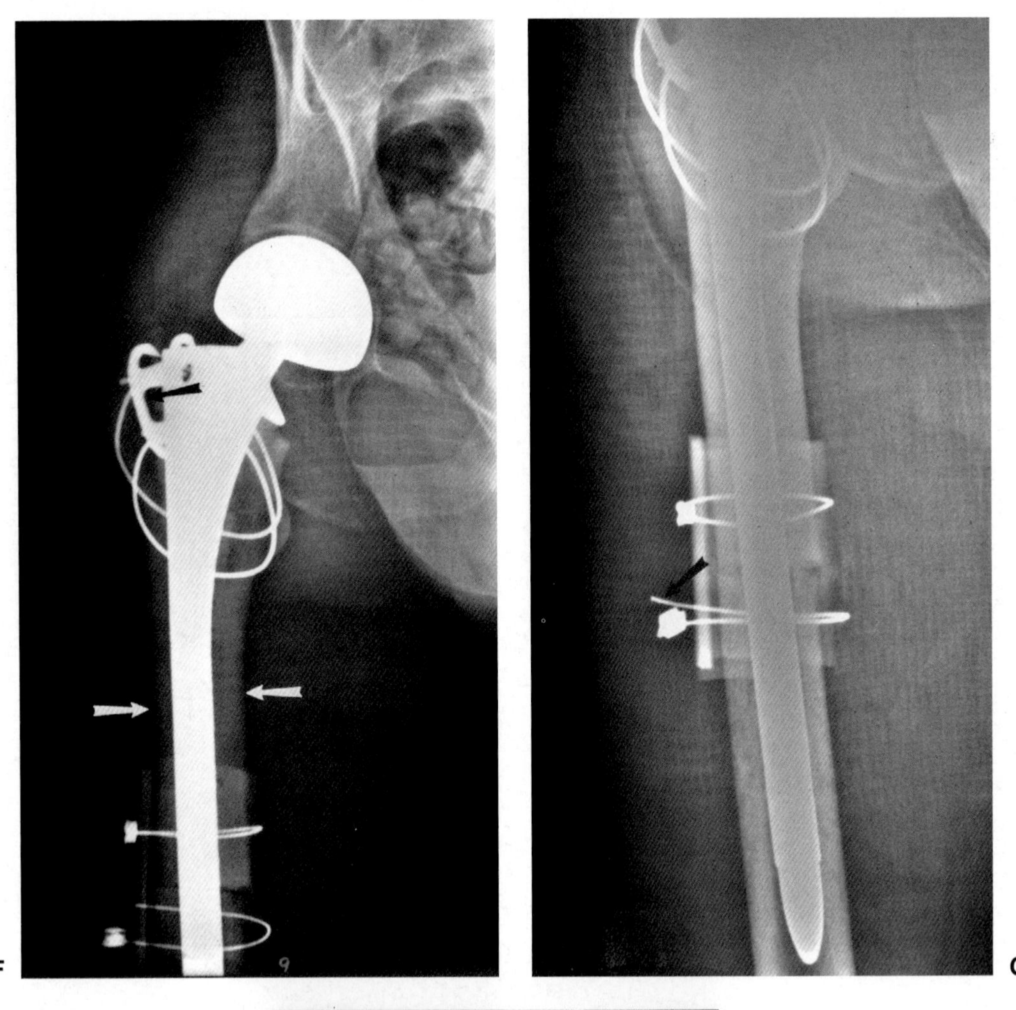


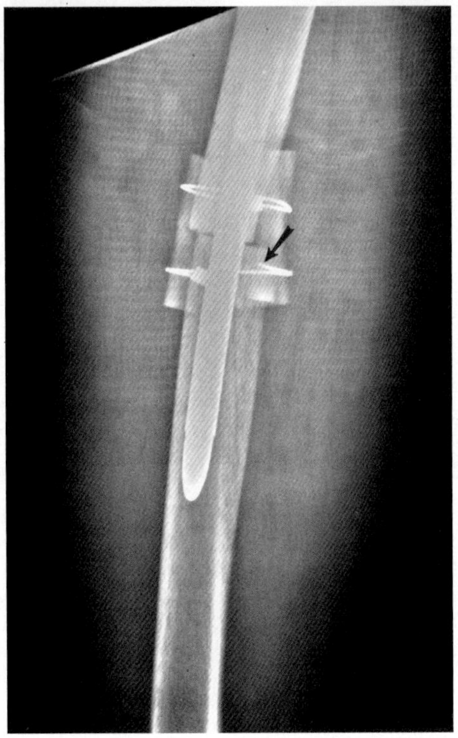


Fig. 14-16 (*Continued*)

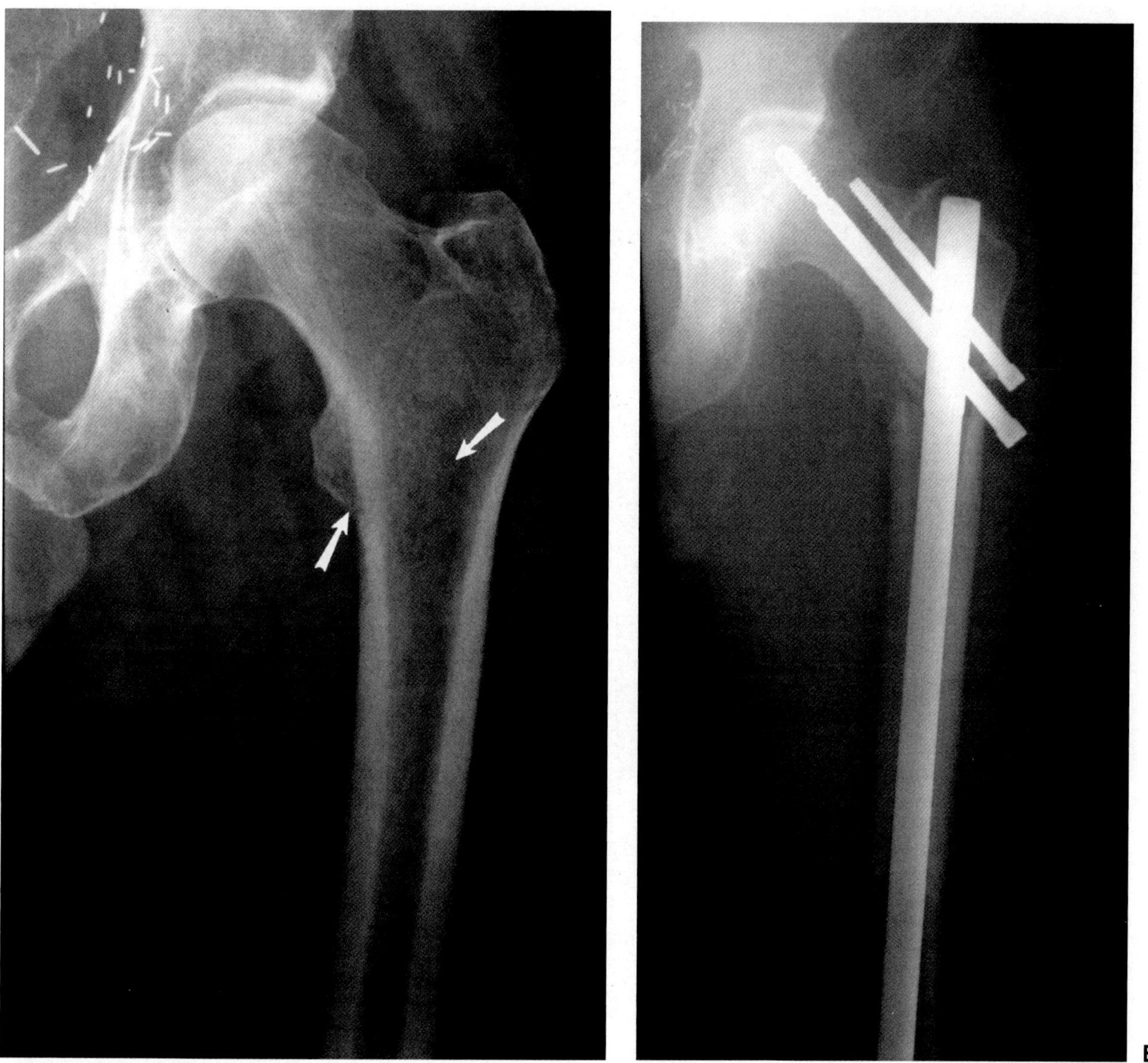


Fig. 14-17 Metastasis to the lesser trochanteric region with pathologic fracture. Initial radiograph (A) demonstrates a permeative lesion in the lesser trochanter and proximal femur (*arrows*). B: Radiograph following pathologic fracture with intramedullary nail for fixation.

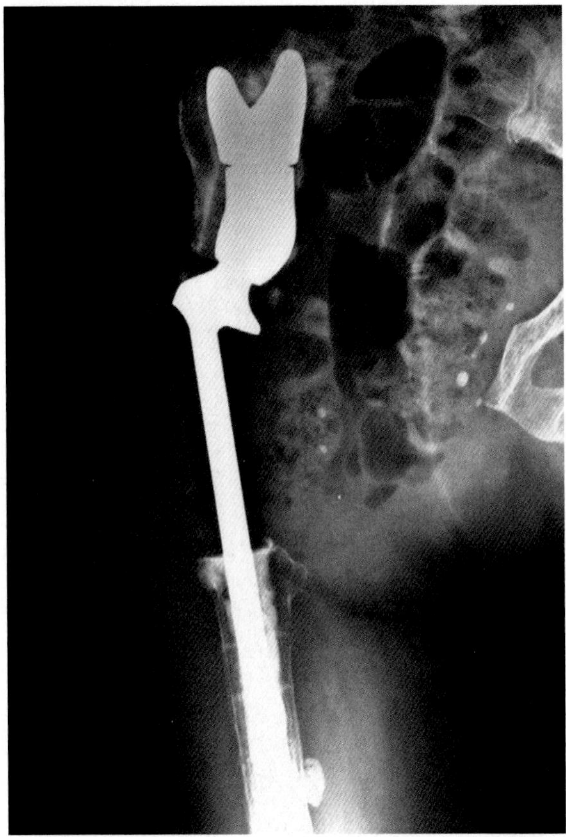

Fig. 14-18 Saddle prosthesis. Resection of the proximal femur, pubic bones, ischium, and acetabulum with a saddle prosthesis and long-stem femoral component.

later date. Spectroscopy can also be used at 1.5 or 3 T, although this is still not a commonly used clinical tool.

## Tumor Recurrence

Recurrence following limb-saving procedures has decreased over the years due to adjuvant therapy, improved patient selection, and the ability to achieve tumor-free margins. Adjuvant chemotherapy tends to create a pseudocapsule around the lesion enhancing the chances for successful wide excision. Recurrence rates for high-grade osteosarcoma are <10% in most series. Higher recurrence rates have been noted with pelvic reconstruction (29%). Radiographs are useful and important for comparison with other modalities, specifically MRI. Bone, soft tissue, and hardware abnormalities may be visible and lead to the next best imaging study to clarify the problem (Figs. 14-15 and 14-21). Regardless of the symptoms, recurrence is always an important consideration during postoperative imaging. MRI or CT may be the best choice, although PET imaging can also be useful for detection of local recurrence or distant metastasis.

When using MRI for follow-up, it is best to obtain a baseline study 4 to 6 weeks after surgery or when the patient can tolerate the procedure. This study serves as a baseline for future comparison and detection of subtle recurrence is more easily accomplished. The subsequent studies should use the same imaging parameters. Typically, T1- and T2-weighted sequences are used with conventional or dynamic gadolinium enhancement techniques. The latter may assist with determining recurrent malignancy from other processes. Spectroscopy may be useful in some settings, but this has not become a commonly used tool clinically.

Image degradation can be a problem with MRI and CT depending on the surgical technique and hardware or prostheses used (see Fig. 14-31). Metal artifact on MR images is common with orthopaedic fixation devices, most of which contain some degree of ferromagnetic material which results in variable degrees of susceptibility artifact depending on the size and configuration of the implants. Pure titanium is not ferromagnetic and causes less image distortion. Multiple approaches to artifact reduction on MR images have been described.

**MR artifact reduction techniques**

Increase frequency-encoding gradient
Aligning frequency encoding along the device
Increase pixels in frequency-encoding direction
Increasing the bandwidth
Use fast spin-echo or fast STIR
Use T1 with gadolinium
Avoid gradient-echo techniques

There are also artifact reduction techniques for CT. Multidetector row CT with advanced hardware and software changes have increased the utility of CT in evaluating patients with orthopaedic implants (Fig. 14-31C and D). Titanium has lower beam attenuation coefficients compared to stainless steel. Therefore, similar to MRI, there is less artifact with titanium devices. Artifact can also be reduced by modifying milliampere-seconds, kilovolt peak, and reconstruction algorithms. Multichannel detectors collect redundant data, which also reduces metal artifact.

# Suggested Reading

Delloye C, Banse X, Brichard B, et al. Pelvic reconstruction with a structural pelvic allograft after resection of a malignant bone tumor. *J Bone Joint Surg.* 2007;89A:579–587.

Douglas-Akinwande AC, Buchwalter KA, Rydberg J, et al. Multichannel CT: Evaluating the spine in postoperative patients with orthopaedic hardware. *Radiographics* 2006;26:S97–S110.

Fayad LM, Barker PB, Jacobs MA, et al. Characterization of musculoskeletal lesions with 3-T proton MR spectroscopy. *AJR Am J Roentgenol.* 2007;188:1513–1520.

Ohashi K, El-Khoury GY, Bennett DL, et al. Orthopaedic hardware complications diagnosed with multi-detector row CT. *Radiology* 2005;237:570–577.

Peh WCG, Chan JHM. Artifacts in musculoskeletal magnetic resonance imaging: identification and correction. *Skeletal Radiol.* 2001;30:179–191.

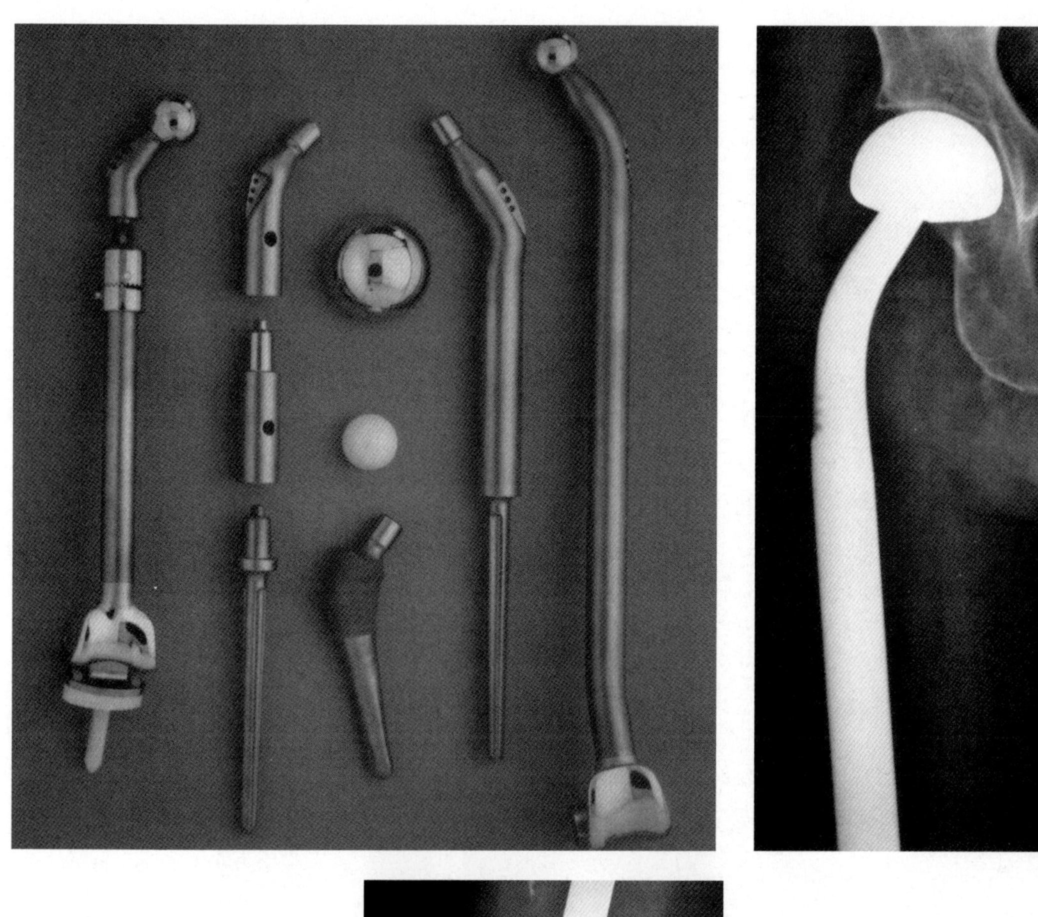

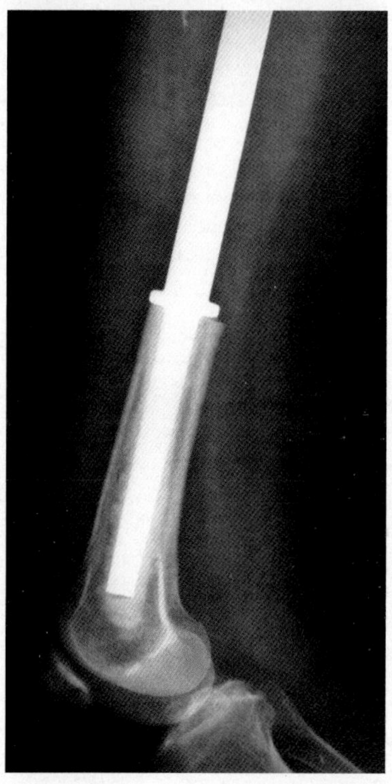

Fig. 14-19 A: Hip and femur custom prostheses. Left—total femoral component with expandable upper shaft and knee articulation, center—modular femoral components, and right—total femoral component. (Courtesy of Wright Medical Technology, Arlington Tennessee.) Radiographs (B and C) of a 70-year-old woman with femoral chondrosarcoma following resection of the proximal two thirds of the femur with custom bipolar prosthesis. The patient was well and using a cane for walking support 11 years later.

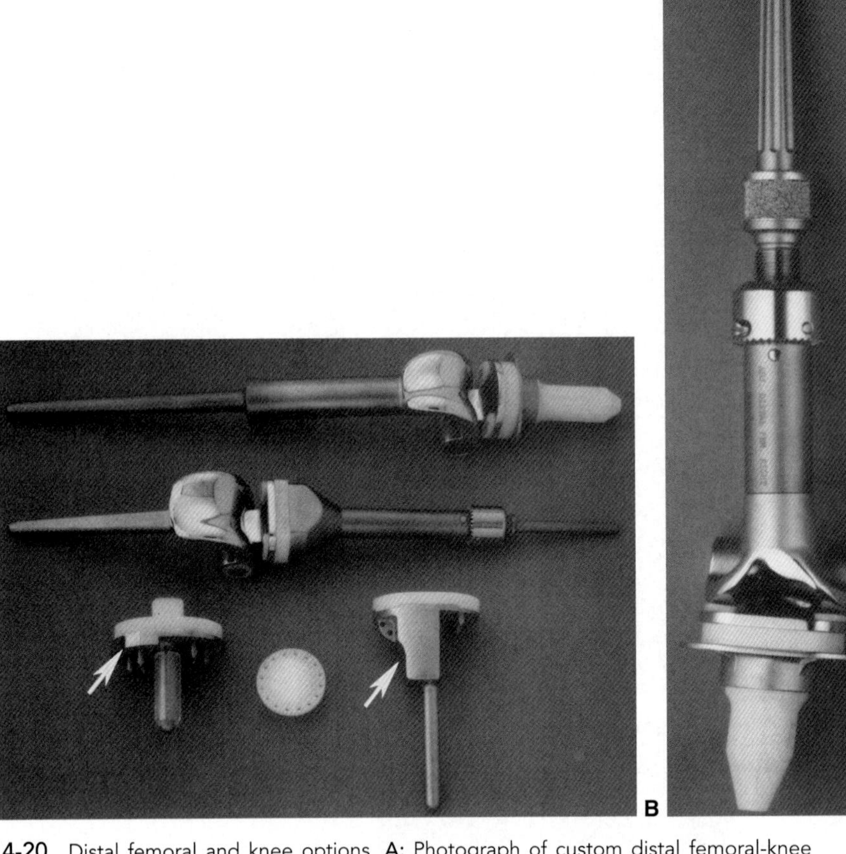

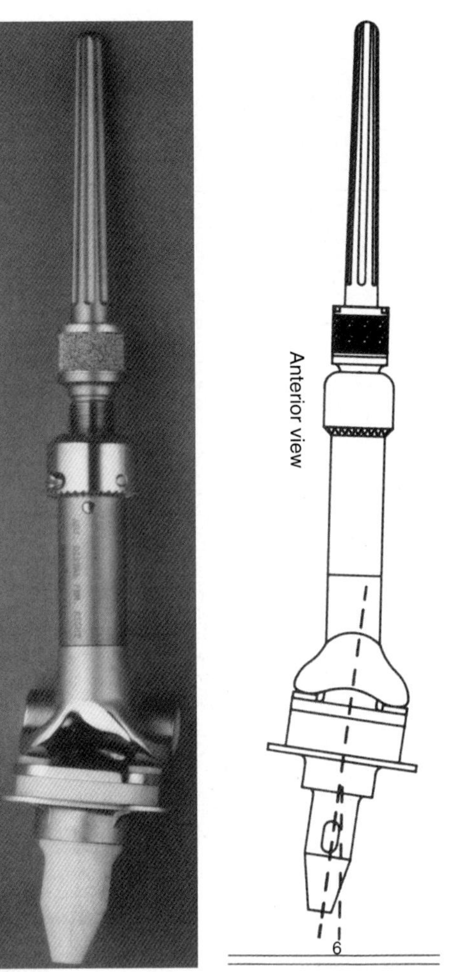


Fig. 14-20 Distal femoral and knee options. A: Photograph of custom distal femoral-knee components. Top—long-stemmed femoral component, center—long-stemmed expandable tibial design, bottom—revision knee systems for tibial bone loss augmentation (*arrows*) and polyethylene patellar component. B: Custom-designed distal femoral component with expansion capability and illustration (C) showing the normal valgus angle of the knee. (Courtesy of Wright Medical Technology, Arlington, Tennessee.)

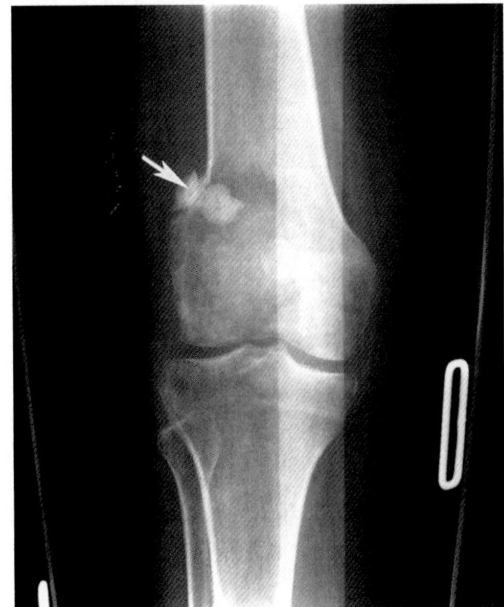

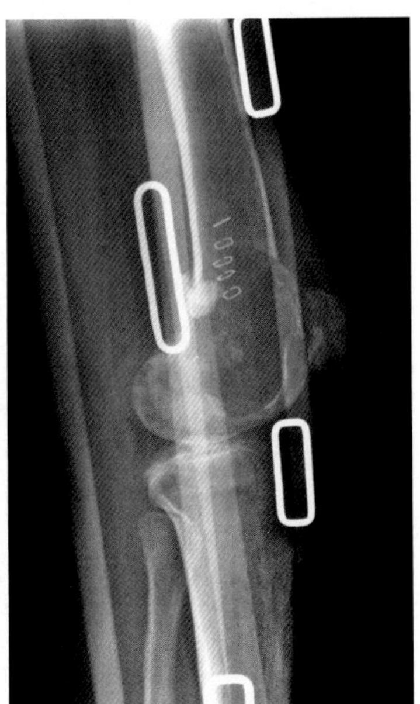

Fig. 14-21 Giant cell tumor of the distal femur. Anteroposterior (AP) (A) and lateral (B) radiographs demonstrate a lytic destructive lesion in the distal femur with a pathologic fracture and methyl methacrylate plug in the biopsy site (*arrow*). The lesion was packed with methyl methacrylate (C and D). E and F: The distal femur was resected and a custom rotating hinge prosthesis placed with supplemental iliac bone graft at the femur-component interface (*arrows*).

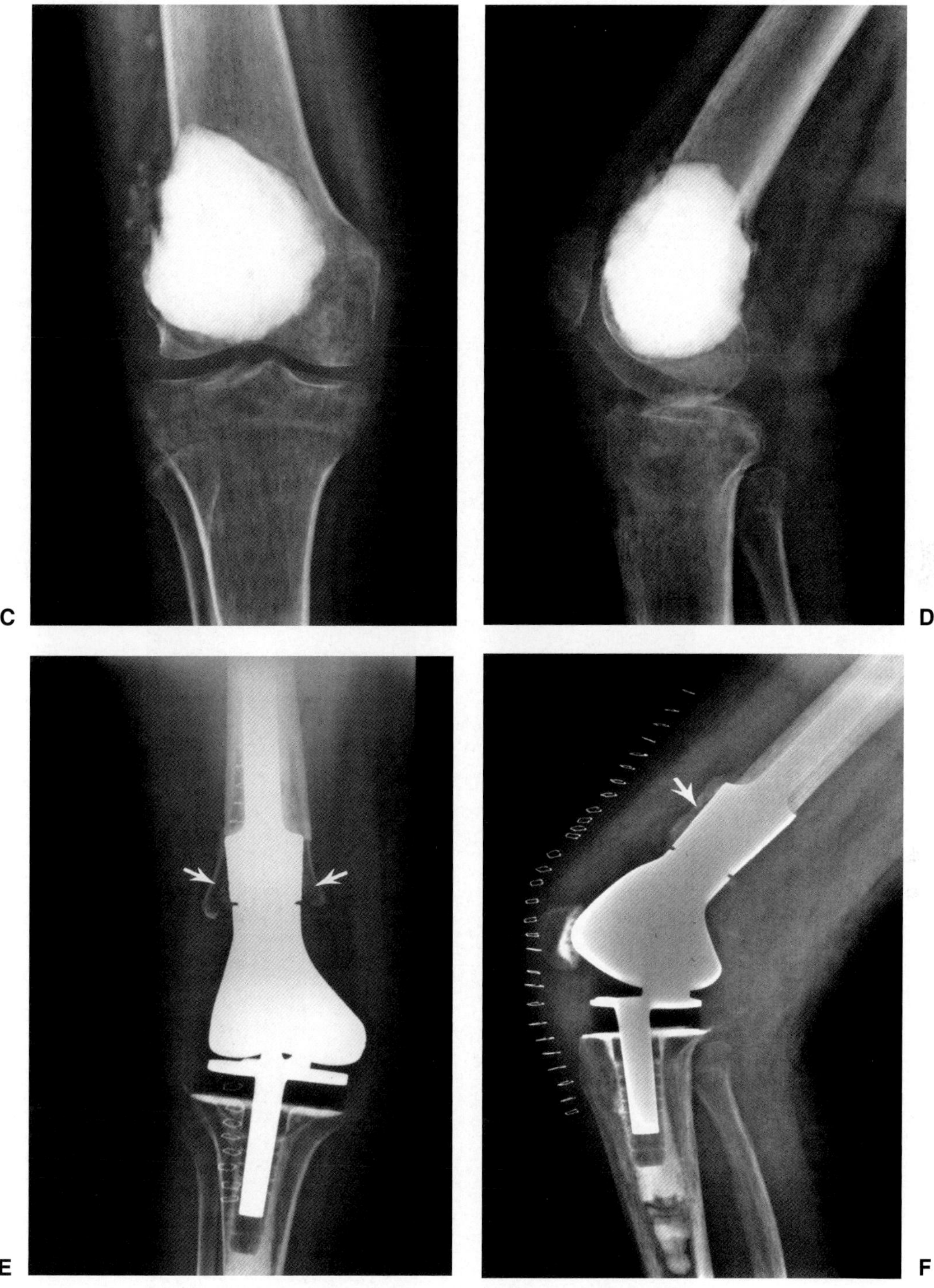


Fig. 14-21 (*Continued*)

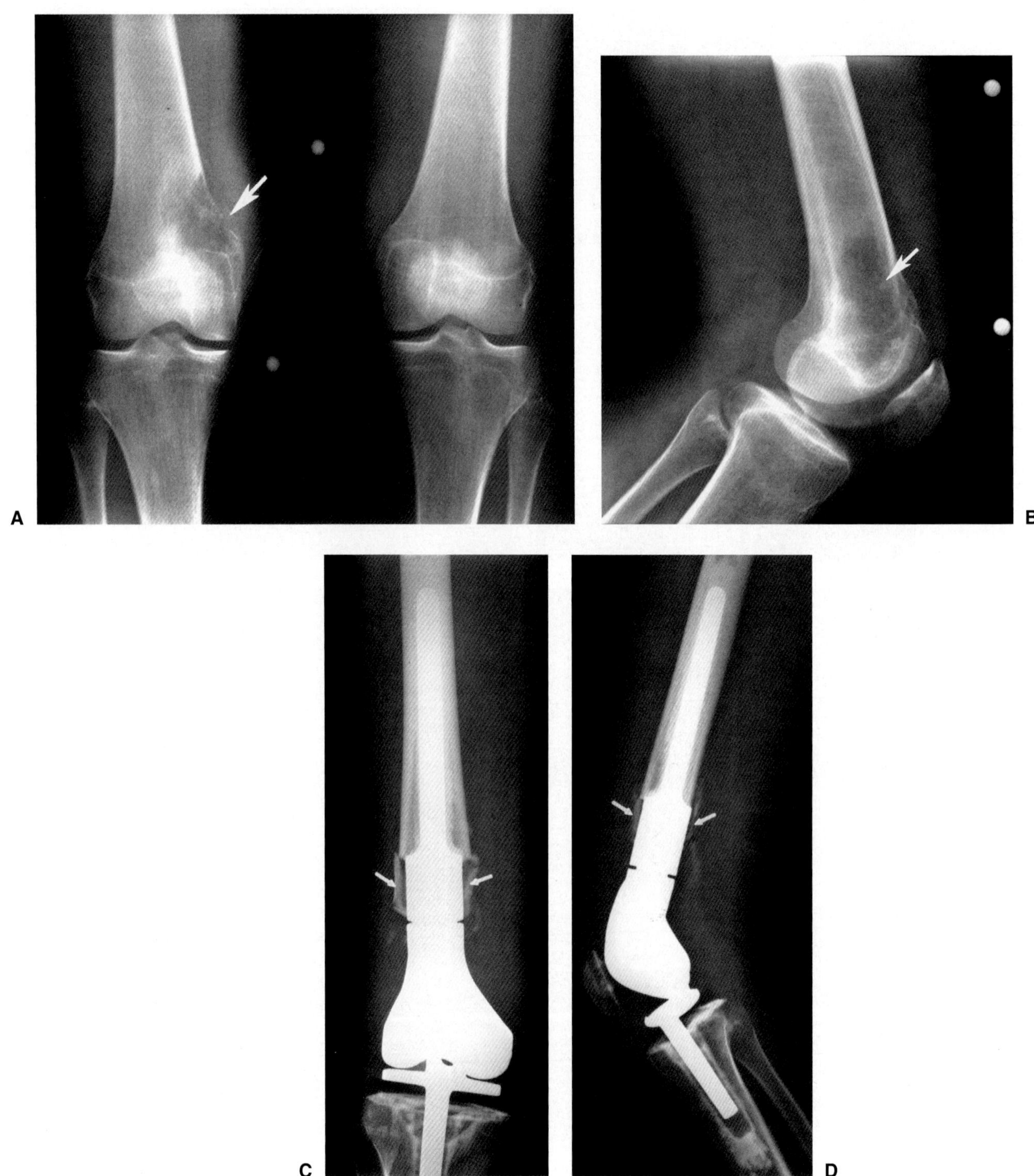


Fig. 14-22 Sixteen-year-old male with an osteosarcoma of the distal femur. Anteroposterior (AP) (A) and lateral (B) radiographs demonstrate a lytic destructive lesion with pathologic fracture and soft tissue mass (*arrow*). Following wide excision with tumor free margins, a kinematic rotating hinge prosthesis was positioned (C and D) with supplemental iliac autograft (*arrows*).

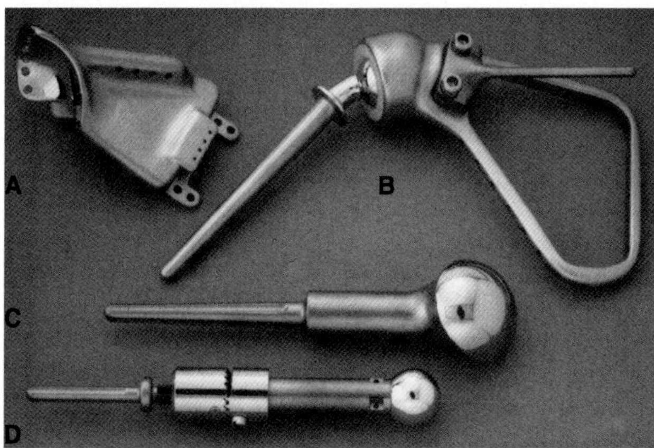


Fig. 14-23 Customized scapular (*A*), total shoulder with endoprosthesis (*B*), conventional (*C*) and expandable endoprosthesis (*D*). (Courtesy of Wright Medical Technology, Arlington, Tennessee.)

Picc P, Sangiorgi L, Bahamonde L, et al. Risk factors for local recurrences after limb-salvage surgery for high-grade osteosarcoma of the extremities. *Ann Oncol.* 1997;8: 899–903.

Vanel D, Shapeero LG, Tardivon A, et al. Dynamic contrast-enhanced MRI with subtraction of aggressive soft tissue tumors after resection. *Skeletal Radiol.* 1998;27:505–510.

## Graft/Hardware and Miscellaneous Complications

Complications related to bone grafts include nonunion or failure to incorporate, delayed union, graft resorption, and infection. As noted in the preceding text, complications may also be related to the type of graft. Autograft harvesting increases operative time and may cause more blood loss, wound infection, chronic pain, or sensory deficit related to the surgical site. Allograft may result in disease transmission or autoimmune response.

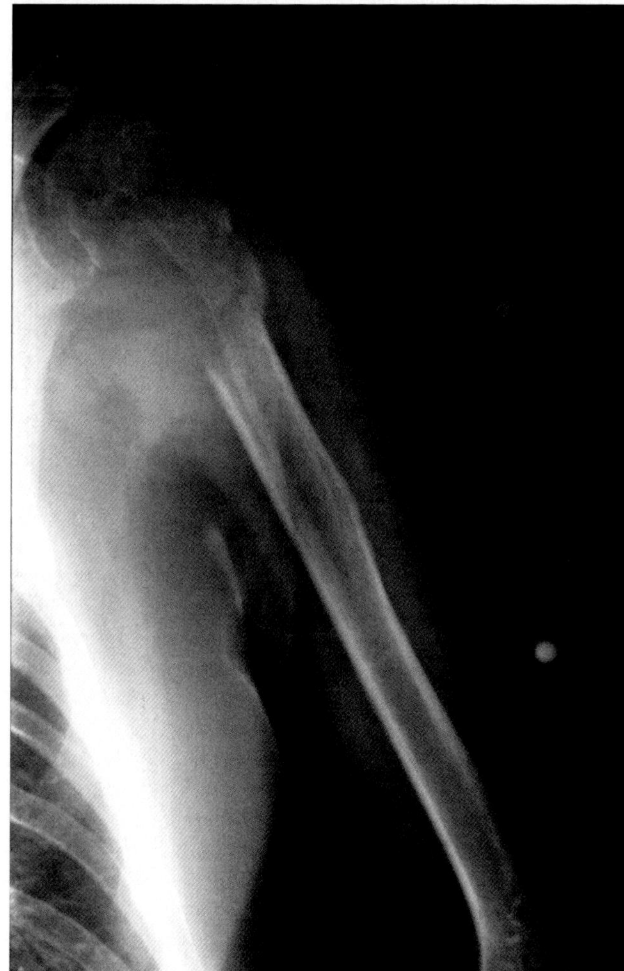


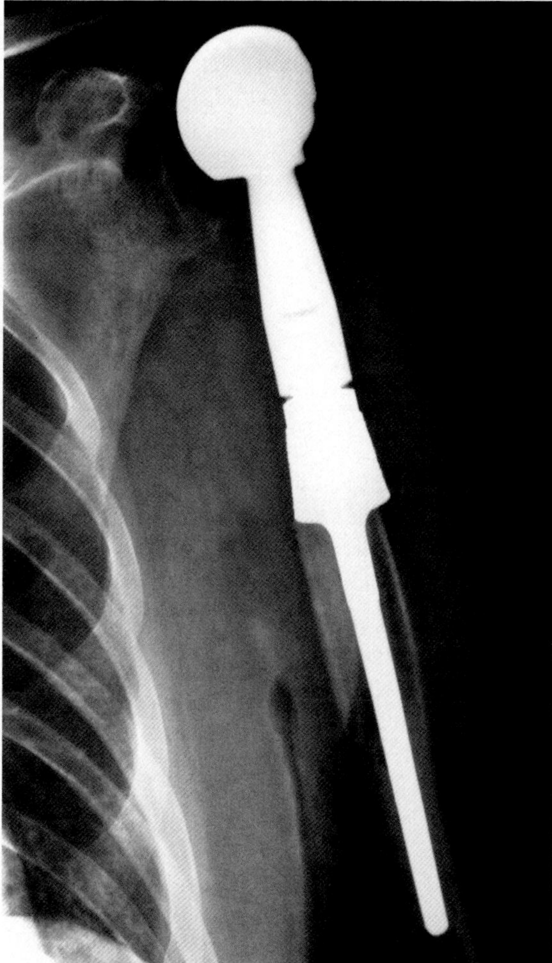


Fig. 14-24 A: Pathologic fracture of the proximal humerus due to metastasis. B: Radiograph following resection of the proximal humerus with a Howmedica custom endoprosthesis.

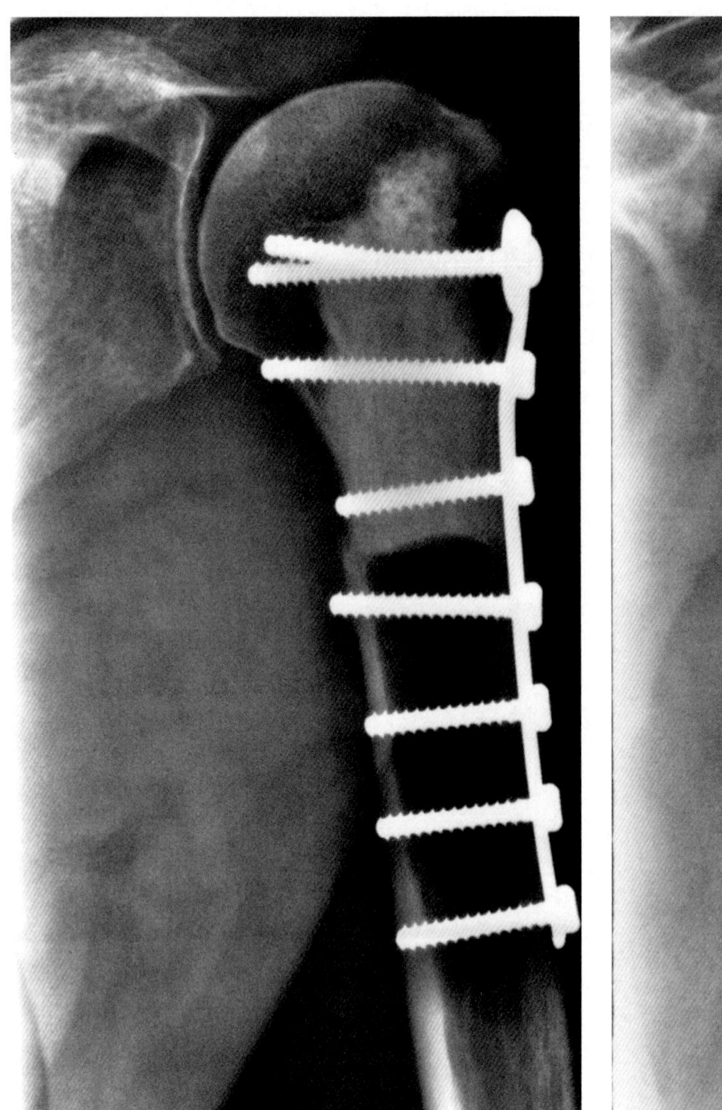


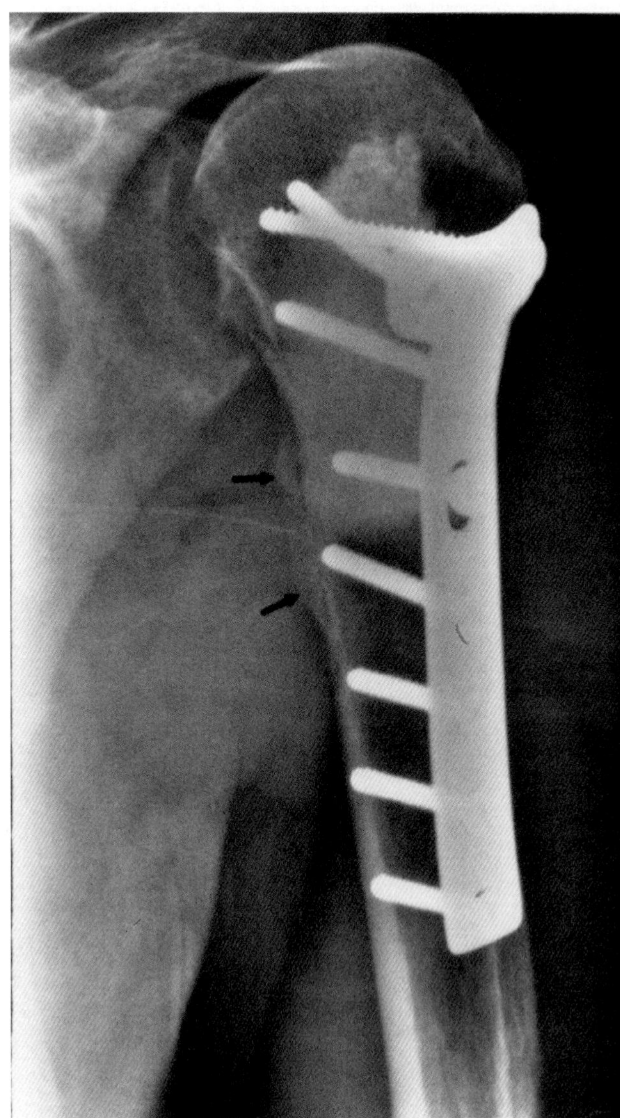


Fig. 14-25 Proximal humeral allograft. Radiographs (A and B) following placement of a proximal humeral allograft with methyl methacrylate and plate and screw fixation. The graft is incorporating (*arrows*).

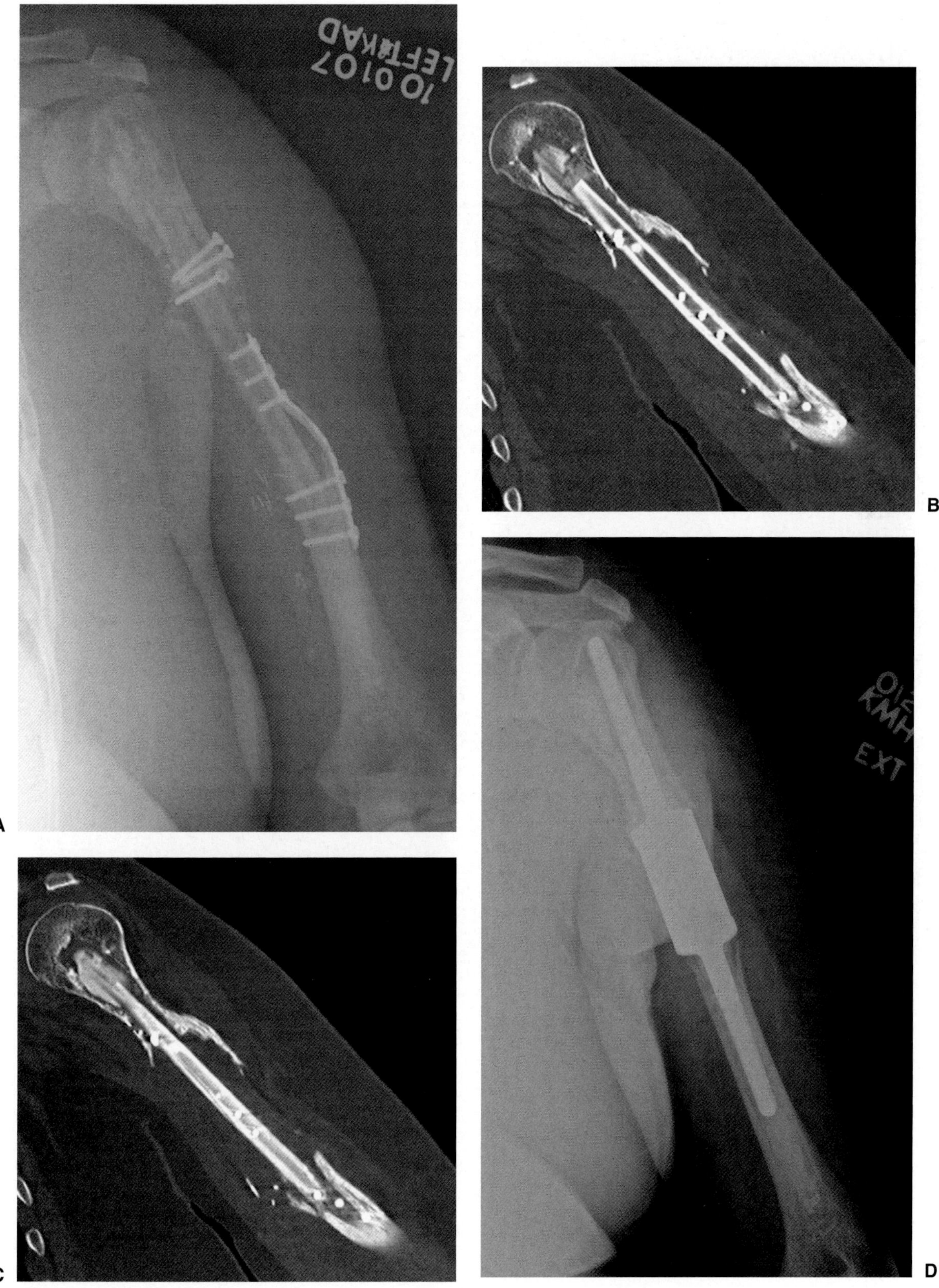


Fig. 14-26 Myeloma with pathologic fracture treated with resection and fibular graft. A: Radiograph demonstrating a fibular spacer with screw fixation proximally and plate and screw fixation distally. Computed tomographic (CT) images in the coronal plane (B and C) demonstrate graft failure and loosening proximally and distally. D: The graft was removed and replaced with a custom spacer.

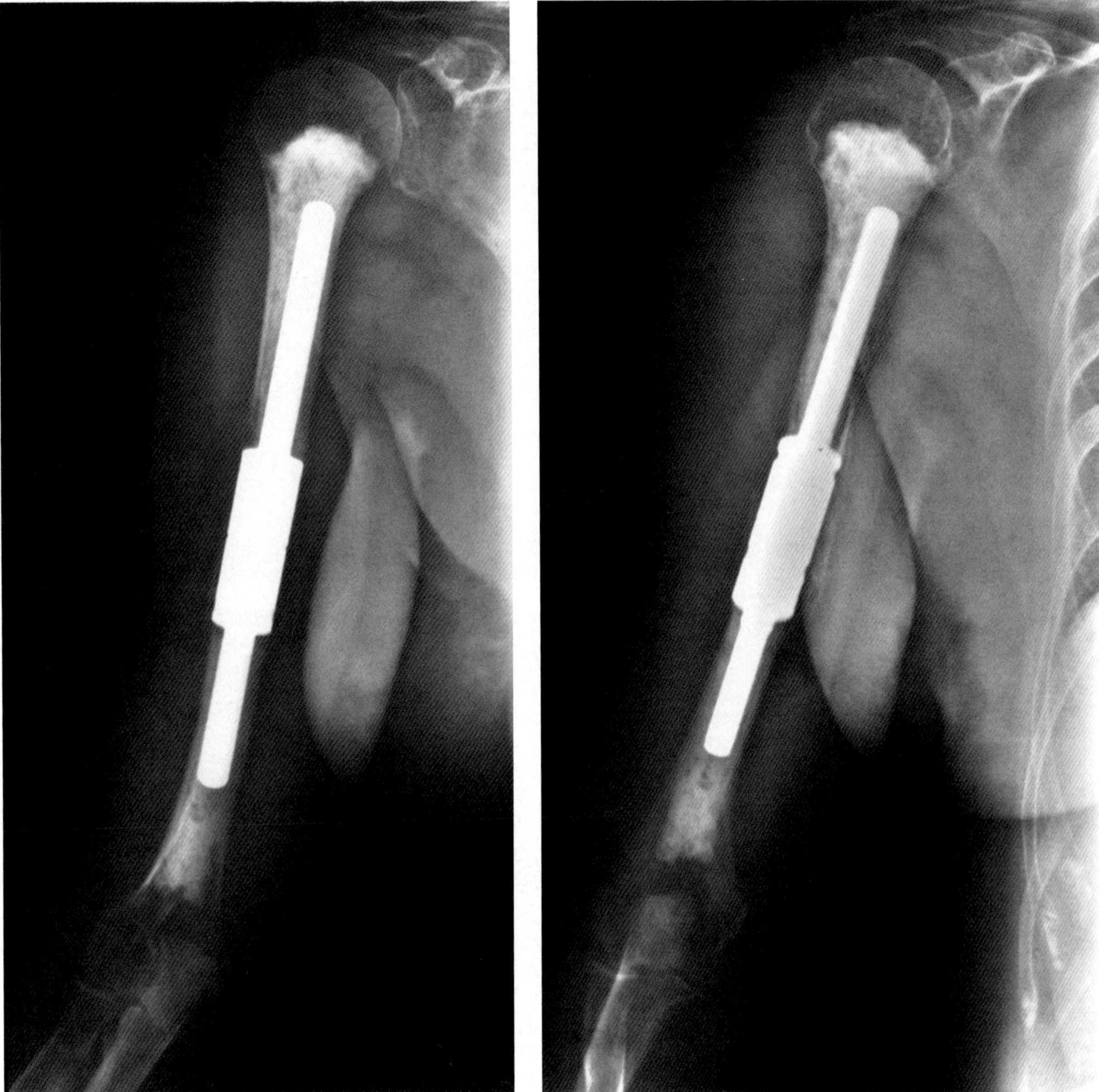


Fig. 14-27 Mid shaft humeral fracture due to plasmacytoma. Radiographs (A and B) demonstrate treatment with a cemented mid humeral spacer.

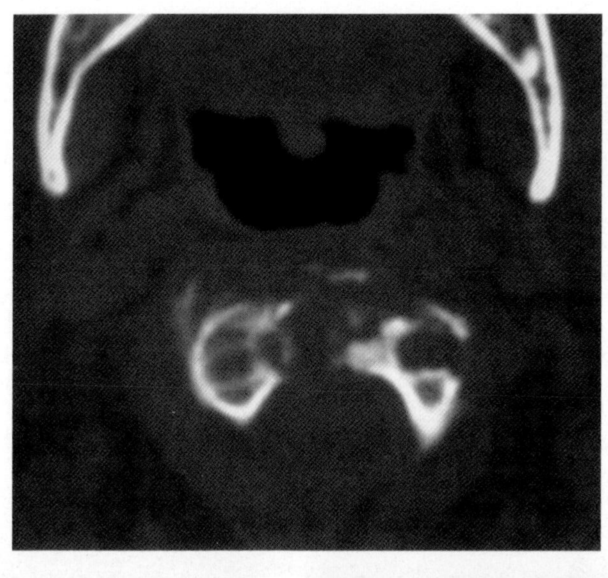

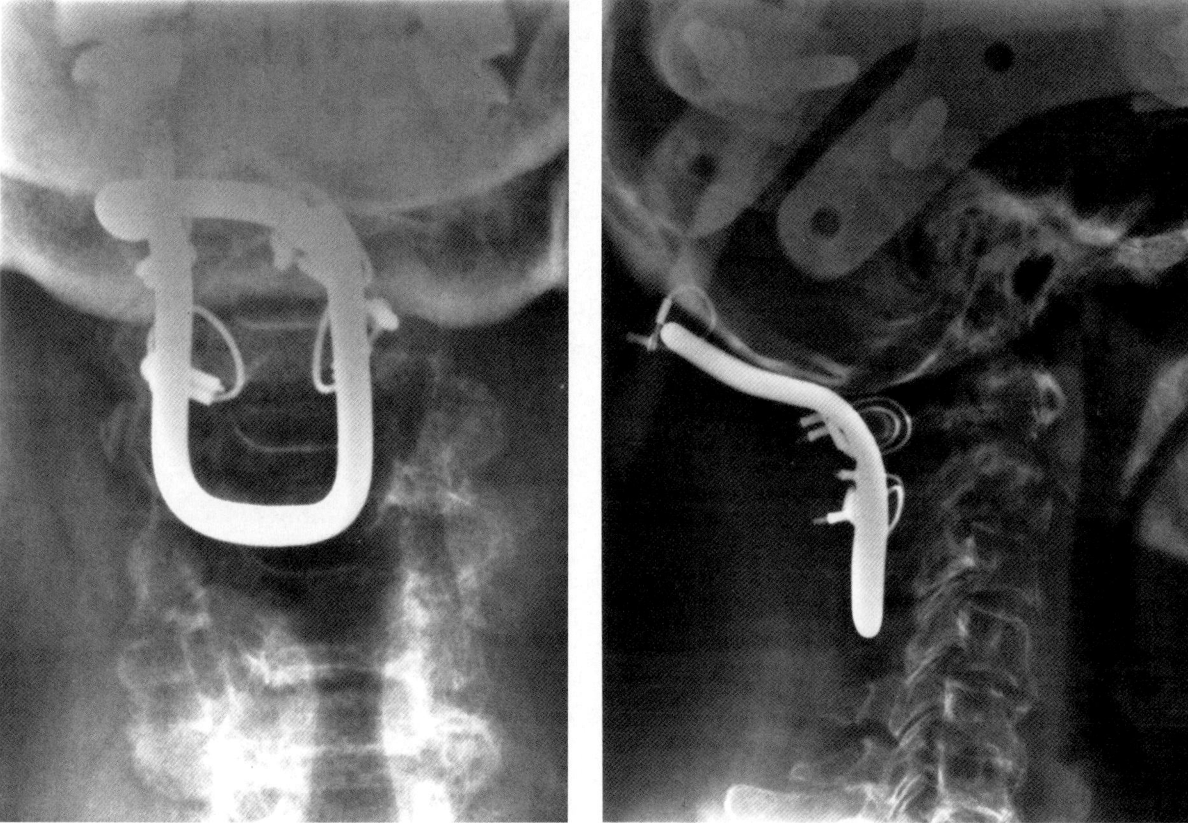

Fig. 14-28 Destruction of C2 due to metastasis. A: Axial computed tomographic (CT) image demonstrates destruction of C2. Anteroposterior (AP) (B) and lateral (C) postoperative images after fusion with a Luque rectangle and Songer cables. There is external support with a Halo device.

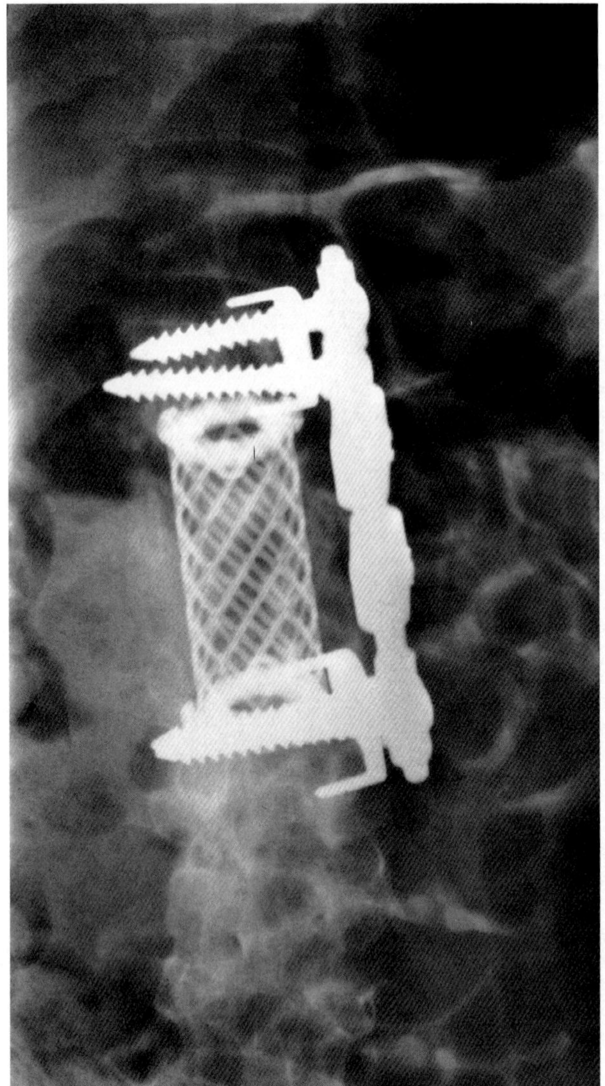

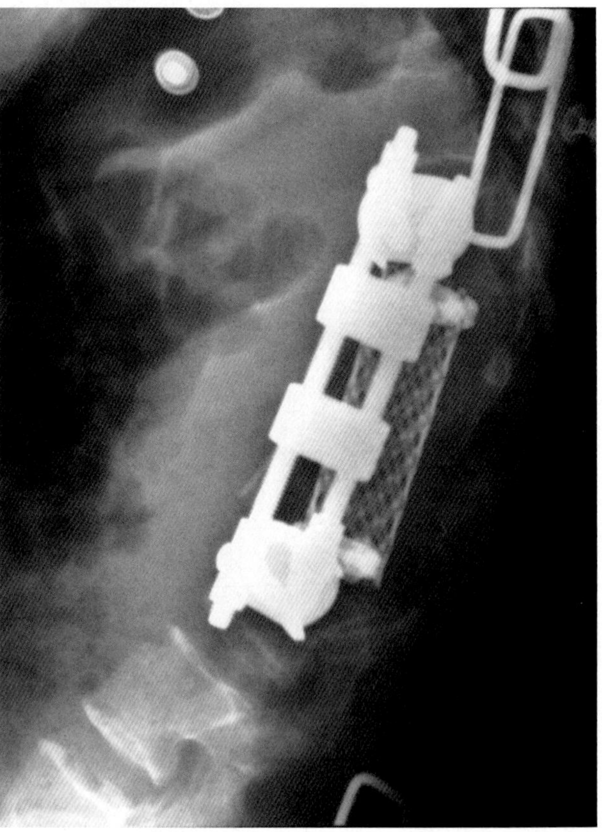

**Fig. 14-29** Upper lumbar destructive lesion with corpectomies of L1-2 and anterior instrumentation. Anteroposterior (AP) (**A**) and lateral (**B**) radiographs following fixation with an anterior cage and Kenada device for T12 to L3.

The incidence of nonunion is 12% to 30%. This may occur at one or both ends of intercalated grafts (Fig. 14-26). There appears to be no significant difference in nonunion related to patient age, gender, or the size of the graft. Location may make some difference as pelvic allograft nonunion is reported at 12%.

The overall incidence of graft fractures is 16%. Fractures of the graft or hardware combined occur in 27% of patients. Graft fractures are categorized into three types. Type I (5% of fractures) is really graft dissolution or resorption. This may in fact be an autoimmune response and typically occurs 6 to 12 months following surgery. Type II (51%) fractures occur in the shaft or at the host-allograft junction and most commonly occur approximately 2 years following surgery. This may require graft removal and revision. Type III (44%) fractures are intra-articular and likely related to avascular necrosis. Type III fractures tend to occur 2.5 to 3 years following surgery. Results following graft revision are good to excellent regardless of the type of fracture.

In addition to fracture (see Fig. 14-32), hardware failure of other types (screw pullout, loosening, soft tissue irritation) can lead to removal or revision in up to 23% of patients (see Fig. 14-33). Graft and hardware failure are usually readily detected on serial radiographs. In some cases, CT or MRI is required for further evaluation.

Deep infection is one of the most feared complications. The incidence following limb-saving procedures is 6% to 12% or comparable to revision arthroplasty. Most infections occur in the first 6 months following surgery. Imaging approaches are similar to those described with other arthroplasty procedures and include radionuclide scans, PET, MRI, and CT. Radionuclide scans are most effective >1 year following surgery.

Other local complications related to surgery include neurologic deficits. Most are nerve palsies diagnosed clinically and

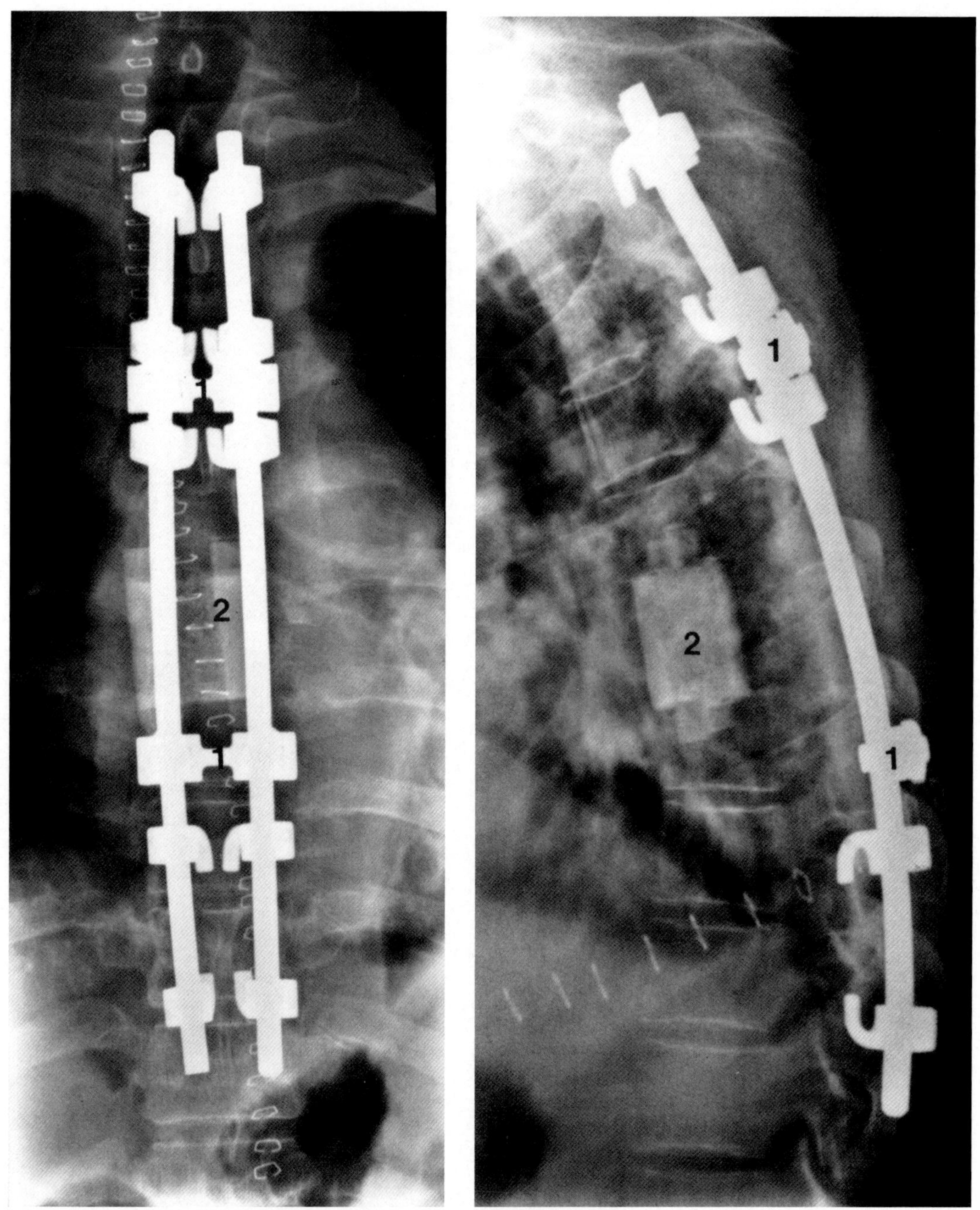


Fig. 14-30 Thoracic chondrosarcoma with previous T6-7 laminectomies. Anteroposterior (AP) (A) and lateral (B) radiographs demonstrate posterior instrumentation with rods, hooks, and cross-links (*1*) and an iliac strut graft at the T6 level (*2*).

**Fig. 14-31** Recurrent fibrous osteosarcoma. **A:** Technetium Tc 99m methylene-diphosphonate (MDP) scan demonstrates multifocal intense uptake about the right humerus with no distant metastasis. **B:** Computed tomographic (CT) scout image demonstrates a mid humeral resection with spacer in place. There is loosening at the proximal and distal ends with a large soft tissue mass. Coronal (**C**) and sagittal (**D**) reformatted CT images demonstrate the extensive soft tissue mass with areas of calcification and periosteal reaction at the spacer margins with loosening. Axial (**E**) and coronal (**F**) conventional T1-weighted images demonstrate the large low-signal intensity mass with areas of hemorrhage posteriorly (bright signal). The spacer causes local artifact. Axial fast spin-echo T1- (**G**) and postcontrast T1-weighted images (**H**), both with fat suppression, result in significant worsening of the artifact from the spacer. There is significantly less artifact with the coronal fast short T1 inversion recovery (STIR) (**I**) image.

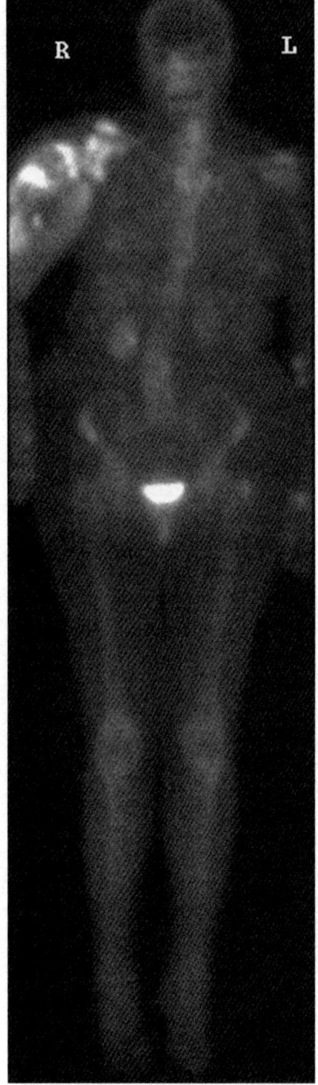

A

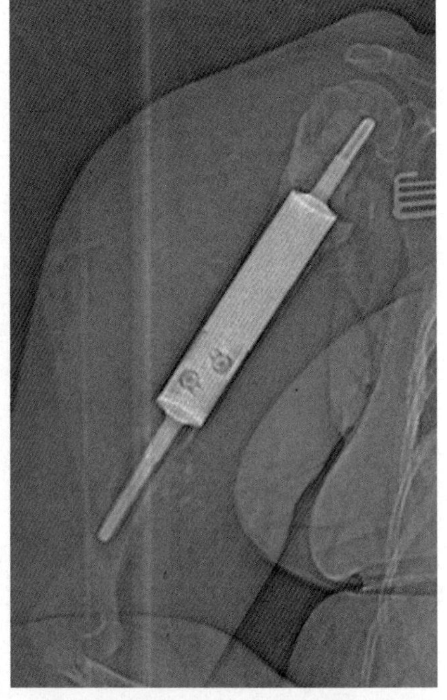
B

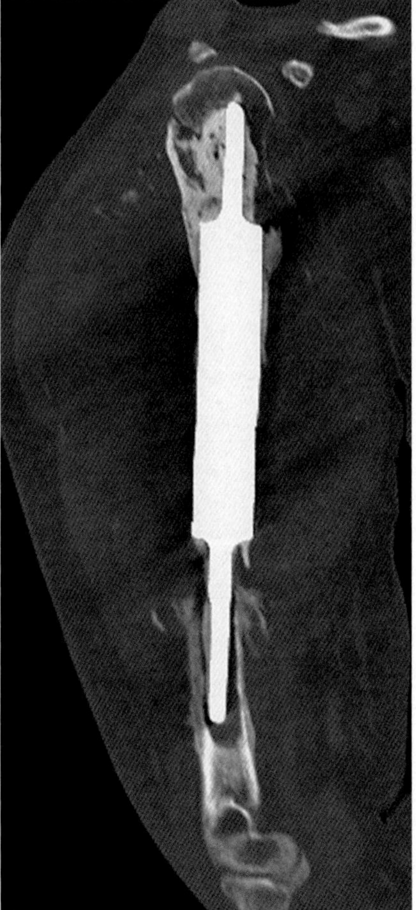
C

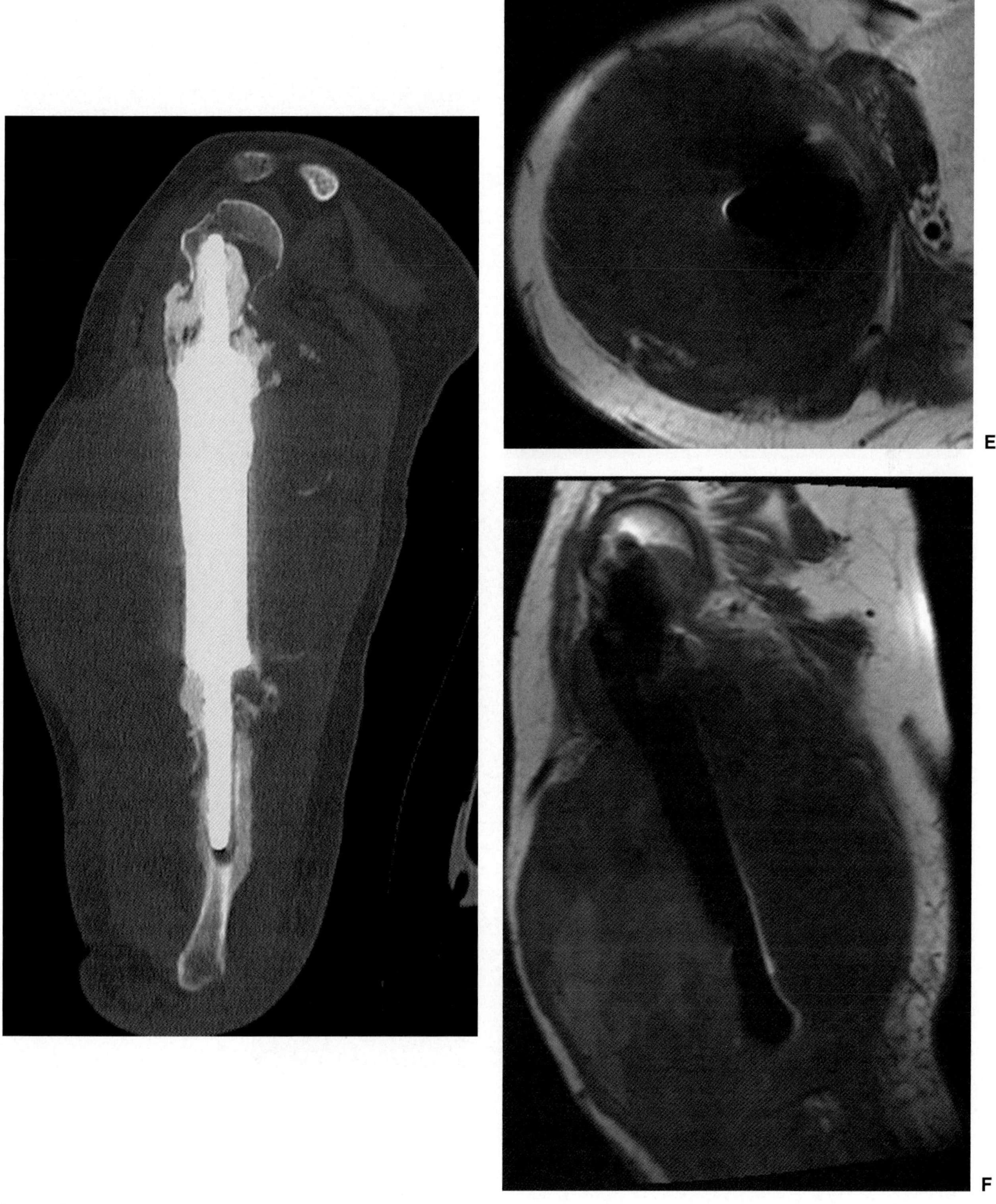


Fig. 14-31 *(Continued)*

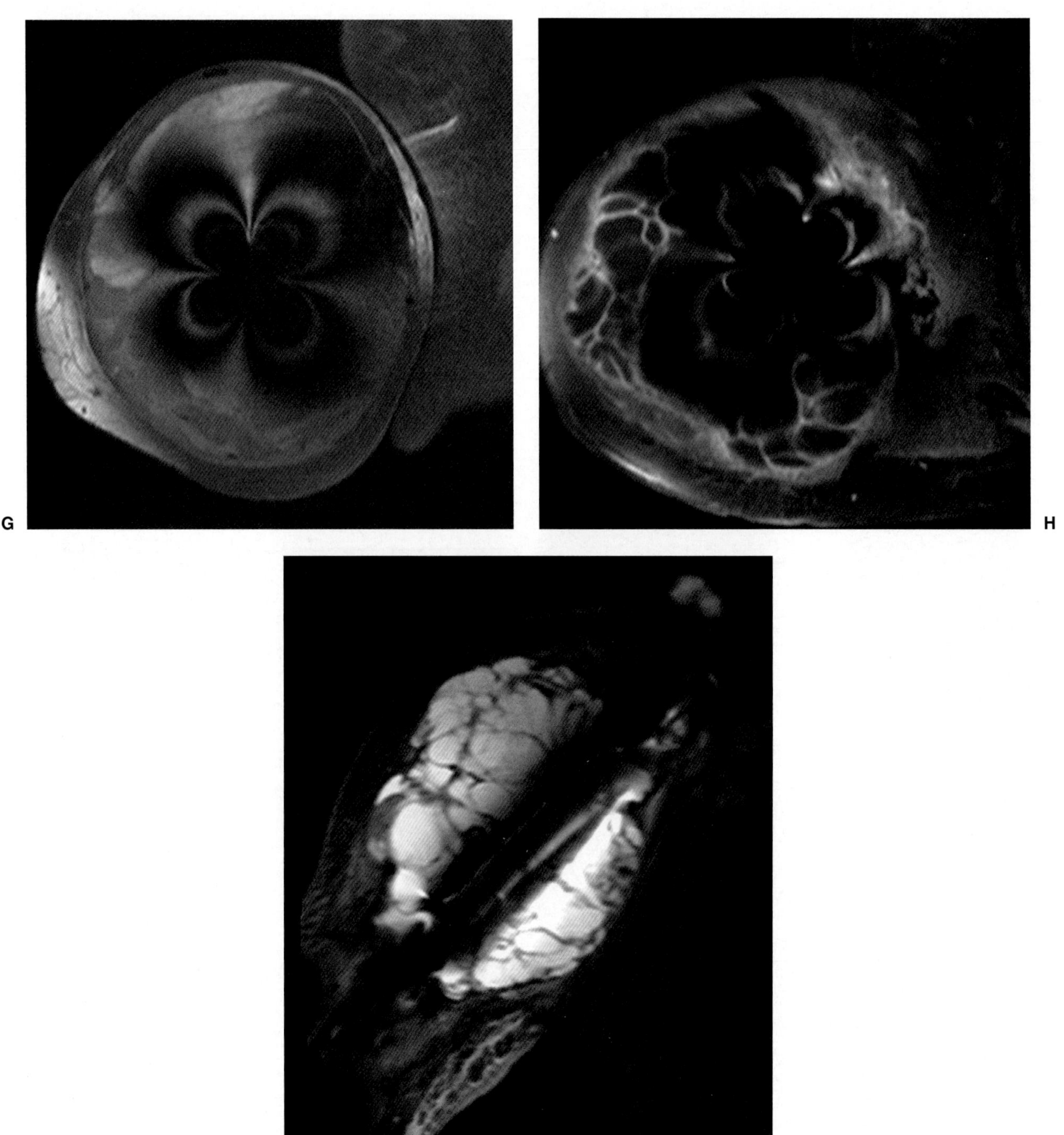


Fig. 14-31 *(Continued)*

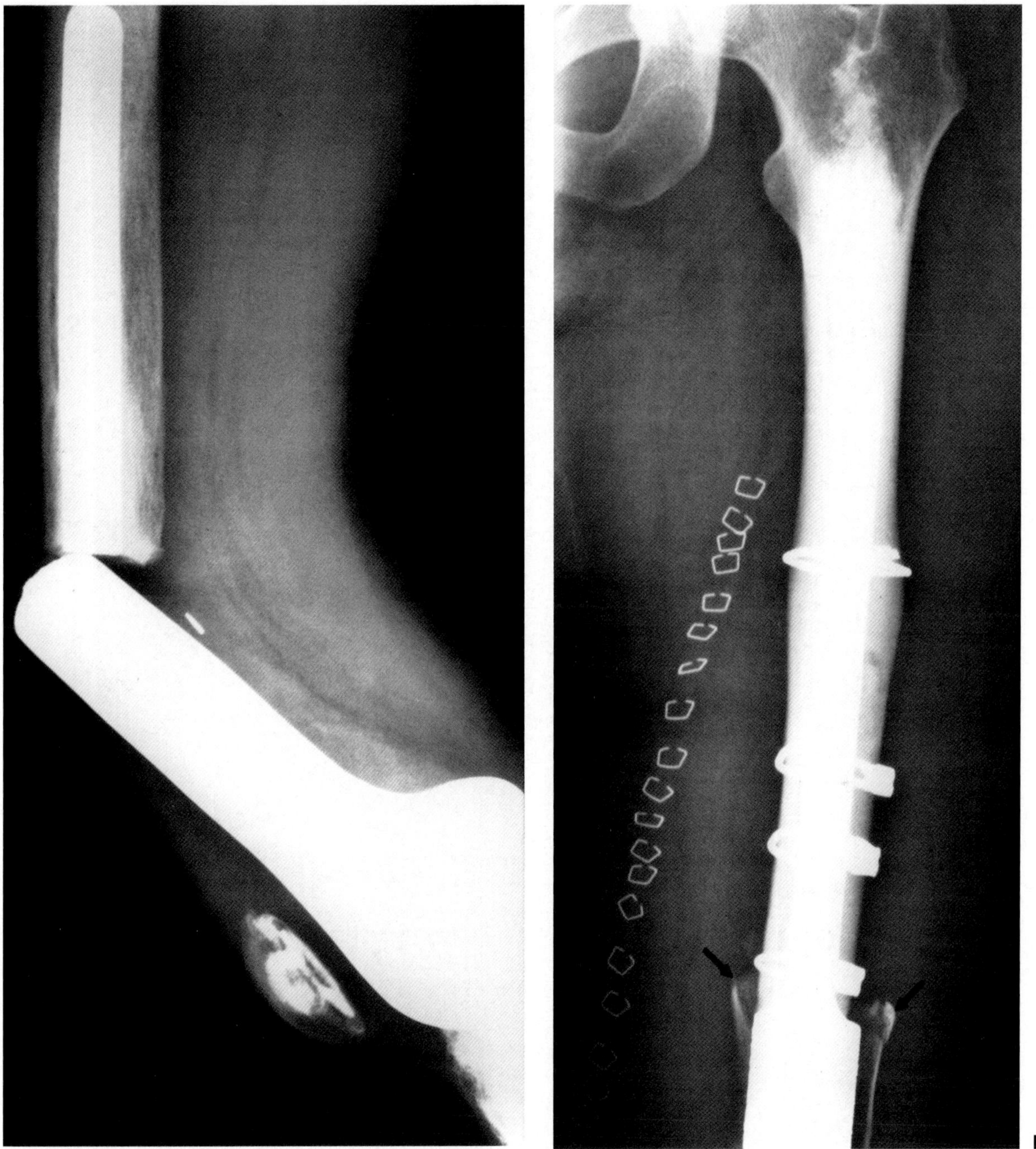


Fig. 14-32 Prosthesis fracture. A: Lateral radiograph demonstrating fracture of the femoral component at the component–bone interface. B–D: The component was revised with a longer femoral stem, supplemental autograft at the component–bone junction and Dall-Miles cables proximally.

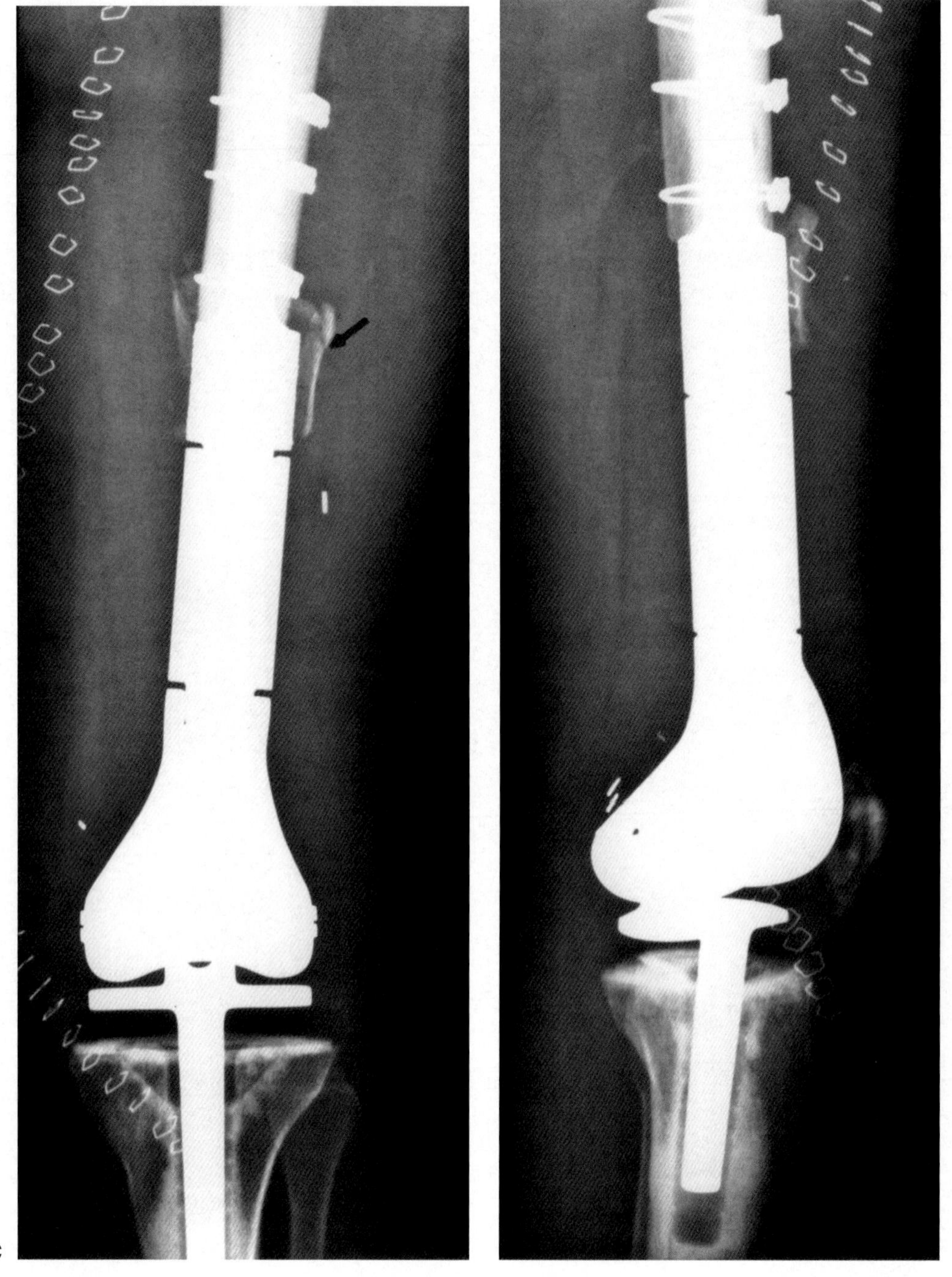


Fig. 14-32 *(Continued)*

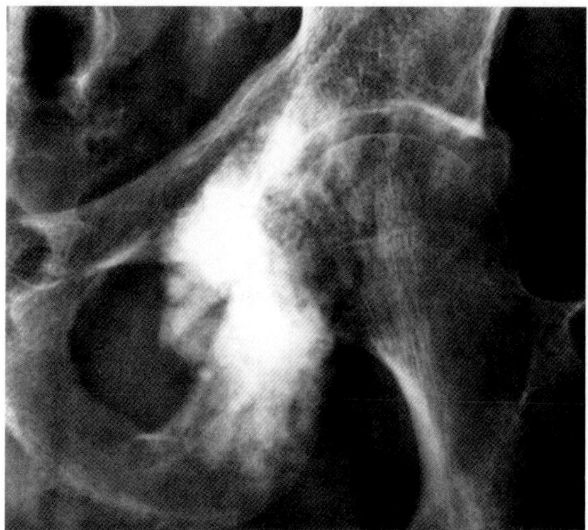

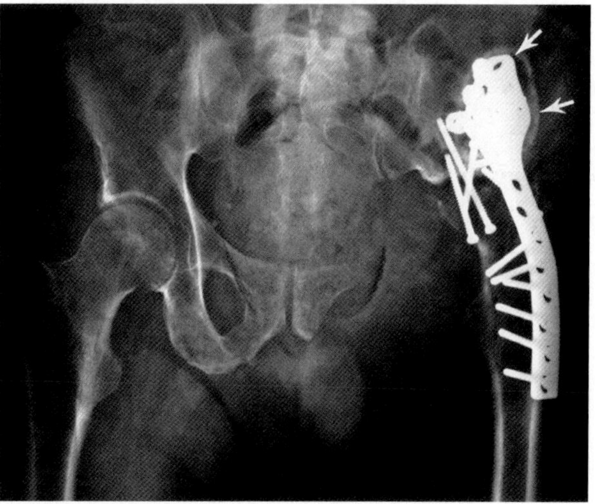

Fig. 14-33 Pelvic osteosarcoma. A: Radiograph demonstrating a dense osseous lesion arising from the central acetabulum. B: The patient was treated with wide excision and arthrodesis with a cobra head plate and screws for fixation. There is sclerosis and lucency about the upper plate due to loosening.

with electromyogram (EMG). This complication is particularly common with pelvic reconstructions where nerve palsy, specifically the sciatic nerve, occurs in up to 25% of patients. These neuropathies are commonly chronic and may not completely resolve.

Other orthopaedic complications include leg length discrepancy that can be evaluated with scanograms or CT. Nonorthopaedic complications include urinary tract infections, pneumonia, pulmonary emboli, and deep venous thrombosis. These complications usually occur in the early postoperative period.

## Suggested Reading


Beaman FD, Bancroft LW, Peterson JJ, et al. Imaging characteristics of bone graft materials. *Radiographics* 2006;26:373–388.

Berrey DH Jr, Lord CF, Gebhardt MC, et al. Fractures of allografts. *J Bone Joint Surg.* 1990;72A:825–833.

Delloye C, Banse X, Brichard B, et al. Pelvic reconstruction with a structural pelvic allograft after resection of a malignant bone tumor. *J Bone Joint Surg.* 2007;89A:579–587.

Griffiths HJ, Andersen JR, Thompson RC, et al. Radiographic evaluation of the complications of long bone allografts. *Skeletal Radiol.* 1995;24:283–286.

Hoeffner EG, Ryan JR, Qureshi F, et al. Magnetic resonance imaging of massive bone allografts with histologic correlation. *Skeletal Radiol.* 1996;25:165–170.

Ortiz-Cruz E, Gebhardt MC, Jennings C, et al. The results of transplantation of intercalary allografts after resection of tumors. *J Bone Joint Surg.* 1997;79A:97–106.

Patel SR, Miller PR, Gross M, et al. Massive bone allografts for limb salvage. *AJR Am J Roentgenol.* 1997;168:543–546.

# Index